D1604622

Foundations of Veterinary Studies

The Cardiorespiratory System

Integration of normal and pathological structure and function

A.S. King

BSc, PhD, DSc, MRCVS
Emeritus Professor of Veterinary Anatomy
University of Liverpool

b

Blackwell
Science

© A.S. King 1999

Blackwell Science Ltd
Editorial Offices:
Osney Mead, Oxford OX2 OEL
25 John Street, London WC1N 2BL
23 Ainslie Place, Edinburgh EH3 6AJ
350 Main Street, Malden
  MA 02148 5018, USA
54 University Street, Carlton
  Victoria 3053, Australia
10, rue Casimir Delavigne
  75006 Paris, France

Other Editorial Offices:

Blackwell Wissenschafts-Verlag GmbH
Kurfürstendamm 57
10707 Berlin, Germany

Blackwell Science KK
MG Kodenmacho Building
7–10 Kodenmacho Nihombashi
Chuo-ku, Tokyo 104, Japan

First published 1999

Set in 9.5/11.5 pt Times
by Best-set Typesetters Ltd., Hong Kong
Printed in the UK by
the Alden Press, Oxford and Northampton
Bound in the UK by
MPG Books Ltd, Bodmin, Cornwall

The Blackwell Science logo is a
trade mark of Blackwell Science Ltd,
registered at the United Kingdom
Trade Marks Registry

DISTRIBUTORS
  Marston Book Services Ltd
  PO Box 269
  Abingdon
  Oxon OX14 4YN
  (*Orders*: Tel: 01235 465500
        Fax: 01235 465555)

USA
  Blackwell Science, Inc.
  Commerce Place
  350 Main Street
  Malden, MA 02148 5018
  (*Orders*: Tel: 800 759 6102
              781 388 8250
        Fax: 781 388 8255)

Canada
  Login Brothers Book Company
  324 Saulteaux Crescent
  Winnipeg, Manitoba R3J 3T2
  (*Orders*: Tel: 204 837 2987
        Fax: 204 837 3116)

Australia
  Blackwell Science Pty Ltd
  54 University Street
  Carlton, Victoria 3053
  (*Orders*: Tel: 03 9347 0300
        Fax: 03 9347 5001)

A catalogue record for this title
is available from the British Library

ISBN 0-632-05024-1

For further information on
Blackwell Science, visit our website:
www.blackwell-science.com

Contents

Preface

This book surveys the normal anatomy and physiology, and closely related pathophysiological and clinical aspects, of the cardiorespiratory system. The autonomic nervous system is included because of its role in regulating cardiac and respiratory functions, and the immune system is also briefly surveyed because of its contribution to the defence of the lung. The book follows the same general approach as that published in 1987 by Oxford University Press under ther title *Physiological and Clinical Anatomy of the Domestic Mammals, Volume 1, Central Nervous System.* It was always intended that these would be the first two volumes of a series, but then in 1997 the project was transferred to Blackwell Science. The CNS volume is now being revised into a second edition, though under the new general title of Foundations of Veterinary Studies. Volumes on the Gestrointestinal System and Urogenital System are being prepared, and it is planned to complete the series by volumes on the Locomotory System and Head.

Veterinary educationalists now recognize that the 'artificial barriers created by autonomous departments should be removed', with 'integration of course components, unimpeded by traditional subject boundaries' (Editorial, *Veterinary Record*, June 17 1995), 'the acute overload of the veterinary curriculum' being relieved by 'a core curriculum with integration of subjects' (*British Veterinary Association Annual Review*, 1994–5). The present volume, like the others in this series, aims to meet these two great objectives for veterinary education, firstly by integrating anatomy (developmental, microscopic, and macroscopic) with physiology and by opening the door into pathophysiology and clinical studies; and secondly, by identifying an indispensable minimum of core material for the preclinical curriculum.

The contents of the book are therefore divided into core text and advanced text. The advanced text is intended to be obviously distinguishable from the core text, and is presented in smaller print and indented. The information in the core text is regarded here as the essential minimum that a preclinical student should actually **know** before proceeding to the clinical part of the curriculum, and could therefore be regarded as examinable material. The identification of such core material is obviously highly subjective, but a lecturer using this book can apply personal judgement by using the numbered headings to guide students selectively through the core and advanced text.

The advanced text is based on major reference works and review articles, supported by references to the sources. Although not mandatory reading, such text is likely to appeal to at least some undergraduate preclinical students, leading to the early exposure to research that should characterize 'a true University education' (Selborne Committee of Enquiry into Veterinary Research, *Veterinary Record*, December 13, 1997). The advanced text should also be useful to undergraduate students as they proceed through the pathological and clinical components of the curriculum. However, the main objective of the advanced text is to contribute to the continuing professional development (CPD) of veterinary graduates, by giving a deeper morphological, physiological, and pathophysiological insight into disease and clinical procedures. In the UK, increasing importance is attached to CPD (Royal College of Veterinary Surgeons, *Guide to Professional Conduct*, 1996).

This appears to be the first time that all of these preclinical objectives have been explicitly adopted in book form in the biomedical sciences, except perhaps for restricted topics such as *Brodal's Neurological Anatomy*. Integrated manuals for preclinical medical students have begun to appear, but their advanced material seems rather sparse and they are therefore of relatively little value after the preclinical course is over.

The text, and especially the core text, has been made as user-friendly as possible. Structures and functions are in bold type or italics, thus enabling topics to be found quickly. Headings and subheadings, with cross-references between them, are designed to make it easy for the reader to explore a subject fully. The core text has been simplified down to the essentials and contains no references to the literature. The *Nomina Anatomica Veterinaria* (4th edn), *Nomina Histologica* (revised 2nd edn), and *Nomina Embryologica* (1992) have been adopted, but English forms (as in Schaller et al., 1992) have been used in the core text and Latin forms are given in the advanced text only. To help readers who are not familiar with Latin, the Latin terms are generally stated in the nominative singular case only, as listed in the Nomina.

This volume arose from in-house versions published by the Department of Veterinary Anatomy, University of Liverpool, in the 1970s and 1980s. The five editions were widely read among English-speaking veterinary students. All the editions had on their cover an illustration of the heart and lungs from *De Humani Corporis Fabrica* by Adrianus Spigelius, 1627, a 'well-known and reputable anatomist' and holder of the Chair of Anatomy and Surgery at Padua. The present edition retains this illustration. To borrow from Spigelius is not too remiss, since most of the plates in his book seem to have been plagiarized from Casserius, a teacher of William Harvey at Padua. At that time, scientific observation was so restricted by scholastic prejudice that Spigelius succeeded in producing a memoir of ninety pages on the tapeworm without discovering its head. Times have changed, but there is still truth in the old medical aphorism that for every mistake made from not knowing, nine are made from not looking.

A.S.K.
Liverpool, 1998

Dedicated to my rather talented cats, Poppy, Hector, and Bismarck, who kept me company during the long watches.

Acknowledgements

Several people have helped me greatly with this volume. My wife, D.Z. King, not only maintained the household while I, like Achilles, 'sulked in my tent' with my word processor, but, as a skilled histologist and electron microscopist, she read and corrected text and illustrations. It has been a particular pleasure to have Professor C.M. Brown of the Department of Veterinary Clinical Sciences of Iowa State University as co-author of the clinical chapters, and Dr. J.B. Dixon of the Department of Veterinary Pathology of the University of Liverpool as co-author of the chapter on immunology. Professor Brown and I shared educational experiments in University teaching 25 years ago that initiated the objectives of this series of books. Dr Dixon generously sacrificed precious time to direct my re-education in immunology; we too had collaborated in the 1980s in developing University teaching. Professor Donald Kelly and Tim Nicholson read passages on the heart and bronchial circulation. Dr. S.C. O'Neill contributed a section on excitation-contraction coupling in the myocardium. Dr. Leslie Hall directed my attention to perfusion-ventilation matching and commented on this topic in earlier manuscripts. Marie Hughes, Leahurst Librarian, performed valuable library searches. G. Martin and A. Bannister helped with illustrations. Dr. Cathy Kennedy of Oxford University Press nobly supported the development of this book and the other books in the series. Finally Antonia Seymour at Blackwell Science, Shahzia Chaudhri and Dr. Janet Pascoe enthusiastically carried the work through to publication.

Part 1
Autonomic Nervous System

Chapter 1
General Principles of the Autonomic Nervous System

1.1 Definitions: somatic and autonomic nervous systems

It has long been customary to divide the nervous system into a somatic or cerebrospinal component which controls the 'body' (soma), and an autonomic or visceral component which controls the viscera. 'Autonomic' means a 'law to itself'. Early anatomists and physiologists really did believe the autonomic nervous system to be completely independent from the rest of the nervous system, both structurally and functionally, but this misconception was finally discarded about 100 years ago. Nevertheless, in order to describe the nervous system it is still convenient to retain the concept of somatic and autonomic components.

The history of anatomical and physiological researches into the autonomic nervous system was reviewed by Mitchell (1953, pp. 1–10). The eighteenth century anatomist Winslow suggested that the sympathetic ganglia function independently from the rest of the nervous system. This idea was developed by Bichat (1801–1803) into a theory proposing the complete structural and functional independence of the sympathetic ganglia. However, by 1840 histologists had demonstrated cell bodies in the ganglia, and had distinguished between the myelinated and unmyelinated nerve fibres in the rami connecting the ganglia to the spinal nerves. In the 1880s, embryologists showed that the primordial ganglion cells come from the neural tube. Finally, the anatomical and physiological studies of Gaskell and Langley at the end of the nineteenth century established the full structural and functional relationships of the sympathetic ganglia to the brain and spinal cord. Despite having completed the demolition of Bichat's independence theory, in 1898 Langley surprisingly suggested the term 'autonomic nervous system' for the entire cranial, thoracolumbar, and sacral outflow to the viscera, but added the warning that 'autonomic' suggested 'a much greater degree of independence of the nervous system than in fact exists'. Later still, it was discovered that centres in the highest parts of the brain, even in the cerebral cortex itself, regulate the functions of the autonomic nervous system (Section 1.5). At this level of the nervous system, somatic and autonomic functions are so closely integrated that distinctions between somatic and autonomic components then become almost imperceptible. Nevertheless, the two terms are still useful for descriptive purposes.

1.2 Somatic and autonomic motor nerves

1.2.1 Tissues innervated

Somatic motor (efferent) nerves supply **skeletal muscle** in the limbs, trunk, head, and tail. Autonomic motor nerves supply **smooth muscle**, **cardiac muscle**, and **glands**, in the great visceral systems of respiration, circulation, digestion, excretion, reproduction, and endocrine function (Fig. 1.1).

1.2.2 Preganglionic and postganglionic neurons

A somatic motor neuron (neuron 4, black, Fig. 2.1) projects its axon (nerve fibre) directly from the neuraxis (brain or spinal cord) to the target tissue (skeletal muscle). On the other hand, in peripheral autonomic motor pathways there are usually **two** efferent (i.e. motor) neurons. The first (neuron 3, green, Fig. 2.3) projects its axon from the neuraxis to a peripheral ganglion; it is therefore known as a **preganglionic neuron**. It makes a synapse in this ganglion with a second type of neuron (neuron 4, also green, Fig. 2.3), which projects its axon from the ganglion to the target tissue (smooth muscle, gland); the second neuron is therefore known as a **postganglionic neuron**. Thus, as a general rule, there is a **preganglionic–**

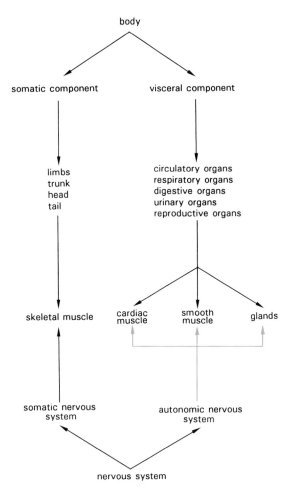

Fig. 1.1 Flow diagram expressing the basic components of the body and their motor innervation. The upper two thirds of the diagram show the basic components of the body at the top, and beneath them are the basic tissues requiring a motor (efferent) nerve supply. The lower third of the diagram shows the motor innervation of the tissues. The somatic components are on the left, and the visceral components are on the right. Efferent (motor) pathways of the somatic nervous system innervate skeletal muscle. Efferent pathways of the autonomic nervous system (green) innervate cardiac muscle, smooth muscle, and glands. The diagram omits striated muscle of the head that is innervated by the special visceral (branchial) motor system.

postganglionic relay in autonomic motor pathways (Fig. 3.1), but never in somatic motor pathways.

In accounts of the pre- and postganglionic neurons of the autonomic nervous system, the terms pre- and postganglionic axons are used interchangeably with the terms pre- and postganglionic fibres. The term 'fibre' is employed more often than 'axon'. It is not clear why this convention came to be adopted. The structure is clearly an axon, and axon must therefore be the proper term; it seems undesirable to have two terms for the same structure. It is apparent, however, that the older classic works on the anatomy of the autonomic nervous system (e.g. Mitchell, 1953) quite consistently used 'fibre' rather than 'axon'. Perhaps this was because in an autonomic ganglion the identity of axons as opposed to dendrites would not have been apparent, whereas 'nerve fibre' would have been safely applicable to either of them. Today, some neuroanatomists use 'fibre' (e.g. Burnstock, 1995, pp. 1292–1309), others use 'axon' (e.g. de Lahunta, 1983, pp. 115–129), and most use mainly 'fibre' but also 'axon'. The *Nomina Histologica* (1994) leaves the matter undecided by advocating both axon and neurofibra. In the first four chapters of this book, axon is used consistently, but elsewhere the common usage of 'fibre' is conceded.

1.2.3 *Special visceral motor nerves*

These nerves supply the striated muscles in the head that come from the **branchial arches** (gills) of lower vertebrates. They include the muscles of the face and jaws, and the muscles of the larynx, pharynx and oesophagus, but not the muscles of the eyeball and tongue since these are derived from somites and not branchial arches. The branchial (special visceral) cranial nerves complete the *motor* part of reflex arcs that originate in autonomic afferent pathways from the larynx, pharynx, and oesophagus (Sections 4.10, 4.15).

The motor nerves of the special visceral system resemble somatic nerves in their anatomy, in that the motor neuron projects from the neuraxis directly to the target tissue of striated muscle so that there is no pre–postganglionic relay.

1.3 The sympathetic, parasympathetic, and enteric nervous systems

The peripheral motor pathways of the autonomic nervous systems are subdivided into two main components, the **sympathetic** and **parasympathetic systems**. This subdivision has both a functional and an anatomical basis. There is a third component of the autonomic nervous system, the **enteric nervous system**. This is shared anatomically and functionally by the other two systems, but has a very large degree of structural and functional independence.

1.3.1 Differences in the general distribution of sympathetic, parasympathetic, and enteric nervous systems

The sympathetic nervous system is the most extensive and physiologically diverse of the three systems, sending axons to all parts of the body. The parasympathetic nervous system supplies relatively few targets, confined to the head and trunk. The enteric nervous system is restricted to the alimentary system, but has great physiological (and clinical) importance.

1.3.2 Functional distinctions between sympathetic and parasympathetic systems

The **sympathetic system** induces the visceral responses which are required for **fight and flight**; it tends to produce massive, widespread responses. The **parasympathetic system**, on the other hand, induces the visceral responses required for **conservation of bodily reserves**; its actions are local rather than widespread. The sympathetic and parasympathetic systems often exert an **antagonistic influence**; where one inhibits function, the other excites it. For example, a smooth muscle cell in the wall of a bronchus could receive a sympathetic axon which inhibits it and a parasympathetic axon which excites it. Most organs receive a **dual innervation** of this kind. On the whole the parasympathetic system plays the dominant role in controlling visceral functions. However, some organs, for example sweat glands, piloerector muscles, and many blood vessels, receive a sympathetic innervation only. The undeniably spectacular actions of the sympathetic nervous system in emotional and physical stress (fight and flight) should not, however, distract attention from the ongoing and essential housekeeping role of many sympathetic pathways in the control of normal body functions.

The two systems act at their postganglionic effector endings through different transmitter substances, **noradrenaline** (or **adrenaline**) being typically released by sympathetic postganglionic

effector endings and **acetylcholine** by parasympathetic postganglionic effector endings. Neurons that release noradrenaline (or adrenaline) at their effector endings are known as **adrenergic neurons**. Those that release acetylcholine at their effector endings are referred to as **cholinergic neurons**.

The functional state of any organ receiving an antagonistic innervation depends on the balance between the impulses delivered by the two opposing systems. Both systems are continually active, the basal rate of activity being known as **sympathetic tone** and **parasympathetic tone**. The activity of an organ can be adjusted by (1) increasing the basal tone, or (2) by reducing the basal tone, of either the sympathetic or the parasympathetic system (for example, see Section 3.2). In general, the two divisions collaborate in the fine adjustment of visceral functions. By this collaboration, they conserve the internal environment of the body in a 'steady state'; thus they maintain within acceptable limits the gases, metabolites, pH, temperature, etc., of the fluids that bathe the cells of the body. This they must do despite the rapid changes in the intercellular fluids which accompany sudden alterations in the activity of the body, such as fluctuations in temperature and in the concentration of metabolic products.

The preservation of the internal environment in a steady state is known as **homeostasis**. The significance of homeostasis can be appreciated by comparing the problems of a simple unicellular animal such as a paramecium in a pond with those of a fibrocyte in a skeletal muscle of a mammal. If the paramecium enters an area of its environment which is uncongenial through low pH, high temperature, or a shortage of nutrition it can swim to another part of the pond. The fibrocyte, on the other hand, is trapped among muscle cells which liberate heat and toxic metabolic products such as lactic acid and CO_2, and compete with it for oxygen. Since many of the cells of man begin to die, especially in the brain, if the fluids around them go outside pH 7.0–7.8 or above a temperature of 45°C (114°F), the fibrocyte has a rather narrow margin of safety. To sum up, the function of the autonomic nervous system is to *preserve homeostasis*, i.e. to *regulate the internal environment*. The function of the somatic nervous system is to enable the body to *control the external envi-*

ronment by taking whatever physical actions are necessary for survival.

As knowledge of the autonomic nervous system (systema nervosum autonomicum) grows, it has become apparent that the **antagonism** between the sympathetic system (pars sympathica) and parasympathetic system (pars parasympathica) is less significant than was originally supposed, and that the sympathetic system is not restricted to the mass actions of fight and flight. In fact, the sympathetic system is involved in the fine tuning of many functions (Williams *et al.*, 1989, p. 1155; Jänig and McLachlan, 1992). For example, the parasympathetic system and the sympathetic system participate together in the neural regulation of the rate and force of contraction of the heart (Section 22.8. 3). In some functions the sympathetic system provides the *only* neural control; thus *vasoconstriction* and *vasodilation* of nearly all blood vessels depend on varying degrees of sympathetic tone without any parasympathetic contribution (Section 13.3.3). In other functions, for instance the control of the bladder, the parasympathetic system is dominant (Section 3.14).

1.3.3   *Anatomical distinctions between sympathetic and parasympathetic systems*

The main anatomical distinction is the difference in the regions of the central nervous system (CNS) from which the peripheral motor pathways emerge. The **sympathetic outflow** from the CNS is limited to the *thoracic* and *lumbar* regions of the spinal cord (Section 2.1, Figs 2.2, 3.1): the **parasympathetic outflow** from the CNS is confined to the *brain* and the *sacral* region of the spinal cord (Section 3.1, Fig. 3.1). The sympathetic system is therefore often called the **thoracolumbar system** and the parasympathetic the **craniosacral system**. The peripheral motor nerves of the somatic nervous system arise from virtually the whole length of the CNS.

1.3.4   *The enteric nervous system*

The enteric nervous system is situated in the wall of the gut from the oesophagus to the anal canal. It consists of two nerve plexuses (the **myenteric plexus** and **submucosal plexus**, Section 3.18), each plexus containing not only numerous axons but very large numbers of nerve cells. Its function is to control gut motility and secretion. Both the

parasympathetic (Section 3.20) and the sympathetic systems (Section 3.21) connect anatomically with the enteric nervous system and can influence its functions. The parasympathetic system has a particularly strong functional influence, and can initiate gut motility and secretion.

For this reason, the enteric system came to be regarded as a postganglionic component of the parasympathetic system. However, this concept has now been abandoned. It has been known since the end of the nineteenth century that the gut can maintain its reflex activities after all connections with the rest of the nervous system have been severed. It has now also been shown that the enteric nervous system contains its own intrinsic sensory receptors, interneurons, and motor neurons, which are integrated into an intrinsic system for co-ordinating gastrointestinal functions. Nevertheless, the enteric system is under the overall command of the central nervous system, mainly through its connections with preganglionic fibres of the vagus (Section 3.20).

The enteric nervous system is known as the **Plexus nervorum intrinsecus (intramuralis)** in the *Nomina Histologica* (1994), and **Plexus entericus** in the *Nomina Anatomica Veterinaria* (1994).

1.4   Afferent pathways in the autonomic nervous system

Probably every student of biology knows that the 'somatic' part of the nervous system operates by reflex arcs. These reflex arcs consist of essentially three neurons: (i) a sensory or **primary afferent neuron**, (ii) one or more **interneurons**, and (iii) a motor or **efferent** neuron (Fig. 2.1). The afferent and efferent neurons in these reflex arcs are known as somatic afferent and somatic efferent neurons. The interneurons are not categorized as somatic. **Somatic reflex arcs** enable an animal to react to its **external environment**.

It has long been clear that the **autonomic nervous system** functions on an anatomical basis of reflex arcs, like any other part of the nervous system. Indeed, nearly all branches of the autonomic nervous system contain some afferent axons and some of them, for example the vagus nerve at the level of the diaphragm, consist mainly of afferent axons. The concept that the autonomic nervous system contains afferent components is therefore widely accepted by contemporary physiologists, pharmacologists, and anatomists, and is adopted here.

Nearly all such afferent autonomic neurons are typical **primary afferent neurons** (the only exceptions being in the enteric nervous system, see Section 3.18). Thus they have their nerve cell bodies (**cell station**) in a **dorsal root ganglion**. The ganglion can be associated with the dorsal root of a *spinal* nerve as in Fig. 2.3. Alternatively it can be a ganglion on the root of a *cranial* nerve; a ganglion of this type is the homologue of the dorsal root ganglion of a spinal nerve. The cell bodies of all primary afferent neurons send a centrally directed axonal process into either the spinal cord or the brainstem. Histologically, these are pseudo-unipolar neurons, with a single axon that divides into two branches (neuron 1, Fig. 2.1).

Autonomic reflex arcs enable an animal to regulate its **internal environment** (i.e. maintain homeostasis) by adjusting the functions of its respiratory, cardiovascular, and alimentary systems. The many varieties of such reflex arcs are surveyed in Chapter 4.

At the end of the nineteenth century, Langley proposed that the autonomic nervous system be divided into sympathetic and parasympathetic components (see Mitchell, 1953). He restricted these terms to the **motor** pathways to the viscera, although fully aware of the presence of afferent fibres in these nerves. His reason for this restriction was that, anatomically, visceral afferent pathways resemble somatic afferent pathways, whereas visceral efferent pathways are distinguished from somatic efferent pathways by the presence of a peripheral synapse (Patton, 1966, p. 353). Subsequently, the term autonomic nervous system itself also came to be restricted to efferent pathways.

Later it was suggested that the term visceral nervous system should be used to cover the combined sensory and motor nerves of the viscera, but that the term autonomic nervous system should continue to be restricted to the efferent pathways only. This is misleading, since it implies that the anatomical branches of the autonomic nervous system contain nothing but motor axons, whereas nearly all of them include numerous afferent axons. Many authorities (e.g. Patton, 1966, p. 353; Weiner and Taylor, 1985, p. 67; Williams *et al.*, 1989, p. 1167) now use the terms 'autonomic' and 'visceral' as synonyms, covering afferent as well as efferent components, and this usage is adopted here.

A traditional distinction is often made between **taste fibres** and other visceral afferent fibres, taste fibres being classified as **special visceral afferents** and the rest as **general visceral afferents**. There seems to be no good reason to set up a special category of taste afferents. They form a typical component of autonomic reflex arcs as in salivation, and like virtually all other visceral afferent fibres in the cranial nerves they project into the **nucleus of the solitary tract**. In this volume and the others in this series, taste fibres are regarded simply as visceral afferent fibres.

A further question is whether sympathetic afferent fibres can be distinguished from parasympathetic afferent fibres. Certainly there are afferent fibres in many sympathetic nerves and in many parasympathetic nerves. The former could be called sympathetic afferents and the latter parasympathetic afferents. But this is seldom done, and usually all these afferents are simply classed as autonomic afferent (or visceral afferent) fibres.

However, all this is only a matter of semantics. The important point is that visceral functions are dominated by afferent information and mediated through reflex arcs, in just the same manner as somatic functions. In recent years, recognition of this principle has compensated for the older tendency to regard the visceral nerves as concerned essentially with motor activity and has led to a much wider understanding of visceral reflex mechanisms (Iggo, 1966).

1.5   Autonomic pathways in the central nervous system

Each of the three great divisions of the brain (the forebrain, midbrain, and hindbrain), as well as the spinal cord, contains components with autonomic functions (see Vol. 1 in this series, on the CNS; King, 1987) for definitions of these and other terms associated with the brain or spinal cord). In the forebrain (cerebral hemisphere, or telencephalon), the **cerebral cortex** itself is linked to lower autonomic centres. For example, recognizing a frightening situation, or even simply thinking about one, can accelerate the heart rate, raise the arterial pressure, and dilate the pupils. However, at the highest levels of the CNS, **homeostasis** is governed by the **limbic system**, an array of autonomic centres within the forebrain and midbrain. Dominant among these is the **hypothalamus**. Visceral functions influenced by the hypothalamus include the *cardiovascular responses to fight and flight, thermoregulation, gut* *motility*, and *emptying of the bladder*. Other functions regulated by the hypothalamus include *reproductive activity*, *circadian rhythm*, *sleep*, and *endocrine functions*.

Autonomic activities are often mediated through so-called '**centres**' in the brain, for example **respiratory**, **cardiovascular**, and **gastrointestinal 'centres'**. As the names of these centres imply, a 'centre' is responsible for co-ordinating the afferent and efferent pathways involved in a particular function. Autonomic centres can be regarded as components of the **reticular formation**, a widespread ascending and descending network of neurons forming the most primitive part, and the largest single component, of the **neuraxis** (brain and spinal cord). A given centre often contains a number of '**nuclei**'. A '**nucleus**' consists of an assembly of nerve cells all sharing an essentially similar anatomical distribution and physiological function. In principle, 'nuclei' are either afferent (sensory) or efferent (motor). The afferent axons that go to an afferent nucleus will typically *ascend* the neuraxis together in a bundle of fibres known as an afferent (sensory) '**tract**': the efferent (motor) axons that leave an efferent nucleus will *descend* the neuraxis together in a bundle of fibres known as an efferent (motor) '**tract**'. It will be observed that 'afferent' and 'sensory' tend to be used interchangeably, as do 'efferent' and 'motor'.

Afferent autonomic pathways ascend the spinal cord in the **spinoreticular** and **spinothalamic tracts**, and make synaptic relays in the **nucleus of the solitary tract** in the hindbrain. The nucleus of the solitary tract has been divided into a series of subnuclei (nine in all), including broncho-pulmonary, cardiovascular, and gastrointestinal sites. Many axons from the nucleus of the solitary tract *project to* (send axons to) the autonomic centres in the hindbrain. Other axons ascend still further, reaching autonomic centres in the **limbic system**, and in the case of pain ascend even to the **conscious cerebral cortex**. Tracts *ascending* the spinal cord often have the prefix 'spino-' (e.g. *spino*reticular), whereas tracts *descending* the

spinal cord have the suffix '-spinal' (e.g. reticulo*spinal*).

The hindbrain autonomic centres project to the **parasympathetic motor nuclei** of the **oculomotor**, **facial**, **glossopharyngeal**, and **vagus nerves** (Section 3.3.1) – the four cranial nerves with autonomic components. The hindbrain autonomic centres also project caudally through the white matter of the spinal cord in the **reticulospinal tracts**. The effector endings of the fibres of the reticulospinal tracts form synapses with the preganglionic neurons of the sympathetic system in the lateral horn of the thoracolumbar segments, and with the parasympathetic preganglionic nerve cell bodies in the sacral segments of the spinal cord.

For further details of the structure and function of autonomic pathways in the brain and spinal cord see specific chapters in the first volume in this series on the CNS (King, 1987).

The **reticular formation** consists of a network of neurons forming the primitive core of the vertebrate neuraxis (see Vol. 1 in this series on the CNS; King, 1987). It extends continuously throughout the whole length of the brainstem and spinal cord, the part in the brain being divided into median, medial, and lateral columns (Williams *et al.*, 1989, p. 989). Its rostral limit is in the diencephalon (including the thalamus and hypothalamus), its middle part lies in the midbrain, and its caudal part is in the hindbrain (pons and medulla oblongata) and spinal cord. It contains ascending pathways projecting afferent information, and descending pathways projecting efferent commands. The ascending and descending systems intermingle intimately and exchange many synaptic contacts; it is a general characteristic of individual neurons of the reticular formation that they form synaptic contacts with many other widely separated neurons. Therefore it is predictable that the autonomic 'centres' (for example the various respiratory 'centres', Section 11.1), are far from being circumscribed clusters of neurons, but actually overlap each other and even overlap other autonomic control centres in the hindbrain.

Afferent fibres from the various thoracic and abdominal viscera appear to arborize over the whole length of the **nucleus of the solitary tract**, indicating a considerable overlap of projections and indistinct viscerotopic organization (Mayer, 1994, p. 932).

Chapter 2
Sympathetic Motor Pathways in the Peripheral Nervous System

I GENERAL PRINCIPLES

2.1 Outflow of sympathetic motor pathways from central nervous system to peripheral nervous system

Throughout the whole length of the spinal cord there are two so-called 'horns' of grey matter on each side, a dorsal horn which is essentially afferent in function and a ventral horn which is somatic efferent in function. In the thoracic and the first few lumbar segments of the spinal cord there is an additional **lateral horn**, which is sympathetic efferent in function (Fig. 2.1). Sympathetic motor neurons in the lateral horn in these restricted thoracic and lumbar segments produce the entire outflow of motor sympathetic pathways from the central nervous system to the whole of the body, by means of the preganglionic–postganglionic relay (Section 1.2.2).

In a stylized mammalian model as in Figs 2.2 and 3.1, there are 15 such restricted segments, from T1 (the first thoracic segment) to L2 (the second lumbar segment) inclusive, which can be divided into three groups each of five segments according to the regions of the body that they supply: (i) segments T1 to T5 inclusive supply the thoracic viscera, the forelimb, the neck, and the head; (ii) segments T6 to T10 supply the abdominal viscera; (iii) segments T11 to L2 supply the pelvic viscera, hindlimb, and tail.

The spinal segments that possess a sympathetic motor outflow vary with the species. The outflow may extend caudally to L3 in man (Williams *et al.*, 1989, p. 1156), to L4 in the cat (Brodal, 1981, p. 701), and to L4 or 5 in the dog (Stromberg, 1993, p. 1042). Some authorities mention an outflow from C8 in the dog (Stromberg, 1993, p. 1042), cat (Brodal, 1981, p. 701), and man (Crosby *et al.*, 1962). The lateral horn (cornu laterale) is strictly a lateral projection of the **intermediolateral grey matter** (substantia intermedia lateralis), the grey matter uniting the dorsal and ventral horns (NAV, 1994, note 8).

Estimates by Jänig and McLachlan (1987, p. 1341) suggested a total of 35 000 to 40 000 sympathetic preganglionic neurons on each side of the spinal cord in the cat. Approximate numbers innervating the various regions are estimated to be the following: head, 6000; forelimb, 4000; abdominal viscera, 15 000; pelvic organs and distal colon, 2300; hindlimb and tail, 4500; trunk, 6000. Surprisingly, the thoracic viscera were omitted from these figures. Perhaps the main value of these estimates lies in revealing the importance of sympathetic motor pathways to the abdominal viscera, many of which are vasoconstrictor and involved in the regulation of arterial pressure and the distribution of blood throughout the body.

2.2 Spinal nerve

A typical **spinal nerve** (Section 8.17) is formed by the union of a dorsal and a ventral root (Fig. 2.1). The **dorsal root** carries afferent (sensory) pathways and the **ventral root** contains efferent (motor) pathways. In the highly schematic somatic reflex arc shown in Fig. 2.1 there are four somatic neurons. The first (no. 1) is a so-called **primary afferent neuron** (Section 1.4); its receptor endings lie in the somatic tissues of the body (skin, in this example), its cell body is in the **dorsal root ganglion**, and its centrally projecting axon passes through the dorsal root to end in the dorsal horn by making synapse with the second neuron. The second and third neurons (nos. 2 and 3) are **interneurons**. The third neuron synapses in the ventral horn with the fourth and final neuron, a **somatic motor neuron** (no. 4).

Peripheral to the union of its two roots, the spinal nerve divides into a **dorsal ramus** (or dorsal division) which is distributed to all somatic re-

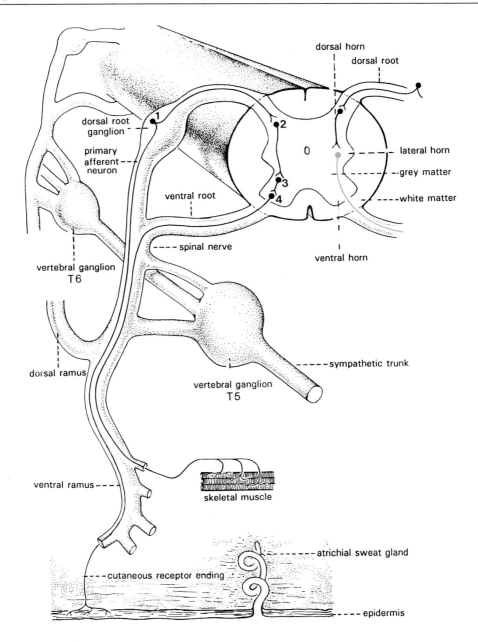

Fig. 2.1   Schematic transverse section through the spinal cord at the fifth thoracic segment, to show a somatic reflex arc and the components of a typical spinal nerve. The somatic reflex arc is on the left side of the diagram. Neuron 1 is a primary afferent neuron with its receptor ending in the skin, and its cell body (cell station) in a dorsal root ganglion; neurons 2 and 3 are interneurons; neuron 4 is a somatic efferent neuron with its cell station in the ventral horn and its effector endings on skeletal muscle fibres. The right side of the diagram shows a part of a sympathetic reflex arc, with a primary afferent neuron, one interneuron, and a preganglionic neuron (green) with its cell body in the lateral horn. A typical spinal nerve has a dorsal root with a dorsal root ganglion, and a ventral root; it also has a dorsal ramus supplying tissues dorsal to the vertebral column, and a ventral ramus supplying tissues ventral to the vertebral column. The sweat gland is not associated with a hair follicle and is therefore an atrichial sweat gland. This type of sweat gland occurs on the foot pads of the cat and dog, and all over the body surface of man; its innervation is cholinergic. Not drawn to scale.

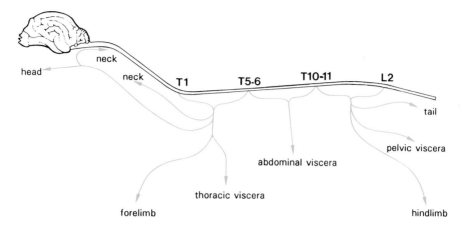

Fig. 2.2 **Diagram summarizing the outflow of preganglionic sympathetic fibres from the neuraxis to the main regions of the body.** The diagram is based on a hypothetical mammal in which a total of 15 segments of the thoraco-lumbar spinal cord contribute to the outflow. These can be divided into three groups, each of five segments. Segments T1–T5 supply the head, neck, forelimb, and thoracic viscera; segments T6–T10 supply the abdominal viscera; segments T11–T12 supply the pelvic viscera, hindlimb, and tail.

gions *dorsal* to the transverse processes of the vertebral column, and a **ventral ramus** (ventral division) to all somatic regions *ventral* to the transverse processes of the vertebral column (Fig. 2.1). The ventral divisions of spinal nerves in the regions of the forelimb and hindlimb form the **brachial plexus** (Section 2.21) and **lumbosacral plexus** (Section 2.27), which innervate the limbs.

2.3 Basic components of sympathetic motor pathways

2.3.1 Preganglionic neuron

The nerve cell bodies that form the lateral horn are known as sympathetic preganglionic neurons, neuron no. 3 in Fig. 2.3 being an example. The neuroanatomical way of expressing this is to state that the preganglionic neuron has its **cell station** (or cell location) in the **lateral horn**.

Embryologically and phylogenetically the nerve cells in the region of the **lateral horn** (cornu laterale) constitute a single cell mass that first appears in a position dorsal and dorsolateral to the central canal (Crosby *et al.*, 1962, p. 70). One group of these cells remains near the central canal to become the **intermediocentral cell column** (substantia intermedia centralis); the other group mi-

grates laterally to form the **intermediolateral cell column** (substantia intermedia lateralis). Both columns run from about T1 to L2, and contain preganglionic sympathetic cell bodies.

2.3.2 White ramus communicans

The axon of each preganglionic neuron leaves the spinal nerve via a white ramus communicans and runs to the vertebral ganglion of the same segment (Fig. 2.3). The ramus communicans is 'white' because the axons of preganglionic neurons are always *myelinated*.

2.3.3 Vertebral ganglion

There is a pair of sympathetic vertebral ganglia (Figs 2.1, 2.3) on the ventrolateral aspect of each vertebra throughout the length of the vertebral column, except in the neck where the number of ganglia on each side is reduced by fusion to three (Section 2.5).

2.3.4 Postganglionic neuron

The sympathetic postganglionic neuron has its cell station in the vertebral ganglion (neuron no. 4 in Fig. 2.3).

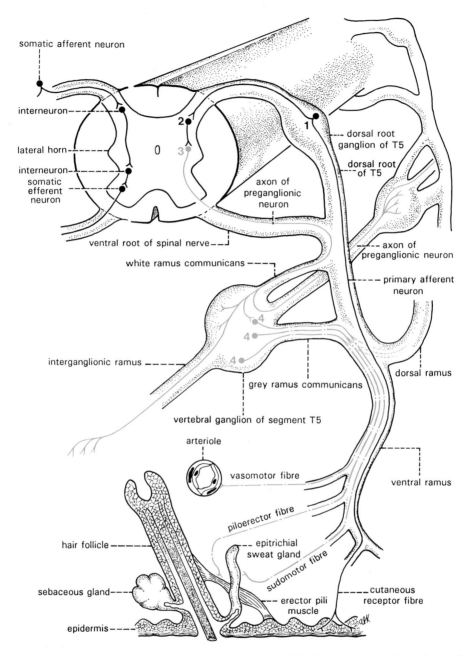

Fig. 2.3 Schematic transverse section of the spinal cord at the fifth thoracic segment, to show a hypothetical sympathetic reflex arc and the distribution of sympathetic motor pathways to the somatic tissues of the body. The sympathetic reflex arc is on the right side of the diagram. Neuron 1 is a primary afferent neuron (pseudo-unipolar) with its receptor endings in the skin and its cell station in a dorsal root ganglion. It could be a thermoreceptor neuron, stimulated by heat. Neuron 2 is an interneuron. Neuron 3 (green) is a preganglionic neuron with its cell station in the lateral horn; its axon extends for several segments up and down the interganglionic rami of the sympathetic chain, making synapses with about 20 postganglionic neurons in the vertebral ganglia. Three postganglionic neurons, no. 4 (also green), are shown with their cell stations in the vertebral ganglion of segment T5. These represent the three functional types of sympathetic postganglionic neurons that innervate tissues in the somatic components of the body: vasomotor, piloerector, and sudomotor neurons. Application of a warm stimulus in the

2.3.5 *Grey ramus communicans*

The grey ramus is formed by axons of the postganglionic neurons that return from the vertebral ganglion to the spinal nerve (Fig. 2.3). This ramus communicans is 'grey' because the axons of postganglionic neurons are always *unmyelinated*.

2.3.6 *Sympathetic trunk*

The successive vertebral ganglia are linked to each other by a series of **interganglionic rami**. The vertebral ganglia and their interganglionic rami form the **sympathetic trunk** (sympathetic chain), which runs the whole length of the vertebral column from the base of the skull to the tail. The interganglionic rami (the links in the chain) are formed by the axons of preganglionic neurons. As is shown in Fig. 2.3, the axon of a typical preganglionic neuron (no. 3 in the diagram) forms several branches in the vertebral ganglion of its own segment. Some of these branches form synapses with postganglionic neurons in this particular vertebral ganglion. Other branches enter the sympathetic chain and pass cranially or caudally to a vertebral ganglion lying one or several segments cranial or caudal to their origin. These branches, therefore, form the *links* of the sympathetic chain, or interganglionic rami; hence the links of the chain consist of the axons of preganglionic neurons.

Having spread cranially and caudally to the vertebral ganglia of several segments, these preganglionic sympathetic branches divide and make synapses in each ganglion with *several* postganglionic neurons. Thus each individual preganglionic neuron makes synapses with *many* postganglionic neurons (20, or even more). This means that the effects of sympathetic motor activity are widespread. In contrast, each preganglionic neuron in the parasympathetic system makes synapse with only about three postganglionic neurons (Section 3.2). These contrasting ratios are the anatomical basis for the *mass action* of the sympathetic system, as opposed to the *localized action* of the parasympathetic system.

> The **ratio of pre- to postganglionic neurons** ranges from about 1:20 (Jänig and McLachlan, 1987, p. 1374) to about 1:200 (Jänig and McLachlan, 1992).

2.3.7 *Prevertebral ganglion*

In the abdomen, there are three pairs of sympathetic prevertebral ganglia (Section 2.13) which lie on the ventral aspect of the aorta (Fig. 2.5). Unlike the vertebral ganglia and rami communicantes they are not segmental. As Fig. 2.5 shows, they receive axons from preganglionic neurons (neurons no. 2 in segments T6 to T10 in Fig. 2.5).

> The distinction between 'white' and 'grey' rami has proved too schematic (Brodal, 1981, p. 708). According to Mitchell (1953, p. 206), in man the white rami in the fresh state appear off-white and opaque and the grey rami greyish pink and semitranslucent, but neurosurgeons contend that the two types cannot be distinguished on the operating table (Brodal, 1981, p. 708). In the monkey, some rami contain both myelinated and unmyelinated axons, and therefore constitute a mixed type (Sheehan and Pick, 1943). According to Stromberg (1993, p. 1043), in the dog most rami are mixed. On the other hand, in the lumbar region of the cat Baron *et al.* (1985) distinguished white from grey rami without reporting mixed rami. In the horse, Dyce (1958) was unable to distinguish white from grey rami in the thorax, but in the first four lumbar segments the grey rami were the more cranial, round in section, and greyish pink and translucent; the white rami were more caudal, wider, and flattened. Clearly, there are species variations.
>
> Small **intermediate ganglia** (ganglia intermedia) lie outside the chain of vertebral ganglia, usually near rami communicantes (Weiner and Taylor, 1985, p. 68).

Fig. 2.3 (Continued) region of the cutaneous receptor ending could reflexly induce inhibition of the vasomotor neuron (vasodilation), inhibition of the piloerector neuron (flattening of hair), and excitation of the sudomotor neuron (sweating). The vasomotor and piloerector fibres are adrenergic. The sudomotor fibre in this diagram innervates a sweat gland associated with a hair follicle unit, and is therefore an epitrichial sweat gland with adrenergic innervation. Epitrichial sweat glands occur all over the body surface of domestic mammals, and in the axillary, pubic, and perianal regions in man. Postganglionic fibres of these three functional types are also distributed throughout the dorsal ramus of the spinal nerve (broken lines). The left side of the diagram shows the neurons of a somatic reflex arc, as in Fig. 2.1. Not drawn to scale.

The existence of **interneurons** in sympathetic ganglia was previously disputed, but has now been confirmed in many mammals (Williams *et al.*, 1989, p. 1157). They are either 'small intensely fluorescent' cells (**SIF cells**) or **chromaffin cells**, both of them containing catecholamines. SIF cells may release dopamine which directly hyperpolarizes the postganglionic neurons in the ganglion, or they may act indirectly by secreting substances into local blood vessels.

In the NAV (1994) the vertebral ganglia are the ganglia trunci sympathici, and the prevertebral ganglia are the ganglia of the autonomic plexuses (ganglia plexuum autonomicorum). Some authorities (e.g. Jänig and McLachlan (1987, p. 1377) use the term paravertebral ganglion instead of vertebral ganglia. The prevertebral ganglia are sometimes called the 'subsidiary' sympathetic ganglia (e.g. Williams *et al.*, 1989, p. 200).

2.4 Sympathetic reflex arc

Figure 2.3 shows a (hypothetical) sympathetic reflex arc. Four neurons are involved. The **afferent neuron** (no. 1 in the figure) has its receptor endings in the skin (and is therefore a somatic afferent); in this example its endings would be sensitive to changes in temperature. The cell body of this **primary afferent neuron** is in the dorsal root ganglion, like almost every other primary afferent neuron of the spinal cord. The central part of its axon projects into the dorsal horn where it makes a synapse with neuron no. 2, an **interneuron**. The latter makes a synapse in the lateral horn with neuron no. 3, this being the **preganglionic neuron** (green). The axon of the preganglionic neuron leaves the spinal cord by a white ramus communicans and synapses with several **postganglionic neurons** (for example neurons no. 4, green). The axons of the postganglionic neurons return to the spinal nerve via a grey ramus communicans, and are distributed peripherally in the dorsal and ventral rami of the spinal nerve to end on various types of effector organs (smooth muscle of a blood vessel, smooth muscle erecting a hair, and a sweat gland).

Transmission through a pre- and a postganglionic neuron is a constant characteristic of all motor autonomic pathways, both sympathetic and parasympathetic. It never occurs in motor somatic pathways.

2.5 Embryology of sympathetic motor neurons

The **preganglionic neurons** of the sympathetic system arise from the ventrolateral grey matter of the thoracolumbar segments of the developing neural tube; the region of the grey matter where they develop is known as the **intermediate grey column**, and is destined to become the **lateral horn** (Section 2.1). The **postganglionic sympathetic neurons** arise from the **neural crest**, and migrate to form the **vertebral** and **prevertebral ganglia**.

In the early embryo there is one pair of primordial vertebral ganglia for every spinal segment, but during development some of the ganglia in the neck and tail fuse. Thus in the neck the primordial eight vertebral ganglia (corresponding to the eight cervical spinal nerves) are reduced to three, forming the caudal, middle, and cranial cervical ganglia (Fig. 2.4). In the sacral region and tail the number of ganglia is erratically reduced by fusion.

In the thoracic and first few lumbar segments of the neural tube, a lateral column of neuroblasts forms in the mantle layer of the **ventrolateral lamina** of the neural tube. These neuroblasts become the **sympathetic preganglionic neurons**. Their axons enter the developing ventral roots of the spinal nerves and then emerge to join the vertebral ganglia of the sympathetic trunk, thus forming the white rami communicantes.

The **source** of the **sympathetic postganglionic neurons** is controversial (Mitchell, 1953, p. 28; Williams *et al.*, 1989, p. 200). The earlier experimental evidence indicated that they come exclusively from the **neural crest** and migrate via the dorsal roots to form the vertebral and prevertebral ganglia. However, more recent evidence suggested that at least some of the postganglionic neurons in these ganglia migrate from the ventral region of the mantle layer of the neural tube, drawing their related preganglionic axons after them; according to this view the preganglionic neuron is really no more than a modified interneuron, the synaptic transmission at the preganglionic effector endings being typical of that between interneurons, i.e. cholinergic (Mitchell, 1953, p. 13). Opinion today clearly favours the neural crest.

Developing sympathetic and parasympathetic postganglionic neurons are evidently **multipotential autonomic nerve cells** (Gabella, 1979; Landis, 1990). When vagal neural crest is grafted into the region of the thoracic neural crest that would normally form the adrenal medulla, it forms adrenal medulla; likewise potential adrenal medullary neural crest grafted into the site of vagal neural crest forms cholinergic enteric neurons (Gabella, 1979). Again, neurons dissociated from the cranial cervical ganglion of new born rats and grown in tissue culture initially synthesize and store catecholamines, but if myocardial cells are included in the culture the neurons acquire cholinergic functions (Landis, 1990). Similarly when developing axons contact the developing **atrichial sweat glands** (Section 2.7.2) in the foot pad of the rat in early postnatal development they are at first adrenergic; they then acquire cholinergic and peptidergic properties (releasing peptides at their effector endings, Section 2.34), and catecholamines disappear (Landis, 1990). Thus the target tissue induces secondary cholinergic properties. It has long been known that target tissues determine the number of neurons that survive during development, but it is now known that target tissues can also determine the phenotypic properties of those neurons that do survive.

II SYMPATHETIC MOTOR PATHWAYS TO SOMATIC REGIONS OF THE BODY

The skin, connective tissues, skeletal muscle, and bones of the limbs, trunk, head, and tail are generally regarded as the **somatic parts of the body**. All of these regions, however, contain **visceral tissues**, namely **smooth muscle** and **glandular tissue**, much of which requires a sympathetic nerve supply. Most of the smooth muscle lies in the walls of blood vessels. The hairs, which coat the body of most mammals, can be raised by the smooth muscle of the piloerector muscles. The glands are mainly cutaneous (e.g. sweat glands), though the head also contains salivary glands, endocrine glands, glands in the mucosal lining of the nasal cavity, and glands associated with the eye.

2.6 Sympathetic preganglionic neuron

The sympathetic preganglionic neuron has its cell station in the lateral horn of segments T1 to L2. The axon projects in the white ramus communicans to the vertebral ganglion of the same segment. Its branches form synapses with postganglionic neurons in that ganglion and in adjacent vertebral ganglia (Fig. 2.3). All preganglionic neurons (not only parasympathetic but

also sympathetic) release acetylcholine at their endings (Section 2.33.2).

2.7 Sympathetic postganglionic neuron: vasomotor, sudomotor, piloerector functions

All sympathetic postganglionic neurons that control tissues in the somatic parts of the body have their cell station in a **vertebral ganglion**. Three functional varieties of postganglionic neuron distribute their axons to the somatic regions of the body (i.e. to the head, limbs, trunk, and tail): (i) **vasomotor**, (ii) **sudomotor**, and (iii) **piloerector neurons** (Fig. 2.3). They innervate, respectively, blood vessels, sweat glands, and hair-erecting muscles. Almost all of the larger nerves in the limbs carry these three varieties of sympathetic motor axons. Their functions are predictable from the requirements of **fight and flight**. Remember that 'axon' and 'fibre' are used interchangeably in most accounts of the autonomic nervous system, pre- or postganglionic fibre being the same as pre- or postganglionic axon (Section 1.2.2).

2.7.1 Vasomotor postganglionic sympathetic neurons

Adrenergic sympathetic vasomotor neurons are of great importance in circulatory physiology. They innervate the smooth muscle in the walls of the arteries and veins in the skeletal musculature and skin, thereby regulating the calibre of these vessels. As a rule, excitation of sympathetic vasomotor neurons, as in '**fight and flight**', causes the smooth muscle to contract giving **vasoconstriction**. Vasoconstriction, however, would not be expected to occur in active skeletal musculature. In fact, in **exercise** there is a marked **vasodilation** of these vessels, the mechanism of which depends primarily on metabolic factors, especially on the local concentration of oxygen in the tissues (Section 13.2.1).

Axons of **cholinergic sympathetic vasodilator neurons** (Section 2.33.2) have been found in the skeletal muscle of some mammalian species (e.g. the cat). They may play a significant role in skeletal muscle at the *onset* of **exercise**, by inducing a *preliminary* **vasodilation** (Section 13.3.4).

2.7.2 *Sudomotor and piloerector postganglionic sympathetic neurons*

Tubular exocrine glands known as **sweat glands**, which secrete in response to heat, are fairly evenly distributed over the skin of the **general body surface** of all of the domestic mammals. These glands are typically arranged in **hair follicle units**. Such a unit (Fig. 2.3) consists of (1) a hair follicle, (2) a piloerector muscle, (3) a sebaceous gland, and (4) a sweat gland; the duct of the sweat gland opens into the hair follicle just superficial to the opening of the sebaceous gland (consequently the sweat is mixed with sebum before being released on the surface of the skin). Because these sweat glands are associated with hairs they are known as **epitrichial sweat glands** (Greek: epi, on; thrix, hair).

There is a second type of sweat gland that is **not** associated with hairs, and is therefore known as an **atrichial sweat gland** (Fig. 2.1). This occurs on the foot pads of the dog and cat, and over all of the general body surface of man; these are areas of skin that are entirely or virtually hairless. Like epitrichial sweat glands, atrichial sweat glands respond to heat.

In **fight and flight** *sweating* is needed for heat loss, and *piloerection* for intimidation as well as thermoregulation. Therefore it is predictable that these functions will be controlled by sympathetic motor pathways, by means of postganglionic **sudomotor** and **piloerector neurons**.

In all the domestic mammals and man, the sympathetic **sudomotor axons** of **epitrichial glands** are essentially *adrenergic*, and the sympathetic **sudomotor axons** of **atrichial glands** are essentially *cholinergic* (Section 2.33). Circulating adrenaline (and to a lesser extent noradrenaline) induces secretion in both types of gland.

Epitrichial sweat glands have been found in the horse, ox, sheep, goat, pig, dog, cat, buffalo, camel, and llama (Jenkinson, 1969, pp. 202, 219). Not all hair follicles have an epitrichial sweat gland; in animals such as the sheep, goat, and dog, in which the hair follicles occur in groups of primary and secondary hairs, only the large primary hairs have sweat glands. Predictably, in man epitrichial sweat glands occur only where there is dense body hair, i.e. in the axillary, scrotal, and perianal regions.

Sweat glands and piloerector organs were presumably evolved for **thermoregulation**, by providing sweat for evaporative cooling and by enabling air to be either trapped within the hairy coat for insulation or excluded for cooling. The sharing of this primordial function is reflected in the combination of sweat glands and piloerector organs in **hair follicle units**. Since thermoregulation is an important aspect of homeostasis (Section 1.3.2), its control lies within the province of the autonomic nervous system. However, thermoregulation by **sweating** is far from universal in mammals. Indeed it appears to be of prime importance only in primates and ungulates (Jenkinson, 1973). Large ungulates such as horses, cattle, camels, and big antelopes, do rely primarily on sweating for heat loss. Small ungulates such as sheep, goats, and small gazelles, and those carnivores that have been studied, employ panting for evaporative cooling (Schmidt-Nielsen, 1990, p. 273); nevertheless, in at least the domestic representatives of these taxa (including the sheep, goat, dog) the sweat glands on the body surface can still respond to heat, with the possible exception of the pig and cat (Jenkinson, 1969). Although the sweat glands on carnivore foot pads can respond to heat, they are not likely to contribute significantly to thermoregulation and have probably been adapted for other functions such as minimizing damage through friction (Jenkinson, 1973). Sweat glands may also have been secondarily adapted in other ways, for example for protecting the skin against bacteria, for excretion, or for production of sexually stimulating scent (Jenkinson, 1969). Birds, which share fully developed endothermic homoiothermy with mammals, totally lack sweat glands and therefore rely mainly on evaporative cooling from the respiratory tract (panting and gular fluttering); like mammals, birds also trap or exclude air in their body coat (feathers). A third method of evaporative cooling is salivation and licking, as in the rat and kangaroo (Schmidt-Nielsen, 1990, p. 273).

Modern textbooks of anatomy and physiology usually follow work dating back to 1917 by classifying sweat glands into **apocrine** and **merocrine** (or **eccrine**) types, but the evidence for the occurrence of apocrine secretion by sweat glands is now widely questioned (Jenkinson, 1973; Bal, 1977, p. 499; Jenkinson *et al.*, 1979; Krstic, 1984, p. 401; Dyce *et al.*, 1987, p. 367; Williams *et al.*, 1989, p. 1226). It would seem to be time to abandon the apocrine–merocrine classification. However, the recognition of two types of sweat gland does seem justifiable, firstly on grounds of differing anatomical relationships to hair follicles, hence epitrichial and atrichial; secondly, these two types differ in their sympathetic innervation, the epitrichial glands being primarily adrenergic and the atrichial type being primarily cholinergic.

Although it is established that sweating in mammals, including the ox, sheep, goat, pig, dog, donkey, horse (Jenkinson, 1973), and man (Jenkinson, 1969; Shields, *et al.*, 1987), is controlled by sudomotor sympathetic postganglionic neurons, the details of the **control mechanism** are still very poorly understood. In the **epitrichial glands** which characterize most species, including the ox, sheep, goat, dog, and horse (Jenkinson, 1969, 1973), the mechanism has been shown to act through sympathetic **adrenergic** neuronal pathways (Jenkinson, 1973). Furthermore the epitrichial sweat glands of all these species respond to some degree to injection of adrenaline, noradrenaline being less effective (Jenkinson, 1969, 1973). The epitrichial glands of man have previously been regarded as not innervated but controlled by circulating adrenaline (Green, 1989, p. 148), or innervated by adrenergic endings (Junqueira and Carneiro, 1983, p. 395), or innervated by both adrenergic and cholinergic endings (Williams *et al.*, 1989, p. 1226), or innervated mainly by cholinergic endings with a minority of adrenergic endings (Shields *et al.*, 1987). However, this account is complicated by the fact that the epitrichial sweat glands of the dog and horse also respond to acetylcholine (Jenkinson, 1973), even though the mechanism controlling the glands in these two species is not essentially cholinergic (Jenkinson, 1969, 1973). Yet another complication in the horse is that its sweat glands respond to exercise, provided that the adrenal medulla and its innervation are intact (Jenkinson, 1969). Furthermore the sweat glands of the horse appear to be directly responsive to increased blood flow, so that in an area that has undergone sympathetic denervation the vasodilation apparently causes profuse sweating (de Lahunta, 1983, p. 117); this can be a feature in clinical cases of sympathetic deficit in horses (Section 2.29). In the **atrichial sweat glands** of man and the foot pads of the dog, cat, and rat, the mechanism appears to operate through sympathetic **cholinergic** neuronal pathways (Jenkinson, 1969; Shields *et al.*, 1987). However, the picture is again complicated by observations showing that the atrichial glands in man show some response to injections of adrenaline (Jenkinson, 1969, 1973; Shields *et al.*, 1987), and that some of the innervation of these glands in man is adrenergic (mainly β-adrenergic, and slightly α-adrenergic) as well as cholinergic (Shields *et al.*, 1987). The atrichial glands in the foot pads of the cat also respond to adrenaline and noradrenaline.

To summarize: (1) **adrenergic** sympathetic neuronal pathways dominate in **epitrichial** glands; (2) **cholinergic** sympathetic neuronal pathways dominate only in the **atrichial** sweat glands of man and the foot pads of the dog and cat; (3) there are indications of both **adrenergic and cholinergic** factors in both **atrichial and epitrichial** glands, suggesting the possibility of a dual innervation of both types of gland. This rather baffling mixture of adrenergic and cholinergic properties in sudomotor axons is considerably clarified by the multipotential attributes of developing sympathetic postganglionic neurons (Section 2.5).

Attempts to clarify the innervation by **histological** and **ultrastructural studies** of the **nerve endings** have so far proved indecisive. Both types of sweat gland possess an inner secretory epithelium covered by a layer of **myoepithelial cells**, and an outer sheath of fibrocytes. The myoepithelial cells could expel secretion or regulate the supply of metabolites to the secretory cells (Williams *et al.*, 1989, p. 1226). In the atrichial glands of man the **secretory cells** are of two types, dark and light (Williams *et al.*, 1989, p. 1226). There are few blood vessels or nerves near the epitrichial glands of the ox, sheep, goat, and cat, and no axonal varicosities within the fibrocyte sheath; these glands therefore appear not to be directly innervated (Jenkinson *et al.*, 1978). On the other hand, many blood vessels (mostly capillaries) and **unmyelinated axons** lie close to the atrichial glands of man and the cat's foot pad, and to the epitrichial glands of the equine body surface (Jenkinson *et al.*, 1978), and there are **axonal varicosities** and capillaries actually inside the fibrocyte sheath of the gland (Jenkinson *et al.*, 1978); therefore, these glands may be directly innervated (Jenkinson *et al.*, 1978, p. 636). The epitrichial glands of man evidently possess both **adrenergic** and **cholinergic endings** (Williams *et al.*, 1989, p. 1226). These findings have been variously interpreted: (1) **adrenergic mechanisms** may control the myoepithelium, leading to **discharge of sweat**, and **cholinergic mechanisms** may control **secretion** (Jenkinson, 1969; Shields *et al.*, 1987); (2) glands that are not directly innervated may be activated by the transfer of transmitter substances by cutaneous blood vessels (Jenkinson *et al.*, 1978).

2.8 Course of sympathetic postganglionic axons to somatic regions of body

In principle, every segment of the body from the head to the tail has a pair of vertebral ganglia and every spinal nerve receives a grey ramus communicans. Therefore each spinal nerve contains an allocation of vasomotor, sudomotor, and piloerector postganglionic sympathetic axons. It is these pathways that enable a cat to raise its fur from the beginning of its neck to the end of its tail. In Fig. 2.4 the grey rami are represented by the green lines that extend upwards from every vertebral ganglion and then turn down towards an arrowhead. The dorsal and ventral rami of the spinal nerves (Section 2.2) carry their postganglionic sympathetic axons to all parts of the head, neck, trunk, limbs, and tail. However, the final distribution of postganglionic axons to the target tissues (blood vessels, sweat glands, and hair erecting muscles) is attained by transfer

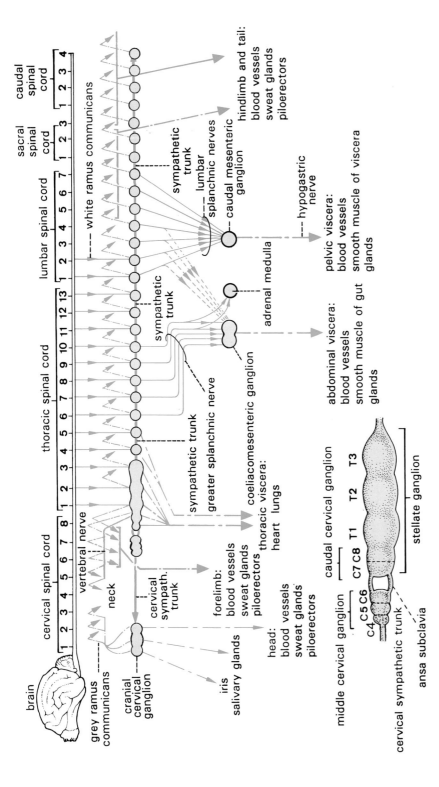

Fig. 2.4 Diagram summarizing the sympathetic motor pathways in a hypothetical mammal. A vertebral ganglion (light green) lies on each vertebra, except in the neck where some ganglia fuse to form the stellate ganglion and the middle and cranial cervical ganglia. The vertebral ganglia are linked, forming the sympathetic trunk (chain). The sympathetic motor pathways are represented by green lines. The outflow from spinal cord to vertebral ganglia of preganglionic pathways (continuous green lines) in white rami communicantes is restricted to segments T1 to L2 inclusive. Postganglionic pathways (green dot-dash lines) return as grey rami communicantes to each spinal nerve, including the spinal nerves that supply the limbs and tail. Arrowheads indicate the direction of motor impulses. Postganglionic pathways project from the stellate ganglion to the heart and lungs, and from the cervical ganglia to the forelimbs and head. Preganglionic pathways project to the prevertebral ganglia (coeliacomesenteric and caudal mesenteric ganglia) in greater splanchnic and lumbar splanchnic nerves. The first few lumbar splanchnic nerves not only supply the caudal mesenteric ganglion (continuous lines) but may also supply the coeliacomesenteric ganglion (broken lines). Postganglionic pathways (green dot-dash lines) project from the prevertebral ganglia to the abdominal and pelvic viscera. The inset shows the derivation of the stellate ganglion from a fusion of the caudal cervical ganglion with the vertebral ganglia T1–T3. The middle cervical ganglion is joined to the stellate ganglion by the ansa subclavia. The cervical and thoracic ganglia that fuse are indicated by C4 to T3.

of these axons to the terminal branches of the **arterial tree**.

This segmental pattern of distribution of sympathetic postganglionic axons to the somatic parts of the body holds good in principle. However, some of the primordial vertebral ganglia become fused in the embryo (Section 2.5), in the neck (Section 2.19) and in the tail (Section 2.25), so that their segmental arrangement is lost.

The **great arteries** near the brachial and lumbosacral plexuses (e.g. the subclavian and iliac arteries) receive postganglionic filaments directly from the adjacent sympathetic ganglia or plexuses (Mitchell, 1953, pp. 232, 298). It was originally believed that these perivascular plexuses continue to the terminal arterial branches, and surgery to relieve arterial spasm in man was based on this view. It was eventually shown that such perivascular pathways in the limbs extend only a short distance (for example, the iliac arterial pathway only reaches the middle of the thigh) and that further distally the pathways are continued in branches of peripheral nerves (Clark, 1965, p. 220).

III SYMPATHETIC MOTOR PATHWAYS TO THORACIC VISCERA

2.9 Sympathetic preganglionic neurons controlling thoracic viscera

The cell station of sympathetic preganglionic neurons controlling the thoracic viscera is the **lateral horn** of the five segments T1–T5 (Fig. 2.2; neuron 1, segment T5, in Fig. 2.5). The axon of the preganglionic sympathetic neuron typically makes synapses with about 20 postganglionic neurons. Most of these synapses are in the stellate ganglion.

2.10 Functions of sympathetic postganglionic neurons innervating thoracic viscera: stellate ganglion

The cell station of sympathetic postganglionic neurons supplying thoracic viscera is mainly in the **stellate ganglion** (cervicothoracic ganglion). The stellate ganglion is formed by fusion of the last

few cervical and first few thoracic vertebral ganglia (Fig. 2.4, inset). It is a large ganglion, lying within the thoracic inlet at the dorsal end of the first intercostal space.

Functionally the postganglionic axons to the thoracic viscera are of four types (Fig. 2.5): (i) motor cardiac axons to the heart, (ii) vasomotor axons to the coronary vessels, (iii) motor axons to the smooth muscle of the bronchial tree, and (iv) motor axons to the bronchial glands. The functions of types (i) and (iii) are predictable from the requirements of **fight and flight**.

In addition to synapses in the stellate ganglion (ganglion cervicothoracicum), the preganglionic neuron may also make synapses in the vertebral ganglia of segments T4 and T5 as shown in Fig. 2.5, or in the middle cervical ganglion (Fig. 2.4, inset).

Species variations in the thoracic ganglia that combine to form the **stellate ganglion** are: horse, T1 and T2 (McKibben, 1975, p. 690); man, T1, with T2 and sometimes T3 and T4 (Williams *et al.*, 1989, p. 1160); dog, T1–T3 (McKibben and Getty, 1968a). In man the preganglionic outflow to the thoracic viscera is from segments T1–T5 (Williams *et al.*, 1989, p. 1161). The ganglion is about 4–6 cm long craniocaudally in the horse (McKibben, 1975, p. 690), 1.5–3.0 cm in the dog (McKibben and Getty, 1968a), and about 1.5–2.5 cm in man (Mitchell, 1953, p. 227).

2.10.1 *Sympathetic postganglionic cardiac neurons*

These are distributed to the conducting system of the heart and to the cardiac muscle cells of the atria and ventricles (Section 22.8.1). They *accelerate the heart rate*, and therefore are sometimes called **cardiac accelerator axons**. They also increase the *force of ventricular contraction*.

2.10.2 *Sympathetic postganglionic vasomotor coronary neurons*

Stimulation of sympathetic cardiac nerves is followed by an increase in **coronary blood flow**. This response appears to show that these are vasodilator nerves, as would be expected from the requirements of **fight and flight**. However, the stimulation of sympathetic nerves to the heart also increases heart rate and arterial pressure, and these changes might indirectly cause the increase in coronary flow. It is now believed that these vasomotor axons are predominantly **vaso-constrictor** in action; the **vasodilation** that occurs in skeletal muscle and in the coronary circulation in exercise is induced by other factors, notably the fall in oxygen tension in the cardiac muscle cells (Section 18.6).

2.10.3 *Sympathetic postganglionic neurons to smooth muscle of bronchial tree and pulmonary vessels*

These axons inhibit the bronchial smooth muscle and therefore dilate the airway. Some axons innervate the pulmonary arterial vasculature, causing a slight vasoconstriction (see Section 17.21.4).

Control of this function varies with the species. In some species, including man, relaxation of the bronchial muscle is attained by circulating catecholamines (Section 6.12.1).

2.10.4 *Sympathetic postganglionic neurons to glands of bronchial tree*

It would be expected that these sympathetic pathways would *inhibit* the secretion of mucus and thus keep the airway clear for fight and flight (Section 6.12.2). However, the action of the sympathetic system on the mucous glands and goblet cells of the tracheobronchial tree is far from clear, earlier observations being negative or equivocal. But it has now been shown that sympathetic stimulation and sympathomimetic amines *increase* tracheal output of mucus, acting mainly or wholly through β-adrenergic receptors (Gallagher *et al.*, 1975).

2.10.5 *Sympathetic postganglionic neurons to branches of the pulmonary arteries and their arterioles*

Stimulation of these motor pathways causes slight pulmonary arterial vasoconstriction, but the sympathetic system has no major function in the control of the pulmonary circulation (Section 17.21.4).

2.11   Course of sympathetic postganglionic axons to thoracic viscera

The postganglionic sympathetic axons pass directly to the **heart** (Fig. 3.1) as a network of **sympathetic cardiac nerves**, lying in the mediastinum. The postganglionic axons to the **lungs** (Fig. 3.1),

also in the mediastinum, pass to the hilus of the lung and follow the bronchial tree.

In the dissection room the **sympathetic cardiac nerves** are less distinct than this description might suggest. Some authors failed to find any at all in the dog and cat, or observed them on the left side only (see McKibben and Getty, 1968a,b, for review), but they are in fact present, though very variably, on both sides. Many such filaments, some relatively large and others quite delicate, arise not only from the sympathetic ganglia but also from the vagus nerve. Of those that arise from the sympathetic ganglia in the dog and cat, the majority spring from the left and right middle cervical ganglia (McKibben and Getty, 1968a,b; these authors call the middle cervical ganglion the 'vertebral' ganglion (see Section 2.19). At least in the dog, the cardiac nerves are nearly always a mixture of sympathetic and vagal axons, no matter which trunk they arise from, and moreover the mixture is very variable (Stromberg, 1993, p. 1041). In the horse several cardiac nerves arise from the left and right stellate ganglia, and from the sympathetic trunk as far caudally as the seventh intercostal space (McKibben, 1975, pp. 691, 693), but as in the dog and cat most of the sympathetic cardiac innervation comes from the middle cervical ganglion (McKibben and Getty, 1969a). In the ox and sheep cardiac nerves arise from the left and right stellate ganglia, but the vertebral ganglia of segments T3–T6 contribute most of the sympathetic cardiac nerves (McKibben, 1975, pp. 1156–1159).

The profuse network of sympathetic and vagal cardiac filaments forms the **cardiac plexus** (McKibben, 1975, p. 693) (Fig. 19.8).

Having reached the heart, sympathetic cardiac axons travel along the coronary vessels to each chamber of the heart and finally disperse to their target tissues in the conducting system and myocardium (Section 22.8.1). The vasomotor coronary axons end on the arteries and arterioles of the coronary vasculature.

Sympathetic bronchial axons are distributed to the lungs mainly in the several **vagal bronchial nerves**. These form the **pulmonary plexus** (Section 6.12) and then enter the hilus of the lung along the bronchial tree.

IV   SYMPATHETIC MOTOR PATHWAYS TO ABDOMINAL VISCERA

2.12   Sympathetic preganglionic neurons controlling abdominal viscera: greater splanchnic nerve

The cell station of preganglionic sympathetic neurons controlling the abdominal viscera is in the lateral horn of the five segments T6–T10 (Fig. 2.2; neuron 2 in Fig. 2.5). The axon passes through the vertebral ganglion of the same segment, and then becomes part of the **greater splanchnic nerve**. The axon ends by entering a **pre**vertebral ganglion, where it forms numerous branches which synapse with postganglionic neurons. The ratio of pre- to postganglionic neurons is therefore about 1:20, as in the vertebral ganglia (Section 2.3.6).

Species variations in the segments of the spinal cord that form the **greater splanchnic nerve** (nervus splanchnicus major) are as follows: man, mainly T5–T10, but sometimes also T1–T4 (Williams *et al.*, 1989, p. 1162); dog, T6–T13; cat, T5–T7 (Ghoshal, 1975, p. 1738); horse, T6–T16 (Dyce, 1958). The nerve is at first smaller and then much larger caudally than the sympathetic chain, which it accompanies closely in passing from the thorax to the abdomen between the crus of the diaphragm and psoas minor muscle (Sisson and Grossman, 1969, p. 854).

One to three ill-defined **lesser splanchnic nerves** (nervi splanchnici minores) arise from the last thoracic and first lumbar vertebral ganglia (Ghoshal, 1975, p. 1734) and lose themselves in the greater splanchnic nerve or in the autonomic plexuses and lesser ganglia associated with the aorta.

The first two to four **lumbar splanchnic nerves** (nervi splanchnici lumbales) (Section 2.16) may also contribute preganglionic axons to the coeliacomesenteric ganglion (Fig. 2.4, broken lines) and to the plexuses on the aorta.

2.13 Sympathetic prevertebral ganglia

The sympathetic prevertebral ganglia arise embryologically from the neural crest (Section 2.5). Paired primordia form on the ventral surface of the aorta. The two members of the pair typically lie on either side of one of the great branches of the aorta; they tend to fuse across the midline, thus enclosing the root of an aortic branch within a ring of ganglionic tissue.

The most important prevertebral ganglia in the abdomen are the **coeliac** (Fig. 2.5), **cranial mesenteric**, and **caudal mesenteric ganglia**, so named according to the three great branches of the aorta (coeliac, cranial mesenteric, and caudal mesenteric) with which they are associated. The coeliac and cranial mesenteric ganglia tend to fuse craniocaudally into a composite **coeliacomesenteric ganglion** (Fig. 2.4). The cell bodies and axons of sympathetic postganglionic neurons form the main constituents of the coeliac, cranial mesenteric, and caudal mesenteric ganglia.

The **coeliac, cranial mesenteric**, and **caudal mesenteric ganglia** supply sympathetic postganglionic axons to the abdominal viscera. These axons reach their target organs by following the arteries with which their ganglia are associated (Section 2.15). The **caudal mesenteric ganglion** innervates the **pelvic viscera** as well as the descending colon (Section 2.17).

The prevertebral ganglia are not restricted to *motor* components of the sympathetic system. They also appear to receive a substantial input of *afferent* axons from the **enteric nervous system** (Section 4.11), particularly from the colon (Jänig and McLachlan, 1987, p. 1393). These have been shown to arise from mechanoreceptors that are activated by distension of the intestinal wall (Gabella, 1987, p. 365). There is evidence of a wide range of **integrative mechanisms** in the **prevertebral ganglia** (Jänig and McLachlan, 1987, p. 1393), presumably founded on this afferent input from enteric receptors. **Pacemaker neurons** have been identified in the caudal mesenteric ganglion (Jänig and McLachlan, 1987, p. 1393).

2.14 Functions of sympathetic postganglionic neurons innervating abdominal viscera

The cell stations of the sympathetic postganglionic neurons that innervate the abdominal viscera are in the **coeliacomesenteric ganglion** and **caudal mesenteric ganglion**. Functionally, these postganglionic neurons are of three main types (see list at bottom right of Fig. 2.5): (i) vasomotor to blood vessels, (ii) motor to the smooth muscle in the wall of the gastrointestinal tract, and (iii) motor to the glands of the gastrointestinal tract. The inhibitory or excitatory functions of all three types of neuron can be largely predicted by the requirements of **fight and flight**. There are also motor neurons innervating the kidneys, ureters, and gonads.

2.14.1 *Functions of sympathetic vasomotor postganglionic neurons innervating splanchnic vasculature*

Sympathetic postganglionic vasomotor neurons innervating the splanchnic vascular bed are very

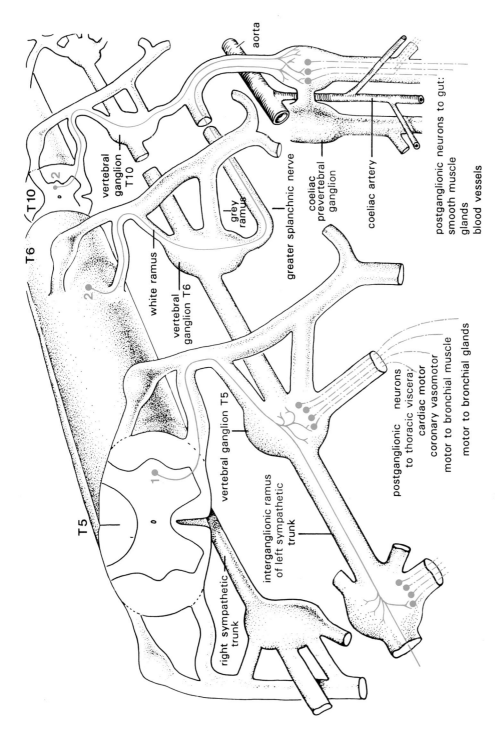

aorta

vertebral ganglion T10

grey ramus

greater splanchnic nerve

coeliac prevertebral ganglion

coeliac artery

white ramus

vertebral ganglion T6

postganglionic neurons to gut:
smooth muscle
glands
blood vessels

vertebral ganglion T5

postganglionic neurons
to thoracic viscera:
cardiac motor
coronary vasomotor
motor to bronchial muscle
motor to bronchial glands

interganglionic ramus
of left sympathetic
trunk

right sympathetic
trunk

T5

T6

T10

Fig. 2.5 Diagram of segments T5 to T10 of the spinal cord to show the sympathetic motor pathways supplying the thoracic and abdominal viscera.
The sympathetic pathways are represented by green lines, the preganglionic fibres being drawn as continuous lines and the postganglionic fibres as dot-dash lines. The pathways to the thoracic viscera are represented by preganglionic neuron 1 in the lateral horn of segment T5 (this outflow really arises from T1–T5). Neuron 1 makes synapses with any one of the four functional types of postganglionic neuron shown with their cell station in vertebral ganglion T5, i.e. cardiac motor, coronary vasomotor, motor to bronchial muscle, or motor to bronchial glands. The pathways to the abdominal viscera are represented by preganglionic neuron 2 in the lateral horn of T6 and T10. The axon of neuron 2 combines with other similar preganglionic axons to form the greater splanchnic nerve. Neuron 2 makes synapses with any one of the three functional types of postganglionic neuron shown with their cell station in the coeliac ganglion, i.e. motor to the smooth muscle of the gut wall, secretomotor to the glands of the gut, or vasomotor to the blood vessels of the gut. Not drawn to scale.

numerous, profusely innervating the arteries and veins of the gastrointestinal tract. The neuronal cell bodies lie mainly in the **coeliacomesenteric ganglion**. The axons are distributed to the branches of the coeliac artery and cranial mesenteric artery, and to the gastrointestinal veins that accompany these arteries. Other postganglionic vasomotor neurons have their cell station in the **caudal mesenteric ganglion**, and distribute their axons to the branches of the caudal mesenteric artery and its associated veins.

These vasomotor neurons are vasoconstrictor in function. They contribute to the control of systemic **arterial pressure**, since they provide a variable **resistance** to the output of the left ventricle. If the systemic arterial pressure falls, for example because of dilation of other vascular beds, reflex vasoconstriction occurs in the arteries and arterioles of the splanchnic bed. Splanchnic arterial vasoconstrictors also provide a mechanism for the **redistribution of blood** according to physiological demands (Section 13.8). For instance, in **exercise** they enable blood to be diverted from the gut to the skeletal musculature; in **haemorrhage** they allow blood to be redirected to the high priority circulations of the brain and heart. Such splanchnic arterial vasoconstriction would reduce the motility of the gut, the rate of secretion of the glands, and the rate of absorption by the gut wall, but digestion is suspended in the interests of the body as a whole.

The **veins of the splanchnic bed** (the hepatic portal vein and its tributaries) are also controlled by abundant vasoconstrictor axons. A large proportion (possibly about 70%) of the **total blood volume** is contained within the veins of the body. The veins of the splanchnic bed are particularly capacious (Section 13.3.5), and therefore form a major **blood reservoir** that can be mobilized in exercise or haemorrhage (Section 12.16.3).

Sympathetic vasomotor axons also constrict the blood vessels of the **spleen**, thus releasing blood into the general circulation (Section 14.18.2). In the domestic mammals there is abundant smooth muscle in both the capsule and the trabeculae of the spleen; this contracts intensely under sympathetic stimulation, thus releasing a relatively large volume of blood and stored red blood cells. Con-

versely, sympathetic inhibition allows the spleen to expand, forming a substantial blood reservoir.

> The coeliac, cranial mesenteric, and caudal mesenteric arteries are richly supplied with noradrenergic axons, right down to the small arterioles. The mesenteric veins, particularly the large ones, also have noradrenergic axons, but their innervation is less dense than that of the arteries, and limited to vessels over 100 μm in diameter (Gabella, 1979).

2.14.2 Functions of sympathetic postganglionic neurons innervating smooth muscle of gut

Postganglionic neurons from the coeliacomesenteric ganglion innervate the muscle in the **wall** and in the **sphincters** of the gut. Their function is predictable from the requirements of **fight and flight**. They *inhibit* the muscle in the **gut wall** causing it to relax, and they *excite* the **sphincter muscles** causing the sphincters to close. The movement of ingesta through the alimentary tract is thus arrested.

> Noradrenergic axons are present in the **myenteric plexus** (Sternini, 1988) and **submucosal plexus** (Gabella, 1979) of the gut wall. Fluorescent histochemical observations suggest that the vast majority of sympathetic postganglionic axons synapse directly with **enteric ganglion cells** (Wood, 1987, p. 103) (Section 3.21). Tracer studies show that some of these come from the prevertebral ganglia (Sternini, 1988) and others from the cranial cervical ganglion via the vagus nerve (Section 2.24.2). Those in the muscle coat are particularly numerous in the sphincter areas, and especially the internal anal sphincter (Gabella, 1979; Sternini, 1988).

2.14.3 Functions of sympathetic postganglionic neurons innervating glands of gastrointestinal tract

The glands of the gastrointestinal tract receive a motor nerve supply from sympathetic postganglionic neurons in the coeliacomesenteric ganglion. As would be expected from the needs of **fight and flight**, these pathways *inhibit* the glands of the abdominal viscera.

> In the gastrointestinal mucosa noradrenergic axons form a network around the basal parts of the glands and the adjacent blood vessels (Gabella, 1979). The noradrenaline released from such axons inhibits the

glandular secretion of the gastrointestinal tract, partly by direct actions on the glandular cells and partly through the indirect effects of vasoconstriction (Sernka and Jacobson, 1983, p. 57).

2.14.4 *Functions of sympathetic postganglionic neurons innervating kidney, ureter, and gonads*

Sympathetic postganglionic neurons in small **renal ganglia** innervate the kidney. They contribute to the **regulation of blood volume** by several mechanisms (Section 22.9.1): (1) Vasomotor sympathetic postganglionic neurons innervating the kidney are mainly *vasoconstrictor*. By regulating the calibre of the **afferent** and **efferent glomerular arterioles**, they adjust the *rate* of renal *filtration* and *reabsorption*. (2) Sympathetic postganglionic neurons control the **juxtaglomerular apparatus**; excitation of these sympathetic pathways causes the apparatus to release **renin**, and this gives rise to **angiotensin** which *constricts* the *efferent* glomerular arteriole. Also angiotensin elicits the secretion of **aldosterone** by the adrenal cortex.

Axons from the greater, lesser, and lumbar splanchnic nerves, and from the coeliac ganglion, form the **renal plexus** (plexus renalis) (Williams *et al.*, 1989, p. 1165). The sympathetic input to the renal plexus may therefore be derived from the sympathetic outflow from anywhere between segments T6 and L2 (in man, mainly from T10–T11).

Within the renal plexus there are several small **renal ganglia**; there is also a larger **aorticorenal ganglion** at the level of the renal artery (Schaller *et al.*, 1992, p. 502). Axons from the renal plexus continue into the kidney around the branches of the renal artery, supplying the vessels, glomeruli, and tubules, and especially the cortical tubules, but most of these axons are vasomotor (Berry *et al.*, 1995, p. 1307). Presumably they are mainly postganglionic sympathetic axons arising from the ganglia in the renal plexus.

The renal plexus also supplies the **ureteric, testicular,** and **ovarian plexuses** (Williams *et al.*, 1989, p. 1165). The testicular and ovarian plexuses, and the more caudal part of the ureteric plexus, are reinforced by parasympathetic axons from the pelvic plexus. Probably the sympathetic axons in the gonadal plexuses are vasoconstrictor, and the parasympathetic axons are vasodilator (Williams *et al.*, 1989, p. 1165). The testicular and ovarian plexuses also contain (sympathetic) *afferent* axons (Williams *et al.*, 1989, p. 1165), which are presumably pain pathways (Section 4.6; Fig. 4.2).

2.14.5 *Functions of sympathetic postganglionic neurons innervating the liver*

In the liver, sympathetic postganglionic *vasomotor* axons constrict both the arterial and the venous vessels (Scott, 1986, p. 88), and *secretomotor* axons stimulate *glycogenolysis* (Section 2.33.1).

2.15 Course of sympathetic postganglionic axons to abdominal viscera: autonomic plexuses

The **coeliac** and **cranial mesenteric ganglia** supply sympathetic postganglionic axons to the abdominal viscera (Fig. 3.1). The **caudal mesenteric ganglion** supplies sympathetic postganglionic axons to the **descending colon** and also to the **pelvic viscera** (Section 2.17).

The *sympathetic postganglionic* axons arising from these ganglia intermingle with *vagal preganglionic* axons to form the great **autonomic plexuses of the abdomen** (Section 3.11.1). (These numerous plexuses are named simply according to the artery that they follow, e.g. **aortic plexus, coeliac plexus, cranial mesenteric plexus,** and **caudal mesenteric plexus,** or according to the organ that they supply, e.g. **hepatic plexus, splenic plexus,** and **renal plexus.**)

The sympathetic postganglionic axons to the abdominal viscera travel to their target organs through the autonomic plexuses. Thus the axons supplying the wall of the stomach travel along the branches of the coeliac artery which supply blood to the stomach. This is shown in principle in the lower right corner of Fig. 2.5.

The **coeliac, cranial mesenteric,** and **caudal mesenteric ganglia** on the two sides of the body are connected along the aorta by two or three irregular longitudinal filaments with many connections across the midline, thus forming the **abdominal aortic plexus** (plexus aorticus abdominalis) in the midline. This plexus can be subdivided into subsidiary plexuses with subsidiary prevertebral ganglia, named according to the branches of the aorta with which they are associated. They include the aorticorenal, phrenic, and renal ganglia, and the coeliac, cranial mesenteric, caudal mesenteric, intermesenteric, hepatic, pancreatic, splenic, adrenal, renal, testicular, ovarian, cranial, rectal, iliac, and femoral plexuses. The term intermesenteric plexus (plexus intermesentericus) (or intermesenteric nerve, Dyce, 1958; Jänig and McLachlan, 1987, p. 1337) is given to the part of the aortic plexus that connects the coeliacomesenteric ganglion to the caudal mesenteric ganglion.

The anatomy of the plexuses varies within and between species, and the precise sources and destinations of their axons are uncertain.

V SYMPATHETIC MOTOR PATHWAYS TO PELVIC VISCERA

The pelvic viscera lie in the entrance to the pelvic canal, and within the canal itself. They include the rectum, bladder, urethra, uterine body, cervix, vagina, and accessory reproductive glands of the male.

2.16 Sympathetic preganglionic neurons controlling pelvic viscera: lumbar splanchnic nerves

The cell station of the sympathetic preganglionic neurons controlling the pelvic viscera lies in the lateral horn of the five segments T11 to L2 (Fig. 2.2). The axons of the preganglionic neurons pass through the segmental lumbar vertebral ganglia and emerge as the seven, segmentally arranged, **lumbar splanchnic nerves** (Fig. 2.4). These axons synapse with postganglionic sympathetic neurons in the **caudal mesenteric ganglion** (Fig. 3.1), which lies on the root of the caudal mesenteric artery.

In an extensive review of the literature, Jänig and McLachlan (1987, p. 1337) concluded that the anatomy of the sympathetic innervation of the pelvic viscera (and the terminal colon) is essentially similar in all the mammalian species so far investigated, although there are minor species differences. In the cat, the animal from which most of the information has come, the **sympathetic motor outflow** to the pelvic viscera generally originates relatively far caudally, from segments L3–L5 of the spinal cord (Jänig and McLachlan, 1987, p. 1338). Most of the preganglionic axons in this outflow pass through their segmental vertebral ganglia and project to the caudal mesenteric ganglion through four or five **lumbar splanchnic nerves** arising from vertebral ganglia L2–L5 (Baron *et al.*, 1985). In man the outflow is from segments T11–L2 of the spinal cord, most of it projecting to the caudal mesenteric ganglion via four lumbar splanchnic nerves from ganglia L1–L4. For details of the outflow

and lumbar splanchnic nerves in the dog and laboratory mammals see Jänig and McLachlan (1987, p. 1338).

Although most of the sympathetic preganglionic outflow to the pelvic viscera projects via the lumbar splanchnic nerves directly to the caudal mesenteric ganglion (where the synapses with the postganglionic neurons occur), there are three other significant pathways (Jänig and McLachlan, 1987, pp. 1333, 1337, 1346). (i) Some of the sympathetic preganglionic axons from the lumbar splanchnic nerves pass through the caudal mesenteric ganglion, and synapse with postganglionic neurons in *subsidiary ganglia* in the abdominal aortic plexus. (ii) Appreciable numbers of sympathetic preganglionic axons pass through the caudal mesenteric ganglion into the hypogastric nerve, and synapse with postganglionic neurons in small ganglia in the **pelvic plexus**; these ganglia are commonly known in the literature as the **pelvic ganglia** (Section 3.13), but this term has not been adopted by the *Nomina Anatomica Veterinaria*. Some of the ganglion cells in the pelvic ganglia receive synapses not only from preganglionic sympathetic, but also from preganglionic parasympathetic, axons (Section 3.13). (iii) Yet other sympathetic preganglionic axons travel caudally in the sympathetic chain, and synapse with postganglionic neurons in the lumbar and sacral vertebral ganglia; their postganglionic axons (forming about 20% of the total) reach the pelvic organs via the **pelvic nerve**.

The distal part of the descending colon joins the rectum at the pelvic inlet and therefore does not belong to the pelvic viscera, but in all mammalian species so far investigated it receives its sympathetic outflow from the same segments of the spinal cord as the outflow to the pelvic viscera (Jänig and McLachlan, 1987, p. 1337). The preganglionic axons synapse in the caudal mesenteric ganglion, and the postganglionic axons project to the colon in the **caudal mesenteric plexus** (Section 2.18).

2.17 Functions of sympathetic postganglionic neurons innervating pelvic viscera

The cell station of the sympathetic postganglionic neurons that innervate the pelvic viscera is in the **caudal mesenteric ganglion** (Figs 2.4, 3.1). The postganglionic axons pass caudally to the pelvic viscera as the **hypogastric nerve** (Fig. 2.4, Section 2.18). These sympathetic postganglionic neurons are of four functional types: (i) vasomotor, (ii) motor to the smooth muscle of the bladder, descending colon, and rectum, (iii) motor to the smooth muscle in the accessory reproductive glands in the male, and (iv) motor to the smooth muscle in the uterine wall. The inhibitory or excitatory functions of the vasomotor axons and of the motor axons to the bladder and rectum can be predicted by the requirements of **fight and flight**.

2.17.1 *Sympathetic postganglionic vasomotor neurons innervating the pelvic organs*

The vasomotor neurons are vasoconstrictors, and will therefore diminish the circulation in the pelvic organs in exercise.

2.17.2 *Sympathetic postganglionic neurons innervating the smooth muscle of the bladder and rectum*

Sympathetic postganglionic axons supplying the smooth muscle of the **wall** of the **bladder** and **rectum** are *inhibitory*, whereas those innervating any smooth muscle that constricts the **neck** of the **bladder** (the region of the **trigone** of the bladder) and the smooth muscle of the **internal anal sphincter** (Fig. 3.4) are *excitatory*. These patterns of innervation *promote filling* and *inhibit emptying* of the rectum and bladder. The main muscular **sphincter mechanism** of the **bladder** is provided by the **urethralis muscle**; this muscle consists of circular striated muscle surrounding the pelvic urethra, and is innervated by *somatic efferent* axons of the **pudendal nerve**.

> It is generally accepted that the filling and emptying of the **bladder** is *mainly* under the control of the *parasympathetic* pathways in the **pelvic nerve** (Sections 3.12, 3.14). The possibility that *sympathetic* postganglionic axons in the **hypogastric nerve** innervate the bladder is controversial. Some observations have indicated that stimulation of the hypogastric nerve inhibits the smooth muscle in the *wall* of the bladder and excites a *smooth muscle* **sphincter** in the neck of the bladder (Mitchell, 1953, p. 306; Taira, 1972; Williams *et al.*, 1989, p. 1167). The noradrenergic sympathetic postganglionic innervation of the smooth muscle of the bladder wall is in fact sparse, except for the superficial muscle in the region of the trigone in some species (Jänig and McLachlan, 1987, p. 1351). Other observations have suggested that the filling and emptying of the bladder are *almost entirely* controlled by its *parasympathetic innervation*, and that the *sympathetic axons* are *mainly vasomotor* in function (White *et al.*, 1952, p. 384; Mitchell, 1953, p. 306; Williams *et al.*, 1989, p. 1167) and have very little effect on bladder contraction (Guyton, 1986, p. 461).

The matter is further complicated by uncertainties about the very existence of bladder sphincters. Some anatomical studies reported a distinctly circular arrangement of muscle bundles at the neck, as in the horse (Sisson and Grossman, 1975, p. 530), and in the human male though not the human female (Dyson, 1995, p. 1840). The structure in the human male is described by Dyson as a complete circular collar of smooth muscle surrounding the neck of the bladder and the preprostatic urethra to which the term internal urethral sphincter could suitably be applied; however, in the human female the corresponding region of the urethra is devoid of a well-defined circular component of smooth muscle, and therefore there is no smooth muscle sphincter. In the female goat there are 'no circular smooth muscle fibres that could possibly constitute a sphincter' (Hartman, 1973, p. 63). In the bitch, a coat of smooth muscle beneath the mucosa (i.e. between the mucosa and the striated urethralis muscle) has been called the **internal urethral sphincter**; excitation of this muscle by sympathomimetic drugs has been successfully employed to control incontinence in the bitch (White and Pomeroy, 1989). However, there is also evidence in the domestic mammals and man that the smooth muscle bundles in the neck of the bladder are directed *towards* the orifice, i.e. *longitudinally* rather than circularly, and should therefore dilate rather than constrict the orifice (Ruch, 1966, p. 1016; Dyce *et al.*, 1987, p. 181); if so, there is *no internal sphincter of the bladder*. According to this view, the neck of the bladder resists the pressure within the filling bladder essentially *passively* because the radius of the lumen of the neck is relatively small and therefore, according to Laplace's law, the narrow neck exerts a relatively great pressure; dilation of the neck by contraction of its *longitudinal* muscle bundles reduces the resistance to flow and micturition occurs (Ruch, 1966, p. 1016). Ruch (1974, p. 537) noted reports that the neck of the bladder in man does contain an exceedingly rich collection of circular elastic fibres that could contribute to closure. The concept that there is *no true internal sphincter of the bladder* is widely accepted (Ruch, 1966, p. 1016; 1974, p. 536; Brodal, 1981, p. 768; Dyce *et al.*, 1987, p. 181).

The so-called '**external sphincter**' of the bladder is in fact the **urethralis muscle**, which consists of circular skeletal muscle surrounding the pelvic urethra in the male and female of the domestic mammals and man (Williams *et al.*, 1989, p. 1422). This muscle is believed to play 'an important active role' in the voluntary restraint of micturition at rest in the human male and female (Williams *et al.*, 1989, p. 1423). Hartman (1973, pp. 63, 91) believed it to be the *only* factor maintaining continence in the female goat; in this animal the urethralis muscle begins about half way between the vesico-urethral junction and the external urethral orifice, and as the bladder becomes distended the proximal part of the urethra forms a funnel-shaped extension of the bladder which gradually advances along the urethra.

The striated urethralis muscle is generally stated to be under the control of **somatic motor axons** of the **pudendal nerve** (e.g. Christensen, 1979, p. 576; Williams *et al.*, 1989, p. 1149). However, it has been claimed that in man the nerve axons travel in the **pelvic nerve** (pelvic splanchnic nerve in the *Nomina Anatomica*, 1989) (Williams *et al.*, 1989, p. 1422). The pudendal nerve is formed by sacral spinal nerves: S3–S4 in the horse; mainly S3, but also S2 and S4 in ruminants; and all three sacral nerves in the dog and cat (Ghoshal, 1975, pp. 686, 1147, 1711, 1722); it definitely innervates the **external anal sphincter** (Fig. 3.4).

A survey by Janssens and Peeters (1997) indicated that **urinary incontinence** may affect middle-aged spayed bitches when deeply relaxed as in sleep, especially in certain docked breeds. Leakage of urine is also distressingly common in multiparous postmenopausal women who had difficult deliveries, the leakage occurring when the intraabdominal pressure is raised during physical stress such as coughing. It is believed that, owing to hormonal deficiencies, the capacity of the striated urethralis muscle to seal the urethral lumen is impaired. In women, damage to the pudendal nerve during labour is a contributory factor. Some improvement of urethral control may be achieved by administration of oestrogens and sympathomimetics, and by a large variety of surgical procedures, but none of these treatments has yielded a high success rate in dogs.

Despite the uncertainties about the possible anatomy of bladder sphincters, it seems to be generally agreed that sympathetic motor axons in the hypogastric nerve activate smooth muscle at the neck of the bladder in the human male during **ejaculation**, which does somehow prevent reflux of semen into the bladder (Williams *et al.*, 1989, p. 1409); standard techniques of transurethral surgery for the relief of an enlarged prostate in man disable this function, with resulting loss of fertility. In the **penis**, noradrenergic sympathetic postganglionic endings occur around most arteries in the corpus cavernosum, but there are few in the corpus spongiosum; **erection** elicited by stimulation of the pelvic nerve may subside on stimulation of the hypogastric nerves (Jänig and McLachlan, 1987, p. 1359). There is no doubt that **seminal emission** is induced by sympathetic postganglionic axons innervating smooth muscle in the male accessory reproductive glands; however, although erection can occur in human males with spinal transection at cervical or thoracic levels, emission and ejaculation almost never happen, and therefore the latter functions must depend on signals descending from the brain (Jänig and McLachlan, 1987, p. 1391).

2.17.3 *Sympathetic postganglionic neurons innervating smooth muscle in male accessory glands*

These postganglionic neurons are involved in ejaculation. They cause sudden contraction of the smooth muscle in the accessory glands; this delivers semen into the pelvic urethra, a function known as **seminal emission**. **Ejaculation proper**, the ejection of semen from the whole length of the urethra, is achieved by the reflex contraction of the striated musculature associated with the pelvic and penile urethra (the **urethralis muscle**), under the control of somatic motor pathways in the **pudendal nerve**. The pudendal nerve is also motor to the external anal sphincter.

2.17.4 *Sympathetic postganglionic neurons innervating smooth muscle of uterine wall*

The postganglionic sympathetic axons supplying the smooth muscle in the wall of the **uterus** cause transient contraction.

The functions of the postganglionic sympathetic motor axons to the **uterus** are uncertain. This is partly because the uterine musculature is strongly affected by circulating hormones (Williams *et al.*, 1989, p. 1136), and also because uterine responses vary in different physiological states (Mitchell, 1953, p. 310). Although there is a diffuse adrenergic innervation of the smooth muscle of the uterine wall, the role of these axons in uterine function remains unknown (Creed, 1979; Jänig and McLachlan, 1987, p. 1393). However, the general impression seems to be that they usually cause contraction of the smooth muscle in the uterine wall, and vasoconstriction (Williams *et al.*, 1989, p. 1167; Mitchell, 1953, p. 310).

Circulating catecholamines in the non-pregnant uterus are usually associated with *relaxation* of the smooth muscle in the uterine wall (Russell, 1966, p. 1140) through β receptors (Section 2.33.1) (Creed, 1979), but oestrogen increases the sensitivity to α excitation (Creed, 1979); the pregnant uterus may be excited by these hormones (Russell, 1966, p. 1140).

The function of the sympathetic uterine innervation is presumably of minor importance, since the *denervated uterus* functions normally during pregnancy and parturition (Crosby *et al.*, 1962, p. 543). Indeed, the use of protein gene product 9.5, which is a general cytoplasmic marker that demonstrates all types of afferent and efferent nerve fibre, has shown that *neuronal degeneration* is almost total in the uterus of the guinea pig at term (Lundberg *et al.*, 1988).

Jänig and McLachlan (1987, p. 1389) pointed out that the sympathetic preganglionic outflow to the pelvic viscera is believed to be slightly larger numerically than the parasympathetic preganglionic outflow to the same viscera, and yet the lumbar sympathetic outflow can apparently be lost without significant impairment of function, with the solitary exception of the failure of seminal emission. Admittedly a substantial part of the sympathetic preganglionic outflow is vasoconstrictor, but there must be a surprisingly large number of preganglionic neurons with nonvascular functions that cannot yet be accounted for.

2.18   Course of sympathetic postganglionic axons to pelvic viscera: hypogastric nerve and pelvic plexus

Sympathetic postganglionic axons reach the pelvic viscera in the paired **hypogastric nerve** (Fig. 2.4), which lies on the ventrolateral aspect of the sacrum parallel with the caudal continuation of the aorta (the median sacral artery). In the pelvic cavity the hypogastric nerve (sympathetic) joins with the **pelvic nerve** (parasympathetic) to form the **pelvic plexus**. The pelvic plexus lies on the lateral aspect of the rectum (Section 3.13). The sympathetic and parasympathetic components of the pelvic plexus co-operate to regulate defaecation, urination, erection, and ejaculation.

The sympathetic postganglionic axons to the descending colon travel through the **caudal mesenteric plexus** (plexus mesentericus caudalis) (the lumbar colonic nerves of Jänig and McLachlan, 1987, p. 1339). In the cat and dog this plexus follows the caudal mesenteric artery and its branches to the descending colon and the cranial part of the rectum (Evans and Christensen, 1979, p. 726).

VI   SYMPATHETIC MOTOR PATHWAYS TO FORELIMB AND CAUDAL PART OF NECK

2.19   Sympathetic preganglionic neurons controlling smooth muscle and glands in the forelimb and caudal part of neck

The cell station of sympathetic preganglionic neurons controlling smooth muscle and glands in the forelimb and caudal part of the neck is in the lateral horn of the five segments T1–T5 (Fig. 2.2). The axons synapse with postganglionic neurons in the **stellate ganglion** (Section 2.10) and in the middle and caudal cervical ganglia.

Some synapses also occur in the **middle cervical ganglion**.

The eight primordial segmental vertebral ganglia in the neck become partly fused during embryonic development (Section 2.5). It is believed that the ganglia corresponding to segments C7 and C8 become the **caudal cervical ganglion**, but this ganglion is itself incorporated into the stellate ganglion (Fig. 2.4, inset). The vertebral ganglia of segments C4, C5, and C6 probably fuse to form the **middle cervical ganglion** (Fig. 2.4, inset). The **subclavian ansa** connects the middle and caudal cervical ganglia. The three most cranial cervical ganglia probably fuse to form the **cranial cervical ganglion** (Fig. 2.4).

The identity of the middle cervical ganglion is controversial. Some authors have interpreted this ganglion as the caudal cervical ganglion. In an attempt to avoid this difficulty it was renamed the **vertebral ganglion** in the dog and cat by McKibben and Getty (1968a,b). In man, however, the term vertebral ganglion is also given to a small ganglion close to the stellate ganglion, which is thought to be a detached portion of the stellate ganglion or of the middle cervical ganglion (Williams *et al.*, 1989, p. 1161). Therefore the term 'vertebral ganglion' is reserved in this chapter as a *general term* for the segmental ganglia that characterize the sympathetic system (Section 2.3.3).

The preganglionic outflow to the forelimb in man probably arises from segments T2–T6 of the spinal cord (Williams *et al.*, 1989, p. 1161).

2.20   Functions of sympathetic postganglionic neurons innervating smooth muscle and glands in the forelimb and caudal part of neck

The cell station of the postganglionic neuron is in the **stellate ganglion** or **middle cervical ganglion** (Fig. 2.4).

The postganglionic sympathetic neurons that innervate tissues in the forelimb and neck have the same general functions as those that are distributed to all other somatic regions of the body, i.e. vasomotor, sudomotor, or piloerector (Section 2.7). These functions are predictable from the needs of **fight and flight**.

2.21   Course of sympathetic postganglionic axons supplying forelimb and caudal part of neck

Postganglionic axons reach the forelimb and caudal segments of the neck via the **vertebral nerve**, which arises from the stellate ganglion (Fig. 2.4). The vertebral nerve is essentially a rolled up bundle of grey rami communicantes (Section 2.3.5) destined for cervical segments. It ascends cranially through the transverse foramina of the last few cervical vertebrae, alongside the vertebral artery. Between each vertebra, a grey ramus peels off the vertebral nerve and joins the spinal nerve of that particular segment (Fig. 2.4). A grey ramus goes directly from the stellate ganglion to spinal nerves T1 and C8 (Fig. 2.4).

The **ventral rami** (ventral divisions) of spinal nerves C6, C7, C8, and T1 form the **brachial plexus** (Section 2.2). The great nerves that arise from the brachial plexus (radial nerve, median nerve, etc.) distribute sympathetic postganglionic axons throughout the forelimb. The axons finally reach their target tissues by accompanying the terminal branches of the arteries of the limb.

> The **vertebral nerve** (nervus vertebralis) begins its ascent of the neck by entering the transverse foramen of the sixth cervical vertebra. It supplies grey rami communicantes to cervical spinal nerves 4, 5, 6, and 7. The **dorsal rami** of these spinal nerves then convey the postganglionic sympathetic axons to the tissues of the caudal part of the neck and of the forelimb.
>
> The **dorsal rami** (divisions) of spinal nerves C6, 7, 8 and T1 carry the postganglionic axons to target tissues in the most caudal part of the neck. Spinal nerves C4 and C5 convey postganglionic axons to the middle segments of the neck.
>
> Species variations modify the distribution of sympathetic postganglionic axons to the forelimb and neck. In the domestic mammals and man, T2 sometimes contributes to the **brachial plexus**, and in man (Williams *et al.*, 1989, p. 1130) and sometimes in the dog (Allam *et al.*, 1952) C5 also contributes to the brachial plexus; these additional nerves will carry sympathetic postganglionic axons to the limb.
>
> The **vertebral nerve** tends to become plexiform on the vertebral artery, and grey rami from the **cranial cervical ganglion** may also contribute to this plexus (Mitchell, 1953, p. 225); consequently the cranial limit of the vertebral nerve is not distinct, and some of its axons may reach the third or second cervical spinal nerves.

VII   SYMPATHETIC MOTOR PATHWAYS TO HEAD AND CRANIAL PART OF NECK

2.22   Sympathetic preganglionic neurons controlling glands and smooth muscle of head and cranial part of neck: cervical sympathetic trunk and cranial cervical ganglion

The sympathetic preganglionic neurons that supply the head and the cranial part of the neck have their cell station in the lateral horn of the first few thoracic segments of the spinal cord (T1–T5 in Fig. 2.2). The axons pass through the stellate ganglion, then continue to the head in the **cervical sympathetic trunk** (Fig. 19.1), and end by synapsing with postganglionic neurons in the **cranial cervical ganglion** (Fig. 2.4).

The cervical sympathetic trunk and vagus nerve in the neck are bound within a common fascial sheath, thus forming the **vagosympathetic trunk**. The vagosympathetic trunk is related to the trachea and common carotid artery on both sides of the neck, and to the oesophagus on the left side (Fig. 5.1).

The spindle-shaped **cranial cervical ganglion** (Fig. 19.2) lies deep between the wing of the atlas and the vertical ramus of the mandible, close to the base of the skull.

> The **ansa subclavia** (Latin, ansa, handle of a bucket or loop of a sandal) is a ring of nerve fibres connecting the **stellate ganglion** (ganglion stellatum) to the **middle cervical ganglion** (ganglion cervicale medium) (Fig. 2.4, inset). The subclavian artery passes through this ring. The postganglionic sympathetic axons that arise in the stellate ganglion and are destined to reach the cranial cervical ganglion, pass through one or other limb of the ansa, and then continue through the middle cervical ganglion to enter the cervical sympathetic trunk.
>
> The **cranial cervical ganglion** (ganglion cervicale craniale) is probably formed in the embryo by fusion of the vertebral ganglia of segments C1, C2, and C3. In the mature animal it is close to the proximal ganglion of the vagus, and to the terminal division of the common carotid artery into the external carotid, internal carotid, and occipital arteries (Fig. 19.1).
>
> Although in mammals generally the **cervical sympa-**

thetic trunk (truncus sympathicus) and **cervical vagus** form a single **vagosympathetic trunk** (truncus vago-sympathicus) (Fig. 19.1), in a few mammals including man and rabbit the two nerves remain separate. Current textbooks do not make it clear whether or not the two nerves are separate in the cat (Fig. 19.2), but Grandage (1988, p. 1110) explicitly states that they are; McKibben and Getty (1968b) show them as separate in the cat in their Fig. 3, yet use the term vagosympathetic trunk in their text. It has been reported (see McKibben, 1975, p. 1723) that slender filaments occasionally arise from the cervical sympathetic trunk and go to the trachea, oesophagus, and great vessels, but this is not confirmed by any other accounts.

2.23 Functions of sympathetic postganglionic neurons innervating glands and smooth muscle of head and cranial part of neck

The cell station is in the **cranial cervical ganglion** (Fig. 2.4). The ganglion distributes postganglionic axons to (i) the glands of the head, (ii) the dilator muscle of the iris, (iii) smooth muscle in the upper and lower eyelids, and (iv) smooth muscle of the third eyelid, and also supplies (v) vasomotor, sudomotor, and piloerector axons throughout the head and upper part of the neck. The functions of these pathways are mostly predictable from the demands of **fight and flight**.

2.23.1 *Sympathetic postganglionic axons innervating glands of head*

Sympathetic postganglionic axons innervating the **salivary glands** (Fig. 3.1) include both vasoconstrictor axons and secretomotor axons. Salivary secretion during the sympathetic activity of 'fight and flight' tends to be thick and viscous. The **lacrimal gland** receives sympathetic post-ganglionic *vasoconstrictor* axons; it is likely that sympathetic axons associated with the **lateral nasal gland, mucous glands of the nasal cavity, thyroid gland**, and **parathyroid gland** are also primarily if not entirely *vasoconstrictor*, and therefore tend to *reduce secretion*. Diminished secretion of nasal mucus keeps the airway clear in fight and flight.

The role of the sympathetic innervation of the **salivary glands** is controversial. The classical view suggested that it inhibits secretion, if only through the activity of *vasoconstrictor* fibres, but a secretomotor function has now been shown in at least some species (Magee, 1966, p. 980; Williams *et al.*, 1989, p. 1298); this function is probably activated through α-adrenoreceptors (Neal, 1992, p. 20). Parasympathetic and sympathetic endings form complex arborizations around the secretory endpieces. Cholinergic and adrenergic endings share the same Schwann cell and the same glandular cell; the sympathetic secretomotor endings also induce contraction of the myoepithelial cells in the ducts and secretory endpieces (Williams *et al.*, 1989, pp. 1297–1298). However, there is considerable species variation.

Saliva formed by *adrenergic* activity differs in quantity and composition from that induced by *parasympathetic* stimulation (Williams *et al.*, 1989, p. 1298). The thick viscous saliva that follows sympathetic stimulation may be due to a reduction in blood flow caused by sympathetic vasoconstriction, rather than the direct effect of the sympathetic axons on the glandular cells (Day, 1979, p. 14). During parasympathetic stimulation, the glandular acini produce a copious primary secretion with ionic concentrations quite similar to extracellular fluid, but the duct system actively secretes potassium and reabsorbs sodium (Guyton, 1986, p. 772). Sympathetic vasoconstriction slows the rate of primary secretion, and this allows the slower flowing saliva to acquire a much higher potassium and lower sodium content than the saliva arising directly from parasympathetic stimulation (Sellers, 1977, p. 241).

It was believed that, unlike the glands elsewhere in the digestive tract, the salivary glands are entirely independent of humoral factors (Magee, 1966, p. 980). It is now known that local hormones (plasma kinins) profoundly affect salivary secretion by maintaining vasodilation after sympathetic stimulation (Williams *et al.*, 1989, p. 1280).

The **thyroid gland** receives sympathetic postganglionic axons, but their distribution suggests a vasomotor, presumably vasoconstrictor, rather than a secretomotor function. Similar axons also occur in the **parathyroid** gland, but some of these have a closer relationship to the secretory cells and may be secretomotor (Stromberg, 1993, pp. 1044–1045).

The role of the sympathetic axons in the **lacrimal gland** is not fully established. They cause vasoconstriction. Any secretory effect is small, but the mucus concentration of the secretion may increase (Tietz and Hall, 1977, p. 683).

2.23.2 *Sympathetic postganglionic axons innervating dilator muscle of iris*

Postganglionic axons from the cranial cervical ganglion supply the **dilator muscle of the iris** (Fig. 3.1) which consists of radially arranged myoepithelial cells. As predictable from **fight and flight**, the sympathetic innervation dilates the pupil.

> Sympathetic postganglionic axons also supply the **ciliary muscle**. Their function is uncertain. In some experimental mammals stimulation leads to flattening of the lens, as in accommodation for far vision (Patton, 1966, p. 229). This may result directly from inhibition of the ciliary muscle, or indirectly from vasoconstriction causing a reduction in the volume of the ciliary body (Williams *et al.*, 1989, p. 1189).

2.23.3 *Sympathetic postganglionic axons innervating smooth muscle of eyelids*

The upper and lower eyelids contain bundles of smooth muscle, constituting the superior and inferior **tarsal muscles**. These receive postganglionic axons from the cranial cervical ganglion, and widen the palpebral opening. Widening is favourable in fight and flight.

2.23.4 *Sympathetic postganglionic axons innervating retractor muscle of third eyelid*

The third eyelid or nictitating membrane (semilunar fold of the conjunctiva) in carnivores is returned to its resting position by the smooth muscle fibres of its retractor muscle, innervated by postganglionic axons from the cranial cervical ganglion. The third eyelid is removed from the field of vision in fight and flight.

> The third eyelid (plica semilunaris conjunctivae) of the cat is very mobile. It is retracted by two thin sheets of smooth muscle, the **medial** and **ventral retractor muscles of the third eyelid**, so-called because they arise respectively from the fascial coats of the medial and ventral rectus muscles of the eyeball; these insert respectively on the dorsal and ventral aspects of the shaft of the cartilage of the third eyelid (Thompson, 1961).
>
> Sharp (1987) maintained that the nictitating membrane of the horse lacks any sympathetic innervation, but this not confirmed by de Lahunta (1983, pp. 118, 217).

2.23.5 *Sympathetic postganglionic vasomotor, sudomotor, and piloerector axons of head*

These axons from the cranial cervical ganglion are distributed to cutaneous and somatic tissues throughout the head and the upper part of the neck. Vasoconstrictor axons also supply the arteries of the **brain** and **retina**. The functions of these pathways are broadly consistent with flight and fight.

> The **intracranial arteries** are abundantly supplied by sympathetic vasoconstrictor axons (Guyton, 1986, p. 340), but the brain is enclosed in a rigid bony box, and therefore the combined volume of tissue, blood, and cerebrospinal fluid must be nearly constant (Scott, 1986, p. 77). Under these conditions the role of vasoconstrictor mechanisms is not immediately obvious. However, it is possible for blood to be redistributed in the brain by constriction of the arteries of a relatively inactive area and dilation in a metabolically active area, as happens in the visual cortex; such vasodilation appears to be induced by release of vasodilator factors (Section 13.2), as in the coronary and skeletal muscle circulation. The sympathetic vasoconstrictor axons seem to have very little tonic activity, and under normal conditions induce negligible effects on blood flow when stimulated. However, a sudden increase in arterial pressure can induce vasoconstriction, suggesting a supportive function for the vascular wall (Scott, 1986, p. 78).

2.24 Course of sympathetic postganglionic axons in head and upper part of neck

The sympathetic postganglionic axons in the head reach their target tissues by two routes: (i) **vascular**, by following the internal and external carotid carotid arteries and their branches; (ii) **nervous**, by joining the cranial nerves and the first few cervical spinal nerves.

2.24.1 *Vascular distribution of sympathetic postganglionic axons in the head*

The vascular route is readily accessible because of the close anatomical relationship of the cranial cervical ganglion to the terminal branching of the common carotid artery into the internal and external carotid arteries. At this point (Fig. 19.1) a large bundle of postganglionic axons (the **internal carotid nerve**) leaves the ganglion and accompanies the **internal carotid artery** into the cranial cavity, continuing along the intracranial arterial branches. A similar bundle of postganglionic axons joins the **external carotid artery** (the **exter-**

nal carotid nerve), and continues as a plexus over the arterial branches supplying the superficial and deep components of the extracranial structures of the head.

These vascular pathways provide a route for the **sudomotor** and **piloerector axons** of the head, and for the general distribution of vasomotor axons both outside and inside the skull. The **salivary glands**, **thyroid gland**, and **parathyroid gland** obtain their sympathetic supply by the vascular route.

> The **external carotid nerve** (nervus caroticus externus) forms an external carotid plexus (Fig. 19.1). Plexuses form on the branches of the external carotid artery. Postganglionic axons detach themselves from the sympathetic plexuses on arteries lying close to the **mandibular** and **sublingual ganglia** and the **otic ganglion** (ganglion mandibulare, sublinguale, oticum); the axons penetrate these ganglia and distribute themselves into the mandibular and sublingual salivary glands, and parotid salivary gland.
>
> The **internal carotid nerve** (nervus caroticus internus) and **internal carotid artery** together enter the **carotid canal** in the tympanic part of the temporal bone. In the canal, the nerve becomes the **internal carotid plexus** on the wall of the artery. At the end of the canal (Evans and Christensen, 1979, p. 677), the artery and its plexus enter the cranial cavity and ramify over the surface of the brain.
>
> In the *horse*, before they enter the carotid canal the internal carotid artery and internal carotid nerve are suspended in a fold of the **diverticulum of the auditory tube** (guttural pouch) and may become involved in infection of the diverticulum, leading to Horner syndrome (Section 2.29).

2.24.2 *Distribution of sympathetic postganglionic axons in cranial and spinal nerves*

The cranial cervical ganglion forms true grey rami communicantes that join the first few **cervical spinal nerves** (Fig. 2.4) and distribute vasomotor, piloerector, and sudomotor axons to the cranial part of the neck. These pathways are complementary to the distribution of such axons to the more caudal part of the neck by the **vertebral nerve** (Section 2.21).

The last four cranial nerves (IX, **glossopharyngeal**; X, **vagus**; XI, **accessory**; XII, **hypoglossal**) receive filaments directly from the cranial cervical ganglion. Strictly these filaments

are not grey rami communicantes, since that term is usually reserved for connections to *spinal* nerves (Section 2.3.5); nevertheless, they consist of postganglionic (unmyelinated) axons, and these cranial nerves are homologous to spinal nerves anyway. These postganglionic sympathetic filaments consist mainly of vasoconstrictor axons, innervating blood vessels in those mucous membranes and skeletal muscles of the head that are innervated by this group of cranial nerves.

Cranial nerves III (**oculomotor**), IV (**trochlear**), V (**trigeminal**), VI (**abducent**), and VII (**facial**) receive their postganglionic sympathetic axons from the plexus that accompanies the internal carotid nerve, mostly from *within* the cranial cavity. These sympathetic postganglionic axons include an important group of motor axons that supply smooth muscle associated with the eye, in the iris and eyelids. All of these postganglionic sympathetic axons supplying the eye make a detour through the **tympanic cavity** and can be damaged there by disease, resulting in **Horner syndrome** (Section 2.29). The filaments that join the facial nerve supply vasoconstrictor axons to the **lacrimal gland** and the **glands of the nasal mucosa** (Fig. 3.1).

> The **vertebral nerve** tends to become plexiform on the vertebral artery, and the cranial cervical ganglion may also contribute to this plexus (Section 2.21). Therefore the boundary between the grey rami supplied to cervical spinal nerves by the cranial cervical ganglion and those supplied by the vertebral nerve is indistinct.
>
> The oculomotor, trochlear, trigeminal, abducent, and facial nerves receive their postganglionic sympathetic components from the **internal carotid plexus** (Williams, 1989, p. 1158). Those to the **facial nerve** arise from the plexus as the **deep petrosal nerve** (nervus petrosus profundus), shortly before the internal carotid nerve and its plexus leave the carotid canal to enter the cranial cavity (Mitchell, 1953, p. 217). The deep petrosal nerve joins the **major petrosal nerve** (nervus petrosus major) (which consists of parasympathetic preganglionic axons of the facial nerve projecting to the **pterygopalatine ganglion** (Section 3.9.1; Fig. 3.2); the combined deep and greater petrosal nerves form the **nerve of the pterygoid canal** (nervus canalis pterygoidei) (McClure, 1979, p. 922). On reaching the pterygopalatine ganglion (which lies on the pterygopalatine branch of the maxillary division of the trigeminal nerve), the sympathetic axons pass through the ganglion and travel with preganglionic axons of the facial nerve to the glands and smooth muscle of the nasal and oral mucosa, paranasal sinuses, and nasopharynx, and to the lacrimal gland (Mitchell, 1953,

pp. 166, 217; Stromberg, 1993, p. 1035) using branches of the maxillary and ophthalmic nerves (trigeminal) as a roadway.

The postganglionic sympathetic components to the **oculomotor, trigeminal, trochlear,** and **abducent nerves** leave the **internal carotid plexus** after it has entered the cranial cavity, and enter the roots from the brain stem of these cranial nerves (Mitchell, 1953, p. 217).

The pathways by which the sympathetic post-ganglionic axons reach their target tissues in the **eye** are not fully established, may vary with the species, and may be multiple (Williams *et al.*, 1989, p. 1194). However, they all begin in the **internal carotid nerve** and its **internal carotid plexus**. It has been known for over 70 years that, on their way to the orbit, they make a detour through the tympanic cavity (Mitchell, 1953, p. 204; Thompson, 1961) by branching from the internal carotid plexus as the **caroticotympanic nerves** (nervi caroticotympanici) and joining the **tympanic plexus** (plexus tympanicus) on the cochlear promontory (Mitchell, 1953, p. 217; Williams *et al.*, 1989, p. 1228). They emerge from the tympanic cavity in a filament which rejoins the internal carotid plexus and enters the cranial cavity (Mitchell, 1953, p. 204). There they form two main components that leave the plexus. One of these joins the **oculomotor nerve** and passes through its **short ciliary nerves** to supply the **tarsal muscles** (musculus tarsalis inferior and superior) (smooth muscle) (Mitchell, 1953, p. 204) and the **blood vessels** of the **retina** (Patton, 1966, p. 229) and of the **eyeball** in general (Williams *et al.*, 1989, p. 1097). The other main component joins the **ophthalmic division of the trigeminal nerve**. Some of these other axons pass through the **nasociliary branch** and its **long ciliary nerve** to inner-vate the **dilator muscle of the iris** (smooth muscle) (Thompson, 1961; Williams *et al.*, 1989, p. 1158). Others continue through the nasociliary nerve and into the **infratrochlear nerve**; they then leave the infratrochlear nerve as a fine filament that supplies the **medial muscle of the third eyelid** (smooth muscle) (Thompson, 1961). A third component of sympathetic postganglionic axons leaves the internal carotid plexus on the ventral surface of the brain and joins the **maxillary division of the trigeminal nerve** and passes through its **zygomatic branch** to innervate the **ventral muscle of the third eyelid** (smooth muscle) (Thompson, 1961). Some sympathetic axons also supply the **ciliary muscle** (smooth muscle) (Williams *et al.*, 1989, p. 1189), but their final pathway into the eyeball is uncertain.

In man, but not the domestic mammals (McKibben and Getty, 1968a,b, 1969a,b), a **cardiac nerve** arises from the cranial cervical ganglion and returns to the thorax (Williams *et al.*, 1989, p. 1161).

Tracer studies in experimental animals (Kirchgessner and Gershon, 1989) show that postganglionic axons from the cranial cervical ganglion join the vagus nerve and are distributed in the myenteric plexus of the gastroin-testinal tract.

VIII SYMPATHETIC MOTOR PATHWAYS TO HINDLIMB AND TAIL

2.25 Sympathetic preganglionic neurons controlling smooth muscle and glands in hindlimb and tail

It will be recalled (Section 2.1) that the **preganglionic outflow** of the sympathetic system from the spinal cord is confined to 15 segments of the spinal cord, and that it is only the last five of these segments that supply the hindlimb and tail (Fig. 2.2). As Fig. 2.4 shows, the axons of the postganglionic neurons in these last five segments must travel caudally a long way along the lumbar, sacral, and coccygeal (caudal) segments of the **sympathetic trunk** (Section 2.3.6), and make synapses with postganglionic neurons in the **vertebral ganglia** of these segments (Section 2.3.3).

The cell station of preganglionic neurons controlling sympathetic projections into the **hindlimb** lies in the lat-eral horn of the five segments T11–L2 (Fig. 2.2). Their axons pass caudally along the sympathetic trunk until they reach the vertebral ganglion of segment L4. Here some of them synapse with postganglionic neurons. The remainder continue caudally in the trunk, making synapses in successive lumbar and sacral vertebral gan-glia of segments as far caudally as S2 (Fig. 2.4).

Preganglionic neurons controlling sympathetic projec-tions into the **tail** also have their cell stations in the lateral horn of segments T11–L2. Their axons again pass caudally along the sympathetic trunk, until they reach the vertebral ganglion of segment S3. The first contin-gent of axons synapses here with postganglionic neu-rons. Other contingents of preganglionic axons continue along the sympathetic chain to synapse with postganglionic neurons in successive **coccygeal ganglia** (ganglia caudalia) (Fig. 2.4).

In the sacral region, the left and right sympathetic trunks move closer together so that (in the dog and cat, for example) variable fusion occurs between the three primordial pairs of sacral ganglia. After the sacral seg-ments the chain continues, in animals with tails, as thin single or paired cords with occasional erratic coccygeal ganglia which may sometimes fuse with each other (Section 2.5).

In man the paired cords end by uniting in the **ganglion impar**, a small median ganglion ventral to the coccyx. In some dogs the sacral sympathetic ganglia are reduced to a single median ganglion which has been regarded as the ganglion impar, but in contrast to man the trunks continue caudal to this ganglion (Stromberg, 1993, p. 1051). They usually go to the third or fourth caudal segment, and then continue as a slender median trunk accompanying the median caudal artery as far as the eleventh caudal segment; coccygeal (caudal) ganglia usually occur up to the seventh caudal segment (McKibbern and Ghoshal, 1975, p. 1740). In the cat the sympathetic trunks on each side fuse at about L7 and separate again after S2 (Baron *et al.*, 1985).

2.26 Functions of sympathetic postganglionic axons innervating smooth muscle and glands in hindlimb and tail

The postganglionic neurons that supply the hindlimb have their cell stations in the six vertebral ganglia of the last few lumbar segments and the first few sacral segments (L4 to S2 in Fig. 2.4). Those supplying the tail have their cell stations in the last sacral vertebral ganglion and the coccygeal vertebral ganglia (Fig. 2.4). These postganglionic axons have the same general functions as those that supply all other somatic regions of the body, i.e. vasomotor, sudomotor, or piloerector. Under conditions of **fight and flight**, the cat shows particularly impressive **piloerection** throughout the whole length of its tail.

2.27 Course of sympathetic postganglionic axons to hindlimb and tail

The hindlimbs are usually innervated by the ventral rami of the five or six spinal nerves from the last lumbar segments and the first sacral segments, which in most species form the **lumbosacral plexus** (Section 2.2). The details vary slightly according to the number of lumbar and sacral vertebrae in each species. Each of these spinal nerves receives a grey ramus communicans from its corresponding vertebral ganglion.

The great nerves formed by the lumbosacral plexus (femoral nerve, sciatic nerve, etc.) carry sympathetic postganglionic axons to all parts of the hindlimb, the final course being completed by

transferring to the terminal branches of the arteries of the limb.

In the domestic carnivores the sympathetic postganglionic axons destined to supply the **hind limbs** arise in six pairs of grey rami, from the vertebral ganglia of segments L4–S2 inclusive (Fig. 2.4). The **dorsal rami** of the same spinal nerves distribute postganglionic axons to the corresponding segments of the back.

The coccygeal (caudal) spinal nerves receive grey rami communicantes (Fig. 2.4), and convey postganglionic sympathetic axons in their branches to the **tail**.

The greatest species difference in these pathways occurs in man, which has the misfortune to lack a tail. Man has a lumbar plexus ranging from L1 to L4, a lumbosacral sympathetic trunk formed by L4 and L5, and a sacral plexus derived from the ventral rami of spinal nerves S1 to S4 inclusive. There is also one coccygeal spinal nerve (Williams *et al.*, 1989, pp. 1140, 1143).

IX PERIPHERAL SYMPATHETIC MOTOR DISORDERS

2.28 Vasomotor, sudomotor, and piloerector disturbances

Disorders in these functions can result from lesions in peripheral sympathetic pathways. An obvious result is vasodilation, due to the loss of vasoconstrictor tone. This is detectable on the surface of the body by the increased warmth of the skin at the affected site, or by the increased redness of mucous membranes.

Horses living in hot humid tropical climates commonly experience a functional anhidrosis (loss of sweating). They lose the ability to sweat, develop hyperthermia, and are unable to work, with serious effects on the racing calendar. The basis for this condition is not understood, but it can be reversed by air-conditioned housing.

Possible causes of sympathetic lesions include trauma of the sympathetic trunk or its vertebral ganglia by fractured vertebrae or ribs, or compression of rami communicantes or ganglia by tumours.

When postganglionic sympathetic axons are cut, or the ganglion containing their cell bodies is removed, the effector organ becomes increasingly responsive to circulating adrenaline or noradrenaline a few days or weeks later. This condition is known as **denervation sensitivity**. For example (Brodal, 1981, p. 720), removal of the stellate ganglion causes immediate vasodilation of the head, neck, and forelimb, through loss of vasoconstrictor tone. During subsequent weeks the flow returns to near normal through increased tone of the vascular smooth muscle. However, a dose of noradrenaline now causes a reduction in flow 2 to 4 times greater than the same dose before denervation. A possible explanation of this supersensitivity is that the disappearance of transmitter substance at the synaptic endings of the postganglionic axons stimulates the formation of many new receptor sites on the cell membrane of the smooth muscle cells (Guyton, 1986, p. 694).

2.29 The Horner syndrome

This group of clinical signs, indicating a sympathetic deficit in the head, is well known in the domestic species and man. The main features are gross constriction of the pupil (miosis), drooping of the upper eyelid, and vasodilation of the face.

The vasodilation can be detected from the warmth of skin especially of the ears, and congestion of the oral and conjunctival mucous membranes. The upper eyelid droops (ptosis) due to paralysis of its smooth muscle (the superior tarsal muscle). Also the third eyelid is extended across the eye because of paralysis of its retractor smooth muscle. In man and ox (particularly on the surface of the bovine nose) there is a loss of sweating on the face; but in the horse there is profuse sweating all over the face, apparently associated with the increased cutaneous blood flow.

A causal lesion may lie anywhere along the peripheral course of the sympathetic pathways to the eye, on the same side as the affected eye. In the dog and cat, infection of the middle ear cavity can be the cause, because of the detour through the cavity made by the sympathetic postganglionic axons to the eye (Section 2.24.2). Infection of the diverticulum of the auditory tube (guttural pouch) that damages the internal carotid nerve (Section 2.24.1) is a possible cause in the horse. Horner syndrome can arise in small animals that have been run over by a car; the impact can force the forelimb caudally and rupture the roots of the brachial plexus, with tearing extending to the region of the stellate ganglion. In the dog the cervical sympathetic trunk can be damaged by a bite. For central lesions causing Horner syndrome, see the Volume on the CNS.

2.30 Dysautonomia

This condition may involve dysfunction of both the sympathetic and the parasympathetic systems. See Section 4.19.

X TRANSMITTER SUBSTANCES IN PERIPHERAL AUTONOMIC PATHWAYS

Because the sympathetic and parasympathetic effector endings share similar features, the following account considers both the sympathetic and the parasympathetic systems.

In the autonomic nervous system, a preganglionic neuron terminates in an axonal ending that releases a chemical neurotransmitter which acts on a postganglionic cell body: likewise the postganglionic neuron terminates in an axonal ending that releases a chemical neurotransmitter, and this acts on a target cell such as a smooth muscle cell. In principle these relationships are essentially similar to the synapse between two successive neurons in the brain, or at the synapse between the motor end-plate of a somatic motor neuron and a skeletal muscle cell. In every case, the first cell requires a chemical transmitter substance to act on the second cell.

Perhaps not surprisingly, however, the processes differ in detail. The actual structural design of the endings varies. The differences in structure have little impact on the functions of these structures, but the functional anatomy of the synapse is so basic that no applied biologist should overlook it. The differences in the neurotransmitter substances are a different matter, since these overflow into physiological differences of potential diagnostic importance and become of pharmacological significance in the treatment of disease.

2.31 Autonomic motor nerve endings

Transmission of a nerve impulse requires a specialized nerve ending to present neurotransmitter substance to the target cell. In the central nervous system, and at the neuromuscular junction between somatic neuron and skeletal muscle fibre, the axonal ending is enlarged into a button-like swelling, the **synaptic bulb**. This goes by many other names, but nearly all of them can be easily recognized (e.g. synaptic end bulb, presynaptic end bulb, synaptic knob, and a French term bouton terminal). The official name is terminal bulb (bulbus terminalis).

Nerve signals are projected from the synaptic

bulb to the target cell across a narrow gap, the **synapse**. Synapses are basically of two types, chemical and electrical, the great majority being chemical. **Chemical synapses** have the useful characteristic of being able to transmit signals in *one direction only*, i.e. from the terminal bulb to the target cell, and this enables signals to be accurately directed to highly specific target cells. However, chemical transmission unavoidably introduces an irreducible delay into the transmission of a reflex. **Electrical synapses** are characterized by **gap junctions**, and are therefore fast but are liable to transmit signals *in either direction*.

Since chemical transmission is in one direction only, structural asymmetry at the synapse is predictable. The synaptic bulb has two vital components, synaptic vesicles and mitochondria. The **synaptic vesicles** contain transmitter substance, which excites or inhibits the target cell. The **mitochondria** provide ATP for the rapid synthesis of new transmitter substance, since transmitter substance acts for only a few seconds after release. The synaptic vesicles release their contents into the synaptic cleft (the space between the bulb and the target cell), when an action potential reaches the synaptic bulb. Release is probably caused by the flow of large numbers of calcium ions into the bulb together with the sodium ions that cause the action potential. The calcium ions bind with protein receptors on the plasmalemma, and this then causes the synaptic vesicles to fuse with the plasmalemma and discharge to the exterior by exocytosis.

Autonomic endings on **smooth muscle cells** take the form of a bare axon with a chain of enlargements, or **varicosities**, like oranges in a stocking. Each varicosity is packed with vesicles containing transmitter substance, and there is also a supporting array of mitochondria. Transmitter substances are released from a varicosity by exocytosis, and must then diffuse across the **junctional cleft** (equivalent to the synaptic cleft), through the intercellular fluid, in order to reach receptor sites on target cells, for example smooth muscle. Once started, the impulse to contract may spread throughout a sheet of smooth muscle by passing from muscle cell to muscle cell at points of low electrical resistance, i.e. at **gap junctions** (often known as nexi), as in the myocardium.

The **synaptic cleft** in a typical classical synapse is about 20–50 nm wide, whereas the **junctional cleft** between a varicosity and a smooth muscle cell is sometimes much wider, varying from 20 nm to 2 μm (Burnstock, 1985).

Usually varicosities lack pre- or postjunctional membrane specializations. Varicosities are about 1–2 μm in diameter, about 10 times the diameter of the intervening lengths of axon. Only a few of the varicosities in a chain seem to release transmitter during a single nerve impulse (Burnstock, 1985).

A preganglionic fibre typically forms a number of terminal branches in several ganglia, making synaptic connections with about 20 or more postganglionic neurons (Section 2.3.6). It is likely that all these postganglionic neurons will be of the same functional type, e.g. sudomotor, vasomotor, etc., thus enabling each preganglionic neuron to act in only one effector system (Williams *et al.*, 1989, p. 1157). The vast majority of synapses in sympathetic ganglia are axodendritic (Weiner and Taylor, 1985, p. 70), but the distribution over the whole surface has not been studied (Jänig and McLachlan, 1987, p. 1345).

2.32 Ligand-activated ion channels

The movement of hydrophilic molecules into or out of a cell is obstructed by the lipid cell membrane (plasmalemma). Ion channels (receptor–channel complexes) in the cell membrane are formed by a **receptor protein molecule** projecting through the surface of a cell; these have a central channel which can be opened or closed when a transmitter substance (the **ligand**) binds to the receptor and thus alters the molecular conformation of the complex. When open, the channel allows the ready transfer of ions down their concentration gradients, into or out of the cell. Such a channel is known as a **channel protein**. It has to have two principal components, namely a *binding component* that binds with the neurotransmitter, and a *channel (ionophore) component* that acts as the ion channel. There are also **carrier proteins** that bind with substances and then transport them to the other side of the membrane.

Two types of ligand-activated channels are particularly important, i.e. sodium and potassium channels. An *inflow* of sodium ions into an excitable cell (nerve cell or muscle cell) *excites* the cell: therefore a transmitter substance that opens sodium channels is an **excitatory transmitter**. On the other hand, an *outflow* of potassium ions *inhibits* the cell, so the transmitter substance that opens potassium channels is an **inhibitory transmitter**.

A transmitter substance may have either

excitatory or inhibitory effects on the same tissue, for example on smooth muscle in different parts of the bladder (Section 2.33): it is the receptor that determines whether the response will be excitation or inhibition.

2.33 Adrenergic and cholinergic transmission

The classical neurotransmitters in motor autonomic nerves are noradrenaline and acetylcholine. Motor endings that release noradrenaline are known as **adrenergic endings** (although 'noradrenergic' would be more appropriate), and those that release acetylcholine are **cholinergic endings**.

2.33.1 *Noradrenaline and adrenoreceptors*

Noradrenaline (synonym, norepinephrine) is the transmitter substance released by the great majority of **postganglionic sympathetic endings**. It acts on the effector organ (the target cell, i.e. a smooth muscle cell, a cardiac muscle cell, or a glandular cell) through ion channels mediated by two types of receptor, **alpha-** and **beta-adrenoreceptors.** In general, the α-*adrenoreceptors* are *excitatory* and the β-*adrenoreceptors* are *inhibitory*, but a notable exception is the excitatory action of β$_1$-adrenoreceptors on the heart (Section 22.8.1).

These two types of adrenoreceptor account for the ability of noradrenaline to excite **smooth muscle** in some tissues and inhibit it in others. For example, the smooth muscle in the wall of the bladder is *inhibited* by β-receptors, whereas the smooth muscle that constricts the junction of the urethra and bladder (Section 2.17) is *excited* by α-adrenoreceptors. As stated in Section 2.32, the binding of noradrenaline to the α-adrenoreceptor of a smooth muscle cell opens the ion channel to Na$^+$ ions, thus depolarizing the cell and leading to contraction: binding with the β$_2$-adrenoreceptor of a smooth muscle cell opens the channel to K$^+$ ions, thus hyperpolarizing the cell and leading to relaxation. For an account of membrane potentials see King (1987).

Other α-**adrenoreceptor** excitatory effects on **smooth muscle** cells include *vasoconstriction* of nearly all blood vessels (Sections 2.7.1; 2.14.1; 13.3.2); *closure of intestinal sphincters* (Section 2.14.2); *contraction* of the smooth muscle of the *spleen* (Section 2.14.1); *dilation of the pupil* (via *contraction* of radially-arranged myoepithelial cells, Section 2.23); and *piloerection* (Section 2.7.3). It will be noticed that all of these effects of α-adrenoreceptors on smooth muscle are predictable from **fight and flight**, with the important exceptions of the smooth muscle of blood vessels in skeletal muscles and the myocardium – vasodilation during flight and fight *does* occur in skeletal and cardiac muscle, but it is activated metabolically by a fall in oxygen tension (Sections 2.7.1; 2.10.2); and not by neuronal activity.

Beta-adrenoreceptors are divided into two types, β$_1$ and β$_2$. Beta$_2$-adrenoreceptors cause *relaxation* of *vascular* (Section 13.3.2), *bronchial* (Section 6.12.1), and *uterine* smooth muscle, and also *inhibit* the smooth muscle of the *gut wall*. Beta$_1$-adrenoreceptors *excite cardiac muscle*, causing both cardiac acceleration and increased force of myocardial contraction. The relaxation of bronchial and gut wall muscle, and the excitation of the heart, are predictable in **fight and flight**.

It is believed that most smooth muscle cells have both α- and β$_2$-receptors, with a preponderance of one or the other. A smooth muscle cell will contract or relax depending on whether α- or β$_2$-receptors predominate. For example, α-receptors generally predominate in **vascular smooth muscle**, and therefore the standard response of blood vessels to sympathetic stimulation is vasoconstriction (Section 13.3.2).

The sympathetic innervation of glandular cells is generally inhibitory, but this may be an indirect effect through vasoconstriction (Section 2.23.1).

As is predictable from the concept of **fight and flight**, the sympathetic system increases the availability of glucose for rapid metabolism. The sympathetic innervation of the **liver** therefore stimulates rapid **glycogenolysis**.

The responses of α- and β-receptors to circulating **adrenaline** and **noradrenaline** (Section 2.34) are essentially similar to their responses to noradrenaline released by sympathetic postganglionic endings.

Adrenaline, noradrenaline, and dopamine (the immediate precursor of noradrenaline), are **cate-**

cholamines. These are **biogenic amines** derived from tyramine (Lackie and Dow, 1989, p. 36). The aromatic part of the molecule is catechol, *o*-dihydroxybenzene. Adrenaline and noradrenaline are chemically identical, except that noradrenaline lacks a terminal methyl group.

Although β_2-adrenoreceptors are the main inhibitors of smooth muscle cells, the smooth muscle of the bronchi is also inhibited by β_1-adrenoreceptors (Section 6.12.1). The smooth muscle of the gut wall is inhibited by both β_1-adrenoreceptors (Neal, 1992, p. 20) and α-adrenoreceptors (Bülbring and Kuriyama, 1972; Tietz and Hall, 1977, p. 682). This inhibitory action on gut muscle by α-adrenoreceptors constitutes an exception to the general rule that α-adrenoreceptors are excitatory to smooth muscle cells.

Vascular β_2-adrenoreceptors appear to be largely restricted to the vascular beds of skeletal muscle and the myocardium (Smith and Hamlin, 1977, p. 105).

Excitatory α-receptors are said to be present on cells of **salivary glands**, and presumably are responsible for producing the thick viscous saliva that characterizes sympathetic activity, though this is uncertain (Section 2.23.1). **Atrichial sweat glands** appear to be essentially activated by sympathetic cholinergic endings (Section 2.7.2).

Some of the physiological and pharmacological characteristics of the contractile response of smooth muscle in the vascular bed of skeletal muscle indicate that the receptors are not of the α-type, and a **gamma-noradrenergic receptor** has been postulated (Hirst *et al.*, 1985). However, the term γ-receptor has also been given to vasodilator receptor sites on vascular smooth muscle cells responding to acetylcholine (Smith and Hamlin, 1977, p. 113).

The sympathetic postganglionic axons that induce *glycogenolysis* by **hepatic cells** act through α-receptors in the rat, and β_2-receptors in man (Hoffman, 1989, p. 98).

2.33.2 Acetylcholine and cholinergic receptors

Acetylcholine is the transmitter substance released by all **preganglionic endings** in both the *sympathetic* and the *parasympathetic systems* (Section 2.6). It is also released by all **parasympathetic postganglionic endings** (Section 3.7). In somatic motor pathways acetylcholine is the transmitter at the **motor end-plate**. Some cholinergic vasodilator sympathetic axons occur in skeletal muscle (Section 13.3.4).

The preganglionic sympathetic axons that control the cells of the **adrenal medulla** also release acetylcholine; however, this is to be expected since the cells of the adrenal medulla are really modified postganglionic sympathetic neurons.

Acetylcholine works through two types of **ligand-activated ion channel** (Section 2.32), known as 'nicotinic' and 'muscarinic' receptors. **Nicotinic receptors** are so called because they respond to nicotine as well as to acetylcholine. They occur at the synapses between pre- and postganglionic axons in *all autonomic ganglia*. They are therefore situated in the postjunctional position, on the plasmalemma (cell membrane) of the dendrites or cell body of the **postganglionic neurons** in these ganglia (i.e. in *both sympathetic and parasympathetic ganglia*), and (predictably) on the *cells of the adrenal medulla*. They also occur on the cell membrane of skeletal muscle fibres at the motor end-plate.

Muscarinic receptors are so called because they respond not only to acetylcholine but also to muscarine, an alkaloid of a poisonous toadstool. They occur in the postjunctional position, on the plasmalemma (cell membrane) of all target cells controlled by the endings of postganglionic parasympathetic axons. Since parasympathetic postganglionic axons have excitatory effects on most of the tissues that they innervate, muscarinic receptors are usually excitatory (Neal, 1992, p. 22). Such receptors occur on *smooth muscle cells* in many organs, and on numerous *gland cells* (nasal and lacrimal glands, bronchial glands, and glands of the oral cavity, stomach, and to a lesser extent intestines). The sympathetic cholinergic sudomotor axons that activate *atrichial sweat glands* (Section 2.7.2) are muscarinic. So also are *sympathetic cholinergic vasodilator* axons in skeletal muscle.

An important exception to the excitatory effect of muscarinic receptors is the **heart** (Neal, 1992, p. 22). Vagal stimulation induces the release of acetylcholine at the sinuatrial node (Section 22.8.2); acting through muscarinic receptors, the acetylcholine opens potassium ion channels, and thus hyperpolarizes the nodal cells, hence *slowing the heart* (Section 3.7). Another example of inhibition by acetylcholine is the inhibition of smooth muscle in the vasculature of **erectile tissue**, resulting in erection; this inhibitory action is carried out by parasympathetic vasodilator axons in the pelvic nerve (Section 3.12), presumably by muscarinic receptors.

On the basis of their nicotinic or muscarinic affinities, specific drugs can be selected in clinical practice to block or stimulate either of these two types of receptor. For example, *atropine* is an antagonist of acetylcholine at muscarinic receptors, and can be used before anaesthesia to reduce airway secretions or as a spasmolytic in equine spasmodic colic.

2.34 Other possible autonomic transmitter substances

It has long been assumed that each neuron liberates the same transmitter from all of its cell processes; known as

Dale's principle, this hypothesis became extended to mean that each neuron liberates only *one* transmitter. The latter view is now seen to be an oversimplification, and many motor autonomic neurons appear to release not only one of the classical transmitters, but also another transmitter, or even several other transmitters (Section 2.37).

There is evidence from immunocytochemical studies and correlation of light and electron microscopy (Burnstock, 1985; Sternini, 1988), that not only acetylcholine and noradrenaline, but many other substances are possible transmitters in the autonomic nervous system. Among these are: *dopamine* (precursor of noradrenaline) and *serotonin* (5-HT), these being amines, as are adrenaline and noradrenaline; *γ-aminobutyric acid* (GABA), an amino acid; two purines, *adenosine-5'-triphosphate* (ATP) and *adenosine*; and about 14 biologically active peptides, notably *vasoactive intestinal peptide* (VIP), *substance P* (SP), *neuropeptide Y* (NPY), and calcitonin gene-related peptide (CGRP) (Sternini, 1988).

Of these (Weiner and Taylor, 1985, pp. 95–96), the *purines* are evidently stored in postganglionic neurones and inhibit peristalsis and gut sphincters, and may exist in other viscera; *serotonin* seems to be excitatory to gut smooth muscle; many of the *peptides* appear likely to be transmitters in autonomic ganglia, some being *modulators*, and others being *afferent transmitters*. Various criteria for establishing transmitters have been devised (e.g. Burnstock, 1985). Sternini (1988) considered that only acetylcholine, noradrenaline, and probably serotonin, satisfy all such criteria at this time, and that GABA, SP, and VIP are likely candidates, but this is a matter of opinion.

Until very recently, the idea that a highly toxic gas might be a physiological intercellular messenger would have been received with extreme scepticism, but it now appears that *nitric oxide* (NO) is an example of such a messenger. An enzyme catalyzes the synthesis of NO from L-arginine. The nitric oxide system has been found to act as a transmitter substance in a wide variety of components in the brain, and particularly in the enteric nervous system (Section 3.20) where it has recently emerged as the major nonadrenergic, noncholinergic, transmitter (Vincent and Hope, 1992). It is also formed by endothelial cells, where it induces vasodilation and thus contributes to the regulation of blood flow (Section 13.6).

The more fundamental part of Dale's principle, i.e. that a neuron liberates the same transmitter from all its cell processes, has been widened in current discussions to take account of the release of multiple transmitters; thus it now proposes that a neuron releases the *same set of transmitters* from all of its terminals. However, recent observations on the mollusc *Aplysia* suggest that in this animal a single neuron can store and presumably release different sets of transmitters from its various endings,

thus challenging the very basis of the principle (Sossin *et al.*, 1990).

2.35   Transmitter vesicles

In synaptic bulbs and the varicosities of axonal endings, transmitter substances are stored in **membrane-bound vesicles** of various shapes and sizes. Electron microscopy (Cook and Burnstock, 1976) suggests that acetylcholine occupies **clear vesicles** about 40–60 nm in diameter. Evidently noradrenaline is contained in **small dense-cored granular vesicles** of similar diameter but with a tiny granule, or (less commonly) in medium-sized dense-cored granular vesicles (60–95 nm). Large dense-cored vesicles, up to 160 nm in diameter, are believed to enclose either purines or serotonin. Axonal endings packed with small mitochondria, but containing only a few vesicles, are believed to be afferent (Taha and King, 1986).

At least eight different types of axonal ending can be identified in the mammalian gut wall (Cook and Burnstock, 1976). Nearly all of them contain more than one type of vesicle (Burnstock, 1985), and immunohistochemistry indicates up to four different transmitters in an ending (Sternini, 1988). However, the problem of reliably relating particular vesicles to particular transmitters is still unresolved (Burnstock, 1985).

The *formation of vesicles* may occur in the neuronal cell body. Such vesicles are conveyed to the axonal ending by fast anterograde axonal transport, together with precursors of vesicles and reserves of synthesized membrane (Schwartz, 1979). However, it is not necessary for all transmitter vesicles to be exported from the cell body, since most vesicles are formed by local recycling in the ending itself.

The *release* of the transmitter substance from vesicles occurs by *exocytosis* (Guyton, 1986, p. 551). The arrival of an action potential depolarizes the plasmalemma of a varicosity or synaptic bulb, and this allows Ca^{2+} ions in the interstitial fluid to enter the ending via calcium channels and also releases Ca^{2+} from intracellular stores. The increased concentration of intracellular Ca^{2+} ions promotes the fusion of transmitter vesicles with the prejunctional membrane, and hence induces the release of the transmitter substance (ligand) by exocytosis. The transmitter substance diffuses across the junctional cleft and binds to the appropriate receptor molecule on the postjunctional membrane. The response depends on whether the receptor is excitatory or inhibitory. If *excitatory*, the binding of ligand to the receptor molecule of the target cell triggers the opening of cation-selective channels; this allows an *inflow* of Na^+ ions from the interstitial fluid into the target cell, and hence leads to *depolarization*, resulting in contraction of a smooth muscle cell or secretion by a glandular cell. If the receptor is *inhibitory*, the binding of ligand to the receptor molecule of the target cell allows an *outflow* of K^+ ions from the intracellular fluid of the target cell; this leads to *hyperpolarization* of the target cell, resulting in relaxation of a smooth muscle cell or inhibition of secretion by a glandular cell.

It has been estimated that a single cholinergic vesicle contains about 3000 molecules of acetylcholine, and that a cholinergic axon terminal has enough vesicles to transmit a few thousand impulses (Guyton, 1986, p. 551).

2.36 Coupling of receptor activation to cellular response

The arrival of a transmitter substance on the plasmalemma of a smooth muscle cell can lead to *excitation–contraction coupling* (Guyton, 1986, pp. 141–145). In the presence of suitable receptors, acetylcholine and noradrenaline may depolarize the plasmalemma, and this response in turn elicits the contraction; the local depolarization may often fail to generate an action potential, but electrotonic spread over the whole surface of the cell is then enough to cause muscle contraction. Excitation–contraction coupling is activated by Ca^{2+} ions as in skeletal muscle, but the calcium comes mainly from the extracellular fluid rather than the relatively sparse sarcoplasmic reticulum.

Some smooth muscle cells (arterial and tracheal; Creed, 1979) contract in response to a low concentration of circulating noradrenaline or adrenaline, or other circulating hormones (Guyton, 1986, p. 145), without any change at all in the membrane potential, though at higher concentrations there is some depolarization but still no spike (Creed, 1979). In such instances (Guyton, 1986, p. 145), the transmitter binds with a receptor that activates a non-voltage mechanism leading to contraction. For instance, the transmitter may activate the enzyme *adenylcyclase*, protruding through the plasmalemma; this enzyme causes the formation of cyclic adenosine monophosphate (cAMP) within the cell; acting as a *second messenger*, the cAMP can release Ca^{2+} ions from the sarcoplasmic reticulum, and can also alter the ATPase activity of the myosin heads, thus changing the degree of smooth muscle contraction (Section 13.4.1).

Excitation–contraction coupling in cardiac muscle cells is surveyed in Section 21.16.

It has been shown that *stimulus–secretion coupling* in several types of cell (e.g. pancreatic acinar cells) works through Ca^{2+}-activated, non-specific cation channels; acetylcholine initiates a small rise in intracellular Ca^{2+} which activates such channels and thus leads to an influx of Na^+ and Ca^{2+} ions, thereby stimulating secretion (Partridge and Swandulla, 1988).

'Second messengers' may couple receptor activation to cellular response. Stimulation of a receptor by a transmitter increases (or, more rarely, decreases) the intracellular concentration of substances which then trigger processes culminating in a cellular response (Neal, 1992, p. 9). Cyclic AMP was the first to be characterized (Lackie and Dow, 1989, p. 53), initiating many intracellular activities (Guyton, 1986, p. 689), but calcium ions now appear to be a more important second messenger. Another is inositol triphosphate (IP_3), which is involved in the activation of smooth muscle by α-adrenergic receptors, by increasing intracellular calcium.

2.37 Neuromodulation of transmitter effects

Transmission can be modulated by postjunctional neuromodulation and prejunctional neuromodulation.

The anatomy of axonal endings and their vesicles in the autonomic nervous system provides several possible mechanisms of *postjunctional neuromodulation*. In all of these, the effects of one transmitter on the target cell could be modulated by the action of another transmitter on the same target cell, by several possible mechanisms (Burnstock, 1985). Adrenergic and cholinergic varicosities often lie side by side, frequently sharing the same Schwann cell; the transmitter substances of both of them could be within range of the same target cell. Or, a single autonomic varicosity usually contains more than one type of vesicle; differential release could be possible at different impulse frequencies (Section 3.7). Or again, more than one transmitter may be contained in one vesicle; the **cotransmitter** may facilitate the action of the other transmitter or inhibit its release.

For instance, in some parasympathetic endings acetylcholine in small clear vesicles has been claimed to coexist with various peptides stored separately in large granular vesicles (Burnstock, 1985). The release and actions of two such **cotransmitters** have been experimentally studied in the salivary glands of the cat. Electrical stimulation of the axons at low frequencies releases acetylcholine, which causes salivary secretion by the glandular cells and weak vasodilation in the gland. Stimulation at higher frequencies releases VIP, which produces strong vasodilation thereby meeting the increased metabolic demands of the tissue. The VIP has no direct effect on the glandular cells, but it enhances the action of the acetylcholine by *postjunctional modulation* of the muscarinic receptors; it also increases the release of acetylcholine by acting on **prejunctional receptors**. Thus the role of this type of cotransmitter may be to enhance secretion during maximum functional demand.

In *prejunctional neuromodulation* the transmitter that activates receptors on the target cell also acts on receptors on the varicosity (or synaptic bulb) that released that transmitter; in other words this transmitter acts both postjunctionally and prejunctionally. Its action on the prejunctional receptor may increase or decrease the release of the transmitter. If it decreases the release, this is *negative feedback*; if it increases release, this is *positive feedback*. An example of negative feedback is offered by a second type of alpha receptor in adrenergic endings. Known as **α_2-adrenoreceptors**, these occur on noradrenergic terminals. By inhibiting adenylcyclase (Section 2.36), and thereby reducing the influx of calcium ions, they diminish the further release of noradrenaline (Neal, 1992, p. 25). In summary, the α_2-receptor is prejunctional and inhibits the release of noradrenaline; the **α_1-adrenoreceptor**, which produces the typical responses at adrenergic endings, is postjunctional.

Reciprocal synapses appear to be another neuromodulation mechanism. For example, it has been suggested (King *et al.*, 1975) that the reciprocal synapses in the carotid body may provide positive feedback between the type I cell and its afferent axonal ending, thus increasing the discharge frequency of the afferent axon in hypoxia, but the role of these synapses is unresolved (Section 19.9.3).

2.38 Removal of transmitter substances

A transmitter substance released into the junctional cleft binds instantly with a matching receptor molecule, and briefly opens or closes its ion channel. The action on the channel is transient, because the transmitter is rapidly removed from the cleft by diffusion into the extracellular fluids, by enzymatic destruction, and by re-uptake into the varicosity or synaptic bulb that released it. Most of the *noradrenaline* released at an adrenergic ending undergoes re-uptake by the ending in a few seconds and is recycled in transmitter vesicles. Most of the *acetylcholine* in the junctional cleft disappears much more quickly (in 1–2 ms), being hydrolysed into choline and acetate by the enzyme *acetylcholinesterase*; much of the choline undergoes re-uptake.

The residue of noradrenaline is destroyed by enzymes, e.g. *monoamine oxidase* (MOA), contained within the ending itself, or by the enzyme *catechol-O-methyltransferase* (COMT) that occurs in all tissues. MOA lies in the outer membrane of mitochondria in the nerve ending, and waits passively to mop up superfluous noradrenaline released into the cytoplasm by a neighbouring dense-cored granular vesicle. *Acetylcholinesterase* is attached to polysaccharide molecules (glycosaminoglycans) associated with the postjunctional (and to a lesser extent the prejunctional) membranes (Neal, 1992, p. 23). Acetylcholine that diffuses into the bloodstream is hydrolysed by non-specific acetylcholinesterase (Tietz and Hall, 1977, p. 678).

2.39 Adrenal medulla

During conditions of **fight and flight**, stimulation of the sympathetic nerves to the adrenal medulla causes the release of large quantities of *adrenaline* and *noradrenaline* into the blood stream. The circulating noradrenaline and adrenaline act on α- and β-receptors throughout the tissues of the body in essentially the same manner as noradrenaline from the sympathetic nerve endings, causing vasoconstriction and increased cardiac activity, but their effects last much longer – minutes, rather than the seconds allowed by the rapid removal of the neurotransmitters. Also the adrenaline and noradrenaline from the adrenal medulla stimulate the very abundant tissues that receive no sympathetic innervation; indeed every cell in the body increases its metabolic rate in response particularly to adrenaline.

The **adrenal medulla** consists of clusters and columns of **medullary endocrine cells** which lie in rows along wide **venous sinusoids**. The base of each cell faces away from the sinusoid and receives synapses from preganglionic sympathetic axons; as in all autonomic ganglia, the synapse is cholinergic (Section 2.33). The cell has many dense-cored vesicles, some of which contain *adrenaline* and others *noradrenaline*. The cells arise from the midthoracic region of the neural crest, and are homologous to postganglionic sympathetic neurons.

Two types of **medullary endocrine cell** occur in some mammals, one secreting *adrenaline* and the other *noradrenaline* (Williams *et al.*, 1989, p. 1469). Both types contain **membrane-bound granular vesicles** about 200 nm in diameter, the granule being more electron dense in the noradrenaline cells. In some mammals, cells containing both adrenaline and noradrenaline are present. The contents of the vesicles are released from the apices of the cells by exocytosis into the perivascular spaces, and pass through the **fenestrated endothelium** into the sinusoids.

The sympathetic preganglionic axons that innervate the endocrine cells are (unexpectedly) mainly unmyelinated, at least in the rat (Williams, 1989, p. 1165). Some similar axons form synapses with scattered multipolar neurons that are probably vasomotor postganglionic neurons.

Both *noradrenaline* and *adrenaline*, when released into the circulating blood, cause **constriction of blood vessels** and increased **cardiac activity**, but there are differences in detail. Noradrenaline acts mainly on α-receptors, and to a lesser extent on β_1-receptors, whereas adrenaline excites α- and β_1-receptors about equally (Guyton, 1986, p. 690). Because noradrenaline has a relatively small effect on β_1-receptors it does not increase cardiac output as much as adrenaline; on the other hand noradrenaline, by acting mainly on α-receptors, causes a much greater vasoconstriction than does adrenaline, and hence increases the peripheral resistance and arterial pressure more than adrenaline (Guyton, 1986, p. 692).

In the arterial tree of skeletal muscle, adrenaline in physiological doses causes a transient increase in blood flow, because of vasodilation acting through the low threshold of β_2-receptors for adrenaline. At higher concentrations adrenaline causes vasoconstriction, because it now activates α-receptors with a higher threshold (Rowell, 1974b, p. 210). The initial vasodilation caused by adrenaline may occur through adrenal medullary secretion when exercise is anticipated, giving a valuable preparatory increase in blood flow (Section 13.3.4).

2.40　APUD system

This name was given to various cell types scattered throughout many tissues of the body, all of them capable of secreting hormones or neurotransmitters; a more recent name is the **diffuse neuro-endocrine system**. Such cells include the **adrenal medullary endocrine cells**, and **SIF cells** and **chromaffin cells** in sympathetic ganglia, secreting *catecholamines*; various cell types in **pancreatic islets**, e.g. **A cells** secreting *glucagon*, **B cells** secreting *insulin*; numerous cell types in the gastric and intestinal epithelium producing various hormones including *gastrin*, *secretin*, and *cholecystokinin*; a range of cells in the hypothalamus, and several in endocrine glands, e.g. **C cells** in the parathyroid gland secreting *calcitonin*, and **M cells** in the pituitary secreting *melanotropin*. Altogether about 40 cell types have been added to this system since it was first established by Pearse in the 1960s (Williams *et al.*, 1989, p. 1466).

The name APUD came from the capacity of these cells for **a**mine **p**recursor **u**ptake and **d**ecarboxylation. Cytologically they are characterized by **membrane-bound dense-cored granules** about 100–200 nm in diameter, as in the cells of the adrenal medulla (Section 2.39). Originally they were believed to arise from the **neural crest**, but some are **endodermal** and others **mesodermal**. The secretions of APUD cells act directly on adjacent cells, or indirectly on remote cells by blood transport, thus reinforcing the autonomic nervous system in controlling homeostasis.

Chapter 3

Parasympathetic Motor Pathways in the Peripheral Nervous System: Enteric Nervous System

I GENERAL PRINCIPLES

3.1 Parasympathetic motor outflow from central nervous system

The parasympathetic motor outflow from the central nervous system (Fig. 3.1) is limited to the brain and the sacral region of the spinal cord (Section 1.3.2) – hence the alternative name of **craniosacral system**.

The **cranial outflow** supplies the viscera of the head by the following cranial nerves: oculomotor (III), facial (VII), glossopharyngeal (IX), and vagus (X). The vagus nerve also supplies the viscera of the thorax and abdomen.

The **sacral outflow** supplies the pelvic viscera by the pelvic nerve.

As in the sympathetic system, the parasympathetic motor outflow from the neuraxis takes the form of a preganglionic–postganglionic relay (Section 1.2.2).

3.2 General functions of parasympathetic motor pathways

As stated in Section 1.3.2, the parasympathetic motor pathways generally induce the visceral responses required for **conservation of bodily reserves**. This principle can be used to predict the effects of parasympathetic activity in individual organs. For instance, cranial nerve III innervates the **iris** of the eye; conservation would suggest constriction rather than dilation of the pupil. An alternative and often easier way to predict the motor functions of the parasympathetic innerva-

tion of an organ is to establish the sympathetic effect on the organ first (fight and flight) and then reverse it. For instance, the requirements of fight and flight suggest that the sympathetic nerves to the iris would dilate the pupil (to admit more light); reversal of this shows that the parasympathetic nerves to the iris should constrict the pupil.

Most organs have both a sympathetic and a parasympathetic motor innervation (Fig. 3.1), but in general the parasympathetic system is responsible for the fine adjustment of visceral functions. This activity is aided by the lower **ratio of pre- to postganglionic parasympathetic neurons**, which is only about 1:3 in the parasympathetic system, as opposed to about 1:20 or more in the sympathetic system (Section 2.3.6). Fine adjustment is also made more flexible by the existence of **basal parasympathetic tone** (Section 1.3.2). For example, gastrointestinal activity can be *directly increased* by stimulating the parasympathetic tone of the vagal innervation of the gut, but it can also be *indirectly reduced* by decreasing the normal basal tone. If there were no basal parasympathetic tone the vagus would only be capable of increasing the activity of the gut.

The **glands** of the oral, pharyngeal, and nasal cavities (salivary and nasal mucosal glands, and lacrimal gland), and the many gastrointestinal glands, are all strongly stimulated by parasympathetic motor nerves and respond with copious secretion. The glands of the oral cavity and stomach are particularly responsive, whereas those of the small and large intestine are controlled mainly by local factors acting chiefly through the enteric nervous system. The parasympathetic system has only one major function in controlling

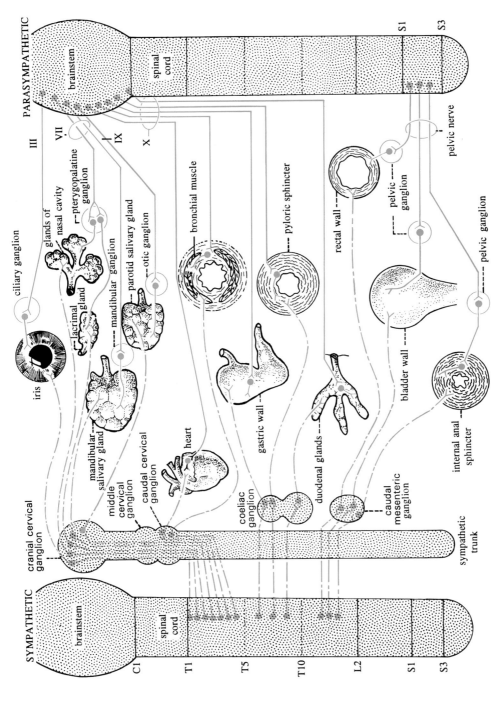

Fig. 3.1 Diagram summarizing the distribution of the main sympathetic and parasympathetic motor pathways to the viscera. Every organ is supplied by a preganglionic–postganglionic relay from both the sympathetic and parasympathetic systems. The pathways to the gastrointestinal tract are simplified by omission of the enteric nervous system, which in principle is interposed between the vago-sympathetic motor pathways and the target tissues in the gut wall. All the nerves are green. Broken green lines, parasympathetic pathways. Continuous green lines, sympathetic pathways. The organs are not to scale.

circulation, namely reducing the rate (and to much smaller extent) the force of contraction of the heart (Section 22.8.2). The motor parasympathetic pathways in the sacral part of the parasympathetic system dominate the reflexes of **micturition** and **defaecation**.

3.3 Parasympathetic preganglionic neuron

3.3.1 *Cranial region*

There are four cranial nerves with parasympathetic motor components: the oculomotor nerve (cranial nerve III), facial nerve (cranial nerve VII), glossopharyngeal nerve (cranial nerve IX), and the vagus nerve (cranial nerve X). The preganglionic neurons of these four cranial nerves have their cell stations in the grey matter of the brainstem, in a discontinuous series of four parasympathetic motor nuclei, one nucleus for each cranial nerve. These nuclei lie in line with each other in the brain stem, in a position which corresponds with the lateral horn of the spinal cord; they are, in fact, homologous with the lateral horn. Each nucleus is named according to the cranial nerve to which it belongs; hence **parasympathetic motor nucleus of the oculomotor nerve**, **parasympathetic motor nucleus of the facial nerve**, **parasympathetic motor nucleus of the glossopharyngeal nerve**, and **parasympathetic motor nucleus of the vagus nerve** (Fig. 3.3). The positions of these nuclei in the brainstem are explained in the first volume in this series on the CNS (King, 1987).

The axons of these preganglionic neurons run at first in the trunk of the parent cranial nerve. Only a *small minority* of the axons in cranial nerves III, VII, and IX are parasympathetic motor axons, and these become isolated into a few relatively slender branches.

The preganglionic parasympathetic motor axons of nerves III, VII, and IX finally form synapses with postganglionic axons in small ganglia close to, or embedded in, their target organs, thus constituting the preganglionic–postganglionic relay that characterizes autonomic motor pathways.

The **vagus nerve** (Section 3.11) does consist *mainly* of autonomic axons, and most of its branches contain numerous parasympathetic preganglionic motor axons. These preganglionic axons make synapses with postganglionic neurons in some organs, thus exemplifying the typical preganglionic–postganglionic autonomic motor relay. In the gut, however, the vagal preganglionic neurons form a major exception to this rule: here, they make synapses not with postganglionic neurons but with nerve cells of the **enteric nervous system** (Section 3.4.1).

The **preganglionic branches** of the oculomotor nerve (cranial nerve III), facial nerve (cranial nerve VII), and glossopharyngeal nerve (cranial nerve IX), are as follows: the **short ciliary nerves** (nervi ciliares breves), belonging to the oculomotor nerve (nervus oculomotorius) (Section 3.8); the **major petrosal nerve** (nervus petrosus major) and **chorda tympani**, belonging to the facial nerve (nervus facialis) (Section 3.9); and the **minor petrosal nerve**, belonging to the glossopharyngeal nerve (nervus glossopharyngeus) (Section 3.10). The two parasympathetic motor branches of the facial nerve join branches of the trigeminal nerve (nervus trigeminus), which they use as a roadway. It has been estimated that 75% of all the parasympathetic motor axons in the body are vagal (Guyton, 1986, p. 687).

The **parasympathetic motor nuclei** (nuclei parasympathici) have the following (unofficial) other names in the literature: the oculomotor parasympathetic nucleus (nuclei parasympathici nervi oculomotorii) is the **Edinger–Westphal nucleus**; the facial parasympathetic nucleus (nucleus parasympathicus nervi facialis) is the **rostral** or **superior salivatory nucleus**; the glossopharyngeal parasympathetic nucleus (nucleus parasympathicus nervi glossopharyngei) is the **caudal** or **inferior salivatory nucleus**; the vagal nucleus (nucleus parasympathicus nervi vagi) is the **dorsal motor nucleus**.

The embryonic derivation of the parasympathetic nuclei is mentioned in Section 3.6.

3.3.2 *Sacral region*

The preganglionic neurons of the sacral part of the parasympathetic nervous system have their cell stations in the grey matter of the sacral segments of the spinal cord. These cell bodies lie between the dorsal and ventral horns. Their site therefore corresponds to the **lateral horn** of the thoracolumbar segments of the spinal cord (Fig. 2.1), except that they do not form a projecting lateral horn.

The preganglionic axons from the sacral out-flow pass through the ventral roots of the related sacral spinal nerves, the precise segments varying with the species. The preganglionic axons leave the ventral roots by passing through the ventral rami (Section 2.2), and form the **pelvic nerve** (Section 3.12), which combines with the **hypogastric nerve** (Section 2.18) to form the **pelvic plexus** (Section 3.13).

The preganglionic sacral parasympathetic axons make synapses either with postganglionic neurons in the characteristic autonomic manner, or (like the vagus) with nerve cells in the enteric nervous system (Section 3.4.1).

The *dog* and *cat* have three sacral segments, the sacral parasympathetic motor outflow being S2–S3 in the dog and S1–S3 in the cat; the *rabbit* has four sacral segments, and a parasympathetic outflow through S2–S4; *man* has five sacral vertebrae, and a parasympathetic outflow through S2–S4 (Jänig and McLachlan, 1987, p. 1338). In large mammals with five (the *horse* and *ox*) or four (*sheep*) sacral segments the main outflow is through S3–S4, with a variable contribution from either S2 or S5, or from both of these (Ghoshal, 1975, pp. 702, 1170, 1174). According to Christensen (1979, p. 576) in the *dog* the parasympathetic axons come from S1–S2, and some-times S3.

3.4 Parasympathetic postganglionic neuron

3.4.1 *Cranial region*

The cell stations of the parasympathetic postganglionic axons of the **oculomotor**, **facial**, and **glossopharyngeal nerves** are located in four small ganglia. These ganglia lie near or in the target organ (see below).

The preganglionic axons of the **vagus** that supply the heart and lungs (Sections 3.11.2 and 3.11.3) form typical preganglionic–postganglionic relays within the target organ. However, the vagal motor pathways to the **gut** break all the rules. In the gut, the vagal preganglionic fibre makes a synapse with a nerve cell in the **enteric nervous system**. It has long been believed (Section 1.3.4) that this **enteric ganglion cell** (enteric nerve cell) must be nothing more than a vagal postganglionic neuron, and that the enteric nervous system is therefore simply the gut part of the vagal motor

pathways. However, the ability of the enteric nervous system to function fully after all of its vagal connections have been cut, and the fact that vast numbers of enteric ganglion cells have no vagal (indeed no parasympathetic) innervation have made this concept untenable. Instead, it is now accepted that the vagal preganglionic fibre in the gut ends by making a synapse on an enteric ganglion cell; the exact identity of this cell is not known, but it certainly receives and distributes enough neuronal contacts within the enteric nervous system to activate complex preprogrammed functions such as peristalsis and segmentation (Section 3.20).

The cell stations of the postganglionic neurons in the head lie in the following ganglia: the **ciliary ganglion** (ganglion ciliare) (nerve III), the **pterygopalatine ganglion** (ganglion pterygopalatinum) and **mandibular ganglion** (ganglion mandibulare) (nerve VII), and the **otic ganglion** (ganglion oticum) (nerve IX) (Fig. 3.1).

3.4.2 *Sacral region*

The cell station of postganglionic sacral para-sympathetic neurons occurs in numerous small **pelvic ganglia** (Fig. 3.1) in the pelvic plexus, or in minute ganglia on or in the walls of some of the pelvic viscera (Section 3.13). For example, postganglionic axons pass from these ganglia to the smooth muscle of the **bladder** and thus form typical autonomic preganglionic–postganglionic relays. However, both preganglionic and postganglionic sacral axons to the **rectum** and **descending colon** make synapses with enteric ganglion cells (Fig. 3.4).

3.5 Afferent axons in parasympathetic nerves

Autonomic afferent axons accompany the parasympathetic efferent pathways. There are taste axons in the **chorda tympani** of the **facial nerve** (Section 4.3.1). The **glossopharyngeal nerve** consists mainly of afferent axons: many of these arise from the mucosa of the oropharynx and tongue in the **pharyngeal** and **lingual** rami of the glossopharyngeal nerve (Fig. 4.3), and are in-volved in the reflexes of **swallowing** and **saliva-tion**; others are cardiovascular afferent axons in the **carotid sinus nerve** (Fig. 4.3), arising from the

carotid body and **carotid sinus** (Section 4.3.2). There are vast numbers of afferent axons in the **vagus** (Section 4.3.3), from the alimentary tract and its associated glands, from the respiratory tract, and from the heart and its great blood vessels, especially the aorta (Fig. 3.3).

Autonomic afferent axons also form a major part of the **pelvic plexus** and **pelvic nerve** (Section 4.3.4). They arise from the pelvic viscera and descending colon, forming the afferent side of the reflex arcs of **micturition** and **defaecation** and also carrying some of the pain pathways from the bladder.

These afferent pathways are discussed more fully in Chapter 4.

3.6 Embryology of parasympathetic neurons

The **preganglionic neurons** of the parasympathetic system develop in the **neural tube**. The **postganglionic neurons** of the parasympathetic cranial nerves arise from the **neural crest**.

The developing **preganglionic neurons** in the **cranial component** of the parasympathetic system assemble into a longitudinal series of four **nuclei** in the midbrain (the oculomotor parasympathetic motor nucleus) and in the hindbrain (the facial, glossopharyngeal, and vagal parasympathetic motor nuclei). These nuclei are related to the developing segments of the head (Lumsden and Keynes, 1989). The **preganglionic neurons** of the **sacral component** of the parasympathetic system arise in the neural tube of sacral segments (Noden and de Lahunta, 1985, p. 130).

The **postganglionic neurons** of the parasympathetic system are derived from the **neural crest** of the **brain stem** and **sacral region** of the neural tube (Noden and de Lahunta, 1985, p. 132). In the avian embryo, the vagal part of the neural crest lies at the level of somites 1–7 (Gabella, 1979). The first five of these somites are occipital somites (Noden, 1984), which correspond approximately with rhombomere 8 of Lumsden and Keynes (1989). The postganglionic neurons that supply the **heart** are derived from neural crest cells at the levels of the first two somites, which correspond to the site of the cardiac primordium at this stage of development (Noden and de Lahunta, 1985, p. 131).

Developing autonomic postganglionic neurons are evidently **multipotential autonomic nerve cells**, capable of differentiating into either sympathetic or parasympathetic postganglionic neurons (Section 2.5).

3.7 Parasympathetic transmitter substances

Acetylcholine is released from the **synaptic bulbs** of all **pre**ganglionic endings in parasympathetic **ganglia**; acetylcholine is also released from **varicosities** on the endings of all parasympathetic **post**ganglionic axons (Section 2.33.2). All of these are **cholinergic endings**.

Nearly all of these cholinergic pathways are *excitatory* to their target cells. Hence they stimulate the smooth muscle of the gut and airways, thus causing increased gastrointestinal motility and bronchial constriction. They excite glandular cells in the alimentary tract and respiratory tract, thus increasing salivary, gastrointestinal, and bronchial secretion. They activate smooth muscles of the eye, thus constricting the iris and inducing accommodation for near vision. They stimulate the smooth muscle of the rectum and bladder, thus causing defaecation and urination.

One group of parasympathetic cholinergic endings is *not* excitatory to its target cell. These are the **vagal cardiac pathways** – an important exception to the rule. The postganglionic endings of this pathway *inhibit* the sinuatrial node, and thus *slow* the heart (Section 22.8.2).

In both the bulbs and the varicosities of pre- and postganglionic parasympathetic axonal endings, the acetylcholine is stored in **clear vesicles** about 40–60 nm in diameter, and released by **exocytosis** induced by an increase in intracellular Ca^{2+} (Section 2.35). The released acetylcholine is rapidly removed from the junctional cleft by **acetylcholinesterase** (Section 2.38).

Acetylcholine works through **nicotinic receptors** in all synapses in parasympathetic ganglia, and through **muscarinic receptors** at all of the target cells innervated by parasympathetic postganglionic endings (Section 2.33.2). **Muscarinic receptors** are usually *excitatory* (Neal, 1992, p. 22), stimulating smooth muscle cells in many organs and glandular cells in the alimentary and respiratory tracts, and especially the glandular cells of the oral cavity and stomach. However, muscarinic receptors do have one particularly important *inhibitory* function, namely inhibition of the cells of the **sinuatrial node**, and thus *slowing the heart rate* (Section 2.33.2). Also the smooth muscle in the walls of the arteries of erectile tissues is inhibited by sacral cholinergic parasympathetic pathways; in the male and female erectile tissues, these pathways cause vasodilation and hence *erection* (Section 3.12). There are also parasympathetic

vasodilator axons in the salivary glands (Scott, 1986, p. 64), and uterus, and perhaps in the prostate and vesicular gland of the male (Section 3.12).

II CRANIAL PARASYMPATHETIC MOTOR PATHWAYS

The following sections summarize the anatomical and functional characteristics of the parasympathetic motor components of the oculomotor, facial, glossopharyngeal, and vagus nerves (Fig. 3.1). Each of these four cranial nerves contains the axons of large numbers of other functional types of neuron, in addition to autonomic motor (efferent) neurons. For example, as just mentioned in Section 3.5, the facial, glossopharyngeal, and vagus nerves include autonomic afferent axons.

The parasympathetic motor pathway of each of these four cranial nerves consists, of course, of a preganglionic neuron and a postganglionic neuron. As stated in Section 3.4, the cell bodies of the postganglionic neurons of the **oculomotor, facial**, and **glossopharyngeal nerves** are assembled in small isolated ganglia close to the glands that they supply. These ganglia are shown in Fig. 3.1. On the other hand, the cell bodies of the postganglionic neurons of the **vagus nerve** are scattered throughout the tissues of the organs that they innervate.

3.8 Oculomotor nerve: parasympathetic motor pathways

The oculomotor nerve consists mainly of somatic motor (efferent) axons innervating the extrinsic muscles of the eyeball, and contains relatively few parasympathetic preganglionic axons. The latter separate themselves from the main trunk of the oculomotor nerve a few centimetres after it leaves the cranial cavity, and enter the parasympathetic ganglion of the oculomotor nerve (the **ciliary ganglion**, Fig. 3.1). In the ganglion, the preganglionic axons synapse with postganglionic axons. The postganglionic axons leave the ganglion and penetrate the wall of the eye to innervate the ciliary

muscle and the circular smooth muscle of the sphincter of the pupil.

Excitation of these parasympathetic pathways causes the **ciliary muscle** to contract. This relaxes the tension on the zonule that suspends the lens and allows the elastic capsule of the lens to make the lens more convex for focusing on close objects. The **sphincter muscle** of the iris contracts in response to parasympathetic stimulation, thus diminishing the aperture of the pupil.

> The oculomotor nerve divides into a **dorsal branch** (ramus dorsalis) that supplies only the dorsal rectus and levator palpebrae muscle, and a much larger **ventral branch** (ramus ventralis) that supplies the other orbital muscles. The **ciliary ganglion** (ganglion ciliare) is small (about 1 mm diameter in the *dog*), but sits prominently on the ventral branch. The parasympathetic postganglionic axons emerge from the ganglion as two or three **short ciliary nerves** (nervi ciliares breves). These accompany the optic nerve, and penetrate the sclera at the back of the eyeball near the attachment of the optic nerve.

3.9 Facial nerve: parasympathetic motor pathways

The facial nerve consists mainly of motor neurons (special visceral motor, Section 1.2.3) that supply the facial muscles. Its relatively small number of autonomic afferent and parasympathetic motor preganglionic axons run in two nerves to the two parasympathetic ganglia of the facial nerve (the pterygopalatine ganglion and the mandibular ganglion).

3.9.1 *Innervation of lacrimal gland, and nasal and palatine glands*

The parasympathetic preganglionic axons to these glands arise in a branch of the facial nerve. This branch ends in a ganglion (the pterygopalatine ganglion in Fig. 3.1). Synapses with postganglionic neurons occur in this ganglion. The postganglionic axons innervate the lacrimal gland, and the many mucous glands that line the nasal mucosa and the mucosa of the palate. Excitation of these pathways induces lacrimation and the copious secretion of mucus in the nasal and oral cavities.

The branch of the facial nerve that distributes these parasympathetic preganglionic axons to the **ptery-gopalatine ganglion** (ganglion pterygopalatinum) is the **major petrosal nerve** (nervus petrosus major). This nerve arises from the main trunk of the facial nerve (Fig. 3.2), as it goes through the facial canal in the wall of the middle ear cavity. It consists mainly of efferent preganglionic parasympathetic axons. The latter pass to

the **pterygopalatine ganglion**, on the **pterygopalatine nerve** of the maxillary division of the **trigeminal nerve**.

The **facial nerve** has a motor and a sensory root, the former being the larger. The sensory root lies between the motor root and the vestibulocochlear nerve, and is therefore called the **intermediate nerve**. The parasympathetic efferent axons are included in the inter-

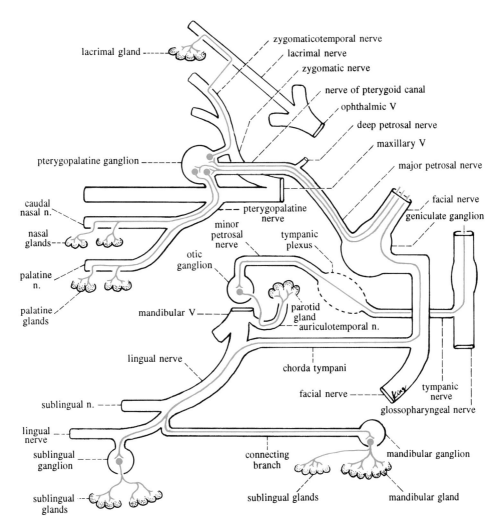

Fig. 3.2   Diagram of the main parasympathetic motor pathways of the facial and glossopharyngeal nerves. In principle, the facial nerve provides preganglionic fibres through the major petrosal nerve and the chorda tympani. The major petrosal fibres synapse in the pterygopalatine ganglion with postganglionic neurons that innervate the lacrimal gland and the glands of the nasal cavity and palate. The preganglionic fibres in the chorda tympani synapse in the mandibular ganglion, and innervate the mandibular and sublingual salivary glands; in some species a relay in the sublingual ganglion supplies part of the sublingual glands, as shown. The glossopharyngeal nerve sends its preganglionic fibres through the minor petrosal nerve, with a synaptic relay in the otic ganglion to the parotid salivary gland. All of these parasympathetic motor pathways use branches of the trigeminal nerve as roadways. The topographical details of these roadways, and the numbers, sizes, and sites of the parasympathetic ganglia, vary with the species (see Sections 3.9 and 3.10).

mediate nerve. The intermediate nerve is not grossly separable in the *dog* (McClure, 1979, p. 922).

The **major petrosal nerve** (McClure, 1979, p. 922) arises from the **geniculate ganglion**, at the **genu** of the facial nerve. After passing through the petrous temporal bone it lies on the osseous auditory tube. It is then joined by the sympathetic **deep petrosal nerve** (nervus petrosus profundus) (Section 2.24.2), to form the **nerve of the pterygoid canal** (nervus canalis pterygoidei) (Fig. 3.2). This nerve emerges from the rostral end of the pterygoid canal and enters the **pterygopalatine ganglion**. The ganglion, which is spindle-shaped and about 2–3 mm long in the *dog*, lies near the main trunk of the maxillary nerve and is closely attached by two or three small branches to the **pterygopalatine nerve** of the **maxillary nerve** (McClure, 1979, p. 916). In the *horse and domestic ruminants* there are several small pterygopalatine ganglia and one or more larger ones several millimetres long, numbering up to about eight in total; the ganglia tend to be linked to each other and to the caudal nasal and palatine nerves by a plexus of fine filaments (for review, see Godhino and Getty, 1975, pp. 654, 1089, 1102, 1118).

Postganglionic parasympathetic axons pass from the pterygopalatine ganglion or ganglia to the **caudal nasal nerve** and innervate the **glands of the nasal mucosa** (Williams *et al.*, 1989, p. 1110); other postganglionic axons enter the **palatine nerves** and innervate the **glands of the palatine mucosa** (Fig. 3.2).

Yet other postganglionic axons from the major petrosal nerve innervate the **lacrimal gland**, but their course is controversial. The classical view (Mitchell, 1953, p. 162; Crosby *et al.*, 1962, p. 526; Williams *et al.*, 1989, p. 1102) is that the axons enter the **zygomatic nerve** of the **maxillary division of the trigeminal** and then the **zygomaticotemporal** branch of the zygomatic nerve (Fig. 3.2); from here they transfer to the **lacrimal** branch of the **ophthalmic division of the trigeminal nerve**, and emerge as fine filaments supplying the lacrimal gland. However, an alternative route is to reach the lacrimal gland by lacrimal filaments from the zygomaticotemporal nerve, omitting the ophthalmic nerve altogether (Mitchell, 1953, p. 162; Williams *et al.*, 1989, p. 1155). The zygomaticotemporal route (omitting the ophthalmic nerve) is given for the *dog* by McClure (1979, p. 916). However, in the *rat* these elaborate pathways via the maxillary and ophthalmic pathways have been denied, and a direct supply of lacrimal rami from a retro-orbital plexus of parasympathetic filaments of the pterygopalatine ganglion has been claimed (Ruskell, 1971; Williams *et al.*, 1989, p. 1155). Stromberg (1993, p. 1035) acknowledged the possibility that in the *dog* the gland is innervated by direct filaments from the pterygopalatine ganglion as well as by pathways through the zygomatic and lacrimal nerves.

There is evidence that the major petrosal nerve supplies **vasodilator axons** to the **cerebral circulation** (Section 13.3.4).

A further complication is the source of the **zygomaticotemporal nerve (ramus)**. It has been stated to be a branch of the ophthalmic nerve in the *horse* (Grau, 1943, p. 939; Godhino and Getty, 1975, p. 652), *ox* (Butler, 1967; Godhino and Getty, 1975, p. 1084), and *sheep* and *pig* (Godhino and Getty, 1975, pp. 1096, 1374); however, it is described as a branch of the maxillary nerve in the *dog* (Godhino and Getty, 1975, p. 1689; McClure, 1979, p. 914) and in *man* (Williams *et al.*, 1989, p. 1102). These variations may be due to species differences, or to uncertainty in resolving the close anatomical relationships of the maxillary and ophthalmic nerves. The NAV (1983, p. A127, footnote 467) placed the zygomaticotemporal nerve with the maxillary nerve in all the domestic species, and implied that confusion arose through the close association of the maxillary and ophthalmic nerves. The nerve currently retains its official position with the maxillary nerve (Schaller *et al.*, 1992, p. 466).

3.9.2 *Chorda tympani*

Most of the axons in the chorda tympani are *taste afferents* from the tongue (Section 4.3.1), but it also contains efferent parasympathetic preganglionic axons. The chorda tympani is so called because it crosses the tympanic membrane in the middle ear cavity. The preganglionic efferent axons enter a ganglion that lies close to the mandibular salivary gland (the mandibular ganglion, Fig. 3.1), and make synapses there with their postganglionic neurons. The postganglionic axons are secretomotor to the mandibular and sublingual salivary glands (Fig. 3.2). Excitation of these pathways induces secretion of copious watery saliva.

The **chorda tympani** arises from the facial nerve while the latter is nearing the end of its course in the facial canal, and enters the middle ear cavity traversing the medial aspect of the handle of **malleus**. It escapes from its canal in the petrous temporal bone by passing through the **petrotympanic fissure**, and joins the **lingual nerve** (Fig. 3.2).

The parasympathetic preganglionic axons leave the lingual nerve and, in the *dog*, form a long preganglionic connecting branch (Fig. 3.2); this passes caudally along the mandibular duct to the **mandibular ganglion**, which lies in the hilus of the mandibular gland (Godhino and Getty, 1975, p. 1690; McClure, 1979, p. 920). The postganglionic neurons have their cell station in the mandibular ganglion, and innervate the mandibular and sublingual salivary glands; in the *dog* there is usually a small **sublingual ganglion** (Fig. 3.2), situated much more rostrally in the angle between the connecting branch and the lingual nerve (Godhino and Getty, 1975, p. 1690; McClure, 1979, p. 920), which presumably innervates the more rostral parts of the sublingual salivary gland. In the *horse* (Godhino and Getty, 1975, p. 657) the preganglionic axons travel in the **sublingual** as well as the lingual nerve. In this species there are numerous (5–12) **mandibular ganglia**, some barely visible to the naked eye and others almost 10 mm long. A rostral group distributes postganglionic axons mainly to the sublingual gland; the postganglionic axons from the caudal group pass along the mandibular duct and supply the mandibular gland. The domestic *ruminants* (Godhino and Getty, 1975, pp. 1089, 1102, 1118) have one or two large (about 6 mm long) and between four and nine small mandibular ganglia interconnected by filaments. The ganglia form postganglionic filaments that pass caudally along the mandibular duct to the mandibular gland; some postganglionic filaments pass rostrally along the mandibular duct to innervate the sublingual glands. Evidently the postganglionic axons from the mandibular ganglion are unusually long in the *horse* and *ruminants*, since they follow the mandibular duct caudally to its gland; in the *dog* the postganglionic axons follow the general rule for the parasympathetic system in being short, since the mandibular ganglion is on the gland itself.

3.10 Glossopharyngeal nerve: parasympathetic motor pathways

The glossopharyngeal nerve consists mainly of autonomic (visceral) *afferent axons* from the tongue and pharynx (hence the name, 'glossopharyngeal') and from the carotid sinus and carotid body (Fig. 4.3). It has only a few parasympathetic motor preganglionic axons. These pass to a ganglion (the otic ganglion) near the parotid salivary gland (Fig. 3.1). Here the preganglionic axons synapse with postganglionic neurons. The postganglionic axons innervate the parotid salivary gland. Excitation causes salivation.

The parasympathetic preganglionic axons of the glossopharyngeal nerve form the **tympanic nerve** (nervus tympanicus). This is the first branch from the main trunk (Fig. 3.2), and arises from the fused **proximal** and **distal glossopharyngeal ganglion** in the *dog* (Godhino and Getty, 1975, p. 1691) or from the distal ganglion in species in which the ganglia are not fused (e.g. *ruminants*; Godhino and Getty, 1975, p. 1091). In the tympanic cavity, the tympanic nerve reaches the cochlear promontory and enters the **tympanic plexus** (to which the sympathetic

caroticotympanic nerve also contributes, Section 2.24.2). The preganglionic axons emerge from the tympanic plexus as the **minor petrosal nerve** (nervus petrosus minor), which joins the **otic ganglion** (Fig. 3.2).

In the *dog* and *ruminants* the **otic ganglion** is always a single large ganglion, lying on or close to the mandibular nerve near the origin of the **buccal nerve** (Godhino and Getty, 1975, p. 1089; Stromberg, 1979, p. 1035). In the *horse* the site is again related to the mandibular and buccal nerve, but the ganglion is small and difficult to find, and is often replaced by a number of minute ganglia in a fine plexus (Godhino and Getty, 1975, p. 656).

Postganglionic parasympathetic axons from the otic ganglion pass by two or three rami to the **auriculotemporal nerve** of mandibular V (Fig. 3.2) and are carried to the **parotid salivary gland** in the *dog* (Stromberg, 1979, p. 1035) and *horse* (Godhino and Getty, 1975, p. 656). In the *horse* and *ruminants* postganglionic axons from the otic ganglion also enter the **buccal nerve**; in the *ox*, these axons are carried to the parotid salivary gland (Habel, 1975, p. 873; Godhino and Getty, 1975, p. 1089); in the *horse* they are carried to the **dorsal buccal salivary glands** (Godhino and Getty, 1975, p. 656). It has been claimed that a large number of the postganglionic axons from the otic ganglion may run in the adventia of the maxillary artery, and that yet others pass to the facial nerve (Stromberg, 1979, p. 1035). In the *ox*, a small number of preganglionic secretomotor axons to the parotid gland may also come from the facial nerve (Habel, 1975, p. 873).

The parasympathetic motor supply to the salivary glands is well known to be strongly secretomotor (Section 2.23.1), but has also been shown to be **vasodilator**. The vasodilator action has been established, for example, in the submandibular gland of the *dog* (Sellers, 1977, p. 240) and the parotid gland of the *ox* (Phillipson, 1977, p. 255), though the degree of vasodilation and the rate of salivary flow are not directly related. Observations on the salivary glands of the *cat* suggest that this dual action may be achieved by the combined action of acetylcholine and VIP, the latter acting as a cotransmitter (Section 2.37). Vasodilation in the mandibular salivary gland of the cat is thus **initiated** neurally. It is then **maintained** by **plasma kinins** formed locally, when **kallikrein** is released by secretory cells stimulated by sympathetic amines (Williams *et al.*, 1989, p. 1297).

Two principal types of protein secretion occur in saliva, a **serous secretion** containing **ptyalin** for splitting starches and a **mucous secretion** for lubrication. Also secreted are **hormones** and other compounds such as a glucagon-like protein and perhaps **serotonin**, and also antimicrobial agents such as **IgA** and **lysozyme** (Williams *et al.*, 1989, p. 1290). Of the three major salivary glands, the parotid is serous and the mandibular and sublingual are mixed serous and mucous. In *mammals* generally the **mandibular gland** secretes only when the animal is feeding, whilst the **sublingual glands** maintain a very slow resting rate of secretion; in *ruminants* the **parotid gland** secretes continuously, but the flow is much faster during feeding and rumination, and is greater on the side in which the bolus is being chewed. The total secretion of saliva in the *ox* in 24 h is 100–200 litres, of which about 50 litres come from the parotid gland (Phillipson, 1977, pp. 254–255).

In *mammals* generally there are numerous **minor salivary glands** (Habel and Biberstein, 1960, p. 159; Phillipson, 1977, p. 254), including the following: **labial glands**, associated with both lips, which are mainly mucous; three clusters of **lingual glands**, associated with the tongue, which are serous, mucous, or mixed according to their location on the tongue; **dorsal**, **middle**, and **ventral buccal glands**, arranged in lines and associated with the cheek, which are serous, mucous, or mixed according to their site and species; two well defined multilobular serous **molar glands** in *ruminants*, associated with the cheek; **palatine glands**, mucous; and **pharyngeal glands**, associated with the pharyngeal wall, which are mucous. The **zygomatic gland** of *carnivores* (mixed, serous and mucous) is homologous to the dorsal buccal glands of *herbivores* (Evans and Christensen, 1979, p. 413). The total mass of the minor glands in the *ox* almost equals that of the parotid, mandibular, and sublingual glands together (Habel, 1975, p. 872).

Details of the **innervation of the minor glands** are hard to find. It is generally agreed that the palatine glands get their parasympathetic efferent supply via the **major petrosal nerve** and pterygopalatine ganglion (Fig. 3.2). The preganglionic pathways of the other minor glands are either the major petrosal nerve, the chorda tympani, or the minor petrosal nerve, depending in principle on the topographical position of any particular gland. Thus the glands in the *rostral* part of the tongue are innervated via the chorda tympani (Crosby *et al.*, 1962, p. 533), whereas those in the *caudal* part are innervated by the glossopharyngeal nerve (Chibuzo, 1979, p. 444) presumably via the minor petrosal nerve; the preganglionic filaments pass from **lingual rami** of the glossopharyngeal nerve (Crosby *et al.*, 1962, p. 533). The **buccal** and **labial glands** are in general supplied via the chorda tympani (Crosby *et al.*, 1962, p. 533), except that the dorsal buccal glands in the *horse* (as just stated) and the homologous zygomatic gland in the *dog* are apparently innervated by the glossopharyngeal nerve via the otic ganglion (Stromberg, 1993, p. 1035). Usually these glands seem to have their own postganglionic cell bodies either singly or in small clusters, as in the glands of the tongue (Chibuzo, 1979, p. 442).

3.11   Vagus nerve

The vagus nerve (Fig. 3.3) consists mainly of autonomic afferent and parasympathetic efferent (motor) preganglionic axons.

The most important of the motor parasympathetic pathways of the vagus are those that innervate the heart, bronchi, stomach, and intestines, as shown in simplified form in Fig. 3.1. Figure 3.3 illustrates the same parasympathetic motor pathways of the vagus in more detail, as a black continuous line, distributed to the lungs, heart, and gastrointestinal tract. Figure 3.3 also

Fig. 3.3   Diagram summarizing the distribution of the vagus nerve. The parasympathetic motor component (continuous black lines) arises from the parasympathetic nucleus of the vagus in the brain stem. It supplies the following: laryngeal glands, via the cranial and recurrent laryngeal nerves; the smooth muscle and glands of the trachea, via tracheal rami of the recurrent laryngeal nerve; any smooth muscle and glands in the cervical oesophagus, via oesophageal rami of the recurrent laryngeal nerve; the bronchial smooth muscle and glands, via the bronchial rami of the vagus; the heart, via the cardiac rami; any smooth muscle and glands in the thoracic and abdominal oesophagus, via vagal oesophageal rami (not shown); and the smooth muscle and glands of the gastrointestinal tract as far as the transverse colon. The diagram shows pre- and postganglionic relays in these pathways.

The vagus also contains a special visceral efferent (branchial motor) component (broken black lines). This component arises in the brain stem from the nucleus ambiguus. It begins its course in the accessory (or spinal accessory) nerve, but almost immediately transfers from the spinal accessory nerve to the vagus. These fibres form the motor innervation of the following: pharyngeal muscles, via the pharyngeal ramus; laryngeal muscles, via the cranial and recurrent laryngeal nerves; and oesophageal striated muscle, via the oesophageal rami.

The vagus consists mainly of autonomic afferent fibres (continuous green lines). These arise from: the laryngeal mucosa, via the cranial and recurrent laryngeal nerves; the lung via bronchial rami; the atria, via cardiac rami; baro- and chemoreceptor afferents from the aortic arch and aortic bodies via the aortic nerve; and mechano- and chemoreceptors from the gastrointestinal tract as far as the transverse colon.

The topographical relationship of the vagal ganglia to the branches of the vagus is not accurately portrayed. The pharyngeal ramus should arise between the two vagal ganglia; the cranial laryngeal nerve should arise from the distal vagal ganglion.

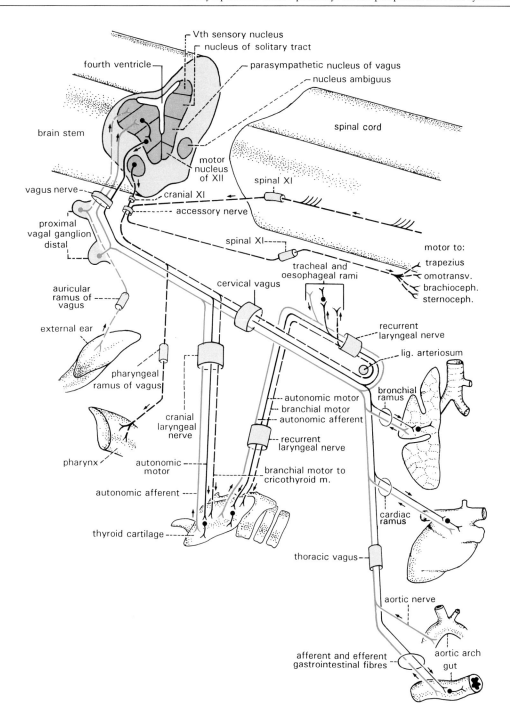

shows some additional vagal parasympathetic motor preganglionic pathways, namely those to the larynx, trachea, and oesophagus, via the recurrent and cranial laryngeal nerves. The functional effects of excitation of these vagal parasympathetic motor pathways are summarized below in Sections 3.11.1–3.11.6.

3.11.1 *Topographical anatomy of vagus nerve*

In the neck, the vagus becomes associated with the cervical sympathetic trunk, forming the **vagosympathetic trunk** (Section 2.22).

After entering the thoracic inlet, the vagus and the cervical sympathetic trunk part company, approximately at the level of the middle cervical ganglion. The right and left vagi pass caudally into the **mediastinum**. There they give rise to the right and left **recurrent laryngeal nerves**, which must now turn back and pass cranially to the larynx. To make this turn, the right recurrent laryngeal nerve goes round the derivative of the embryonic right fourth aortic arch, namely the right subclavian artery; the left recurrent laryngeal nerve goes round the derivative of the left sixth arch, namely the ligamentum arteriosum. **Cardiac rami** arise from the recurrent laryngeal nerves (Fig. 19.5) and from the left and right vagus nerves.

On both sides of the thorax, the vagus nerves pass over the dorsal aspect of the root of the lung, giving several **bronchial rami** to the lung (Figs 3.3, 19.5).

Immediately caudal to the hilus of the lung, the right and left vagus nerves divide into a dorsal and a ventral branch (Fig. 19.5). The right and left ventral branches fuse to form the **ventral trunk of the vagus**; the right and left dorsal branches combine to form the **dorsal trunk of the vagus**. The dorsal and ventral vagal trunks lie in the midline on the dorsal and ventral surfaces respectively of the oesophagus, and pass through the diaphragm at the **oesophageal hiatus**.

Within the abdomen the dorsal and ventral vagal trunks immediately form **gastric branches**, but caudal to that point the two vagal trunks totally lose their gross anatomical individuality by breaking down into plexiform branches that combine with the great sympathetic plexuses of the abdomen. These sympathetic plexuses are associated with the branches of the abdominal aorta along which they travel (e.g. the **coeliac plexus**), and with the individual abdominal organs that they eventually supply (e.g. **hepatic plexus**, **splenic plexus**) (Section 2.15).

The vagal preganglionic axons to the gut make synapses with **enteric ganglion cells** in the **myenteric plexus** of the **enteric nervous system** (Sections 3.4.1, 3.20).

The main trunk of the vagus emerges from the cranial cavity through the **jugular foramen**. Its **proximal ganglion** occurs in the foramen, and from this ganglion arises the **auricular ramus** (Fig. 3.3) which contains the only *somatic afferent axons* in the vagus (distributed to the external ear). The **cranial component** of the **accessory nerve** is transferred to the vagus immediately peripheral to the proximal vagal ganglion (Fig. 3.3). The **distal vagal ganglion** occurs a short distance peripheral to the union with the cranial component of the accessory nerve. The **pharyngeal ramus** of the vagus (not shown in Fig. 3.3) arises between the two ganglia, and is motor to the pharyngeal muscles; the **cranial laryngeal nerve** arises from the caudal end of the distal vagal ganglion (Figs 19.1, 19.2) (in Fig. 3.3, it arises caudal to the correct site). The **cranial laryngeal nerve** consists almost entirely of autonomic afferent axons from the rostral part of the larynx (Section 4.3.3).

By receiving the **cranial component** of the **accessory nerve** (from the **nucleus ambiguus**, Fig. 3.3), the vagus acquires a substantial number of **special visceral efferent (branchial motor)** axons from the **accessory nerve**. These innervate the striated musculature of the pharynx (by the pharyngeal branch of the vagus), of the larynx (by the cranial and caudal laryngeal nerves of the vagus), and of the oesophagus (by the recurrent laryngeal nerve) (Fig. 3.3).

The relative numbers of afferent and efferent axons in the main trunk of the vagus vary with the site, but the proportion of efferent axons is always small (probably less than 20%).

3.11.2 *Vagal parasympathetic innervation of the larynx, oesophagus, and trachea*

The **recurrent laryngeal nerve** provides a parasympathetic motor innervation to the glands of the laryngeal mucosa (Figs 3.3, 19.5). It also forms **oesophageal** and **tracheal rami** (Fig. 3.3), which supply a parasympathetic preganglionic motor innervation to any smooth muscle and glands in the cervical part of the oesophagus, and the smooth muscle and glands of the trachea.

Smooth muscle and glands in the thoracic and abdominal oesophagus receive a direct parasympathetic motor innervation via **oesophageal rami** of the vagus; these arise from the main trunk of the left and right vagus nerves before they divide into their dorsal and ventral branches, and from the dorsal and ventral vagal trunks after the division has occurred.

Oesophageal musculature: cardiac sphincter: oesophageal glands

The **oesophageal muscle** in the cranial third of the oesophagus is striated in all domestic species and man. In several species (*dog*, *ox*, and *pig*), striated muscle extends almost the whole length of the oesophagus. This striated muscle is branchial arch musculature, and therefore its motor innervation is not parasympathetic, but **special visceral motor** (Section 1.2.3) from the cranial component of the spinal accessory nerve, by means of the oesophageal rami of the recurrent laryngeal nerve (Fig. 3.3), and those of the vagus (Fig. 19.5). The **pharyngeal muscles** for swallowing, and the **laryngeal muscles** with the all-important function of controlling the laryngeal airway (Section 4.15), are also branchial (i.e. striated) musculature; they, too, are innervated by **special visceral motor** axons from the cranial component of the spinal accessory nerve, via the **pharyngeal ramus** of the vagus and the **cranial** and **recurrent laryngeal nerves** (Fig. 3.3).

In the **tunica muscularis** (muscle layer) of the **oesophagus**, the transition from striated to smooth muscle in the *horse*, *cat*, and *man* takes place somewhere in the middle or caudal third of the oesophagus, whereas in the *pig* it occurs just cranial to the cardia (Habel and Biberstein, 1960, p. 178; Crosby *et al.*, 1962, p. 534). In *ruminants* and the *dog* the entire tunica muscularis has been said to be striated (Habel and Biberstein, 1960, p. 178). In the *dog*, however, smooth muscle appears in the tunica muscularis immediately **after** the oesophagus has gone through the diaphragm; it then increases progressively, and finally forms about two thirds of the tunica muscularis immediately before the gastric mucosa begins (C. Vaillant, personal communication, 1996). De Lahunta and Habel (1986, p. 206) stated that in the *dog* the last 1–2 cm of the middle layer are smooth muscle.

Only the **smooth muscle** of the oesophagus, including that of the **muscularis mucosa** along the whole length of the oesophagus, is supplied by **vagal preganglionic parasympathetic axons** (Crosby *et al.*, 1962, p. 533). The preganglionic axons synapse with neurons in the **enteric ganglia** (Section 3.20), starting at the most cranial level of the oesophageal smooth muscle; stimulation of the vagal preganglionic axons causes *oesophageal peristalsis* (Crosby *et al.*, 1962, p. 533).

Despite consisting of striated muscle and therefore lacking the enteric nervous system, the tunica muscularis

of the *cranial part* of the oesophagus in *mammals generally*, and the tunica muscularis of almost the whole of the oesophagus in the *ruminant* and *dog*, generates typical *peristaltic waves*. The cell bodies of the special visceral motor neurons that control this striated muscle lie in the **nucleus ambiguus** of the brainstem, and their axons lie in **oesophageal branches** of the **recurrent laryngeal nerve** (Fig. 3.3). These neurons fire in overlapping sequence, causing the contraction to proceed aborally in a peristaltic wave. In the oesophagus of the *dog*, the peristaltic wave immediately caudal to the diaphragm is taken over by the smooth muscle and its enteric nerve supply. The enteric nervous system then supplies the all important mechanism for opening and closing the gastro-oesophageal junction without allowing gastric reflux.

There is something of a mystery about the presence or absence of a **cardiac sphincter** at the junction of the oesophagus with the stomach. Non-anatomists (e.g. Blood and Studdert (1988, p. 639) for *domestic animals* generally, and Waterman and Hashim (1991) for the *dog*) deny the presence of an anatomical sphincter. Anatomists tend to use the term 'cardiac sphincter', but appear to do so with confidence for the *horse* only (see Nickel *et al.*, 1973, p. 181; Sisson, 1975, p. 479; Dyce *et al.*, 1987, p. 511). In the *horse*, towards the cardia the tunica muscularis of the oesophagus 'reaches an extraordinary thickness', but the actual cardiac sphincter is supposed to be formed by the interlocking of internal oblique gastric muscle bundles (the 'cardiac loop') with circular gastric muscle bundles (Nickel *et al.*, 1973, p. 181); de Lahunta and Habel (1986, p. 232) state that in the *horse* 'the cardiac sphincter is much thicker and better defined than in the other animals', but without making it clear whether this refers to the oesophageal wall, the gastric bundles, or both together. No matter what it consists of, this sphincteral structure is supposed to prevent eructation and vomiting in the *horse*, though vomiting does occur sometimes; however, acute gastric distension can lead to rupture of the stomach. In *ruminants* the circular muscle of the oesophagus, a short distance cranial to the diaphragm, is said to combine functionally (though not structurally) with bundles of gastric musculature to 'act as a caudal oesophageal sphincter' (Nickel *et al.*, 1973, p. 147). In the domestic *carnivores*, the oesophageal wall is reported to get progressively thicker caudally, being thickest a few centimetres cranial to the cardia where there is a constriction of the lumen (Nickel *et al.*, 1973, p. 122). Evans and Christensen (1979, p. 456) stated that, in the *dog*, the oesophageal wall is thickest where it joins the stomach, but attributed the existence of a 'feeble cardiac sphincter' to a thickening of the inner circular muscle layer of the stomach at the cardia (Evans and Christensen, 1979, p. 477). According to histologists, the inner oblique layer of the gastric tunica muscularis 'forms the sphincter cardiae' apparently in mammals generally (Habel and Biberstein, 1960, p. 196); another view is that 'the junctions of the oesophagus with the pharynx and stomach are not marked by anatomic thickenings that serve as sphincters' (Banks, 1981, p. 385). In *man*, attempts to find aggregations of muscle qualifying anatomically as a sphincter have failed (Williams *et al.*, 1989, p. 1333). However, many other anatomical factors have been postulated to explain sphincteric control of the oesophageal-gastric junction in man. These include the obliquity of the oesophageal entrance, combinations of spiral and longitudinal muscle, mucosal folds, and relationships between the circular muscle of the oesophagus and the muscle of the right crus of the diaphragm, but none of these has been convincing (Williams *et al.*, 1989, p. 1333).

There is, of course, no doubt whatever about the presence in man and mammals generally of a mechanism at the gastric end of the oesophagus that very effectively restricts the reflux of gastric contents into the oesophagus. The acid and proteolytic enzymes of the contents of the simple stomach are not good for the oesophageal mucosa. **Gastro-oesophageal reflux** can cause destruction of oesophageal tissue, formation of scar tissue, and stricture leading to a form of **oesophageal achalasia** (Section 3.23.1). Such reflux is prevented by what is probably best termed an 'oesophageal sphincter zone', in which the circular smooth muscle in the abdominal part of the oesophagus is tonically contracted, presumably by the myogenic drive of pacemaker muscle cells; as in gut sphincters in general (Section 3.22), the sphincter zone is opened by relaxation of its circular muscle by inhibitory enteric neurons, for instance during **eructation** or the entry of ingesta into the stomach during **oesophageal peristalsis**. Appropriate mechanoreceptor mechanisms for co-ordinating the muscle in the sphincter zone are known to exist (Section 4.11.1).

The frequency and serious consequences of **disorders of the oesophageal sphincter zone** in man and domestic mammals have stimulated various investigations into the length and site of the zone. In the *cat*, for example, it has been found that some standard anaesthetic drugs tend to relax the sphincter zone, leading to reflux and resulting later in **oesophageal stricture** (Hashim and Waterman, 1991). In the *dog* and *man*, manometry has shown the sphincter zone to be about 4 or 5 cm long, lying caudal to the diaphragm (Waterman and Hashim, 1991). This agrees with the observations by Vaillant mentioned above (C. Vaillant, personal communication, 1996), showing that, caudal to the diaphragm, smooth muscle takes over the tunica muscularis of the oesophagus of the dog. Debate about whether or not there is an **anatomical** cardiac sphincter is really irrelevant. As pointed out by Gabella (1987, p. 335), the functional characteristics of the gut sphincters depend on the relationship between the myogenic drive and the inhibitory innervation of the circular muscle by the enteric nervous system, rather than on an anatomical arrangement of muscle fibres: on this basis, there **is** a cardiac sphincter at the gastric end of the oesophagus.

Oesophageal glands, mucous in type, occur along the whole length of the oesophagus of the *dog* and *man*, but are restricted in the *horse*, *ruminants*, and *cat* to the pharyngoesophageal junction (Habel and Biberstein, 1960, p. 177; Williams *et al.*, 1989, p. 1333). Presumably these glands receive a vagal secretomotor preganglionic parasympathetic innervation; the preganglionic axons synapse with enteric ganglion cells (Section 3.20). It is to be expected that this innervation would be strongly excitatory, as it is for the other glands in the upper part of the alimentary tract (Guyton, 1986, p. 691). Lubrication by the mucus from the glands at the beginning of the oesophagus protects the mucosa from excoriation by the incoming ingesta; the mucous secretion at the caudal end of the oesophagus protects the mucosa from minor reflux of gastric juices of simple stomachs (Guyton, 1986, p. 774).

3.11.3   *Vagal parasympathetic innervation of the heart*

Preganglionic parasympathetic **cardiac rami** arise from the recurrent laryngeal nerves and from the vagus nerves, and are distributed over both atria (Fig. 3.3). The preganglionic endings make synapses with postganglionic neurons in the walls of both atria. The postganglionic endings are concentrated mainly around the **sinuatrial node**, and to a lesser extent around the **atrioventricular node** (Section 22.8.2). Stimulation of these endings decreases the heart rate.

The vagal cardiac rami also distribute parasympathetic vasodilator axons to the **coronary arterial vasculature**, but their effect on the *normal* coronary circulation is almost negligible.

The **parasympathetic cardiac rami** from the recurrent laryngeal nerves and the vagal trunks join with the **sympathetic cardiac nerves** to form the **cardiac plexus** (Godhino and Getty, 1975, pp. 662, 1092). At least in the dog, both the 'vagal' cardiac rami and the 'sympathetic' cardiac nerves of the cardiac plexus usually contain both parasympathetic vagal preganglionic axons and sympathetic postganglionic axons (Section 2.11).

In *man* (Mitchell, 1953, pp. 181, 247, 250) the **cardiac plexus** is a midline meshwork of nerves comprising both vagal and sympathetic cardiac axons from both sides of the body; all of its components (vagal, sympathetic, and bundles of left and right sided axons) lose their individual identities. The plexus contains clusters of nerve cell bodies, forming small **ganglia**; these are considered to be largely, if not exclusively, parasympathetic motor neurons (Salmons, 1995, p. 1500).

3.11.4 *Vagal parasympathetic innervation of the lungs*

The preganglionic parasympathetic **bronchial rami** (Figs 3.1, 3.3, 19.5) enter the hilus of the lung and follow the bronchial tree. The postganglionic cell bodies occur in small groups in the bronchial walls. The postganglionic axons are excitatory to the **bronchial smooth muscle** (Section 6.12.1), and are therefore bronchoconstrictor in action. They are also secretomotor to the **bronchial glands** (Section 6.12.2). Some of the axons in the bronchial rami are afferent (Section 4.16). The pulmonary arteries and veins receive some vagal vasomotor axons.

> The preganglionic axons of the vagal bronchial rami mingle with sympathetic postganglionic axons from the stellate ganglion to form the **pulmonary plexus** at the root of the lung (Sections 2.11, 6.12). Numerous plexiform branches of this plexus follow the bronchial tree and the associated blood vessels into the substance of the lungs (Godhino and Getty, 1975, p. 663). The preganglionic vagal axons synapse in the **bronchial ganglia** of the pulmonary plexus and its branches. The postganglionic axons are excitatory to the **bronchial smooth muscle** and **bronchial glands**. Postganglionic vagal fibres have a weak dilator action on **pulmonary blood vessels** (Crosby *et al.*, 1962, p. 531; Williams *et al.*, 1989, p. 1165); they cause a slight fall in resistance to blood flow when stimulated, but it is doubtful that they contribute significantly to the control of pulmonary blood flow (Guyton, 1986, p. 289) (Section 17.21.4).

3.11.5 *Vagal parasympathetic innervation of the stomach*

Having passed through the oesophageal hiatus, the dorsal vagal trunk and the ventral vagal trunk immediately form **gastric rami** to supply the stomach (Fig. 3.1). These are not lost in plexuses shared with the sympathetic system, but remain distinctively vagal as they ramify over the surface of the stomach. The preganglionic axons synapse with **enteric ganglion cells** in the myenteric plexus (Section 3.20). These pathways promote gastric motility and copious gastric secretion (Section 3.20), and the opening of the pyloric sphincter (Section 3.22).

The vagal pathways to the smooth muscle and glands of the oesophagus, stomach, and intestines break the rule laid down in Section 1.2 that peripheral motor autonomic pathways project through both a pre- and a postganglionic neuron. In these vagal pathways the postganglionic neuron is replaced by an **enteric ganglion cell** (Section 3.20).

> The distribution of the gastric branches is in principle the same in the simple and the complex stomach (de Lahunta and Habel, 1986, p. 239), since the dorsal and ventral vagal trunks run side by side along the lesser curvature of both types of stomach. The dorsal vagal trunk supplies the visceral surface of the simple stomach. However, the development of the rumen, primarily from an area supplied by the dorsal trunk, causes a great increase in the size and number of the branches of the dorsal trunk (Habel, 1970, p. 41). In the *ruminant* it supplies the rumen, both the visceral and parietal surfaces of the omasum, and the visceral (left) surface of the abomasum, all these being essentially dorsal parts; it also supplies the visceral surface of the reticulum (Habel, 1970, p. 43). The **ventral vagal trunk** supplies the parietal surface of the *simple* stomach; in the *ruminant* it supplies the reticulum, the parietal surface of the omasum, and the parietal surface of the abomasum (essentially ventral parts), but not the rumen.
>
> The stomach responds to vagal stimulation by increased motility and secretion. The **gastric glands** secrete pepsinogen from their chief cells, acid from their parietal cells, and mucus from their mucous cells. Vagal stimulation also activates type G cells (Section 2.40) in the pyloric glands to secrete **gastrin**, which acts on the gastric glands and causes them to secrete additional highly acid gastric juice.
>
> At the origins of the gastric branches, **hepatic branches** to the liver arise from the dorsal and ventral vagal trunks (Stromberg, 1993, p. 1040) and end in ganglia at the hepatic porta and in the walls of the gall bladder, cystic duct, and bile duct. Postganglionic axons have been traced to the smooth muscle in the wall of the bile duct, including the sphincter; opinions differ as to whether there are secretory axons to the hepatic cells (Crosby *et al.*, 1962, p. 537).

3.11.6 *Vagal parasympathetic innervation of the pancreas*

The **pancreas** receives an extensive vagal innervation. Axons pass to the pancreas from the ventral vagal trunk along the right gastric and pancreaticoduodenal arteries (Stromberg, 1993, p. 1040). Postganglionic vagal axons arise from postganglionic neurons in ganglia on and within the pancreas; the axons end on the exocrine acinar cells and the cells of the endocrine islets, and also on the smooth muscle of the pancreatic ducts (Crosby *et al.*, 1962, p. 537). Vagal activity causes secretion of enzymes into the pancreatic acini, where they are temporarily stored. The arrival of acid ingesta in the small intestine causes the release of **secretin** and **cholecystokinin** from cells in the mucosa of the small intestine (Section 2.40). These local hormones are absorbed into the blood, and on reaching the pancreas stimulate it to produce copious secretion with a high concentration of bicarbonate ion (the effect of secretin) and large quantities of digestive enzymes (the effect of cholecystokinin) (Guyton, 1986, p. 780).

3.11.7   *Vagal parasympathetic innervation of the intestines*

After giving off the gastric branches, the dorsal and ventral vagi blend with the **sympathetic plexuses** that accompany the aorta and its branches (Section 2.15), and consequently can no longer be followed by dissection. The vagal preganglionic axons follow the aortic branches that supply the intestine, notably the cranial mesenteric artery, and thus supply the **small intestine** and the **large intestine** approximately to the end of the **transverse colon**. The axons end by making synapses with **enteric ganglion cells** in the **myenteric plexus** (Section 3.20). These vagal pathways are secretomotor to the glands of the intestine, and excitatory to the smooth muscle in the walls, except the caecal sphincters which they inhibit (Section 3.22). As just stated (Section 3.11.5), the enteric ganglion cell replaces the postganglionic neuron in this vagal pathway.

Details of the distribution of the vagus caudal to the stomach are scarce (Stromberg, 1993, p. 1041). The **dorsal vagal trunk** appears to form the major link with the sympathetic **aortic plexus** by projecting its preganglionic parasympathetic axons directly into the sympathetic **coeliac** and **mesenteric plexuses** (Ghoshal, 1975, p. 1736; Stromberg, 1979, p. 1041). Sympathetic postganglionic and vagal preganglionic axons accompany the branches of the coeliac and cranial mesenteric arteries (for example, the ileocolic artery; Evans and Christensen, 1979, p. 725). It seems to be generally agreed that in the *dog* vagal axons reach at least as far caudally as the end of the transverse colon (Ghoshal, 1975, p. 1736; Stromberg, 1993, p. 1041). The density of vagal innervation is relatively low in the small intestine, and high in the proximal half of the large intestine (Guyton, 1986, p. 757). The

glands of the small and large intestine are controlled principally by local factors in the intestines, operating mainly through the **enteric nervous system** (Section 3.18.3) rather than by parasympathetic and sympathetic nerves (Guyton, 1986, p. 691).

3.11.8   *Vagal parasympathetic innervation of other thoracoabdominal organs*

Crosby *et al.* (1962, pp. 538–546) reviewed evidence for the presence of vagal pre- and postganglionic axons in the testis, ovary, kidney, ureter, adrenal gland, spleen, and thymus; however, the functions of such innervation were not clear, although vasomotor actions (usually vasodilator) seem the most likely. There is little, if any, evidence for vagal secretomotor functions in these tissues. Sacral parasympathetic pathways may also be vasodilator to the testis and ovary (Section 3.12).

III   SACRAL PARASYMPATHETIC MOTOR PATHWAYS

3.12   Pelvic nerve

The sacral parasympathetic **preganglionic axons** emerge from the ventral rami (divisions) of two or three sacral spinal nerves (Section 3.3.2), and combine to form the **pelvic nerve** on each side of the body (Fig. 3.1). These axons supply the pelvic viscera and descending colon. The pelvic nerve also contains many autonomic afferent axons from the pelvic viscera (Section 4.3.4). The pelvic nerve joins the **hypogastric nerve** (Fig. 3.4) to form the **pelvic plexus** (Section 3.13).

Many of these sacral parasympathetic **preganglionic axons** in the pelvic nerve synapse with parasympathetic **postganglionic neurons** in either the **pelvic ganglia** (Fig. 3.1) (Section 3.13), or in minute ganglia on or in the walls of the pelvic viscera (Fig. 3.4). These **postganglionic neurons** are *excitatory* to the smooth muscle in the wall of the **bladder**, *inhibitory* to any smooth muscle that constricts the neck of the bladder (Section 2.17.2), *vasodilator* to the **erectile tissues** of the penis and clitoris, *excitatory* to the smooth muscle (Fig. 3.4) and glands of the wall of the **rectum** and **descending colon** (by making synapses with enteric ganglion cells, Section 3.20), and *inhibitory* (Fig. 3.4) to the **internal anal sphincter** (by synapsing with inhibitory enteric ganglion cells, Section 3.22).

Many other sacral parasympathetic **preganglionic axons** in the pelvic nerve also have an *excitatory* action on the smooth muscle and glands in the walls of the **rectum** and **descending colon**, and an *inhibitory* action on the **internal anal sphincter**, but these **preganglionic axons** synapse with **enteric ganglion cells** instead of with postganglionic parasympathetic neurons (Fig. 3.4). Such sacral preganglionic parasympathetic axons therefore resemble the **vagal** axons that project to the walls of the oesophagus, stomach, and intestines (Sections 3.11.5, 3.11.6), which are likewise **pre**ganglionic and synapse *directly* with **enteric ganglion cells** instead of postganglionic neurons.

To *summarize*, both **pre-** and **postganglionic** sacral parasympathetic axons of the pelvic nerve make synapses with **enteric ganglion cells** (Section 3.4.2).

The **external anal sphincter** consists of skeletal muscle, and is innervated by the somatic motor axons of the **pudendal nerve** (Fig. 3.4).

> The **pelvic nerve** is also known as the **pelvic splanchnic nerve** or **nervus erigens**.
>
> In the *dog*, there may be either one or two pelvic nerves on each side, though the two may unite into a single nerve (Evans and Christensen, 1979, p. 1018); the pelvic nerve or nerves accompany the prostatic/vaginal artery as far as the lateral surface of the rectum, and there merge with plexiform branches of the hypogastric nerve to form the **pelvic plexus** (Christensen, 1979, p. 566; de Lahunta, 1983, p. 124). In the *horse* there are usually five or six pelvic nerves on each side; in the *ox* the pelvic nerves are represented by fine filaments varying in their numbers and courses; in the *sheep* about five pelvic nerves descend to the pelvic plexus as separate nerves on each side (Ghoshal, 1975, pp. 702, 1170, 1174). The pelvic nerves also contain **sympathetic postganglionic axons** with their cell stations in the lumbar and sacral vertebral ganglia of the sympathetic chain (Section 2.16).
>
> The sacral parasympathetic motor pathways are definitely *excitatory* to the smooth muscle of the wall of the **bladder**, **descending colon**, and **rectum**, and *inhibitory* to the smooth muscle of the **internal anal sphincter**. They also innervate the end of the transverse colon in man (Williams, 1989, p. 1156), and have been traced throughout the whole length of the large intestine of the dog (Stromberg, 1993, p. 1042). Their possible role in preventing the escape of urine from the bladder is controversial in view of the uncertainties about the anatomical basis for this mechanism (Sections 2.17, 3.14).

Knowledge of neuronal elements of the processes regulating the **reproductive organs**, especially in the female, is still minimal (Jänig and McLachlan, 1987, p. 1391). In the male, only the mechanism of **erection** is understood. Dense cholinergic and VIP terminals occur around most of the arteries of the **penile vasculature** and in the corpus cavernosum penis, though there are only a few in the corpus spongiosum penis (Jänig and McLachlan, 1987, p. 1351). Erection normally takes place by excitation of these nerve terminals through a sacral reflex arc; hence erection can occur after transection of the cervical or thoracic spinal cord. However, the neuronal pathways even of erection are not entirely clear, since complete interruption of the sacral parasympathetic supply to the pelvic organs does not necessarily abolish erection; it seems that the sympathetic outflow to the reproductive organs can take over the function of the sacral parasympathetic outflow (Jänig and McLachlan, 1987, p. 1391). One possible explanation of this is the convergence of sympathetic preganglionic axons of the hypogastric nerve and preganglionic parasympathetic axons of the pelvic nerve on the same postganglionic neuron (Jänig and McLachlan, 1987, p. 1380) in pelvic ganglia (Section 3.13).

It has been reported that sacral parasympathetic motor pathways supply the **prostate**, **vesicular gland** (**seminal vesicle**), **ductus deferens**, and **uterus**, and all these pathways are believed to be *vasodilator* in function; it is thought likely that the pathways to the male accessory reproductive glands are *secretomotor*, but firm evidence for this is scarce (Crosby *et al.*, 1962, pp. 541–543). *Vasodilator* sacral parasympathetic pathways have been reported in the **testis**, **ovary**, and **uterine tube** (Williams *et al.*, 1989, p. 1156), and there is also evidence for vagal vasodilator pathways in the **testis** and **ovary** (Section 3.11.8). There are secretomotor endings in the **endometrium** that probably contain acetylcholine and VIP, and definite vasodilator nerves in the extrauterine arteries (Jänig and McLachlan, 1987, p. 1351).

The pudendal nerve is formed from the ventral divisions of sacral spinal nerves (S3–S4 in the *horse* and *ruminants*, and S1–S3 in *carnivores*, Section 2.17.2).

3.13 Pelvic plexus and pelvic ganglia

The **pelvic plexus** consists of a network of parasympathetic and sympathetic axons, lying on the lateral surface of the rectum. It is formed by the blending of the **pelvic nerve** and the **hypogastric nerve** (Section 2.18). Ganglia are scattered in the plexus where the blending occurs; these are known as the **pelvic ganglia** (Figs 3.1, 3.4). Other ganglia are situated on or in the walls of the pelvic viscera. The pelvic ganglia, and the

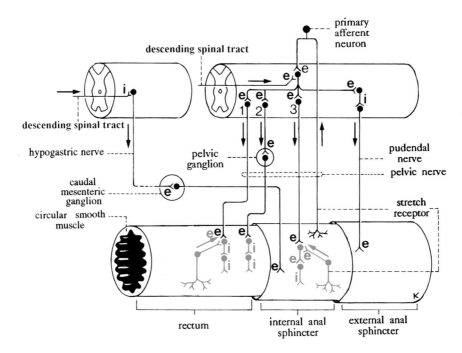

Fig. 3.4 Reflex pathways of defecation. Defecation is initiated by stretch receptors in the wall of the rectum. A primary afferent neuron in such a stretch receptor reflex is represented by the nerve cell body shown (black) at the top of the diagram on the right. The cell body would be in a dorsal root spinal (sacral) ganglion. The receptor ending of this neuron lies in the wall of the internal anal sphincter, and its afferent axon is labelled stretch receptor. In the spinal cord, this primary afferent stretch receptor neuron is shown synapsing with an interneuron that is excitatory (e) to three preganglionic parasympathetic motor neurons (numbered 1, 2, and, 3, in black) in the intermediolateral grey matter of the sacral spinal cord. Of these three preganglionic motor neurons, 1 and 2 each activate *two **inhibitory** enteric motor ganglion cells in series (i and i, green)*, in the wall of the rectum. Preganglionic neuron no. 1 makes this connection directly, going without interruption from the spinal cord to the wall of the rectum. Preganglionic neuron no. 2 makes this connection indirectly, via a pre–postganglionic synapse in a pelvic ganglion. The more *peripheral* of the two inhibitory enteric motor ganglion cells (the one further away from the spinal cord) inhibits the circular smooth muscle of the rectum, thus preventing the rectal muscle from contracting in response to pacemaker muscle cells in the rectal wall. The more *central* of the two inhibitory enteric motor ganglion cells (the one nearer to the spinal cord) inhibits the more peripheral inhibitory enteric motor ganglion cell. This releases the circular smooth muscle of the rectal wall from inhibition, thus allowing it to respond to the tonic myogenic drive of pacemaker muscle/cells. **Peristalsis** of the rectum results. Inhibition of an inhibitory effect is disinhibition. Here, disinhibition has induced rectal peristalsis.

Peristalsis can also be activated by a simple stretch reflex arc that operates *entirely within the gut wall*. This reflex arc consists of only three very short enteric neurons (green, shown furthest to the left in the rectal wall). The first of these three neurons is a stretch receptor afferent neuron, with its cell body in the wall of the rectum. The arrow shows the direction of its impulses. Both the second and the final neuron in the arc are inhibitory enteric motor ganglion cells. Activation of the arc causes disinhibition, and thus allows the pacemaker muscle cells to cause peristalsis.

The parasympathetic motor neuron no. 3, in the sacral spinal cord, induces **relaxation of the internal anal sphincter**. Its motor ending enters the internal anal sphincter. Here it synapses with an *excitatory* enteric motor ganglion cell (e, green). This excitatory neuron synapses with an *inhibitory* enteric motor ganglion cell (i, green). Activation of this inhibitory neuron inhibits the tonic myogenic drive of the muscle pacemaker cells, thus allowing the internal anal sphincter to relax during defecation. Relaxation of the internal anal sphincter is also attained by a simple reflex arc operating entirely within the rectal wall. It consists of only three very short neurons (green, shown furthest to the right, in the internal anal sphincter). The first neuron in this arc is a stretch receptor afferent neuron with its cell body in the wall of the internal anal sphincter. The arrow indicates the direction of its impulses. The second neuron is excitatory, activating the inhibitory third neuron. Activation of the inhibitory neuron blocks the drive of the muscle pacemaker cells and thus allows the sphincter to relax in defecation. The inhibitory third neuron is usually silent, thus allowing the pacemaker drive to maintain tonic contraction of the internal anal sphincter and keep the sphincter closed.

At the extreme right end of the diagram, a somatic motor neuron in the spinal cord sends its axon, via the pudendal nerve, into the external anal sphincter (e, black). This pathway closes the **external anal sphincter** by conscious control. The segment of ganglia on or in the walls of the pelvic viscera, are the cell station of the sacral parasympathetic postganglionic neurons in pelvic nerve pathways (Section 3.4.2).

In *man*, the **pelvic plexus** (plexus pelvinus) is usually known as the **inferior hypogastric plexus**.

The position of the pelvic plexus is variably described, in three main sites: (i) 'on the pelvic wall' (Christensen, 1979, p. 576), 'subperitoneal' (Dyce *et al.*, 1987, p. 324), 'within the connective tissue layers overlying the pelvic organs' (Jänig and McLachlan, 1987, p. 1339), or 'in the extraperitoneal connective tissue' (Williams *et al.*, 1989, p. 1166); (ii) 'on the ventrolateral aspect of the rectogenital pouch' (Ghoshal, 1975, pp. 701, 1170, 1737); (iii) 'on the lateral surface of the rectum' (Stromberg, 1993, p. 1051). These three apparently different positions reflect different levels in the pelvic canal. Where it is first formed, by the blending of the pelvic and hypogastric nerves, the pelvic plexus lies on the pelvic wall subperitoneally. Some of its axons are destined to reach the walls of organs that are suspended by peritoneum (intraperitoneal organs), but others go to organs that are retroperitoneal. For example, the more cranial part of the rectum is intraperitoneal, but the terminal part is entirely retroperitoneal. Components of the plexus that are destined for the intraperitoneal part of the rectum must reach their target by leaving the lateral pelvic wall and passing between the two peritoneal sheets that form the floor of the rectogenital pouch; components of the plexus that go to the retroperitoneal part of the rectum can get there by travelling directly along the pelvic wall, i.e. retroperitoneally. Other pelvic organs are partly intraperitoneal and partly retroperitoneal, such as the prostate in the dog which is entirely retroperitoneal at 8 months and entirely intraperitoneal at 10 years (de Lahunta and Habel, 1986, p. 294). The bladder is mostly extraperitoneal when empty and mostly intraperitoneal when full (in the larger species) (Dyce *et al.*, 1987, p. 180).

Precise definition of the beginning and end of the pelvic plexus is, moreover, virtually impossible. The hypogastric nerve and pelvic nerve may become plexiform before they blend into a single pelvic plexus; the periphery (ends) of the pelvic plexus extends into subsidiary plexuses of progressively finer filaments that disperse into their target organs. These subsidiary plexuses are named according to the organs that they innervate, the main ones being the **middle** and **caudal rectal**, **prostatic**, **deferential**, and **uterovaginal plexuses**, and the **plexus** of the **corpus cavernosum** of the **penis** and **clitoris** (Ghoshal, 1975, p. 702).

In some species the **pelvic ganglia** (ganglia pelvina) are submacroscopic, the ganglion cells being scattered throughout the pelvic plexus and its subsidiary plexuses (*horse*, and *ruminants*; Ghoshal, 1975, pp. 702, 1170, 1174, 1179). In *man* the plexuses contain small and numerous ganglia (Williams *et al.*, 1989, p. 1166). In the *dog*, there may be one or more macroscopic ganglia in the pelvic plexus (Stromberg, 1993, p. 1042), as well as minute ganglia. Postganglionic cell bodies are also assembled into small ganglia on or in the walls of the pelvic viscera (Jänig and McLachlan, 1987, p. 1346).

Large numbers of **sympathetic** postganglionic neurons project through the pelvic plexus onto the pelvic viscera and descending colon. The corresponding number of **parasympathetic** postganglionic axons in the pelvic plexus is unknown but is thought to be considerably smaller. Most of the sympathetic postganglionic axons in the pelvic plexus (Section 2.16) have their cell station in the **caudal mesenteric ganglion** and send their axons through the **hypogastric nerve** to the pelvic plexus. Others (about 20% of the total) have their cell stations in the lumbar and sacral ganglia of the **sympathetic chain**, and project their sympathetic postganglionic axons through the pelvic nerve to the pelvic plexus. In addition, appreciable numbers of sympathetic preganglionic axons pass through the caudal mesenteric ganglion, onward through the hypogastric nerve, and so into the pelvic plexus, where they synapse with postganglionic neurons in the

---

Fig. 3.4 (Continued)   spinal cord on the *right* carries an excitatory descending pathway (e, black). This organizes defecation: firstly it activates excitatory neurons 1 and 2, thus stimulating peristalsis of the rectum; secondly it also activates neuron 3, and thus relaxes the internal anal sphincter; and thirdly (shown at the extreme right hand end of the spinal cord) it activates an inhibitory neuron in the cord (i, black), and this inhibits the somatic motor neuron in the pudendal nerve that excites the external anal sphincter, thus activating relaxation of the external anal sphincter during defecation.

The segment of spinal cord shown on the left of the diagram contains the cell body of a *preganglionic motor sympathetic* neuron (black). The axon of this neuron excites a postganglionic sympathetic neuron in the caudal mesenteric ganglion. This postganglionic sympathetic neuron excites (e, black), and therefore *closes*, the **internal anal sphincter**. The sympathetic preganglionic neuron with its cell body in the spinal cord is itself inhibited by an inhibitory motor neuron descending in the spinal cord (i, black, arrow indicating direction of transmission). This inhibitory descending neuron thus provides a motor pathway that enables voluntary *opening* of the internal anal sphincter during defecation.

Arrows indicate afferent and efferent fibres. Stretch receptor signals are projected to the brain by ascending spinal pathways (not shown).

pelvic ganglia. **Anatomically**, therefore, the **pelvic plexus** is predominantly sympathetic. The **pelvic ganglia** had previously been regarded as predominantly para-sympathetic, and most of the larger ganglia, which are extramural in position, are indeed parasympathetic; however, in the *cat* 40% of the intramural ganglia are parasympathetic and 40% sympathetic, the remaining 20% receiving their preganglionic axons from **both** systems (Crosby *et al.*, 1962, p. 539). Nevertheless, the pelvic plexus is clearly dominated **functionally** by the sacral parasympathetic system. Indeed elimination of the sympathetic pathways to the pelvic viscera causes no significant impairment of function, except for the loss of seminal emission (Section 2.17). However, the sacral parasympathetic outflow is essential for normal micturition (Section 3.14), and though not strictly essential is also highly important for normal defecation (Section 3.14).

There is clear evidence (Jänig and McLachlan, 1987, p. 1333) that both sympathetic and parasympathetic preganglionic axons may form synapses with the **same ganglion cell** within the pelvic ganglia. Such convergence may explain the ability of the sympathetic system to activate parasympathetic pelvic functions, such as inducing erection after destruction of the sacral segments of the spinal cord (Section 3.12). Moreover, only some of the postganglionic axons innervate their target organs directly; others control their target organs indirectly, e.g. through the enteric nervous system. Therefore it is not clear whether neurons in the pelvic ganglia can be reliably designated as sympathetic or parasympathetic. Jänig and McLachlan (1987, p. 1389) suggested that it might be better to regard them as an altogether separate class of neuron.

3.14 Micturition and defecation

The sacral parasympathetic motor pathways are definitely excitatory to the smooth muscle of the wall of the bladder, descending colon and rectum, and inhibitory to the smooth muscle of the internal anal sphincter. However, their role in preventing the escape of urine from the bladder remains obscure, largely owing to the doubt about the existence of an 'internal sphincter' of smooth muscle on the neck of the bladder (Section 2.17.2). Nevertheless, it is certain that the sacral parasympathetic motor outflow is essential for micturition and very important for defecation.

Micturition and defecation are controlled by essentially similar peripheral and central neuronal pathways. Both processes are initiated by

mechanoreceptors responding to stretch and pressure in the walls of the bladder and rectum respectively (Section 4.14.1). These primary afferent neurons project through the **pelvic plexus** and **pelvic nerve** to sacral segments of the spinal cord (Fig. 3.4). There they make neuronal links that complete reflex arcs with the parasympathetic preganglionic neurons in the intermediolateral grey matter (Fig. 3.4). The preganglionic axons that supply the muscular wall of the **bladder** make the return journey to the bladder via the pelvic nerve, and form synapses with postganglionic neurons in the **pelvic ganglia** or in the wall of the bladder; these are excitatory to the smooth muscle in the bladder wall and cause the bladder to empty. The preganglionic axons forming the sacral parasympathetic pathway to the **rectum** and **descending colon** also return via the pelvic nerve. Some of these preganglionic axons to the rectum and descending colon make synapses in the pelvic ganglia with postganglionic neurons that project to enteric ganglion cells (Fig. 3.4); other preganglionic axons project directly on enteric ganglion cells (Fig. 3.4) (Sections 3.4.2, 3.12, 3.20). Many of these pre- and postganglionic axons of the pelvic nerve activate the circular muscle of the descending colon and rectum, producing rectal peristalsis; others inhibit the **internal anal sphincter** (Section 3.22).

Some primary afferent neurons from the bladder and rectum project through **ascending pathways** in the spinal cord to the brainstem and from there ultimately to the conscious **cerebral cortex**, informing the brain that the organs are filling. Motor pathways project from the cortex, through the brainstem, and down the spinal cord via **descending pathways** to the sacral preganglionic neuron (Fig. 3.4), enabling conscious control of the emptying mechanisms.

Distension of the bladder or rectum initiates a **spinal micturition reflex** or **spinal defecation reflex** via the sacral segments of the spinal cord, resulting in (i) contraction of the bladder or contraction of the rectal wall (Fig. 3.4), and (ii) simultaneous reflex inhibition of any **sphincter mechanisms** that the **bladder** may possess (especially the **pudendal nerve** to the **urethralis muscle**, Section 2.17), or of the **internal** and **external anal sphincters** (Fig. 3.4). These reflexes can be inhibited or facilitated by the central control of the cerebral cortex (via descending spinal pathways, Fig. 3.4), enabling micturition or defecation to occur at appropriate times and places in the house-trained dog or cat, or when socially acceptable in man. Male and female ponies can be readily trained by bribery with suitable delicacies to micturate on command, although they tend to be inhibited by strangers and to be generally bashful about performing in public (J.S. King, personal communication, 1997).

In addition to the spinal defecation reflex operated by the pelvic nerve there is also an **intrinsic defecation reflex**. The latter is a function of the enteric nervous system (Section 3.22). When faeces enter the rectum, stretch receptors (Fig. 3.4) reflexly activate enteric ganglion cells to cause peristalsis of the rectum and colon, and relaxation of the internal anal sphincter. The intrinsic defecation reflex is weak, and needs to be reinforced by the parasympathetic defecation reflex.

Fortunately, the basic excitatory arc of the **micturition reflex** is unmistakable – the afferent limb goes into the sacral spinal cord by the **pelvic nerve**, and the efferent parasympathetic limb goes out to the bladder by the same nerve. But almost every other aspect of micturition is more or less controversial. The existence of an internal sphincter of smooth muscle in mammals in general is doubtful (Section 2.17.2). The possible inhibitory effect on micturition of the numerous sympathetic post-ganglionic axons in the **hypogastric nerve** is dubious (Section 2.17.2); indeed these abundant hypogastric axons are looking for a function (Section 4.14).

The transmission of impulses from the sacral spinal cord to the brain, reporting filling of the bladder, is also unassailable, but Brodal (1981, p. 770) concluded that 'the pathways for afferent impulses from the bladder within the central nervous system are incompletely known'. At that time, clinical experience from human **cordotomy** patients seemed have indicated that sensations of fullness of the bladder, giving rise to the desire to micturate, ascend the spinal cord in the same region as the sensation of pain from the bladder and urethra; this region is the superficial ventral part of the *lateral funiculus*, which could be consistent with *spinoreticular* or *spinothalamic pathways*. However, it seems now to be generally agreed that, after ventrolateral cordotomy, patients still retain awareness of the need to micturate, and it is therefore apparent that some of these axons must ascend the cord in the *dorsal funiculus*, in the *gracile fascicle* (Dyson, 1995, p. 1841), inherently improbable though this may seem since the dorsal funiculus is mainly concerned with mechanoreceptor projections from the limbs (Guyton, 1986, p. 583; King, 1987, Sections 7.3, 7.4; Berry *et al.*, 1995, pp. 989, 998). Further evidence for a pathway from the bladder ascending in the dorsal funiculus comes from clinical cases of **tabes dorsalis**, a condition in man in which the spirochaete of syphilis selectively destroys the axons of the dorsal funiculus; this damages the micturition reflex, with resulting incontinence (Ruch, 1974, p. 537). De Lahunta (1983, p. 125) supported the view that the stretch receptor pathway from the bladder ascends to the conscious cortex primarily via the spinothalamic system, but also via the gracile fascicle. However, Berry *et al.* (1995, p. 993) noted that spinoreticular axons are intermingled with those of the spinothalamic tracts, and this would make it virtually impossible to identify this pathway from the bladder as spinothalamic as opposed to spinoreticular. Further light is thrown on the ascending bladder pathways by the *functionally similar* pathways from the *gastrointestinal tract*. Many afferent axons from the gut are carried to the thoracolumbar spinal cord by the **splanchic nerves**; the second order neurons of these pathways are believed to project to the brainstem via the *spinoreticular* and *spinothalamic tracts*, and also by the *dorsal columns* (Mayer, 1994, p. 933).

A particularly searching review of the anatomy and physiology of micturition was made by Ruch (1974, pp. 525–545), himself an active contributor to research in this field. The ascending spinal pathway (or pathways) activate(s) a sequence of at least four control regions in the brain that successively inhibit and excite bladder contraction in alternation. In descending order these are, **cerebral cortex** (inhibitory), **hypothalamus** (excitatory), **midbrain** (inhibitory), and **pons** (excitatory). Also stimulation of the globus pallidus, red nucleus, and substantia nigra inhibits contraction. There is even an excitatory and inhibitory input from the cerebellum, as well as several other brain areas. Ruch (1974, p. 543) marvelled that 'such a simple act as micturition, which can only start, continue, and stop, should have and presumabably require such manifold representations', though he did concede that 'the matter is of considerable importance to the individual'. The trigger of the whole mechanism, which decides when it will operate, is the cerebral cortex.

The multiplicity of the areas of cerebral cortex and brain stem that influence micturition mean that the descending spinal pathways are likely to be complex; not surprisingly, therefore, they are in doubt (Ruch, 1974, p. 542). It has been suggested that the descending pathway mediating the conscious voluntary control of micturition may belong to the corticospinal tract (Brodal, 1981, p. 770). There is evidence that the reticulospinal tracts participate (Ruch, 1974, p. 541). Several descending pathways have been found in the lateral funiculus (Ruch, 1974, Fig. 28-20). Current accounts of human neuroanatomy (e.g. Berry *et al.*, 1995) seem to contain no additional information.

IV PERIPHERAL PARASYMPATHETIC MOTOR DISORDERS

3.15 Cranial parasympathetic outflow disorders

3.15.1 *Oculomotor nerve*

Unilateral interruption of the parasympathetic efferent pathways in the oculomotor nerve causes gross and persistent dilation of the pupil on the affected side, with no response when light is directed into either eye. If the destructive lesion involves the whole of the main trunk of the oculomotor nerve there will also be a somatic efferent deficit in the form of a 'down and out' (lateral and ventral) deviation (**strabismus**) of the affected eye.

> Complete dilation of the pupil is known as **mydriasis**. Asymmetry of the pupils is known as **anisocoria**. See Section 2.29 for sympathetic lesions causing gross constriction of the pupil (**miosis**). An expanding space-occupying lesion such as a neoplasm may directly compress the oculomotor nerve causing mydriasis; the parasympathetic function is usually affected before the somatic efferent function (de Lahunta, 1983, p. 121).

3.15.2 *Facial and glossopharyngeal nerves*

Theoretically, interruption of the parasympathetic efferent pathways in either of these two cranial nerves could cause abnormalities of **salivation**. This can be tested in man by eliciting reflex responses from the salivary glands, but this is not routinely attempted in the neurological examination of domestic mammals. A loss of **lacrimal secretion** through interruption of the parasympathetic pathways of the facial nerve to the lacrimal gland (Section 3.9.1) can be potentially serious, since drying of the cornea can lead to a corneal ulcer. For information on other neurological deficits arising from lesions of the facial and glossopharyngeal nerves see King (1987).

3.15.3 *Vagus nerve*

Interruption of the main trunk of the vagus nerve, immediately distal to the point where it receives its special visceral (branchial) motor component from the **accessory nerve**, paralyses the laryngeal and pharyngeal muscles by eliminating these motor pathways in the **pharyngeal rami** and the **cranial** and **recurrent laryngeal nerves**. It also paralyses the striated muscle in the tunica muscularis of the oesophagus (Section 3.11.2). Serious neurological deficits result, including **dysphagia** (difficulty in swallowing) and obstruction to breathing (**roaring** in horses).

The many **parasympathetic** motor components of the vagus would also be paralysed. However, it is only disorders of the vagal innervation of the gut that are recognizable clinically; furthermore, these are largely concealed by the extraordinary ability of the enteric nervous system to maintain the motility and secretomotor reflexes of the gut after all connections with the central nervous system have been cut (Section 3.20). **Bilateral vagotomy** (strictly vagotomy of the dorsal and ventral vagal trunks) at the level of the terminal oesophagus can be survived by mammals with a simple stomach; in ruminants, however, the integration of the motility of the stomachs is too complex to be managed by the enteric nervous system without vagal control, and total vagotomy is therefore fatal (Section 3.20).

> Clinical signs similar to those resulting from vagotomy are observed in cattle with naturally occurring lesions near the vagal trunks where they pass over the oesophagus or the compartments of the stomachs, and these led to the concept of '**vagus indigestion**'. However, it seems likely that most of such cases involve the enteric nervous system rather than the vagus nerves (Section 3.23.3).

3.16 Sacral outflow disorders

Disorders of micturition and defecation can be predicted from the innervation of the bladder and the colon and rectum (Section 3.14).

3.16.1 *Lesions of spinal cord cranial to the sacral outflow*

Causes include fractured vertebrae, and in the *dog* a severe prolapse of an intervertebral disc especially at T13–L1. These result in loss of voluntary control of micturition and defecation, and therefore **incontinence**. The **bladder** becomes distended, and urine tends to dribble out. After a few days or weeks typical (sacral parasympathetic) micturition reflexes reappear, culminating in **spontaneous micturition**. There may be some retention of faeces in the **rectum**, but the **intrinsic defecation reflex** (Section 3.14) usually still operates giving involuntary evacuation. In *man* a small daily enema is needed to induce adequate defecation.

3.16.2 *Destruction of sacral spinal cord or pelvic nerve*

Causes include fractures at the lumbosacral junction. The **bladder** is distended, and dribbling may be continuous. Eventually reflex micturition may establish itself, but is presumably not neurogenic but myogenic through contraction of the smooth muscle stimulated by stretching; for this to happen, the smooth muscle in the bladder wall must be kept healthy, but even then evacuation is only partial. The **rectum** has the advantage, compared with the bladder, of possessing the enteric nervous system and its intrinsic defecation reflex; in domestic animals this usually maintains evacuation, only occasional enemas being necessary; however, in man large enemas are usually needed. Destruction of the sacral spinal cord paralyses the **pudendal nerve** and relaxes the **external anal sphincter**, but destruction of the pelvic nerve does not.

V   ENTERIC NERVOUS SYSTEM

3.17 Smooth muscle of gut

The principal layer of smooth muscle in the alimentary tract is the **muscular tunic** (tunica muscularis). It extends from the oesophagus to the anal canal; it consists of an outer **longitudinal layer** and an inner **circular layer**, reinforced by oblique layers in the stomach. At the junctions between major segments of the gut the muscle may be rearranged into a distinct anatomical sphincter, though the sphincter properties generally depend on the physiology and innervation of the muscle rather than its anatomical arrangement.

Of crucial importance functionally are structural adaptations on the surfaces of the muscle cells. These consist of (i) **direct attachments** between cells, and (ii) **gap junctions** (**nexi**) with channels allowing exchange of ions and small molecules between the two cells, and thus permitting electrical coupling between the two cells. Mechanical cooperation and electrical communication are achieved by these junctions. *Nexuses are much more abundant in the circular than the longitudinal muscle.*

Two fundamental physiological properties of the enteric nervous system have been proposed. The first is that *the circular muscle functions as an electrical syncitium, from the oesophagus to the internal anal sphincter*. The second is that organized excitation of the electrically coupled circular muscle cells is *initiated myogenically by pacemaker circular muscle cells, and not neuronally* (Section 3.22).

A much thinner layer of smooth muscle cells is formed by the **muscularis mucosa**. This variable structure forms part of the mucous membrane (tunica mucosa) from the beginning of the oesophagus to the anus. When present, it separates the connective tissue of the lamina propria from that of the submucosa. It probably influences the local topography of the mucous membrane, thus varying the calibres of blood vessels and squeezing secretion from glands.

The two fundamental properties of the enteric nervous system just mentioned were put forward by Wood (1987, p. 94), but the concept of the circular muscle as a continuous electrical syncitium from oesophagus to anus may need to be somewhat qualified. There are well-attested reports (Bass *et al.*, 1961) that, immediately peripheral to the pyloric sphincter, a connective tissue septum separates the gastric circular muscle from the duodenal circular muscle. Moreover, Kelly (1981) stated that at this site about three-fourths of the longitudinal muscle turns towards the lumen, into the circular muscle, thus interrupting the circular muscle by a series of septa. Edwards and Rowland (1986) accepted the existence of this break in the continuity of the circular muscle across the pyloric sphincter.

3.18 Nerve plexuses and ganglion cells

The enteric nervous system co-ordinates the processes of gastrointestinal secretion and absorption, independently of the central nervous system.

It lies in the wall of the gut, starting at the point where smooth muscle first appears in the muscle tunic of the oesophagus, and ending in the anal canal (Section 1.3.4).

It consists of two nerve plexuses, the myenteric plexus and the submucosal plexus. Each plexus is composed of dense networks of nerve axons containing enormous numbers of ganglion cells. The **myenteric plexus** (Auerbach's plexus) lies between the longitudinal and circular layers of smooth muscle of the tunica muscularis. The **submucosal plexus** (Meissner's plexus) lies between the tunica muscularis and the muscularis mucosa (i.e. in the **submucosa**). The two plexuses communicate by axons passing through the circular muscle layer.

The plexuses contain afferent neurons, interneurons, and efferent (motor) neurons. The afferent neurons mostly have mechanoreceptor or chemoreceptor endings. The interneurons integrate the afferent information, and control the motor neurons. The motor neurons project to the smooth muscle, glands, and blood vessels in the gut wall. The cell bodies of the afferent neurons, interneurons, and motor neurons tend to be assembled into groups constituting the **enteric ganglia**, the nerve cells being known as **enteric ganglion cells**.

Because these afferent neurons do not have their cell stations in dorsal root ganglia, and do not project to the central nervous system, they do not qualify as **primary afferent neurons** (Sections 1.4, 4.2.3).

The enteric nervous system has its own, entirely independent, capacity for the **integration** of afferent information from the gut into appropriate local secretomotor, muscular motor, and vasomotor reflexes; it can also generate complex stereotyped patterns of activity, such as **segmentation**, **peristalsis**, **retroperistalsis**, and the **intrinsic defecation reflex**. It maintains these reflexes and complex activities after nearly all connections with the central nervous system have been severed (Sections 1.3.4, 3.15.3).

Despite its capacity for independent function, the enteric nervous system is under the overall command of the central nervous system. This control is activated mainly through **parasympathetic** motor projections of the **vagus** and **pelvic nerve** to the enteric ganglia (Section 3.20), and to a much

smaller extent through motor projections of the **sympathetic system** to the enteric ganglia (Section 3.21). Obviously, however, the central nervous system must first receive comprehensive afferent information about what is going on in the gut. This afferent information is transmitted mainly in the vagus nerve, by mechanoreceptor and chemoreceptor axons with their sensory endings in the gastrointestinal tract as far as the transverse colon (Section 4.11); similar afferent information from the descending colon and rectum is transmitted by the **pelvic nerve** (Section 4.14).

The **integration** of the enteric system is believed to have the following anatomical basis (Wood, 1987).

3.18.1 *Sensory receptors*

Mechano-, **chemo-**, and **thermoreceptors** (Section 4.11) continually monitor the state of the gut wall and the contents of the lumen, and project to interneuronal processing centres in the enteric ganglia (Wood, 1987, pp. 67, 93). Other mechano-, chemo-, and thermoreceptors project to the central nervous system mainly by the **vagus** and to a lesser extent by the **pelvic nerve**, in particular to the **nucleus of the solitary tract** and from there to **gastrointestinal 'centres'** in the **reticular formation** of the brainstem. The afferent projections to the central nervous system, particularly the vagal projections, enable the strategic commands from the central nervous system to the enteric system to be modified appropriately in response to changes within the gut lumen. In addition to projections to the central nervous system, substantial numbers of enteric receptor neurons project to the sympathetic **prevertebral ganglia**, wherein a wide range of integrative mechanisms are believed to take place (Section 2.13). For further discussion of the ability of the nervous system to monitor events in the gut, see Sections 4.11 and 4.14.

3.18.2 *Interneuronal circuitry*

The interneuronal circuitry (the 'central computer') is based on synaptic connections between interneurons within the enteric ganglia. Such circuitry *processes* and *integrates* the afferent information, and then *generates commands* to motor neurons in the ganglia. For example, tactile stimulation of the intestinal mucosa induces a relatively simple reflex secretion of mucus and fluid into the lumen (Wood, 1987, p. 93). Alternatively, the interneuronal output can trigger much more complex preprogrammed patterns of stereotyped motor behaviour, such as **segmentation**, **peristalsis**, or **retroperistalsis**, which may then continue automatically without depending on further afferent input (Wood, 1987, p. 98). Sensory input, circulating hormones, and commands from the central nervous system may all contribute to the appropriate selection by the interneuronal circuitry of one or other of the various complex motility patterns (Wood, 1987, p. 98).

Enteric ganglion cells that may be involved in the *integrative functions* of the enteric nervous system are multipolar neurons that are silent, or fire tonically and are then refractory (Weyns, 1988, p. 78). There is evidence that one of the processes of such a multipolar integrative neuron may be utilized to inform the central nervous system of what this cell is doing in the integrative circuitry of the enteric nervous system (Wood, 1987, pp. 95–96). See Section 4.11 for discussion of the several mechanisms by which the nervous system may monitor events taking place in the gut.

3.18.3 *Motor neurons*

Motor neurons in the **enteric ganglia** activate specific effector systems (Wood, 1987, p. 96). Such effector systems include: a *cholinergic excitatory pathway* from the myenteric plexus to the **longitudinal muscle**; an *inhibitory* (probably VIP, rather than ATP) pathway from the myenteric plexus to the **circular muscle** (Section 3.22); and an *excitatory pathway* from neurons in the myenteric plexus to **secretomotor neurons** in the submucosal plexus which innervate the mucosal and submucosal glands (Kirchgessner and Gershon, 1989). By regulating these effector systems the enteric ganglia can make moment-to-moment adjustments of local gastrointestinal activity. Blocks of motor neurons, integrated together, are responsible for triggering preprogrammed patterns of activity such as **segmentation**, etc.

3.19 Embryology of enteric nervous system

The neurons of the enteric nervous system arise from the neural crest of the head and sacral region.

The neurons of the **enteric nervous system** have been attributed to many possible developmental sources, including the gut mesoderm, the endoderm, the neural tube, and the neural crest (Gabella, 1979, pp. 178–181). The more recent experiments, however, have shown that, in the avian embryo, most of the enteric neurons originate from the vagal neural crest with a small additional contribution from the sacral neural crest. These precursor cells migrate into the wall of the gut at an early embryonic stage. In the embryos of some mammalian species there is evidence of a similar dual origin, i.e.

vagal and sacral neural crest, but in others there seems to be no sacral source, and therefore the precursors from the vagal neural crest must then migrate craniocaudally along the entire length of the alimentary tract.

3.20 Relationship of enteric nervous system to parasympathetic motor pathways

The enteric nervous system had long been regarded as no more than an outpost of the parasympathetic nervous system (Section 1.3.4). Its ganglion cells were thought to be parasympathetic postganglionic neurons of the vagus or pelvic nerve, forming the final efferent relay for controlling the secretomotor functions and motility of the gut and its sphincters.

The ability of the enteric system to continue its reflex functions *after all connections with the central nervous system have been cut* cast doubt on this concept. It also became apparent that the number of enteric ganglion cells in the enteric system is immensely greater than the number of preganglionic parasympathetic axons that connect with it. Therefore the notion that the enteric ganglion cells are vagal postganglionic neurons has been abandoned.

Despite the ability of the enteric nervous system to function independently of the central nervous system it does not normally do so. Command signals from the central nervous system are transmitted to the enteric system along parasympathetic (and, less importantly, sympathetic) motor pathways.

The **parasympathetic pathways** are mainly **preganglionic axons** in the **vagus** (Sections 3.11.1, 3.11.5, 3.11.7); their function is to stimulate gastrointestinal motility and secretion, and the opening of gut sphincters. This they do by making synapses with enteric ganglion cells in the myenteric plexus. At first sight, such enteric ganglion cells may therefore appear to be postganglionic vagal neurons, but they are anatomically indistinguishable from the vast numbers of other enteric ganglion cells in the myenteric plexus that do **not** receive synapses from vagal preganglionic axons. This fact, together with the proven ability of the enteric system to function after all connections with the vagus have been cut, has destroyed the classic concept of the preganglionic–postganglionic relay in vagal motor pathways to the gut (Section 3.4.1). Instead, an individual vagal preganglionic fibre to the gut is now regarded as synapsing with a single **command neuron** in the enteric nervous system that activates and integrates a **subset** of neural circuits in the enteric nervous system. Such subsets are preprogrammed to carry out complex motor functions such as **segmentation**, **peristalsis**, and **retroperistalsis**.

There is also a **sacral parasympathetic motor pathway** to the gut in the **pelvic nerve** via the **pelvic plexus** (Section 3.12). Like the vagal projections to the gut that have just been described, an individual sacral parasympathetic axon typically ends on an enteric ganglion cell. Its function is to reinforce mass contraction of the descending colon and rectum during **defecation** (Section 3.14).

Unlike the vagal parasympathetic pathways to the gut (Sections 3.11.1, 3.11.5, 3.11.7), the **sacral parasympathetic efferent axons** in the pelvic nerve and pelvic plexus that enter the gut wall include both *preganglionic* and *postganglionic axons*. Thus some of the preganglionic axons in the pelvic nerve synapse with postganglionic nerve cell bodies in the **pelvic ganglia**; the postganglionic fibre enters the gut wall and ends by making a synapse with an enteric ganglion cell (Fig. 3.4). Other preganglionic axons in the pelvic nerve continue directly into the wall of the gut, and end by making a synapse with an enteric ganglion cell (Fig. 3.4).

The relationship between the parasympathetic and enteric nervous systems can be summarized as follows. The central nervous system delivers **strategic** commands to the enteric system, via the **vagus** and **pelvic nerves**. As stated in Section 3.18, these strategic commands are activated by afferent information reaching the brain from the gut through mechano- and chemoreceptors of the vagus and pelvic nerves. Thus central control determines the *general strategy* of gut motility and secretion, and the opening of sphincters. But the enteric system carries out its local, i.e. *tactical*, responses to these commands as a totally independent system.

There seems to be only one gut function that cannot be managed by the enteric nervous system without the participation of the central nervous system, and that is the integrated function of the compartments of the **complex stomach of rumi-nants**. Total **vagotomy** so dislocates the elaborate reflexes of these compartments that the animal dies within a month. **Defecation** is also somewhat precarious without control by the central nervous system (Section 3.16.2).

The **vagus** of man at the level of the diaphragm contains less than 2000 efferent axons, but it has been estimated that the small intestine of the cat contains about 100 million enteric ganglion cells (Wood, 1987, p. 103). It is inconceivable that so few platoons of vagal preganglionic axons could make synapses with such an army of enteric ganglion cells.

The available evidence indicates that the preganglionic axons of the vagus reach the **myenteric plexus**, but not the **submucosal plexus** (Kirchgessner and Gershon, 1989); in the myenteric plexus, they are more numerous in the stomach than in the small intestine, declining sharply and progressively distally, and ending caudally at the ileocolic junction in the rat (Kirchgessner and Gershon, 1989) and at the rectum in the cat (Wood, 1987, p. 103). In the myenteric plexus they innervate ganglion cells, but the proportion of ganglion cells so innervated is extremely low, i.e. as already stated vast numbers of enteric ganglion cells have no parasympathetic (or sympathetic) innervation. Vagal axons can reach the caudal end of the small intestine by passing longitudinally through the myenteric plexus without interruption, as well as by using the more obvious route from the **dorsal vagal trunk** and **coeliacomesenteric plexus** (Section 3.11.6).

The functional organization of the **enteric ganglion cells** with which preganglionic **vagal axons** synapse is not known (Wood, 1987, p. 67). However, it has been postulated (Wood, 1987, pp. 98, 103) that command signals from the brain are transmitted along vagal axons to interneuronal circuitry in the enteric nervous system; perhaps, in the ideal concept, the command signals may be transmitted to single 'command neurons' in the enteric system. The relevant internuncial circuitry, or the single command neurons if such exist, activates a block or **subset of neural circuits** in the enteric system that is preprogrammed to carry out a complex stereotyped sequence of motor events such as *peristalsis* or *segmentation*, etc. The resulting motor events can continue automatically without sensory input, but can also be modulated by sensory input. Furthermore, it is likely that the subsets of neural circuits are interconnected in order to achieve optimal performance of the gut as a whole (Wood, 1987, p. 67). This model explains the powerful influence of the relatively minuscule number of vagal axons on motility and secretion over such vast lengths of the alimentary tract (Wood, 1987, p. 103).

The capacity of the enteric ganglia to *process information* and *integrate* complex patterns of motor activity far exceeds that of any other autonomic ganglia and is indeed even 'brain-like' in its characteristics (Wood,

1987, p. 69). Perhaps this should not be too surprising, since the *number of neurons in the enteric system is estimated to be about the same as the number of neurons in the spinal cord* (Wood, 1987, p. 68). It was pointed out by Wood (1987, p. 68) that a striking example of the *integrating* capacity of the enteric system is the ability of **raptor birds** to swallow a mouse, add gastric juices, crush and grind the victim's body in the stomachs, empty the liquid content into the duodenum by peristalsis, form the bones and hair into a pellet, and eject the pellet by retroperistalsis. The manoeuvres of the complex compartments of the **ruminant stomach** are even more sophisticated, requiring coordination of the ruminoreticular contraction cycle, the omasal cycle transporting ingesta from reticulum to abomasum, regurgitation during rumination, eructation, closure of the reticular groove in suckling, and abomasal motility and secretion. However, it is beyond the powers of the enteric system to sustain unaided all these elaborate and interrelated motility patterns shown by the compartments of the ruminant stomach. Command signals from the vagus are found to be essential, since **vagotomy** of the dorsal and ventral vagal trunks on the terminal oesophagus is fatal within a month. The abomasum continues to empty, but ruminal and reticular activities cease; however, a ruminant animal can survive section of either the *dorsal* or the *ventral* trunk *alone*, indicating the remarkable powers of **integration** possessed by the enteric system (de Lahunta and Habel, 1986, p. 239). In mammals with a simple stomach, bilateral **vagotomy** at the end of the oesophagus is not fatal, and has even been used to treat peptic ulcers in man, though it causes a distressing reduction of gastric motility (Guyton, 1986, p. 801); nevertheless, gastric secretion and peristalsis eventually return (Crosby *et al.*, 1962, p. 536).

It has recently been shown that a major population of neurons in the enteric nervous system uses nitric oxide as the main nonadrenergic, noncholinergic transmitter substance (Section 2.34).

3.21   Relationship of enteric nervous system to sympathetic motor pathways

The **sympathetic pathways** to the enteric system are postganglionic axons from the **coeliacomesenteric ganglion** and **caudal mesenteric ganglion**. They inhibit enteric ganglion cells, thus shutting down gastrointestinal blood flow and motility as in **fight and flight**.

Several lines of structural and functional evidence all indicate that the vast majority of **sympathetic** postganglionic axons to the gut make synapses directly with enteric ganglion cells (Jänig and McLachlan, 1987, p. 135; Wood, 1987, p. 103) (Section 2.14.2). At these synapses they release noradrenaline which acts presynaptically to suppress cholinergic and perhaps serotonergic synaptic transmission between myenteric neurons. Thus the sympathetic system shuts down gut activity by preventing the release of excitatory transmitter substances within the interneuronal circuits of the enteric nervous system (Wood, 1987, p. 103).

3.22   Innervation of longitudinal and circular smooth muscle of gut

The **longitudinal muscle** contracts only when it is stimulated by cholinergic enteric ganglion cells in the myenteric plexus. Neuronal tone, perhaps parasympathetic tone (Section 3.2), presumably maintains a modest degree of contraction all the time, but basically the muscle is relaxed.

The **circular muscle** operates in an entirely different manner. It is excited **myogenically**, not neuronally. The source of this excitation is 'pacemaker muscle cells' in the circular muscle, these being continually active. Therefore (in the absence of appropriate innervation) the circular muscle would be *continually contracted*, and this would cause intestinal obstruction; moreover, because the circular muscle functions as an electrical syncitium (Section 3.17) such obstruction could be widespread. In fact, the muscle does have a nerve supply: common sense suggests that it should be **inhibitory**, and indeed it is (Fig. 3.4). At rest, these inhibitory neurons, which lie in the ganglia of the myenteric plexus, are **tonically active**; consequently, at rest, the circular muscle is continually relaxed. But, during segmentation or peristalsis, the circular muscle must be allowed to contract. For this to happen, the inhibitory ganglion cell that silences the circular muscle must itself be inhibited. Therefore the enteric ganglia contain **inhibitory ganglion cells** that synapse with the inhibitory neurons (Fig. 3.4). Inhibition of the inhibitory neuron releases the circular muscle, and allows it to respond to the excitatory myogenic stimulus.

In the central nervous system, inhibition of an inhibitory control mechanism, allowing an excitatory influence to dominate, is known as **disinhibition** (see King, 1987) and this term is also used for the control mechanism of the circular muscle. This elaborate mechanism of (i) a basic **myogenic** drive, (ii) an **inhibitory neuron** restraining this drive, and (iii) a **disinhibitory neuron** allowing the muscle to respond to the myogenic drive, seems vulnerable to functional disorders (Section 3.23).

Readers encountering the myenteric neuronal control of the **smooth muscle of the gut wall** for the first time will have noticed that the **longitudinal muscle** has the standard **control mechanism**, i.e. its contraction is *directly initiated* by **cholinergic neurons**. In marked contrast, the **control mechanism** of the **circular muscle** is unusual and complex, but the way to understand it is to *begin with the continuous myogenic drive*. Because of its numerous gap junctions, the circular muscle functions as an electrical syncitium. Consequently the continuous myogenic drive would constrict the entire length of the gut, and bring movement of ingesta to a standstill. To prevent this from happening, the circular smooth muscle must be controlled by tonically acting *inhibitory motor neurons*. But tonic inhibition would paralyse the gut, and this too would bring the movement of the ingesta to a standstill. To overcome this difficulty, *disinhibitory motor neurons* are required to inhibit the inhibitory neurons, and thus allow the circular muscle to contract under the influence of the myogenic drive. Integration by the neuronal circuitry of the myenteric plexus regulates the disinhibition so as to allow **waves** of contraction to pass along the gut (**peristalsis**), or **localized** concentric contractions to occur (**segmentation**).

The myogenic drive on the circular muscle can also be harnessed to operate the **sphincters of the gut**. This mechanism requires a different relationship between inhibitory neuron and circular smooth muscle, compared with the rest of the gut. The first design requirement of a gut sphincter is that it should be able to remain *continuously closed* by continuous contraction of its circular muscle. This is achieved by the tonic myogenic drive. The other design requirement of a sphincter is obviously that it should be *able to open* when this is physiologically advantageous. When the sphincter is to be opened, the inhibitory neuron becomes active and the circular muscle therefore relaxes. The inhibitory neuron can be activated (in order to open the sphincter) by an excitatory preganglionic fibre of the vagus or pelvic nerve

(Fig. 3.4), thus allowing the sphincter to be controlled by autonomic nuclei in the brain stem or (as in the case of the internal anal sphincter) by the conscious activity of the cerebral cortex. The inhibitory neuron can also be activated by the enteric ganglia. In this instance the activation would be by a local reflex starting from a stretch receptor neuron with its afferent endings in the wall of the gut in the immediate vicinity of the sphincter (Fig. 3.4); this is the basis of the **intrinsic defecation reflex** (Section 3.14).

The contraction of the **longitudinal muscle** in the gut wall appears to be initiated solely by acetylcholine released from motor neurons of the ganglia of the myenteric plexus, acting via muscarinic receptors (Wood, 1987, pp. 94, 96). Thus strips of longitudinal muscle devoid of the myenteric plexus cannot be activated by electrical stimulation. The longitudinal muscle evidently receives no inhibitory innervation.

The responsiveness of the **circular muscle** to the pacemaker cells is controlled by the **inhibitory** motor neurons in the enteric ganglia of the myenteric plexus; the **inhibitory transmitter substance** of these inhibitory motor neurons is **VIP** (rather than ATP, as first supposed), VIP being one of the few neuropeptides that hyperpolarize and therefore relax intestinal smooth muscle (Wood, 1987, p. 96). Contraction of the circular muscle must be initiated by an inhibitory neuron that inhibits the tonically active peptidergic (VIP) inhibitory neurons (i.e. by disinhibition). The first neuron in the disinhibitory chain is a **cholinergic neuron**, which inhibits the second neuron via **nicotinic receptors**. The presence of nicotinic receptors in these particular enteric ganglion cells is consistent with nicotinic receptors in parasympathetic ganglia (Section 3.7).

Inhibitory (VIP) neurons in the myenteric ganglia have the additional function of mediating the action of the **vagus** and **pelvic nerve** in *opening* the **sphincters** of the gut (Wood, 1987, p. 97). In such a pathway, a preganglionic parasympathetic fibre of the vagus or pelvic nerve activates an excitatory motor neuron in the myenteric plexus; this neuron excites an inhibitory motor neuron (Fig. 3.4), which inhibits the circular muscle in the sphincter and thus allows the sphincter to relax. But this mechanism requires (i) the circular muscle in the sphincter to be tonically active, and (ii) the inhibitory motor neurons in the ganglia to be normally silent at rest; this is the direct opposite to the mechanism that operates in the circular muscle other than in the sphincters, where (i) the inhibitory neuron is tonically active, and (ii) the circular muscle is normally inhibited at rest. The ganglia in the myenteric plexus can also reflexly open a sphincter without parasympathetic intervention, in response to stimulation by stretch receptors in the gut wall (Wood, 1987, p. 97). This reflex arc again requires two motor neurons in series, the first being an excitatory interneuron (acting by nicotinic cholinergic or perhaps serotonergic receptors), and the second being a normally silent inhibitory neuron which releases VIP to inhibit the tonically active sphincter muscle.

The relative importance of neuronal and myogenic control mechanisms in the **muscularis mucosa** remains to be established (Gabella, 1987, p. 361).

3.23   Disorders of enteric nervous system

The peculiar mode of operation of the circular muscle, with its myogenic drive and its inhibitory and disinhibitory neurons (Section 3.22), appears to be vulnerable to malfunction. Its disorders are of two types, loss of the inhibitory control and loss of the disinhibitory control. The first of these results in **spasm** of the circular muscle, and the second in **loss of motility** of the circular muscle known as **ileus**. Both of these conditions can produce a life-threatening interruption of gastrointestinal activity.

3.23.1   *Spasm*

The inhibitory neurons in the myenteric plexus of a segment of intestine stop working. This allows the myogenic pacemakers to trigger a maximum contractile response of the circular muscle, which spreads within the electrical syncitium. The affected segment behaves like a sphincter with no capacity for relaxation. The region immediately proximal to the constriction becomes dilated, leading for example to **megaoesophagus** or **megacolon**.

The segment affected by spasm may be at the junction between two major components of the gut and is then known as **achalasia**, meaning failure to relax (Blood and Studdert, 1988) (Greek: apo, absence of; chalasao, I loosen). In **oesophageal achalasia** the distal end of the oesophagus and the cardiac sphincter in animals with a simple stomach are in spasm, causing distension of the oesophagus (**megaoesophagus**). In **pyloric achalasia** the spasm is at the pylorus. In **aganglionic megacolon** the spasm occurs in the distal colon. A well known example of the latter is Hirschsprung's disease in *man* and piebald *mice* in which the inhibitory neurons are congenitally absent from the rectum. Similar forms of congenital megacolon occur in the *horse, dog*, and *cat*. In *ruminants*, **achalasia of the reticulo-omasal sphincter** and **pyloric achalasia** can be a factor in **vagus indigestion**. Although several of these conditions can be congenital, they can

also arise from inflammatory destruction of myenteric neurons (Wood, 1987, p. 100).

3.23.2   *Ileus*

Ileus is the opposite to spasm. There is no motor activity in the intestine, and therefore there is no peristalsis. The effect is the same as that of acute intestinal obstruction. The immediate cause is continuous activity of the inhibitory neurons in the ganglia of the myenteric plexus (i.e. the terminal neurons that inhibit the circular muscle fibres and thus prevent the muscle fibres from responding to the myogenic drive). But the indirect cause is presumably failure of the **disinhibitory neuron** (which, in normal circumstances, allows the muscle to respond to the myogenic drive).

Ileus can be caused by an array of abdominal disasters, including acute peritonitis, severe abdominal trauma, excessive handling of the gut during surgery, or acute inflammation of the kidney or urinary bladder. In *horses* it can be a major postoperative problem after surgery for colic.

The **gut paralysis** that occurs in **ileus** reflects a *continuous activity* of the *inhibitory neurons* in the myenteric circuitry that inhibits the circular muscle fibres (Wood, 1987, p. 100). It is possible that *sympathetic reflex activity* may sometimes be involved in causing ileus (Guyton, 1986, p. 769; Wood, 1987, p.100). The afferent pathway of such reflexes is by *nociceptors* (Section 4.4.5) projecting, for example, from the visceral peritoneum to the prevertebral sympathetic ganglia or to the spinal cord, with efferent noradrenergic projections via the sympathetic ganglia to the gut. Similar nociceptor reflexes projecting from the kidney or bladder may explain ileus in acute inflammation of the urinary system. Noradrenaline suppresses cholinergic and perhaps serotonergic synaptic transmission within the interneuronal circuits of the enteric system, by acting presynaptically (Section 3.21); this may inactivate the cholinergic (nicotinic) neurons that inhibit the inhibitory (VIP) neurons of the circular muscle. If so, cholinergic or serotonergic agonists might offer some relief to clinical cases of ileus. Alternatively pharmacological agents that stimulate the release of serotonin may help, and empirical observations on equine postoperative ileus encourage this view.

3.23.3   *Vagus indigestion in cattle*

The fatal results of cutting the **dorsal** and **ventral vagal trunks** immediately cranial to the diaphragm in cattle have been mentioned (Section 3.15.3). Ruminoreticular and omasal activity cease, though the abomasum empties slowly. If the dorsal and ventral vagal trunks are cut immediately distal to the origin of the nerves to the rumen, the ruminoreticulum continues to contract but the animal dies from omasal atony. Clinical signs similar to these are seen in clinical conditions (notably traumatic reticuloperitonitis resulting from penetrating foreign bodies) involving peritonitis or abscesses near the dorsal and ventral vagal trunks. These observations led to the concept of 'vagus indigestion', the term suggesting an essentially **vagal** cause. However, it seems more likely that the disorder arises mainly in the **enteric** nervous system rather than in the vagus, and that these are examples of spasm or ileus precipitated by peritonitis or trauma.

> In a survey of **vagus indigestion** de Lahunta and Habel (1986, p. 239) pointed out that the vagal-enteric pathways are vulnerable at all levels, i.e. mucosal and submucosal receptors, afferent projections up the vagus, centres in the brain stem, efferent projections down the vagus, and the neuronal circuitry of the enteric nervous system. Only rarely have specific lesions such as abscesses been correlated post mortem with significant degeneration of vagal nerve axons, and many cases show no lesion involving a vagal trunk.
>
> Disorders of the myenteric nervous system appear sometimes to affect the **abomasum** alone, without any evidence of traumatic peritonitis. An example is right-sided dilation of the abomasum in adult dairy cows soon after calving (Buchanan *et al.*, 1991). The aetiology is not clear, but the condition may result from spasm of the pylorus or from primary atony of the abomasal musculature, the latter being regarded as the more likely cause.

3.24 Regeneration of enteric nervous system

The treatment of gastrointestinal disorders often involves the total transection and subsequent reattachment of parts of the alimentary tract. Although inevitably damaged by such necessary procedures, the enteric nervous system recovers functionally.

> Surgical transection followed by end-to-end anastomosis induces degenerative changes and neuron loss in the enteric nervous system, but subsequent regeneration

leads to almost complete functional recovery (Karaosmanoglu *et al.*, 1996).

A final tribute to the enteric nervous system

The following note appeared in the Introduction of a report on haemorrhoidectomy written by W.C. Bornemeier and was published in the *American Journal of Proctology*, February 1960. With thanks to the author for permission to publish.

'The prime objective of a hemorrhoidectomy is to remove the offending varicosity with as little damage as possible to the patient. Of all the structures in the area, one stands out as the king. You can damage, deform, ruin, abuse, amputate, maim, or mutilate every structure in and around the anus except one. That structure is the sphincter ani. There is not a muscle or structure in the body that has a more keenly developed sense of alertness and ability to accommodate itself to varying situations. It is like the goalie in hockey – always alert.

'They say man has succeeded where the animals fail because of the clever use of his hands yet, when compared to the hands, the sphincter ani is far superior. If you place into your cupped hands a mixture of fluid, solid, and gas and then, through an opening at the bottom, try to let only the gas escape, you will fail. Yet the sphincter ani can do it. The sphincter apparently can differentiate between solid, fluid, and gas. It can apparently tell whether its owner is alone or with someone, whether standing up or sitting down, whether its owner has his pants on or off. No other muscle in the body is such a protector of the dignity of man, yet so ready to come to his relief. A muscle like this is worth protecting.'

Although conceived in praise of the richly deserving anal sphincter, the hidden hero is really the enteric nervous system – which tells the sphincter how to do it.

Chapter 4
Afferent Pathways in the Autonomic Nervous System

I GENERAL ORGANIZATION OF AUTONOMIC AFFERENT PATHWAYS

4.1 The existence of autonomic afferent neurons

Like all other parts of the nervous system, the autonomic nervous system is based on reflex arcs, and it is now generally accepted that it includes the *afferent components* of such arcs (Section 1.4). In many autonomic nerves, the afferent axons outnumber the efferent; the vagus nerve, for instance, is about 90% afferent at the level of the diaphragm. There are also very large numbers of afferent axons in sympathetic nerves such as the splanchnic nerves.

> The physiological characteristics of autonomic afferent axons have been exhaustively studied electrophysiologically by recording the impulses travelling towards the central nervous system. This began with an investigation by Adrian in 1933 of pulmonary inflation receptors signalling through afferent axons in the vagus nerve, and since then has been extended to single axon recordings of many cervical, thoracic, abdominal, and pelvic afferent autonomic pathways (Iggo, 1966, p. 122).
>
> Attempts to find the actual receptor endings of afferent autonomic axons by light and electron microscopy were for a long time inconclusive. However, technical advances such as anterograde neural tracing techniques combined with confocal microscopy have now made it possible to identify some structural details of vagal gastrointestinal afferent endings (Mayer, 1994, p. 930) (Section 4.11.1).
>
> The total number of afferent axons in the abdominal vagus is about 15 000, and a similar number occurs in the thoracic splanchnic nerves (Mayer, 1994, pp. 930, 933).

4.2 General functional characteristics of autonomic afferent axons

4.2.1 Non-pain autonomic afferent axons

Large numbers of afferent autonomic axons are present in both parasympathetic and sympathetic peripheral nerves. **In general**, those in the **parasympathetic nerves** are concerned with all visceral functions *except pain*, and serve most visceral reflexes. The great majority of such non-pain afferents are more or less continuously involved in intensive **mechanoreceptor** or **chemoreceptor activities**, which monitor organ conditions in minute detail and induce the visceral reflexes needed to maintain **homeostasis** of the internal environment (Section 1.3.2). **Thermoreceptor** activities also occur in some organs. Very few of these myriads of afferent signals ever reach conscious levels of perception, but some do induce general visceral sensations such as *hunger, nausea,* the feeling of *fullness* of the stomach, rectum, and bladder, and the sensations that occur during *micturition* and *defecation*.

4.2.2 Pain autonomic afferent axons

In complete contrast, the main function of the afferent axons in **sympathetic nerves** is to transmit the sensation of **visceral pain** from the thoracic and abdominal organs.

The general rule is that parasympathetic pathways are *not* responsible for the transmission of visceral pain, but there are three exceptions: (1) the **pelvic nerve** (Section 3.12) carries pain pathways from the **pelvic viscera**; (2) the **vagus nerve** transmits pain sensations from the **respiratory tract** and **oesophagus**; and (3) the

glossopharyngeal nerve mediates pain pathways from the pharynx. Furthermore, some thoracic and abdominal organs receive a **somatic innervation** from the body wall (Section 4.9).

There is a striking difference in the activity of pain and non-pain pathways from the viscera. The non-pain pathways are *continuously active*, but *hardly any of their signals reach consciousness under physiological conditions*: the pain pathways are *completely silent for long periods*, but when activated by mucosal irritation *their signals can reach consciousness all too clearly*.

4.2.3 *Autonomic primary afferent neurons: cell stations*

Typical autonomic afferent neurons are **primary afferent neurons** (Section 1.4). They therefore have their cell stations in one of two possible sites: either (1) in the **afferent** (i.e. sensory) **ganglion** on the *root* of a parasympathetic *cranial nerve*, for example the vagus; or (2) in a **dorsal root ganglion** of a *spinal nerve*. It will be recalled that these two types of ganglia are homologues, and that their nerve cells are pseudounipolar neurons (Section 1.4). These neurons send their centrally continuing axons directly into the neuraxis (Section 1.4).

Non-pain autonomic primary afferent axons in the head travel in *cranial nerves*, i.e. the **facial**, **glossopharyngeal**, and **vagus nerves**. They therefore have their cell stations in the homologous 'dorsal root ganglia' of these three cranial nerves, i.e. the **geniculate ganglion** (of the facial nerve (Fig. 3.2) so called because it occurs on the knee-like bend of the facial nerve), the **distal glossopharyngeal ganglion** (Fig. 4.3), and the **distal vagal ganglion** (Fig. 3.3).

Pain autonomic primary afferent axons arising from thoracic and abdominal viscera travel in *peripheral sympathetic nerves* such as the **cardiac nerves** and **splanchnic nerves**. They therefore have their cell stations in the dorsal root ganglia of thoracolumbar spinal nerves.

Autonomic primary afferent axons arising from the **pelvic viscera**, whether **non-pain** or **pain** in function, travel in sacral peripheral nerves and therefore have their cell stations in the dorsal root ganglia of sacral spinal nerves.

4.2.4 *Autonomic primary afferent neurons: central projections*

The **non-pain**, autonomic primary afferent pathways in *cranial nerves* (notably the vagus nerve) project into the **nucleus of the solitary tract** (Section 11.7), as in Fig. 3.3.

The **pain**, autonomic primary afferent neurons with their cell bodies in the dorsal root ganglia of thoracolumbar spinal nerves (see Section 4.2.3) project into the **spinoreticular** or **spinothalamic tracts** of the spinal cord.

These two great pathways (1, the cranial nerves and the nucleus of solitary tract; and 2, the spinoreticular and spinothalamic tracts) distribute to the brain *nearly all* of the incoming information carried by both *pain* and *non-pain* autonomic afferents from the viscera.

Non-pain afferent information transmitted through the nucleus of the solitary tract is further projected to the **autonomic centres** in the hindbrain and **limbic system** (Section 1.5), and sometimes also to the **conscious cerebral cortex** (e.g. the sense of fullness of the stomach, pleasant or unpleasant).

Pain afferent information in the spinoreticular and spinothalamic tracts is projected to the thalamus (via the spino*thalamic* tract), and from there to the **conscious cortex**.

The afferent neurons in the **enteric nervous system** are not primary afferent neurons (Section 1.4). They have their cell stations in the **enteric ganglia** in the gut wall, as in Fig. 3.4, and do **not** project directly into the neuraxis.

There is electrophysiological evidence (Mayer, 1994, p. 933) for significant convergence and reciprocal interactions in the brainstem, midbrain, and hypothalamus, between vagal afferents and the spinothalamic and spinoreticular afferent pathways from the abdominal viscera. Many of the spinothalamic and spinoreticular afferent pathways arise from **mucosal receptors** in the gastro-intestinal tract (Section 4.5), and are conveyed to the spinal nerves via the splanchnic nerves (Section 2.12); the main function of these pathways seems to be to act as **nociceptors** (pain receptors), but they only do this when the mucosa is irritated (hence the term 'sleeping nociceptors'). They also function as rapidly adapting **mechanoreceptors**, being extremely sensitive to light stroking, though not responsive to distension, contraction, or compression. They appear to contribute to the reflex control of gastric emptying, even in the absence of noxious stimuli. (See Section 4.4.5 for the polymodal characteristics of these receptors.)

However, the exact spinal pathways by which afferent axons from the abdominal and pelvic viscera reach the brainstem are not completely established. Although it is believed that gastrointestinal afferents in the splanchnic nerves project their second order neurons to the brain stem via the spinoreticular and spinothalamic tracts, there is also evidence that some of them project through the dorsal columns (Mayer, 1994, p. 933). Clinical observations indicate that at least some of the afferent pathways conveying the sense of fullness of the bladder also project through the dorsal column (Section 3.14).

Autonomic reflexes are not initiated solely by autonomic afferent pathways (Williams *et al.*, 1989, p. 1168). Some sympathetic reflexes are induced by the special senses or by stimulation of somatic receptors, especially in the skin. For example, painful stimulation of the skin can cause a reflex rise in arterial pressure and dilation of the pupil. See also the hypothetical reflex arc in Fig. 2.3. Conversely, autonomic afferent pathways can evoke a somatic motor reflex response. For instance, painful stimuli of some (though not all) hollow organs in the abdomen can reflexly induce a marked protective rigidity of the abdominal wall by contraction of the rectus abdominus muscle (Ruch, 1966, p. 359; Williams *et al.*, 1989, p. 1168).

4.3 Non-pain autonomic afferent pathways in parasympathetic nerves

The parasympathetic nerves that carry **non-pain** afferent autonomic axons from the viscera are the **facial nerve**, **glossopharyngeal nerve**, **vagus nerve**, and **pelvic nerve** (Fig. 4.1). These autonomic afferent axons are primary afferent neurons. As stated in Section 4.2, the cell stations of the axons of these three cranial nerves are respectively in the **geniculate**, **distal glossopharyngeal**, and **distal vagal ganglia**. They then project into the **nucleus of the solitary tract**, and from there to the autonomic centres in the hindbrain (e.g. gastrointestinal, respiratory, and cardiovascular centres), and thence to the higher centres of the limbic system.

4.3.1 Facial nerve

The facial nerve (Section 3.9) conveys autonomic afferent axons from taste buds (on the rostral two thirds) of the tongue (Fig. 4.1). The pathway is in the **chorda tympani**, with the cell station in the **geniculate ganglion** (Section 4.10.2).

4.3.2 Glossopharyngeal nerve

The glossopharyngeal nerve (Section 3.10) carries taste afferent and general autonomic afferent pathways (Fig. 4.1) from the tongue (the caudal third) by its **lingual rami** (Fig. 4.3). General autonomic afferents are conveyed from the pharynx by its **pharyngeal ramus** (Fig. 4.3) (Sections 4.10.1, 4.10.2). Arterial baro- and chemoreceptor axons are carried from the carotid sinus and carotid body via the **carotid sinus nerve** (Fig. 4.3) (Section

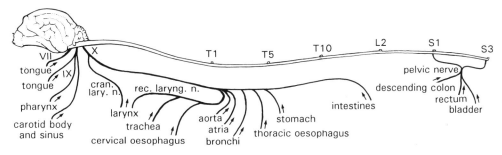

Fig. 4.1 Diagram summarizing the principal non-pain autonomic afferent pathways in parasympathetic nerves. The facial nerve (VII) carries taste afferents from the tongue (rostral two thirds) in the chorda tympani. The glossopharyngeal nerve (IX) conveys taste afferents and general autonomic afferents from the tongue (caudal third) in its lingual rami, general autonomic afferents from the pharynx in its pharyngeal ramus, and baro- and chemoreceptor afferents in the carotid sinus nerve. The vagus (X) nerve conducts autonomic afferent fibres of many functional types from the respiratory tract, the heart and its great arteries, and the alimentary tract as far as the descending colon. The pelvic nerve carries all autonomic afferent pathways (pain as well as non-pain) from the pelvic part of the descending colon, from the rectum and bladder, and from all other pelvic viscera except the vagina.

4.17). The cell stations of all these various types of afferent pathways are in the distal glossopharyngeal ganglion. Central projections go to the nucleus of the solitary tract (labelled AA, for 'autonomic afferent', in Fig. 4.3).

4.3.3   *Vagus nerve*

The vagus nerve (Section 3.11) is responsible for the autonomic afferent innervation of the *respiratory tract*, the *heart* and its *great arteries*, and of the *alimentary tract* starting at the oesophagus and ending approximately at the descending colon (Fig. 4.1). The **cranial laryngeal nerve** is the main afferent nerve of the *larynx* (Section 4.15). The **recurrent laryngeal nerve** supplies autonomic afferent axons to the *trachea* and the *cervical oesophagus*, by its **tracheal** and **oesophageal rami** (Figs 3.3, 4.1). The *thoracic* and *abdominal oesophagus* are innervated by the **dorsal** and **ventral trunks** of the vagus, via its **oesophageal rami** (Sections 3.11.2, 4.10). The *stomach* (Section 4.11) sends its afferent axons through the vagal **gastric rami** (Section 3.11.5). The *intestines* as far down as the descending colon (Section 4.11) send their afferent vagal axons through the great plexuses of the abdomen (Section 3.11.1), e.g. the **coeliacomesenteric plexus**. Afferent autonomic axons from the *lung* (Section 4.16) ascend the bronchial tree and join the vagus by means of its **bronchial rami** (Section 3.11.4). The aortic *baro-* and *chemoreceptor axons* (Section 4.17) travel through an independent branch of the vagus (the **aortic nerve**), or in the main trunk of the vagus. *Atrial volume receptors* (Section 4.18.1) project into the **vagus** via its **cardiac rami** (Section 3.11.3).

All of these afferent axons have their cell stations in the **distal vagal ganglion**. Central projections are to the **nucleus of the solitary tract**.

4.3.4   *Pelvic nerve*

The pelvic nerve (Section 3.12) transmits autonomic afferent pathways, pain (Section 4.8.3) as well as non-pain (Section 4.14), from the **pelvic viscera** and (probably) from the pelvic part of the **descending colon** (Fig. 4.1). The cell stations of all these axons are in the dorsal root ganglia of sacral spinal nerves. Both pain pathways, and non-pain pathways signalling fullness of the bladder and rectum, project through ascending tracts in the spinal cord to the hindbrain, and thence to the conscious cerebral cortex, thus enabling **micturition** and **defecation** to be consciously controlled. (See Section 3.14 for further discussion of these pathways.)

4.4   Visceral pain

The viscera are not normally exposed to the all too frequent stimuli that excite cutaneous pain receptors, and therefore have not evolved similar sensitivity. Surgeons performing abdominal operations such as **rumenotomy** under nothing more than local anaesthesia of the body wall can handle and cut, and even crush and burn, the abdominal organs without causing any sensation; biopsy excisions and cautery of the human cervix uteri are held not to cause pain. But *stretching* of the rumen or cervix is painful. Evidently the viscera have evolved pain sensitivity appropriate to their own environment. Visceral pain can be fiercely intense, as in a horse with acute colic.

4.4.1   *The adequate stimuli for visceral pain*

The basic adequate stimuli for the conscious perception of pain from viscera are: (1) *sudden and severe distension* of a hollow organ; (2) *excessive tension in smooth muscle*, as in violent contraction (spasm) of the smooth muscle in the wall of a hollow organ, often experienced as rhythmical surges of cramping pain as in diarrhoea or menstruation; (3) *ischaemia* (inadequate blood supply); (4) *stretching of mesentery*; and (5) *chemical irritants*.

Combinations of these basic stimuli can occur. For example, violent contraction of a hollow organ may obstruct the blood flow, and the resulting ischaemia may strongly augment the pain. The area of stimulated tissue is significant. For instance, mechanical stimulation (handling) of a small area may be painless, but can become painful if spread over a broad area; an escape of proteolytic acid gastric juice through a perforated gastric or duodenal ulcer can damage a broad area of visceral peritoneum, leading to extremely severe pain. A concurrent **inflammation** can markedly lower the threshold of pain axons, so that a stimulus such as distension that would otherwise be imperceptible becomes acutely painful.

> The accumulation of lactic acid from anaerobic metabolism could account for the pain of **ischaemia**. Products of cell injury such as *bradykinin, histamine, prostaglandins,* and *proteolytic enzymes* could damage pain endings. Bradykinin and some of the prostaglandins can directly stimulate pain nerve axons without actually damaging them (Guyton, 1986, p. 594). Bradykinin is one of the most potent algogenic substances known to man (Jänig and Morrison, 1986, p. 100).

4.4.2 *Particularly sensitive visceral structures*

Among the most sensitive visceral structures are the **visceral peritoneum** and the **mesenteries**. The latter are acutely sensitive to stretching, a stimulus that induces the strongest visceral pain sensations in both man and other mammals. The mesenteries have sympathetic afferent pathways that arise from **Pacinian corpuscles** (Section 4.12.1) and project to the spinal cord through the **splanchnic nerves**. However, the **roots of the mesentery** and structures such as the **broad ligament** arise from the body wall, and thereby collect a **somatic innervation** in the form of free nerve endings (Section 4.9). This somatic innervation may account for the special sensitivity of such mesenteries. It is not known whether the visceral pleura is acutely sensitive to stretching.

4.4.3 *Relatively insensitive visceral structures*

A few viscera are supposed to be relatively insensitive to all forms of noxious stimuli. Notable among these are the *parenchyma* of the *liver* and the *alveoli* of the *lung*. However, the *capsule* of the *liver* is very sensitive to stretch, though this is to be expected from its attachment to visceral peritoneum, and unpleasant sensations do sometimes arise from the lung.

4.4.4 *Parietal serosa*

For good anaesthesia, it must be appreciated that the **parietal peritoneum** and **parietal pleura** are **somatic** *not* visceral structures. They therefore receive an afferent innervation from the intercostal nerves, from the phrenic nerve, and from lumbar segmental nerves. Consequently all parietal serosa are acutely sensitive to all the familiar painful stimuli that assail the outside of the body. Thus puncturing the parietal peritoneum in the imperfectly anaesthetized abdominal wall of a cow deserves a well aimed kick. Likewise the spread of an inflammatory pathological state from the visceral to the parietal serosal lining of the peritoneal and pleural cavities can greatly accentuate the pain of visceral disease.

> Inflammation of the parietal peritoneum is accompanied by sensitivity to pressure applied externally to the abdominal wall. For example, external pressure is greatly resented in colic in the horse, when leakage of gastrointestinal contents through an intestinal perforation has caused inflammation of the parietal peritoneum. The acuteness of the pain depends on how much of the peritoneal cavity is involved and on the type of leakage. Release of acid contents from a ruptured stomach is much worse than leakage from the small colon or rectum (Johnston, 1992).

4.4.5 *Visceral nociceptor axons*

It is believed that the sensation of **visceral pain** transmitted from thoracic and abdominal viscera by **sympathetic nerves**, and from the pelvic viscera by the **pelvic nerve**, is *not* conveyed by specialized axons dedicated exclusively to nociception. The axons appear to be a homogeneous population of general purpose autonomic afferents, which respond to several types of stimuli. Hence they cannot be subdivided into functional types. For example, the afferent axons from the bladder in the pelvic nerve cannot be classified into 'micturition axons' or 'pain axons', since any one these axons can convey both types of sensation – one can speak only of 'bladder afferents'. The discharge patterns of these generalized visceral afferent axons evidently encode the various events in the bladder that (a) give rise to non-painful and painful sensations, (b) initiate a number of bladder reflexes, and (c) contribute to the general regulation of the bladder. It is the job of the central nervous system to decode these visceral afferent signals and generate the appropriate peripheral responses.

The vagus may transmit the sense of pain from the lung, but otherwise is not involved in pain pathways from the thoracic, abdominal, or pelvic viscera.

The identity of **visceral nociceptor axons** was reviewed by Jänig and Morrison (1986). The term 'nociceptor' was introduced by Sherington in 1906 to denote sensory receptors sensitive to damaging or potentially damaging stimuli. The existence of somatic nociceptors in the skin, muscles, and joints, has been established in a number of mammals including man. However, there seems to be no conclusive evidence for a class of dedicated visceral nociceptors in the many sympathetic nerves that transmit the sensation of pain from the thoracic and abdominal viscera, or in the pelvic nerve which transmits the sensation of pain from the pelvic viscera. Possible exceptions include the gall bladder, from which pain appears to be the only sensory experience, whereas other organs such as the colon or bladder can give rise to a range of sensations from mild fullness to frank pain (Cervero and Jänig, 1992).

Adequate stimuli are touch, distension, smooth muscle contraction, tension, intra- or extravascular chemical stimulation, ischaemia, and the application of heat. Thus the axons are *polymodal*. Mayer (1994, p. 941) emphasized their mechanoreceptor characteristics. Biological mechanical stimuli include gastrointestinal, respiratory, or circulatory movements. Afferents in the pelvic nerve respond to the same wide range of stimuli, and seem to differ only in not being tonically active.

This functional homogeneity of these visceral afferent axons in the thoracic and abdominal sympathetic nerves and pelvic nerve requires that both painful and non-painful events in their viscera be encoded in the intensity of discharge of these visceral afferent neurons. The conscious recognition of these visceral afferent discharges, as, say discriminating between a normal sensation of fullness of an organ and the sensation of pain in that organ, must then depend on decoding by central neurones.

The actual mechanisms of *central neuronal decoding* of these signals are not known, but they probably involve neuronal gating influences (Jänig and Morrison, 1986, p. 108). Cervero and Jänig (1992) have speculatively envisaged the broad types of peripheral and central pathways that could operate mechanisms of this kind. They also widened the concept by suggesting that there are *two groups* of visceral afferent pathways in **abdominal sympathetic nerves** and the **pelvic nerve**. The first group would be *low threshold visceral receptors* which normally regulate the activity of viscera. These project into central pathways that control regulatory reflexes and give non-painful sensations; they also project into central pathways that evoke the sensations of pain. At most physiological levels of stimulation their pain activity is subliminal. The second group of receptors project only into central pain pathways. These are *high threshold visceral receptors*. They are activated by events such as the intense contraction of a hollow organ, or hypoxia or inflammation of

tissue. The resulting central excitability causes acute and persistent visceral pain. An important aspect of this central hypersensitivity is that the activity of the low threshold receptors (which normally give non-painful sensations) now evokes visceral pain. Thus the normal regulatory activity of the viscera not only becomes conscious (to a human patient) but may also be painful.

Mayer (1994, pp. 933, 941, 944) seemed to regard these high threshold and low threshold characteristics as multiple manifestations of a *single type of receptor*. According to this view, the numerous afferent axons in the thoracic splanchnic nerves (as numerous as the afferent axons in the vagus) have a *dual function*. In addition to their nociceptive role, they also have mechanoreceptor properties enabling them to interact with vagal afferent pathways in the reflex control of gastric function (Mayer, 1994, pp. 933, 941). Mayer referred to them as 'sleeping nociceptors' (Section 4.2.4), since they only develop their nociceptor function when the viscera are irritated (Section 4.11).

4.5 Course of pain axons in sympathetic nerves

The receptor endings of pain pathways are believed to be free nerve endings in the visceral walls. They lead into **C axons** (unmyelinated axons), similar to those that typically conduct the sensation of *true pain* (as opposed to *pricking pain*) from the *somatic* parts of the body (see the first volume in this series on the CNS; King, 1987).

The axons from the receptor endings tend initially to follow local arteries. In the abdomen, they then pass through the prevertebral ganglia and continue centrally in the **splanchnic nerves**. They traverse the segmental vertebral ganglia of the sympathetic trunk and enter a **white ramus communicans**. After continuing briefly in the spinal nerve they pass through the **dorsal root** to the **dorsal root ganglion**. Here they have their cell station, like virtually all other primary afferent neurons.

Ascending projections through the **spinothalamic** and **spinoreticular tracts** distribute autonomic pain signals to the brain, including the conscious cerebral cortex.

The receptor endings seem not to have been identified microscopically. The axons are mainly C fibres, but there are also Aδ axons (Mayer 1994, p. 933). They contain a significant peptide component (in contrast to vagal afferents). It is assumed from their physiological characteristics that the endings lie in, or immediately beneath, the mucosal epithelium. There seem to be large numbers of these axons. The total number of such afferent axons in the splanchnic nerves seems to be similar to vagal afferent axons.

4.6　Segmental distribution of sympathetic pain pathways

Afferent axons in peripheral sympathetic nerves project segmentally into the spinal cord (Fig. 4.2). They enter the spinal cord at the thoracolumbar segments that form the sympathetic preganglionic motor outflow to the same organs. Consider, for example, the **heart**: the motor efferent sympathetic outflow comes from segments T1 to T5 (Fig.

2.2, thoracic viscera), and the afferent pain input goes to the same segments, T1–T5 (Fig. 4.2). Likewise the efferent sympathetic output to the **stomach** and **small intestines** is from T6 to T10 (Fig. 2.2), and the afferent pain input from these organs is to T6–T10 (Fig. 4.2). Again the efferent sympathetic outflow to the kidney, ureter, testis, and ovary includes segments T10–L2, and these organs have afferent pain projections to T10–L2 (Fig. 4.2). However, the kidney and ureter probably get their main pathways from somatic nerves (Section 4.9).

The segmental input of pain pathways from the various abdominal organs of man has been established by the surgical removal of sympathetic nerves for the relief of hypertension or intractable pain.

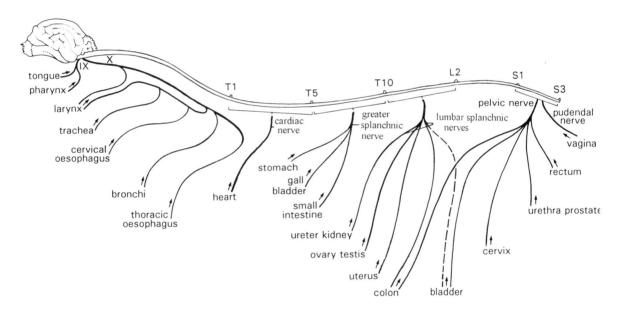

Fig. 4.2　Diagram summarizing the principal autonomic pain pathways. The thoracic, abdominal, and pelvic part of the diagram is based on surgical observations in man; the pathways seem likely to be similar, at least in carnivores. The glossopharyngeal nerve (IX) carries pain pathways from the tongue (caudal third) in its lingual rami, and from the pharynx in its pharyngeal ramus. Pain pathways from the rostral part of the larynx as far caudally as the vocal folds are transmitted by the cranial laryngeal nerve of the vagus nerve (X); the recurrent laryngeal nerve of the vagus (X) carries pain pathways from the rest of the larynx. Pain pathways from the trachea and cervical oesophagus run in the tracheal and oesophageal rami of the recurrent laryngeal nerve. Pain fibres from the bronchial tree are conveyed by the bronchial rami of the vagus (X). The thoracic and abdominal oesophagus project pain fibres through the oesophageal rami of the vagus. Pain fibres from the heart pass through sympathetic cardiac nerves to the dorsal roots of spinal nerves T1–T5. The sympathetic greater splanchnic nerves conduct pain fibres from the stomach and small intestine to spinal nerves T6–T10. Lumbar splanchnic nerves carry pain pathways to segments T10–L2 from the kidney, ureter, the body of the uterus, the gonads, and most of the large intestine; the pelvic end of the descending colon projects through the pelvic nerve to S1–S3. The bladder receives some sympathetic afferents, possibly pain, from segments T10–L2, but most of its pain pathways are in the pelvic nerve. The other pelvic viscera project their pain pathways through the pelvic nerve, except the vagina which sends them through the pudendal nerve.

4.7 Referred visceral pain

It is known that, in man, pain from an organ deep within a body cavity may be felt on the surface of the body, and this is known as referred pain. **Referred pain** plays little part in veterinary diagnosis, but on neuroanatomical grounds its occurrence in lower mammals is likely and might be actively misleading.

The pain axons in the dorsal root of a typical thoracolumbar spinal nerve will contain pain axons from the somatic structures of that particular segment of the body; it will also contain pain axons from a thoracic or abdominal organ. For example, the dorsal root of spinal nerve T7 will contain cutaneous pain axons from the seventh intercostal space. It will also contain some of the pain axons from the stomach (Fig. 4.2). Eventually both of these pain inputs will project through the multineuronal relays of the spinothalamic and spinoreticular tracts (see Vol. 1 on the CNS; King, 1987) to the thalamus and cerebral cortex, where they are recognized as pain.

However, this is not a one-to-one series of neuronal projections. On the contrary, the central nervous system is parsimonious, and often requires a neuronal pathway higher up in the neuraxis to carry more than one type of sensation from the periphery; in other words, two separate neuronal pathways from the periphery may converge on one neuron in the spinal cord. There is some evidence that the pain axons in the dorsal roots outnumber the pain axons in the tracts; if so, *several pain axons must converge on, i.e. share, one tract axon.*

As stated in Section 4.2.2, pain pathways from the viscera are mainly silent, but pain signals from the surface of the body occur often. Consequently when the cerebral cortex receives pain signals from a *shared* spinothalamic pathway, it recognizes the common rather than the uncommon source of the signals. Therefore gastric pain signals entering the spinal cord through the dorsal root of spinal nerve T7 are interpreted by the cortex as pain from the surface of the body at segment T7. This surface region of a segment of the body is known as a **dermatome**. Since the gastric pain pathways enter segments T6–T10, referred gastric pain extends over dermatomes T6–

T10. In man these dermatomes have their cranial limit at the level of the nipples and their caudal limit at the umbilicus. Referred pain from the stomach does indeed extend between these limits. Referred pain is often accompanied by local tenderness of the skin itself.

In addition to the well-defined referred visceral pain on the surface of the body, visceral disease can cause vague agonizing pain, much deeper and somewhere near the organ itself though poorly localized. This is known as **unreferred visceral pain** (or splanchnic pain).

It can be difficult to distinguish sensations arising through frankly pathological processes, from sensations associated with somewhat exaggerated but essentially normal activity. For example, in man, transient 'abdominal pain' caused merely by strong intestinal contraction is commonplace.

Referred pain can be diagnostically misleading in veterinary practice, (Iggo, 1977, p. 607) since it may cause an animal to attend vigorously to, even to the extent of gnawing, an area of skin that is in itself perfectly normal.

In human medicine a knowledge of referred pain is diagnostically important. The matter has been well studied (Ruch, 1966, pp. 360–362). Information on **gastrointestinal referred pain** has been obtained by inflating a balloon at various levels of the tract in volunteers, medical students appropriately enough. The pain is usually ventral (anterior) but is sometimes dorsal. It is usually in the midline. It moves caudally as the stimulus descends through the tract. Jejunal and ileal projections are all in the umbilical region and variations of several feet in length in the site of the balloon along the intestine have no appreciable effect on the localization. The pain is precisely localized and sharp or cramp-like. The pain from the large intestine is more diffuse and less intense, always below the umbilicus, and tends to be to one side of the midline.

Since the commonest cause of death in the developed world is **ischaemic heart disease** caused by insufficient *coronary blood flow* (Guyton, 1986, p. 299) there is particular interest in *cardiac pain* (known as *angina pectoris*). Usually, agonizing **unreferred pain** occurs deep to the cranial part of the sternum, and **referred pain** is localized on the surface of the left shoulder and the medial aspect of the left arm. Probably it is usually the left arm because the left side of the heart is much more often affected by coronary disease than the right, but occasionally the right arm is involved and often the left side of the neck, and even the left side of the face (Guyton, 1986, pp. 302, 600).

4.8 Visceral pain pathways in parasympathetic nerves

Parasympathetic nerves are not primarily involved in pain pathways from the viscera (Section 4.2.2), but there are the following exceptions to this rule.

4.8.1 Glossopharyngeal nerve

Pain axons from the **tongue** (caudal two thirds) project through the **lingual rami** (Fig. 4.2; Section 4.10.4). The pain pathway from the pharyngeal wall passes through the **pharyngeal ramus** and **pharyngeal plexus** of the glossopharyngeal nerve. The cell station of both of these pathways is in the **distal glossopharyngeal ganglion**.

4.8.2 Vagus nerve

Pain is perceived in the **larynx**. The axons project through the **cranial** and **recurrent laryngeal nerves** (Fig. 4.2). The cranial laryngeal nerve, which guards the entrance to the larynx as far as and including the vocal folds (Section 4.15.4), is probably the main supply. The cell stations are in the **distal vagal ganglion**.

Pain from the **oesophagus** is projected through the **oesophageal rami** of the recurrent laryngeal nerve and of the main trunk of the vagus (Fig. 4.2). Unpleasant sensations from the **trachea** and **bronchi** (Section 4.16), verging on pain, are an all too familiar experience in ordinary infections of the upper respiratory tract. They evoke the *cough reflex* and other responses. These pain pathways are not conducted by sympathetic nerves, but by the vagus. The pathways reach the vagus via the **bronchial rami**, and via the **tracheal rami** of the **recurrent laryngeal nerve** (Fig. 4.2).

4.8.3 Pelvic nerve: pudendal nerve

The **pelvic nerve** is the main exception to the general rule that pain pathways from the viscera travel in sympathetic nerves (Section 4.2.2). Thus pain pathways from the **cervix**, **prostate**, **pelvic urethra**, the pelvic part of the **descending colon**, **rectum**, and most of the **bladder** travel in the pelvic nerve (Fig. 4.2), which is a parasympathetic nerve.

The cell stations of all afferent axons in the pelvic nerve are in the **dorsal root ganglia** of **sacral spinal nerves**, probably the same sacral spinal nerves as those that form the parasympathetic motor outflow into the pelvic nerve.

The afferent pathways from the **vagina** differ from those from the other pelvic viscera. They all travel in the **pudendal nerve**, and are regarded as *somatic afferents*, not autonomic afferents. The pudendal nerve supplies afferent axons not only to the vagina but to the **external genitalia** in both sexes and to the **anal mucosa**. The cell stations of all the afferent axons in the pudendal nerve are in the same sacral dorsal root ganglia as those that belong to the pelvic nerve. The pudendal nerve also carries the somatic motor axons that innervate the skeletal muscle of the **external anal sphincter** and **urethralis muscle** (Section 2.17.2).

Central projections of all the above pain pathways continue by neuronal relays in the spinoreticular and spinothalamic tracts, culminating in the conscious cerebral cortex.

It is useful in veterinary clinical practice to be able to block by local anaesthesia the afferent pathways that travel in the **pudendal nerve**. In the ox, the pudendal nerve can be blocked directly by injecting it as it crosses the lateral pelvic wall (**pudendal nerve block**). It can also be blocked indirectly at its dorsal root ganglia or at the dorsal roots of its sacral spinal nerves by **epidural anaesthesia** (see volume on the CNS; King, 1987), but this technique also blocks the somatic motor pathways in these spinal nerves, thus causing incoordination of the hind limbs. Pudendal nerve block is used for surgery of the external genitalia of the bull. It anaesthetizes and relaxes the **penis** without incoordinating the hindlimbs; surgery on the penis is easier if the animal stays on its feet. In the cow epidural anaesthesia is used to arrest voluntary straining during birth. **Straining** is initiated reflexly by the entrance of the fetal membranes or fetus into the **vagina**, as in the second stage of labour (Section 16.12). Epidural anaesthesia indirectly blocks the afferent limb of this reflex arc. Control of straining makes it easier to rectify an incorrect presentation of the fetus. It is not necessarily inconvenient if the animal goes down.

4.9 Visceral pain pathways in somatic nerves

As already stated (Section 4.4.4), the **parietal pleura** and **parietal peritoneum** have a typical somatic sensory innervation which makes them acutely sensitive to all injurious stimuli. These somatic pain pathways extend for a short distance into the reflections of the parietal peritoneum from the body wall. Thus the **root of the mesentery** and the **broad ligament** of the uterus receive a somatic pain innervation, as well as a typical visceral pain innervation via sympathetic nerves. This may explain the acute sensitivity of the mesentery to stretching (Section 4.4.2).

As retroperitoneal organs, the **kidney** and **ureter** are believed to get most of their pain pathways from somatic nerves in the body wall, sympathetic pathways to T10–L2 being in the minority (Section 4.13).

> In severe coronary ischaemia in man, as during the acute phase of coronary thrombosis, intense **unreferred** pain sometimes occurs immediately adjacent to the sternum as well as being *referred* to the other regions mentioned in Section 4.7. This sternal pain may be explained by somatic pain axons passing from the heart through the pericardium, where the pericardium is reflected over the great vessels (Guyton, 1986, p. 600), or it may be accounted for by somatic pain axons passing from the pericardium through the reflection of the ventral mediastinum from the parietal pleura on the adjacent ventral (anterior, in man) wall of the thoracic cavity (Fig. 6.1). On its course through the mediastinum, the **phrenic nerve** (Section 8.17.3), which of course is a somatic nerve (mainly motor to the diaphragm), gives afferent branches to the **mediastinal pleura** and **parietal pericardium** (Williams *et al.*, 1989, p. 1129), and is therefore another possible avenue for cardiac pain; it may perhaps be involved in cardiac pain referred to the neck (Section 4.7), since the phrenic nerve joins the neuraxis at cervical segments C3, C4, and C5 in man (C5, C6, and C7 in the dog; Evans and Christensen, 1979, p. 978).

II AUTONOMIC AFFERENT RECEPTORS AND REFLEXES OF VARIOUS ORGANS

4.10 Receptors of the tongue, pharynx, and oesophagus, and their reflexes

4.10.1 *Mechanoreceptors*

The **tongue** is richly supplied with autonomic tactile receptors which help it to manoeuvre a bolus into the pharynx for swallowing. The axons run from the tongue (caudal third) in the **lingual rami** of the **glossopharyngeal nerve** (Fig. 4.3).

Tactile **deglutition receptors** in the mucosa of the wall of the oral pharynx (Fig. 4.3) are stimulated when the tongue has forced a bolus from the oral cavity into the pharynx. The receptors induce the **swallowing reflex**. Swallowing (deglutition) takes the form of a peristaltic wave that, once initiated, cannot be arrested. As would be expected, the rostral region of the oral pharynx is the most sensitive zone for initiating the swallowing reflex.

The pathways for most of these pharyngeal autonomic afferent axons run in the **glossopharyngeal nerve**, via its **pharyngeal ramus** and the **pharyngeal plexus** (Fig. 4.3). (A few pharyngeal pathways from the most caudal part of the pharyngeal mucosa, adjoining the epiglottis, are in the **vagus nerve**.)

Tactile **retching receptors** are also present in the pharyngeal wall. When stimulated by a foreign body in the food, or a probe, they induce not swallowing but **retching**. This reflex response is known as the **gag reflex** in clinical neurology, and is used to test the afferent pathways of the **glossopharyngeal nerve** (see King, 1987).

Stretch receptors in the wall of the oesophagus respond to distension by inducing **oesophageal peristalsis**. The axons are in the **oesophageal rami** of the **recurrent laryngeal** and **vagus nerves**.

The cell stations of pharyngeal afferents are in the **distal glossopharyngeal ganglion**. Those of oesophageal afferents are in the **distal vagal ganglion**.

> The receptors for the swallowing reflex have not been identified histologically (Widdicombe, 1986a, p. 375).
>
> In addition to the swallowing and gag reflexes there is a third pharyngeal reflex, the **aspiration reflex**, also known as the **sniff reflex** (Widdicombe, 1986a, p. 372). It consists of repeated short powerful sniff-like inspiratory efforts, reflexly evoked by *mechanical* rather than chemical stimulation of the nasal pharynx. Effective stimuli are a solid object like a catheter, a jet of air, water, and (presumably) mucus. The glottis remains open. The result is to draw material from the upper respiratory tract in general and nasal pharynx in particular into the oral pharynx where it would be swallowed, or to the larynx where it would be coughed out. The reflex is strong in cats, occurs in dogs, rats, mice, and pigs, and

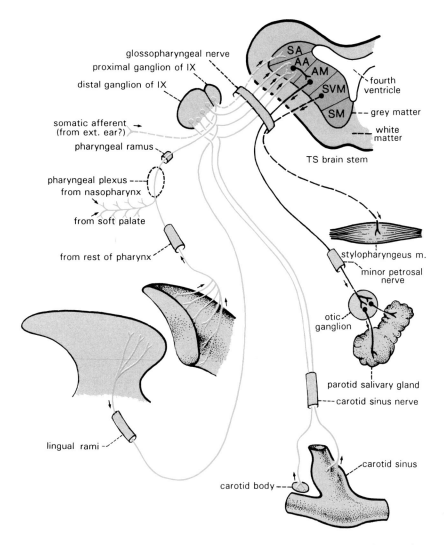

Fig. 4.3 **Diagram summarizing the distribution of the glossopharyngeal nerve.** The glossopharyngeal nerve (IX) is mainly afferent. Its motor fibres are limited to the parasympathetic innervation (AM, autonomic motor) of the parotid salivary gland via the minor petrosal nerve (axons represented by black continuous lines), and to the special visceral (branchial) motor innervation (SVM) of the stylopharyngeus muscle (axon represented by black broken line). There is a small somatic afferent component (SA) which probably supplies the external ear (axon represented by green broken line). The rest of the glossopharyngeal nerve is autonomic afferent (AA) (the axons are all represented by continuous green lines). General autonomic afferent fibres innervate the nasopharynx and soft palate via the pharyngeal ramus, and the tongue (caudal third) via the lingual rami. The lingual rami also carry taste fibres. Baro- and chemoreceptor fibres are conveyed from the carotid sinus and carotid body by the carotid sinus nerve. The proximal and distal glossopharyngeal ganglia are fused in most of the domestic mammals. The proximal ganglion is restricted to somatic afferent neurons; the distal ganglion is the cell station of all the autonomic afferent neurons.

is weak in rabbits and man. The peripheral afferent pathway is via the **glossopharyngeal nerve**.

The stimuli that elicit the aspiration reflex also cause reflex laryngeal dilation by the abductor muscles of the larynx, bronchodilation, and mucosecretion into the lower respiratory tract (Widdicombe, 1986a, p. 375).

Weyns (1988, pp. 76–79) has reviewed **oesophageal receptors**. **Mucosal receptors** in the oesophagus of the sheep and cat are activated by strong and rapid **distension**, **tactile** stroking, and strong and rapid **flow** of saline solution. Their function may be to monitor the mechanical consistency of the ingesta. **Distension receptors** in the muscle tunic seem to be concentrated at the oral and gastric ends of the thoracic oesophagus; they may recognize the passage of a bolus by either the distension it causes or by the contraction that propels the bolus towards the stomach. Three types of mechanoreceptor have been identified in the region of the **cardiac sphincter** (Section 3.11.1) of the cat and sheep, i.e. mucosal receptors, serosal receptors, and receptors in the muscle tunic. It is believed that all three types are likely to be transiently stimulated by **gastro-oesophageal regurgitation**, and may therefore be involved in coordinating the sphincter zone.

4.10.2   Chemoreceptors

Taste buds contain chemosensitive taste cells. The **taste receptor cell** is a spindle-shaped cell embedded with other cells in a taste bud, and making synaptic contact with an autonomic afferent axonal ending. The receptor cells respond to salt, acid, bitter, and sweet solutions, and to distilled water, depending on the species. Taste buds on the cranial two thirds of the tongue are innervated by the **facial nerve** (Fig. 4.1), via the **chorda tympani** (Section 3.9.2); the buds on the caudal third are supplied by the **glossopharyngeal nerve**, via its **lingual rami** (Fig. 4.3).

The cell stations are in the **geniculate ganglion** of the facial nerve, and the **distal glossopharyngeal ganglion**.

Taste buds on the palatal mucosa are supplied by the **major petrosal nerve** of the **facial nerve** (Section 3.9.1).

Taste axons are often classified as special visceral afferents, but are treated here as ordinary autonomic afferent axons (Section 1.4).

Taste buds occur in fungiform, vallate, and foliate papillae in the dog (Chibuzo, 1979, pp. 423–444) and in man (Williams *et al.*, 1989, pp. 1169–1170). The afferent axons from taste buds in the **fungiform papillae** on the rostral two thirds of the tongue lie in the **chorda tympani** of the **facial nerve**, and have their cell station in the **geniculate ganglion**. The **lingual rami** of the **glossopharyngeal nerve** supply the taste buds in the **foliate** and **vallate papillae** on the caudal third of the tongue (Chibuzo, 1979, p. 444). The small number of taste buds on the epiglottis and adjacent pharyngeal wall are innervated by the **vagus** (Crosby *et al.*, 1962, p. 140; McClure, 1979, p. 928), presumably via its **cranial laryngeal nerve**. In man, at least, there are a few taste buds on the oral surface of the soft palate (Williams *et al.*, 1989, p. 1169), probably innervated by the **glossopharyngeal nerve**.

There are essentially three types of spindle-shaped cells in a **taste bud**, though other types, which are probably variants on these, have been described (e.g. Chibuzo, 1979, pp. 433–436). (1) **Basal cells**, which differentiate into other taste bud cells (Krstic, 1984, p. 410). (2) **Supporting cells** (type I of Chibuzo, 1979), which are the most numerous, are wrapped round the other types of cell and around the axons in the bud. (3) The **taste receptor cell** (type III of Chibuzo, 1979) is the only cell in the bud that makes synaptic contact with an afferent axonal ending, and is therefore interpreted as the taste receptor component. The receptor cells have a very short life span, being replaced after about 10 days (Krstic, 1984, p. 410). They die if their afferent axon is cut. **Dense cored granular vesicles** are present in supporting cells and receptor cells.

At least five functional **types of taste axon** have been identified electrophysiologically (Iggo, 1977, p. 593): distilled water axons, salt axons, acid pH (sour) axons, bitter axons, and sweet axons, but no axon is completely specific. Each afferent axon synapses with receptor cells in several buds, and may therefore respond to more than one type of chemical stimulus. Hence, the conscious identification of a particular taste is likely to be the result of analysis within the gustatory areas of the brain (Williams *et al.*, 1989, p. 1170). All vertebrates so far examined have salt and acid axons, and bitter axons have been found in all mammals; water axons are absent in man, rat, ruminants, and fish; sweet axons are present in the dog, rabbit, and rat, but not in the cat (Iggo, 1977, p. 594).

Taste stimuli, especially sour, reflexly induce copious **salivation** (Guyton, 1986, p. 773).

4.10.3   Thermoreceptors

The tongue and pharynx have acute *thermal sensitivity*. The pathways from the tongue are as follows: somatic afferents from the rostral two thirds of the tongue, in the **lingual nerve** of the **trigeminal nerve**; autonomic afferents from the caudal third, in the **lingual rami** of the **glossopharyngeal nerve** (Fig. 4.2). The pharyngeal pathway is in the **pharyngeal ramus** of the **glossopharyngeal nerve**.

Thermoreceptors in the oesophagus are less obtrusive but are present, as an incautious gulp of ice-cold beer or boiling-hot tea will show. The afferent pathways are the **oesophageal rami** of the **recurrent laryngeal nerve** from the cervical oesophagus, and the **oesophageal rami** of the vagus from the thoracic oesophagus.

The cell stations of afferent axons in the glossopharyngeal nerve will be in the **distal glossopharyngeal ganglion**. Those of vagal afferents will be in the **distal vagal ganglion**.

4.10.4 *Nociceptors*

Pain sensations from the tongue and pharynx, including the raw pain of a severe 'sore throat', are all too familiar. Pain sensations can also arise in the oesophagus of man, and presumably also in lower mammals. Their pathways (Fig. 4.2) are the same as for the thermoreceptors just described.

> In man pain sensation from the thoracic oesophagus can be referred to the midline along the length of the sternum. It may therefore overlie the heart, without in any way indicating cardiac disease. Pain from the distal end of the oesophagus is a burning sensation, known as heartburn.
> **Heartburn** is usually attributed to regurgitation of acid ingesta from the stomach. The accuracy of this assumption has been reviewed by Ruch (1966, p. 360). Experiments on conscious volunteers revealed that the same burning sensation is caused by inflating a balloon in the distal end of the oesophagus, or simply by the presence of water.
> Sometimes the sensation runs up the oesophagus, but without gastric contents entering the mouth; radiographic observations suggest that this sensation is caused by a retroperistaltic wave. It seems likely that all heartburn sensations are caused by abnormal neuromuscular activity, and that the chemical nature of any regurgitated fluid is of little importance.

4.11 Receptors of the gastrointestinal tract and their reflexes

Several types of receptor ending, including **mechanoreceptors**, **chemoreceptors**, **thermoreceptors**, and **nociceptors**, lie in the walls of the gastrointestinal tract, especially in the muscular tunic and the mucous membranes. They are organized in three systems.

(1) Many receptors belong to neurons that have their cell stations in **enteric ganglia**, and operate entirely within the **enteric nervous system**, contributing to the **local reflexes** of the enteric nervous system. Their role is to optimize the local processes of digestion and absorption.

(2) Other gastrointestinal receptor endings belong to chemoreceptor and mechanoreceptor **vagal afferent neurons**. These endings extend as far down the tract as the descending colon. They belong to typical primary afferent neurons, with their cell stations in the **distal vagal ganglion**. Their central projections go to the nucleus of the solitary tract. From there, they project by further neuronal relays to the **gastrointestinal centres** in the brainstem. These pathways promote the **central regulation** of gut functions.

(3) The third system is formed by large numbers of dual purpose afferent axons ('sleeping nociceptors') in the sympathetic splanchnic nerves (Section 4.4.5). Many of these belong to primary afferent neurons, with their cell stations in thoracolumbar dorsal root ganglia. Neuronal relays continue up the spinal cord to the brainstem and higher brain levels. These serve as pain axons after mucosal irritation, but appear also to act as mechanoreceptors of the normal gastrointestinal tract, thereby contributing to the reflex regulation of gastric function.

> As just stated, many of the receptor endings in the gut wall project to enteric ganglion cells (Wood, 1987, p. 93), and are therefore integral components of the **enteric nervous system** (Section 3.18.1) remaining entirely within the gut wall. Other gut receptors belong to the axons of primary afferent neurons that run through the **splanchnic nerves**. These have their cell stations in the thoracolumbar spinal ganglia, and project through neuronal relays in the spinal cord to the brainstem, transmitting nociceptor and mechanoreceptor impulses (Section 4.4.5). Some of these splanchnic neurons are known to project collaterals that synapse with sympathetic postganglionic neurons in the **prevertebral ganglia** (Gabella, 1987, p. 365); there is evidence for a wide range of **integrative mechanisms** in prevertebral ganglia (Jänig and McLachlan, 1987, p. 1393). Yet others of these gastrointestinal receptors project to the central nervous system via primary afferent neurons in the **vagus** and **pelvic nerves** (Section 3.18.1).
> Thus the state of the gut is monitored at least at *three levels*, i.e. by the enteric nervous system itself, by the prevertebral ganglia, and by the brainstem (Wood, 1987, p. 95; Gabella, 1987, p. 365). Furthermore, projections from integrative enteric ganglion cells to the central nervous system (Section 3.18.1) may enable the nervous system to monitor events at a fourth level by receiving direct information about the activity in the integrative circuitry of the enteric nervous system (Wood, 1987, pp. 95–96).
> Considerable convergence and reciprocal interaction of all these afferent pathways has been demonstrated in the brainstem (Mayer, 1994, p. 930).

4.11.1 *Gastrointestinal mechanoreceptors*

Distension receptors signal the volumes of the stomach and intestine. **Pressure receptors**, responding to compression of the gut wall, register the presence and movement of ingesta. **Tactile receptors** cause reflex contraction and relaxation of the gut wall proximal and distal, respectively, to the stimulus, thus inducing **movement of the ingesta**. Fast adapting mechanoreceptors respond to the **mechanical properties** (roughage, etc.) of the ingesta.

Mechanoreceptors can induce **secretomotor, muscular,** and **vasomotor reflexes** entirely within the **enteric nervous system**, thus perfecting the details of gut function. Enteric mechanoreceptors also contribute to the more complex reflex activities of the enteric nervous system, such as **segmentation, peristalsis,** and **retroperistalsis** (Section 3.18). The mechanoreceptor neurons in the enteric nervous system are very short neurons. Their cell stations are in the **enteric ganglia**, and their axonal projections are restricted to the myenteric and submucosal plexuses. Therefore they are not true **primary afferent neurons** (Section 4.2.3).

Several types of **mechanosensitive neurons** belonging to the enteric nervous system have been demonstrated electrophysiologically in the **myenteric ganglia**. Among these are mechanosensitive neurons that discharge during contractions of the circular smooth muscle, but these are not conclusively known to be mechanoreceptors (Wood, 1987, p. 95). Mechanoreceptors with cell bodies in both the submucous plexus and the myenteric plexus respond to *distension*; their endings appear to be respectively in the mucous membrane and the muscle tunic (Weyns, 1988, p. 77). There is also evidence for **pressure receptors** in the intestinal mucosa, sensitive to pinching. They appear to signal *movement of the mucosa* through contraction of the muscularis mucosa, and also the *presence* and *movement of ingesta* (Weyns, 1988, p. 76). Stroking the mucosa of the small intestine of the dog induces the '**mucosal reflex**', in which the proximal side of the gut is excited and the distal inhibited (Weyns, 1988, p. 76).

Other **mechanoreceptor neurons** project to the central nervous system via the **vagus nerve**, and therefore are true primary afferent neurons. Important examples are **slowly adapting vagal stretch receptors** from the **stomach** and **small intestine**. Their endings lie entirely in the outer layers of the muscle tunic of the gut wall. **Vagal gastric receptors** of this type have been described in the rat, cat, goat, and sheep, and evidently they normally signal the degree of *distension* of the stomach caused by the progressive arrival of ingesta (Weyns, 1988, p. 77). These slowly adapting vagal gut receptors fire continuously at low frequency when the tract is at rest, and at progressively faster frequencies during increasing distension. They also fire at a higher frequency during muscular contraction (Wood, 1987, p. 95). This is because the endings in the outer muscle layers are **in series** rather than in parallel with the smooth muscle cells (Iggo, 1966; Wood, 1987, p. 95).

It was pointed out by Iggo (1966) that this system of **slowly adapting, 'in series' mechanoreceptors** in the external muscle layers is a *basic characteristic* of the hollow abdominal and pelvic organs. In the normal organ, such receptors induce propulsive movements. Their slowly adapting activity during filling of the organ can account for a variety of familiar conscious sensations, including pleasant fullness of the stomach after a good meal and fullness of the bladder. In conscious man, *slow* distension of the stomach goes unnoticed, but *rapid distension to the same volume* evokes a sense of fullness (Iggo, 1966), a point exploited by Chinese cuisine in which an extended series of *many small items* is gradually eaten.

However, if the lumen is obstructed, the slowly adapting 'in series' mechanoreceptors may initiate very powerful and prolonged isometric contractions (Iggo, 1966). These can account for the acute pain of **obstruction** of the alimentary tract, and also obstruction of the bile duct, urethra, and salivary ducts by calculi, excessive tension in smooth muscle being one of the adequate stimuli for visceral pain (Section 4.4.1). Incidentally, there is no way by which the brainstem can distinguish between distension or obstruction as the cause of such severe mechanoreceptor activity. Iggo (1977, p. 595) remarked that this increases the difficulty of diagnosing abdominal disorders; presumably this is because it may be impossible to differentiate diagnostically between obstruction and distension, although in practice the obstruction of a hollow organ will usually be followed by distension with either fluid or gas.

Fast adapting vagal gastrointestinal receptors occur in the epithelium, mucosa, and myenteric plexus of the rabbit, cat, and sheep. They are believed to signal the *mechanical properties* of the ingesta and changes in the *passage of ingesta* (Weyns, 1988, p. 78).

Serosal mechanoreceptors responding to *probing, stretching,* and *distension* have been found in the **duodenal serosa** (Weyns, 1988, p. 79).

Little is known about the **structure** of any of the **mechanosensitive endings** involved in these afferent mechanisms (Gabella, 1987, p. 365), apart from a general suspicion (one might say 'gut feeling') that the complex networks of free axons that are regularly seen in the mucosa must be involved. Mayer (1994, p. 931, Fig. 1), however, surveyed accounts of investigations with the confocal microscope of labelled vagal afferent axons in the stomach of the rat. Each axon had two supposedly sensory components: (i) *intraganglionic laminar endings,* comprising a succession of about four short collaterals each forming terminal arborizations on the surface of an enteric ganglion, with branches extending into the periganglionic collagen; (ii) *intramuscular terminal branches,* comprising long collaterals running between the muscle bundles of the outer longitudinal muscle, and forming spiny appositions on fibrocytes surrounding the bundles. The intramuscular endings were believed to be gastric tension receptors, but no function was suggested for the intraganglionic endings. It is clear that other mechanoreceptor endings, and also chemoreceptors, lie in or immediately beneath the gastric epithelium, since they stop functioning in the presence of topical local anaesthetics (Mayer, 1994, p. 940).

4.11.2   *Gastrointestinal chemoreceptors*

Vagal *acid* and vagal *alkali* **receptors** are present in the gastric mucosa, and vagal receptors responding to *glucose, amino acids, NaCl,* and *fatty acids* occur in the small intestine. These receptors project via cell stations in the **distal vagal ganglion** (Fig. 3.3), and neuronal relays in the nucleus of the solitary tract, to the **gastrointestinal centres** in the brainstem. Similar receptors project locally to **enteric ganglia**, and induce **enteric reflexes** that move the ingesta along the gut.

The *functions of gut chemoreceptors* have been well reviewed by Weyns (1988, p. 75). The enteric nervous system responds to chemical stimulation by **enteric reflexes**, in which **contraction** is induced **proximal** to the stimulus and **inhibition distal** to it, thus reflexly inducing local movement of ingesta. These enteric receptors react to certain fats and organic acids, and are also **osmoreceptors**.

Gastric chemoreceptors innervated by the **vagus nerve** respond to *acidic* (pH 3) or *alkaline* (pH 8) solutions (Wood, 1987, p. 95). However, the response to acids is not related to pH per se, but rather to titratable acidity and molecular weight (Weyns, 1988, p. 75).

There are very slowly adapting vagal *glucose* **receptors** mainly in the duodenum and proximal jejunum. Slowly adapting *amino acid* **receptors** occur in the small intestine. Vagal receptors responding to hypertonic *fatty acids*, hypertonic *NaCl,* and *organic acids* have been found in the small intestine. In the sheep there are probably receptors in the reticuloruminal mucosa that respond to the *acetate* anion and reflexly inhibit *ruminal movements*, and others that induce or inhibit *eructation* (Iggo, 1977, p. 595). *Acid* **receptors** in the abomasum excite *motility* of the **forestomachs** (de Lahunta and Habel, 1986, p. 240).

4.11.3   *Gastrointestinal thermoreceptors*

In man, *cold* and *heat* are consciously perceived from the stomach, though less well than from the oesophagus. The cell stations are in the distal vagal ganglion.

This topic has been reviewed by Weyns (1988, p. 79). In man, stimuli of the gastric mucosa above 40°C and below

18°C are recognized, respectively, as hot and cold. Heat stimuli can modify gastric motility.

Vagal afferents in the **duodenum** of the cat can be stimulated by *warm* (38–51°C) and *cold* (10–36°C) solutions; these receptors are not mechano- or chemosensitive. Application of *heat* (over 46°C) to the wall of the **small intestine** of the cat causes local inhibition of the intestinal wall. *Intra-abdominal heat* in the sheep (42–44°C) causes *thermoregulatory changes*, the pathways being in the **splanchnic nerves**. **Peritoneal mechanoreceptors** also respond to *heat stimuli*, and therefore thermosensitive endings in the abdomen may not always be specific thermoreceptors.

4.11.4   *Gastrointestinal nociceptors*

Provided they receive an **adequate stimulus** (*distension, spasm, ischaemia, stretching, chemical irritation*, Section 4.4.1), the stomach, small intestine, and the colon at least as far as the transverse colon, transmit consciously perceived pain via sympathetic peripheral nerves (Fig. 4.2). The cell stations of these axons are in the **dorsal root ganglia** of segments T6–T10.

The pelvic part of the descending colon probably projects its pain pathways via the pelvic nerve (Fig. 4.2; Section 4.14.2). The cell stations will then be in the **dorsal root ganglia** of sacral spinal nerves.

'In series' mechanoreceptors (Section 4.11.1) play a major part in the acute pain caused by obstruction of tubular organs.

The general characteristics of visceral pain receptors are considered in Section 4.4.5.

4.12   Receptors of the mesenteries and their reflexes

4.12.1   *Mesenteric mechanoreceptors*

Pacinian corpuscles are scattered about the mesenteries. They are also seen in large numbers in histological sections of the pancreas in many species. Their very rapidly adapting mechanosensitive characteristics are well known, but such functions in this site are not understood.

These structures are macroscopically visible on the mesentery alongside the blood vessels as small oval objects up to 2 mm in diameter (Iggo, 1977, p. 595), and are often excited by arterial pulsations (Iggo, 1966). Their afferent pathways go through the **splanchnic nerves** (Mitchell, 1953, p. 124), which raises the possibility of pain transmission (Section 4.12.3).

The cell stations of the afferent axons are in **thoracolumbar dorsal root ganglia**.

Intra-abdominal heat receptors, and mechanosensitive receptors in the mesenteries that also respond to heat, are discussed in Section 4.11.3.

4.12.2 *Mesenteric nociceptors*

The mesenteries are acutely sensitive to pain caused by stretching. The pathways are mainly sympathetic, in the **splanchnic nerves**. They are probably also **somatic**, in branches of lumbar spinal nerves. The axons enter through the **root of the mesentery** or from the parietal peritoneum into structures such as the **broad ligament** (Section 4.9).

As stated at the beginning of this section, **Pacinian corpuscles** in the mesentery project through the **splanchnic nerves**. Although these structures are primarily mechanosensitive, they may perhaps become nociceptive, depending on the intensity of discharge (Section 4.4). There are also **free nerve endings** in the mesenteries, and these are suspected of being the **somatic pain axons** projecting through lumbar spinal nerves (Mitchell, 1953, p. 124); their cell stations would be in **lumbar dorsal root ganglia** (Section 4.9).

4.13 Nociceptors of kidney and ureter, testis and ovary, and body of uterus

Pain pathways from these organs pass through the sympathetic **lumbar splanchnic nerves** (Mitchell, 1953, p. 285; Ruch, 1966, p. 354), into segments T10–L2 (Fig. 4.2). The cell stations will be in the **dorsal root ganglia** of these spinal nerves. However, as retroperitoneal organs the kidney and ureter are believed to get most of their pain axons from **somatic** lumbar spinal nerves (Guyton, 1986, p. 601) (Section 4.9). The uterus also receives possible somatic pain pathways via the broad ligament (Section 4.12.2). The acute pain caused by obstruction of the bladder and ureter by urinary calculi is probably transmitted by 'in series' mechanoreceptors (Section 4.11.1), which initiate prolonged, powerful, and painful contractions

of the smooth muscle of these organs (Section 4.4.1).

4.14 Receptors of the pelvic viscera and their reflexes

Nearly all of the functionally important **afferent pathways from the pelvic viscera**, whether for pain or other modalities, travel in the **pelvic nerve**. The organs concerned are the bladder, terminal descending colon, rectum, uterine cervix, pelvic urethra, prostate, and vesicular gland. Intact afferent, as well as efferent, pathways in the pelvic nerve are of prime importance in the proper function of the three principal organ systems within the pelvic canal, i.e. the **urinary bladder** (Section 3.14), the **male reproductive organs**, and the **descending colon** and **rectum**.

The only major exception is the **vagina**, which projects all its afferent pathways via the somatic **pudendal nerve** (Section 4.8.3).

Afferent pathways projecting in both the **pelvic** and the **pudendal nerves** have their cell stations in the **dorsal root ganglia** of **sacral spinal nerves**.

Large numbers of afferent autonomic axons arise from the **pelvic viscera** via **sympathetic nerves** (see Jänig and McLachlan, 1987, pp. 1333, 1335, 1357). The afferent pathway for these sympathetic axons from the true pelvic organs is the **hypogastric nerve**. The axons from the **descending colon** project through the **lumbar splanchnic nerves**. The sympathetic axons from the **bladder** and **urethra** have their cell stations in the **dorsal root ganglia** of segments T10–L2 (Fig. 4.2), and those from the **descending colon** and **rectum** have theirs in L2–L3, with minor species variations.

The presence of these numerous **sympathetic afferent axons** from the **pelvic viscera** (besides the well known **parasympathetic pathways** from the pelvic viscera in the pelvic nerve) seems to occur generally in all the mammalian species so far investigated. The functions of the **sympathetic component** remain, however, entirely mysterious. Denervation of these sympathetic pathways yields no serious disturbances of visceral sensation. They appear at present to be functionally of little importance (Jänig and McLachlan, 1987, p. 1335), but this almost certainly means only that the right questions have not yet been asked. Brodal (1981, p. 767) noted that they are generally assumed to be concerned mainly with pain.

Yet other afferent neurons in sympathetic nerves have their cell stations in ganglia within the **myenteric** and **submucosal plexuses** of the distal colon. They project their axons into the **prevertebral sympathetic ganglia** and synapse there with postganglionic neurons. They are presumed to have integrative functions. Since their cell stations are *not* in dorsal root ganglia, and their ongoing axonal projections do *not* reach the spinal cord, these afferent neurons are not true **primary afferent neurons**. It is not known whether such afferent pathways also occur in the pelvic viscera proper (Jänig and McLachlan, 1987, p. 1334).

4.14.1 *Mechanoreceptors from bladder and rectum*

Afferent components of the reflexes of **micturition** and **defecation** have been discussed in Section 3.14. Both of these reflexes are initiated by stretch receptors in the wall of the organ. The axons of these primary afferent neurons are in the **pelvic nerve**, the cell stations being in **sacral dorsal root ganglia**.

The *stretch receptor signals* from the **neck of the bladder** are particularly strong, and are the main factor *initiating* the reflexes of **micturition** (Section 3.14). *Completion* of the emptying of the bladder is achieved by two other groups of receptors (Gans and Mercer, 1977, pp. 489–490). One group is apparently in series with muscle fibres in the bladder. These are distorted during contraction of the muscle, and their discharges to the brainstem via the **pelvic nerve** maintain excitation of the motor centres controlling micturition. The other group of receptors lies in the wall or the mucosa of the **urethra**. These probably project via the **pelvic nerve**, and certainly do so from the prostatic part of the urethra (Crosby *et al.*, 1962, p. 542). The afferent pathway has been attributed to the **pudendal nerve** (e.g. Iggo, 1977, p. 595; Ruch, 1974, p. 536), but this would probably only be correct for the **penile urethra**. The urethral receptors are stimulated by the flow of urine, and recruit additional micturition activity in the centres of both the brain stem and the sacral spinal cord. Whatever their pathway may be, these receptors supply a *positive feedback* mechanism in micturition.

Possible afferent nerve endings have been shown by light microscopy in the muscle and mucous membrane of the bladder (Crosby *et al.*, 1962, p. 540).

4.14.2 *Nociceptors from pelvic viscera*

Most of the pain pathways from the *bladder, pelvic urethra, prostate, cervix*, the *pelvic part of the descending colon*, and the *rectum* pass through the **pelvic nerves** (Fig. 4.2; Section 4.8.3), and have their cell stations in sacral **dorsal root ganglia**. The acute pain caused by

obstruction of the bladder or pelvic urethra by urinary calculi is probably projected by 'in series' mechanoreceptors in the external muscle layers (Section 4.11.1). Pain pathways from the *anal canal* travel mainly in somatic afferent axons of the **pudendal nerve**.

Surgical experience in man suggests that there are three **pain pathways** from the **bladder**, i.e. the parasympathetic **pelvic nerve**, the sympathetic **hypogastric nerve**, and the somatic **pudendal nerve** (Mitchell, 1953, p. 119). However, those in the pudendal nerve appear to be restricted to the **neck** of the bladder and presumably reach the pudendal nerve via the reflections of the parietal peritoneum forming the ligaments of the bladder. Moreover, cutting the sympathetic pathway in the hypogastric nerve has been reported to make no appreciable difference to chronic pain from the bladder, and therefore it has been concluded that the *principal pain pathways* travel in the **pelvic nerve** (Crosby *et al.*, 1962, p. 540; Williams *et al.*, 1989, p. 1420). On the other hand, Ruch (1974, p. 526), a major authority on bladder innervation, concluded that painful impulses from the dome of the bladder are conducted by the hypogastric nerve, and that the pelvic nerve conveys pain impulses only from the trigone.

Pain pathways in man from the **uterine cervix**, pelvic (sigmoid, in man) part of the **descending colon**, and **rectum**, resemble those from the bladder. They pass mainly through the **pelvic nerve** (Ruch, 1966, Fig. 11 on p. 354), but some also lie in the **pudendal nerve** (Mitchell, 1953, pp. 126, 196). All of these organs possess sympathetic afferent axons, but as for the bladder they appear to contribute little or nothing to the transmission of pain (Mitchell, 1953, p. 126; Crosby *et al.*, 1962, p. 542). The sympathetic afferent axons from the **rectum** travel not only in the **hypogastric nerve** but also along the arteries of these pelvic organs (Williams *et al.*, 1989, p. 1375).

Pain pathways from the **prostate** and **pelvic urethra** probably lie mainly in the **pelvic nerve** (Ruch, 1966, Fig. 11 on p. 354; Mitchell, 1953, p. 126), but some authorities attribute them to the hypogastric nerve (Jänig and Morrison, 1986, Fig. 7 on p. 102; Williams *et al.*, 1989, p. 1168), or in the case of the urethra to both the pelvic nerve and the hypogastric nerve (Jänig and Morrison, 1986, p. 106).

4.14.3 *Receptor pathways of the anal canal*

The ectodermal **cutaneous zone** of the **anal canal** (lined by stratified squamous epithelium) receives a cutaneous somatic nerve supply from the **pudendal nerve**. The endodermal **columnar zone** has an autonomic afferent innervation by both the hypogastric and the pelvic nerves. Fortunately these receptors confer the ability to distinguish reliably between flatus and faeces in the anal canal, except when the faeces are watery as in acute diarrhoea.

> The cutaneous zone is supplied by the **perineal nerves** (inferior rectal nerve in man), which are branches of the pudendal nerve in the dog (Evans and Christensen, 1979, p. 1014) and man (Williams *et al.*, 1989, p. 1373). Pain impulses from the endodermal zone, at least in man (Williams *et al.*, 1989, p. 1373), are transmitted by both the hypogastric and the pelvic nerves.

4.15 Receptors of larynx and their reflexes

The essential design requirements of the larynx are the following: (1) to prevent the entrance of swallowed, and (worse still) vomited, material into the lower airways; (2) to allow the ready access of air during inspiration and expiration without undue resistance to flow; and (3) to permit the removal of mucus from the trachea. To meet these somewhat conflicting requirements the larynx is equipped with a formidable array of receptors and reflexes, including *mechanoreceptor, chemoreceptor, thermoreceptor*, and *nociceptor* capabilities. In addition many mammals, especially man, have adapted the larynx for phonation.

Most of these receptors are situated in the rostral region of the laryngeal wall, i.e. the **vestibule** and **glottis**. They extend caudally to include the **vocal folds**. They are therefore well placed to give early warning of the invasion of oropharyngeal or oesophageal material into the larynx. Their axonal pathway (Fig. 3.3) is in the **cranial laryngeal nerve**. The **recurrent laryngeal nerve** supplies the afferent innervation of the **infraglottic cavity** (Fig. 3.3), i.e. the laryngeal cavity caudal to the vocal folds.

Afferent axons in the **cranial** and **recurrent laryngeal nerves** have their cell station in the **distal vagal ganglion** (Fig. 3.3).

> The *main afferent pathways* from the larynx run in the **cranial laryngeal nerve**, and these are responsible for most of the reflex responses of the larynx including coughing and bronchoconstriction. The afferent innervation of the infraglottic cavity by the recurrent laryngeal nerve is of only minor importance (Karlsson *et al.*, 1988), since there are only a few afferent axons from laryngeal

receptors in this part of the larynx (Widdicombe, 1986b, p. 53).

Although there are so many laryngeal receptors there are no convincing correlations between the microscopy of autonomic afferent nerve endings and electrophysiological activity from laryngeal structures, and only a few indications of correlations between axon activity and reflex effect (Widdicombe, 1986a, pp. 375–387). Plexuses of **free nerve endings**, myelinated and unmyelinated, lie in the mucosa and submucosa, and these may be afferent, though some at least could equally well be efferent. There are also claims of specialized endings, including structures like taste buds around the epiglottis in the lamb and dog, and small encapsulated endings in the submucosa. There are few electron microscopic observations on any laryngeal nerve endings. However, the clinical importance in man of **sleep apnoea**, **sudden infant death syndrome**, and **gastro-oesophageal aspiration syndrome** has stimulated active research into correlations between the histology of receptor endings and axon activity, and between axon activity and reflex effect (Widdicombe, 1986a, p. 375).

4.15.1 *Laryngeal mechanoreceptors*

Tactile receptors at the entrance to the larynx respond instantly to stimulation by inducing the **laryngeal closure reflex (laryngeal constrictor reflex)**. This closes the laryngeal airway by activating the **adductor muscles of the glottis** (especially the *cricoarytenoidalis lateralis*). Stronger mechanical stimulation evokes the **cough reflex** instead of the constrictor reflex. Sustained mechanical stimulation, caused for example by the lodging of a small foreign body in the glottis (in man, in the **laryngeal sinus**, which is the homologue of the **laryngeal ventricle** in the domestic mammals), can maintain the laryngeal closure reflex to the point of suffocation. The laryngeal entrance of the *cat* is particularly sensitive to tactile stimuli and can respond by violent laryngeal spasm during attempts at intubation for anaesthesia. On the other hand, in the *horse* the threshold of sensitivity is so high that a bronchoscope can be inserted through the larynx without any anaesthesia at all.

Deeper in the laryngeal cavity, mechanical stimulation of the **vocal folds** initiates the **expiration reflex**.

The **cough reflex** and **expiration reflex** are designed to clear the airway by an expiratory effort. But the cough reflex begins with an inspiration, and this might draw material into the lower airways and thus lead to **aspiration pneumonia**. The expiration reflex consists of an expiratory effort, which may be followed by coughing or apnoea. Arising as it does from the vocal folds, the expiration reflex is the last line of defence against the entry of oropharyngeal or oesophageal material into the trachea. The **vocal folds** are said to be exquisitely sensitive to mechanical stimuli.

Of the **mechanosensitive receptors** (Widdicombe, 1986a, pp. 375–387), the tactile receptors probably lie very near the surface of the mucosa. Mechanical irritation of the larynx causes the **closure reflex** even if the stimulus is too weak to cause coughing. Puppies, and human babies at birth, lack the **laryngeal closure reflex** and this may be a factor in the **aspiration syndrome** in the newborn.

When evoked by stronger stimulation of the laryngeal tactile receptors, the **cough reflex** begins with a weak inspiration and is followed by the familiar explosive effort to clear the airway. The **expiration reflex** consists of a brief expiratory effort without a preceding inspiration. Its site of origin is specifically the **vocal folds**; mechanical stimulation of the vocal folds causes not coughing but the expiration reflex. Presumably, the role of the expiration reflex is to prevent aspiration of material that touches the vocal folds, whereas the cough reflex might initially draw such material into the lower airways. Thus the expiration reflex may be important in preventing conditions such as **aspiration pneumonia**.

There are many **laryngeal pressure receptors**. These may be less spectacular functionally than the tactile receptors, but they induce an important **upper airway dilator reflex**. The receptors are tonically active. Most of them are excited by a *fall in pressure* in the laryngeal cavity (as in inspiration). Others are stimulated by a *rise in pressure*. Excitation arising from a fall in pressure induces reflex stimulation of the **dilators of the larynx** (notably the **cricoarytenoidalis dorsalis** muscle), and also of the **dilators of the pharynx** (notably the **genioglossus**) and **dilators of the nostrils**. Thus the upper airway dilator reflex enhances the patency of the upper airway.

Other mechanosensitive receptors are '**drive**' **receptors**. These fire in response to *distortion* of the laryngeal wall, particularly during activity of the dilator muscles of the larynx, and probably include receptors in the **laryngeal joints** and **laryngeal muscles**.

Both mechanical and chemical irritation of the larynx can induce reflex **bronchoconstriction**. Coughing and bronchoconstriction are airway reflexes that share the function of protecting the lung from noxious agents (Karlsson *et al.*, 1988).

The peripheral axonal pathway of *all the laryngeal reflexes* described above is presumed to be in the cranial laryngeal nerve. The cell station of the afferent neurons is in the distal vagal ganglion. The receptors themselves have not been identified microscopically.

4.15.2 *Laryngeal chemoreceptors*

The **cough reflex** can be evoked by strong stimulation of **irritant-sensitive chemoreceptors** by irritant gases. Weaker stimulation causes the **laryngeal closure reflex**.

The pathway of these afferents is mainly in the **cranial laryngeal nerve** but is also partly in the **recurrent laryngeal nerve**, the cell stations being in the **distal vagal ganglion**.

Irritant-sensitive chemoreceptors in the larynx are sensitive to *cigarette smoke, ammonia, sulphur dioxide*, and a range of *other irritant gases*; they also respond to *mechanical deformation* (Widdicombe, 1986a, pp. 377, 381).

Laryngeal **water receptors** (responding to distilled water) have been found in the dog, cat, rabbit, and various newborn mammals. The idea of water receptors may seem strange, but is not particularly remarkable since such receptors also occur in lingual taste buds of some species (Section 4.10.2). Laryngeal endings stimulated by water respond primarily to a deficiency in permeant anions, especially chloride, rather than to the low osmolarity of water. In adult mammals the laryngeal water receptors can induce the **cough reflex**, for example by inhalation of aerosols of water. If the stimuli are too weak to cause the cough reflex, they can induce the **laryngeal closure reflex**. The **apnoeic reflex** to water is weak or absent in mature mammals. Other chemical stimuli including cigarette smoke and ammonia can evoke the apnoeic reflex in adults.

In **neonatal mammals** the water receptors evoke the **apnoeic reflex**. This has been found in puppies, newborn lambs, and other mammalian neonates. It can be fatal in anaesthetized neonates. The pathway is in the **cranial laryngeal nerve**, since electrical stimulation of this nerve causes apnoea in most species including man, and cutting it eliminates apnoeic reflexes. Activation of the apnoea reflex from the larynx, perhaps sensitized by inflammation, is a possible mechanism of the **sudden infant death syndrome**.

Contact of water with the epiglottis or larynx can also elicit the **swallowing reflex** (Widdicombe, 1986b, p. 55). This occurs simultaneously with a brief apnoea, and therefore it is likely that the same stimuli and reflex axonal pathway are involved. The maturity and condition of the animal may determine whether the response is swallowing, apnoea, or both.

As stated in Section 4.15.1, stimulation of laryngeal chemoreceptors can induce reflex **bronchoconstriction**.

4.15.3 *Laryngeal nociceptors*

The pain pathways from the rostral part of the larynx as far as the vocal folds are transmitted by the **cranial laryngeal nerve**, and from the rest of the larynx by the **recurrent laryngeal nerve** (Fig. 4.2). The cell stations are in the **distal vagal ganglion**.

> In man, inflammation and irritation of the larynx can cause subjective sensations of irritation, tickling, a desire to cough, rawness, burning, and pain, but it is difficult to correlate these with observations on experimental animals (Widdicombe, 1986b, pp. 49–64). Some irritant stimuli (e.g. ammonia and sulphur dioxide) may initially be restricted to the airway epithelium, but tissue damage may lead to deeper diffusion of mediators and products of cellular breakdown such as histamine, prostaglandins, and bradykinin.
>
> The receptors and their axonal projections are not known. For example, when irritation of the larynx causes both a cough and a sense of rawness it is not known whether or not the two responses share the same afferent axon. There is no evidence of a sympathetic afferent innervation of the larynx, and therefore the cranial and recurrent laryngeal nerves must provide the laryngeal pain pathways.

4.16 Receptors of the tracheobronchial tree and lungs, and their reflexes

There are several types of autonomic afferent pathways from the trachea and lungs, including stretch receptors and irritant receptors. They are all **vagal** (Section 4.3.3). The afferent axons from the trachea enter the vagus via the **tracheal rami** of the **recurrent laryngeal nerve** and of the main trunk of the **vagus nerve** (Section 3.11.2; Fig. 3.3). The afferent axons from the bronchial tree and alveoli join the main trunk of the vagus through the **bronchial rami** (Fig. 3.3). The cell stations of all these pathways are in the **distal vagal ganglion**. Central projections proceed through the **nucleus of the solitary tract** to the **medullary respiratory centre** in the brainstem (Section 11.2; Fig. 11.1).

The **stretch receptors** are of particular importance, since they play a major role in controlling the pattern of **eupnoea** (resting breathing) in mammals generally (though not in man). The receptor endings are in the walls of the trachea and the larger bronchi. They are therefore often known as **bronchial stretch receptors**. When these airways are dilated during inspiration, the receptors are deformed. Their resulting discharges project signals to the **medullary respiratory centre** in the brainstem, reflexly inducing the **inflation reflex** or **Hering–Breuer reflex**. This reflex inhibits inspiration (Section 11.4).

There are also **irritant receptors**. One group lies superficially in the epithelium of the **trachea** and **larger bronchi**. These receptors are sensitive to very fine particles such as dust, and to irritant gases. They also respond to substances produced by cell injury (e.g. histamine). They defend the upper tracheobronchial airways by reflexly inducing *coughing*, *laryngeal closure*, and *mucus secretion*. Another group of irritant receptors (**C-fibre receptors**) extends into the **alveoli**. These respond to similar stimuli, and defend the lower airways by inducing similar reflexes. They also induce *bronchoconstriction*. Bronchoconstriction protects the exchange tissue by increasing the resistance to air flow.

The lung is supposed to be rather insensitive to **pain** (Section 4.4.3), but in man unpleasant sensations are common in respiratory infections and during inhalation of irritant gases, and are also experienced during tracheal and bronchial endoscopy. Lower mammals are unlikely to be exempt from similar sensations.

> Three main groups of receptors in the tracheobronchial tree and alveoli have been extensively studied (Widdicombe, 1977; 1986b, pp. 56–59): **slowly-adapting bronchial stretch receptors**, **rapidly-adapting irritant stretch receptors**, and **C-fibre (J) receptors**. All three are more or less polymodal: the first is primarily mechanosensitive, but also chemosensitive; the second is about equally mechanosensitive and chemosensitive; the third is primarily chemosensitive, but also mechanosensitive. A fourth type of receptor, associated with **neuroepithelial bodies**, has a less well defined physiological role. A few afferent sympathetic pulmonary axons have been encountered, but the sensory innervation of the tracheobronchial tree and alveoli is predominantly vagal (Widdicombe, 1986b, p. 57).

4.16.1 *Slowly-adapting bronchial stretch receptors*

These are responsible for the **Hering–Breuer inflation reflex** (Widdicombe, 1977). The receptor ending is believed to be in the smooth muscle of the trachea and the larger bronchi. A reconstruction from electron micrographs suggests that the ending consists of a compactly branching bare axon closely entwined with collagen fibrils and smooth muscle cells.

The receptors fire during *inflation*, adapting only slowly to maintained distension of the airway. Collapse of the airway may either inhibit or stimulate them. Their volume threshold is low, and many of them are tonically active. Contraction of the adjacent smooth muscle increases their activity, indicating possible vago-vagal feedback control. Their overall action is to *inhibit inspiration* and *prolong expiration*. Besides these mechanosensitive activities, they show some response to endogenous chemicals; bronchoconstrictor drugs such as acetylcholine and histamine increase their activity, probably primarily through contraction of the adjacent smooth muscle.

These slowly-adapting stretch receptors are an important factor in the normal control of eupnoeic breathing in lower mammals (Widdicombe, 1986b, p. 59). However, in man they only act when the tidal volume increases to about three times its resting value, and therefore their function in man seems to be to *prevent over-inflation of the lung* (Guyton, 1986, p. 505). There is no evidence that their signals reach conscious levels.

4.16.2 *Rapidly-adapting irritant stretch receptors*

These occur throughout the **trachea** and larger bronchi, with the greatest concentration at the tracheal **carina** and few or none in the smaller bronchi (Widdicombe, 1977, p. 100). At least some branches are close to the airway lumen (Widdicombe, 1986b, p. 56), probably in the form of bare **intraepithelial axonal endings** which lead into myelinated axons. Both inflation and deflation evoke rapidly-adapting discharges, often with a strong off-response. Responsiveness to light touch and inhaled dust suggest a superficial site in the mucosa. They also respond to irritant gases, and to chemical mediators such as histamine, prostaglandins, and acetylcholine. Their sensitivity increases in pathological conditions including embolism, congestion, and pneumothorax. These are **polymodal receptors**, responding to physiological and pathological conditions (Widdicombe, 1986b, p. 58).

The main reflex responses to stimulation of the rapidly-adapting irritant stretch receptors are *cough* and cough-associated reflexes from the **carina** and **large bronchi**, and *hyperpnoea* from the small bronchi. The cough associated reflexes include *bronchoconstriction, laryngeal closure*, and *mucus secretion*. Some species (mouse and ferret) lack intraepithelial tracheobronchial nerve endings and have no tracheobronchial cough reflex. In general, the irritant receptors contribute to the physiological control of breathing, and also play a role in responses to pathological conditions (Widdicombe, 1986b, p. 59).

4.16.3 *C-fibre receptors*

These (also known as J-fibre receptors) comprise two groups of similar receptors, named **pulmonary** and **bronchial C-fibre receptors** according to their sites, the pulmonary variety being at the alveolar level and the bronchial type in the smaller bronchi (Widdicombe, 1986b, pp. 56, 59). Unmyelinated axons (C-fibres) have occasionally been found actually in the walls of alveoli.

C-fibre receptors respond primarily to endogenous mediators such as *bradykinin, prostaglandins, histamine,* and *acetylcholine*. Some inhaled gases stimulate them. They are also excited by various lung pathologies, especially *pulmonary congestion* (i.e. a rise in pulmonary capillary pressure), *pulmonary oedema, pneumonia,* and *pulmonary embolism*. Furthermore, they are activated by strong *inflation* or *deflation*, depending on the species (Widdicombe, 1986b, p. 59).

The reflex response in most mammals to the stimulation of C-fibre receptors, by either exogenous chemicals or pathological conditions, is *apnoea* followed by *tachypnoea* (rapid shallow breathing). There is also reflex *laryngeal constriction, bronchoconstriction, secretion of tracheal mucus, hypotension,* and *bradycardia,* but apparently not coughing. Thus these receptors yield widespread and profound defensive responses (Widdicombe, 1986b, p. 59).

4.16.4 *Neuroepithelial bodies*

Neuroepithelial bodies (Lauweryns and co-workers, 1974, 1977) consist of clusters of about 10–80 (Krstic, 1984, p. 287) respiratory endocrine cells embedded in the bronchial and bronchiolar epithelium, occurring throughout the entire length of the bronchial tree and even including alveolar ducts (Sections 6.3.1 and 6.12.1); they also occur as single cells. They are much more common in neonates, but do occur in adult mammals, though the incidence varies with the species. The cells are tall columnar, extending from the basal lamina to the airway. The cytoplasm is characterized by **dense-cored granular vesicles** about 100–200 nm in diameter, some of which contain *serotonin*. The cells show a capacity for *amine uptake, decarboxylation,* and *storage* (Breeze and Wheeldon, 1977), thus resembling **APUD cells** (Section 2.40). At their base the cells are innervated by putative afferent and efferent axonal endings, some with synaptic thickenings of a type clearly suggesting efferent innervation (Lauweryns *et al.*, 1974). **Fenestrated capillaries** are close to the bases of the cells.

Exposure of the animal to *hypoxia* or *hypercapnia* decreases the intracellular content of serotonin and promotes exocytosis of the dense-cored granules from the base of the cells. It is suggested that the cells are chemosensitive to the composition of the respiratory gases, and could activate their afferent axonal endings by the release of serotonin, thus inducing respiratory re-flexes through the brainstem (Lauweryns *et al.*, 1977). However, this afferent pathway has not been investigated and its role has not so far been defined (Widdicombe, 1986b, p. 57). The released serotonin could also have a local effect. It is postulated that, by entering the fenestrated capillaries and draining through the bronchopulmonary veins to the pulmonary veins, it could perhaps mediate the **pulmonary vasoconstriction** that is known to be induced by hypoxia or hypercapnia in the neonatal and adult lung (Lauweryns and co-workers, 1974, 1977). Such vasoconstriction could regulate the perfusion:ventilation ratio (Section 6.29) by shunting blood from poorly to better ventilated regions (Lauweryns *et al.*, 1977) (Section 17.21).

Interest in the possible functions of the neuro-epithelial bodies has been further stimulated by the discovery that the cells of the bodies are electrically excitable (Lopez-Barneo, 1994). They possess O_2-sensitive K^+ channels, the activity of which is inhibited by low P_{O_2}, thus showing a remarkable similarity to the granular cells of the carotid body. It has therefore been suggested that the neuroepithelial bodies might complement the well-known arterial chemoreceptor mechanism of the carotid body, particularly in the homeostasis of respiration during the transition from fetal to neonatal life (Lopez-Barneo, 1994).

4.16.5 *Nocisensitive pathways from the tracheobronchial tree*

The very existence of *pain perception* from the **lung** is controversial. It has long been maintained from stimulation experiments in the cat that there are no pain pathways in the vagus caudal to the recurrent laryngeal nerves (see Ruch, 1966, p. 355), and this would exclude the bronchial rami from transmitting pain. Iggo (1977, p. 606) stated that the lungs are not a source of pain. According to Ruch (1966, Fig. 11 on p. 354) the pulmonary (visceral) pleura is 'insensitive'. Williams *et al.* (1989, p. 1271) confirmed that the visceral pleura is insensitive to thermal and tactile stimuli, but that is to be expected from any truly visceral structure; presumably the visceral pleura *is* sensitive to adequate stimuli for visceral pain, such as stretching and chemical irritants. The alveoli of the lungs have been listed as entirely insensitive to pain of any type (Guyton, 1986, p. 599).

However, there is no doubt that unpleasant sensations can be derived from lung receptors (Widdicombe, 1986b, pp. 60–61). Indeed, distressing respiratory sensations during *respiratory infections* and *asthma* must be one of the commonest of all noxious visceral experiences. Insertion of a *tracheal* or *bronchial endoscope* causes a burning sensation that is abolished by anaesthetizing the airways. *Tracheitis* or inhalation of *irritant aerosols* gives an uncomfortable raw feeling, and this too can be eliminated by local anaesthesia of the airways. The sense of tightness suffered during an asthmatic attack is also eliminated by anaesthetizing the airways or the vagus nerve. *Inflation of a collapsed lung* causes an unpleasant tearing sensation. In man, small *pulmonary emboli* may produce no symptoms, but large emboli can cause sharp chest pain that is worse during breathing. Electrical stimulation of the dorsal wall of the left or right main bronchus in man causes pain in the ventral wall of the thorax or in the ventral part of the neck (Comroe, 1975, p. 262). In domestic mammals, pleuritic pain (Blood and Studdert, 1988, p. 313) is found in cattle after thrombosis of the caudal vena cava (Dalgleish, 1991), though the pain may arise from involvement of the pleura rather than the exchange tissue itself.

Healthy young men subjected to high altitude (Paintal, 1995) experience unpleasant sensations in the throat and upper chest, essentially of choking and pressure and occasionally 'burning', inducing a dry cough. It is concluded that these sensations must be transmitted by C-fibre receptors (Paintal's J-receptors).

The pathways for unpleasant pulmonary sensations must be vagal, via either the irritant stretch receptors, or the C-fibres, or both, but the problem is not yet resolved. Whatever axons are involved will join the vagus via the bronchial rami and perhaps via the tracheal rami (Fig. 3.3). The cell stations will be in the distal vagal ganglion. If such nociceptive pathways are confirmed as vagal, they will be the only exception to the principle that pain pathways from the thoracic and abdominal viscera are transmitted by sympathetic nerves (Sections 4.2.2).

4.17 Receptors of the great arteries and their reflexes

Mechano- and chemoreceptors occur on the roots of the embryonic aortic arches (Section 19.2). Since only the third, fourth, and sixth arches persist in mammals, the receptor sites are confined to the derivatives of these arteries: the roots of the left and right internal carotid arteries, the aortic arch, the root of the right subclavian artery, and the root of the pulmonary trunk. The mechanoreceptors respond to stretch. In these sites they are often referred to as **baroreceptors**. The baroreceptor site on the root of the internal carotid artery is known as the **carotid sinus**.

4.17.1 *Arterial baroreceptors*

There are large numbers of baroreceptor endings in the wall of the carotid sinus and aortic arch, concentrated mainly in the adventitia. The receptors are slowly adapting. The higher the pressure in the artery the greater the distension of its wall, and therefore the greater the firing frequency of the receptors (Section 19.4). Increased baroreceptor activity reflexly inhibits the 'cardiovascular centre' in the brain stem, and excites vagal motor neurons in the **parasympathetic motor nucleus of the vagus**. The result is a reflex fall in arterial pressure (Section 19.4).

The peripheral nerve pathway from the carotid sinus is in the **carotid sinus nerve** of the **glossopharyngeal nerve**, the cell station being in the **distal glossopharyngeal ganglion** (Figs 4.3, 19.8). The pathway from the aorta (Figs 3.3, 19.8) and subclavian artery is in the cervical trunk of the **vagus nerve**, or in a separate branch of the vagus known as the **aortic nerve** (depressor nerve), depending on the species. The cell station is in the **distal vagal ganglion** (Fig. 3.3).

Proving that a particular axonal ending responds to a particular stimulus requires electrophysiological recording from the receptor and subsequent identification of the actual ending by electron microscopy. These two steps have only been achieved for very large receptor structures such as encapsulated mechanoreceptors in the skin. However, it has been possible to identify presumptive **aortic baroreceptor endings** by their **ultrastructural characteristics**. These include a greatly expanded diameter of the ending, dense packing with many mitochondria, a surface largely bare of Schwann cell covering, and a close association with elastic or collagen axons. There are also unusual numbers of atypical organelles such as dense bodies and myelin bodies, consistent with rapid turnover of axoplasm due to the continuously repeated deformation of the arterial wall at each heart beat. These features have been consistently observed in both aortic arch (Krauhs, 1979) and carotid sinus endings (e.g. Knoche *et al.*, 1980).

Presumptive **efferent endings**, aminergic or peptidergic, also occur in the wall of the aortic arch and pulmonary trunk (Kienecker and Knoche, 1978) and carotid sinus (Knoche and Kienecker, 1977). These endings are typified by small or large **dense cored vesicles**. They often share the same Schwann cell as the presumptive baroreceptor endings, and could modulate the stimulus threshold of the baroreceptor ending (Knoche and Addicks, 1976). This would be an example of postjunctional neuromodulation (Section 2.37).

The functional characteristics of arterial baroreceptors are considered in Section 19.4. Below a variable threshold of about 30–60 mmHg (4.0–8.0 kPa) a receptor is silent. Above the threshold the firing rate increases roughly in proportion to the increase in pressure, reach-

ing a maximum rate at about 220 mmHg (29.3 kPa). If phasic changes in pressure are applied experimentally by an external hydraulic system, the receptors fire fastest during the most rapid change. Thus the receptor senses both the pressure level and its rate of change.

4.17.2 Arterial chemoreceptors

In mammals the main sites are the left and right **carotid bodies** (Figs 4.3, 19.1–19.3) on the roots of the left and right internal carotid arteries (Section 19.7), and the cluster of **aortic bodies** (Fig. 19.5) between the aortic arch and the pulmonary trunk (Section 19.10).

The carotid and aortic bodies consist of **granular cells** which make synaptic contacts with autonomic afferent axonal endings; there are also supporting cells known as **sustentacular cells** (Fig. 19.6). The afferent axons from the carotid body pass via the **carotid sinus nerve** to the glossopharyngeal nerve, the cell stations being in the **distal glossopharyngeal ganglion** (Fig. 4.3). Those from the aortic bodies run in the **aortic nerve** of the **vagus**, with the cell station in the **distal vagal ganglion** (Figs 3.3, 19.8). Further projections go via the **nucleus of the solitary tract** to the **medullary respiratory centre** in the brainstem (Fig. 19.8).

The axonal endings are excited by a fall in the P_{O_2} of the blood, and also by a rise in the P_{CO_2} or the concentration of hydrogen ions, causing a strong reflex increase in respiration and a minor increase in arterial pressure (Section 19.9).

The granular cells are now believed to be the actual chemoreceptor element in the carotid and aortic bodies (Section 19.9.3).

4.18 Receptors of the heart and their reflexes

4.18.1 Atrial volume receptors: regulation of blood volume

Low pressure stretch receptors in the walls of the left and right atria contribute to the **regulation of blood volume**. The receptors act as **volume receptors**, responding to the varying distension of the atrial walls that accompanies an increase or decrease in blood volume. The axons travel in the

cardiac rami of the vagus (Fig. 3.3). They have their cell stations in the **distal vagal ganglion**, and thence project to the **nucleus of the solitary tract**. From there, neuronal relays connect to the **cardiovascular centre** in the brainstem (Fig. 19.8), and to the **neurohypophysis**.

An *increase in blood volume* stimulates the atrial volume receptors. This reflexly increases glomerular filtration, decreases tubular reabsorption, and inhibits the secretion of antidiuretic hormone. A *decrease* in blood volume has the reverse effects. These mechanisms are considered more fully in Section 22.9.

4.18.2   *Atrial receptors: Bainbridge reflex*

Stretch receptors in the wall of the right atrium and great veins send their axons through vagal cardiac branches. They respond to a rise in venous pressure by inducing a reflex cardiac acceleration (the Bainbridge reflex, Section 22.10).

4.18.3   *Cardiac nociceptors*

In man, these project through **sympathetic cardiac nerves** via the spinal nerves of segments T1–T5 (Fig. 4.2, Sections 4.6, 4.7). The cell stations are in the dorsal root ganglia of these thoracic segments.

4.19   Pan-dysautonomia

This term means a generalized dysfunction of the autonomic nervous system. It is considered at the end of the four chapters on the autonomic nervous system because it can involve autonomic reflex arcs at any point, i.e afferent, integrative, or efferent components.

Pan-dysautonomia is well known as a generally fatal condition in the cat (*feline dysautonomia*) and horse (*equine dysautonomia*, or *grass sickness*), and has also been recorded in the dog and man. The clinical signs suggest widespread involvement of *all three components* of the autonomic nervous system, i.e. the sympathetic, parasympathetic, and enteric nervous systems. However, the disturbances express themselves differently in the various species, depending on

which components are most severely affected. Consequently few prominent clinical features are shared by all species.

One of the most basic signs is *gastrointestinal involvement*. This presents as virtually *complete stasis* in the **horse** (Edwards, 1987), *severe constipation* and inability to defecate in the **cat** (Nash, 1987), and manageable *constipation* in **man** (Mathias, 1987). These disturbances almost certainly arise from failure of the enteric nervous system, but they may be accentuated by deficits in the parasympathetic system, or by hyperactivity of the sympathetic system as in some forms of ileus.

Megaoesophagus (a deficit of the enteric nervous system, Section 3.23.1) is conspicuous in the **cat** (Griffiths and Pollin, 1987), **horse** (Greet and Whitwell, 1987), and **dog** (Schrauwen *et al.*, 1991), but does not occur in **man** (Mathias, 1987). Protrusion of the *nictitating membrane* (sympathetic deficit, Section 2.23.4) is seen in the **cat** and **dog**, but not in the **horse**. *Distension of the bladder* (parasympathetic deficit) occurs in the **cat** (Nash *et al.*, 1982) and **dog** (Schrauwen *et al.*, 1991).

It is evident that in the cat and dog there are extensive indications of *parasympathetic deficits* (dryness of the nose, oral mucosa, and eye; dilated pupil; distended bladder) (Nash, 1987; Schrauwen *et al.*, 1991), whereas in the horse accelerated heart rate (tachycardia) and high levels of circulating catecholamines indicate *sympathetic over-activity* (Edwards, 1987). In man the opposite applies, with a *severe sympathetic deficit* causing postural hypotension (Weyns, 1988, p. 97).

The one feature that seems to be shared by all species is the presence of widespread neuronal and axonal lesions throughout the ganglia and central components of the autonomic and enteric nervous systems (Sharp, 1987).

In both feline and equine dysautonomia there is degeneration not only in sympathetic and parasympathetic ganglia generally, but also in autonomic nuclei in the brainstem and in the intermediolateral grey matter of the spinal cord (Griffiths and Pollin, 1987; Gilmour, 1987). The lesions affect both neuronal cell bodies and axons (Sharp, 1987; Gilmour, 1987). Lesions have also been found in the enteric ganglia in feline (Griffiths and Pollin, 1987) and equine dysautonomia (Gilmour, 1987), and in cases of feline dysautonomia a marked depletion of neuropeptides has been shown in the enteric ganglia even when there was little evidence of neuronal lesions (Vaillant, 1987). Lesions are not confined to the autonomic nervous system, but involve somatic motor components in the neuraxis (e.g. oculomotor and hypoglossal nuclei, and ventral horn) and afferent components (e.g. dorsal root ganglia and vestibular nuclei) (Griffiths and Pollin, 1987; Gilmour, 1987).

Plasma catecholamine levels are markedly higher in grass sickness than in normal horses, and parasympathomimetics have only a very transient effect on gut motility (Edwards, 1987). Increased plasma catecholamines in grass sickness may be an example of the increased sympathetic reflex activity that may con- tribute to ileus (Section 3.23.2). On the other hand, in man there is a substantial reduction in catecholamines in relevant tissues, with hypotension (Mathias, 1987), and in the cat there is bradycardia (Nash, 1987).

Part 2
Respiratory System

Chapter 5
Trachea and Lungs

The respiratory system can be divided into the **upper respiratory tract** and **lower respiratory tract**. The upper respiratory tract consists of the **nasal cavity** and **larynx**. The lower respiratory tract is formed by the **trachea** and the **lungs**.

I EMBRYOLOGY

5.1 Embryology of tracheobronchial tree

A midline furrow, the **laryngotracheal groove**, arises in the floor of the embryonic pharynx. In much the same way as the neural groove forms the neural tube, so the laryngotracheal groove deepens and its lips fuse to form the **laryngotracheal tube**, except at the rostral end where it opens into the pharyngeal cavity. The closure of the lips of the laryngotracheal groove forms two compartments in the embryonic pharynx, namely the larynx and trachea ventrally and the oesophagus dorsally.

The **larynx** develops at the rostral end of the laryngotracheal tube. Caudal to the larynx, the laryngotracheal tube forms the **trachea**. The caudal end of the laryngotracheal tube becomes bifid, and thus gives rise to left and right diverticula which become the left and right **lung buds**. The first divisions of the lung buds form *four* masses in the *right* lung bud and *two* in the left, thus foreshadowing the **cranial**, **middle**, **caudal**, and **accessory lobes** of the **right lung**, and the **cranial** and **caudal lobes** of the **left lung** (Section 5.6.1). Subsequent divisions form the epithelial precursors of the rest of the **bronchial tree** and the **alveoli**.

Since the embryonic pharynx is a part of the foregut, its epithelium is derived from the **endoderm**, and therefore the epithelial lining of the laryngotracheal tube is also endoderm. Consequently the entire epithelial lining of the larynx, trachea, bronchial tree, and alveoli is endoderm.

The epithelium of the tracheobronchial tree acquires a covering of **splanchnic mesoderm**; this forms the smooth muscle and elastic connective tissue of the tracheobronchial tree, and it also develops the profuse capillary plexus that becomes the alveolar blood supply. The capillary plexus gets its blood from the pulmonary arteries, which arise from the sixth arterial arch (Section 15.5).

As the developing **lung buds** (gemmae pulmonales) rapidly enlarge, they migrate caudally and bulge into the pleural coelomic cavity from the dorsal body wall, and thus become covered with splanchnic mesoderm (mesoderma splanchnicum). The mesothelial surface of the coelomic splanchnic mesoderm covering each bulging lung becomes its **visceral pleura**.

The bifid lung bud develops initially into the left and right **principal (primary) bronchus**. Each principal bronchus then divides into two daughter branches, a process referred to as **dichotomy** (Weibel, 1984, p. 217). It is generally assumed that dichotomy is repeated until the whole of the branching bronchial tree has been formed. The number of dichotomous branchings varies with the species, there being at least 23 dichotomous generations in the human lung (Weibel, 1984, p. 277) but only 7–9 in the mouse (Krahl, 1964, p. 254). As just stated, the first order branches are the two **principal bronchi**. The second order branches are, of course, the branches of the principal bronchi: they form the **lobar bronchi**, including the **tracheal bronchus** in the ruminants and pig. The third order branches become the **segmental bronchi**.

This simple description of the branching of the bronchial tree conceals a multitude of complications. The word 'dichotomy' may suggest a division into two *equal* branches, but the word means simply 'division into two' and conveys no information about the *form* of the two daughter branches. Hare's (1975) drawings of teased lungs from the adult horse, ox, pig, and dog, show that, in fact, the daughter branches are often dissimilar in diameter, and that the larger one often goes straight on and the smaller one comes off at an angle. Weibel (1984, p. 274) designates such a system of unequal branching as **irregular dichotomy**, as opposed to **regular dichotomy** in which the two daughter branches *are* the same size. Furthermore, as Krahl (1964, p. 255) pointed out, the mode of branching is by no means uniform; it is indeed often dichotomous, but it can also be **trichotomous** (division into three daughter bronchi). The trichotomous formation occurs when a parent bronchus forms two daughter branches, one on each side, the parent bronchus going straight on. This is probably what is meant by the term 'monopodial branching', as used by Amis and McKiernan (1986) in their account of *bronchial endoscopy* in the dog (Section 5.10.1). **Monopodium** is a botanical term meaning 'single foot'; it is defined as a single primary axis from which all main lateral branches develop. A poplar tree is a good example. This monopodial system describes quite well the architecture of the bronchial tree within, for example, the caudal lobe of the lung of the **pig** (Hare, 1975, Fig. 41-11, and p. 1296); here, the principal bronchus runs axially through the lobe, giving off branches at irregular intervals from all its sides, dorsal and ventral as well as lateral. Thus it does resembles a poplar tree, in which the main trunk is straight and gives off branches on all sides. The arboreal allusion to bronchial 'tree' still holds good, but it has to be the right sort of tree. 'Monopodial' is not an ideal term, since 'single foot' means little in the lung, but no better alternative seems to be available. For further discussion of the patterns of bronchial branching in the adult, see Section 6.1.

It is customary to distinguish three stages in the development of the lung, **glandular** (pseudoglandular), **canalicular**, and **alveolar**, in that order (Williams *et al.*, 1989, p. 239). These are not the happiest of terms, since 'canalicular' suggests canalization and therefore implies that the 'glandular' stage consists of solid cords. Both stages are tubular, but the epithelium is tall and the lumen narrow in the glandular stage, whereas the reverse applies to the canalicular stage (Weibel, 1984, pp. 220–221). Alveoli form in the alveolar stage (Latshaw, 1987, p. 120).

The **alveoli** arise as solid cords of cuboidal epithelial cells, which are eventually invaded by the lumen of the **bronchioles** (Noden and de Lahunta, 1985, p. 282). The branching of the bronchial tree is virtually complete at birth in domestic mammals (Latshaw, 1987, p. 121), but continues postnatally in man (Williams *et al.*, 1989, p. 239). Alveoli continue to form postnatally in mammals generally. The more active the neonate the more advanced is its alveolar development at birth (Latshaw, 1987, p. 120); thus of the domestic mammals the ruminants are the most advanced, next the horse and pig, and then the carnivores, and less advanced than all of these are man and rodents.

In utero, the tracheobronchial tree and alveoli are filled with **lung fluid**. This is probably formed by secretion from the epithelium of the conducting airways and transudation from the blood plasma, and appears to flow steadily into the amniotic fluid (Weibel, 1984, p. 223).

Surfactant (Section 6.25) first appears in the lung fluid of man between the 18th and 25th weeks of gestation (Weibel, 1984, p. 264). Sometimes it is sufficiently abundant by the 26th or 28th week to enable a newborn baby to survive in a protected environment. In sheep, surfactant is first produced at 125–130 days (Noden and de Lahunta, 1985, p. 283). Insufficiency of surfactant in neonates is a major factor in the **respiratory distress syndrome of the newborn** (Section 16.26.1).

Shortly after the laryngotracheal tube arises, its lumen becomes obliterated by adherence of the walls (Williams *et al.*, 1989, p. 238) or by an epithelial plug (Latshaw, 1987, p. 118). However, when the components of the larynx begin to differentiate the tube is recanalized.

II   TRACHEA

5.2   Topographical anatomy of trachea

The trachea runs in the midline from the larynx to the root of the lung, and therefore has a cervical part and a thoracic part.

The **cervical trachea** lies parallel to the cervical vertebral column, but is always widely separated from the vertebrae by the massive **longus colli** muscle which covers the vertebrae ventrally (Fig. 5.1). At the cranial end of the neck, the **oesophagus** is dorsal to the trachea (Fig. 5.1, C2). In the rest of the neck the oesophagus is on the left of the trachea (Fig. 5.1, C4). Ventrally the trachea is covered by the paired strap-like **sternohyoideus** and **sternothyroideus muscles**. In the midline of the caudal part of the neck the trachea is also covered by the much thicker and wider **sternocephalicus muscle**. However, from the middle of the neck cranially (Fig. 5.1, C4), the left and right sternocephalicus muscles progressively diverge dorsolaterally (Fig. 5.1, C2) and this makes it easier to palpate the trachea in the *cranial* part of the neck. Dorsolaterally the trachea is related on each side to the **vagosympathetic trunk**, the **common carotid artery**, the lymphatic **tracheal trunk**, the **internal jugular vein** (in species that have it), and the **recurrent laryngeal nerve** (Fig. 5.1). Except at the cranial end of the neck, these vessels and nerves are displaced laterally on the left side by the oesophagus (Fig. 5.1, C4).

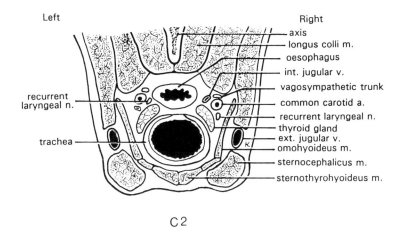

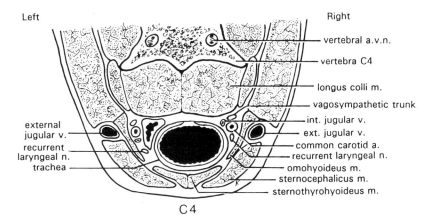

Fig. 5.1 Caudal views of transverse sections through the neck of a horse at the levels of the second and fourth cervical vertebrae, to show the relations of the trachea. At the cranial end of the neck (C2, second cervical vertebra) the oesophagus lies between the trachea and the vertebra. In the middle segments of the neck (e.g. C4, fourth cervical vertebra) the oesophagus lies on the left of the trachea, and the trachea is in contact with the longus colli muscle. The sternocephalicus muscle overlies the trachea in the ventral midline, caudal to C4. At C4, sternocephalicus is beginning to diverge dorsolaterally, allowing exposure of the trachea for tracheotomy. At C2 the divergence is greater, making palpation of the trachea easier. At C4 on the right side the trachea is related to the common carotid artery and its satellite nerves and vessels. On the left side these vessels and nerves are displaced laterally by the oesophagus. The recurrent laryngeal nerve is relatively closely related to the trachea on the right side, and to the oesophagus on the left.

The **thoracic trachea** begins at the **thoracic inlet**. At this point the trachea reaches its most ventral level (Fig. 25.2). Therefore fluids introduced artificially into the trachea as in **transtracheal aspiration** (Section 25.7) tend to pool in this pendent segment of the trachea and can be aspirated from there. As the trachea passes through the thoracic inlet, it is sandwiched between the oesophagus on the left and the first rib on the right. Caudal to the thoracic inlet both the trachea (Fig. 18.1) and the oesophagus ascend dorsally as they pass through the **cranial mediastinum** (Fig. 9.1). The oesophagus climbs dorsally more than the trachea, and on reaching the level of the heart (Fig. 9.1) has returned to its original position in the midline, dorsal to the trachea. Both the trachea and oesophagus pass to the right of the aortic arch (Fig. 19.5), as would be expected since the mammalian aortic arch arises in the embryo from the *left* fourth arterial arch (Section 15.5).

Having reached the dorsal aspect of the base of the heart (Fig. 19.5), the trachea ends at the **tracheal bifurcation**, where it divides into the left and right **principal bronchi** (primary bronchi). The tracheal bifurcation lies at about the level of the fifth rib or fifth intercostal space (Section 5.4.2; Fig. 25.2). The division is marked by the **carina** (Section 5.3.1). The division is unequal, the *right principal bronchus* having a *greater diameter* than the left (Fig. 25.3A), as is predictable from the greater size of the right lung. The left principal bronchus diverges laterally more than the right lung. These relationships affect the entrance of *foreign bodies* into the lungs (Section 5.10.2).

In the pig and ruminants the trachea gives off the tracheal bronchus (Fig. 5.4, Section 5.6.1) to the cranial lobe of the right lung a substantial distance before it bifurcates into the left and right principal bronchi; this affects the length of an *endotracheal tube* used for *anaesthesia* (Section 5.4.3), since it is necessary *not* to block the entrance to the tracheal bronchus by using a tube that is too long.

The position of the trachea relative to the oesophagus at the thoracic inlet seems to vary. A short distance cranial to the inlet, the oesophagus may regain its position dorsal to the trachea, or it may do this a short distance after entering the thorax. Within the actual inlet the oesophagus usually lies somewhat to the left of the trachea, and dorsal to the cranial vena cava.

In the ox, sheep, goat, and pig, the tracheal bronchus (bronchus trachealis) arises from the trachea at about the level of the third rib (Hare, 1975) (Section 5.4.3).

In the horse, the tracheal bifurcation may be slightly more caudal than in the other species, being related to the fifth or sixth intercostal space (Hare, 1975, p. 521).

The trachea is attached at its cranial end to the cricoid cartilage of the larynx (by the cricotracheal ligament). At its caudal end, it is attached to the lung by the two principal bronchi; it is also attached to the dorsal surface of the fibrous pericardium and to the diaphragm by connective tissue. Because of its attachments at each end, the trachea is kept under constant elastic tension.

The diameter of the trachea changes during breathing. In deep inspiration, the thoracic trachea becomes slightly wider because of the fall in pressure in the pleural cavity, while the cervical trachea become slightly narrower because of the fall in intratracheal pressure (von

Hayek, 1960, p. 69); the reverse happens in forced expiration (de Lahunta and Habel, 1986, p. 202).

The length of the trachea also varies during breathing, and with the movements of the larynx in swallowing (Hare, 1975, p. 134). The tracheal bifurcation moves caudally during inspiration and cranially during expiration. Strongly extending the head moves the bifurcation cranially with the larynx.

The movements of the trachea have been quantified in man (von Hayek, 1960, p. 72). The larynx moves cranially about 3 cm during swallowing and about 7 cm when the head is tilted far backward; the latter movement shifts the bifurcation of the trachea about 1 cm cranially (von Hayek, 1960, p. 72). During deep inspiration the bifurcation of the trachea moves caudally in man from the level of the cranial border of the fifth thoracic vertebra to the sixth (Williams *et al.*, 1989, p. 1259). The attachment to the diaphragm probably contributes substantially to this inspiratory movement, though the elastic traction of the bronchi must help (von Hayek, 1960, p. 73).

The attachment to the diaphragm in man takes the form of a continuous sheet of collagenous connective tissue caudal to the tracheal bifurcation. This sheet spreads out between the two bronchi, both lungs, and the tendinous centre of the diaphragm (von Hayek, 1960, pp. 70–72). Most of its fibres run longitudinally into the dorsal wall of the fibrous pericardium, the caudal vena cava, and the diaphragm; oblique fibres run criss-cross from the principal bronchus to the pulmonary ligament of the opposite side of the body.

The craniocaudal motility of the trachea affects radiographic interpretation, at least in man, as does the position of the body. In man in the supine position the entire thoracic trachea lies near the vertebral column, separated from it only by the oesophagus. In the prone position the bifurcation moves about 2 cm from the vertebral column, thereby stretching the dorsal mediastinum. Comparable studies of the effects of breathing and posture on the site of the trachea in domestic mammals seem not to have been reported.

The recurrent laryngeal nerve is sometimes regarded as being enclosed within the carotid sheath together with the common carotid artery, vagosympathetic trunk, and internal jugular vein, but it can be incorporated within the fascia of the trachea on the right side and that of the oesophagus on the left (de Lahunta and Habel, 1986, p. 169).

5.3 Structure of trachea

The trachea consists of horse-shoe shaped 'rings' of hyaline cartilage. The incomplete dorsal gap of each 'ring' is closed by fibrous tissue, which also links adjacent rings. The lumen is lined by mucosa.

5.3.1 *Tracheal cartilages*

Being incomplete dorsally (Fig. 5.2), the cartilages tend to spring open at the top because of their inherent elasticity, and this keeps the membranous dorsal wall under tension. The dorsal gap

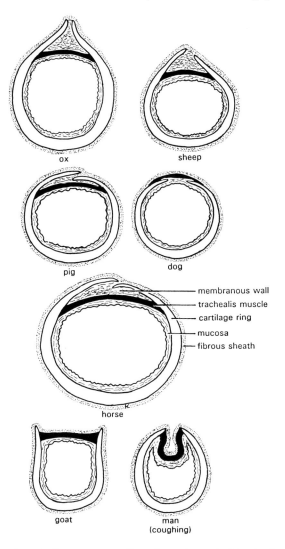

ox
sheep
pig
dog

- membranous wall
- trachealis muscle
- cartilage ring
- mucosa
- fibrous sheath

horse
goat
man
(coughing)

Fig. 5.2 Transverse sections through cervical tracheal rings, fixed in situ, of ox, sheep, pig, dog, horse, and goat together with a semi-schematic transverse section of a human thoracic tracheal ring during coughing. These shapes are a general guide to the characteristics of each species, but can vary in unfixed specimens and in different parts of the trachea. The human thoracic tracheal ring shows the reduction in lumen caused by infolding of the dorsal membranous wall, resulting in increased linear velocity of expelled air during coughing.

can be narrowed by the **trachealis muscle**, which consists of smooth muscle (Fig. 5.2). The elasticity of the cartilages assures the patency of the trachea, but at the same time allows the trachealis muscle to adjust the dead space of the trachea and its resistance to air flow. The flexibility of this design is therefore functionally superior to that of some other vertebrates, such as birds, in which the tracheal cartilages are complete rings.

The most caudal tracheal cartilage is modified to form the **tracheal carina** (Latin: carina, the keel of a ship), at about the fourth to sixth intercostal space (fifth or sixth, in the horse). The carina is a median vertical ridge of cartilage, its sharp edge projecting cranially; it extends from the dorsal to the ventral wall of the last tracheal ring, and thus splits the tracheal airway into the left and right principal (primary) bronchi. The first bronchial cartilage of the left and right **principal bronchus** is attached by an annular ligament to the last tracheal cartilage and also to the carina, thus founding the tubular framework of the two principal bronchi.

The **shapes** of the tracheal cartilages (cartilagines tracheales) seem to vary rather unpredictably within a species, but the differences are nevertheless used to identify the species in the dissection room, abattoir, and post-mortem room. The lumen of the **ox** and **sheep** tends to be narrowed transversely, and the cartilages may have a dorsal ridge (Fig. 5.2). In the **horse** (Figs 5.1, 5.2) the lumen is generally narrowed dorsoventrally. In the **pig** and the **carnivores** (Fig. 5.2) the cartilages are more nearly circular; in the pig and sometimes in the horse, the tips of the cartilages just overlap, but in the carnivores the tips are quite widely separated. The carnivores differ from the other species in that the trachealis muscle is visible on the *dorsal* surface of the trachea (Fig. 5.2). In **man** and the **goat** (Fig. 5.2) the cartilages are U-shaped.

The different **shapes** of the tracheal cartilages are useful as a rough guide to the species, but are not entirely reliable because they may vary within a species. In the **ox** and **sheep** a dorsal ridge is said to be more prominent in a fresh specimen than in a specimen fixed in situ (Nickel *et al.*, 1973, Figs 341–349; Hare, 1975, p. 927). In the **horse** the relationships are reported to be the other way round, since the dorsal tips of the cartilages are supposed to overlap in the specimen fixed in situ (Fig. 5.2), but to be separated by a substantial gap in the fresh specimen (Nickel *et al.*, 1973, Fig. 349). Yet in illustrations of transverse sections of the horse's neck, which were almost certainly obtained from fixed specimens (e.g. Popesko, 1972, Vol. 1, Figs 165–168; de Lahunta and Habel, 1986,

Fig. 7-1; Dyce *et al.*, 1987, Fig. 18-28) the tracheal carti-lages show a large dorsal gap, as in Fig. 5.1.

One possible cause of such variations in the shapes of the tracheal cartilages is the **trachealis muscle** (musculus trachealis), which when contracted draws the tips of the cartilages together but when relaxed allows the gap be-tween the tips to widen. This may be one reason why fresh specimens apparently differ from fixed specimens, and could explain the dorsal overlapping in fixed equine specimens; on the other hand, the diminished promi-nence of the dorsal ridge in fixed ruminant specimens is the opposite from what would be expected. However, specimens fixed in situ are presumably affected by the action of the fixative on surrounding tissues as well as on the trachealis muscle, and this may create further differ-ences. Apparently the effects of fixation have not been tested.

The shapes of the tracheal cartilages also vary along the series of cartilages (Ackernecht, 1943, p. 475). For instance in the **sheep** the more cranial rings tend to resemble the drawing of the sheep's ring in Fig. 5.2, whereas in the middle of the series they tend to be U-shaped like those of the **goat** (Fig. 5.2), and in the caudal third of the trachea the tips overlap as in the pig (Fig. 5.2) (Hare, 1975, p. 928). In the **horse** the most cranial cartilages are almost circular (Fig. 5.1, C2), but as the series progress caudally they soon become flattened dorsoventrally (Fig. 5.1. C4) giving transverse to dorsoventral diameters at a ratio of about 1.4:1; in the thoracic trachea the diameters once again become nearly equal and sometimes the dorsoventral diameter is the greater (Hare, 1975, p. 512).

The cartilage of the **carina** (carina tracheae) may be derived from the most caudal tracheal cartilage, the most cranial bronchial cartilage of the left and right principal bronchus, or a combination of both (Hare, 1975, p. 134). In some species there is no cartilage but only fibrous tissue, and this is known as a membranous carina (Hare, 1975, p. 134).

The **number** of rings varies between species and within species. In the pig there are 32–36 rings, in the cat 38–43, in the dog 42–46, and in the horse and ruminants 48–60; adjacent rings may fuse partly or completely, this being commonest in the pig and least common in rumi-nants, and in the horse several small cartilage plates are interposed between the tips of the last few cartilages before the bifurcation (Ackernecht, 1943, p. 476).

The elasticity of the tracheal cartilages contributes to the efficacy of **coughing**. Coughing is an important de-fence mechanism of the lung (Section 7.6.2). It begins with a deep inspiration followed by closure of the glottis. Forcible contraction of the expiratory muscles then raises the pressure in the pleural cavity. This compresses the bronchi and thoracic trachea. Radiographic studies show that in man, and presumably in other species in which the cartilages of the thoracic trachea gape widely

at their tips (e.g. goat), the area of the lumen is greatly reduced by the inwards buckling of the dorsal soft tissues (Fig. 5.2) (Hayek, 1960, p. 69); there is evidence that in man the aperture can be reduced to a mere slit by the additional tucking of one cartilage lip under the other (Comroe, 1975, p. 230). Compression of the lungs is believed to reduce the bronchial lumens to slits (Guyton, 1986, p. 475). Sudden opening of the glottis allows the air in the lungs and thoracic trachea to explode outwards, thus blasting foreign matter through the laryngeal outlet. The compression of the lumens of the thoracic trachea and bronchi contributes to a very high linear velocity of the escaping air (up to $100 \, \text{mile} \, \text{h}^{-1}$ ($160 \, \text{km} \, \text{h}^{-1}$) in man) (Guyton, 1986, p. 475).

In the large herbivores, **vascular canals** occur in the hyaline cartilage (Hare, 1975, p. 132). In old animals the cartilage may undergo **calcification** and **ossification**.

5.3.2 *Fibrous components*

The cartilage rings are enclosed in a fibrous sheath (tunica adventitia), which extends over the outer and inner surfaces of the rings and fuses with the perichondrium. The sheath also forms the **annular ligaments** (tracheal ligaments, ligamenta annularia) which join the successive cartilages, and the **membranous wall** (paries membranaceus) (Latin: paries, wall) that fills the dorsal gap between the tips of each cartilage.

The fibrous sheath consists mainly of collagen but includes some elastin. The **collagen fibres** cross *diagonally*, thereby allowing *changes* in the *diameter* of the lumen and in the *lengths* of the annular ligaments. The elastic fibres provide *elastic recoil* after stretching (Section 6.9).

5.3.3 *Mucous membrane*

The surface of the mucosa has many **longitudinal folds**, which permit *dilation* of the lumen. The lining is a typical **respiratory epithelium**, com-prising pseudostratified columnar ciliated cells and goblet cells (Fig. 6.3A), contributing to the **mucociliary escalator** that defends the lung (Sec-tion 7.2). The lamina propria comprises loose con-nective tissue, but with many elastic fibres. Most of the tubular **mucoserous glands** and **lymphoid nodules** lie in the submucosa. The mucoserous glands contribute **tracheobronchial secretions** (Section 7.3) to the mucous carpet of the mucociliary escalator.

The epithelial lining of the trachea also includes **brush cells (microvillous epitheliocytes), respiratory endocrine cells** (Feyrter cells, neuroendocrine cells), and **epithelial serous cells**. For the characteristics of these cells see Section 6.3.1.

5.3.4 *Innervation of trachea*

Motor **parasympathetic** pathways supply the smooth muscle of the trachea via **tracheal rami** from the recurrent laryngeal nerve and tracheal rami from the main trunk of the vagus (Section 3.11.2; Fig. 3.3). The goblet cells and mucoserous glands receive an excitatory motor innervation from both vagal and sympathetic nerves, the latter being, if anything, the more productive (Section 6.12.2). The tracheal rami also carry **afferent pathways** from the trachea; these include stretch receptors mediating the Hering–Breuer inflation reflex (Section 4.16.1, 11.4), as well as irritant receptors and nociceptors (Sections 4.16.2 and 4.16.5).

5.4 Applied anatomy of trachea

The trachea can be **palpated** in the live animal. In the horse and ox this is easier at the cranial end of the neck, where the left and right **strenocephalicus muscles** have diverged laterally from the trachea leaving it covered only by the sternohyoideus and sternothyroideus muscles (Fig. 5.1, C2). In the dog it is possible to get the tips of the fingers around the dorsal surface of the trachea and feel the flattened membranous dorsal wall. The divergence of the sternocephalicus muscles is a good site for **tracheotomy** in the horse (Sections 5.4.2, 25.6).

Intubation of the trachea for anaesthesia is in general use in small and large animals (Section 25.6). The diameter and length of the tube are important. A tube should not be so narrow that it creates an avoidable resistance to airflow, nor should it be so long that it seals off the entrance into the tracheal bronchus in a pig or ruminant or blocks one of the two principal bronchi.

The pendent part of the trachea at the thoracic inlet allows the pooling of fluid introduced for lavage of tracheal secretions, and is therefore convenient for transtracheal **aspiration** (Section 25.7).

5.4.1 *Palpation of thyroid gland*

The thyroid gland of the live horse can be palpated at the cranial end of the trachea, immediately caudal to the larynx (see Fig. 5.1, C2). If the sternocephalicus muscle is displaced laterally, the thyroid gland can be seized between the fingers. The gland is mobile and slips readily from the grasp. The gland can also be palpated in the live dog, especially when the gland is enlarged. It is the only exclusively endocrine gland that can be palpated during a physical examination.

5.4.2 *Site for tracheotomy*

In the horse, the divergence of the sternocephalicus muscle provides a good site for tracheotomy (Hare, 1975, p. 511) (Section 25.6). By palpation, the tracheal rings can be counted from the larynx to rings 4–6, where tracheotomy is conveniently performed in this species (de Lahunta and Habel, 1986, p. 69). The left and right parts of the sternothyrohyoideus muscle can be separated in the midline to expose the trachea.

5.4.3 *Intubation*

Endotracheal tubes have been in general use for balanced anaesthesia in small and large animals since the 1950s. The selection of a suitable endotracheal tube depends on the anatomy of the laryngeal and tracheal airway, and dead space and resistance to gas flow (Lodge, 1969).

The position of the opening from the trachea into the tracheal bronchus in relation to the thoracic cage is important in intubation of the pig and ruminants (see immediately below). In the ox the opening occurs about 15 cm cranial to the bifurcation into the left and right principal bronchi (bronchus principalis) (Lodge, 1969). Hare (1975, p. 934) estimated the distance from the tracheal bronchus to the bifurcation to be about 10 cm in the ox, and 5 cm in the sheep and goat. Hare (1975) noted that, in the ox, sheep, goat and pig, the opening into the tracheal bronchus lies at about the level of the third rib (Section 5.2).

The position of the tracheal bifurcation (bifurcatio tracheae) into the left and right principal bronchi in relation to the rib cage is even more important. In all the domestic species and man the bifurcation lies at the level of about the fifth rib or fifth intercostal space, or in the horse the sixth intercostal space (Fig. 25.2), (Hare, 1975, pp. 134, 521, 1294, 1572; Sisson and Grossman, 1969, pp. 535, 550; Williams *et al.*, 1989, p. 1259). The bifurcation may move caudally during inspiration (Section 5.2).

The length of an endotracheal tube is therefore critical. A tube that is too long and projects from the mouth increases the dead space needlessly; the 'to and fro' soda lime absorption system is particularly likely to create dead space (Taylor, 1988). If a tube is too long and is inserted too far into the trachea, it can seal off the entrance to the tracheal bronchus in a pig or ruminant (Lodge, 1969), thereby creating a major venous-to-arterial shunt in the cranial lobe of the right lung (Fig. 6.9B, Section 6.30). If pushed yet further, an over-long tube could even block one of the two principal bronchi (Lodge, 1969), thus depriving a whole lung of ventilation. In view of the relationships of these major bronchi to the thoracic cage, the caudal end of an endotracheal tube should therefore not pass beyond the level of the first rib (Lodge, 1969).

The diameter of an endotracheal tube is also critical. A tube with a diameter that is too small can greatly increase the resistance to gas flow, since resistance is inversely proportional to the fourth power of the radius (Section 6.14). When a normal animal is anaesthetized it can tolerate a modest increase in resistance, but an animal with a respiratory disorder may be unable to do so. Anatomically, the limiting factor in horses is simply the internal diameter of the trachea, since a tube that fills the trachea can be easily passed through the larynx. But in the ox a tube that perfectly fills the trachea will not go through the larynx, and therefore the limiting factor in this species is the transverse diameter of the rima glottidis (Lodge, 1969). Any gap between the tube and the tracheal wall is closed by an inflatable cuff.

The passage of a tube through the nasal or oral cavity, and the profound species variations in the mechano-sensitivity of the laryngeal mucosa, are discussed under bronchoscopy in Section 25.8.

5.4.4   *Transtracheal aspiration*

This technique is discussed in Section 25.7. The pendent part of the trachea, at the thoracic inlet, pools the fluid introduced for lavage of tracheal secretions and is therefore convenient for aspiration.

5.4.5   *Compression and collapse of trachea*

The natural transverse narrowing of the tracheal rings in the ox is said to make the trachea vulnerable to lateral compression by local forces (Dyce *et al.*, 1987 p. 612). In young calves, callus formation on a fractured first rib can compress the trachea and cause inspiratory dyspnoea (Gasthuys *et al.*, 1992). In the dog, collapse of

tracheal rings or the membranous dorsal wall occurs mainly at the thoracic inlet, and can also happen to the thoracic trachea (de Lahunta and Habel, 1986, p. 202). On palpation, the cartilages feel flaccid and can be easily compressed; in advanced stages the cartilages become extremely flattened dorsoventrally (Reif, 1971, p. 77). This condition usually affects miniature or toy breeds, causing a functional stenosis with reduced exercise tolerance and a cough (Blood and Studdert, 1988, p. 925). Radiographs taken during inspiration, expiration, and coughing may be needed for diagnosis (de Lahunta and Habel, 1986, p. 202). A similar dorsoventral collapse is regarded as not uncommon in the horse (Carrig *et al.*, 1973). Instead of being more or less circular in cross section, the cartilages of the cervical trachea become abnormally flattened dorsoventrally and the dorsal membranous wall is thinly stretched, the cartilage looking like the shaft of a bow and the membrane the string. The lumen may be reduced to a thin slit, so that mild exercise causes marked dyspnoea. A possible cause is paralysis of the trachealis muscle.

5.4.6   *Transection of trachea*

Transection of the trachea can occur from trauma, particularly from hyperextension of the head and neck in cats (Blood and Studdert, 1988, p. 926).

5.4.7   *Spread of infection*

At the thoracic inlet, the trachea (with the oesophagus) is covered with the loose fascia of the neck which continues into the cranial mediastinum. This fascia provides a pathway for the spread of fluids and infection (Section 9.4) of particular importance in leaking wounds of the oesophagus (Dyce *et al.*, 1987, p. 630).

5.4.8   *Radiographic anatomy*

An acute angle, open caudally, is formed as the thoracic vertebrae arch dorsally from the tracheal bifurcation. This angle is diagnostically important in thoracic radiology in the dog (Section 24.9.1), but varies with the breeds (de Lahunta and Habel, 1986, p. 202).

III   GROSS ANATOMY OF THE LUNG

5.5   External features

The **texture** of the lung is soft, spongy, and elastic, and crepitates when squeezed. After removal from the unpreserved body the normal postnatal lung still contains some air and therefore floats on water. Its light weight reflects its name, which comes from the Old English word 'lungen' meaning light. In the meat trade, the lung is still known as 'lights'. A lung that is filled with fluid from pathological processes will sink. Likewise the lung of a fetus or a new-born animal that has not breathed feels firm and will not float.

When the unfixed lung is removed from the body it contracts. It can be reinflated, but instantly collapses again when the inflationary pressure is removed. About one third of this **elastic recoil** is caused by elastic fibres (Section 6.9), and most of the rest comes from surface tension (Section 6.25).

The **colour** of the normal lung depends on how much blood it contains. If the animal was bled out at death the colour is pale pink, though with a yellowish tinge due to its very abundant elastic tissue. In an animal that has not been bled out at death the colour is a dark pink-red. The blood typically takes about 3–5 hours to clot. If the lungs are not removed immediately after death the blood gravitates (**hypostasis**) from the upper to the lower levels of a lung, and even from the upper to the lower lung if the cadaver is on its side, the lowest parts are then dark red and the upper parts light red. In dogs and cats living in towns the lungs have a greyish colour due to permanent deposits of inhaled carbon particles in **interstitial macrophages** (**anthracosis**) (Section 6.20); the carbon is inert and small amounts produce no significant adverse effects. Similar deposits in the bronchial lymph nodes can make them black.

The **dimensions** of the right lung are greater than those of the left in all species, and especially in the ruminants and the pig. The relatively large size of the right lung displaces the heart somewhat to the left side (Fig. 25.1).

The **root** of the lung is the cluster of structures that together enter the medial surface of the lung. The components of the root are the **principal bronchus**, the **pulmonary blood vessels**, **bronchial blood vessels**, **bronchial lymphatic vessels**, and the **pulmonary plexus** consisting of the sympathetic and parasympathetic **bronchial nerves** (Sections 2.10.3, 2.10.4, 3.11.4, and 6.12). The principal bronchus is the first order of branching of the tracheobronchial tree. The zone on the medial surface of the lung where these structures actually penetrate the lung tissue is known as the **hilus** of the lung (Fig. 5.3).

The **ventral border** of the lung (Fig. 5.3) separates the costal (lateral) surface from the medial surface of the cranial, middle, and caudal lobes. It is thin, and slides into the **costomediastinal recess** at each inspiration (Section 9.6.2). At the level of the heart, the ventral border forms the **cardiac notch** (Section 5.6.2). The **basal border** (the green line in Fig. 5.3) separates the **diaphragmatic surface** of the lung (green in Fig. 5.3) from the **costal surface**. The basal border is thin, and slides in and out of the **costodiaphragmatic recess** (Section 9.6.1) during breathing. The basal border is important clinically, in the physical examination of an animal, because its position at the end of expiration forms the caudoventral boundary of the area of percussion and auscultation of the lung (Section 23.7). The movements of the ventral and basal borders into their recesses play a major role in ventilating the lungs during breathing (Section 5.7).

In the horse the right lung (pulmo dexter) is, as usual, larger than the left lung (pulmo sinister), but the difference (which is due mainly to the greater mediolateral thickness of the right lung) is smaller than in the other domestic species (Dyce *et al.* 1987, p. 496). Ackerknecht (1943, pp. 497, 502) reported that the right lung exceeds the left in the horse by about 15% in weight and about 33% in volume; in the adult ox and calf the right lung exceeds the left by about 45% in weight.

The formal description of a lung recognizes an apex, a base (or diaphragmatic surface, facies diaphragmatica), two other surfaces (costal and medial, facies costalis and medialis), and three borders (dorsal, margo dorsalis; ventral, margo ventralis; and basal, margo basalis) (Fig. 5.3) (Hare, 1975, pp. 135, 518). The terms apex (apex pulmonis) and base (basis pulmonis) arise from the resemblance of each lung to half a cone, the two lungs together making a complete cone that fits the conical thoracic cavity. The **apex** is the cranial end of the lung, and occupies the **pleural cupola** (Section 9.6.5). The **base** of the lung, i.e. the **diaphragmatic surface** of the lung (green in Fig. 5.3), fits over the dome of the diaphragm. The **medial surface** has two parts, vertebral (pars vertebralis) and mediastinal (pars mediastinalis) (Fig. 5.3). Its **vertebral part** is in contact with the bodies of the thoracic vertebrae. The **mediastinal part** of the medial surface faces the mediastinum. In specimens *fixed in situ* the mediastinal part moulds itself to the

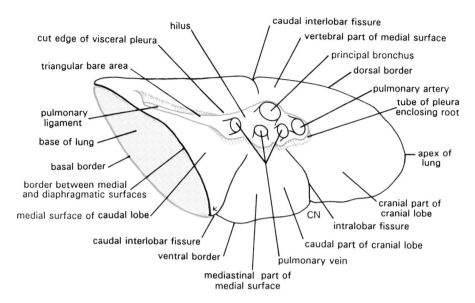

Fig. 5.3 Diagram of the medial surface of the left lung of the dog, to show the lobes, hilus, pulmonary ligament, root, and basal border. The hilus is an area bare of visceral (pulmonary) pleura. The visceral pleura is reflected along the border of the hilus, forming a tube of pleura (green) that encloses the root and passes medially to become continuous with the mediastinal pleura. The pleural tube around the root is incomplete caudally, where it contributes to the pulmonary ligament. A triangular bare area on the medial surface of the lung extends caudally from the hilus. The visceral pleura is reflected from this area as a dorsal and a ventral sheet; these sheets fuse to form the pulmonary ligament (green). The root is formed by the principal bronchus, arteries, veins, and nerves that penetrate the medial surface of the lung at the hilus. CN denotes the region of the cardiac notch, which is barely detectable in the left lung of this species. The medial surface of the lung is divided into a vertebral part which is dorsal and in contact with the thoracic vertebrae, and a mediastinal part which is in contact with the mediastinum. The diaphragmatic surface is green. The basal border (green) separates the diaphragmatic surface from the costal surface. The relationships of the hilus, the components of the root, and the basal border, are similar in the other domestic species and man, but there is no true pulmonary ligament in the ox. The relationships are also essentially similar in the right lung.

organs in the mediastinum, and therefore has cardiac, aortic, and oesophageal **impressions** (impressio cardiaca, aortica, oesophagea). The **ventral border** (Fig. 5.3) separates the costal surface from the medial surface of the cranial, middle and caudal lobes. The **basal border** (margo basalis) (Fig. 5.3) separates the diaphragmatic surface from the costal surface. This definition of the basal border is the one intended by the *Nomina Anatomica Veterinaria* (Habel, 1992, p. 190), and is in general use by clinicians. In his otherwise definitive account of pulmonary anatomy, Hare (1975, pp. 135, 520) defined it as separating the diaphragmatic surface not only from the costal but also from the medial surface, thus making it the entire oval rim around the diaphragmatic surface.

The **hilus** of the lung (hilus pulmonalis) (Fig. 5.3) is an area of the medial surface of the lung, dorsal to the cardiac impression, which is not covered by pleura (Section 9.2). At this bare area, the left lung is directly attached to the right lung by mediastinal connective tissue.

The **root** of the lung (radix pulmonalis) is formed by the **principal bronchus** and its accompanying vessels and nerves. In all species the bifurcation of the trachea lies at about the fifth rib or fifth intercostal space, but may reach the sixth intercostal space in the horse (Section 5.4.3). The distinction between the root and the hilus is not obvious, but the essential difference is that the root consists of a bundle of structures that 'root' themselves into the lung, whereas the hilus is the area on the medial surface of the lung where the root actually goes in. In all the domestic species and in man the components of the root are orientated around the principal bronchus (Fig. 5.3), in essentially the same relationships (Hare, 1975, pp. 519, 932, 1293, 1571; Williams *et al.*, 1989, Fig. 8.34B). The **principal bronchus** is dorsal in the root (and of course in the hilus). Cranial or cranioventral to the principal bronchus is the **pulmonary artery**. The **pulmonary veins** surround the principal bronchus and pulmonary artery ventrally and ventrocaudally. The bronchial artery (or arteries) lies on the principal bronchus. The **pulmonary lymphatics** surround the principal bronchus.

The nerves form the **pulmonary plexus** (Section 6.12), which is divided into dorsal and ventral parts; the dorsal part lies on the dorsal aspect of the principal bronchus, and the ventral part lies cranioventral to the principal bronchus in association with the pulmonary artery. The pulmonary plexus contains the autonomic afferent pathways from the lungs (Section 4.16), and vagal parasympathetic preganglionic fibres (Section 3.11.3) and sympathetic motor postganglionic fibres (Sections 2.10.3 and 2.10.4).

These relations of the bronchus to the vessels and nerves also hold in the mediastinum (Hare, 1975, p. 136). In the ruminants and pig, the tracheal bronchus of the right lung (Section 5.6) forms a second smaller root (Dyce *et al.*, 1987, p. 157). Also associated with the root of the lung are the tracheobronchial lymph nodes (Section 7.9.1).

The bronchus, vessels, and nerves that form the **root** are all embedded in connective tissue. The whole root complex is contained in a tube of pleura that passes from the mediastinal pleura to the visceral pleura on the medial surface of the lung. However, this pleural tube is incomplete on its caudal surface; here, the pleura is reflected caudally as the pulmonary ligament.

The **pulmonary ligament** (ligamentum pulmonale) (Fig. 5.3) is a double membrane of pleura that is stretched horizontally and caudally between the root of the lung, the mediastinum, and the medial surface of the lung. It attaches to the mediastinum simply by becoming continuous with the mediastinal pleura (Fig. 9.5). Its attachment to the medial surface of the lung is associated with a triangular area on the medial surface of the lung, caudal to and continuous with the hilus, that (like the hilus) is not covered by pleura (Fig. 5.3). Along the dorsal and ventral borders of this bare triangular area, the visceral pleura is reflected off the medial surface of the lung as a dorsal and a ventral horizontal sheet (Fig. 5.3). These dorsal and ventral sheets pass medially, converge, and become continuous with the double pleural sheet of the pulmonary ligament (Hare, 1975, p. 131) (Fig. 5.3). At its caudal end, the pulmonary ligament has a curved, falciform, free border (Ackerknecht, 1943, Fig. 911; Williams *et al.*, 1989, p. 1270).

The **right pulmonary ligament** becomes continuous with the mediastinal pleura that covers the oesophagus (Williams *et al.*, 1989, p. 1270); its attachment extends caudally as far as the oesophageal hiatus of the diaphragm, where it ends by becoming continuous with the diaphragmatic pleura (Dyce *et al.*, 1987, p. 400). The **left pulmonary ligament** becomes continuous with the mediastinal pleura that covers the aorta (Dyce *et al.*, 1987, p. 400). The pulmonary ligament occurs in the horse (Sisson and Grossman, 1969, p. 536; Hare, 1975, p. 517); a distinct pulmonary ligament is also present in the pig, dog, and man, but a true ligament is absent in the ox (Ackerknecht, 1943, p. 333).

5.6   The lobes of the lung: lobar bronchi

In all the domestic species the lungs have lobes. The lobes are separated by deep **fissures** or indentations, except in the horse (Fig. 5.4); because of the absence of fissures, the lobes are not distinctly defined in the horse. The fissures are deepest in the carnivores, giving the impression that the lobes dangle loosely from the hilus.

The trachea divides asymmetrically at the **carina** into the left and right **principal bronchi** (Section 5.2, Fig. 25.3A). Each lobe is supplied by a **lobar bronchus**, which arises directly from the principal bronchus. Since the principal bronchus is the first order branch of the tracheobronchial tree, the lobar bronchus is a second order branch (or a second order bronchus). The concept of 'order of bronchus' becomes important when defining bronchi in **bronchoscopy** (Sections 5.10.1, 25.8). Accompanying the lobar bronchus within its lobe are a pulmonary artery, a pulmonary vein, and a bronchial artery. (For lung lobectomy, see Section 25.11.)

5.6.1 *Species variations in lobes*

In all the domestic species except the horse, the **right lung** has four lobar bronchi (1–4 in Fig. 5.4) supplying four lobes, namely the **cranial**, **middle**, **caudal**, and **accessory lobes**. In **ruminants** the right lung looks as though it has five lobes, but as is shown in Fig. 5.4, the two most cranial of these are supplied by the same lobar bronchus (no. 1); these are therefore named the **cranial** and **caudal parts** of the **right cranial lobe**. In the **ruminants** and the **pig** the lobar bronchus (no. 1) that supplies the right cranial lobe arises from the trachea, and is known as the **tracheal bronchus** (Section 5.2).

The right lung of the horse appears at first sight to be fundamentally different from that of the other domestic species. It may appear to lack lobes altogether; however, the lobes are there, although the fissures between them are not well-defined. But even after the existence of lobes is recognized, there appears to be one lobe missing from both the left and the right lung (the middle lobe). In the **horse** a fissure in the right lung

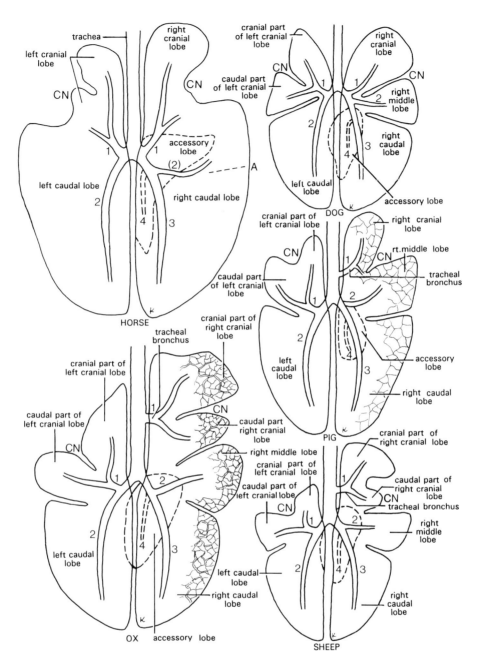

Fig. 5.4 Dorsal view diagrams of the lungs of domestic species to show the lobes of the lungs and the lobar bronchi that supply them. The trachea bifurcates into the left and right principal bronchi. The lobar bronchi are branches of the principal bronchus, except that in the ruminants and pig the lobar bronchus 1 to the right cranial lobe arises from the trachea and is known as the tracheal bronchus. In all species except the horse, the right lung has four lobes (cranial, middle, caudal, and accessory) supplied by lobar bronchi 1 to 4, respectively. In the horse the middle lobe is nearly always absent. The broken line, A, across the caudal lobe of the horse, indicates where the fissure between the middle and caudal lobes would be if the middle lobe were present; in the absence of the middle lobe, bronchus (2) of the horse contributes to the caudal lobe. In the ruminants the cranial lobe is divided into cranial and caudal parts (both parts being supplied by bronchus 1), giving the appearance of one more lobe than in the pig. The accessory lobe is ventral and largely invisible from this view, and is therefore shown in broken lines. The left lung has two lobes in all species, cranial and caudal (supplied by lobar bronchi 1 and 2 respectively, but note that 1 and 2 in the left lung are not intended to indicate homology with lobar bronchi 1 and 2 in the right lung). In all species except the horse the left cranial lobe is divided into cranial and caudal parts. The fissures between the lobes are deepest in the dog and cat. Connective tissue septa give the surface of the lung a marbled appearance, known as lobulation. This is particularly obvious in the ox and only slightly less so in the pig (shown only on the edge of the lung in the diagrams). In the sheep and horse it is very much less conspicuous, and in the dog it is entirely indistinct.

between the middle and caudal lobes (indicated at A, in Fig. 5.4) is usually not developed; thus the right lung of the horse nearly always has only three lobes, i.e. cranial, caudal, and accessory, supplied by the three lobar bronchi 1, 3, and 4 in Fig. 5.4. Nevertheless, bronchus 2 is still there in the right lung of the horse, but instead of supplying its own lobe (the middle lobe in the other species) it contributes to an enlarged caudal lobe.

The presence of the **accessory lobe** on the right lung only is one reason why the right lung is bigger than the left. The accessory lobe lies more or less in the ventral midline, sandwiched between the caudal lobes of the right and left lungs. It occupies its own private pocket of pleura, the **mediastinal recess**, formed between the mediastinum and the **plica vena cava** (Section 9.6.3).

In all the domestic species including the horse the **left lung** has only two lobar bronchi (1 and 2 in Fig. 5.4), supplying only two lobes, the **cranial** and **caudal lobes**. However, in all except the horse the cranial lobe is clearly divided into two parts, both parts being supplied by the same bronchus (no. 1 in Fig. 5.4); these are named the **cranial part** of the **left cranial lobe** and the **caudal part** of the **left cranial lobe**.

The **terminology** of the lobes is now based on the bronchi, but used to be based on the fissures. The earlier names are still employed in some clinical literature. The cranial lobes (lobus cranialis) were previously known as the **apical lobes** (the right apical lobe of ruminants being named as two parts, cranial and caudal, just as the right cranial lobe is now named as two parts), the caudal lobes (lobus caudalis) were the **diaphragmatic lobes**, and the accessory lobe (lobus accessorius) was the **intermediate** or **mediastinal lobe**. These older alternatives are unlikely to be troublesome, since both the old and the new terms are equally meaningful topographically. Confusion can arise, however, over the lobes in the middle. What is now the right middle lobe (lobus medius, pulmonis dextri) was previously called the **right cardiac lobe**; the lobe of the left lung that is now the caudal part of the left cranial lobe (pars caudalis, lobus cranialis, pulmonis sinistri) was known as the **left cardiac lobe**. The old terminology is topographically valid, since these two 'lobes' are related to the heart in both the right and the left lung; however, as Fig. 5.4 shows, these lobes arise from different lobar bronchi on the right and left sides.

In the **horse** a fissure between the middle and caudal lobes of the right lung (indicated at A, in Fig. 5.4) is usually not developed (Hare, 1975, p. 135). However, a relatively large bronchus (no. 2, in Fig. 5.4) arises from the right principal bronchus and supplies a cranioventral segment of the caudal lobe of the right lung (cranial to line A in Fig. 5.4); this segment corresponds fairly well in position and size with the middle lobe of the right lung in the other species (Hare, 1975, p. 521). Ackerknecht (1943, p. 478) also specified a 'ramus bronchialis cardiacus for the middle lobe' of the horse, despite omitting a 'middle lobe' in the lobation of this species. This bronchus of Hare and Ackernecht, labelled (2) in Fig. 5.4, may be the homologue of lobar bronchus 2 in the right lung of the other species. From experience of bronchoscopy in the horse, Derksen (1990, p. 78) remarked on the close correspondence of this bronchus to the bronchus of the right middle lobe in other species, and named it the 'middle segmental bronchus'.

In man the accessory lobe of the right lung is absent (Hare, 1955). Hence the right lung usually has a cranial (superior), middle, and caudal (inferior) lobe, and the left lung has a cranial (superior) and caudal (inferior) lobe.

The right principal bronchus in man has a larger diameter and deviates less from the axis of the trachea than the left bronchus (Krahl, 1964, p. 247), factors which affect the direction taken by foreign bodies (Section 5.10.2). The right principal bronchus has a greater diameter than the left in the horse (Fig. 25.3) (Dyce *et al.*, 1987, p. 501), and the left one diverges from the trachea at a greater angle (Derksen, 1990, p. 78). Since the right lung is so much larger than the left in all the domestic species, the right principal bronchus is presumably always greater in diameter than the left. This could cause foreign bodies to enter the right principal bronchus rather than the left (Section 5.10.2).

The relationships of a lobar bronchus to its accompanying pulmonary artery and pulmonary vein vary with the species. In the ruminants, pig, and horse, the three structures are close together, but in the cat, dog, and monkey, the pulmonary vein runs an independent course through the lobe to the hilus (McLaughlin *et al.*, 1961).

5.6.2 *Cardiac notch*

The **cardiac notch** is a gap in the **ventral border** of the left and right lungs (CN in Figs 5.3 and 5.4), which allows the pericardium to make contact with the thoracic wall.

Its position varies slightly between the species, but in principle is predictable from the general position of the heart, which lies between the third and sixth ribs (Section 20.5); thus the notch on both the left and the right side is typically centred on the ventral quarter of about the fourth rib (Fig. 5.5).

As might be expected from the slight displacement of the heart to the left side by the greater

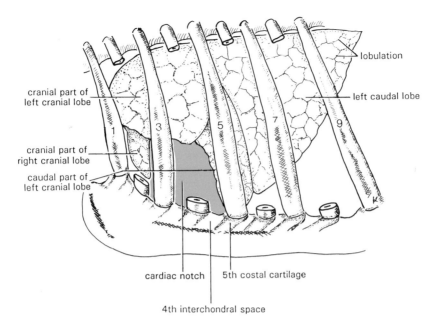

cranial part of left cranial lobe

cranial part of right cranial lobe

caudal part of left cranial lobe

lobulation

left caudal lobe

cardiac notch | 5th costal cartilage

4th interchondral space

Fig. 5.5   The left cardiac notch of an adult ox, drawn from a preserved cadaver. The region of the notch is shown green. The cranial boundary of the notch lies under rib 3 and the caudal boundary lies at the cranial edge of rib 5. The cranial boundary is formed by the cranial part of the cranial lobe of the right lung, which extends to the left side of the thorax. The surface of the heart is framed by the notch. (Redrawn from material kindly supplied by Dr. W.C.D. Hare.)

size of the right lung, the notch is generally more extensive on the left side (though in the dog it is more extensive on the right side). The heart should make contact with the left and right thoracic walls at the cardiac notch, at least during the expiratory phase of breathing. However, the notch is markedly reduced during inspiration when the ventral border of the lung expands into the **costomediastinal recess**. Nevertheless, it provides a valuable 'acoustic window' to the heart for **echocardiography** (Section 24.15). The question whether or not the cardiac notch also affects the **area of cardiac dullness** when the heart is percussed is discussed in Section 23.9.2.

The **cardiac notch** (incisura cardiaca pulmonis dextri, sinistri) is a distinct feature in the preserved cadaver, in which the lungs have been fixed in full expiration. It can then usually be recognized in both the left and the right lungs of the horse, ox, sheep, pig, dog, and cat. In all these species except the dog, the **left** notch has a substantially wider area than the right. Essentially this is because in the horse, ruminants, and pig the cranial part of the right lung is much more bulky than the cranial part of the left lung. Thus in the ruminants and pig the right

cranial lobe and middle lobe have together a much greater volume than the left cranial lobe, and in the horse the right cranial lobe is much bigger than the left (Fig. 5.4); consequently in all these species the heart has less contact with the thoracic wall on the right side than the left.

The wider area of the left cardiac notch would seem to be consistent with the observation of clinicians that the **area of cardiac dullness** (Section 23.9) is greater on the left side of the thorax than the right. In the dog, however, the area of the right cardiac notch is greater than the left; nevertheless, in this species, as in the others, the area of cardiac dullness is larger on the left side presumably because of the thinness of the intervening lung tissue. Moreover, in all species the area of the notch must change from moment to moment during breathing, and is markedly reduced, even on the left side, when the thin ventral border of the lung expands into the **costomediastinal recess** during inspiration. See Section 23.9 for discussion of the **area of cardiac dullness** in **cardiac percussion**.

Fortunately, in view of the growing interest in echocardiography (Section 24.15), Hare (1975) supplied a thorough account of the topographical anatomy of the **cardiac notch** in the various species, as seen in the typical preserved cadaver. In the **horse** (Hare, 1975, p. 519) the left cardiac notch is exceptionally large, allowing the pericardium to lie in direct contact with the thoracic wall from the third to the fifth intercostal space. The shape of the left notch is roughly quadrilateral. It extends dorsally from the ventral ends of ribs three to six, reaching about 10 cm from the ventral end of the fourth rib. On the right side the notch is much smaller, extending from the third rib to the fourth intercostal space. The shape of the right notch is usually triangular, the apex being about 8–10 cm dorsal to the ventral ends of ribs three and four. In the **ox** (Hare, 1975, p. 932), the left notch is extensive, spreading over the ventral third of the third rib, third intercostal space, fourth rib, and fourth intercostal space (Fig. 5.5); its cranial border is formed by the caudal edge of the cranial part of the cranial lobe of the *right* lung, which comes over to the left side of the thorax. The right notch is small and variable in size, permitting a small area of contact between the heart and thoracic wall in the ventral part of the fourth rib and the adjacent intercostal spaces. In the **sheep** and **goat** (Hare, 1975, p. 932), the left notch lies on the ventral part of the fifth rib and fifth intercostal space. In the **pig** (Hare, 1975, p. 1294), the left notch is shallow dorsoventrally but wide craniocaudally, and includes the ventral third of the second and third intercostal spaces and the ventral end of the fourth intercostal space. As in the ox, the cranial end of the space is bounded by the cranial lobe of the *right* lung. The right notch is deep dorsoventrally but narrow craniocaudally, allowing the heart to contact the right thoracic wall in the region of the ventral end of the fourth rib and the adjacent intercostal spaces. In the **dog** (Hare 1975, p. 1572) the right notch is much more extensive than the left, but even then it only allows the heart in its pericardium to be related to the thoracic wall over a small area. On both sides it lies opposite the ventral ends of the third, fourth, and fifth intercostal spaces. In the **cat** (Hare, 1975, p. 1572), the right notch is moved one space caudally, i.e. to the fourth, fifth, and sixth intercostal spaces; on the left side it lies at the fourth, fifth, sixth, and seventh intercostal spaces. It will be apparent that in all of these species, except perhaps the cat, the cardiac notch will be covered by the triceps brachii muscle (Fig. 23.1, Section 23.3). Therefore, to use the cardiac notch as an acoustic window in echocardiography, the limb must be drawn forward.

5.7 Movements of the lung during breathing

In resting breathing, the main movement of the lung as it expands during breathing is by the caudal lobe into the **costodiaphragmatic recess** (Section 9.6.1). At the end of a resting expiration, this recess is only a potential space in the pleural cavity, where the dome of the diaphragm lies against the thoracic wall. When the diaphragm contracts, its dome pulls away from the thoracic wall (Fig. 10.3C); this opens the recess (Section 10.6.3), and the **basal border** of the caudal lobe of each lung moves in, though without filling the recess completely. If a transparent window were made in the thoracic wall, caudal to the so-called **area of auscultation**, e.g. about half way down rib 9 in the ox (Fig. 23.2B) and dog (Fig. 23.2C), the basal border of the lung would be seen to slide caudoventrally into the costodiaphragmatic recess during inspiration and to disappear craniodorsally on expiration. In the intact live animal, the peripheral limit of the costodiaphragmatic recess is the **costodiaphragmatic line of pleural reflexion** (Section 23.8), since it is along this line that the costal (parietal) pleura becomes continuous with the diaphragmatic (parietal) pleura.

A similar potential space in the pleural cavity lies between the mediastinum and the thoracic wall, the **costomediastinal recess** (Section 9.6.2; Fig. 9.1). The increase in the transverse and dorsoventral diameters of the thorax during inspiration (Section 10.6) opens this recess and draws in the ventral border of the lung, probably obliterating the cardiac notch.

The movements of the lung into the costodiaphragmatic and, though to lesser extent, into the costomediastinal recess are a major factor in ventilating the lung during breathing.

The changing position of the basal border of the lung during inspiration has to be taken into account when attempting to hear the sounds of the living lung (**auscultation**) through the thoracic wall (Section 23.7.1).

The medial surface of the lung moves very little, owing to the attachments of the root and hilus, and the relative immobility of the mediastinum during breathing. The dorsal border and apex of the lung also move only slightly, since the vertebral column and pleural cupola are relatively immobile. It seems to be generally believed that the separation of the lobes by deep fissures lubricated by serous membranes allows the lobes some freedom to move individually (Hare, 1975, p. 136; Dyce *et al.*, 1987, p. 158), and thereby to occupy instantly whatever space is made available by the respiratory movements of the thoracic cage. Although such movements have been observed in man, opinions differ about their characteristics (von Hayek, 1960, p. 104), and descriptions are far from clear.

5.8   Lobules of the lung: interlobular septa

On the surface of the lung a mosaic of polygonal areas is visible through the visceral pleura, giving a marbled appearance known as 'lobulation'. The boundaries of these areas are formed by septa of pulmonary connective tissue, the interlobular septa. The septa extend from the depth of the lung to its surface, where they are more or less obvious depending on the species.

In the ox the septa are very thick, causing the lobulation to be prominent both on the superficial surface of the lung (Fig. 5.4) and on the cut surfaces of slices of the lung. In the pig lobulation is again conspicuous (Fig. 5.4), but less so than in the ox. In the sheep, goat, and horse, lobulation is very much less distinct. In the carnivores it is almost invisible, septa being represented by only incomplete strands of connective tissue. The degree of lobulation is an aid to identifying the species from which a lung may have come.

The lobulation seen on the surface of the lung has no agreed structural relationship to the airways in either the domestic mammals or man, and there is much confusion about such relationships.

Some anatomical and histological reference books make little or no attempt to define a lung lobule in terms of the airway on which it is based (e.g. Krahl, 1964, p. 241 in his seminal review of lung morphology). Junqueira and Carneiro (1983, p. 369) recognized a 'pulmonary lobule'; this is supplied by a bronchiole, leading into the apex of a pyramidal area of pulmonary tissue enclosed by connective tissue septa which admittedly are often incomplete. Others distinguished a **primary (principal) pulmonary lobule** which is based on a particular component of the airway, and a much larger **secondary pulmonary lobule** which embraces a number of primary lobules and is enclosed by the connective tissue septa visible on the surface. The component used for the basis of the **primary lobule** ranges from a single alveolar duct (Miller, 1947, p. 41) to a single terminal respiratory bronchiole (Krstic, 1984, p. 4).

The *Nomina Histologica* (1992, p. 37) bravely takes the plunge and clearly defines a **primary pulmonary lobule** (lobulus pulmonis primarius) as a respiratory bronchiole (Section 5.14) with all of its associated alveolar ducts, alveolar sacs, and alveoli. But some mammals, for example the mouse, have no respiratory bronchioles (Krahl, 1964, p. 254). However, basing the primary pul-

monary lobule on a respiratory bronchiole is physiologically sound, since as Weibel (1984, p. 273) pointed out, the primary pulmonary lobule is then the all-important unit of airways that is actually responsible for gas exchange. True to this principle, Weibel (1984) widened the definition by basing the primary pulmonary lobule not merely on a single respiratory bronchiole, but on a **first order** respiratory bronchiole; in some species such as man and dog, one primary pulmonary lobule could then contain three or more generations of respiratory bronchioles, with all their alveolar ducts, alveolar sacs, and alveoli. (Weibel (1984) and others use the term respiratory **acinus** as a synonym for the primary lobule of the lung.)

The definition of a **secondary pulmonary lobule** (lobulus pulmonis secundarius) remains confused (Williams *et al.*, 1989, p. 1276). The confusion has not been resolved by the *Nomina Histologica* (1994, p. 37), which states only that a secondary lobule contains 'about 50 primary lobules and is delineated by interlobular septa'.

Von Hayek (1960, p. 111) found it impossible to identify any reliable structural principles for defining the relationship between the airways and the **septa** (and hence the secondary lobules) in the human lung, because of the total lack of structural uniformity. Enormously varying volumes of lung are enclosed by septa; in some parts of the lung there are no septa at all, so that the tissues of adjacent zones blend; some large areas receive one and sometimes even two substantial bronchi yet are not correspondingly subdivided by septa; some small areas bounded by septa receive only a single small respiratory bronchiole.

The lungs of seven mammalian species were explored in some detail by McLaughlin *et al.* (1961) and Tyler *et al.* (1971), and three more mammalian species were mentioned by Tyler *et al.* (1967). In the ox, sheep, and pig, the **interlobular septa** are thick, complete, and fuse to a thick visceral pleura, thus completely enclosing secondary lobules. In these species, the interlobular septa presumably account for most of the lobulation (marbling) that is so conspicuous on the surface of the lung. In the horse and man, the septa are thick but haphazardly arranged and incomplete, and therefore the secondary lobules are incompletely developed; the visceral pleura is thick. In the dog, cat, Rhesus monkey, rabbit, rat, and guinea pig, there are no septa but only incomplete strands of connective tissue, so that secondary lobules are absent; the visceral pleura is extremely thin. For further discussion of the structure and vascularity of the pleura see Sections 9.7 and 9.9.

In the sheep and goat, lobulation on the surface is clearly visible only on the cranial and middle lobes of the right lung, and the cranial lobe and the basal border of the caudal lobe of the left lung (Hare, 1975, p. 934).

5.9   Bronchopulmonary segments: segmental bronchi

A bronchopulmonary segment is supplied by a **segmental bronchus**. A segmental bronchus is defined as a third order branch of the tracheobronchial tree, the first order being the principal (primary) bronchus itself and the second order being a lobar bronchus branching off the principal bronchus (Section 5.6). A segment is a wedge-shaped piece of lung, the apex of the wedge forming the junction with the segmental bronchus and the base forming part of the surface of the lung. Adjacent segments are separated by planes of connective tissue which are continuous with the visceral (pulmonary) pleura.

The concept of the bronchopulmonary segment is useful in human pulmonary surgery, where resection of diseased segments is practised (Section 25.11). The term is also used by bronchoscopists in veterinary medicine, but otherwise has limited currency.

The segmental bronchi of the dog are shown diagrammatically in Fig. 9.3.

The definition of a segmental bronchus as being a third order bronchus is that used by Hare (1975, p. 136). A segmental bronchus can also be defined as a primary branch of a lobar bronchus (Williams *et al.*, 1989, p. 1261), which is of course the same as the previous definition. (See also Section 5.10.1, for a different usage of the term 'segment' in bronchoscopy.)

A bronchopulmonary segment, or lung segment, is a relatively large and more or less independent area within the lung. It represents an anatomical, ventilatory, and pathological unit, of which the orifice lies in a large lobar bronchus and is recognizable in bronchoscopy. However, because of **collateral ventilation** (Section 6.3.2), segments are not totally isolated during ventilation.

A segment can be isolated in either the fresh or fixed lung by breaking down its intersegmental connective tissue septa (Hare, 1955). Such **intersegmental septa** are recognizable in the sheep (Hare, 1955) and man (Williams *et al.*, 1989, p. 1263), and are very thick in the ox (Dyce *et al.*, 1987, p. 626). Details of variations in the density of the septa have not been reported in other species, but presumably they are best developed in species with well-defined interlobular septa (ox, sheep, pig, horse and man).

On the basis of defining a segment as a unit supplied by a primary branch of a lobar bronchus, Hare (1955) found 12 segments in the right lung of the sheep, and

eight in the left lung. Segments can be identified in the horse (Hare, 1975, p. 521). The pig is reported to have 14 segments in the right lung and ten in the left (Jericho, 1968), or ten and six (Hare, 1975, p. 1295) (Fig. 17.4). In man there are ten segments in the right lung and ten in the left (Williams *et al.*, 1989, pp. 1261–1263; *Nomina Anatomica*, 1989, p. A45).

Because the intersegmental septa reach the surface of the lung, they contribute to the marbling known as lobulation, but they are not solely responsible for it. Interlobular septa (Section 5.8) are presumably the main cause of marbling.

5.10   Applied anatomy of the lung

Percussion and auscultation of the lungs in the physical examination of an animal are considered in Sections 23.5–23.7. The anatomy of the lung as revealed by radiography and other imaging techniques is surveyed in Chapter 24. Bronchioscopy is considered in Chapter 25.

5.10.1   *Bronchoscopy*

The flexible fibreoptic endoscope has opened the bronchial tree of large and small domestic mammals to various diagnostic and therapeutic procedures (Section 25.8), and standard texts on veterinary medicine now contain information on bronchoscopy. The need to communicate bronchoscopic data, so that sites observed by a bronchoscopist can be accurately found at a second examination, has understandably prompted the reconsideration of bronchial terminology. Amis and McKiernan (1986) proposed a system for identifying canine airways in which letters and numerals designated the order of origin and orientation of 'segmental' and 'subsegmental' bronchi; 'rudimentary' bronchi were also mentioned. Unfortunately, although the proposed system is no doubt workable, none of these terms was discussed or defined, and it appears that the term 'segment' was not confined to third order bronchi (the usual anatomical definition, Section 5.9); herein lies the seed of future confusion, bronchial branchings being already quite complex enough.

Anyway, Amis and McKiernan (1986) observed bronchoscopically a number of 'segmental' bronchi arising from the lobar bronchus of each of the cranial, middle, caudal, and accessory lobes of the right lung, and the cranial and caudal lobes of the left lung, of the dog. For example, in the **lobar bronchus of the right caudal lobe**, the first 'segmental' bronchus arose from the dorsal wall at about the level of the lobar bronchus of the accessory lobe. Caudal to this point, a series of 'segmental' bronchi arose from the dorsal and ventral wall, totalling 5–15. In the **lobar bronchus of the left caudal lobe**, 4–13 'segmental' bronchi arose from the dorsal and ventral wall. All the 'segmental' bronchi of the lobar bronchi of the cranial and caudal lobes of the right and left lungs had either a dorsal or a ventral orientation, thus offering an anatomical basis for the ventral (i.e. pendent, see Section 5.10.3) parts of the lung as predilection sites for disease. The authors reported that, in the small or medium-sized live dog of 25 ± 7 kg, seven 'segmental' bronchi in the right lung and six in the left could be entered readily with a bronchoscope 4.9 mm in diameter.

A diagrammatic view of the canine bronchial tree, based on the bronchoscopic observations of Amis and McKiernan (1986) is shown in Fig. 9.3.

5.10.2 *Foreign bodies*

In man, foreign bodies enter the right principal bronchus more often than the left (Krahl, 1964, p. 247), because the right principal bronchus has a greater diameter and deviates less from the trachea. In the horse (Fig. 25.3), the right principal bronchus has a larger diameter and is less oblique (Sisson and Grossman, 1969, p. 535; Derksen, 1990, p. 78), and in the dog (Amis and McKiernen, 1986) the right principal bronchus appears bronchoscopically to be an almost direct continuation of the trachea, whereas the left deviates more acutely. It might be expected that foreign bodies would preferentially enter the right bronchus in domestic mammals also. Foreign bodies can be removed during bronchoscopy (Section 25.8).

5.10.3 *Pendent drainage*

In the dog the lobar bronchus to the right middle lobe arises ventrally from the principal bronchus, and is therefore particularly subject to **pendent** drainage and infection (de Lahunta and Habel, 1986, p. 200). In general, secretions tend to pool in the most ventral regions of the lung, notably in the ventral parts of the cranial and middle lobe in the domestic mammals. These regions need special attention during **auscultation** of the lung (Section 23.6.1). **Bronchiectasis** (Section 24.9.8) usually involves the pendent parts of the lung (Blood and Studdert, 1988, p. 130).

5.10.4 *Segmental and lobular isolation of infection*

Some **infections** and **bronchiectasis** may be confined to individual **bronchopulmonary segments** or even to **secondary lobules**. This may occur in the ox, where the septa between segments and secondary lobules are particularly well-developed (Section 5.8) and may become even thicker or oedematous in disease (Dyce *et al.*, 1987, p. 627); in the pig pneumonic lesions are often (though not always) confined to the segments by a sharp line of demarcation (Jericho, 1968). On the other hand, channels of collateral ventilation (Section 6.3.2) tend to promote the spread of infection between the small and large units of the lung. In man one or several diseased segments can be resected (Williams *et al.*, 1989, p. 1263), but this is not yet a significant procedure in veterinary practice (Dyce *et al.*, 1987, p. 158).

5.10.5 *Torsion of lobe*

The capacity for movement of individual lobes (Section 5.7) allows the possibility of **torsion** of a lobe (Dyce *et al.*, 1987, p. 400). Although uncommon, this occurs in the dog and cat, mainly of the middle lobe, either spontaneously, or after trauma, or in association with pleural effusion (Blood and Studdert, 1988, p. 543). The particularly loose attachments of the lobes at the hilus (Section 5.6) could favour torsion in carnivores. Torsion of a lobe can be resolved by **lobectomy** (Section 25.11).

Chapter 6
Airways of the Lungs

I CONDUCTING AND RESPIRATORY AIRWAYS

6.1 Airway design

The airways in the mammalian lung consist of a branching tree of entirely blind-ending tubes. This design creates physiological problems, since it is impossible to empty the airways completely at expiration, and therefore a mammal must inspire its fresh air into an inconvenient cushion of residual air low in oxygen. If you have ever wondered how a bar-headed goose can fly over the summit of Mount Everest, which in terms of human energetics is equivalent to riding a bicycle at full speed at 30 000 feet (above 9 km), look for a different lung design and you will find it: there are no blind-ending tubes in the avian lung. However, that is another story, and the mammal must make do with what it has got. For a comparison of the energetics and gas exchange mechanisms of birds and mammals, see King and McLelland (1984), and Section 6.26.

The airways of the mammalian **lung** are divided into conducting airways and respiratory airways. The **conducting airways** are concerned only with carrying air to and from the respiratory airways. The **respiratory airways** are responsible for the gaseous exchanges with the blood. The components are as follows (Fig. 6.1):

> conducting airways of the lung
>   bronchus
>   bronchiole
> respiratory airways of the lung
>   respiratory bronchiole
>   alveolar duct
>   alveolar sac
>   alveoli

Oxygen moves through this system of dichotomously branching tubes by a combination of **mass flow** (convection) and **diffusion**. During resting breathing, movement by mass flow alone occurs only as far as the beginning of the first respiratory bronchioles (Fig. 6.1). The respiratory bronchiole is the start of a transitional stage where mass flow and diffusion combine to shift oxygen, and this continues through the alveolar duct. The alveoli on the walls of the respiratory bronchiole and alveolar duct get their oxygen by diffusion. In the alveolar sac, oxygen moves solely by diffusion.

The respiratory airways are also known as the **exchange tissue**.

Opinions differ on the level at which **diffusion** is the only mechanism. Hildebrandt (1974, p. 300) puts it at the beginning of the alveolar duct: Weibel (1984, Fig. 10.6) attributes it to the alveolar sac.

The numbers of **generations of branches** vary greatly in different species. Small mammals such as the mouse have only 7–9 generations altogether (Krahl, 1964, p. 254), whereas man has about 23 (Weibel, 1984, p. 277). The **respiratory bronchioles** (bronchuli respiratorii) are particularly variable. Three or more well-developed respiratory bronchioles are present in man, dog, cat, and Rhesus monkey, whereas in the ox, sheep, pig, and horse, respiratory bronchioles are rare and poorly developed with only minimal alveolar budding (McLaughlin *et al.*, 1961). It has been claimed that in the horse there are no respiratory bronchioles at all (see Dixon, 1992). The rat, guinea pig, and rabbit, have only one very short one, and the mouse has none (Krahl, 1964, p. 254).

During development, the airways form by monopodial, trichotomous, or dichotomous branching (Section 5.1). The drawings by Hare (1975, Figs 19–28, 30–26, 41–11, 52–17, 52–18) of the teased lungs of the adult horse, ox, pig, and cat, indicate that the **principal bronchus** (bronchus principalis) runs axially through the lung, giving off the lobar bronchi from its sides at varying angles and varying intervals; this is the **monopodial pattern**, resembling the axial trunk and oblique and irregular branches of a poplar tree. The **lobar bronchi** (bronchi

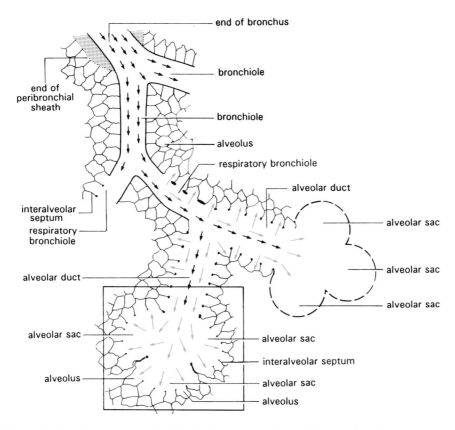

Fig. 6.1 Diagram to show the arrangement of the terminal airways. The peripheral end of a bronchus is shown, including the tapering end of its peribronchial sheath (stipple). The bronchiole has no peribronchial sheath. The respiratory bronchioles have alveoli opening from one side. The alveolar ducts have alveoli opening from all sides. The tips of the septa of alveoli opening from respiratory bronchioles and alveolar ducts are guarded by knob-like bundles of smooth muscle, very large in respiratory bronchioles. The alveolar ducts open into alveolar sacs; the square at the bottom of the diagram encloses the end of an alveolar duct, and three alveolar sacs. The septa between the atrial sacs are exaggerated for clarity. The tips of the septa of alveoli opening from the alveolar sacs are not guarded by smooth muscle, but are slightly enlarged by the presence of fibres of the fibrous continuum. The arrows indicate the movements of gas during inspiration. The black arrows represent mass flow (convection), and the green arrows diffusion. Mass flow accounts for all movement of gas as far down as the beginning of the respiratory bronchiole. From here to the end of the alveolar duct, movement is by a combination of mass flow and diffusion. Movement of gas in the alveolar sac and all alveoli is by diffusion only.

lobares) again run axially through a lobe, giving off **segmental bronchi** (bronchi segmentales) (Section 5.9) in a similar monopodial pattern (Fig. 17.4). Some of these monopodial branchings in the lobes are frankly **trichotomous**. This means that the axial lobar bronchus simultaneously forms a pair of equal branches on either side, rather like a trifid toasting fork except that the central prong then goes straight on; this trifid pattern may be repeated two or three times along the course of a lobar bronchus. It seems to be the lateral (i.e. segmental) branches formed by such trichotomy that then begin to divide by regular **dichotomy**, i.e. forking into two equal

and similar daughter bronchi. Hence the monopodial system seems to persist for the first half dozen or so generations of branches, and it is only then that regular dichotomy appears. This impression is confirmed by the observations on the canine lung by bronchoscopists (Amis and McKiernan, 1986), which revealed monopodial characteristics through at least six airway generations; even after that, the dog 'appears to have many patterns of airway branching'. Perhaps the truth is that genuine regular dichotomy is only a characteristic of the airways at the microscopic level, but this would be difficult to establish.

6.2 Bronchus

The bronchus is lined by a **mucous membrane**. Its epithelium is a typical pseudostratified respiratory epithelium, consisting of **ciliated columnar cells** with **goblet cells** (Fig. 6.3A). Beneath the narrow layer of connective tissue under the epithelium lie well-developed spiral bands of **bronchial smooth muscle** (Figs 6.2, 6.3B; Section 6.10). Outside the bronchial muscle there are irregular plates of **bronchial cartilage** (Fig. 6.3B). Between the smooth muscle and cartilage plates are **bronchial glands** (Fig. 6.3B); these are mucoserous glands, containing both mucous and serous elements. In the connective tissue immediately under the epithelium there are many **lymphoid nodules**, **lymphocytes**, and **plasma cells** (Sections 7.9.2, 7.9.3).

A bronchus has another special structural feature, the **peribronchial sheath** (green in Fig. 6.3B). The sheath contains a rich plexus of blood capillaries (the outer bronchial vascular plexus) and a network of lymphatic vessels (Fig. 6.3B; Section 6.13). This highly vascular sheath has the important function of isolating the bronchial airway from the varying tensions caused by the elastic continuum during inspiration and expiration (Section 6.13). This in turn allows the spiral bronchial muscle to regulate the volume of the bronchial lumen.

Although the **epithelial lining** of the first generations of bronchi is a pseudostratified columnar ciliated epithelium (epithelium pseudostratificatum columnare ciliatum), very similar to that of the trachea (Krstic, 1984, p. 55), the height and complexity of the epithelium progressively diminish with the bronchial branchings. Hence the lining of a last generation of bronchi is reduced to a simple columnar ciliated epithelium, which passes without abrupt transition into the high cuboidal epithelium of the first generation of bronchiole (Krahl, 1964, p. 250). However, as Krahl (1964, p. 250) pointed out, the height of the cells in histological sections varies with the contraction or relaxation of the bronchial smooth muscle, and this may vary with fixation; when the muscle contracts strongly, the cells are squeezed into a long thin shape in their long axis, but when the muscle relaxes they become shorter and wider.

Histological terms are available for the layers of the bronchial wall (Krstic, 1984), and may be convenient for precise description of pathological tissues. The layer of loose connective tissue beneath the epithelium is the lamina propria (Fig. 6.3B). The epithelium and lamina propria together form the **tunica mucosa respiratoria** (respiratory mucosa). Outside the spiral bronchial muscle (**tunica muscularis**) is another layer of loose connective tissue, the **tela submucosa** or submucosa (Latin: tela, a web – in weaving) (Fig. 6.3B). The glands are in the submucosa. The next layer is the **tunica fibrocartilaginea** (the fibrocartilaginous layer), consisting of the plates of hyaline cartilage and dense connective tissue. The outermost layer (forming the peribronchial sheath of the bronchus) is the **tunica adventitia**. These terms are essentially similar to those of other tubular organs, as might be expected, since the respiratory tract arises from the foregut (Section 5.1). However, they are modified from those of the intestine in that, (a) the main muscular component, the spiral muscle, is in the same site as the muscularis mucosa of the gut, whereas the massive tunica muscularis of the gut (its principal muscle layer) would appear to be missing in the bronchus, and (b) the bronchus has a tunica fibrocartilaginea.

In mammals generally (Krahl, 1964, pp. 247–252) the **lobar bronchi** resemble the trachea structurally, in that a transverse band of smooth muscle covers the tips of the C-shaped **bronchial cartilages** dorsally, like the **trachealis muscle** in the trachea. Medium-sized bronchi (**segmental bronchi**) have irregular plates of cartilage and abundant glands, with **bronchial smooth muscle** (musculus spiralis) in typical spiral bands (Section 6.10). Smaller bronchi have reduced remnants of cartilage and fewer glands, but retain well-developed spiral bands of bronchial smooth muscle. The **peribronchial sheath** is still present in small bronchi, but is thinner. In mammals generally, the **terminal bronchus** is the last airway to contain both cartilage and glands. In very small species, such as the mouse, there is no cartilage beyond the principal bronchus (Krahl, 1964, p. 253).

The secretory terminals of a typical **bronchial gland** (glandula bronchialis) consist of approximately equal numbers of mucous tubules and serous acini (Krahl, 1964, p. 250). The **serous glandular cells** contain **lysozyme** (Breeze and Wheeldon, 1977, p. 751) (Section 7.8.5).

The epithelial lining of bronchi includes **brush cells** (microvillous epitheliocytes, epitheliocytus microvillosus) (Section 6.3.1) and also serous cells.

The **epithelial serous cell** has only recently been recognized as a specific cell type, occurring in the trachea and bronchi (Breeze and Wheeldon, 1977, p. 715L). It is a columnar cell, reaching the airway lumen, with an electron-dense cytoplasm containing large membrane-bound, electron-dense, secretory granules (which are not osmiophilic). The function is unknown, but it is suggested that it might contribute to the **periciliary fluid** beneath the tracheobronchial mucus (Section 7.2). There is also evidence that this cell contains **lysozyme**, and that it is involved in the production of the **secretory component** of secretory IgA and the transepithelial transfer of **secretory IgA** (Section 14.29.4) (Breeze and Wheeldon, 1977, p. 716).

Neuroepithelial bodies are embedded in the epithelium at all levels of the tracheobronchial tree (Section 6.3.1). They consist of clusters of **respiratory endocrine cells**. These cells also occur singly in the airway epithelium.

6.3 Bronchiole

The bronchiolar **epithelium** is typically reduced to cuboidal, and in the normal animal it possesses **no** mucus-secreting elements (i.e. it has no goblet cells and no mucoserous submucosal glands). **Ciliated cells** are still present, but are progressively reduced in number and finally disappear altogether. **Cartilage** is absent. The **spiral bronchial muscle** is very well-developed, and can virtually close the airway altogether. There are many **lymphoid nodules** just beneath the epithelium; **plasma cells** and **lymphocytes** are abundant in and below the epithelium (Section 7.9.3).

An essential functional feature of the bronchiole is that it lacks a vascular sheath corresponding to the peribronchial sheath. Therefore it is not isolated from the varying tensions on its wall, but is inescapably expanded during inspiration and contracted during expiration (Section 6.13).

6.3.1 *Structure of bronchioles*

Krahl (1964, pp. 249, 254) considered the **epithelium** of the first generation(s) of bronchiole (bronchulus) to be high cuboidal, progressing to simple cuboidal. Krstic (1984, p. 55) regarded the epithelium as simple columnar, becoming cuboidal at the respiratory bronchiole. These minor differences in the description of the epithelium, and those of the bronchial epithelium also (Section 6.2), are probably influenced by fixation, and perhaps also by species variations.

The relatively delicate structure of the last generation of bronchiole, i.e. the terminal bronchiole, retains the basic histological layers of epithelium plus **lamina propria** (Fig. 6.3B), forming a **tunica mucosa**, but the tela submucosa is not recognizable.

Of all the airways, the bronchioles have the greatest proportion of **smooth muscle** in their walls relative to the diameter of the lumen (Krahl, 1964, p. 253); hence the powerful constrictor action of this muscle on the airway (Comroe, 1975, p. 128).

Although its functional significance is substantial, the presence or absence of a **peribronchial sheath** is not reliable for distinguishing bronchi from bronchioles in histological sections. In large or medium-sized bronchi the sheath is often distinct, whereas in bronchioles it is often clearly absent, but in the smaller bronchi the sheath becomes gradually reduced. Therefore at the borderline between bronchus and bronchiole it is difficult to decide whether a sheath is present or not.

The presence or absence of **cartilage** is also not a reliable criterion for distinguishing a bronchus from a bronchiole in all mammals (Krahl, 1964, p. 253), since (Section 6.2) the smallest laboratory mammals have no cartilage beyond the first bronchial division. Sometimes it is arbitrarily stated that a bronchiole can be distinguished by having a lumen that is less than 1 mm in diameter. However, this is not a useful criterion in small laboratory mammals such as the mouse since only its larger bronchi exceed 1 mm; moreover, in all species the diameter of the bronchiolar lumen is strongly influenced by the action of fixative on the smooth muscle in its wall.

Whilst **goblet cells** (exocrinocytus caliciformis) are not a general characteristic of normal bronchioles, they are very occasionally found in man and probably in most other mammals, but in disease their number increases greatly (Breeze and Wheeldon, 1977, p. 711).

In mammals generally, **ciliated cells** progressively disappear at the borderline with respiratory bronchioles, but according to Dixon (1992) ciliated cells are more numerous in the horse than in any other species, persisting up to the bronchoalveolar junction.

Almost all of the non-ciliated cells interspersed between the ciliated cells of bronchioles are **exocrine bronchiolar cells** (**Clara cells**) (exocrinocytus bronchiolaris). It has been generally believed that this cell is confined to the most distal bronchioles, but they may be present throughout the conducting airways (Peao et al., 1993). The structure and function of this cell have attracted much interest (Breeze and Wheeldon, 1977, pp. 730–773). It is taller than the ciliated cells. Its apex is crowned by a projecting dome which consists of an amorphous electron-lucent matrix, containing disintegrating smooth endoplasmic reticulum, mitochondria virtually devoid of cristae, and electron-dense membrane-bound inclusions. It is agreed that the cell is secretory. The suggestion that the secretion is the main source of **pulmonary surfactant** is both strongly supported (e.g. Smith et al., 1974) and much criticized (see Breeze and Wheeldon, 1977, p. 737), but the source appears now to be settled in favour of the granular epithelial cell (Section 6.25). Perhaps the exocrine bronchiolar cell secretes the surfactant that is known to line bronchioles, thus stabilizing bronchioles against surface tension; alternatively it may secrete the **periciliary fluid**, the watery medium (sol) bathing the cilia of bronchioles (Section 7.2) (Breeze and Wheeldon, 1977, p. 737). Possibly it may secrete surfactant which has been demonstrated directly or indirectly elsewhere in the conducting airways, i.e. between the gel and sol layers of the mucous carpet and along the mucous surface of the whole of the tracheobronchial airway (Section 7.3.4).

Two other epithelial cell types are found in the epithelial lining of bronchioles. These are the **brush cell** and the **respiratory endocrine cell** (Breeze and Wheeldon, 1977, p. 730).

Brush cells (epitheliocytus microvillosus) (also known as the alveolar type III cell) are scattered throughout the tracheobronchial tree and alveoli, but their exact distribution varies greatly in different species (for review see Dormans, 1985). Thus this cell is confined to the trachea in the mouse and guinea pig, to the bronchi in the calf, and to the proximal bronchioles in the pig; in man it occurs (controversially) in the trachea and bronchi. In the rat it is found in all parts of the tracheobronchial tree and also in the alveoli, but especially in the **alveolar ducts**. The cell is basic columnar, but characterized by (1) a pronounced brush border of blunt thick microvilli about 1–2 μm long, (2) bundles of fine filaments extending from the microvilli deep into the cytoplasm, and (3) many micropinocytotic vesicles; also (4) synapses with intraepithelial axons have been reported. The function of brush cells in unknown, but it may be absorption of epithelial transudate (suggested by the structural similarity to intestinal cells), or contraction in response to local changes in airway gases, or receptor activity in response to physical or chemical stimuli (Dormans, 1985).

Respiratory endocrine cells have many synonyms including Feyrter cells, K cells (Kultschitzky-like cells), argyrophil cells, granular cells, neuroendocrine cells, and neuroepithelial cells. Despite their possible functional importance, the respiratory endocrine cells (neuroepithelial cells) seem to have been omitted from the *Nomina Histologica* (1994). They occur singly or in clusters (**neuroepithelial bodies**) (Sections 4.16.4, 6.12.1) at all levels of the tracheobronchial tree, down to and including the alveolar ducts (Breeze and Wheeldon, 1977, p. 721). They occur in several mammalian species, and are particularly numerous in the fetus and neonate. They show the ultrastructural and cytochemical characteristics of APUD cells (Section 2.40), notably the capacity for *amine uptake*. Their possible function in respiratory reflexes (Section 6.12.1), or in mediating the pulmonary vasoconstriction of hypercapnia or hypoxia (Section 17.21.1) by releasing serotonin, is discussed in Section 4.16.4. Several **peptides** have now been found in these cells, including gastrin-releasing peptide, calcitonin, leu-enkephalin, and calcitonin gene-related peptide; gastrin-releasing peptide could play a role in *bronchoconstriction, vasoconstriction,* and *monocyte chemotaxis* (Miller, 1989). Respiratory endocrine cells are present in large numbers (hyperplasia) in children with certain diseases including **cystic fibrosis** and **bronchiectasis**, and in adults with **chronic bronchitis** and **emphysema**; moreover gastrin-releasing peptide is a growth factor for both epithelial cells and fibroblasts, and therefore a role in **airway repair** as well as development has been postulated (Miller, 1989).

The **neuroepithelial bodies** are embedded in the bronchiolar epithelium (Section 4.16.4).

6.3.2   *Collateral ventilation of bronchioles*

Experiments have shown that smoke blown into one bronchus can emerge from another bronchus. Admittedly, this can be partly explained by interalveolar pores (Section 6.23), but it seemed likely that larger channels of collateral ventilation must exist. For example, there could be bronchiolar–alveolar channels between bronchioles and the alveoli that lie in contact with their walls; in Fig. 6.1, these could exist along the walls of the bronchiole (not respiratory bronchiole), and connect with the alveoli belonging to other bronchioles.

Such pathways escaped detection until the 1950s, but bronchiolar–alveolar channels passing through the bronchial wall and into the adjoining alveoli have now been found in the lungs of man, cat, and rabbit (Krahl, 1964, p. 266). The channels have a diameter of about 30 μm, i.e. about thrice that of interalveolar pores, and they remain open when the bronchial muscle is obviously contracted. Because of its potential importance in the pathogenesis of **obstructive airway disease** (Section 7.17), collateral ventilation has attracted much interest. It has been found that considerable movement of gas can occur by collateral ventilation, but the precise anatomical pathways are still not fully clarified (Hildebrandt, 1974, p. 301).

6.4   Respiratory bronchiole

A respiratory bronchiole has a few alveoli scattered irregularly along its wall (Fig. 6.1), allowing limited gaseous exchanges. Most of the wall is lined by a typical bronchiolar epithelium, i.e. cuboidal, with no goblet cells or glands and no cilia. At the entrance to an alveolus the cuboidal epithelium changes abruptly to thin simple squamous cells. Stout knob-like bundles of bronchial smooth muscle guard the entrance to each alveolus (Fig. 6.1), but compared with ordinary bronchioles the wall as a whole has relatively few smooth muscle cells.

Small laboratory mammals have no respiratory bronchioles (bronchiolus respiratorius) or only one generation. Respiratory bronchioles are also rare in the large domestic mammals; only in carnivores and primates are several well-developed generations present. A first generation respiratory bronchiole is almost completely lined with cuboidal epithelium, but peripherally the alveoli become progressively more numerous and the cuboidal epithelium is restricted to a strip occupying about a half or third of the circumference (Krahl, 1964, p. 256). The first alveoli may be shallow and small, but most of them are typical alveoli like those of alveolar ducts or alveolar sacs. Respiratory bronchioles contribute far less to gas exchange than alveolar ducts, which have alveoli on all their walls. The **spiral bronchial muscle** continues along the respiratory bronchiole, giving off windings that form the stout knobs of muscle guarding the entrances to its alveoli.

Brush cells and **respiratory endocrine cells** may occur in respiratory bronchioles, at least in some species.

6.5 Alveolar duct

The alveolar duct has alveoli which open on all its sides, rather like a corridor with doorways in not only its sides, but also its ceiling and floor. Hence the alveolar duct has no wall as such: its 'wall' is formed by the openings of its alveoli. The openings into the alveoli are guarded by rings or windings of smooth muscle (Fig. 6.1), which are continuous with the spiral bronchial and bronchiolar muscle. By contracting, these rings of smooth muscle enable gas to be redistributed from alveoli with poor blood perfusion to alveoli with good blood perfusion (Section 6.30.3). The calibre of the alveolar duct is substantially greater than that of the respiratory bronchiole (Section 6.8).

Alveolar ducts (ductus alveolaris) are devoid of **brush cells** (Section 6.3) in most mammals, but in the rat these cells encircle the lumen in a ring-like array (Dormans, 1985). **Respiratory endocrine cells** (Section 6.3) occur in alveolar ducts (Breeze and Wheeldon, 1977, p. 721).

Various authors have reported a further subdivision of the terminal airway, i.e. the **atrium** (atrium alveolare) This was said to be an irregular space between the alveolar duct and alveolar sacs, but is believed to be an artefact (Krahl, 1964, p. 258).

6.6 Alveolar sac

This is a rotunda-like area on the end of the alveolar duct, bearing alveoli on all its walls like the alveolar duct (Fig. 6.1). Usually there is a cluster of alveolar sacs at the end of one alveolar duct. The **alveolar sac** should not be confused with the **alveolus**.

The septa associated with alveolar sacs (sacculus alveolaris) have slightly enlarged tips, due to the presence of fibres of the fibrous continuum; these small enlargements can be contrasted with the bulkier tips of the septa along the alveolar duct, which contain smooth muscle cells as well as connective tissue fibres (Krahl, 1964, p. 257).

6.7 Alveolus

Every alveolus is ventilated by a respiratory airway (Section 6.1), i.e. by either a respiratory bronchiole, an alveolar duct, or an alveolar sac. Gaseous exchanges take place in the alveoli, and consequently the alveoli are known collectively as the **exchange tissue** of the lung.

6.7.1 *Shape of alveoli*

The alveoli are minute polygonal chambers.

Alveoli resemble the tiny polygonal bubbles that occur in froth (Weibel, 1984, p. 340). Like the bubbles in froth, adjacent alveoli share their walls; once this is appreciated, it becomes obvious that alveoli cannot be spheres but must, in principle, be polygons, with flat or slightly curving walls like the walls of bubbles in froth. This is how the alveolar walls appear if the lungs are fixed under tension during inspiration: when the lungs are fixed in expiration, or when partly or completely collapsed, the walls are undulating (Krahl, 1964, p. 259) or even crumpled (Weibel, 1984, p. 327).

6.7.2 *Alveolar dimensions*

The diameter of alveoli changes with inflation and deflation of the lung. The diameter also varies with the size of the animal. In small mammals they are too small to be visible to the naked eye, but in a large mammal like a man they can just be seen.

If fixed during inspiration, the diameter of alveoli in the smallest mammals is only about 35 μm (about five times the diameter of a standard erythrocyte).

In the adult human lung each **primary lobule** (Section 5.8) has about 2000 alveoli, the total **number** of alveoli in the entire lung being about 300 million (von Hayek, 1960, p. 87; Weibel, 1984, p. 339). The total **surface area** of the alveoli is at least 100 m^2, almost the area of a tennis court; yet the distance from the outside air to the alveolar surface in a man is only about 40–50 cm (Weibel, 1984, p. 340). The capillary network is fed by about 300 million arterial end branches, and drained by a similar number of veins (Weibel, 1984, p. 341).

Alveolar diameter is in general greater as **body mass** increases. For example, the smallest diameter (about $35\,\mu m$) is found in the shrew (Tenney and Remmers, 1963), but in the dog the diameter is about $122\,\mu m$ (Siegwart *et al.*, 1971), and in man it reaches about $250\,\mu m$ (Weibel, 1984, p. 339). Smaller mammals have a higher oxygen consumption per unit body mass (mass-specific oxygen consumption) than larger mammals, because their bodies have a larger mass-specific surface area and therefore lose heat relatively faster (Section 6.26). Some small mammals are also particularly energetic (e.g. shrews, bats, and the Japanese waltzing mouse), and these have very small alveoli (Tenney and Remmers, 1963; Geelhaar and Weibel, 1971); the energetic advantage of small alveoli is that the pressure gradient of oxygen (which constitutes the driving force for oxygen during diffusion) is higher than in large alveoli (Weibel *et al.*, 1981).

The dimensions of the alveoli apparently vary according to their positions in the lung. It has been shown that the alveoli at the cranial end of the human lung (the 'top' of the lung, in the standing position) are relatively large (West *et al.*, 1993), and it is assumed that this applies to the alveoli in the dorsal regions of the lung in quadrupeds. These regional differences are attributed to distortion of the lung under its own weight.

To be meaningful, measurements of **alveolar diameter** must standardize the degree of inflation or deflation of the lung, and regulate the possible shrinkage of fixed material. Inflation and deflation can be controlled by methods devised by Weibel and his co-workers; thus the lungs are collapsed (after death) by pneumothorax, and then, by means of tracheal infusion of fixative at a constant head of pressure (usually $25\,cm\ H_2O$ or $2.5\,kPa$), are re-expanded to resting levels and simultaneously fixed. Shrinkage is minimized by using fixatives of appropriate osmolarity (for review, see Maina and King, 1984, and Maina *et al.*, 1989).

6.7.3   *The alveolar wall defined*

The alveolar wall is like a very thin irregular sandwich (Fig. 6.6A). The two outermost surfaces of the sandwich are two flat membranes, formed by two extremely thin **alveolar epithelial cells**. The structural and functional characteristics of the alveolar wall are considered more fully in part II of this chapter.

A wall that separates two adjacent alveoli should strictly be called an **interalveolar septum** (septum interalveolare) (Fig. 6.6A), but is commonly known simply as the **alveolar wall**.

6.7.4   *Pulmonary capillaries*

A network of pulmonary (alveolar) blood capillaries (Section 17.14) is the main filling in the sandwich between the two alveolar epithelial cells (Fig. 6.6A). Since the polygonal surfaces of the alveolar wall are more or less flat, the pulmonary capillary network is also essentially a flat sheet between two flat membranes. Therefore the flow through the capillary network is virtually in the form of a thin flat film of blood. The sheet-like disposition of the pulmonary capillary network is visible in the three-dimensional view obtained by a scanning electron micrograph of the surface of an alveolar wall (Fig. 6.6B).

This is the richest capillary network in the entire body. The capillaries anastomose with each other so profusely and continuously that any gaps remaining between them are often smaller than the diameters of the capillaries themselves (Fig. 6.6B).

When cut in section, as in the drawing of a transmission electron micrograph in Fig. 6.6A, the alveolar wall looks like a string of blood capillaries. Many of the individual capillaries are exposed to two different alveoli, which may be ventilated by two different alveolar ducts (or respiratory bronchioles). Other capillaries, like the one in Fig. 6.7, project from the alveolar wall into a single alveolar cavity; most of the outer surface of such a capillary is separated from alveolar gas by only the very thin alveolar epithelial cell. This part of this particular capillary is available for gas exchange. Here, the tissue separating blood from gas is reduced to the cytoplasm of the endothelial cell, a single basal lamina, and the very thin alveolar epithelial cell: this is the **blood–gas barrier** (Section 6.24).

The sheet-like **capillary network** is not limited to one wall of one alveolus but is continuous with the networks in adjoining alveolar walls (Fig. 6.6B).

Although the capillary network in the alveolar wall is reckoned to be the richest in the body, it is nevertheless restricted to two dimensions. There are other candidates for the richest capillary network, including the myocardium (Section 18.3) and carotid body (Section 19.7.2), and these networks are in three dimensions.

6.7.5   *Fibre 'skeleton' of alveolar wall*

The pulmonary capillary network is not the only filling of the sandwich formed by the alveolar wall.

There are also connective tissue cells and fibres, which are collectively known as the **alveolar interstitium** (Section 6.20). The alveolar interstitium includes a connective tissue 'skeleton' of **collagen fibrils** and **elastic fibres** (Figs 6.6A, 6.7), which are a part of the **fibrous continuum** of the lung (Section 6.9). These fibres form a framework which supports the alveolar wall.

Between the fibres lie **alveolar interstitial channels** that provide essential drainage for alveolar interstitial fluid (Section 6.20).

In principle, the *design of the alveolar wall* demands the reduction of its supporting tissues to the absolute minimum, to allow optimal diffusion of gas between the blood in the capillaries and the air in the alveoli. Nevertheless, reduction of supporting tissue cannot be carried too far, since the alveolar walls might then tear during maximum inspiration. An even greater hazard from making the alveolar wall too thin is that the pulmonary capillaries may burst when the pulmonary arterial pressure rises during very severe exercise (Section 6.24).

The fibrous framework provides guy ropes that tether alveoli to each other by means of their walls, thus making the alveoli **interdependent** and providing them with a certain degree of mechanical stability. This potential stability becomes important in disease conditions such as the **respiratory distress syndrome of the newborn**, where there is a tendency for alveoli to collapse (Section 16.26.1). The fibre framework also suspends the capillary network within the alveolar wall.

6.8   Calibres of airways

The calibre of the airways is of great importance in the resistance to the flow of oxygen (Section 6.14). The many generations of dichotomous branchings of the airways provide a method for maintaining the resistance to flow at a constant level. This is achieved by adjusting the airway diameter at each branching. Thus the combined cross-sectional area of the two daughter airways slightly exceeds the cross-sectional area of the parent airway. Because of this, the resistance to flow remains constant.

The combined cross-sectional area of the two tubes produced by each **branching** of a **bronchus** or a **bronchiole**

(the conducting airways, Section 6.1) is about *1.4 times greater* than the cross-sectional area of the parent airway (Comroe, 1975, p. 125). The resistance incurred during the **mass flow** of gas along a tube depends critically on the diameter of the tube (Section 6.14). When the incremental factor at branches is 1.4, the resistance to mass flow per unit length remains constant (Comroe, 1975, p. 125). Thus the diameters of the *conducting airways* are adapted to allow the mass flow of air to proceed with minimal loss of energy (Weibel, 1984, p. 277). These relationships are based on the assumption that **laminar flow** occurs in bronchi and bronchioles (Section 6.14).

The **branching** of a **respiratory bronchiole** and an **alveolar duct** (the respiratory airways) produces in each case two daughter branches, both of which have much the same diameter as the parent. Thus the total cross-sectional area *nearly doubles* with each division (Weibel, 1984, p. 278). This is efficient, since **diffusion** is much more important than mass flow for moving oxygen in these *respiratory airways* (Section 6.1, Fig. 6.1), and diffusion is promoted by a large cross-sectional area (Weibel, 1984, p. 278).

Airway design is therefore optimal for oxygen transport, both by mass flow and by diffusion.

6.9   The elastic continuum and fibrous continuum

The elastic continuum consists of a three dimensional network of branching and anastomosing **elastic fibres** that spread throughout all components of the airways, i.e. both the bronchial tree and the exchange tissue (Fig. 6.2). It begins at the root of the lung, on the principal bronchus. It is particularly dense *longitudinally* in the walls of the bronchi and bronchioles (Fig. 6.2). At the alveolar ducts (and respiratory bronchioles if present) the fibres become *spiral* and act as a powerful spring when stretched (Fig. 6.2).

Collagen fibres are interwoven among the elastic fibres. The combined meshwork of elastic and collagen fibres is known as the **fibrous continuum**.

The elastic continuum suspends the bronchi, bronchioles, respiratory bronchioles, and alveolar ducts, by means of their **peribronchial sheaths** (Section 6.13). Also it ramifies in and supports the walls of the alveoli (Section 6.7.5); it incorporates the **periarterial sheaths** of the blood vessels that ramify in the parenchyma (tissue) of the lung (Section 6.13); it attaches to the tributaries of the pulmonary vein (Section 6.13); and it links with the connective tissue **septa** that form the

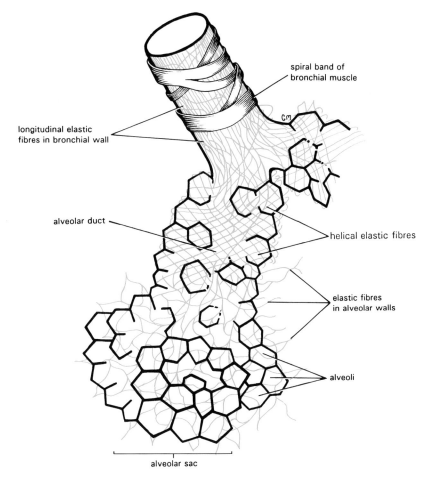

spiral band of
bronchial muscle

longitudinal elastic
fibres in bronchial wall

alveolar duct

helical elastic fibres

elastic fibres
in alveolar walls

alveoli

alveolar sac

Fig. 6.2 Diagram to show the distribution of elastic fibres in the conducting and respiratory airways. Branching and anastomosing elastic fibres (green) ramify throughout the walls of the tracheobronchial tree and alveoli, forming the three dimensional elastic continuum. Many of the very numerous elastic fibres in the bronchi and bronchioles run longitudinally. Those in the alveolar ducts are helical, and have a spring-like action. The elastic fibres in the alveolar walls run in all directions. The elastic continuum applies longitudinal, radial, and three-dimensional traction to all parts of the airways, both conducting and respiratory, during the respiratory cycle.

lobulation of the lung (Section 5.8). Finally it ends by becoming continuous with the connective tissue of the **visceral pleura** (Section 9.7).

When the thorax and lungs are at rest and not moving, as during the expiratory pause (the brief pause at the end of a resting expiration), the passive traction generated by the elastic fibres in the fibrous continuum is transmitted from the visceral (pulmonary) pleura to the airways, alveoli, and blood vessels, thus tending to hold all of them open. When the thorax and lungs expand during the next inspiration, the elastic fibres of the con-

tinuum apply active traction from the visceral pleura to the airways, alveoli, and blood vessels, thus tending to expand them beyond their resting levels. Since the elastic continuum is three dimensional, this expansion is both longitudinal (the airways and vessels becoming *longer*) and transverse (the airways and vessels becoming *wider*). Note, however, that the transverse expansion of bronchi and arteries is modulated by the **peribronchial** and **periarterial sheaths** (Section 6.13).

Energy is stored in the elastic fibres when they are stretched during inspiration, particularly in the longitudinal and spiral fibres of the bronchi and alveolar ducts. This energy is used to supply about one third of the forces needed for **resting expiration**; most of the remaining energy for this comes from surface tension (Section 6.25, 10.2.2).

The main role of the **collagen fibres** in the elastic continuum is to set the limits of distension of the airways and blood vessels, and particularly of the alveoli. In the interests of optimal gas exchange the tissues in the alveolar walls are reduced to a minimum, but the collagen fibres are needed to protect the alveolar walls from being torn during forced inspiration.

Elastic fibres have low tensile strength but great extensibility, allowing them to be stretched to more than twice their resting length before they rupture: collagen fibres are virtually inextensible (less than 2%), but have great tensile strength (a collagen fibre 1 mm in diameter can support a 500 g weight) (Weibel, 1984, p. 316). When the lung is partly deflated, as in the expiratory pause, the collagen fibres are seen to be wavy, i.e. partly folded. The elastic fibres cause the thin alveolar wall to become folded during expiration, just as a paper bag can become crumpled (Miller, 1947, p. 45); the folding of the wall folds the collagen fibres, particularly in the creases of the crumpled alveolar wall. During inflation, the elastic fibres in the elastic continuum are easily stretched, but only until the collagen fibres are unfolded and drawn taut; after that, the collagen fibres resist stretching very strongly. The collagen fibres would seem to restrict the compliance of the lung as a whole. However, an analogy is a nylon stocking, which has high compliance because of its knitted constitution although its individual fibres are very difficult to stretch (West, 1975, p. 93).

Much of the 'elastic recoil' of expiration probably comes from the **longitudinal elastic fibres** in the *bronchial and bronchiolar walls* (Krahl, 1964, p. 267). An even larger contribution is thought to be provided by the helical fibres encircling the *alveolar ducts and respiratory bronchioles*; this action is believed to be derived from the coiling and uncoiling of the helical fibres (analogous to a spring) rather than to the stretching and contraction of individual fibres (Hance and Crystal, 1975, p. 694).

A particularly heavy ring of elastic fibres surrounds the mouth of each alveolus, at its opening from the alveolar ducts and alveolar sacs (Radford, 1964, p. 441). These rings are thought to preserve the shape of the individual alveoli during inflation, preventing the alveolar ducts and sacs from being converted into smooth-walled cavities by the tension in their walls.

There are also numerous **reticular fibres** throughout the fibrous continuum (Krahl, 1964, p. 269). They appear to be associated mainly with the capillary walls. It has been suggested that they help the capillaries to withstand excessive dilation and linear stretching; this is consistent with the structure of reticular microfibrils, which consist either of chemically modified tropocollagen (tropocollagen being the fundamental element of collagen) or mature collagen (Krstic, 1984, p. 359).

The main source of strength of the blood–gas barrier, however, is a layer of type IV collagen in the single **basal lamina** shared by the endothelial cell and the alveolar epithelial cell (Section 6.24).

The different physical characteristics of elasticity and compliance should be recognized in biology (Bock, 1974, p. 144). **Elasticity** is the property of resuming the original shape and dimensions when stress is removed. **Compliance** (Section 6.31) is the property of being deformed under stress. Thus a steel ball has high elasticity and low compliance: a tennis ball has high compliance and moderate elasticity. Collagen fibres (and hence tendons and typical ligaments) have low compliance and high elasticity: elastic fibres (and hence ligaments such as the ligamentum nuchae that consist of elastic fibres) have high compliance and moderate elasticity.

6.10   Smooth muscle of the airway walls

The bronchial muscle (musculus spiralis) consists of spiral bands of smooth muscle. These bands wind with a steep pitch, criss-cross, in both right and left spiral turns around the large and small bronchi, continue on the bronchioles, and finally disperse around the alveolar mouths on the walls of the alveolar ducts (Fig. 6.2).

They are particularly well-developed in the walls of bronchioles. Here they form the highest proportion of smooth muscle relative to the diameter of the lumen throughout the entire airway (Section 6.3), to such an extent that the walls consist mainly of smooth muscle. In respiratory bronchioles they form conspicuous knobs of muscle at the openings of the alveoli (Fig. 6.1). The windings continue even onto alveolar ducts where they form smaller knobs, again guarding the alveolar openings.

The spiral design of the bronchial muscle provides the airway with a mechanism for actively reducing both its length and its diameter. The presence of muscle that constricts the airway may appear wholly disadvantageous, especially to a sufferer from asthma (Section 7.20). However, by regulating the diameter of the conducting division of the airways, it enables the *normal lung* to balance *anatomical dead space* against *resistance to air flow* (Section 6.16).

Alveolar **hypoxia**, and especially alveolar **hypercapnoea**, have a direct action on the smooth muscle of bronchioles, causing it to relax (Scott, 1986, p. 73). This provides the *airways* with a mechanism of **autoregulation** for adjusting airway resistance. Furthermore, alveolar hypoxia and to a lesser extent alveolar hypercapnoea, provide the *pulmonary microcirculation* with an **autoregulatory mechanism** that shunts blood away from poorly ventilated alveoli (Section 17.21.1).

According to Comroe (1975, p. 129) it has been suggested by Widdicombe that there may be *continuous* regulation of bronchiolar tone in order to provide the optimum combination of airway resistance and anatomical dead space. Furthermore the bronchial muscle plays an important general role in ensuring an even distribution of air flow in the normal lung (Weibel, 1984, p. 286).

There are numerous gap junctions between the muscle cells, suggesting that each muscle bundle may coordinate its individual muscle cells into a single functional unit (Laitinen and Laitinen, 1987).

6.11   Mucus secretion

Goblet cells are present within the pseudostratified columnar ciliated epithelium of the trachea and larger bronchi (Fig. 6.3A), and in the columnar ciliated epithelium of the smaller bronchi. The trachea and the large and small bronchi also possess **mucoserous glands**. The goblet cells and the mucous elements of the mucoserous glands secrete mucus. There are *no* goblet cells or mucoserous glands in normal bronchioles (Section 6.3), respiratory bronchioles, or alveolar ducts.

Tracheal and bronchial mucus play an essential role in the defence of the lung by the **mucociliary escalator** (Section 7.2).

The composition, physical properties, and cellular formation of mucus are surveyed in Section 7.3.2.

Goblet cells are not under nervous control, but discharge in response to local mechanical or chemical stimuli (Comroe, 1975, p. 224). They vary substantially in number from one individual to another, even in apparently normal lungs.

The **bronchial glands** (Krahl, 1964, p. 250) range from

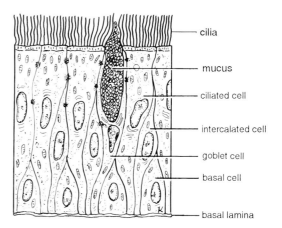

Fig. 6.3A   Diagram showing the cellular components of a pseudostratified ciliated columnar epithelium. This type of epithelium is typical of the respiratory tract in all the larger airways including typical bronchi. There are essentially three types of cell, basal cell, intercalated cell, and columnar ciliated cell ('ciliated cell'). All three rest on the basal lamina but are of different lengths, only the columnar ciliated cell reaching the surface of the airway. The nuclei therefore lie at three different levels. The basal cells are a reserve for regeneration of the epithelium. The intercalated cells are differentiating into columnar ciliated cells. Goblet cells are usually present as well, extending from basal lamina to the surface. As the bronchi get smaller the epithelium decreases in height and complexity, ending as a simple columnar ciliated epithelium. At the first generation of bronchioles, goblet cells disappear, ciliated cells become progressively less numerous, and the epithelium diminishes without abrupt transition into a simple high cuboidal or simple columnar epithelium with only a few cilia.

simple tubules to compound glands. They are particularly numerous in medium-sized bronchi, and progressively decrease in smaller bronchi. There are about equal numbers of mucous tubules and serous acini.

Both the goblet cells and the bronchial glands increase greatly in number in chronic irritation or infection of the tracheobronchial tree (Section 7.17.1).

6.12   Autonomic innervation of the lung

The sympathetic motor postganglionic fibres to the lung arise mainly from the **stellate ganglion** (Section 2.10). Parasympathetic motor preganglionic fibres to the lung are carried in the **bronchial rami** of the **vagus** (Section 3.11.4). These sympathetic and parasympathetic fibres combine into a nerve plexus (the **pulmonary plexus**) which enters the **root of the lung** (Section 5.5). The vagal preganglionic fibres synapse with postganglionic neurons in small ganglia in the bronchial walls (Section 3.11.4).

These autonomic pathways provide motor control of bronchial smooth muscle and bronchial glands. Ciliated cells function without nervous control.

6.12.1 *Bronchial smooth muscle*

The parasympathetic fibres dominate the autonomic motor regulation of the smooth muscle throughout the tracheobronchial tree. They are excitatory to the bronchial smooth muscle, causing it to contract. Sympathetic inhibitory pathways to the bronchial muscle exist. However, their ability to dilate the bronchi varies greatly in different species, and in general they have surprisingly little effect and in some species (notably man) no detectable effect at all.

Some mechanism for obtaining bronchial relaxation is obviously essential for **fight and flight**. This is indeed provided by circulating **adrenaline**. Acting on **β-receptors** on the smooth muscle cells (Section 2.33.1), adrenaline relaxes the smooth muscle of bronchi, bronchioles, respiratory bronchioles, and alveolar ducts. The resulting dilation of these lower airways thus promotes increased gas exchange in the alveoli.

The **afferent autonomic pathways** from the lung are vagal. *Stretch receptors* in the trachea and larger bronchi activate the Hering–Breuer *inflation reflex* (Sections 4.16, 11.4). *Irritant receptors* (Section 4.16) in the tracheobronchial tree, including the alveoli, initiate reflex closure of the larynx, coughing, mucus secretion, and bronchoconstriction (Section 7.6).

Research extending over almost a century seemed to have established that the diameter of the airways in mammals is controlled by parasympathetic excitatory and sympathetic inhibitory pathways (Doidge and Satchell, 1982), and everything seemed straightforward and simple. Prompted by the great clinical importance of **asthma** in human medicine, recent researches have now revealed a baffling array of species variations and many unresolved problems in bronchomotor control. This topic is also important in equine medicine (Sections 7.19, 7.20), since some ponies and horses react to a barn environment and hay by developing **spontaneous obstructive pulmonary disease** (**heaves** or **broken wind**, accompanied by **bronchial constriction**; Scott *et al.*, 1988).

Vagal innervation is confirmed as the dominant neuronal factor, causing **bronchoconstriction**. Vagal innervation is particularly dense in the guinea pig, but rather less dense in the ox, dog, and man (Davis and Kannan, 1987); acetylcholine is released from the axon varicosities of short postganglionic fibres. In man, the bronchoconstriction caused by this cholinergic innervation occurs throughout the tracheobronchial tree, but is most pronounced in the smaller bronchi (1–5 mm diameter). In yet smaller airways (bronchioles less than 0.5 mm) the effect of stimulation is less significant, and alveolar ducts are apparently not affected at all by vagal stimulation (Laitinen and Laitinen, 1987). The neuropeptide **substance P** has been found in postganglionic vagal fibres in the lung, and causes bronchoconstriction when administered *in vivo*; a major part of vagal bronchomotor tone may be the result of release of substance P from vagal postganglionic endings (Leff, 1988).

There is evidence for bronchial relaxation in man through **presynaptic inhibition** of the vagal motor endings by sympathetic postganglionic endings (Davis and Kannan, 1987).

In most mammals (Zaagsma *et al.*, 1987) the upper part of the tracheobronchial tree, i.e. the trachea itself, has quite a dense **adrenergic innervation**, but the lower part (small bronchi, bronchioles) evidently tends to have a much less dense adrenergic innervation as in the guinea pig. Stimulation of these adrenergic pathways can induce relaxation. They act mainly through β_2-adrenoreceptors, but in the tracheal smooth muscle there are usually quite numerous β_1-adrenoreceptors which also induce relaxation (Section 2.33.1).

The two most extreme variants of adrenergic innervation seem to be in the cat (and possibly the dog) in which the noradrenergic innervation is particularly dense (Zaagsma *et al.*, 1987), and in man in which the entire tracheobronchial tree has been regarded as completely devoid of adrenergic innervation (Leff, 1988, p. 1201). However, sympathetic motor endings have been seen in human bronchial smooth muscle (Pack and Richardson, 1984; Laitinen and Laitinen, 1987). Nevertheless the main inhibitory neuronal pathway in man is held to be the nonadrenergic noncholinergic pathway probably mediated by the peptide **VIP** (Laitinen and Laitinen, 1987). VIP (Section 2.34) is a potent relaxant of smooth muscle, but it has not yet been possible to evaluate its contribution to airway tone (Laitinen and Laitinen, 1987). However, despite the presence of these possible inhibitory nerve pathways, stimulating them produces no bronchomotor response in lung strips from the guinea pig, rat, rabbit, monkey, and man, suggesting a lack of functional inhibitory innervation of any kind in the fine airways of these species (Doidge and Satchell, 1982).

In man relaxation of the airways, including the bronchioles, is believed to be entirely mediated by **circulating catecholamines** (Leff, 1988, p. 1201), and this is regarded as a major defence against bronchial spasm (Zaagsma *et al.*, 1987). Both **adrenaline** and **noradrenaline** would appear to be potential mediators, acting solely through β_2-**receptors** (Zaagsma *et al.*, 1987), but there is evidence that the concentrations of circulating noradrenaline in the plasma are too low to influence bronchomotor tone, and that circulating adrenaline remains the only effective source of sympathetic bronchodilation in man (Leff, 1988, p. 1201).

Like smooth muscle cells in other tissues (Section 2.33.1), those in the bronchial walls have α-**adrenoreceptors** as well as beta. Alpha-adrenoreceptors have been demonstrated in many species, including the horse (Scott *et al.*, 1988). The α-adrenoreceptors are capable of causing bronchoconstriction under experimental conditions, but the strong preponderance of β-receptors results in net relaxation (Leff, 1988, p. 1205). However, if airway obstruction in man is already present, treatment by catecholamines may aggravate the obstruction via α-receptors.

The possibility that the spontaneous bronchoconstriction in horses exposed to a hay environment may be mediated by α_1-adrenoreceptors was investigated by Scott *et al.* (1988), but it was found that the role of such α-receptors is probably minimal.

Another possible factor in airway regulation is the release of **amines** from **APUD cells** lying individually within the airway epithelium or in **neuroepithelial bodies** (Section 4.16.4). These cells may be stimulated neuronally or directly from the airway lumen, causing contraction of the bronchial muscle (Laitinen and Laitinen, 1987). It has recently been shown (Section 19.9.3) that the cells of the neuroepithelial bodies are electrically excitable (Lopez-Barneo, 1994). They have oxygen-sensitive K^+ channels that are inhibited by hypoxia, thus leading to electrical excitation of the cell. It is also suggested that the enzyme NADPH oxidase (Section 19.9.3) is the oxygen sensor, as in the granular cells of the carotid body.

Mediators released from mast cells and other inflammatory cells can also cause bronchoconstriction in man, thus contributing to airway obstruction (Zaagsma *et al.*, 1987).

6.12.2 *Innervation of mucus-secreting elements*

The **vagus nerve** provides secretomotor fibres to the **bronchial glands**. For a long time it was believed that the **sympathetic pathways** in the lungs failed to reach the mucus-secreting elements of the airways, and that neither the sympathetic innervation of the airways nor circulating catecholamines had any significant effect on tracheal or bronchial secretion of mucus. Indeed the requirements of **fight and flight** might suggest the need for sympathetic inhibition, rather than excitation, of mucus secretion in order to keep the airways clear. However, it is now apparent that both the vagal and the sympathetic systems induce the secretion of mucus in the trachea and bronchi, the sympathetic being if anything the more productive. Whilst this may not fit too well with the need for optimal ventilation of the exchange tissue during fight and flight, it has to be remembered that the **mucociliary escalator** (Section 7.2) is a vital defence against invasion of the lung by noxious particles including pathogenic microorganisms, and this may take priority over the demands of exercise.

It has been known for over half a century that stimulation of the **vagus** and the application of parasympathomimetic agents increase both the volume of mucus secretion and the amount of glycoprotein secreted by the respiratory tract, but investigations into the possible influence of the **sympathetic system** have previously given ambiguous or negative results (Gallagher *et al.*, 1975). There seemed to be no evidence either for the presence of sympathetic adrenergic endings in bronchial glands or for the ability of sympathomimetic drugs to alter the rate of mucus secretion (Pack and Richardson, 1984).

However, **sympathetic** nerve endings associated with **glandular acini** have now been found in the bronchus of man (Pack and Richardson, 1984) and several other mammals, and efferent fibres have been demonstrated in association with the **goblet cells** of the rat trachea (Jeffery and Reid, 1973). The submucosal glands have also been shown to possess β_2-adrenoreceptors and a few β_1-type receptors (Zaagsma *et al.*, 1987). Moreover the neuropeptide **substance P** has been identified in nerve fibres in airway epithelium, where it is thought to stimulate the secretion of glycoprotein from mucous glands (Leff, 1988, p. 1203).

Finally it has been shown (Gallagher *et al.*, 1975) that in the cat, electrical stimulation of the caudal stump of the **cervical sympathetic trunk**, and the **stellate ganglion**, causes a substantial increase in the output of tracheal mucus, the increase being similar to that obtained from stimulation of the **vagus**. Direct contact of the tracheal mucosa with **adrenaline** and **noradrenaline** induces even greater increases in tracheal mucus, this being mediated mainly, if not entirely, by β-**receptors**. The secretion produced by parasympathetic activity probably originates from the mucous and serous cells of the submucosal glands, rather than from the goblet cells (Gallagher *et al.*,

1975). On the other hand, it is thought that the secretions induced by sympathetic activity may come from the goblet cells. There is a resting level of secretion which is not under nervous control, and also a resting tone in the autonomic pathways which seems to originate in the postganglionic neurons. Both the parasympathetic and the sympathetic secretomotor pathways to the trachea run in the **recurrent laryngeal nerves**.

6.13 Peribronchial and periarterial sheaths

The **peribronchial sheath** is a vascular sleeve, enclosing the bronchial airway. The **periarterial sheath** is a similar vascular sleeve enclosing the branches of the pulmonary artery. These sheaths form adjustable cushions which make the bronchial and arterial lumens largely independent of inspiration and expiration.

All the tubes within the parenchyma of the lung, i.e. those of both the bronchial tree and of the blood and lymphatic vessels, are subjected to both longitudinal and transverse traction during inspiration (Section 6.9); ('transverse' traction may be more clearly expressed as radial or circumferential). When thus stretched longitudinally or transversely during inspiration, all of these tubes contribute to the **elastic recoil** of the lung during expiration, although the densely arranged longitudinal elastic fibres in the walls of the bronchi and bronchioles and the coiled spring-like elastic fibres encircling the alveolar ducts contribute the most to this recoil.

The natural tendency of this longitudinal and radial traction is to *increase* the volume of the airways and blood vessels during *inspiration*, whereas the recoil during *expiration* tends to *decrease* their volume. The peribronchial and periarterial sheaths insulate the bronchi and arterial vessels against this tendency.

Both types of sheath, i.e. peribronchial and periarterial, have an essentially similar structure (Fig. 6.3B). The lumen of the tube (whether airway or arterial blood vessel) is enclosed in a framework of loose connective tissue, founded on the meshwork of elastic and collagen fibres of the **fibrous continuum** (Section 6.9). In this framework is suspended a plexus of **lymphatic vessels**. In the peribronchial sheath there is also an **outer** and **inner bronchial blood-vascular plexus** (Fig.

6.3B). These blood-vascular plexuses consists of blood capillaries and venules (Section 17.6). The channels of the lymphatic and blood-vascular plexuses are able to open widely and fill: thus they allow *bronchoconstriction* and *arterial vasoconstriction*, even during inspiration when the bronchi and arteries are undergoing radial traction.

The blood in the bronchial blood-vascular plexuses is supplied by branches of the **bronchial arteries** (Section 17.6). The lymphatic plexuses in the peribronchial and periarterial sheaths belong to the **peribronchovascular lymphatic pathway** (Section 7.8.1).

Thus the filling or emptying of the lymphatic and/or blood-vascular plexuses in the peribronchial and periarterial sheaths imparts *hydraulic 'give'* to the walls of the bronchi, arteries, and arterioles; this degree of 'give' enables important adjustments of bronchi and arterial vessels, particularly in diameter and to some extent even in length. It is therefore possible for the **smooth muscle** in the bronchial and arterial walls to *regulate* the internal diameter and hence the volume of their tubes (Section 6.16) independently of the inherent tendency for expansion of the lumen during inspiration and reduction of the lumen during expiration.

The **fibrous continuum** also attaches in three dimensions to the **bronchioles**, **respiratory bronchioles**, **alveolar ducts**, and the tributaries of the **pulmonary veins** (Section 6.9). Therefore these smaller airways and the veins are subjected to the same longitudinal and radial forces during inspiration, and the same recoil during expiration, as the larger airways and arterial vessels. However, these smaller airways and the veins (and of course the alveoli) have no insulating vascular sheaths. Consequently their volumes are compelled to expand during inspiration and decrease during expiration.

The **pulmonary veins** and their tributaries are, in fact, suspended in loose connective tissue sheaths, but as just stated *the venous sheath has no vascular plexus, and consequently lacks the hydraulic 'give' that characterizes the periarterial sheath.* Therefore the volumes of the pulmonary veins and their tributaries are dominated by the respiratory cycle, just as are the volumes of the smaller airways: during *inspiration* the veins *fill* –

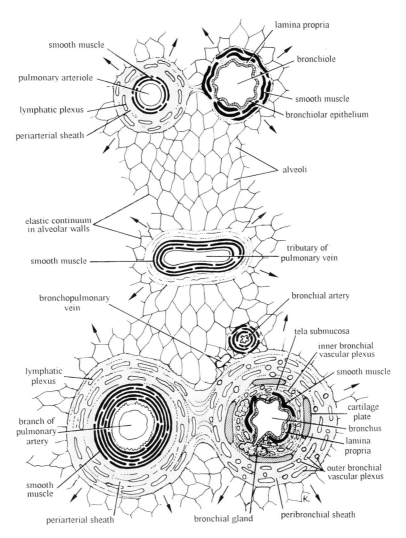

Fig. 6.3B Diagram to show the peribronchial and periarterial sheaths. The peribronchial and periarterial sheaths (green) enclose the bronchus and the branch of the pulmonary artery and arteriole in a framework of loose connective tissue in which is suspended a vascular plexus.

The **peribronchial sheath** contains an outer bronchial vascular plexus external to the cartilage plates, and an inner bronchial vascular plexus between the cartilage plates and the bronchial epithelium. The outer bronchial vascular plexus consists of an outer blood-vascular plexus of arterial and venous blood capillaries, intermingled with a plexus of lymphatic capillaries. The inner bronchial vascular plexus consists of an inner blood-vascular plexus of arterial and venous blood capillaries, intermingled with a plexus of lymphatic capillaries. The **periarterial sheath** forms the outer part of the wall of the vessel, external to the smooth muscle of the tunica media. The periarterial sheath contains a plexus of lymphatic capillaries.

The vascular plexuses in the peribronchial and periarterial sheaths fill during radial traction (arrows) exerted by the fibrous continuum during inspiration. This hydraulic 'give' enables the bronchial, arterial, and arteriolar smooth muscle to regulate the bronchial, arterial, and arteriolar lumen independently of radial traction during inspiration. The bronchiole and the vein lack vascular sheaths. Therefore they must dilate during the radial traction of inspiration, and contract when this traction is released during expiration. The bronchiole has relatively well-developed spiral bronchiolar smooth muscle that is strong enough to close the lumen.

The peribronchial and periarterial sheaths tend to fuse. In some species (dog, cat, man) the tributaries of the pulmonary veins travel alone through the exchange tissue, as in this diagram. In the ruminants, pig, and horse the veins closely accompany the branches of the pulmonary arteries and bronchi.

Branches of the bronchial arteries follow the bronchi. They supply the blood vessels of the outer and inner bronchial vascular plexuses. The bronchial vascular plexuses drain into bronchopulmonary veins that accompany the bronchi.

during *expiration* blood is *ejected* from the veins. The same mechanism acts on the large pulmonary lymphatic vessels: during inspiration the lymphatics fill – during expiration lymph is propelled towards the hilus of the lung (Section 14.8).

> The concept of the **peribronchial** and **periarterial sheaths** and their hydraulic functions was expounded by Krahl in his seminal review of the anatomy of the mammalian lung in the *Handbook of Physiology* (1964, pp. 250–253, 270–271). The terms he used for the peribronchial and periarterial sheaths were '*peribronchium*' and '*periarterial sleeves*'. Strictly, the vascular plexus between the bronchial cartilage and the bronchial epithelium (i.e. the *inner* bronchial blood-vascular plexus) was *not* a part of Krahl's 'peribronchium'. However, he explicitly envisaged (p. 251) that this inner blood-vascular plexus contributes to the insulation of the bronchi against radial traction. For further details of the *structure* and *function* of the peribronchial and periarterial sheaths, and the less well-endowed **venous sheath**, consult Krahl's account.
>
> The branches of the pulmonary artery lie close to the bronchial tree, so that the peribronchial and periarterial sheaths fuse (Fig. 6.3B). In some mammalian species (Section 17.15) the tributaries of the pulmonary veins run separately in the exchange tissue, as in Fig. 6.3B.

6.14 Laminar flow: resistance to fluid flow

When a fluid (i.e. a gas or a liquid) passes along a smooth straight tube, an exceedingly thin layer in contact with the wall remains motionless. Next to this stationary layer there is a thin layer or lamina of gas (or liquid) which *is* moving. Further additional laminae occur, layer by layer, up to the central axis of the tube, each lamina moving slightly faster than the one peripheral to it, the fastest being in the central axis of the tube. Since these laminae are travelling at different speeds, shearing stresses develop as the laminae slide over each other: these shearing stresses are the source of resistance to flow. The resistance of the fluid to this relative motion within itself is its **viscosity**; Newton defined viscosity as 'a lack of slipperiness between adjacent layers of fluid'.

Stress arises when two equal but opposite forces act on a body. It is expressed as force per unit area. If the forces lie on the same line of action and are directed away from each other the body is subjected to **tension**, but when such forces

are directed towards each other the body is subjected to **compression**. If the two forces are applied to a body in the same plane as its upper and lower surfaces, then they place a **shearing stress** on the body. For example, as those of us who enjoyed a misspent youth will know, if a pack of playing cards is placed neatly on a card table, a push applied to the top of the pack causes the cards to slide one upon another, thus distorting the pack; the cards have experienced shearing stress. The laminae of fluid sliding over each other at different velocities in a tube are undergoing shearing stress like the playing cards. **Strain** is the distortion shown by a body subjected to stress; it is expressed as the ratio of the dimensional change to the original dimension, and may be a ratio of lengths, areas, or volumes.

The flow of gas or liquid in a smooth straight tube, as described above, is known as **laminar flow**. The **resistance** during laminar flow is *directly proportional to the length* of the tube (i.e. if the length increases four-fold, the resistance increases four-fold). Furthermore, the resistance is *inversely proportional to the internal radius* of the tube (i.e. as the radius goes down the resistance goes up); however, this inverse relationship is to the *fourth power* of the radius. Therefore a small decrease in internal radius can produce a large increase in resistance (Fig. 6.4). For example, halving the internal radius increase the resistance 16-fold.

The relationships between the dimensions of the tube and its resistance to laminar flow can also be expressed in terms of **flow** and **pressure**. Thus, to maintain a constant flow rate (volume of gas or liquid per unit time), if the length is doubled the pressure must be doubled, or if the radius is halved the pressure must be increased 16-fold. If the pressure remains constant, doubling the length halves the flow rate, and decreasing the radius by half diminishes the flow to one sixteenth of its previous value.

Gas (or liquid) flow in tubes is not always laminar. It may become **turbulent** or there may be **eddy formation**, and then a much greater pressure is needed to maintain the flow rate. During laminar flow the pressure is directly proportional to the flow rate; thus in a tube of constant length and radius, to obtain a flow of three arbitrary units down the tube per unit time a pressure of three arbitrary units is required; in order to double the flow rate the pressure must also be doubled. If the flow should suddenly become turbulent, however, the pressure needed to produce that flow varies with the **square** of the flow rate; thus to maintain a flow rate of three units if the flow has become turbulent, a pressure of nine units will now be required. Eddies may occur in the normal lung at the branchings of the conducting airways (Section 23.6.2).

In smooth straight tubes, flow changes from laminar to turbulent only at high **linear velocity**. In normal healthy airways this is only likely to happen during **hyperpnoea**, as during strong exercise, and then only in the trachea and the first generations of bronchi. In the subsequent generations of airways, the total air flow has been divided among so many small tubes that the linear velocity within each individual tube is relatively low. Consider, however, the velocity at a **constriction** of a medium-sized bronchus, caused for example by a projecting mass of mucus or an inflammatory swelling of the wall. The linear velocity of the gas will greatly increase as it passes through the bottleneck: therefore at this point, turbulence will tend to occur. **Eddies** also tend to occur where there are irregularities of the wall of the airway, as caused by accumulations of mucus or ridges of scar tissue. The extra pressure required to maintain eddy flow is about the same as for turbulent flow.

The **conducting airways** are nicely designed so as to avoid turbulent flow during nearly all normal flow rates. (For reasons which emerge in Section 6.15, it would be disadvantageous to increase the radii of all the normal airways to such an extent that the critical linear velocity for turbulence could never be reached.) In fact, as already stated, turbulence can be reached in the normal animal during maximum breathing. Thus the conducting airways are so constructed that, in many of them, conditions of turbulence are closely approached in quite normal conditions. Consequently a small constriction or obstruction in the wall of such an airway can lead to turbulence even at medium flow rates. If such obstructions of the airways are widespread (Section 7.17) (for example plugs of excess mucus, or inflammatory swelling of the bronchial wall as in Fig. 6.4), or if there is bronchoconstriction (Section 7.20), then turbulence and eddies may become widespread. Abnormally high pressure gradients will then be required to maintain adequate flow rates in cases of severe **obstruction of the airways**, leading to **dyspnoea** (distressed breathing) and an excessive energetic cost of breathing (Section 10.13).

Turbulence in a fluid (for example, in gas as in the airways, or in a liquid such as blood in blood vessels) causes **vibration** which may become detectable as sound. Laminar flow in a gas or liquid is necessarily silent; the laminae slide silently over each other. On the other hand, turbulence is oscillatory, pulsatory, or vibratory, and thus creates sound.

In pathological cases, the clinician, using a stethoscope, can hear an extraordinary variety of abnormal **lung sounds**, from gurgles to crackles and whistles (Section 23.6.2). They may be due to various causes, including the movements of inflammatory fluids or perhaps even the popping open of small airways previously completely collapsed. These sounds are largely caused by **turbulent flow**, which has been induced by narrowing of airways through excessive mucus, swelling of the wall by oedema, or abnormal bronchial constriction caused by spasm of the bronchial muscle as in asthma or by scar tissue as in chronic bronchitis. (See Section 23.10.2 for discussion of **cardiac murmurs**, which are also derived from turbulence.) Some sounds are generated even in the normal lung (Section 23.6.2), probably because eddies develop at the branchings of the normal airway.

Poiseuille's law describes the **laminar flow** of a fluid (i.e. a gas or a liquid) through a straight cylindrical tube. Poiseuille was a physician in France in the nineteenth century (Feigl, 1974, p. 15). He established that flow is directly proportional to the pressure gradient and the fourth power of the radius of the lumen, and inversely proportional to the length of the tube and the viscosity of the fluid. In a system of branching distensible tubes such as the bronchial tree or arterial blood vessels there may be normal turbulence, but Poiseuille's equation is a useful approximation. Its main value is that it shows the crucial influence of radius upon flow.

The application of Poiseuille's equation to the actual measurements of airway diameters suggests that the resistance to mass flow down the bronchial tree is nearly constant up to the *beginning* of the respiratory airways (respiratory bronchioles and alveolar ducts), indicating a nearly uniform pressure gradient (Hildebrandt, 1974, p. 299). As noted in Section 6.8, the gases in the *respiratory airways* move mainly by diffusion and not by mass flow.

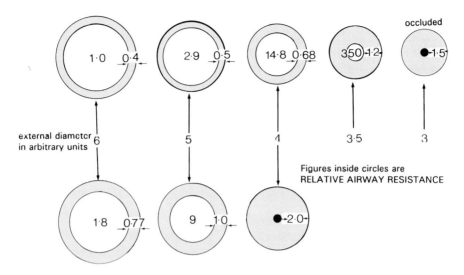

Fig. 6.4   Diagram to illustrate the increase in airway resistance as the internal diameter of a bronchus is progressively reduced. The diagram also shows the adverse effect on airway resistance of a thickening of the bronchial wall. In bronchi, airflow is laminar rather than turbulent, except in the largest airways during hyperpnoea. However, eddies may develop at branches or at partial obstructions caused by inflammation. During laminar flow, resistance is directly proportional to the length of the tube, and inversely proportional to the fourth power of the internal radius. Thus if the length is doubled the resistance is doubled, but if the radius is halved the resistance increases 16-fold. Resistance is even greater with turbulence or eddies.

The **upper row of circles** shows a transverse section of a bronchus which is 6 arbitrary units (e.g. mm) in external diameter, with an internal diameter of 5.2 units and a wall thickness of 0.4 units. Constriction of this bronchus to an external diameter of 5 units (second circle from left) changes the internal diameter to 4 units; the wall becomes *thicker* (0.5) because the *total cross-sectional area* of the bronchial wall must remain *constant, regardless of the degree of dilation or constriction*. When the external diameter is 4 units (third circle from left), the internal diameter is sharply reduced to 2.64 units. At an external diameter of 3 units the bronchus is occluded, the wall thickness now being 1.5 units.

Assuming laminar flow, the resistance to air flow in the first four bronchi would rise from 1.0 arbitrary units of resistance to 2.9, 14.8, and finally (in the fourth circle) to 350 units. Thus, as the external diameter is progressively reduced, the changes in internal diameter and resistance are small at first. But, because the volume of the wall remains constant, the thickness of the wall progressively increases; this reduces the internal diameter very much more than the external diameter. So the increase in resistance becomes enormous.

The **lower circles** show what happens if the wall starts by being thicker, say 0.77 units. This could happen through inflammatory oedema of the bronchial wall due to infection; an increase in the thickness of the mucous carpet would also produce an effective thickening of the bronchial wall. Although the external diameter starts at 6 units as in the upper circles, the lumen now becomes occluded when the external diameter is reduced to only 4 units.

A combination of increased thickness of the bronchial wall and obstruction caused by mucus or spasm of the bronchial muscle can produce a huge rise in airways resistance.

Redrawn from Freedman (1972), with permission of the author and *Bulletin de Physiol-Pathologie Respiratoire.*

6.15   Pulmonary volumes and anatomical dead space

The total volume of fresh air that is taken in during inspiration or expelled during expiration is called the **tidal volume**. In a man, during resting breathing, the normal tidal volume is about 450–500 ml.

Anatomical dead space is an airway in which no appreciable gas exchange can occur. Air cannot undergo gaseous exchanges while in the **conducting airways**, so the internal volume of the conducting airways is known as the **anatomical dead space**. The anatomical dead space is the volume of the airways from the oral and nasal openings, to the last generation of bronchiole of both of the lungs. (The *respiratory bronchiole* carries out

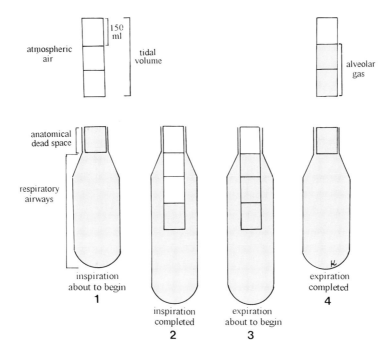

Fig. 6.5 Highly schematic diagram to show the effect of anatomical dead space on the inspired air in man, during normal resting breathing. The total tidal volume is 450 ml, expressed as three blocks of gas each 150 ml in volume. The neck of the flask represents the volume of the conducting airways from the oral and nasal openings to the terminal bronchioles of both lungs, and is therefore the anatomical dead space, 150 ml in volume. The rest of the flask represents the combined respiratory airways of both lungs together, including all alveoli, and it is only here that gaseous exchanges can occur. White blocks, fresh air inspired from the atmosphere; green blocks, alveolar gas.

Before inspiration begins, one block of alveolar gas occupies the anatomical dead space (diagram 1). During inspiration, (diagram 2) this 150 ml block of dead space gas re-enters the respiratory airways, followed by two 150 ml blocks of fresh air. The fresh air that enters the respiratory airways mixes almost instantly with alveolar gas (diagram 3), but the third 150 ml block of fresh air remains stranded in the anatomical dead space and contributes nothing to gas exchange. During the next expiration (diagram 4) the block of fresh air in the anatomical dead space is immediately pushed out by alveolar gas, and replaced by alveolar gas at the end of expiration. Thus in this mammalian species only two thirds of the resting tidal volume contributes to gas exchange: the remaining third is wasted by dead space.

gaseous exchanges: therefore it is a part of the *respiratory airways* as defined in Section 6.1, and does not contribute to the anatomical dead space.) The total anatomical dead space in a man is about 150 ml.

As Fig. 6.5 shows, during a normal **inspiration** during resting breathing in man, 150 ml of dead space gas is the first gas to enter (strictly, *re-enter*) the respiratory airways. This is followed by the first two-thirds (300 ml) of the 450 ml tidal volume of fresh air, which enter the alveoli and mixes almost instantly with **alveolar gas** (Section 6.28); the alveolar gas exchanges oxygen and carbon dioxide with the blood. The last third (150 ml) of

the tidal volume of fresh air remains stranded in the anatomical dead space, and contributes nothing to the gaseous exchanges with the blood. In other words, during resting breathing 450 ml of gas enter the alveoli during inspiration, but of this volume only 300 ml (66%) are fresh air.

At the beginning of **expiration** (Fig. 6.5), the 150 ml of fresh air that were stranded in the conducting airways are expelled, followed by 300 ml of alveolar gas. At the end of expiration, 150 ml of alveolar gas again remain stranded in the conducting airways; this expired air is obliged to re-enter the respiratory airways at the beginning of the next inspiration.

The pulmonary volumes can be expressed by various parameters (Fig. 10.5). The **inspiratory tidal volume** can be greatly increased. A man can inspire an extra 3000 ml in addition to his normal tidal volume of 450 ml. This extra volume is called the **inspiratory reserve volume**. Likewise a man can expire an extra 1100 ml in addition to his normal tidal expiration. This extra volume is known as the **expiratory reserve volume**.

After the most forceful possible expiration, a man still has about 1200 ml in his lungs, and this volume is named the **residual volume**.

The normal mammal has a very large margin of safety in the volume of air that can be inspired. After making the greatest possible expiration a man can inspire over 4 litres of air (the **vital capacity**, see immediately below). Such a maximum inflation necessarily increases the anatomical dead space (from 150 ml to about 230 ml), because the conducting airways are now fully elongated and dilated by the traction of the fibrous continuum (Section 6.9). Nevertheless, 3770 ml (94%) of this huge tidal volume would now reach the respiratory airways and be available for gas exchange with the blood.

Despite this very substantial reserve excess of tidal volume over anatomical dead space in the healthy individual, the margin of safety can be dangerously eroded under pathological conditions, such as **chronic alveolar emphysema** (Section 7.19).

Alveolar dead space and **physiological dead space** are discussed in Section 6.28.2.

The pulmonary volumes mentioned immediately above can be expressed as **pulmonary capacities** (Guyton, 1986, p. 470). The inspiratory tidal volume (450–500 ml) plus the inspiratory reserve volume (3000 ml) is the **inspiratory capacity** (3500 ml) (Fig. 10.5). The expiratory reserve volume (1100 ml) plus the residual volume (1200 ml) is the **functional residual capacity** (2300 ml); this is the volume of gas remaining in the lungs after a normal expiration. The inspiratory reserve volume (3000 ml), plus the inspiratory tidal volume (450 ml), plus the expiratory reserve volume (1100 ml), is the **vital capacity** (4550 ml); this is the maximum volume of gas that can be expelled from the lungs after a maximum inspiration. The vital capacity plus the residual volume is the **total lung capacity** (5750 ml).

6.16   Balance between resistance and volume in conducting airways

Clearly there are two conflicting design requirements in the conducting airways. On the one hand, the internal **radius** of the conducting airways must not be too small, since this would directly increase the **resistance** to air flow and also make **turbulence** more probable; on the other

hand, the **volume** of the conducting airways must not be too great, since this would enlarge the **anatomical dead space**. The design of the conducting airways therefore has to be a compromise between low resistance and small volume.

The **bronchial muscle** (Section 6.10) plays a valuable part in this compromise by providing a fine adjustment of the resistance and volume of the airways, under the control of the autonomic nervous system (Section 6.12.1). The functional significance of the **peribronchial sheath** (Section 6.13) now becomes plain: without the *hydraulic give* conferred by the sheath, the muscular regulation of airway calibre would lose effectiveness.

II   THE ALVEOLAR WALL

6.17   Alveolar epithelial cell

The alveolar wall (Section 6.7.3) is lined by alveolar epithelial cells. This is a simple squamous cell, but so thin that in transverse section it is beyond the resolution of the light microscope (i.e. it is less than 250 nm, or 0.25 μm, in thickness), and is therefore visible only with the electron microscope. It spreads as a thin leaflet over the alveolar wall (Figs 6.6A, 6.7) like an egg in a frying pan, the only thick part of the cell being the site of the nucleus (the yolk of the egg). Because of the exceptionally large area covered by each cell, few nuclei and only occasional junctions between adjacent cells are visible in EM sections (in Fig. 6.6A there are only three nuclei and six cell junctions). The cells are strongly attached by tight junctions, in contrast to the junctions of the underlying endothelial cells which are quite leaky (Section 6.19). However, although the alveolar epithelial cells are so closely attached to each other, there are always *some* quite large gaps between the junctions. Through these gaps, large quantities of water and electrolytes, and even protein molecules, can pass. This helps to maintain a thin layer of fluid on the alveolar surface (Section 6.21).

Both sides of the alveolar wall **are lined by the same individual cell**, the two leaflets being connected by pillars of cytoplasm passing through the alveolar wall (Weibel, 1984, p. 253). Two such **cytoplasmic connections** are shown in Fig. 6.6A; one of these is within the square area of the diagram, and is therefore seen more clearly in Fig. 6.7. Thus the alveolar epithelial cell is not a simple squamous cell in a single plane, but a complex cell consisting of two plates joined by connecting stalks. The structure of the cell therefore resembles the two wings of an old-fashioned biplane aircraft, the wings being connected by struts. This design enables the cell to transfer metabolites from its perinuclear region to its two very extensive but very thin surfaces, thus providing maintenance pathways over long distances without sacrificing thinness.

The alveolar epithelial cell is known officially as the **respiratory epithelial cell** (epitheliocytus respiratorius). Common synonyms are type I epithelial cell and small alveolar cell.

Alveolar epithelial cells are estimated to constitute 75% of all lung cells, and to cover 95% of the alveolar surface (Weibel, 1984, p. 267).

In order to maintain the extreme thinness of the cell for optimal gas diffusion, the nucleus is small and the cytoplasm contains scarcely any organelles. The one exception is the presence of quite numerous **micropinocytotic vesicles** (Fig. 6.7); these reflect the transcellular transport of macromolecules, and may help to remove **pulmonary oedema** (Section 17.26.8) from the luminal surface of the blood–gas barrier (Weibel, 1984, p. 252). They may also transport inhaled dust particles from the alveolar lumen into the alveolar interstitium, to be engulfed by **interstitial macrophages** (Section 7.7.2).

The repair or replacement of a cell with such a complex form would appear difficult. It turns out that alveolar epithelial cells have lost the power of mitosis (Weibel, 1984, p. 255), and can only be replaced by mitosis of the granular epithelial cell, and then only slowly.

6.18   Granular epithelial cell

This is a cuboidal epithelial cell, projecting from the alveolar wall (Fig. 6.6A). Its main structural feature is the presence of many laminated **osmiophilic bodies** consisting of phospholipids. These bodies are believed to be released from the cell surface by exocytosis (arrow in Fig. 6.7). On the surface of the alveolar wall the phospholipid laminae are thought to unravel and become **surfactant** (Section 6.25).

Synonyms for this cell are type 2 alveolar cell, and great alveolar cell. 'Great' is a misnomer, for the volume of this cell is only about half that of the alveolar epithelial cell (Weibel, 1984, p. 255).

The **granular epithelial cell** (epitheliocytus granularis) usually occurs at the junction of several alveolar walls

and near an alveolar pore (Gillespie and Tyler, 1967), as in Fig. 6.6A. It has the cellular characteristics that suggest *substantial metabolic activity*, i.e. abundant mitochondria, rough endoplasmic reticulum, Golgi apparatus, and multivesicular bodies, all of which tend to be arranged in a complex and may be involved in the formation of dipalmitoylphosphatidylcholine (DPPC), a lecithin that constitutes the main **surfactant phospholipid** of the lung (Weibel, 1984, p. 257).

The identity of the main **source of surfactant** in the lung is controversial. One view is that the **exocrine bronchiolar cell** (**Clara cell**) (Section 6.3) is the main source (Smith *et al.*, 1974), and that the function of the granular epithelial cell is not to make, but to remove, surfactant by phagocytosis (Niden, 1967). Alternatively the granular epithelial cell may produce *alveolar surfactant*, and the Clara cell may produce *bronchiolar surfactant* (Section 6.25).

It has recently been shown (see Drake and Gabel, 1995) that the granular cell actively pumps sodium from the fluid in the alveolar lumen and into the alveolar interstitium; water follows by osmosis. In this way, the granular cell plays an important part in the clearance of fluid from the alveoli, and hence in the defence against pulmonary oedema (Section 17.26.6).

6.19   Endothelial cell

The pulmonary blood capillaries of the alveolar wall (Fig. 6.6B) (Section 6.7.4) are lined by endothelial cells. Transport of substances across the endothelial cell occurs by the usual mechanisms (Section 14.2), i.e. via direct diffusion, the intercellular cleft, and numerous micropinocytotic vesicles. The intercellular cleft in particular allows the exchange of water, solutes, and small macromolecules of protein between the blood plasma and the alveolar interstitium.

The **intercellular clefts** are sealed by many zonulae occludentes, which narrow the cleft to not more than 4 nm (Lauweryns and Baert, 1977, p. 641). Whilst this is big enough to allow the passage of small macromolecules, it less readily admits larger particles such as carbon.

Nevertheless, the alveolar capillaries are relatively leaky to protein molecules (Guyton, 1986, p. 371), so that the **oncotic pressure** of the **alveolar interstitial fluid** is *unusually high*, i.e. about 14 torr (Section 17.19.2); the value for the interstitial fluid in other tissues of the body, such as subcutaneous tissue, is only about 6 torr (Section 14.4).

The endothelial cell must be as thin as possible to allow maximal gas exchange. But it has to be strong

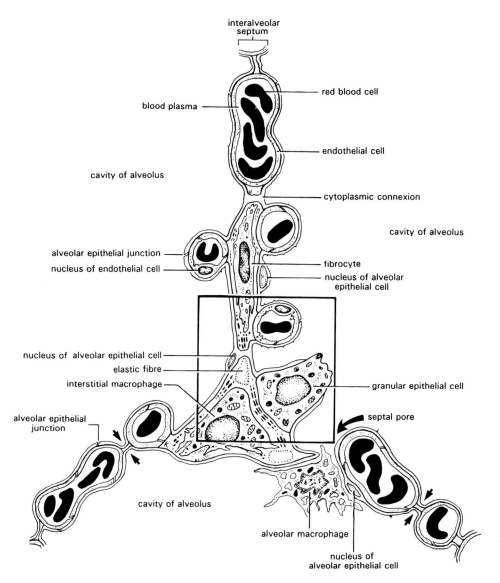

Fig. 6.6A Semidiagrammatic section through the interalveolar septa shared by three alveoli, as seen by transmission electron microscopy. The interalveolar septum is a very slim sandwich, of which the outer surfaces are two sheets of extremely thin alveolar epithelial cells, and the filling is formed mainly by pulmonary capillaries and also by the alveolar interstitium. The two sheets of epithelial cells are joined by stalk-like epithelial cytoplasmic connections. Two such cytoplasmic connections are shown, one in the box and the other above the box. Many of the capillaries are so perfectly incorporated into the interalveolar septum that they are exposed to the gas in two alveoli, one on one side of the interalveolar septum and one on the other side. Other capillaries project from only one side of the interalveolar septum, especially from thick parts of the septum, and are therefore exposed to the gas in only one alveolus. In the lower part of the figure, four arrowheads indicate intercapillary pits. A granular epithelial cell, cuboidal in shape, projects from the surface where several interalveolar septa join, near an alveolar pore. An alveolar macrophage is nosing its way into the pore. In the interstitium there is an interstitial macrophage, a fibrocyte, collagen fibrils, and elastic fibres. The area in the square is enlarged in Fig. 6.7.

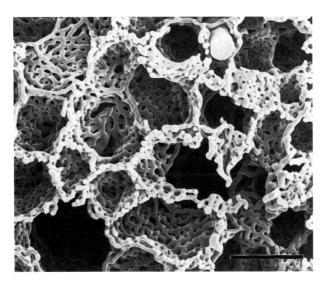

Fig. 6.6B   Scanning electron micrograph of a cast of the pulmonary capillaries of a rat, showing the sheet-like arrangement of the capillary networks. A slice has been cut from the cast, and the cut surface of the slice is shown. The cavities of 20–30 alveoli are visible. The sheet-like networks of pulmonary capillaries represent the alveolar walls. Each sheet consists of pulmonary capillaries that anastomose so profusely that the gaps between capillaries are smaller than the capillaries themselves. The bar is 100 μm. This lung had some degree of emphysema (elastin induced), so that the alveoli are somewhat enlarged.

From Schraufnagel (1987), with permission of the author and Scanning Microscopy International, Chicago, IL 60666, USA.

enough to resist the stress caused by the increase in pulmonary arterial pressure during strenuous exercise; in some species, and particularly in the racehorse, this rise in pressure is very great. The component that provides this strength is the **basal lamina** which the endothelial cell shares with the adjacent alveolar epithelial cell (Section 6.24).

6.20   Interstitium of the alveolar wall: alveolar interstitial channels

The interstitium of the alveolar wall (or alveolar interstitium) is the zone in the thicker parts of the alveolar wall that is occupied by connective tissue elements and alveolar interstitial fluid. The **connective tissue elements** (Fig. 6.7) consist of **fibrocytes**, together with **collagen fibrils** and **elastic fibres**; these fibres belong to the **fibrous continuum** of the lung (Section 6.9). There are also occasional **interstitial macrophages** (Section 7.7.2), some of which store particles of carbon dust permanently (**anthracosis**, Section 5.5).

In the normal lung, **interstitial fluid** in the alveolar wall is minimal in volume. This is because, along the whole length of the pulmonary capillary, the hydrostatic pressure inside the capillary is less than the oncotic pressure of its blood plasma (Section 17.19). This is in marked contrast to the capillaries of the systemic circulation, in which the hydrostatic pressure exceeds the oncotic pressure at the arterial end so that filtration occurs there; reabsorption occurs *only in the venous end* of the systemic capillary, where oncotic pressure exceeds hydrostatic pressure. In the alveolar wall, reabsorption occurs along the *whole length* of the pulmonary alveolar capillary. Indeed the oncotic forces pulling fluid into the alveolar capillaries are so strong that the interstitial space is reduced to almost nothing. This maintains at a minimum the distance across the blood–gas barrier, over which oxygen must diffuse. Nevertheless, at any given moment there is always some interstitial fluid in the alveolar wall.

The design requirements of the **blood–gas**

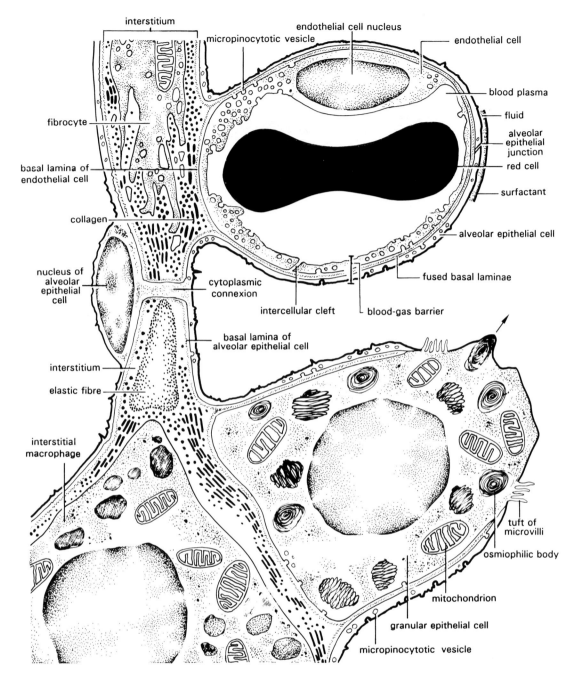

Fig. 6.7 Semidiagrammatic section through the interalveolar septum within the square in Fig. 6.6A. The alveolar epithelial cell spreads as a thin leaflet over the surface of the interalveolar septum. The only inclusions in the alveolar epithelial cell are the nucleus (left) and micropinocytotic vesicles. A cytoplasmic connection joins the perinuclear region of the alveolar epithelial cell to its cytoplasmic leaflet on the right side of the interalveolar septum. Thus this single alveolar cell lines both sides of the interalveolar septum. The cuboidal granular epithelial cell projects from the interalveolar septum. Tufts of microvilli encircle its crown. Its laminated osmiophilic bodies are extruded by exocytosis (arrow), and unravel on the alveolar surface to form surfactant. The endothelial cell has many micropinocytotic vesicles and leaky intercellular clefts. The interstitium contains a fibrocyte, an interstitial macrophage, elastic fibre, and collagen fibrils. The blood–gas barrier consists only of alveolar epithelial cell, endothelial cell, and a single shared basal lamina. The alveolar surface is covered by a thin layer of fluid with surfactant.

barrier (Section 6.24) demand that the thickness of the alveolar wall be minimal. Therefore there can be *no* room for **lymphatic capillaries** in the interstitium of the alveolar wall (Section 7.8). Yet the need for instant removal of interstitial tissue from the alveolar wall is equally imperative, since the accumulation of fluid is a potentially life-threatening event because it slows gas exchange across the barrier.

How, then, can the interstitium remove interstitial fluid if it has no lymphatics? Any interstitial fluid that does form can percolate into irregular anastomosing **alveolar interstitial channels** between the longitudinal collagen fibrils and elastic fibres of the interstitium. Since these fibres are a part of the **fibrous continuum**, the interstitial channels between the fibres are necessarily continuous as well. The channels wind their way through the alveolar walls until they reach the nearest respiratory bronchiole. Here the channels at last encounter the blind ends of the first (i.e. the most peripheral) **lymphatic capillaries** in the lung. The endothelial cells that line lymphatic capillaries are not sealed by intercellular junctions, but have wide **intercellular clefts** (Section 14.6). Therefore, the fluid in the alveolar interstitial channels becomes directly continuous, through the intercellular clefts, with lymphatic fluid in the lymphatic capillaries. In turn, the lymphatic capillaries in the walls of respiratory bronchioles discharge into the profuse network of the **peribronchovascular lymphatic pathways** (Section 7.8.1) in the **peribronchial** and **perivascular sheaths**.

What are the forces that move the fluid through the pulmonary lymphatics? Probably the main forces are **active pumping** by the smooth muscle cells in the walls of collecting lymphatic vessels, and **passive pumping** by the expansion and contraction of the lung during breathing (Section 14.8). With the aid of valves in the lymphatic vessels, these forces drive the lymph to the hilus of the lung, and onward into the **bronchial lymphocentre**, **right lymphatic duct**, and **thoracic duct** (Sections 14.34, 14.36).

The channels in the alveolar interstitium were described by Weibel (1984, p. 333), who in the same work reported that most of the fibrocytes in the alveolar interstitium are contractile **myofibrocytes**, since they are rich in bundles of actomyosin filaments. Weibel regarded these conspicuous structures (myofibrocytes) as being 'in search of a function'; since their long slender contractile cell processes span the interstitial space, he suggested that they could **actively** regulate the compliance of the interstitial space in response to fluid accumulation.

6.21 The alveolar surface

The outer surface of the alveolar epithelial cell, i.e. the surface facing the lumen of the alveolus, is lined by a thin layer of fluid (Fig. 6.7). Floating on this fluid, and therefore in contact with alveolar gas, is a film of surfactant (Fig. 6.7).

The **fluid layer** is essentially aqueous, consisting of water and solutes; it provides wetness for facilitating the diffusion of oxygen and carbon dioxide across the blood–gas barrier.

The **surfactant** helps to control surface tension (Section 6.25).

Accounts sometimes refer to the alveolar wall as dry (Guyton, 1986, p. 292), or 'dry' in inverted commas (Weibel, 1984, p. 252). It could not be really dry, if only because alveolar air is saturated with water vapour. Furthermore, the gaps between the alveolar epithelial cells (Section 6.17) enable alveolar interstitial fluid to reach the alveolar lumen. The term 'dry' is used only relatively, in the context of pulmonary oedema (Section 17.25), and is more safely placed in inverted commas.

A thin layer of lining fluid covering the free surface of the alveolar epithelial cell is, in fact, visible in electron micrographs. It consists of two basic components (Weibel, 1984, p. 325): an aqueous layer of variable thickness called the **hypophase**, and a thin film of **surfactant** on the surface of the hypophase. The constituents of the hypophase are still poorly understood, but they seem to include proteins and mucopolysaccharides, and also substantial amounts of reserve surfactant material. The latter is known as '**tubular myelin**'. It consists of a latticework of leaflets which are continuous with the film of surfactant on the alveolar surface; it is therefore assumed that tubular myelin is folded surfactant that can be unravelled and spread over the air–surface interface when needed.

Where the alveolar wall covers a capillary it bulges into the alveolar lumen, but between the capillaries (Fig. 6.6A, arrowheads) the wall forms concave **intercapillary pits** (Weibel, 1984, p. 332). In life, these pits are filled with hypophase, which may exert a considerable hydrostatic pressure gradient and thus influence the movement of fluid across the alveolar wall (Section 17.19.5).

6.22   Alveolar macrophage

Alveolar macrophages are large phagocytic cells, wandering over the alveolar surface (Fig. 6.6A) by amoeboid movement, and engulfing bacteria and inhaled particles of dust or carbon (Section 7.7.1). They are sometimes known as **dust cells**. They are derived from the haemopoietic tissue of the bone marrow, and are delivered to the interstitium by the blood stream. They then penetrate the alveolar epithelium. They are eventually removed by entering a bronchus and stepping onto the mucociliary escalator.

The **derivation** and **removal** of alveolar phagocytes (macrophagocytus alveolaris) are controversial (Section 7.7.1). The great majority of these cells come from the bone marrow, but not by direct migration of monocytes across the alveolar wall as was previously believed; they differentiate by division and maturation in the interstitium. Some may be derived from alveolar epithelial cells or interstitial macrophages. Their removal is probably achieved solely by the mucociliary escalator.

6.23   Interalveolar pores

Adjacent alveoli are connected by round or oval openings in the interalveolar septa, called interalveolar pores, in mammals generally. The diameter of these pores is about the same as that of a red blood cell. They seem to be peculiarly attractive to alveolar phagocytes, which are quite often caught in the act of going through the hole (Fig. 6.6A).

Although the diameter of alveolar pores (porus septi) is typically about 10 μm, their sizes and shapes depend on the condition of the components of the fibrous continuum that encircle them (Krahl, 1964, p. 265). Rupture of elastic and collagen fibres of the continuum may allow normal pores to expand into the much larger openings that typify the destruction of alveolar walls in some forms of alveolar **emphysema** (Section 7.19.3).

Alveolar pores may have the beneficial effect of ventilating an adjacent bronchiole which has become occluded, but may also have the disadvantage of promoting the spread of infection between neighbouring bronchioles (Krahl, 1964, p. 265).

6.24   Blood–gas barrier

The blood–gas barrier (also known as the blood–gas pathway) is where the tissue of the alveolar wall separating blood from gas is reduced to its minimum. It is across this narrow barrier (Fig. 6.7) that gas exchange occurs by diffusion through the tissues.

The **design requirements** of the blood–gas barrier are (1) *extreme thinness* for maximal gas exchange by *diffusion*, and (2) *sufficient strength* to withstand the *stress* (force per unit area) when the pressure across the capillary wall (transmural pressure) rises to a maximum during exercise.

There are only three structural components in the barrier: (i) the **alveolar epithelial cell**; (ii) the **endothelial cell** of the pulmonary blood capillary; and between them (iii) a single shared **basal lamina**, formed by the fusion of the basal lamina of the epithelial cell with that of the endothelial cell (Fig. 6.7). About 80% of the outer surface of the capillary shown in Fig. 6.7 is separated from the alveolar gas by only these three components.

The two cells of the barrier, and especially the alveolar epithelial cell, are of minimum thickness in order to promote **gas exchange**. The **strength** of the barrier lies in its (shared) basal lamina. Under maximal stress, as in the extreme rise in pulmonary arterial pressure that occurs in a galloping Thoroughbred (Section 17.18.2), one or both of the cells may rupture, but even when that happens the basal lamina often remains continuous. The main constituent of the basal lamina is a network of **collagen molecules**, of a type possessing a tensile strength nearly as great as the collagen molecules in tendon.

The inner surface of the pulmonary capillary is separated from the erythrocyte by a layer of **blood plasma** of varying thickness, which adds a further barrier to gas exchange between air and blood (Section 6.26.5). However, Fig. 6.6A shows that the internal diameter of the capillaries is similar to or less than the diameter of the erythrocytes, so that the red cells have to buckle in order to squeeze their way through the lumen. Therefore their surfaces are often in contact with the endothelium.

Four molecules form the main constituents of the basal lamina of the blood–gas barrier (West and Mathieu-Costello (1994): **type IV collagen** provides the strength; **laminin** attaches the basal lamina to the overlying cells; **entactin** binds the laminin to the type IV collagen; and **proteoglycans** regulate permeability. The collagen molecules are joined together in a meshwork similar to wire netting, thus combining great strength with permeability. Indeed the tensile strength of the (shared) basal lamina evidently approaches that of the very strong type I collagen in tendon. The collagen elements form the **lamina densa** of the basal lamina, the **lamina lucida** on either side of the lamina densa being formed by the other elements.

The Thoroughbred racehorse fails on both of the **design requirements** of the blood–gas barrier (West and Mathieu-Costello, 1994). It is not thin enough to achieve maximal gas exchange, since the galloping Thoroughbred typically develops arterial hypoxaemia. It is not strong enough to prevent rupture of the barrier at peak pulmonary arterial pressures, since haemorrhage commonly occurs from pulmonary capillaries in racehorses and other racing mammals (camel and greyhound) during maximal exercise, giving exercise-induced pulmonary haemorrhage (Section 17.28).

6.25   Surface tension and surfactant

Surface tension is the tendency for the interface between gas and liquid to contract to a minimum area.

The force exerted by the surface tension of a film of liquid inside a sphere is directly proportional to the surface tension of that particular liquid and inversely proportional to the radius of the sphere. Thus as the radius *decreases* the force *increases*, so that smaller spheres have greater forces of surface tension than larger spheres.

For consideration of surface tension, the alveoli of the mammalian lung may be regarded as small spheres lined by liquid. Therefore they develop large forces of surface tension, and this in turn creates functional problems. Firstly, since the average human alveolus expands and contracts over 15000 times a day, the total **energetic cost** of overcoming pulmonary surface tension is substantial. Secondly, since the radii of alveoli are not uniform in any individual animal, the smaller alveoli should empty themselves into the larger ones, the forces of surface tension being greater in the smaller than the larger alveoli; the whole system of alveoli therefore is *potentially unstable*.

A powerful detergent-like **surface active agent** or **surfactant** (a lipoprotein), lies on the surface of the alveolar wall, facing the alveolar lumen. It is released from the **granular epithelial cells** (Section 6.18). By decreasing surface tension, this substance reduces to reasonable proportions the **energetic cost** of repeatedly inflating the alveoli. Secondly it introduces **stability** into the potentially unstable system of alveoli of varying radii. This is because the extent to which the surfactant reduces surface tension is proportional to its concentration at the interface. In a contracted alveolus the radius is reduced and the forces of surface tension should therefore be increased; however, in a contracted alveolus the surfactant becomes more concentrated, and this offsets the tendency for an increased surface tension as the radius decreases. The reverse happens in a dilated alveolus.

Surfactant has several other functions in the normal lung. (1) It restricts the **filtration of fluid** from the blood plasma into the alveoli. Surface tension produces forces *favouring* filtration: by reducing surface tension the surfactant reduces filtration. (2) It facilitates gas transport between the gas and liquid phases at the alveolar surface. (3) It has bactericidal properties (Section 7.15.3) that contribute to the non-immunological defence of the alveoli against bacterial invasion (Section 14.31.5).

About two thirds of the energy needed for a **resting expiration** are supplied by the forces of surface tension within the alveoli; the elastic continuum accounts for most of the remaining third (Section 10.2.2).

The surfactant forms a thin film lying on the surface of the aqueous layer known as the **hypophase**. Substantial reserves of surfactant are contained in the hypophase in the form of 'tubular myelin' that apparently unravels on the surface when needed (Section 6.21).

According to the **Laplace equation**, the pressure arising from surface tension in a sphere (for instance, in a bubble) equals twice the surface tension of the fluid that lines the sphere, divided by the radius of the sphere. If the surface tension of alveolar fluid is assumed to be the same as that of blood plasma (Comroe, 1975, p. 107), i.e. $50 \, dyn \, cm^{-1}$ ($1 \, dyn = 10 \, \mu N$), and if at the end of a normal expiration the alveolar radius is about $50 \, \mu m$ ($0.005 \, cm$), then the *pressure* in the alveolus due to surface tension should be approximately:

$$\frac{2 \times 50}{0.005} = 20000 \text{ dyn/cm}^{-2} \ (2\,\text{kPa})$$

A value of $20000\,\text{dyn}\,\text{cm}^{-2}$ ($2\,\text{kPa}$) is equivalent to a pressure of about $20\,\text{cmH}_2\text{O}$, since the pressure exerted by $1.0\,\text{cmH}_2\text{O}$ is $980\,\text{dyn}\,\text{cm}^{-2}$. (A pressure of $1\,\text{dyn}\,\text{cm}^{-2}$ is expressed in SI units as 0.1 pascal; the pressure exerted by $1\,\text{mmH}_2\text{O}$ is $9.806\,\text{Pa}$, or $0.0098\,\text{kPa}$; Baron, 1994.)

Such calculations of the effect of surface tension on the pressure in a fully inflated lung agree reasonably closely with actual measurements in fully inflated lungs. But at functional or intermediate lung volumes the estimated effect of surface tension turns out to be five to ten times too great. This means that the surface tension must vary with the degree of inflation, being relatively low at small lung volumes, i.e. about $5\text{–}10\,\text{dyn}\,\text{cm}^{-1}$ ($0.005\text{–}0.01\,\text{N}\,\text{m}^{-1}$) instead of $50\,\text{dyn}\,\text{cm}^{-1}$ ($0.05\,\text{N}\,\text{m}^{-1}$) (Clements, 1974, p. 172).

These comparisons show that the effect of surface tension in the normal living lung at expiration must be greatly diminished by the presence of a detergent-like wetting agent, or **surfactant**, at the interface between gas and liquid. As with soaps or detergents, its molecules will have weaker forces of mutual attraction for each other and for other adjacent molecules, and therefore the increased concentration of these weaker attractive forces at the interface of a *contracted alveolus* will especially reduce the surface tension.

Lung washes and extracts indicate that the **composition** of lung surfactant (surface active agent) is a mixture of phospholipids, mainly **lecithins** (Hildebrandt, 1974, p. 309). The principal surfactant is dipalmitoylphosphatidylcholine (DPPC) (Weibel, 1984, p. 257).

The main **source of pulmonary surfactant** has long been controversial. Both the **granular epithelial cell** (Section 6.18) and the **exocrine bronchiolar cells** (**Clara cells**) in the epithelium of the bronchioles (Section 6.3) have been strongly supported; according to the latter view, the **osmiophilic bodies** seen in the granular pneumocytes are surfactant which, far from being extruded onto the alveolar surface, is actually being **removed** from the surface. However, experimental evidence (Nicholas, 1993) (radiolabelling, culture of isolated granular epithelial cells, and observations on isolated perfused lungs) has shown that the granular epithelial cell is the source. Evidently the stimulus to release is mechanical distortion of the cell caused by increased lung volume, the increase in release being massive and instantaneous. The frequency of breathing has no effect. The cells are not innervated, but a variety of agonists and antagonists may modulate their response to mechanical stimulation. After release, about 85% of surfactant is rapidly taken back by the granular epithelial cells and reutilized; in the alveolus, the half-life of its main component is only about 85 minutes.

Pulmonary surfactant has various other functions besides alveolar stabilization and fluid balance (Nicholas, 1993, p. 12). Thus it appears to have a chemotactic attraction for alveolar macrophages, and a bacteriolytic effect. It may also opsonize bacteria, rendering them vulnerable to alveolar macrophages.

Surfactant is first formed in the lung during the last part of pregnancy (Section 5.1).

The concept of the inherent *instability of alveoli* because of surface tension has recently been modified (Hildebrandt, 1974, p. 310). As first presented, the concept was based on the principle that each alveolus is a separate bubble that can expand or contract entirely independently of its neighbours; if this were correct, small alveoli (bubbles) would indeed tend to empty into larger ones, as described above. However, an individual alveolus shares its **interalveolar septa** with adjacent alveoli in an interconnected meshwork of alveoli (Section 6.7.1); the collagen and elastic fibres in these shared interalveolar septa (alveolar walls) act as supporting guy ropes. These tethers tend to prevent an alveolus from collapsing when the transpulmonary pressure is low, and during inflation a collapsed alveolus opens more readily when its tethers exert significant stresses. Thus there is a fundamental *interdependence of alveoli*, which provides a mechanically stabilizing effect. Nevertheless, despite this stabilizing effect whole groups of alveoli do empty simultaneously if surface properties are substantially changed, for example in the **respiratory distress syndrome of the newborn** (Section 16.26.1). Thus the concept of bubble instability is still significant in lung mechanics, but it has to be balanced against the concept of alveolar interdependence.

6.26   Designing the perfect exchange tissue

The design of the gas exchange structures is adapted to the oxygen demands of their owner, and these demands depend particularly on body mass and energetics. All comparisons of the relative oxygen demands of various species have to be standardized against body mass: a dog has a much greater *absolute* oxygen consumption than a bat, but a much smaller *relative* oxygen consumption when standardized against body mass. A parameter that has been standardized against body mass is known as **mass-specific**.

Body mass is an important factor in gas exchange, because the bodies of small mammals have a much greater surface area per unit body mass than large mammals. For example the mass-specific oxygen consumption of a mouse weighing $20\,\text{g}$ is ten-fold greater that that of a cow weighing $500\,\text{kg}$. This is because the smaller animal loses heat from its surface relatively faster than the larger mammal, and this loss has to be paid for by a correspondingly greater oxygen consumption per unit body mass. (In very large mammals like the elephant the problem is removing heat, not retaining it, and hence the large ears that act as radiators.)

Energetics are obviously an important factor in gas exchange. Some mammals have a **life style** that is not energetically demanding, whilst others have one that is extremely energetically demanding. For example, a horse and a cow have a similar body mass, but the energetic demands of the horse far exceed that of the cow, and therefore the mass-specific oxygen consumption of the horse is more than twice that of the cow.

The following paragraphs consider the design requirements of a gas exchange apparatus with the **optimum** capacity for gas exchange.

6.26.1 *Mass-specific lung volume*

Common sense suggests that a relatively large lung would be a good start, since this would make it possible to pack in an abundance of the tissues that actually carry out the gas exchange.

The mass-specific volume of the lung of the horse is 20% greater than that of the dog and man, and that of the dog and man is twice that of the cow (Gehr *et al.*, 1981). However, lung volume is a crude comparator, since it is possible to design a relatively small lung that is a highly efficient gas exchanger.

The greatest known mass-specific lung volume in all mammals occurs in **bats**. In the epauleted fruit-bat (Maina *et al.*, 1982) the value is nearly twice that of the horse, and in the insectivorous bat *Tadarida mops* (Maina and King, 1984) the value is 30% greater than in the horse. The enormous lungs in these bats are related to the huge development of the thorax, at the expense of the abdomen; thoracic enlargement also provides the extensive attachments required by the flight muscles.

6.26.2 *Mass-specific surface area of the blood–gas barrier*

It is obviously desirable that the blood–gas barrier should have the largest possible mass-specific surface area. In fact surface area is one of the two anatomical factors that have the greatest influence on the capacity of a lung for gas exchange.

In some pathological conditions, notably **alveo-lar emphysema** (Section 7.19), there is extensive destruction of alveolar walls. This reduces the surface area available for gas exchange, and can therefore make an important contribution to **respiratory insufficiency** (Section 17.29).

The mass-specific surface area of the horse is about one third greater than that of the dog, whilst that of the dog is about twice that of man and cow (Gehr *et al.*, 1981).

The highest values occur in **bats** (Maina and King, 1984) and very small mammals such as the smallest species of **shrew** (Gehr *et al.*, 1981). These mammals have values about one third greater than that of the horse.

6.26.3 *Thickness of the blood–gas barrier*

This is the most critical anatomical estimator of gas exchange capacity: the thinner the barrier the greater the diffusion.

In the pathological conditions of **alveolar emphysema** (Section 7.19) and **pulmonary oedema** (Section 17.25.4), the blood–gas barrier becomes thicker, thus diminishing its capacity for gas exchange. These changes, too, can be a major cause of **respiratory insufficiency** (Section 17.29).

When the *rate* of an event is considered, the harmonic mean rather than the arithmetic mean should be employed, and therefore the **harmonic mean thickness** of the blood–gas barrier is used to express the diffusing ability of the barrier. The harmonic mean thickness of the barrier in the smallest, and very active, **shrew** is $0.26\,\mu m$. That of the mouse is about $0.3\,\mu m$, mongoose $0.4\,\mu m$, dog and cow $0.5\,\mu m$, horse and man $0.6\,\mu m$ (Gehr *et al.*, 1981), and pig $0.7\,\mu m$ (Meban, 1980). These values are rather nicely graded, relative to the size and energy of the species, except for the unexpectedly thin barrier of the cow. The thinnest barrier of all occurs in **bats**. In a specimen of the pipistrelle, the harmonic mean thickness was only $0.18\,\mu m$ (Maina and King, 1984); thus the barrier in man is about 32 times thicker than the barrier in this tiny, yet exceedingly athletic bat.

6.26.4 *Volume of blood in the pulmonary capillaries*

The volume of pulmonary capillary blood is clearly important, since it would be no good providing a very extensive and very thin surface for diffusion without adequately perfusing it with blood.

The pathological destruction of alveolar walls in **alveolar emphysema** entails the loss of pulmonary capillaries (Section 7.19). This decreases the total volume of blood in the pulmonary capillaries, thereby contributing to **respiratory insufficiency** (Section 17.29).

The mass-specific volume of pulmonary capillary blood of a horse exceeds that of the dog by about 10%. The value for the dog is about 25% greater than that of the cow, and (disconcertingly, for any of us who consider man to be an athletic mammal) the value for the cow is about one third greater than that of man.

The highest value so far found in any mammal occurs in a **bat**, the epauleted fruit-bat (Maina *et al.*, 1982), and this is almost twice that of the horse. In other bats the values are similar to that of the horse (Maina and King, 1984).

6.26.5   *Total anatomical diffusing capacity of the lung for oxygen*

To go from air to haemoglobin, a molecule of oxygen has to diffuse through three structural components in series. The first is the **blood–gas barrier**. The second is the layer of **blood plasma** in the pulmonary capillary. The third is the **erythrocyte** in the pulmonary capillary.

The surface area and thickness of the blood–gas barrier and plasma layer, and the volume of blood in the pulmonary capillaries, determine the rate of diffusion of oxygen through these components. These parameters can be measured (see below), and can then yield an estimate of the total capacity of the left and right lungs together for diffusing oxygen. The value so obtained is known as **the total anatomical pulmonary diffusing capacity for oxygen**. Like all these values, it has to be standardized against the size of the animal, and is therefore expressed per unit body mass.

The **total anatomical** diffusing capacity for oxygen is based on the assumption that alveolar ventilation and pulmonary blood perfusion are maximal, and perfectly matched (Section 6.29), throughout the whole of both the left and the right lung. For various reasons (Section 6.27), this is something that never actually happens in the living animal, and therefore the **total anatomical** diffusing capacity is essentially a theoretical value. Nevertheless, the total anatomical diffusing capacity for oxygen is a valuable parameter, since it expresses the *potential* capacity for gas exchange in a given species. It shows how well a species is

adapted structurally for gas exchange, and is therefore very useful for comparing one species with another. It can also be used to compare one group of animals with another, for example bats with non-flying mammals, or mammals with birds (Fig. 6.8).

These estimates of surface area, thickness, and volume have been obtained by recently developed methods of quantitative biology, known as **morphometry** or **stereology**. In principle, they depend on laying a lattice of horizontal and vertical lines on a transmission electron micrograph. The surface of a component such as the blood–gas barrier will intersect the horizontal lines of the lattice relatively often if the surface area is great, and relatively seldom if the surface area is small. After taking into account the total length of the horizontal lattice lines and the magnification of the micrograph, and possible shrinkage of the tissue during processing, the surface area can be estimated from the number of intersections. Likewise the volume of a component, for example red cells in the pulmonary capillary blood, will be reflected in the number of times the cross points on the lattice hit red cells.

Provided that rigorous precautions are taken to ensure that the electron micrographs are sampled at random, repeatable results can be obtained on a small number of samples. The techniques of stereology have revolutionized the anatomical study of biological tissues by making it possible to quantify observations. They were pioneered in biology by Weibel and Gomez (1962) and in lung pathology by Dunnill (1962), and further refined for the normal lung in a long series of publications by Weibel and his colleagues (see Weibel, 1984, p. 71).

The mass-specific total anatomical diffusing capacity for oxygen for the horse is about 10% greater than that of the dog, and the value for the dog exceeds that for the cow by about 50%. The cow has been found to exceed man by about 33% (Gehr *et al.*, 1981) though other estimates (Gehr *et al.*, 1978) showed the value for the cow to be inferior to that of man. There is no doubt, however, that the total anatomical diffusing capacity for man is similar to that of mammals of low physical activity (Gehr *et al.*, 1978).

The mass-specific total anatomical diffusing capacity is very much greater in some very small mammals. For instance the value in a species of **shrew** (Gehr *et al.*, 1980), which has a mean body mass of only 2.6 g, is about 50% greater than that of the horse. Even higher mass-specific total anatomical diffusing capacities occur in **bats**. The highest value in any mammal has been found in the epauleted fruit-bat (Maina *et al.*, 1982), and is about $2\frac{1}{2}$ times greater than that of the above species of shrew (Maina *et al.*, 1989, p. 40).

The supremely high values in bats (especially in small species of bat) (Maina *et al.*, 1991) are explained ana-

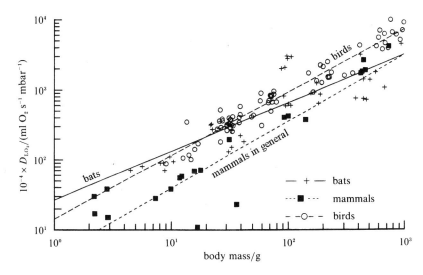

Fig. 6.8 **Comparison of the total anatomical diffusing capacity of the lung for oxygen in non-flying mammals, bats, and birds, based on double logarithmic regression lines.** In birds of all sizes, the diffusing capacity is much higher than that of non-flying mammals of comparable body mass. Small and intermediate sized bats have a diffusing capacity as high as, or even higher than, that of birds of similar body mass, but the largest bats have a diffusing capacity as small as that of non-flying mammals of equivalent body mass.

From Maina *et al.* (1991), with permission of the authors and the Royal Society, London.

tomically by their extremely large mass-specific lung volume (Section 6.26.1), their very extensive mass-specific surface area for gas exchange (Section 6.26.2), their exceptionally thin blood–gas barrier (Section 6.26.3) (Maina *et al.*, 1989), and (in some species) their great pulmonary blood capillary volume (Section 6.26.4). These structural characteristics of the bat's lung represent the upper limits of design in the mammalian respiratory system (Maina *et al.*, 1991). They can be correlated with the fact that bats are the only mammals to have mastered **continuous powered flight**, the most energy-demanding form of vertebrate locomotion (Brackenbury, 1984). The **maximum aerobic capacity** (maximum oxygen consumption) of a flying bat is about twice that of a running mammal of similar size (Maina *et al.*, 1991). Moreover some of the smaller species of bat can **hover**, and this is the most energy-demanding form of flight. The very severe oxygen demands of continuous powered flight testify to the extreme selective pressures during the evolution of bats. Linked to this huge aerobic capacity in bats, is the great size of the heart and the large stroke volume, and the very high haematocrit in these flying mammals (Section 20.4).

The only other extant vertebrate that has mastered continuous powered flight is of course the **bird**. Bird flight requires a metabolic rate well above the maximum attained during exercise by small terrestrial mammals (Thomas and Suthers, 1972). At its most economical speed during horizontal flight, a budgerigar uses 50%

more oxygen than a mouse of the same body mass running hard in an exercise wheel (Tucker, 1968). Steady-state powered flight in birds requires an increase in metabolic rate (oxygen consumption) of at least ten times more than its resting metabolic rate; for example, the humble budgerigar, flying horizontally in a wind tunnel in steady state at its most economical speed, increases its oxygen consumption about 13-fold. This would be heavy work for a man. A well-trained human athlete, such as a racing cyclist of 77 kg body mass, also raises his oxygen consumption about 13-fold in steady state when racing; swimming a fast crawl in steady state requires a 12-fold increase; boxing (which feels like very hard work, as those who have tried it will know) costs a 10-fold increase (McArdle *et al.*, 1981, p. 489).

Section 6.1 mentioned that the **avian lung** is designed on different anatomical principles from that of mammals. Unlike mammals, birds have no blind-ending airways in their lungs, but pump air *through* the lung in the same direction during both inspiration and expiration by means of air sacs, thus largely solving the problem of anatomical dead space; also the relationship between blood flow and air flow in the exchange tissue is more efficient than in mammals, being cross-current (though not counter-current, which would be optimal).

Besides these fundamental anatomical differences in design, the stereological characteristics of the **avian lung** are superior to those of the mammalian lung (Maina *et al.*, 1989, pp. 31, 35, 38, 41, 56). The mass-specific lung volume of birds is about 27% smaller than in mammals of similar body mass. However, the **air capillaries** of birds, which are analogous to the alveoli of mammals, are only about 10 μm in diameter, whereas the alveoli in the smallest mammals are about 35 μm in diameter and in man about 250 μm (Section 6.7.2). These very small diameters in birds cause the mass-specific surface area for gas exchange to be about 15% greater than in mammals, despite the relatively small mass-specific lung volume in this vertebrate class. Furthermore the thickness of the avian blood–gas barrier is only about half that of the mammal. Also the mass-specific volume of pulmonary capillary blood is about 22% greater in birds than in mammals of similar body mass. These stereological differences endow birds in general with a total anatomical diffusing capacity for oxygen (Fig. 6.8) that is at least 20% greater than that of mammals (excluding bats), and may be as much as 80% greater depending on which physical constants are used.

6.27 Physiological diffusing capacity of the lung for oxygen

The **physiological diffusing capacity** of the lung for oxygen is the actual rate of oxygen uptake by the living lungs. It is defined as the volume of oxygen that diffuses from alveolar gas to the pulmonary blood per minute, when the difference between the partial pressure of oxygen in the alveoli and the partial pressure of oxygen in the pulmonary capillary blood is 1 mmHg (0.13 kPa) (i.e. there is a pressure gradient of 1 mmHg). During **severe exercise**, both alveolar ventilation and pulmonary blood flow are increased (the latter by **capillary recruitment**, Section 6.29), so that the physiological diffusing capacity for oxygen increases to about three times its value during resting breathing.

As stated in Section 6.26.5, the **total anatomical diffusing capacity** of the lung for oxygen is based on the assumption that alveolar ventilation and pulmonary blood perfusion are optimal throughout the whole of the exchange tissue of both lungs, but such conditions could only be approached during exercise of extreme severity, and are unlikely to be attained even then. It is therefore to be expected that, in any given animal or species, the anatomical value will substantially exceed the physiological. Comparisons of the anatomical estimate with the physiological measurements in mammals during heavy exercise show that the

anatomical estimate is about twice as great as the physiological measurement.

> The total anatomical diffusing capacity of the lung for oxygen expresses the **potential** capacity for gas exchange in a given species. It is likely that it includes a **safety margin** which is not normally utilized even in the most extreme conditions (i.e. that there is an **inherent redundancy**, a principle found in many organs), and that this contributes to the discrepancy between the anatomical and physiological values (Weibel, 1984, p. 363). The discrepancy may also arise to a greater or lesser extent from inadequate assumptions in the techniques for determining the two values. Measurement of the maximum physiological value is anyway difficult, since it depends on maximum exercise by the subject; this may be attainable by a human subject, but a bat in a wind tunnel or a cooperative quadrupedal mammal obliging enough to run on a treadmill may be reluctant to drive itself to the limit for the sake of even the most enthusiastic experimentalist. However, the anatomical value has the advantage that it can be readily estimated in any available mammal or bird, and with repeatable results. Thus it forms a valuable comparator of the **potential exercise capacity** of mammals, birds, and other vertebrates.

6.28 Alveolar gas: dead space

6.28.1 *Partial pressures of alveolar gases*

In dry air at sea level, the partial pressures in mmHg (kPa) of the constituent gases are: P_{O_2}, 159.1 (21.2); P_{CO_2}, 0.3 (0.04); P_{H_2O}, 0.0 (0.0); P_{N_2}, 600.6 (80.1); total P, 760 (101.3). Very soon after entering the respiratory tract, inspired air rapidly becomes saturated with water vapour, thus changing the partial pressures as follows: P_{O_2}, 149.2 (19.9); P_{CO_2}, 0.3 (0.04); P_{H_2O}, 47.0 (6.3); P_{N_2}, 563.5 (75.1); total P, 760.0 (101.3).

In the alveoli, the partial pressures are changed to those of **alveolar gas**. The new values arise firstly because the alveolar gas is not completely replaced at each breath by fresh air, owing to the anatomical dead space (Section 6.15), and secondly because oxygen is constantly being removed from the alveolar gas and carbon dioxide added.

During normal resting breathing in man at sea level, the partial pressure of **oxygen in alveolar gas** is maintained continuously at about 104 mmHG (13.9 kPa), and that of **carbon dioxide** at about 40 mmHg (5.3 kPa). (Nitrogen and water are about 569 and 47 mmHg (75.9 and 6.3 kPa), respectively.) These values for oxygen and carbon dioxide are of paramount importance, since they govern the P_{O_2} and P_{CO_2} of arterial blood. The **mixed venous blood** that reaches the alveolar capillaries through the pulmonary arteries has a P_{O_2} of about 40 mmHg (5.3 kPa) and a P_{CO_2} of about 45 mmHg (6 kPa) (Fig. 6.9A). This blood becomes arterialized by coming into equilibrium with alveolar gas; thus it leaves the alveolar capillaries as arterial blood, with a P_{O_2} of 104 mmHg (13.9 kPa) and a P_{CO_2} of 40 mmHg (5.3 kPa). Factors that vary the uptake of oxygen by haemoglobin are considered in Section 14.3.

At expiration, the first air that is expelled from the mouth is the fresh air that occupied the anatomical dead space at the end of inspiration; after that, alveolar gas is expelled from the mouth (Section 6.15). Samples taken towards the end of expiration are known as **end-expired air**. These necessarily have the same P_{O_2} and P_{CO_2} as alveolar gas. It therefore follows that end-expired air has the same P_{O_2} and P_{CO_2} as arterial blood leaving the alveoli.

The movement of gas in the alveoli is entirely by **diffusion** (Section 6.1, Fig. 6.1). Diffusion is caused by the kinetic motion of gas molecules. The velocity of this motion is so great, and the distance from bronchiole to alveolar wall so short, that the gases make their remaining journey across the alveoli in only a fraction of a second.

The **pressure gradient** for diffusion of oxygen from alveolar gas to pulmonary capillary is $104 - 40 = 64$ mmHg ($13.9 - 5.3 = 8.6$ kPa). This gradient is sufficient to complete the exchange of oxygen between gas and blood by the time that the red cells have passed the first third of the capillary (Section 17.20). The pressure gradient for exchange of CO_2 is only $45 - 40 = 5$ mmHg ($6 - 5.3 = 0.7$ kPa). This gradient is effective despite being so much smaller than the oxygen gradient, the reason being that CO_2 diffuses about 20 times faster than O_2. Like oxygen, the exchange of carbon dioxide is completed after the blood has traversed the first third of the capillary.

Not all of the blood that leaves the lungs in the pulmonary veins has been through the capillaries of the blood–gas barrier. About 20% (perhaps more) goes through the **bronchial circulation** (Section 17.10), supplying arterial

blood to the smooth muscle and connective tissue of the conducting airways, to the visceral (pulmonary) pleura, and to the relatively bulky connective tissues (in some species, Section 5.8) of the interlobular septa (Section 17.3). The bronchial flow is therefore not oxygenated in the blood–gas barrier. When it leaves the lung it has a typical venous P_{O_2} of about 40 mmHg (5.3 kPa). Most of it drains into the pulmonary veins; consequently it acts as a venous-to-arterial (*right-to-left*) shunt, diluting the arterial blood with a small volume of venous blood. A similar small venous-to-arterial shunt arises from the **coronary circulation** (Section 18.8). The P_{O_2} of arterial blood entering the aorta is therefore not 104 mmHg (13.9 kPa) but about 95 mmHg (12.7 kPa) (Guyton, 1986, p. 494).

6.28.2 *Alveolar ventilation: alveolar and physiological dead space*

The volume of gas that reaches the alveoli is the **inspiratory tidal volume** minus the volume of the **anatomical dead space**. In a normal man this would be about $450 - 150 = 300$ ml. Multiplying this value by the respiratory frequency (say 12 per minute) gives the **alveolar ventilation** (3600 ml min^{-1}).

If alveoli are only partly functional because some of their capillaries are closed (Fig. 6.9C), they contribute to dead space. This is known as **alveolar dead space**. Normally such alveolar dead space can be corrected by **capillary recruitment** (Section 6.29). Alveolar dead space can also arise in the normal animal from *postural mismatching of ventilation and perfusion* (Section 6.30.2), but this can be redressed by compensatory mechanisms (Section 6.30.3). However, alveolar dead space may be greatly increased if many capillaries have been lost by pathological destruction of alveolar walls, as in alveolar emphysema (Fig. 6.10C) (Sections 7.19.2, 7.19.3).

The **total dead space** is the anatomical dead space plus the alveolar dead space. (Unfortunately the total dead space is usually known as the **physiological dead space**, even though it often includes dead space of *pathological* origin.) If the total dead space were to equal tidal volume, no fresh air at all would reach the alveoli, i.e. alveolar ventilation would be zero.

Comroe (1975, p. 180) pointed out that the term 'physiological' dead space is a misnomer, because it includes dead space resulting from disease. This pathological component occurs especially in the commonest of all

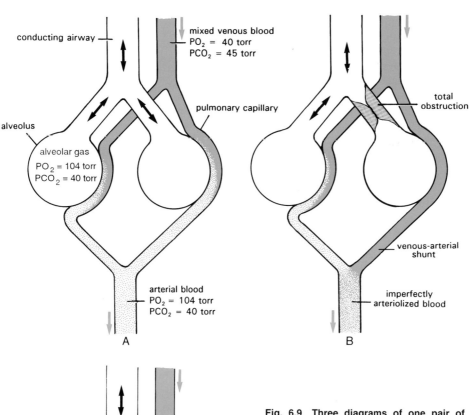

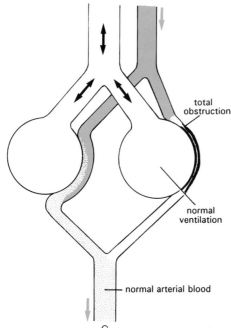

Fig. 6.9 Three diagrams of one pair of alveoli to show matching and mismatching of ventilation and perfusion. The pulmonary capillaries of each alveolus are represented by a single vessel. Venous blood, dark green; arterial blood, light green. Arrows indicate gas flow and blood flow.

A. Normal ventilation and perfusion of both alveoli. This gives a normal ventilation/perfusion ratio (in man, 4:5) and normal arteriolization of the blood.

B. Left alveolus normally ventilated and normally perfused: right alveolus normally perfused, but not ventilated. The right alveolus is normally perfused, but its airway is totally blocked, allowing no ventilation. Therefore the blood to the right alveolus undergoes no gas exchange, and continues unchanged as mixed venous blood directly into the arterial blood, forming a venous-to-arterial shunt. The ventilation/perfusion ratio of the right alveolus has decreased to zero. Hypoxaemia and hypercapnia result.

C. Left alveolus normally ventilated and perfused: right alveolus normally ventilated, but not perfused. The ventilation/perfusion ratio of the right alveolus has increased to infinity. The right alveolus represents alveolar dead space. Hypoxaemia and hypercapnia result.

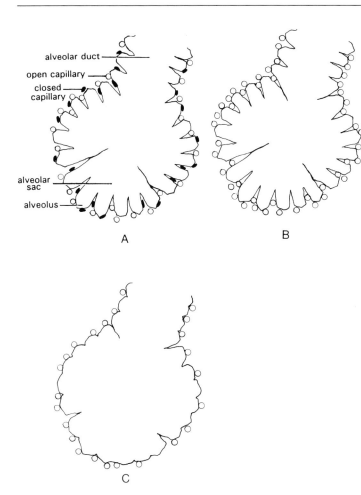

Fig. 6.10 Highly schematic sections through three alveolar ducts and their alveolar sacs and alveoli, to show the changes in their blood capillaries.

A. Normal alveolar duct, alveolar sacs, and alveoli, during resting breathing. About half of the capillaries are open, and the rest are closed, in reserve.

B. The same airways as in A, but with all the capillaries open as in exercise.

C. The same airways as in A and B, after destruction of interalveolar septa (alveolar walls) as in chronic alveolar emphysema. Adjacent alveoli have coalesced, and the three alveolar sacs have also almost coalesced. When such fusions occur these terminal airways appear enlarged. More than half of the blood capillaries have been lost.

serious lung diseases in man, namely pulmonary emphysema caused by smoking (Guyton, 1986, p. 518).

6.29   Matching of gas and blood: capillary recruitment

If the alveolar ventilation in millilitres per minute is divided by the alveolar blood flow in millilitres per minute, the value obtained is the alveolar **ventilation/perfusion ratio**.

Ideally every alveolus should be uniformly ventilated by a normal volume of gas and perfused by a normal volume of blood. Ventilation and perfusion would then be perfectly matched, and this would give an optimal ventilation/perfusion ratio. Under such conditions all of the blood leaving all of the pulmonary capillaries would have a normal P_{O_2} (104 mmHg, 13.9 kPa) and a normal P_{CO_2} (40 mmHg, 5.3 kPa).

Not all of the capillaries in normal alveolar walls are fully perfused at all times; some are kept in reserve. For example, in exercise such reserve capillaries open up and are perfused (Fig. 6.10b; Section 17.21.2), and capillaries that were already open become dilated. These changes are known as **capillary recruitment**. To maintain the proper matching of ventilation and perfusion, recruitment of blood capillaries must be accompanied by an increase in alveolar ventilation.

In a resting healthy man (Comroe, 1975, p. 172), with normally uniform ventilation and perfusion, the oxygen consumption is about 250 ml min^{-1} and CO$_2$ production is about $200 \, \text{ml} \, \text{min}^{-1}$. Under these conditions an alveolar ventilation of about $4000 \, \text{ml} \, \text{min}^{-1}$ will just arterialize 5000 ml of mixed venous blood; precise matching of gas and blood has then been achieved. This gives a **ventilation/perfusion ratio** of **4:5**, or **0.8**, for the whole lung. Ideally this optimal ratio should hold good in each individual alveolus as well as in the entire lung. Scientigraphic observations on the normal horse (Section 19.17) suggest that the ratio in this species is about 1.0 (O'Callaghan, 1991a).

6.30   Mismatching of ventilation and perfusion: venous-to-arterial shunt

If the alveolar ventilation rate is normal but the alveolar perfusion rate decreases, the ventilation/perfusion ratio becomes higher; if the perfusion rate falls to zero, the ratio increases to infinity. If ventilation decreases but perfusion remains normal, the ratio falls; if there is no ventilation at all, the ratio falls to zero. All mismatching impairs gas exchange.

Mismatching of ventilation and perfusion can occur in the normal animal, but has by far its greatest importance in pathological conditions of the lung.

6.30.1   *Mismatching in lung pathology*

In many diseases of the lung, ventilation and perfusion are mismatched. Some areas of alveoli may be normally ventilated, but have a very poor blood flow; other areas of alveoli may have a normal blood flow, but very poor ventilation. In both of these conditions, gas exchange could be seriously impaired, leading to severe respiratory distress.

These principles can be illustrated by two extreme cases. In Fig. 6.9B, the alveolus on the left has normal ventilation and normal perfusion. The alveolus on the right has normal perfusion but no ventilation (its ventilation/perfusion ratio is zero); its incoming venous blood fails to undergo any gas exchange, and therefore continues as unaltered venous (deoxygenated) blood directly into the systemic arterial (oxygenated) blood. This is a **venous-to-arterial shunt** (*right-to-left shunt*), i.e. the shunting of deoxygenated venous blood into the oxygenated arterial blood. If this happens in a

large number of alveoli, the arterial blood will be extensively diluted by venous blood. The P_{O_2} of the arterial blood will then fall drastically, giving severe **hypoxaemia** (deficient saturation of haemoglobin), and the P_{CO_2} of arterial blood will rise (**hypercapnia**).

Defective ventilation can arise from obstruction of bronchi or bronchioles through many causes, including abnormal quantities of mucus, ciliary dysfunction, and bronchial spasm, as in the various forms of **chronic obstructive pulmonary disease** (Sections 7.17, 7.20).

The other extreme case is shown in Fig. 6.9C. Here the left alveolus is again normally ventilated and perfused. The right alveolus also has a normal ventilation, but no perfusion (its ventilation/perfusion ratio is infinity). The ventilation of the right alveolus therefore contributes nothing to the arterialization of the blood: it is therefore equivalent to the ventilation of the conducting airways; i.e. it is **alveolar dead space** (Section 6.28.2). The ventilation of alveolar dead space costs energy because it requires the action of the respiratory muscles, but it achieves nothing towards the supply of oxygen and the removal of carbon dioxide. If it occurs in many alveoli, it will again lead to hypoxaemia and hypercapnia.

Failure of perfusion arises from plugging of arterial vessels by **pulmonary embolism** (Section 17.24), or destruction of the alveolar walls, as in **alveolar emphysema** (Section 7.19).

A **venous-to-arterial shunt** (Comroe, 1975, p. 174) is also known as a **physiological shunt**, or a **venous admixture** (West, 1975, p. 70).

Deficient alveolar ventilation can be caused by various pathological changes (Comroe, 1975, p. 168). **Increased resistance** to gas flow leads to reduced ventilation of alveoli. Causes of regional increases in resistance include all those many factors which may reduce the lumen of the conducting airways; examples are **inflammatory thickening of the bronchial wall, mucus accumulation, bronchial muscle spasm** in response to respiratory allergens or irritant gases (Sections 7.17, 7.20), and compression of bronchi by **tumours**. Many bronchioles may become totally plugged, so that the numerous alveoli peripheral to the obstructions are entirely unventilated. Accumulation of fluid in alveolar sacs and their alveoli as a result of **pulmonary oedema** (Section 17.25.1) can also obstruct alveolar ventilation. Partial or complete collapse of a lung by **pneumothorax** (Section 10.3) or **pleural effusion** (Section 17.27) will prevent the normal dilation of the airways during inspiration, thus impairing alveolar ventilation. **Decreased compliance** of the lung (i.e. increased 'stiffness') (Section 6.31) caused by scar tissue in **chronic alveolar emphysema** (Section 7.19) can also reduce the ventilation of alveoli. Decreased compliance can also arise from the presence of **hard tumours** or **abscesses** in the lung.

Pathological causes of **deficient blood perfusion** (Comroe, 1975, p. 171) include **pulmonary embolism** (Section 17.9.4), occlusion of arterioles by **arteriosclerotic lesions** of the vascular wall, or destruction of pulmonary capillaries as in **alveolar emphysema** (Section 7.19).

Smoking causes **alveolar emphysema** in man (Section 7.19), and this leads to a deficiency in both ventilation and perfusion (Guyton, 1986, pp. 491, 518). Many bronchioles become blocked (Section 7.19.1), causing a fall in the ventilation/perfusion ratio and venous-to-arterial shunts in some parts of the affected lung; in other parts of the lung there may still be some ventilation but many capillaries are destroyed, giving a high ratio and greatly increased alveolar dead space. The result is **chronic obstructive pulmonary disease**, currently the commonest cause of pulmonary disability in man.

Obstructive lung diseases, though arising from a variety of causes, are the major **respiratory diseases of horses**, commonly known under the general term of 'broken wind' or 'heaves' (Sections 7.19, 7.20). Pulmonary diseases in general are the commonest illnesses of adult horses (Dixon, 1992).

6.30.2 *Mismatching in the normal animal due to posture*

Regional reductions in blood flow can occur in certain regions of the lung, depending on the posture of the body (Section 17.23). Thus in the normal man when standing erect, gravity causes the more cranial ('upper' lobes) to be less well perfused than the 'lower' lobes. Likewise in large quadrupeds when standing, because of gravity the dorsal parts of the lung are less well perfused than the ventral parts. Alveoli which are inadequately perfused with blood because of the posture of the animal augment the **alveolar dead space** (Section 6.28.2).

Mismatching because of posture becomes clinically important in large farm animals such as the horse and cow during **lateral recumbency**, as in general anaesthesia or in morbid conditions (Gillespie and Tyler, 1969; it appears to be especially important in the horse during dorsal recumbency for surgery (Section 10.8). Because of gravity (Section 17.23) the lower lung (the 'down' lung) has a much greater perfusion pressure than the upper lung. However, the weight of the animal prevents the 'down' thoracic wall from moving properly during

breathing, and in addition the lower lung bears the weight of the other thoracic viscera and to some extent the weight of the abdominal viscera transmitted through the diaphragm; these forces cause collapse of alveoli (**atalectasis**), and hence hypoventilation, of the lower ('down') lung. The result is a gross mismatching of ventilation and perfusion in that lung, with a major *venous-to-arterial shunt*.

6.30.3 *Mechanisms compensating for mismatching*

Autoregulation by metabolic factors adjusts the *perfusion of pulmonary capillaries* from moment to moment (Section 17.21.1). Thus the low P_{O_2} (and probably also the high P_{CO_2}) in a poorly ventilated alveolus cause vasoconstriction of the local pulmonary arterioles; this increases the resistance to blood flow in the poorly ventilated alveolus, and thus enables the blood to be redistributed to better ventilated alveoli.

Similar metabolic *autoregulation* adjusts the *ventilation of alveoli*. The low P_{CO_2} in an alveolus with inadequate blood flow causes the rings of smooth muscle guarding the alveolar openings in the alveolar ducts (Section 6.5) to contract; this increases the 'stiffness' (reduces the compliance) of these alveoli, thus causing gas to be redistributed to alveoli with a better blood flow and therefore restoring the matching of perfusion and ventilation.

Recent observations by the patch–clamp technique, which enables low-resistance electrical accessibility to the cell's interior without severely damaging the cell membrane, have shown that K^+ currents recorded from cultured myocytes from the rat pulmonary artery are inhibited by exposure to low P_{O_2} (Lopez-Barneo, 1994). This response contributes to the pulmonary vasoconstriction that restores perfusion–ventilation matching in hypoxic alveoli. It is also believed to be the major cause of **pulmonary hypertension** in **mountain sickness** and **right heart disease**.

6.31 Compliance of lung

The compliance of the lung (pulmonary compliance) is the reverse of its stiffness, and therefore reflects the stretchability of the lung. Thus a decrease in compliance is an increase in stiffness and a loss of stretchability. It is established by measuring the pressure required to inflate the lung to a given volume.

The principal cause of decreased compliance is destruction of elastic fibres in the alveolar walls and replacement with fibrous scar tissue, as in **chronic alveolar emphysema** (Section 7.19). Reduced pulmonary compliance increases the energetic cost of breathing. It also decreases alveolar ventilation and causes *mismatching* of alveolar ventilation and perfusion, with a reduction in the ventilation/perfusion ratio and a *venous-to-arterial shunt*.

Lung compliance is decreased by any pathological change that destroys the **elastic fibres** of the alveolar walls and leads to replacement by collagenous **scar tissue**, as in the alveolar emphysema of **chronic obstructive pulmonary disease** (Section 7.19). A pathological increase in **resistance** to air flow in the conducting airways, caused by bronchial **spasm**, excessive bronchial **mucus**, or **oedema** of the airway walls, also lowers lung compliance (Guyton, 1986, p. 469).

The **thoracic cage** also shows compliance (Section 10.2.1), and this may be decreased by arthritic disorders.

Compliance is expressed as the relationship between volume and pressure. Thus if the combined volume of the lungs and thorax increases by 130 ml when the alveolar pressure is increased by 1 cmH_2O (98 Pa), their compliance together is 130 ml $(cmH_2O)^{-1}$ $(1.331 kPa^{-1})$. The lungs alone have about twice the compliance (about 220 ml $(cmH_2O)^{-1}$ $(2.241 kPa^{-1})$ in man) of the lungs and thorax together; this is a clear reminder that work is needed to move the bones and joints of the thoracic cage during breathing.

Values for lung compliance in various mammalian species were given by Crosfill and Widdicombe (1961). Absolute lung compliance is about 40 ml $(cmH_2O)^{-1}$ $(0.411 kPa^{-1})$ in the dog and 13 ml $(cmH_2O)^{-1}$ $(0.131 kPa^{-1})$ in the cat. When expressed as compliance per unit total lung volume at functional residual capacity level, there is little interspecific difference. Koterba *et al.* (1988) regarded the lung compliance of the horse, when standardized against body mass, as similar to that of other species.

Chapter 7
Defence of the Lung

I DEFENCE MECHANISMS

7.1 Defence strategies: exclusion and elimination

No component of the body is so extensively exposed to the external environment as the lung. In man, the surface area of the alveoli alone amounts to almost the area of a tennis court. Despite this huge exposure to noxious agents, including pathogenic organisms and toxic gases, the normal tracheobronchial and alveolar system protects itself successfully. How does it do it?

The mucous membranes of the tracheobronchial tree and the walls of the alveoli have adopted different defensive strategies. These can be summed up as **exclusion** of infective and inert particles from the tracheobronchial mucosa, and **elimination** of such particles from the alveoli. One of the principal devices for protecting a mucous membrane by exclusion is to line it with a physical barrier of mucus, but this is ruled out for the alveoli since the lining would obstruct gas exchange. The alveoli have therefore evolved a unique system of elimination by phagocytosis, which is, however, so efficient that it comes very close to exclusion.

The ideal method of **exclusion** is to prevent the particles from ever contacting the epithelial cells that line the airways. In the tracheobronchial tree this is achieved by the lining of mucus. If microorganisms do make contact with the epithelium despite the mucous carpet (some microorganisms counter this defence by synthesizing mucolytic enzymes), they must then be denied **adhesion** to the epithelial cells. In viral infections, adhesion leads to the **absorption** of virus by molecular receptors on the epithelial surface, the essential

prelude to pathogenicity; in bacterial infections, adhesion is the prerequisite for **colonization**, colonization being followed by **penetration**. If the mechanisms of exclusion fail and the tracheobronchial epithelial cells do absorb virus particles, or are colonized and penetrated by bacteria, the invading micro-organism and its toxins must then be **eliminated** by local or systemic defences.

These various defences are accomplished by the mucociliary escalator of the tracheobronchial airway, reflexes such as coughing, alveolar phagocytosis, pulmonary lymphatic drainage and lymphoid tissue, and the immune and non-immune defence mechanisms, all of these mechanisms being integrated to achieve tracheobronchial and alveolar clearance.

7.2 The mucociliary escalator

The tracheobronchial tree, including the smallest bronchi, is lined by a **mucous carpet** which is continuously swept by cilia towards the pharynx; hence the term mucociliary escalator. In the pharynx the mucus is coughed out or swallowed, generally unnoticed.

The mucociliary escalator plays a vital part in the defence of the lung by **exclusion** of infective and inert particles. Infective particles include viruses and bacteria; inert particles range from harmless carbon to highly dangerous asbestos. Any such particles that collide with the carpet of mucus during breathing should stick to it and be carried to the oropharynx, so it acts like a continuous and constantly moving fly-paper. Not only does the escalator carry particles right out of the tracheobronchial tree, but it also restricts the time available for pathogens to adhere to, colonize, and penetrate the cells that line the tract. The mucociliary escalator in the respiratory tract therefore parallels the anticolonization defences that are made available in the intestine by peristalsis, and by the rapid migration of enterocytes from the crypt to be shed from the summit of the villus.

Bronchioles, respiratory bronchioles, alveolar ducts, and alveoli normally have no mucus, and there are only a few ciliated cells in normal bronchioles (except in the horse, where ciliated cells are claimed to be relatively numerous, Section 6.3.1). Therefore these terminal airways, from the bronchioles to the alveoli inclusive, must rely primarily on alveolar phagocytes for defence against noxious and infective particles (Section 7.7). However, alveolar phagocytes that have engulfed and killed such foreign particles must themselves be removed, and for this to happen they must somehow make the journey to the mucous escalator. The mechanism of this journey is not fully understood (Section 7.7.1).

The mucociliary carpet strictly comprises two layers. One is a sol, the **periciliary fluid**, and the other is a gel, the **mucus** itself; these layers must interact with the **cilia**. A proper balance between the sol, the gel, and the cilia is essential for optimal function.

The periciliary fluid is a watery layer lying on the luminal surface of the epithelium. The cilia of the ciliated cells project into it. Its low viscosity enables the cilia to beat efficiently within it. The periciliary fluid is formed by the underlying epithelium.

The mucociliary transport system has been reviewed by Dunnill (1979, p. 224). Both the periciliary fluid and the mucus are derived very largely from **tracheobronchial secretions**.

The thickness of the periciliary layer is about $5\,\mu m$. It seems likely that the periciliary fluid is not moving at the epithelial surface, but is mobile at its interface with the mucus (Dixon, 1992).

The exact source of the **periciliary fluid** is uncertain. One suggestion is that it may be produced by the **exocrine bronchiolar cells (Clara cells)** (exocrinocytus bronchiolaris) of the bronchiolar wall (Section 6.3.1). Another suggestion is that it comes from the microvilli of the ciliated cells (Breeze and Wheeldon, 1977, p. 710). The **epithelial serous cell** of bronchi (Section 6.2) may also contribute (Breeze and Wheeldon, 1977, p. 716).

7.3   Mucus

The mucous layer lies on the sol layer, and is exposed to the lumen of the airway. It is firm in consistency despite containing much water, and therefore behaves partly as a solid and partly as a fluid. Its gel-like structure is essential for efficient coupling of the mucus with the claw-like tips of the cilia (Section 7.4).

The mucus is secreted by **goblet cells** and **mucoserous glands** of the trachea and bronchi (Section 6.11). It consists of 95% water. **Mucin** is the main non-aqueous component. Its mucin content determines its **viscosity** (i.e. its resistance to flow, Section 6.14), high viscosity being bad for efficient flow.

The mucous layer is of paramount importance in the defensive strategy of **exclusion**. Firstly, it is a physical barrier between the airway epithelium and infective and inert particles, and noxious gases. Secondly, being sticky and moving to the oropharynx, it entraps particles and expels them when they reach the oropharynx. Thirdly, it limits the time available to microorganisms to adhere to, colonize, and penetrate the epithelium. Furthermore, the mucous layer is a hostile environment to a pathogen, since it contains antibodies of the immune system (especially IgA, Section 7.13) and antimicrobial enzymes (e.g. lysozyme, Section 7.15).

The mucous layer is about $2\text{--}5\,\mu m$ thick in the bronchi, and $10\text{--}12\,\mu m$ thick in the trachea (Gehr and Schürch, 1992). It has much greater visco-elasticity than the sol layer. The cilia only touch it with their tips. It seems to be impermeable to water and therefore normally prevents dehydration of the underlying epithelium. Also it gives the epithelium some protection from noxious gases.

The normal resting **output of mucus** is not dependent on the autonomic nervous system. Local secretion seems to be stimulated by mechanical contact of an inhaled particle with the mucosa. Nevertheless, secretion is normally increased by both **vagal** and **sympathetic** stimulation (Section 6.12.2). The total daily output is very uncertain but is undoubtedly small, being probably of the order of 10–100 ml per day in an animal of medium size.

The **time taken for clearance** of the mucociliary carpet depends on its length and rate of movement. If its length is estimated to be about 20 cm in a small mammal and 100 cm in a large mammal, and if the rate of transport is conservatively estimated at 5 mm per minute, in theory a particle might reach the oropharynx in about 40 minutes in small animals and about $3^1/_2$ hours in large animals. It is estimated that 90% of particles can be cleared from the tracheobronchial tree within 1 hour. Complete clearance is believed to take about 24 hours. A microbial pathogen must establish colonization and penetration within these time limits.

7.3.1   *Physical properties of airway mucus*

The **physical properties** of airway mucus, and especially its flow and deformation characteristics, are of particular importance clinically, because they dominate the all-important interaction between the mucus and the cilia. The flow properties of mucus depend largely on three physical characteristics, **viscosity**, **elasticity**, and ability to form **stable threads** (Dixon, 1992).

In the genetic disorder of man known as **cystic fibrosis**, the mucus of the airways and intestines is excessively viscous and fails to flow properly. The condition is characterized by chronic lung infections (and deficient alimentary absorption) and is sometimes known as 'mucoviscidosis'; before the advent of antibiotics it was generally fatal in early childhood.

7.3.2   *Secretion of mucus*

In most species the **mucous layer** is formed mainly by the combined output of **goblet cells** (exocrinocytus caliciformis) and the mucous glandular tubules of the **mucoserous bronchial glands** (glandula bronchialis), but in the horse goblet cells are believed to be the main source (Dixon, 1992). Both the goblet cells and the bronchial glands increase greatly in number in chronic irritation of the tracheobronchial tree caused by infection or irritant particles (Krahl, 1964, p. 250; Comroe, 1975, p. 224; Breeze and Wheeldon, 1977, p. 711; Dixon, 1992)) (Section 7.17.1).

It is generally accepted from observations on a wide range of mammalian species that **goblet cells** (exocrinocytus caliciformis) are numerous in the tracheal and bronchial epithelium. However, it has been reported that, in specific pathogen-free adult rats, goblet cells are so rare that they form less than 1% of the epithelial cells throughout the trachea and bronchi (Breeze and Wheeldon, 1977, p. 711). Presumably goblet cells increase in response to the presence of the microorganisms that are constantly challenging the normal free-living animal. This would be consistent with the marked increase in goblet cells in chronic irritation and infection.

Mucus secretion takes the form of small globules that expand several hundredfold within seconds and are later drawn out into fine threads, which become intertwined

(Dixon, 1992). The capacity to form stable threads is referred to as 'spinnability', and appears to be critical for the effective transport of airway mucus.

7.3.3   *Composition of airway mucus and tracheobronchial secretions*

The **composition of airway mucus** is complex; attempts to evaluate it are impaired by the near impossibility of obtaining clearly defined and consistent samples. According to Dixon (1992), 'airway mucus' normally consists of 95% water and 5% a combination of glycoproteins, proteoglycans, lipids, carbohydrates, and minerals. The chief non-aqueous constituent of mucus is **mucin** in the form of the intertwined threads just mentioned (Dixon, 1992). Mucin is a **glycoprotein** (mucopolysaccharide). The predominant glycoprotein produced by goblet cells and mucous cells is sulphated; there is some firm evidence that the serous cells of the mucoserous glands also produce a sulphated glycoprotein. The **viscosity** of mucus is determined by its sulphated glycoprotein content (Gallagher *et al.*, 1975). The correct viscosity is essential for effective transport; an increase in the glycoprotein content of mucus increases its viscosity, and thus reduces the effectiveness of transport. Various factors increase the viscosity of mucus (Section 7.17.1). Some respiratory viruses secrete an enzyme (**neuraminidase**) that decreases the viscosity of mucus to such an extent that the epithelial cells are laid bare to the virus.

The mucus molecule appears to possess components that mimic the molecular receptor sites for bacteria on epithelial cells, and this may enhance bacterial entrapment. The mucous layer also appears to act as a medium for a variety of other antimicrobial substances, including **IgG** and **IgA** (Sections 7.12, 7.13), and **lysozyme** and **lactoferrin** (Section 7.15) (Stokes and Bourne, 1989, p. 167), which all enter the mucus from the underlying mucosa.

Breeze and Wheeldon (1977, p. 749) reviewed the total composition of '**tracheobronchial secretions**' (perhaps not quite the same thing as airway mucus). According to their account, these secretions consist of **mucosubstances** formed by the **mucoserous glands**, **goblet cells**, and **epithelial serous cells** (Sections 6.2, 6.3). These secretions are reinforced by variable amounts of serum transudate. It is agreed that the mucosubstances govern the physical properties of the secretion. Biochemically, the recoverable secretion in man is 95% water, and 1% each of protein, carbohydrate, lipid (which includes surfactant), and inorganic substances. The main **protein constituents** of 'respiratory fluid' are said to be albumin, secretory IgA and IgG, components of the complement system (Section 14.28.3), and trace amounts of bactericidal proteins including lysozyme and lactoferrin (Section 7.15).

The roles of the various bronchial cell types in secreting these many constituents of the mucous carpet are not well known. However, the **epithelial serous cell** (Section 6.2) seems to be involved in the production of **lysozyme**. **IgA** predominates in the upper respiratory tract; **IgG** increases in proportion in the more distal parts of the tract, and predominates in **bronchoalveolar secretions** (Stokes and Bourne, 1989, p. 174). Much of the IgA appears to be synthesized locally by plasma cells in the walls of the tract; the IgG in the exchange tissue is a 'secretory type' also locally produced, but in the upper airways the IgG is the classical 'circulatory type' that comes from serum transudation (Section 14.28.1).

Although the constituents of respiratory mucus have been intensively studied in human pulmonary diseases, little information is available for the horse in either health or disease (Dixon, 1992).

7.3.4 *Surfactant and airway mucus*

Observations reviewed by Gehr and Schürch (1992) indicate that the periciliary fluid and the mucous layers are separated by a layer of **surfactant**. Measurements of surface tension show indirectly that a layer of **surfactant** also lines the free surface of the mucous carpet of the tracheobronchial airways, though this layer has not been directly demonstrated by electron microscopy. Experiments by Gehr and Schürch (1992) suggest that these layers of surfactant enable surface forces to displace at least some particles (including bacteria) because of their hydrated surfaces, through the mucus and sol layers and into direct contact with the epithelial cells. The subsequent clearance of such particles would necessarily be much slower than removal of particles lying on the mucus surface. This would be inimical to the strategy of defence by exclusion. On the other hand, the layer of surfactant between the mucus and sol layer may be needed to facilitate the sliding of the mucus on the periciliary fluid (Gehr and Schürch, 1992).

7.3.5 *Organization of the mucous carpet*

Formerly, it was generally accepted that the gel layer, i.e. the mucus itself, completely covered the entire upper and lower respiratory tract as far distally as the end of the bronchi (Proctor, 1964, p. 323). There is now evidence that this is not so (Dunnill, 1979, p. 225), and that mucus is transported in separate streams (Van As and Webster, 1974) or discontinuous flakes (Dixon, 1992).

This discovery seems to have revived a mystery about the **thickness of the mucus layer** (Van As and Webster, 1974). If the circumferences of all the bronchi in a man are added together, the total width of the bronchial mucous carpet would be about 30 metres. These innumerable bronchial tributaries of mucus have to be narrowed

in the trachea into a veritable torrent only about 50 mm wide. Some evaporation presumably occurs in the larger airways, and the flow does change proximally from a discontinuous to a continuous stream. Even so, to accommodate the predicted flow of this huge volume of mucus in the trachea, both the velocity and thickness of the carpet would have to be vastly increased. In man, tracheal velocity is about $11–22\,\text{mm}\,\text{min}^{-1}$ (see Dixon, 1992) which is about three to five times faster than bronchial velocity (about $4\,\text{mm}\,\text{min}^{-1}$), but it is estimated that even an eightfold increase in velocity would not compensate. The difficulty is enhanced by the openings of bronchial branches, where the effective bronchial circumference can be reduced by as much as 80%; moreover it is difficult to visualize the visco-elastic mucous carpet dividing in order to go round these openings (As and Webster, 1974).

Similar problems may affect the **arrangement of the sol layer**, which is apparently being formed continuously in the bronchioles, bronchi, and trachea. One hypothesis is that the sol layer is absorbed by the microvilli of the ciliated cells (Section 7.3.5) (Dunnill, 1979, p. 225). However, these microvilli are also believed to be a source of the sol layer. In partial resolution of the possible pile-up of the sol layer, it has been pointed out that, unlike the gel layer, the sol layer may not move very much (Dunnill, 1979, p. 225). If so, it may be sufficient to postulate a simple turnover of sol at the surface of the ciliated cell, formation being somehow balanced against resorption.

7.4 Cilia

Ciliated cells are by far the commonest cells in the epithelium of the normal trachea and bronchi, outnumbering goblet cells by at least five to one. The **cilium** has the same structure as cilia in animals generally, except that its tip has very fine claw-like projections.

Most of the cilium is bathed in the watery sol layer, the **periciliary fluid**, but the **claws** actually penetrate, and thus grasp, the gel layer on the effective forward stroke of the cilium. On the slower recovery stroke, the cilium bends, so that its tip glides past the gel layer. Adjacent cilia beat consecutively (metachronically), as in the Mexican wave of the football terraces, and without neuronal control (also like the terraces).

The cilium has the typical nine microtubular **doublets** surrounding the two central microtubules. One member of each doublet has two rows of **dynein arms**, projecting towards the next doublet. Dynein is an ATP-splitting enzyme similar to myosin, and is essential for ciliary movement.

The ciliated cells of the tracheobronchial tree have numerous **microvilli**, as well as cilia, on their luminal surface. Typically a cell has about 250 cilia about 6 μm long, with about half that number of microvilli about 2 μm long interspersed between them (Breeze and Wheeldon, 1977, p. 707).

The cilia can only beat in the watery sol of low viscosity, and are only effective when the pH, salt concentration, and temperature of this medium are correct (see Dunnill, 1979, p. 224). When these conditions are optimal they beat at the remarkable rate of 25 beats per second. This gives the mucous carpet in the trachea a velocity of about 1.5 cm min^{-1}, but this is the fastest rate. In the dog, the velocity builds up from 1.6 mm min^{-1} in distal bronchi, through 4.0 mm min^{-1} in segmental bronchi, to 8.3 mm min^{-1} in lobar bronchi. Other observations (see Dixon, 1992) estimated human tracheal flow at 1.1–2.2 cm min^{-1} and human bronchial flow at 4 mm min^{-1}.

Little is known about the physiological regulation of ciliary activity. There is some evidence that cholinergic drugs may cause a slight increase in mucociliary transport (Camner *et al.*, 1974). Also β-adrenergic agonists (such as clenbuterol) evidently improve ciliary activity (Section 7.17.3), but this is probably due to bronchodilation which stretches and thins the mucous layer (Dixon, 1992). Electrical stimulation of the nerves that innervate the airways appears to have no clear and consistent effect. The general view (Brody *et al.*, 1972; Comroe, 1975, p. 222) is that nerves are not needed for ciliary motion. The coordination of the beating is based on the mechanical coupling of adjacent cilia, the bending of one initiating the beating of the next (Williams *et al.*, 1989, p. 32).

The possible role of the ciliary cells in the formation and absorption of the sol layer is discussed in Section 7.2.

7.5 Deposition of particles and droplets in the lower respiratory tract

During breathing, dust particles and droplets tend to collide with the mucous carpet, especially at the *branches* of the bronchial tree. At these points the direction of the air stream changes, and the **inertia** of relatively large particles causes them to crash into the wall. There is also a tendency for eddies to disturb the laminar air flow at branches. Lymphoid nodules are concentrated at these branches (Section 7.9.2) a site that is clearly advantageous for immune defences (Section 7.11).

The **diameter** of inspired particles is critical to their site of deposition. Particles larger than 10 μm diameter undergo **inertial collision** with the walls of the **nasal cavity** and **trachea**, stick to the mucus, are filtered out there, and do not reach the bronchi. Particles between 10 and 3 μm are mainly filtered out by inertial collisions in the **bronchi**. Particles which are less than 3 μm penetrate into and beyond the alveolar ducts, and therefore reach the quiet backwaters of the alveoli where diffusion replaces convective air flow (Section 6.1). Here, **sedimentation** (gravitational settling) takes control of particles between 2 and 0.5 μm in diameter. Deposition of very small particles of less than 0.2 μm on the alveolar walls is achieved through **diffusion**.

Fungi, bacteria, and virus particles occur in aerial suspension. Some of these potentially infective organisms are attached to **dust particles** and others are incorporated into **liquid droplets**. The size of dust particles depends on the electrostatic charges of their components. They tend to be between 10 and 3 μm, and therefore are deposited mainly in the *upper* respiratory tract and tracheobronchial tree.

An explosive **sneeze** or **cough** forcibly expels up to a million liquid droplets. The size of these droplets depends on the ambient temperature and humidity, and is therefore much influenced by ventilation of the ambient air. Droplets resulting from a sneeze or cough are about 100 μm in diameter. These remain in the air for several hours before gravitating to the ground. The drier and warmer the air the smaller the droplets become because of evaporation, finally leaving residues about 0.5–5 μm in diameter, some of which contain microorganisms. If droplets of this size enter the respiratory tract, the great majority will penetrate into the alveoli. It is these particles that form the main source of **alveolar infection**.

The concentration of these particles and droplets, and the diameter of the droplets, in the ambient air at any one time depends on the number of animals (or people) per unit volume of air space, on the temperature and humidity, and on the dusty or relatively dust-free nature of bedding or foodstuffs (mouldy hay being a prime offender). Therefore housing of animals, ventilation of the housing, and management of foodstuffs, are crucial factors in controlling the concentration of particles or droplets. Four air changes per hour are considered necessary in a stable.

7.6 Defensive reflexes

The laryngeal closure reflex, cough reflex, and reflex bronchoconstriction, tend to prevent noxious particles from reaching the exchange tissue. A reflex increase in mucus secretion defends by augmenting the mucous carpet. Therefore all these reflexes contribute to the defence of the **tracheobronchial tree** by the strategy of **exclusion** (Section 7.1).

7.6.1 *Closure of the larynx*

Reflex closure of the larynx occurs through the stimulation of **laryngeal mechanoreceptors** (Section 4.15.1), and through excitation of **laryngeal chemoreceptors** by irritant gases (Section 4.15.2). **Tracheal irritant receptors** (Section 4.16) also induce reflex laryngeal closure in response to dust particles as well as irritant gases. **Irritant receptors** in the **bronchi** and **alveoli** (**C-receptors**) respond similarly to dust particles and irritant gases, inducing reflex laryngeal closure (Section 4.16). Laryngeal closure obviously protects the entire tracheobronchial tree by preventing airway access altogether.

7.6.2 *Coughing*

Reflex coughing is evoked by stimulation of the **laryngeal mechanoreceptors** by touch (Section 4.15.1). Reflex coughing also results from the excitation by dust particles and irritant gases of **laryngeal chemoreceptors** (Section 4.15.2), and **tracheal** and **bronchial irritant stretch receptors** (Section 4.16), and **alveolar irritant receptors** (**C-fibre receptors**; Section 4.16). Coughing is an important reserve mechanism for the clearance of mucus.

> Coughing can expel excess respiratory secretions, even down to the fourth or fifth generation of bronchi. In chronic bronchitis in man, it accounts for about 50% of the removal of respiratory secretions. If cilia are lost it may become the main, if not the only, mechanism of removal. In equine pulmonary disease the secretions are

invariably increased; the cough reflex is valuable for removing these secretions, and therefore antitussive agents should be used cautiously in horses (Dixon, 1992).

7.6.3 *Mucus secretion*

In response to dust particles and irritant gases, the **tracheal** and **bronchial irritant receptors** reflexly activate the secretion of tracheobronchial mucus (Section 4.16).

7.6.4 *Bronchoconstriction*

Reflex bronchoconstriction results from the stimulation by dust particles and irritant gases of the **alveolar** (**C-fibre**) **receptors** (Sections 4.16, 7.20).

7.7 Alveolar phagocytosis

There are three main types of phagocyte in the exchange tissue: the alveolar macrophage, the interstitial macrophage, and the neutrophil granulocyte. These cells collaborate in the defence of the **alveoli** by the strategy of **elimination** (Section 7.1).

7.7.1 *The alveolar macrophage*

The alveolar macrophage (Section 6.22) plays a key role in alveolar defence. It has no equivalent in the defensive systems of any other epithelial surface.

These cells arise from the **bone marrow**. They eventually reside on the luminal surface of the alveolar wall, where they are strictly outside the body. The arrival of inert or infective particles on the alveolar wall causes a rapid and very large increase in the number of alveolar phagocytes.

Movement on the alveolar wall is by amoeboid **pseudopodia**. In infections, the alveolar macrophages are presumed to be attracted towards the foreign materials by chemotactic substances; these substances may well include **lymphokines** released by **helper T cells** (Section 14.30). The alveolar macrophages then ingest, kill, and digest inhaled pathogens that have reached the alveolar wall. **Endocytosis** and **lysosomal di-**

gestion of living bacteria, fungi, and spores, are so effective that, despite the continual deposition of infective particles, the alveolar surface is normally sterile; ingestion of non-living particles and debris is equally effective. Alveolar macrophages also contain another surprise for invading micro-organisms in the form of intracellular **lysozyme**, a bactericidal enzyme (Section 14.31).

Alveolar phagocytes that have engulfed and killed foreign particles are removed by the mucociliary escalator.

Alveolar phagocytes interact with other defence mechanisms. They respond to the presence of specific antibody, IgG (Section 7.12), by a marked enhancement of phagocytic activity. If there is inflammation they release a chemotactic factor that attracts **neutrophils** (Section 7.7.4). In the **infected** exchange tissue it is the neutrophil that predominates; in the normal animal subjected to the daily challenge of the environment, neutrophils are relatively rare in the exchange tissue and alveolar macrophages are relatively abundant. The alveolar macrophages are the policemen on the beat; if things get out of hand (inflammation, infection), they call in the neutrophil riot squad.

In the 'normal' lung the **number of alveolar macrophages** (macrophagocytus alveolaris) is said to range from extremely low to practically nil (Lauweryns and Baert, 1977, p. 660). However, the experimental introduction into the alveoli of inert particles (e.g. carbon), or aerosols of bacteria, immediately mobilizes a vast increase in alveolar macrophages; the numbers become so great that about a million can be recovered from the airways of the rat or cat in 1 hour (Lauweryns and Baert, 1977, p. 668). In every-day life, it is 'normal' for the lung to be continually challenged by dust particles and aerosols, many of which carry potentially pathogenic micro-organisms. It is therefore virtually certain that alveolar macrophages will be abundant in a healthy free-living animal.

Helper T cells have the capability of attracting and stimulating macrophages by releasing **lymphokines** (Section 14.30.3). Since T-lymphocytes are quite abundant in **bronchial lavage** (Section 7.9.3), helper T cells seem likely to be a factor in the rapid mobilization of alveolar macrophages.

The haematopoietic **origin** of the great majority of **alveolar macrophages** has been firmly established by the use of chromosome markers, but it remains a possibility that at least some arise by the desquamation of **alveolar epithelial cells** and yet others from **interstitial macrophages** that migrate through the alveolar wall (Lauweryns and Baert, 1977, pp. 662–663).

It has been shown that the alveolar macrophages of haematopoietic origin do not arise by a direct migration of monocytes across the alveolar wall, as was formerly accepted. The precursor cells from the haematopoietic tissue are transported to the lung by the blood. Having reached the **interstitium** of the alveolar wall they do not go immediately through the alveolar wall and become alveolar macrophages, but have been shown by autoradiography to undergo division and maturation in the alveolar interstitium. During this process, they become biochemically and functionally distinct from blood monocytes and macrophages elsewhere in the body.

Activation of alveolar macrophages by **cytokines** (lymphokines), e.g. *interferon-γ* produced by helper T cells and also by cytotoxic T cells (Section 14.31.2), occurs on the surface of the alveoli (Lauweryns and Baert, 1977, p. 663). Furthermore, their phagocytic activity is greatly enhanced in the presence of specific antibody (Stokes and Bourne, 1989, p. 174). Alveolar macrophages also produce a **chemotactic factor** (*chemokine*, Section 14.31.2) that recruits **neutrophils** to the alveoli in large numbers when there is alveolar inflammation (Stokes and Bourne, 1989, p. 174); leucocyte chemotaxis may also result from activation of **complement** (Section 14.28.3) found in tracheobronchial secretions (Section 7.3.3). Furthermore neutrophils are activated by *lymphotoxin* released by helper T cells and cytotoxic T cells, and by *tumour necrosis factor* released by cytotoxic T cells and macrophages (Section 14.31.2). The killing and digestion of organisms phagocytosed by macrophages is based on enzymes within **lysosomes**.

The **lysosome** (Guyton, 1986, p. 15) is a spherical organelle, about 250–750 nm in diameter, formed by the Golgi apparatus and scattered throughout the cytoplasm of neutrophil granulocytes and macrophages. Its typical bilipid membrane encloses small granules consisting of protein aggregates of **hydrolytic enzymes** that digest proteins, nucleic acids, mucopolysaccharides, lipids, and glycogen. Once released, these enzymes can split organic substances that have been phagocytosed, breaking them down into amino acids, glucose, and other diffusable substances.

The life span of alveolar macrophages is about 7–35 days.

The mechanism by which alveolar macrophages **penetrate the alveolar wall** remains something of a mystery. The particular problem is how they cross the alveolar epithelial cells, which are noted for their tightly closed intercellular junctions (Section 6.17). In histological sections, migrating macrophages have been seen in all stages of transition, from a bulge in the alveolar wall to being deeply undercut and almost free of their moorings (Krahl, 1964, p. 264). On the other hand, according to the review by Lauweryns and Baert (1977, p. 663), despite many attempts only two groups of researchers had by then published electron micrographs catching macrophages red-footed in the act of migrating through the epithelium. In view of the vast numbers of cells that must make this journey, that is rather difficult to understand. The best that can be said is that the transepithelial migration must be remarkably rapid.

The mechanism for **removal of alveolar phagocytes** also remains highly controversial (Lauweryns and Baert, 1977, p. 669). The best view is that they leave the alveoli only via the **mucociliary escalator** of the tracheobronchial tree. To do this, they have to cross the gap between the alveolar surface and the beginning of the escalator at the peripheral end of the bronchi (Section 7.2). This is a long and tortuous journey, especially in mammals with several generations of bronchioles and respiratory bronchioles (Section 6.4), and its mechanism is obscure. One possibility is amoeboid movement of the macrophages, but the most likely explanation is that the mucociliary escalator drags the fluid on the alveolar surface towards the bronchioles, carrying the macrophages passively with it.

7.7.2 The interstitial macrophage

Interstitial macrophages (Section 6.20) participate in the clearance of the alveolar interstitium. Thus they phagocytose particles that have traversed the alveolar epithelial cell. What happens to them after that is once again a mystery. They probably migrate in the interstitial fluid to the nearest bronchial or bronchiolar lymphatic capillary, and enter its lumen through an open intercellular junction (Section 7.8). They would then end up in a **pulmonary** or **tracheobronchial lymph node**, where they could deposit their cargo of particles (e.g. anthracosis, Section 5.5). They arise from bone marrow monocytes.

7.7.3 Intravascular macrophage

This variety of macrophage is attached to the endothelial cell lining a pulmonary capillary. It may contribute to the filtering out and removal of small emboli by the pulmonary circulation (Section 17.24).

Another pulmonary macrophage, again belonging to the mononuclear phagocyte system and of monocyte origin, has recently been described (Winkler, 1988; Atwal and Minhas, 1992) under the term 'pulmonary intravascular macrophage'. These cells are claimed to occur in the lungs of ruminants, horse, pig, and cat. This cell is attached to the luminal surface of the endothelial cell of a pulmonary blood capillary by cell junctions that are said

to resemble a zonula adherens. Because of its size, it may almost completely plug the capillary. Functionally, the cell is believed to behave like the stellate macrophagocyte (Kupffer cell) of the liver, which also projects into the lumen of a blood vessel and is involved in the clearance of particulate debris from the blood. It is tempting to speculate that this may be one way by which small emboli are filtered out and removed by the pulmonary circulation (Section 17.24).

7.7.4 Microphages

In the respiratory tract this term can be applied to actively motile **neutrophil granulocytes**. These cells appear in large numbers in the alveolar lumen soon after the arrival of inert particles, especially carbon, and appear to be a normal reaction to severe alveolar pollution. They phagocytose the particles, and also release lysozyme (Section 7.15). Inflammation and infection of the alveoli also attract very numerous neutrophils, in response to a chemotactic factor (*chemokine*, Section 14.31.2) released by alveolar macrophages. As already stated, neutrophils are the predominant cell in infection of the exchange tissue. Neutrophils also appear in the pus that forms in the conducting airways during tracheobronchial inflammation and infection. Their presence can be demonstrated by **bronchoalveolar lavage** (Section 25.8).

The term 'microphage' is not officially recognized by the *Nomina Histologica* (1994), but seems to have currency among pathologists (Blood and Studdert, 1988, p. 582) and a few histologists (Krstic, 1984, p. 260). It is defined as a group of small phagocytes capable of phagocytosing small particles such as bacteria, viruses, and cell debris, and some extracellular substances such as fibrin. It applies particularly to actively motile neutrophil granulocytes. Eosinophilic granulocytes are also included, but according to Krstic (1984, p. 180) they are phagocytic only in the presence of antibacterial antibodies.

It is assumed (Lauweryns and Baert, 1977, p. 671) that **neutrophils** enter the alveolar cavity by migrating rapidly through the alveolar epithelium, but as with alveolar phagocytes no one has published morphological evidence of this process. The mechanism of removal of neutrophils from the alveolar cavity, like alveolar phagocytes, is uncertain, but there is no evidence that they return through the alveolar epithelium and escape to lymphatics via the alveolar interstitium. It is believed that they are drawn to the mucociliary escalator by the presumed movement of the alveolar fluid.

7.8   Pulmonary lymphatics

Profuse lymphatic vessels and abundant lymphoid tissue are typical of all organs which are severely exposed to the external environment, including the intestinal tract, reproductive organs, and skin, as well as the respiratory tract. Metabolically more active organs such as the kidney and liver have less lymphatic tissue.

Pulmonary lymphatics are of particular importance in two defensive functions, removal of pulmonary oedema and clearance of inspired particles. Pulmonary oedema is the abnormal accumulation of fluid in the conducting and respiratory airways; fluid in the conducting airways obstructs the movement of air during breathing, and fluid in the respiratory airways diminishes gas exchange across the alveolar walls, sometimes fatally (Section 17.25).

The lung has three systems of lymphatic pathways, peribronchovascular, pleural, and juxta-alveolar. All three systems are capable of draining both the conducting and the respiratory airways. Valves direct all of this lymphatic flow towards the **hilus** of the lung, where the three systems converge and interconnect.

The **conducting airways** are **directly** served by the peribronchovascular lymphatic system. The lymphatics of the peribronchovascular system reach the respiratory bronchioles, but that is the peripheral limit of their distribution on the bronchial tree.

The **alveoli** have no **direct** lymphatic drainage, because there are no lymphatics in the alveolar walls. However, in the thicker parts of the alveolar walls there is quite a wide **interstitium** (Fig. 6.7) containing **alveolar interstitial channels** (Section 6.20); these channels convey **alveolar interstitial fluid** towards the conducting airways.

The blind ends of lymphatic capillaries first appear in the walls of respiratory bronchioles; here, the interstitial fluid in the alveolar interstitial channels enters the lymphatic capillaries by passing through the loose intercellular junctions of the **lymphatic endothelial cells**. Flow continues towards the hilus of the lung in the lymphatic vessels of the **peribronchial sheath** and **periarterial sheaths**, which together constitute the **peribronchovascular lymphatic pathway**.

This rather improbable drainage pathway through the alveolar interstitial channels and thence into the peribronchovascular lymphatic pathway, probably maintains the steady removal of alveolar interstitial fluid. It also appears to be one of the principal mechanisms protecting the body against **pulmonary oedema** (Section 17.26.2).

The flow of interstitial fluid through the interstitial space in the thicker parts of the alveolar walls, and then into the lymphatic capillaries, also provides a possible escape route for the defence cells in the alveolar interstitium (**interstitial macrophages**; Section 7.7.2).

Until recently there was little evidence on how fluid in the alveolar lumen is absorbed into the alveolar interstitium, but it is now clear (Drake and Gabel, 1995) that the **granular epithelial cell** actively pumps sodium from the alveolar fluid into the alveolar interstitium, and that water follows the sodium by osmosis (Section 6.18).

The abundant researches on the **clearance of particles** from the alveoli by vascular pathways have been reviewed by Lauweryns and Baert (1977, p. 639). Removal is mainly by the **mucociliary escalator** (Section 7.2). However, carbon particles and metallic tracer particles that have been introduced into the alveoli are eventually found in the **lymph nodes** at the hilus of the lung, and they can only have got there by the **lymphatics**. Such particles do pass through the alveolar epithelium into the interstitial fluid of the alveolar wall (Section 7.10); from there they enter the **lymphatic capillaries** and in some instances the blood capillaries also. Morphological data about the precise cellular pathways by which the particles reach the lumen of the lymphatic capillaries are scarce, but the only way the particles can do it is via the **alveolar interstitial channels** (Section 6.20) and finally through the wide **lymphatic intercellular junctions**; endocytosis by the lymphatic endothelial cells is apparently a less significant pathway.

The **endothelial cells** of the pulmonary **blood capillaries** seem to be much less permeable than the walls of the lymphatic capillaries. The blood capillaries are perhaps important only for the removal of water and electrolytes, to which they are freely permeable; the narrow intercellular gaps and zonulae occludentes between the endothelial cells of the alveolar blood capillaries (Section 6.19) can only admit small particles such as peroxidase, and are impermeable to larger particles such as ferritin. Nevertheless ferritin particles are transported by micropinocytotic vessels through the endothelial cells of the blood capillaries, some of the particles being intercepted by secondary lysosomes; however, carbon is not endocytosed by blood endothelial cells, perhaps indicating a selective mechanism of endocytosis.

Those particles that do gain the interstitial space in the alveolar wall have rather a long way to go before they reach the **lymphatic capillaries** in the respiratory bronchioles. Presumably the pulmonary blood capillaries must participate in the clearance of at least the smaller particles, to avoid their accumulation in the alveolar interstitium; for example, ferritin is absorbed by blood capillaries as well as by lymphatic capillaries, though much more by the latter. However, despite the long distance between the alveolar wall and the lymphatics in the respiratory bronchiole there is no doubt that the lymphatic capillaries are much more important than the blood capillaries in alveolar clearance.

7.8.1 *Peribronchovascular lymphatic pathway*

The peribronchovascular lymphatic pathway is formed by the lymphatic plexuses of the **peribronchial** and **periarterial sheaths** (Section 6.13; Fig. 6.3B). These lymphatic plexuses consist of lymphatic capillaries and lymphatic collecting vessels. They appear to drain lymph continuously from the exchange tissue. The **peribronchovascular lymphatics** extend peripherally to the level of the respiratory bronchioles, but do not ramify over the alveolar walls.

In the walls of the respiratory bronchioles, the blind ends of the terminal lymphatic capillaries meet the ends of the **alveolar interstitial channels**, as just described. The peribronchial components of these lymphatic channels receive small lymphatic vessels that drain the numerous **bronchial lymphonodules** (Section 7.9.2).

As the bronchi become larger, the peribronchial lymphatic channels coalesce into **bronchial lymphatic collecting vessels** accompanying the bronchi. These prenodal vessels drain into the inconstant **pulmonary lymph nodes**, and then, near the root of the lung, into the **tracheobronchial lymph nodes** (Section 7.9.1).

Lymph from the lung is propelled by the combination of an active (intrinsic) pumping mechanism and a passive (extrinsic) mechanism. **Active pumping** is provided by the **smooth muscle** in the lymphatic walls, as in tissues generally (Section 14.8). The **passive mechanism** is provided by the pressure changes that occur during **breathing**. During inspiration, radial traction on the peribronchial sheath and periarterial sheath dilates the peribronchial lymphatics and transmits a

fall in pressure to their lymphatic fluid; simultaneously, the contraction of the diaphragm during inspiration raises the intra-abdominal pressure. The resulting pressure gradient from abdomen to thorax causes the peribronchial lymphatics to fill during inspiration. Expiration compresses the peribronchial lymphatics, driving the lymph towards the hilus under the direction of the lymphatic valves.

The peribronchial lymphatic vessels contribute to the **hydraulic 'give'** that enables the diameters of bronchi and pulmonary arteries to be adjusted despite the pressure changes caused by breathing (Section 6.13).

The 'peribronchovascular' and 'pleural lymphatic pathways' are not formally named by the NAV. They simply belong to the **vasa lymphatica afferentia** of the **lymphocentrum bronchale** (NAV, 1983, p. A108) (Section 14.32.4).

Active pumping is believed to be particularly important in maintaining the flow of lymph from normal lungs, but the **passive mechanism** is apparently more important in pulmonary oedema (Drake and Gabel, 1995).

7.8.2 *Lymphatics of the pulmonary pleura*

The lymphatics of the pulmonary (visceral) pleura form a wide-meshed polyhedral network of profusely anastomosing channels, with blind-ending side branches, around the 'lobulated' areas visible on the surface of the lung (Section 5.8). They run all over the surface of the lung and converge on the **root of the lung**. There they drain into **bronchial lymphatic vessels** accompanying the principal bronchus (Section 5.5).

The lymphatics of the pulmonary pleura drain the pleural fluid, maintaining it at a minimum level in the normal lung (Section 9.7) and removing excess fluid from the pleural cavity if pleural effusion forms (Section 17.27.4).

Drake and Gabel (1995) concluded that the **pleural lymphatics** are very effective in maintaining the *volume of pleural fluid* in the pleural cavity at a minimum in the normal animal. However, they called attention to disagreements about the possible role of pleural lymphatics in contributing to the clearing of *lung fluid* via the pleural cavity in the normal animal. Most investigators believe that little, if any, *lung fluid* is removed from the normal lung via the pleural cavity. However, their own laboratory has shown that such movement of fluid can occur under pathological conditions; if there is pulmonary oedema, a large volume of *lung fluid* is cleared through the **pulmonary pleura**, though it takes several hours to do so.

7.8.3 *Juxta-alveolar lymphatics*

As Fig. 6.3 shows, the outer surfaces of the peribronchial and periarterial sheaths are continuous with the walls of surrounding alveoli. The lymphatic capillaries in the outermost regions of the sheaths are in contact with adjacent alveolar walls, and are therefore known as juxta-alveolar lymphatics. These lymphatics can drain fluid from the adjacent alveoli into the peribronchovascular lymphatic pathway. The concept of 'juxta-alveolar lymphatics' was introduced by Lauweryns and Baert (1977, p. 633).

7.8.4 *Structure of pulmonary lymphatic vessels*

The **lymphatic capillaries** (Section 14.6.1) form a network that drains into larger lymphatic collecting vessels (Section 14.6.2). The capillaries have walls of minimal thickness, lined by naked endothelial cells with large spaces between adjoining cells and an incomplete basal lamina. They are therefore highly permeable to solutes and cells.

The **lymphatic collecting vessels** are less permeable, particularly to cells. They have valves and circular smooth muscle, and are capable of the active pumping of lymph (Section 14.8).

The **lymphatic capillaries** are lined by endothelial cells, which in some places are joined by junctional complexes, but elsewhere have open intercellular junctions that do not even overlap, rendering the endothelial lining discontinuous (Lauweryns and Baert, 1977, p. 633). Micropinocytotic vesicles are present. The basal lamina is thin and interrupted, being absent over large areas. The vesicles and discontinuous basal lamina are consistent with endocytosis. However, the significance of transcellular transport in the drainage of pulmonary lymph has recently been minimized and the open intercellular junctions are now regarded as the main drainage pathway in the lung (Lauweryns and Baert, 1977, p. 647).

7.8.5 *Summary of lymphatic drainage pathways in the lung*

Lymphatic drainage is one of the main mechanisms protecting against pulmonary oedema (Section 17.26.2). To keep the blood–gas barrier as thin as possible, lymphatic capillaries are banned from the alveolar walls. Alveolar fluid must travel within the alveolar wall until it reaches the respiratory bronchiole. There it encounters lymphatic capillaries. From here onwards it will be carried to the hilus of the lung by the peribronchovascular lymphatics, and this will be the principal pathway for removal of pulmonary fluid. The lymphatics of the pulmonary pleura drain some fluid from the normal lung, but become a major drainage pathway if pulmonary oedema has occurred.

7.9 Pulmonary lymphoid tissue

7.9.1 *Pulmonary and tracheobronchial lymph nodes*

Along the course of the lymphatics that accompany the lobar bronchi and principal bronchi, and therefore buried in the substance of the lung, there are occasional **pulmonary lymph nodes**. They are small, inconstant, and vary with the species. Their afferent vessels are from the peribronchovascular lymphatics. Their efferent vessels continue as bronchial lymphatic vessels along the main bronchi to the root of the lung. At the root of each lung, the pleural and peribronchial lymphatics drain into the much larger **tracheobronchial lymph nodes** (Section 14.32.4); the efferent vessels from these nodes drain into the **mediastinal lymph nodes**, or directly into the **thoracic duct** (Section 14.34).

Lymph nodes (Section 14.17) act as biological filters, intercepting foreign materials, damaged cells, and particularly macrophages that have phagocytosed foreign material including microorganisms and inert particles. In the **outer cortex** there are lymphatic nodules. Immunocompetent cells in the lymph nodes and spleen become activated, and produce antibodies against microorganisms. Accumulations of carbon particles may make the nodes dark in colour (anthracosis, Section 5.5).

In the *horse* and *carnivores* there are several erratic **pulmonary nodes** (lymphonodi pulmonales), but in the *domestic ruminants* there is only a single (inconstant) pulmonary node (Saar and Getty, 1975, pp. 625, 1059, 1656). The flow from the pulmonary node or nodes drains into the **tracheobronchial lymph nodes**, where it is joined by the flow from the pleural lymphatics.

In the *sheep*, the tracheobronchial nodes drain both lungs mainly into the **thoracic duct**, the rest entering the **right lymphatic duct**: in *man*, most of the flow from the two lungs drains into the right lymphatic duct, and only a minority goes into the thoracic duct (Lauweryns and Baert, 1977, p. 630).

7.9.2 *Tracheal and bronchial lymphonodules*

Abundant lymphonodules (Section 14.15) are present just below the epithelium throughout the length of the tracheobronchial tree, including the terminal bronchioles. They constitute the so-called **bronchus-associated lymphoid tissue (BALT)**. The greatest concentrations occur at the **branches** of the bronchi, these being the places where particles in the inspired air are most likely to collide with the bronchial walls (Section 7.5).

The lymphatic cells within these nodules are involved in the immune defences against pathogens. Abundant resting (uncommitted) B-lymphocytes in the local lymphatic nodules become antigenically stimulated, and activated by T helper cells, to give rise to cells of the **plasma cell series** (Section 14.14) which produce antibodies locally (particularly **IgA**; Sections 7.13, 14.29) specifically against these pathogens. Also T-lymphocytes are activated to produce a cell-mediated immune response (Section 7.14).

> **Aggregated lymphonodules** are large and multiple; **solitary lymphonodules** are small and single.
>
> The largest **aggregated bronchial lymphonodules** (lymphonoduli bronchales) are structurally and functionally analogous to the aggregated lymphonodules of the small intestine (**Peyer's patches**) (Dunnill, 1979), the latter now being widely known as gut-associated lymphoid tissue (GALT) (Stokes and Bourne, 1989, p. 176) (Section 14.15). In fresh lungs, the bronchus-associated lymphoid tissue (Stokes and Bourne, 1989, p. 176) can be seen under the dissecting microscope, and if fixed appropriately is visible to the naked eye as white spots on the mucosal surface (Breeze and Wheeldon, 1977, p. 753).
>
> A **solitary lymphonodule** beneath the bronchial epithelium consists of a spherical accumulation of lymphocytes. It may be surrounded by a capsule consisting of a thin layer of reticular cells, but if so, the capsule is not visible in ordinary preparations and anyway is obscured by infiltrating lymphocytes (Krstic, 1984, p. 237). Central **postcapillary venules** (Section 12.14) may

be present (Breeze and Wheeldon, 1977, p. 755). The **germinal centre** (Section 14.16) contains a mixed population of macrophages, multiplying and differentiating B-lymphocytes and B cells, and some plasma cells. It also contains relatively small numbers of T-lymphocytes and their differentiating T cells, of which helper T cells are the most numerous (Breeze and Wheeldon, 1977, p. 753). The nodule may extend right through the peribronchial sheath, contacting the lymphatic vessels of the sheath; otherwise it will come close to the bronchial epithelium.

About 50% of the lymphocytes in these various lymphonodules are **B cells**, 20% are **T cells**, and the rest cannot be categorized (Breeze and Wheeldon, 1977, p. 755).

The **bronchial epithelium** covering a lymphonodule is specialized. It takes the form of nonciliated columnar or cuboidal cells, with an interrupted basal lamina. Judging by the apparent function of the similar specialized phagocytic epithelial cells (**M cells**, Section 14.29.3) covering intestinal lymphonodules (Stokes and Bourne, 1989, p. 181), the specialized bronchial epithelial cells have the function of ingesting antigen and then transporting it to the lymphocytes in the underlying nodule. This encourages the antigenic stimulation of **B-lymphocytes**; after activation by helper T cells, the resulting B cells multiply and differentiate into plasma cells which secrete mainly immunoglobulin A (Section 14.29). The lymphonodule is the most important site of antibody formation by B-lymphocytes and their plasma cells (Section 14.14).

7.9.3 *Free lymphocytes and plasma cells*

Individual **lymphocytes** and **plasma cells** are plentiful in the lamina propria of the tracheobronchial mucosa. Lymphocytes are also present in the tracheobronchial epithelium. Yet others find their way into the mucous layer, and quite large numbers are recovered by **bronchoalveolar lavage**. All of these are examples of 'free' lymphocytes. Many of them have migrated to the airway surface from the underlying lymphonodules, particularly through the specialized bronchial epithelium covering the lymphonodules. Presumably some of these lymphocytes become immunely activated during their exposure on the airway surface, and return to their lymphonodules to differentiate into plasma cells, and helper or cytotoxic T cells.

Lymphocytes and plasma cells are also found around the acini of the bronchial and tracheal mucous glands (Breeze and Wheeldon, 1977, p. 756). Stokes and Bourne (1989, p. 174) reported up to 40% lymphocytes in the 'free' cell population of the lung, presumably in domestic mammals. Most of the plasma cells contain IgA; a few contain IgG, IgM, or IgE. The lymphocytes are mostly T cells, B cells being the minority (Breeze and Wheeldon, 1977, p. 756).

Bronchoalveolar lavage recovers large numbers of cells, so there is obviously an extensive traffic of cells into the airways. There are species variations, but in man most of them (about 70%) are alveolar macrophages, less than 20% are lymphocytes, and the rest are plasma cells, neutrophils, and eosinophils. The lymphocytes obtained from bronchial lavage are mainly T cells, B cells still being in the minority (Breeze and Wheldon, 1977, p. 756) though present in significant numbers (Stokes and Bourne, 1989, p. 174). The presence of quite abundant T cells is consistent with the activation of alveolar phagocytes and neutrophils through secretion of **lymphokines** (e.g. interferon-δ and lymphotoxin, Section 14.31.2) by helper T cells on the alveolar surface (Section 14.30.2).

7.10   The alveolar epithelium

The fact of **alveolar clearance of particles** by the pulmonary lymphatics and pulmonary blood vessels suggests that some particles somehow manage to pass through the alveolar epithelium and its basal lamina. Since the cell junctions of alveolar epithelial cells are closely sealed by tight junctions, large particles such as ferritin and carbon are unable to pass through the intercellular junctions. However, it is known that such particles can go through the alveolar epithelial cell by endocytosis, to be released into the alveolar interstitial fluid. Here they are engulfed by **interstitial macrophages** (Section 7.7.2), or are carried by fluid flow to the lymphatic capillaries.

The alveolar epithelial cell has lost the power of **regeneration**. After injury it is replaced, though slowly, by mitosis of **granular epithelial cells** (Section 6.17).

7.11   Antigens and antibodies

The airways are affected by a variety of **antigens**, including viruses, the capsules and toxins of bacteria, and plant derivatives such as fungal spores and pollen. The excretory and secretory products of parasitic lungworms are antigenic. The cell membranes of protozoa are significant antigens in some body systems, but not in the respiratory tract. The faeces and fragments of dead house-dust mites are important respiratory antigens in man, capable of causing asthma. Such antigens are commonly foreign proteins, or peptides that form the constituent parts of proteins. Some of them are particulate (e.g. bacteria and spores) and others are soluble (e.g. bacterial toxins).

The tracheobronchial and alveolar airways have immune defences that are highly specific to antigens, and can therefore be targeted at particular pathogens or toxins. There are also equally important non-specific defences that act without involving antigens, and therefore defend the host against a relatively wide range of pathogens (Section 14.31). The specific and the non-specific defences combine with the mucociliary escalator in the strategy of defence of the *tracheobronchial tree* by **exclusion** of pathogens and toxins. The specific and non-specific mechanisms defend the *exchange tissue* (alveoli) by **elimination** of pathogens and toxins.

Pathogenic micro-organisms commonly enter the respiratory system by being inhaled and adhering to the mucous carpet, or by being deposited on the alveolar walls. Adherence is most likely to happen at the *branches of the bronchial tree* (Section 7.5); at these points, **lymphonodules** are particularly numerous in the respiratory mucosa, forming the so-called **bronchial-associated lymphoid tissue (BALT)** (Section 7.9.2).

In the lymphonodules of the tracheobronchial mucosa, antigens derived from micro-organisms bind to **B-lymphocytes**, thus initiating a sequence of cell differentiations that culminates in the production of immunoglobulins by plasma cells specifically against the invading pathogens or toxins. Presumably *free* **B-lymphocytes** wandering in the tracheobronchial mucosa can also be activated. The activated B-lymphocytes differentiate into **plasma cells**, and it is these cells that secrete the various types of immunoglobulins. **Immunoglobulin G (IgG)**, and to a much greater extent **immunoglobulin A (IgA)**, provide the immune defence of the lung (Section 14.29). **Immunoglobulin E (IgE)** takes part in several mechanisms protecting the host against parasites in the gut, and is also involved in allergic airway responses to pollen and fungal spores. All classes of immunoglobulins can exist as cell-surface receptors incorporated in the surface membrane of a cell, and also in a water-soluble secreted form.

Immune responses can be divided into two broad classes (Section 14.22). In **humoral immunity** the antibodies circulate in the body fluids: in **cell-mediated immunity** specialized cells react with and destroy other cells that carry foreign antigen on their surface.

7.12   Immunoglobulin G

In the body in general, the main product of the immunoreactive **B cell** and its progeny of **plasma cells** is immunoglobulin G (IgG), which is the principal **circulating antibody** in the blood plasma (Section 14.28). IgG is therefore essentially a *systemic* rather than a local defence mechanism. Nevertheless, *circulating* IgG does enter the submucosa and mucous carpet of the tracheobronchial tree by passive transudation from the blood plasma. Therefore it does participate in the local immunological defence of the **tracheobronchial tree**, but only in a relatively minor role. In the **alveoli** IgG is more abundant, and makes a relatively greater contribution to defence, particularly by enhancing the activity of alveolar phagocytes, but also by inhibiting bacterial adhesion and by antiviral actions.

IgG is formed in response to the respiratory antigens mentioned at the beginning of Section 7.11. A protein antigen, for example a bacterium or a bacterial toxin, passes from the airway lumen through the mucous carpet and tracheobronchial epithelium. During this journey, or when it has arrived in the lamina propria, the antigen binds with a resting B-lymphocyte (Section 14.28). The B-lymphocyte, now antigenically stimulated, then interacts with a helper T cell. The B-lymphocyte is then fully activated to become a B-immunoblast. This proliferates B cells, which differentiate into plasma cells secreting IgG.

Presumably *circulating* IgG diffuses out of the tracheobronchial mucosa at inflamed locations. In addition to enhancing phagocytic activity and inhibiting bacterial adhesion, it would interact with complement (Section 14.28.3). It would thus co-operate with the essentially *local* immune defence of the tracheobronchial airways that is provided (Section 14.29) by **IgA** (Murray, 1973). Furthermore, IgG can combine with viruses or bacterial toxins and prevent them from binding to mo-

lecular receptor sites on their target cells. Hence circulatory IgG could contribute to the defence of the airways by the strategies of *both elimination and exclusion*.

On the other hand, the **inflammatory response** produced by IgG (Section 14.28.3) might damage the epithelial lining of a mucous membrane (Stokes and Bourne, 1989, p. 171). Consistent with this proposition, the tracheobronchial mucosa is not extensively defended by IgG; nor, indeed, are any of the other major systems of mucous membranes in the body. Instead, mucous membranes generally, including those of the tracheobronchial tree, are defended mainly by a strategy of immune *exclusion* by **IgA** (Section 14.29).

This raises the question, why is IgG relatively abundant in the **exchange tissue**, where the epithelial lining is the exquisitely delicate alveolar epithelial cell? The main defence of the alveoli is, of course, *phagocytosis* (Section 7.7), and IgG improves the phagocytic properties of alveolar macrophages and their supporting neutrophils. This is because part of the IgG molecule forms receptors on the surface of the phagocytic cell; these receptors in turn bind to the IgG that contacts the surface of micro-organisms.

The IgG in the alveoli is not classical circulatory IgG but a locally synthesized 'secretory' IgG (Stokes and Bourne, 1989, pp. 171, 174). Secretory IgG is a minor component of gut secretions in most species, but in the gut of the rat and ruminants it is a major secretory immunoglobulin and is evidently capable of mucosal exclusion by inhibition of bacterial adhesion and by antiviral activities (Stokes and Bourne, 1989, p. 171). Presumably secretory IgG has similar exclusion properties in the exchange tissue. Even so, the secretory form of IgG is a complement-fixing antibody (Stokes and Bourne, 1989, p. 174), and is therefore potentially damaging to the fragile alveolar wall.

7.13   Immunoglobulin A

There is also a powerful, independent, *local* antibody response by B cells. Immune defence of the tracheobronchial tree, and indeed of mucosal surfaces throughout the body, is largely dependent on a locally secreted antibody, immunoglobulin A (IgA), thus constituting a **common mucosal system** (Section 14.29). A specific antigen, for example a bacterium or a soluble toxin, makes contact with the tracheobronchial mucosa. There it may be ingested, transported across the epithelium, and delivered close to a B-lymphocyte in the lamina propria of the mucosa, thus enabling the B-lymphocyte to be *antigenically stimulated* (Section 14.28). Or the antigen may be engulfed by a **mononuclear phagocyte** (Section 14.10); this may act as an **antigen presenting cell** and *activate* a helper T-lymphocyte in the lamina propria (Section 14.30). Interaction between the B-lymphocyte and the helper T cell then causes the B-lymphocyte to proliferate and differentiate into **plasma cells** which locally synthesize IgA specifically against this particular antigen (Section 14.29).

The IgA is then transported through the epithelium and across the mucous carpet, to lie on the *luminal* surface of the mucus. There it blocks the absorption of microbial toxins and inhibits the adherence of micro-organisms to the epithelium. It thus provides the predominant component of the immune defence of the tracheobronchial mucosa. At the same time, it collaborates with the purely physical barrier of the mucociliary escalator to execute the strategy of defence by *exclusion*.

7.14   Cell-mediated immunity: T cells

Pathogens that penetrate the epithelium of the tracheobronchial tree may also activate cytotoxic T-lymphocytes (Section 14.30).

Cytotoxic T cells protect the host against viruses and tumours (Section 14.30). In the respiratory tract, influenza viruses are of particular importance in human medicine, and also in veterinary medicine because of their adverse effects on the performance of racehorses.

Although cell-mediated immunity is of the greatest possible significance in the protection of the body in general against infection and tumours, its role in the defence of the airways in particular has not been extensively investigated (Stokes and Bourne, 1989, p. 172). However, in view of the prevalence of highly pathogenic respiratory viruses, it must be assumed that cytotoxic T cells contribute to the defence of both the tracheobronchial tree and the exchange tissue by the strategy of *elimination*.

7.15   Non-immunological antimicrobial defence

A bactericidal enzyme, **lysozyme**, is present in many body fluids, including tears and saliva. It is secreted beneath respiratory mucus and then diffuses into the mucus carpet, where it forms a first line of defence against bacteria (Section 14.31.1).

> **Surfactant** has also been shown to have a bactericidal action (Junqueira and Carneiro, 1983, p. 378). **Lactoferrin** is another bactericidal agent found in tracheobronchial secretions (Section 14.31.1).

7.16   Alveolar and tracheobronchial clearance

Clearance means the removal of micro-organisms and noxious dust particles from the tracheobronchial tree and exchange tissue. Although the respiratory tract is wide open to invasion by these particles, its defences are normally remarkably efficient.

Potentially infective fungi, bacteria, and viruses, can be attached to dust particles 3–10 µm in diameter, or incorporated into liquid droplets which may evaporate from 100 µm down to 0.5 µm in diameter or less. Those between 10 and 3 µm collide with the bronchial mucous carpet, and those less than 3 µm are deposited on the alveolar walls (Section 7.5). Nevertheless, in a normal man and adult horse the lung is reportedly sterile beyond (caudal to) the first bronchial division (Dixon, 1992). Indeed, it is estimated that 90% of material deposited in the tracheobronchial tree can be physically cleared within 1 hour (Stokes and Bourne, 1989, p. 169).

Alveolar phagocytes remove invading bacteria from the alveolar wall very quickly, and the alveolar surface is sterile under normal conditions (Lauweryns and Baert, 1977, p. 665). If mice are subjected for 30 minutes to a fine aerosol spray of virulent staphylococci, the bacteria penetrate throughout the whole respiratory tract. Because of the small size of the aerosol particles, many of them less than 3 µm in diameter, large numbers of the bacteria reach the alveoli. However, 4–6 hours later 95% of the bacteria have disappeared from the alveoli (Jericho, 1968; Cohen and Gold, 1975). Nearly all of them have been phagocytosed by alveolar phagocytes, and most of these phagocytes have reached the **mucociliary escalator** to be swept out.

The figures for clearance of the tracheobronchial tree and alveoli are an astonishing tribute to the integrated exclusion–elimination defences of the airways by the mucociliary escalator, defensive reflexes, phagocytosis, and immune and non-immune antimicrobial defences.

II   DISEASE PROCESSES

7.17   Failure of the mucociliary escalator: obstructive airway disease

Transport of mucus by the mucociliary escalator is impaired in many pulmonary diseases. It results in the accumulation of mucus and obstruction of the airway. Particularly striking failures occur in man and the horse. For example, in **asthma** or **cystic fibrosis** in man, transport can be reduced by up to 90%; the deficit has not been similarly quantified in the horse, but disruption of mucociliary transport is a major problem in **chronic obstructive pulmonary disease** in that species. In such conditions, the cause can be an abnormal quantity or quality of *mucus*, abnormal *periciliary fluid*, impairment of *cilia*, or combinations of these elements. The relative contributions of such factors have not been established in any species, including even man.

The obstruction of bronchi caused by a failure in mucociliary transport can cause a severe reduction in alveolar ventilation. This leads to pronounced mismatching of ventilation and perfusion, with a low ventilation/perfusion ratio and a serious venous-to-arterial shunt (Section 6.30.1). The obstruction also causes a serious increase in the energetic cost of breathing (Section 10.13).

7.17.1   *Mucus*

The **volume of mucus** must remain within a normal range. Chronic bronchitis (including **chronic obstructive respiratory disease** in horses), or chronic irritation by dust particles or noxious gases (including tobacco smoke), provokes an increase in the number of goblet cells and mucoserous bronchial glands in the tracheobronchial tree, and also induces the occurrence of goblet cells in bronchioles. The **ciliated cells** are

then unable to remove the increased volume of mucus at the proper rate. Mucus tends to pile up at bronchial branches. During its slower movement, and particularly if it stops moving, the mucus has time to absorb high concentrations of toxic substances, which may then diffuse through the gel and sol layers and injure the ciliated cells beneath. A further adverse effect of the increased number of goblet cells is that they crowd out the ciliated cells, so that not only is there more mucus but there are less ciliated cells to remove it, as in chronic bronchitis in man and chronic obstructive pulmonary disease in horses.

The **physical properties of mucus** must also remain within a normal range. Excessively viscous mucus is poorly transported, and may then be dried by evaporation and therefore become even less mobile. Some noxious gases in animal houses, and pulmonary infections, make the mucus too viscous, thus slowing its transport towards the larger airways.

A comment by Dixon (1992) clarifies the general principles of pulmonary pathology in the **horse**. In this species, inflammatory responses are in general extreme, examples being the tendency to excessive post-surgical inflammation and the massive loss of fluid intraluminally from intestinal obstruction. The pulmonary inflammatory response in equine respiratory diseases is equally intense and constant, with excessive production of respiratory secretions and a consequent threat of overwhelming the clearance mechanisms.

Hypertrophy of the mucoserous bronchial glands accounts for most of the extra mucus that is produced in chronic pulmonary disease in man, but in **chronic obstructive respiratory disease** in the horse hyperplasia of goblet cells is the main factor (Dixon, 1992). It is believed that secretion is increased by the direct action of inflammatory mediators (e.g. leukotrienes, prostaglandins, and histamine) on goblet cells and mucoserous glands, as well as by increased autonomic stimulation of the mucoserous glands (Section 6.12.2).

Of the **physical properties** of mucus, **elasticity** and 'spinnability' (Section 6.11) have to be kept within very narrow limits for effective transport (Dixon, 1992). **Viscosity** can vary over a relatively wide range without disturbing mucociliary transport. However, mucus with excessively **increased viscosity** becomes so difficult for the cilia to transport that it lodges in the airways; on the other hand, mucus with very low viscosity is also poorly transported because it gravitates towards the alveoli (Dixon, 1992). Mucus that gets stuck in the airways tends to become inspissated by evaporation. In **chronic ob-**

struction, including **chronic obstructive pulmonary disease in horses**, inspissated mucus forms coiled basophilic plugs known as Curschmann's spirals, which can be found in sputum and transtracheal aspirates (Section 20.7). Viscosity is notably increased during pulmonary infections (Dixon, 1992); this may be caused by the release of nuclear DNA into the mucus, resulting from the destruction of leucocytes and respiratory epithelial cells. (Yellow or green discoloration of respiratory secretions is not due to pathogenic chromogenic bacteria but to an enzyme (myeloperoxidase) released by leucocytes, or to high eosinophil levels.) Some **noxious gases** are known to increase the **viscosity** of the mucus, notably vaporized **ammonia compounds**. The high ammonia concentration in pig houses (Jericho, 1968), and in cattle and poultry houses (Veit and Farrell, 1978), is therefore a potential hazard (Jericho, 1968). Viscosity is increased and elasticity reduced in mucus that is purulent, thus slowing transport (Dunnill, 1979, p. 225; Dixon, 1992); serum proteins, present in the airway exudate because of acute inflammation, also alter the visco-elasticity of the mucus adversely (Dixon, 1992).

Reduced viscosity occurs locally after influenza virus has been deposited on the mucus. A **neuraminidase** on the virus particle probably contributes to penetration of the mucous barrier by rapidly reducing the viscosity of the mucus and thus exposing the epithelial cellular receptor sites that the virus needs for penetration of the cell wall (Cohen and Gold, 1975, p. 329).

Extensive research into the relationship between smoking and cancer of the lung in man has shown that the bronchial branchings are a predilection site of **bronchial carcinoma**. It is here that the excess mucus from proliferating goblet cells and bronchial glands accumulates. While piled up, it has time to absorb high concentrations of carcinogenic compounds from the smoke. These compounds then diffuse into the underlying bronchial epithelium.

7.17.2   *Cilia*

Normal ciliary function is essential for the clearance of mucus by the mucociliary escalator. If the beat is defective, or cilia are lost, or if the ciliated cells are actually destroyed, mucus accumulates. In the larger bronchi and trachea the mucus can still be removed by **coughing**, but the smaller airways readily become blocked and this can lead to a **venous-to-arterial shunt** as in Fig. 6.9B (Section 6.30.1). **Air pollutants** can disrupt ciliary activity, and in some instances stop it altogether (see below). Some viruses, such as those of influenza, cause the cilia to disintegrate, or the virus may actively kill the ciliated cells.

Gaseous factors that interfere with **ciliary action** have been reviewed by Dunnill (1979, p. 225). In **anoxia** cilia do not function at all. However, 100% oxygen is also ciliotoxic, as is 7.5% carbon dioxide. **Air pollutants** in general, and sulphur dioxide and cigarette smoke in particular, disrupt ciliary co-ordination and severely retard tracheal mucociliary clearance in both man and lower mammals. **Anaesthetics**, including intravenous barbiturates, are an important cause of ciliary dysfunction.

Dixon (1992) has reviewed the causes of ciliary dysfunction in horses. In **equine influenza** ciliated cells temporarily shed their cilia or actually disintegrate, significantly disrupting mucociliary clearance for up to a month after clinical signs of influenza have been resolved. In equine **chronic obstructive pulmonary disease** the macrophages initially phagocytose cilia, and then the ciliated epithelium undergoes metaplasia into an undifferentiated non-ciliated epithelium, especially in the smaller airways. The severity of equine obstructive pulmonary disease appears to be correlated with the degree of loss of ciliated cells. Xylazine **sedation** decreases mucociliary clearance, but it is not known whether this is caused by the action of the drug on cilia. The ultrastructure of cilia seems to be more variable in horses than other species.

Congenital ciliary dyskinesia, due to defective or absent **dynein arms**, occurs in man and dogs.

7.17.3   *Therapeutic promotion of mucociliary transport*

Beta-adrenergic agonists have been used successfully in equine pulmonary disease to relieve bronchial spasm by inhibiting the bronchial smooth muscle (Section 6.12.1). These drugs simultaneously increase ciliary activity, probably by stretching the bronchial wall and thinning the mucous layer.

Dixon (1992) has surveyed the efficacy of pharmaceutical agents in promoting mucociliary transport. Only β-adrenergic agonists (Section 6.12.1) emerge favourably. Although they stimulate goblet cells and the resulting mucus seems to be more viscous than normal mucus, these agents also increase ciliary activity (as just stated), and the overall result is a pronounced improvement in mucus transport. Furthermore these drugs inhibit bronchial smooth muscle, and have therefore proved to be an effective relief for bronchospasm and dyspnoea in chronic obstructive pulmonary disease in horses. Finally, they have a significant antiflammatory action, stabilizing mast cells. Of the available drugs, clenbuterol (favoured by over-enthusiastic Olympic athletes suffering suddenly from asthma) is outstandingly good in all these actions. On the other hand, clenbuterol and all other bronchodilators can worsen perfusion–ventilation imbalances by dilating the airways and diverting ventilation to non-functional parts of the lung.

7.18 Defective alveolar phagocytosis

The alveoli form about 95% of the total lung surface, and depend primarily on phagocytosis for defence. Under normal conditions this defence is admirably successful. Unfortunately, however, alveolar macrophages are vulnerable to a very wide range of adverse factors. Some of these are encountered mainly in human subjects, for example cigarette smoke.

Other factors affect veterinary as well as human subjects. Among these are starvation, cold, hypoxia, disorders of acid–base balance leading to metabolic acidosis, and pulmonary viral infections. All of these impair phagocytosis.

Multiple factors that disable alveolar phagocytosis have been reviewed by Dunnill (1979, pp. 227–228).

Irradiation, and **immunosuppressive** and **cytotoxic drugs**, are relatively obvious factors. Lowered resistance to pulmonary infections occurs in **alcoholics**. The adverse effect of **cigarette smoke** is notorious; this can be demonstrated experimentally both *in vitro* and *in vivo*, and severe lower respiratory infections are about nine times more common in smokers than non-smokers.

Under experimental conditions, **cold** and **starvation** delay bacterial clearance. So also does **corticosteroid therapy**, though to a much smaller degree. Unfavourable hygienic conditions during the cold and wet months of the year increase the incidence of pneumonia in pigs (Jericho, 1968). An extreme and apparently unique sensitivity of human alveolar macrophages to **hypoxia** has been demonstrated *in vitro*; this has led to the suggestion that increased susceptibility to pneumonia in patients with chronic bronchitis or collapsed alveoli may be due to deficient phagocytosis in hypoxic regions of the lung. **Metabolic acidosis** has been shown experimentally to weaken the phagocytic defences, and pulmonary infections are known to be common in **diabetic ketosis** and **renal failure**. Experimental **viral** influenza **infections** in mice reduce the capacity to clear inhaled staphylococci. Staphylococci reaching other organs by the intravenous route are dealt with adequately, and this indicates that the defect is local to the lung. In man, viral infections, and especially influenza, are often complicated by secondary bacterial infections. In the pig, viruses are known to enhance a pneumonic process (Jericho, 1968).

7.19 Destruction of alveolar walls: alveolar emphysema

Emphysema is a pathological accumulation of gas in tissues. In **alveolar emphysema** (**pulmonary emphysema**) the gas accumulates in the alveoli, the underlying change being the loss of alveolar walls. It occurs in all the domestic mammals, but is of the greatest importance in man and the horse. In horses, alveolar emphysema is associated with '**broken wind**' or '**heaves**'; these are vernacular names for **chronic obstructive pulmonary disease**, which is a particular problem in this species.

Alveolar emphysema begins when the interalveolar septum (alveolar wall) between two adjacent alveoli begins to break down, so that the two alveoli coalesce. When this process has affected all the alveoli of an alveolar sac, the alveolar sac becomes a simple cavity with virtually smooth walls. Finally, adjacent alveolar sacs coalesce (Fig. 6.10C). These changes convey the impression of an abnormal enlargement of the air spaces distal to the terminal, non-respiratory, bronchiole.

Since the alveolar wall normally contains a profuse **capillary network** (Section 6.7), loss of the wall means loss of alveolar capillaries (Fig. 6.10C) and consequently a reduction in alveolar perfusion; this amounts to a corresponding reduction of the surface area available for gas exchange, and a decrease in the volume of pulmonary capillary blood. The result is a **pathological** increase in **alveolar dead space** (Section 6.28), and severe mismatching of ventilation and perfusion with a high ventilation/perfusion ratio (Section 6.30.1). All these changes contribute to a severe **pulmonary insufficiency** (Section 17.29). Furthermore, the loss of alveolar capillaries increases the resistance of the pulmonary vasculature and therefore leads to **primary pulmonary hypertension** (Section 17.22).

Destruction of the interalveolar septa necessarily disrupts the **elastic** and **collagen fibres** that support the alveolar walls. The elastic fibres break, and the ends retract. Lacking fibrous support, the coalescing airways expand still further. Because of the loss of elastic fibres the **compliance** of the lung increases (Section 6.31) and therefore less energy is needed during inspiration, but this gain is lost because the **alveolar dead space** (Section 6.30.1) is so greatly enlarged. Eventually (in the horse) collagen fibrils are laid down in the surviving alveolar walls. This thickens the remaining blood–gas barrier and still further diminishes gas exchange. The substitution of collagenous scar tissue for elastic tissue now reduces the **compliance** of the lung and correspondingly reduces the resting (and maximum) tidal volume. The anatomical dead space and tidal volume are brought closer and closer together, so that a progressively smaller proportion of the inspired air reaches the respiratory airways. For example, if the total dead space be increased to 200 ml and the tidal volume be reduced to 250 ml, only 20% of the gas arriving at the respiratory airways will be fresh air. The decrease in lung compliance greatly increases the energetic cost of breathing (Section 10.13).

Alveolar emphysema has been extensively studied and reviewed by Gillespie and Tyler (1967, 1969), Tyler *et al.* (1971), and Nowell *et al.* (1971).

Pulmonary emphysema occurs in one form or another in almost all mammals (see also **interstitial emphysema**, below), but alveolar emphysema is probably a major respiratory disease only in the horse and man; **chronic alveolar emphysema** is second only to heart disease as a cause of disability in working men in the USA.

The lungs of man and horse appear to have much in common. The lung of the horse is considered to be anatomically similar to that of man, and both species are susceptible to **asthma** or asthma-like conditions (Section 7.20), the **respiratory distress syndrome of the newborn** (Section 16.26.1), and viral influenza, as well as alveolar emphysema (Gillespie and Tyler, 1967).

Chronic obstructive pulmonary disease in the horse is a combination of chronic bronchitis and bronchiolitis, *supplemented* by alveolar emphysema. It is one of the oldest documented causes of reduced performance in racehorses (Halliwell, 1993). However, in the horse, bronchitis, bronchiolitis, and alveolar emphysema can all occur separately as well as concurrently (Gillespie and Tyler, 1969, p. 59). These conditions can lead to an abnormally dilated lung at the end of expiration, which can be detected by **percussion** of the thoracic wall (Section 23.5.2).

The **aetiology of alveolar emphysema** is unknown, and its **pathogenesis** is not fully understood (Gillespie and Tyler, 1969) in either man or horse, despite intensive research. The aetiology may well be multifactorial, with participation of the following factors, all of which have an anatomical basis.

7.19.1 *Airway obstruction*

Bacterial infection, perhaps superimposed on viral infection or on irritation by noxious dust particles and tobacco smoke, causes bronchial and bronchiolar obstruction by excess mucus and/or ciliary dysfunction (Section 7.17), or by thickening of the airway wall (Section 6.14); the obstruction may be initiated or augmented by **bronchoconstriction** of allergic origin (Section 7.20), from feeding mouldy hay. Collateral ventilation (Section 6.3.2) beyond the obstruction admits gas that then becomes trapped in distal alveoli. Forced expiratory efforts, as in coughing, raise the pressure in the trapped gas and burst the alveolar walls.

7.19.2 *Inflammatory destruction of the alveolar epithelial cell*

In principle, alveolar epithelial cells are likely to be all too vulnerable to inflammation and infection because their exposure to the air is more extensive than that of any other group of cells in the body (Weibel, 1984, p. 265). The alveolar epithelial cell is indeed known to be immediately responsive to **irritant particles** and **noxious gases**, including pure oxygen. Within hours of exposure to such agents, the hitherto invisible cells become clearly visible with the light microscope, suggesting a rapid hypertrophy (Krahl, 1964, p. 262). The flanges of the cells contract, exposing the collagen and elastic fibres of the interstitium to attack. Death of the alveolar epithelial cells ensues. The exposed interstitial fibres are disrupted and new collagenous scar tissue is laid down. Presumably similar inflammatory destruction of the alveolar epithelial cell and alveolar wall is at least a possibility through **bacterial** or **viral action**, if the alveolar phagocytic defences are overwhelmed. However, the evidence for **inflammatory alveolitis** as a factor initiating **alveolar emphysema** seems to be controversial in both man and horse, and has evidently attracted relatively little support.

Repair of the epithelial surface is a slow process. The alveolar epithelial cell has lost the capacity for mitosis (Section 6.17), and replacement is by division of the **granular epithelial cells**. These form a rather thick cuboidal lining, with a high resistance to gas exchange, and it takes several weeks for the cells to transform into alveolar epithelial cells of typical thinness (Weibel, 1984, p. 266).

7.19.3 *Atrophy of the alveolar wall*

This mechanism of causing alveolar emphysema differs from the preceding one in not being associated with inflammation from microbial infection or irritant materials. It appears to be associated with progressive enlargement of pre-existing **interalveolar pores** (Section 6.23), or the formation and enlargement of new pores. Enlargement of pre-existing pores may begin with disruption of the elastic fibres and collagen fibrils that normally encircle the rims of pores (Krahl, 1964, p. 265). The most constant early microscopic feature of this condition is the presence of large holes (fenestrations) in the alveolar walls. Inevitably, the blood capillaries are progressively obliterated, and elastic and collagen fibres are destroyed, as the fenestrations enlarge.

The cause of these atrophic changes is not clear. One possibility is **ischaemia** of the alveolar wall, arising from obstruction of either the **bronchial arterial supply** (Section 17.7) or the alveolar capillaries. The significance of the involvement of the bronchial arteries depends on the extent to which the bronchial arteries supply the alveolar capillary beds. McLaughlin *et al.* (1961) suggested that in the horse (and perhaps also in man) the bronchial arteries supply blood directly to the alveolar capillaries (Section 17.3). However, the evidence that ischaemia caused by obstruction of the bronchial arteries is a major factor in alveolar emphysema does not seem to be strong. Widespread destruction of alveolar epithelial cells, followed by typical slow regeneration, is known to occur in acute peripheral circulatory failure (**hypovolaemic shock**) arising from severe haemorrhage (Weibel, 1984, p. 266). Under such conditions the blood capillaries in the alveolar walls become leaky, causing the further problem of **alveolar oedema**.

Another possible primary cause of the atrophy considered by Gillespie and Tyler (1969, p. 68) is a disorder of **elastic tissue** or **collagen**. Pulmonary emphysema has been produced experimentally by intratracheal or intravenous papain. Such **proteolytic enzymes** that degrade elastin form a group known as 'elastases'. **Elastases** have been found in leucocytes, macrophages, and microorganisms (Hance and Crystal, 1975, p. 676). Gillespie and Tyler (1969, p. 68) cited authorities who regarded a primary disorder of elastic tissue 'as the least likely cause' of alveolar emphysema, but Hance and Crystal (1975, p. 689) suggested that enzymatic attack on elastin remained 'a strong possibility'.

7.19.4 *Interstitial emphysema*

This condition is caused by the escape of gas into the interstitial tissue of the alveolar wall through ruptured alveoli, and is a typical lesion in **acute bovine pulmonary emphysema** (Gillespie and Tyler, 1969, p. 60).

7.20 Bronchial spasm

Bronchial spasm is the excessive contraction of the bronchial, and particularly bronchiolar, smooth muscle. This contributes to many of the various forms of **chronic obstructive pulmonary disease** by causing severe resistance to airflow (Section 6.14).

Autonomic afferent **irritant receptors** in the trachea, bronchi, and alveoli, respond to fine dust particles, irritant gases, and substances produced

by cell injury (e.g. histamine); the receptors reflexly induce bronchoconstriction (Section 4.16). Such reflex bronchoconstriction has been evolved to defend the lung against further incursion of noxious agents in the inspired air, but unfortunately a price has to be paid for this defence since widespread bronchoconstriction is itself a potential cause of respiratory distress.

Allergic responses to airborne allergens such as pollen and fungal spores are another major cause of bronchoconstriction. The allergens cause the local release of **histamine** from **mast cells** lying along the blood vessels in the walls of the small bronchi and bronchioles. The histamine acts directly on the local smooth muscle cells of the small bronchi and bronchioles, resulting in obstructive constriction. Notable examples are **allergic asthma** in man and **chronic obstructive pulmonary disease (heaves) in horses**. In these conditions the increased resistance to air flow caused by bronchial constriction is so great that, in a man suffering from asthma, a 20-fold increase in pressure may be needed to maintain adequate ventilation. If ventilation fails, the result is a severe mismatching of ventilation and perfusion, with a low ventilation/perfusion ratio and a pronounced venous-to-arterial shunt (Section 6.30.1).

Non-allergenic irritant dust particles and noxious gases, as found in the unpleasant gaseous cocktail known as smog, also induce a direct local obstructive constriction of bronchial and bronchiolar muscle, presumably through the release of histamine.

The cause of **chronic obstructive pulmonary disease** in horses has long been controversial, but there is evidence that it is an allergic reaction to mouldy hay (Halliwell, 1993). **Allergic asthma** in man and **anaphylaxis** are caused by essentially similar mechanisms (Neal, 1992, p. 28). **IgE** forms in response to the allergens, and attaches itself to **mast cells** and **basophils**. In allergic individuals the levels of IgE are excessive (up to 100 times above normal). On further exposure to the same allergen, the allergen reacts with the IgE that is already attached to a mast cell. This triggers the release of granules from the mast cell. The granules (and the cytoplasm immediately surrounding them) contain various **mediators**, including **histamine, serotonin, prostaglandins, leukotrienes**, and **bradykinins**. The local release of mediators (for example, from mast cells in the airway walls) induces contraction of local smooth muscle, giving the obstructive constriction of the airways, particularly of bronchioles, that characterizes **allergic asthma**. A massive general release of mediators (from mast cells in the tissues and from circulating basophils) may produce the profound circulatory changes of **generalized anaphylaxis (anaphylactic shock)** (Section 14.27.6). These changes arise from venous dilation, arteriolar dilation, and greatly increased capillary permeability, which combine to induce a life-threatening reduction in venous return (Guyton, 1986, p. 332).

Chapter 8
Thoracic Walls

8.1 Thoracic cavity

The **walls** of the thoracic cavity are formed by the thoracic vertebrae dorsally, the ribs and costal cartilages laterally, and the sternum ventrally. The dorsal and lateral walls are reinforced by the vertebral musculature and intercostal muscles. The caudal wall is formed by the diaphragm. The informal term '**rib cage**' is descriptively useful for indicating the bony components of the thoracic cavity, particularly when discussing their movements during breathing.

The thoracic cavity is cone-shaped. The apex of the cone is formed by the **thoracic inlet**, the narrow vertical opening between the left and right first ribs. The trachea and oesophagus, and the great blood vessels and lymphatics, compete for space at the thoracic inlet, forming a potential bottleneck for oesophageal obstruction (Section 25.12).

In the domestic mammals the thoracic cavity is laterally flattened whereas in man it is dorsoventrally flattened, causing the mere human to envy the comfort enjoyed by a cat asleep on its side. In the dog, the shape of the thorax varies with the breed. The beagle-type dog may be regarded as an average representative of the species the two extreme forms being breeds such as the greyhound with a slender deep thorax and the barrel-chested bulldog. These breed differences in the dog cause variations in the shape and slope of the heart, which in turn affect the interpretation of thoracic radiographs (Section 24.6.1).

The thoracic cavity contains the left and right pleural cavities, and the thoracic viscera enclosed within the pleural membranes. The thoracic viscera so enclosed are the heart, lungs, thymus, and lymph nodes. The pleural membranes also enclose structures that partly or completely traverse the thoracic cavity; these include the thoracic trachea, thoracic oesophagus, and various vessels and nerves (aorta, cranial vena cava, caudal vena cava, veins of the azygos system, thoracic duct, and the phrenic, vagus, recurrent laryngeal, and sympathetic nerves).

However, because the diaphragm is domed cranially, the abdominal viscera also extend a long way within the rib cage. Therefore when a stethoscope is applied to the caudal regions of the lateral thoracic wall it picks up sounds from the abdominal viscera; sounds from the thoracic viscera can only be heard reliably from the more cranial regions of the thoracic wall.

The thoracic cavity (cavum thoracis) is lined by the **endothoracic fascia** (fascia endothoracica) (Section 9.8), which is connective tissue that attaches the costal and diaphragmatic pleura to the underlying bones and muscles. This layer is homologous to the **transversalis fascia** that attaches the parietal peritoneum to the abdominal walls, and thereby completes the homologous structure of the thoracic and abdominal walls (Section 8.9.1).

The **design requirements of a thorax** are diverse and conflicting. It must protect the vitally important organs that it encloses. It must also relay to the rest of the body the forces arising in the forelimb from posture and locomotion, since the forelimb has no direct bony articulation with the vertebral column – unlike the hindlimb which articulates directly with the pelvis. These requirements demand *strength* and *rigidity*. At the same time the thorax has to be capable of increasing and decreasing its volume for breathing. This demands not only *mobility* but also *minimal mass*, so that the lifelong repetitive movements of *breathing* are not too energetically expensive (Section 10.13.)

Mammalian species differences in thoracic architecture reflect an animal's skeletal adaptation to its body mass, posture, locomotion, and habitat (Krahl, 1964, p. 228). When the body mass is shared by all four limbs as in *quadrupedal mammals* the cranial end of the thorax tends to be laterally compressed, thus allowing the heavily loaded forelimbs to be brought close together beneath the body; the caudal end is relatively rounded to provide the greatest possible volume for the visceral contents. The ribs are directed essentially dorsoventrally, in order to suspend the weight of the thoracoabdominal viscera from the arching thoracolumbar vertebral column, like the weight of a suspension bridge. In contrast, mammals that adopt a *bipedal posture* and support little or none of the body mass on their forelimbs tend to have a more rounded or dorsoventrally flattened thorax (kangaroo, monkey). *Aquatic mammals* have a rounded thorax, especially deep-diving species that withstand high external pressures.

The thoracic inlet (apertura thoracis cranialis) is more spacious in man than the domestic animals, thus giving relatively greater tolerance of space-occupying lesions (Section 23.2).

8.2   Thoracic vertebrae

Thoracic vertebrae are readily recognizable, except perhaps at the beginning and end of the series where they share features with the cervical and lumbar vertebrae, respectively. A typical thoracic vertebra has a very tall **spinous process** and a **short body** (Fig. 8.1); the spines of the first thoracic vertebrae are particularly tall, forming the **withers** in the interscapular region. The dorsal tips of the spines are the only parts of the thoracic vertebrae that can be palpated in the live animal (Fig. 8.1). The vertebral canal (Fig. 8.2) contains the spinal cord.

Since all thoracic vertebrae carry ribs (Fig. 8.2), **costal articular facets** for the head and tubercle of a rib are also distinctive features (Fig. 8.3). The head of a typical rib lies between the bodies of *two* vertebrae, articulating with both of them. The head of the first rib lies between C7 and T1. Hence throughout the series, the **head** of a rib with a particular number **precedes** the thoracic vertebra of the same number; for example, the head of rib 2 articulates with the first and second thoracic vertebrae, but is immediately cranial to the second thoracic vertebra. On the other hand, the **tubercle** of a rib always articulates with the transverse process of the thoracic vertebra of the same number; thus the tubercle of rib 2 articulates with the second thoracic vertebra (Fig. 8.7). The **transverse process** is smaller than that of cervical and particularly lumbar vertebrae; this is predictable because the transverse processes of cervical and

lumbar vertebrae are augmented embryologically by incorporating the remnant of a rib.

There are typically thirteen thoracic vertebrae in the ox (Fig. 8.1), sheep, dog (Fig. 8.1), and cat, fourteen or fifteen in the pig, and eighteen in the horse (Fig. 8.1). In man there are twelve.

Thoracic vertebral osteology has been carefully surveyed by Barone (1986, pp. 365–377). The **vertebral body** (centrum) of thoracic vertebrae is particularly short craniocaudally in species such as the horse which have many thoracic vertebrae. Compared with cervical vertebrae, the articular surface of the **cranial extremity** is less convex, and that of the **caudal extremity** is less concave, thus reducing mobility. The **ventral crest** (crista ventralis) is only a simple ridge.

The **spinous processes** at first slope caudally, and then cranially (Fig. 8.1); at the level where the slope changes there tends to be one vertebra in which the spinous process is almost vertical, the **anticlinal vertebra** (arrow in Fig. 8.1C). This vertebra is usually clear in the dog, at the eleventh thoracic vertebra, but in the other domestic species it may be difficult to identify any one vertebra with a truly vertical spinous process, and in the ox all the thoracic spinous processes tend to slope caudally (Fig. 8.1).

The cranial and caudal **costal facets** (fovea articularis cranialis, caudalis) (Fig. 8.3) enable the head of each rib to articulate with two vertebrae (Fig. 8.7). Because the head of the rib gets progressively smaller throughout the series, the costal facets in the vertebrae are also progressively reduced in size (Fig. 8.7). In the most caudal one, two, or three thoracic vertebrae, however, the caudal facet in particular becomes progressively smaller and may be absent altogether (Fig. 8.7); thus the ribs have moved somewhat caudally in relation to the vertebrae. The last thoracic vertebra must always lack a caudal facet, since at this level there are no more fully developed ribs. In a vertebra such as T13 in Fig. 8.7, the rib of the same number articulates solely with the vertebra of the same number, i.e. both the tubercle and the whole of the head of rib 13 articulate with vertebra T13.

The **transverse process** carries a **facet** for the **tubercle of the rib** (fovea costalis processus transversi) (Fig. 8.3). Towards the end of the thoracic series, the facet for the tubercle becomes progressively reduced, and approaches (Fig. 8.3) and finally blends with the cranial costal facet (rib 13 in Fig. 8.7), in agreement with a corresponding reduction and blending of the tubercle with the head of the rib (Section 8.4). Apart from the first few thoracic vertebrae, the dorsal surface of the transverse process also bears a dorsally projecting **mamillary process** (processus mamillaris) (Fig. 8.3) which gets bigger in the last thoracic vertebra.

As in all vertebrae, the **vertebral arch** (arcus vertebrae) is formed by the **pedicle** (pediculus arcus vertebrae) laterally and the **lamina** dorsally (Fig. 8.2). The

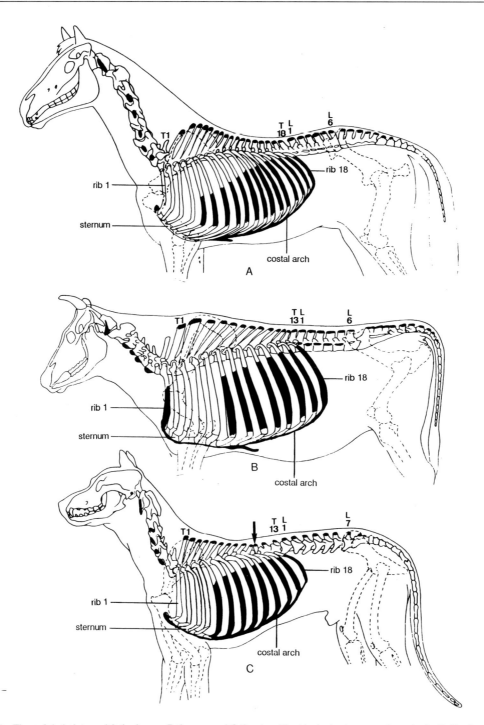

Fig. 8.1 **The axial skeleton of A the horse, B the ox, and C the dog.** The black structures can be palpated in the live animal.

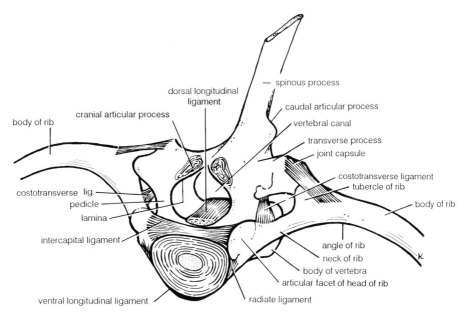

Fig. 8.2 **Dorsocranial view of the ninth thoracic vertebra of a dog.** The intervertebral disc has been cut in transverse section. The articulations of the ninth pair of ribs are shown. The 'articular facet of the head of the rib' is the cranial part of the facet, which articulates with the caudal extremity of the body of the eighth thoracic vertebra. The angle of the rib is the relatively sharp bend between the neck and body of the rib. In the dog the intercapital ligament occurs between the heads of the second to the tenth ribs, becoming progressively more slender at the caudal end of the series. The intercapital ligament shown here is the penultimate one, and should be much more slender.

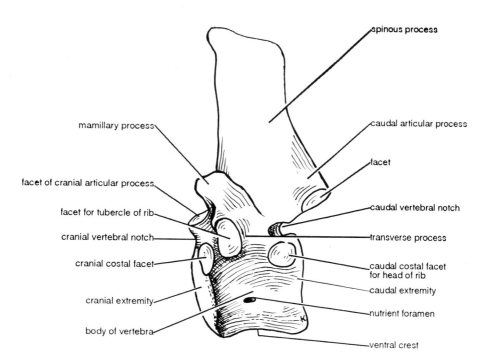

Fig. 8.3 **Left lateral view of the sixteenth thoracic vertebra of a horse.** The facets of the cranial and caudal articular processes are small and flat. The cranial facet faces almost directly dorsally, and the caudal facet ventrally. The facet for the tubercle of the rib has almost blended with the cranial costal facet.

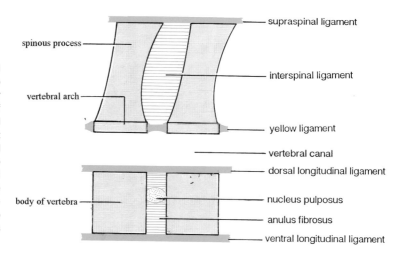

spinous process

vertebral arch

body of vertebra

supraspinal ligament

interspinal ligament

yellow ligament

vertebral canal

dorsal longitudinal ligament

nucleus pulposus

anulus fibrosus

ventral longitudinal ligament

Fig. 8.4   Highly schematic vertical section in the midline through two thoracic vertebrae showing their principal ligaments. The fibres of the ligaments are longitudinal, and make attachments to the vertebrae at all points of contact. The dorsal and ventral longitudinal ligaments also blend with the dorsal and ventral surfaces of the anulus fibrosus. The fibres of the anulus fibrosus are essentially longitudinal, but being also oblique should strictly appear as dots in this section.

vertebral canal (canalis vertebralis) (Fig. 8.2) contains the spinal cord (Fig. 24.8); since the spinal cord is of small diameter in the thoracic region (Vol. 1 of this series on the CNS; King, 1987) the vertebral canal of the thoracic vertebrae is correspondingly narrow. The **cranial** and **caudal vertebral notches** (incisura vertebralis cranialis, caudalis) (Fig. 8.3) combine to form the **intervertebral foramen** (foramen intervertebrale), through which the segmental spinal nerve escapes from the vertebral canal after the union of the dorsal and ventral roots (Fig. 2.1). In the ox and pig, and sometimes in the horse, the caudal notch may become a true intervertebral foramen.

In general, the **mobility** of the thoracic vertebral column is limited by the great size of its spinous processes and the presence of the ribs. The cranial and caudal **articular processes** articulate by only small flat facets. The facets tend to be essentially in the horizontal plane (the cranial facet facing dorsocranially, Figs 8.2, 8.3), thus favouring some lateral bending of the vertebral column; at the caudal end of the thoracic series, however, the facets tend to be more in the vertical plane, thus promoting a somewhat greater degree of dorsal extension and ventral flexion. There may be one vertebra towards the caudal end of the series with its cranial pair of facets in the horizontal plane, and its caudal facets in the vertical plane, this being known as the 'diaphragmatic vertebra'.

8.3   Ligaments of thoracic vertebrae

8.3.1   *Intervertebral disc*

The bodies of successive vertebrae are strongly attached to each other by the intervertebral disc.

The disc comprises an anulus fibrosus and a nucleus pulposus.

The **anulus fibrosus** consists of short collagen fibres that are firmly embedded at each end in the bony extremities of the two adjacent vertebral bodies (Fig. 8.4).

The **nucleus pulposus** of the disc is a remnant of the **notochord**, and in the young animal consists of an embryonic jelly with few cells. Its fluid properties distribute forces evenly throughout the anulus fibrosus when the disc is distorted by compression or movement.

Under abnormal conditions the nucleus pulposus may cause a bulge in the relatively thin dorsal part of the anulus fibrosus, or may actually burst right through, damaging the spinal cord. This is known as **dorsal protrusion** of the **intervertebral disc**.

The fibres of the **anulus fibrosus** of the **intervertebral disc** (discus intervertebralis) are arranged in about 25–30 concentric **lamellae**, one inside the other (Fig. 8.5). The fibres are oblique, their direction alternating in successive lamellae (Fig. 8.6). The obliquity allows some movement between the bodies of two adjacent vertebrae.

The position of the **nucleus pulposus** is dorsally eccentric, so that the dorsal part of the anulus fibrosus is thinner than the ventral part (Fig. 8.5). With advancing age, the nucleus pulposus changes into fibrocartilage. Having thus lost its fluid qualities, it no longer distributes forces evenly throughout the anulus, and therefore great forces develop at particular points within the anulus during distortion of the disc (King, 1956b). During extreme

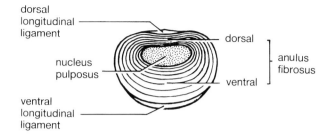

dorsal longitudinal ligament

nucleus pulposus

ventral longitudinal ligament

dorsal

ventral } anulus fibrosus

Fig. 8.5 Thoracic intervertebral disc of a dog in semidiagrammatic transverse section. The rings represent the 25–30 laminae of the anulus fibrosus. The laminae are much thinner dorsally than ventrally, causing the nucleus pulposus to be dorsally eccentric in position.

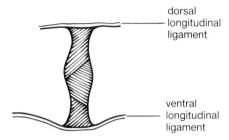

dorsal longitudinal ligament

ventral longitudinal ligament

Fig. 8.6 Lateral view of an intervertebral disc. The two outermost laminae have been partly dissected away, revealing successively deeper laminae with their collagen fibres passing obliquely to each other, in alternating directions. Every collagen fibre is embedded at each end in the adjacent vertebral body.

In the **cat** (King and Smith, 1958), dorsal protrusions of types 1 and 2 occur with much the same frequency as in the dog. As in the dog, dorsal protrusions seldom occur in thoracic discs covered by the intercapital ligament. Otherwise, the distribution of protrusions is altogether different from that in the dog. Thus in the cat cervical protrusions are more common than lumbar protrusions, the thoracolumbar junction is little affected, and lumbar protrusions are commonest in the mid-lumbar region. The most striking difference between the two species is that, in the cat, these protrusions rarely cause compressive myelopathy with clinical signs (de Lahunta, 1983, p. 186).

In **man**, disc protrusion is commonest at the lumbosacral junction.

The thoracic intervertebral discs have the thinnest craniocaudal measurements in the cervical, thoracic, and lumbar series (King and Smith, 1955) This contributes to the limited mobility of the thoracic part of the vertebral column.

ventral flexion of the vertebral column the thin dorsal part of the anulus may bulge or even burst, and thus release material from the nucleus pulposus which compresses the spinal cord, a condition known as **disc protrusion**. Hansen (1952) classified the bursting type as a **type 1 protrusion**, and the bulging variety as a **type 2 protrusion**. Type 1 protrusions tend to occur explosively, striking the ventral aspect of the spinal cord a violent blow. The result is severe mechanical damage directly to the spinal cord, and also major injury to the blood vessels of the cord thus leading to extensive ischaemic necrosis.

In **nonchondrodystrophoid breeds** of **dog** the cartilage conversion of the nucleus pulposus starts at about 4 or 5 years of age, but in **chondrodystrophoid breeds** (dachshund, pekinese, French bulldog, beagle) it can begin in the first year of life, thus explaining the much earlier onset of disc protrusions in these breeds (de Lahunta, 1983, p. 186).

Surveys by Hansen (1952) and Hoerlein (1953) showed that dorsal disc protrusions in the dog are common in the cranial lumbar region, and commonest of all at the thoracolumbar junction. Protrusions in these regions may cause **paresis** or **paraplegia**. The **intercapital ligament** (Section 8.5) appears to protect the first eight discs of the nine discs that it covers dorsally.

8.3.2 *Longitudinal ligaments*

The **ventral longitudinal ligament** runs along the ventral surface of the vertebrae (Fig. 8.4). Its fibres attach to the vertebrae, and blend with the ventral surface of the anulus fibrosus (Fig. 8.2). The **dorsal longitudinal ligament** lies on the floor of the vertebral canal (Fig. 8.4), attaching to the vertebrae and fusing with the dorsal surface of the anulus fibrosus. The **interspinal ligament** passes between the spinal processes (Fig. 8.4). The **yellow ligament** consists of yellow elastic fibres connecting the vertebral arches (Fig. 8.4). The **supraspinal ligament** attaches to the tips of the spinous processes (Fig. 8.4).

The ventral and dorsal longitudinal ligaments and the supraspinal ligament are all powerful structures, but the ventral ligament fades out cranial to the mid-thoracic region. The supraspinal ligament (lig. supraspinale) and interspinal ligament (lig. interspinale) become the **nuchal ligament** (lig. nuchae) in the cervical region.

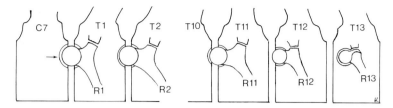

Fig. 8.7 Highly schematic diagram showing the general relationships of ribs to thoracic vertebrae. This hypothetical mammal has thirteen ribs and thirteen thoracic vertebrae. At the cranial end of the series, the head of the rib (circle) articulates with two vertebrae. Thus the head of rib 1 articulates with the caudal costal facet (arrow) of vertebra C7 and the cranial costal facet of T1. Caudally the head of the rib gets smaller and therefore the costal facets get smaller. In the last three thoracic vertebrae the ribs also move caudally in relation to the vertebrae, and this reduces the caudal facet still more, until it disappears in T11 and T12. The last thoracic vertebra never has a caudal costal facet, since the ribs have ended. The tubercle of the rib articulates always with the transverse process of the vertebra of the same number. The neck of the rib and the tubercle are progressively reduced at the caudal end of the series. The virtual loss of the neck (rib 13) causes the articular surface of the tubercle to blend with that of the head of the rib; likewise, the costal facet on the vertebra blends with the facet on the transverse process.

8.3.3 *Articular processes*

These joints are synovial and are secured by joint capsules.

8.4 Ribs

The number of ribs possessed by each species is the same as the number of thoracic vertebrae (13 in the ox, sheep, dog, and cat; 14 or 15 in the pig: 18 in the horse).

The mammalian rib (costa) has two parts, one bony and the other cartilaginous. The proximal bony part, the **rib proper**, is attached at the **costochondral junction** to the distal cartilaginous part, the **costal cartilage** (Fig. 8.8). The costal cartilages of the first eight pairs of ribs (with minor species variations) articulate with the sternum; these ribs are known as **sternal ribs**. The costal cartilages of the remaining ribs articulate with the costal cartilages of the ribs that immediately precede them, thus forming the **costal arch** (Figs 18.3, 18.4); these ribs are known as **asternal ribs**. In some species the last rib or ribs may fail to reach the costal arch, and are then referred to as **floating ribs** (Fig. 8.25).

The rib proper consists of a more or less rounded head, a narrow neck, a tubercle, and a body (Fig. 8.2). Typically, the **head** is placed between two vertebrae. Its articular surface then articulates with the cranial and caudal costal facets

(Fig. 8.3) of two vertebral bodies (Fig. 8.7). The head of the first rib articulates with the last cervical and the first thoracic vertebra (Fig. 8.7); thus it is the more **caudal** of these two vertebrae (T1) that bears the same number as the rib itself (rib 1). The **tubercle** of the rib articulates with the vertebra of the same number, via an articular facet on the transverse process (Figs 8.2, 8.7). Most of the rib is formed by the curved **body** (Fig. 8.2), which is usually flattened and blade-like (Fig. 8.1).

The **costal cartilage** is a rod of fibrocartilage, joining the distal end of the rib at an angle (Figs 5.5, 8.1). The cartilages of sternal ribs articulate with the body of the sternum by synovial joints (Fig. 8.8). Those of the asternal ribs are attached by connective tissue to the costal cartilage of the preceding rib, thus forming the flexible **costal arch** (Figs 8.23, 23.3, 23.4). To provide movement during breathing with minimal loss of energy through friction, every rib requires a mobile joint at each end.

The space between two adjacent ribs is an **intercostal space**. The space between costal cartilages may be known conveniently as an **interchondral space**, though this term is not recognized by the NAV (1994).

In the last one or two ribs the head blends with the tubercle (Fig. 8.7).

The **horse** has eight sternal ribs and ten asternal; the **ox** has eight sternal and five asternal; the **pig** has seven sternal and seven or eight asternal, and rib 15 is often

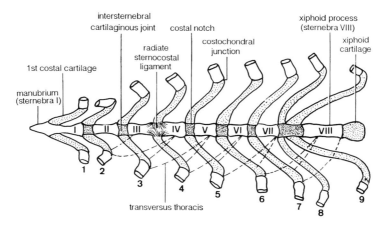

Fig. 8.8   Dorsal view of the sternum of a dog. The sternum in this species is rod-like but is also slightly flattened laterally. The body of the sternum is formed by eight sternebrae (I–VIII). The manubrium is fused to the first sternebra, and the xiphoid process to the eighth sternebra. The costal cartilages of the nine sternal ribs (1–9) articulate by synovial joints with the intersternebral cartilage (dark stipple) at costal notches, the last two costal cartilages sharing one intersternebral cartilage. The radiate sternocostal ligament spreads between the distal end of each costal cartilage and the dorsal and ventral surfaces of the body of the sternum, the dorsal part of one such ligament being shown at rib 4. All cartilage is stippled. The outlines of the fascicles of the left half of the transversus thoracis muscle are shown by broken lines. This muscle covers most of the dorsal surface of the sternum and costal cartilages, from the second sternebra to the caudal end of the xiphoid process.

floating; the **dog** and **cat** have nine sternal and four asternal, the last often floating; **man** has seven sternal and five asternal, the last two floating (Barone, 1986, pp. 423–427).

Throughout the whole class of **mammalia** (Krahl, 1964, p. 229), the number of ribs ranges from nine pairs in armadillos (*Edentata*) to 25 pairs in sloths (also *Edentata*). The *Perissodactyla* (horses, tapirs, rhinoceroses), elephants, and *Sirenia* have from 18 to 20 pairs. But in the majority of mammals the range is from 11 to 16 pairs. Usually seven pairs articulate directly with the sternum, but certain whales and the manatee have only one to three pairs of sternal ribs.

As in **modern fishes**, **ancestral tetrapods** carried ribs on every vertebra from the atlas to the base of the tail (Romer, 1962, p. 173). In **modern amphibians** the ribs are much reduced; they never reach the sternum, and are entirely absent in most frogs and toads except for a sacral rib. In **modern reptiles** the ribs vary greatly. In snakes a pair of vertebral ribs articulates with every vertebra (except the first few), the distal ends being attached to the skin and the sternum being absent. Apart from limbless forms and tortoises and turtles (Williston, 1925, p. 123), most reptiles possess a sternum, with which ribs in the thoracic region articulate by cartilaginous sternal ribs corresponding to mammalian costal cartilages (Bellairs and Attridge, 1975, p. 28). In **birds** the thoracic vertebrae have vertebral ribs, and also sternal ribs (again homologous with mammalian costal carti-

lages) that are ossified and articulate with the sternum (King and McLelland, 1984, p. 56).

8.5   Ligaments of ribs

The **costovertebral articulations** of the head of the rib with the costal facets on the vertebral body, and those of the tubercle of the rib with the transverse process, are all synovial joints and supported by a **joint capsule** and several other ligaments (Fig. 8.2, and see below).

The **intercapital ligament** is a strong thick band, running from the head of one rib to the head of the corresponding rib on the other side. It passes tightly over the dorsal surface of the anulus fibrosus but without fusing with it. It is of particular interest in the dog, since it reinforces the dorsal surface of the intervertebral disc against **dorsal disc protrusion** (Section 8.3.1). However, it occurs between only nine pairs of ribs, from the second to the tenth ribs inclusive. It therefore supports only the nine intervertebral discs that occur between the first and the tenth thoracic vertebrae.

The distal end of the rib is united by cartilage to

the costal cartilage. The sternocostal articulation is mentioned in Section 8.6.

The dorsoventral thickness and craniocaudal width of the **intercapital ligament** (lig. intercapitale) in the dog increase progressively from the first to the fifth ligament, and decrease progressively from the sixth to the ninth ligament (King, 1956b). The first and last ligaments in the series are about one third as thick and wide as the fifth, the first ligament being the least substantial of all. In Fig. 8.2, the intercapital ligament, which is the penultimate ligament in the series, is much too massive.

It was originally suggested that the intercapital ligaments protect the canine disc against dorsal **disc protrusion** (Section 8.3.1). Such disc protrusions are indeed very rare in the dog from any of the first eight discs of the nine that are covered by the ligament, i.e. the discs between the first and ninth thoracic vertebrae (Hansen, 1952; Hoerlein, 1953). The intercapital ligament probably does contribute substantially to the protection of these eight discs. However, a substantial number of protrusions occurs at the ninth disc (between vertebrae T9 and T10). Some other factor, such as mobility, must also contribute to the distribution of protrusions from discs possessing an intercapital ligament (King, 1956b).

The **radiate ligament** (lig. capitis costae intra-articulare) (Fig. 8.2) spreads from the ventral surface of the head of the rib to the bodies of the two adjacent vertebrae. The **costotransverse ligament** (lig. costo-transversarium) (Fig. 8.2) runs between the transverse process and the neck of the rib.

Evidently the costochondral joints (between the ribs and their costal cartilages) are usually united by cartilage. However, synovial intrachondral joints apparently occur within the cartilages of ribs 2 to 5 in the pig, ribs

2 to 10 in ruminants, and sometimes in older carnivores (Schaller *et al.*, 1992, p. 82).

8.6 Sternum

The sternum (Figs 8.8, 8.9) consists of three bony parts, the **manubrium**, the **body**, and the **xiphoid process**. The xiphoid process is extended caudally by the **xiphoid cartilage**. The body is formed by a series of bony sternebrae, united by blocks of cartilage or bone. Each pair of **costal cartilages** articulates by synovial joints at the junction of two sternebrae.

The shape of the **body of the sternum** (corpus sterni) varies, being somewhat laterally flattened in the domestic species but dorsoventrally flattened in man. In the dog (Fig. 8.8) and cat the flattening is not pronounced, so that the sternum is 'rodlike' (Dyce *et al.*, 1987, p. 41). In the horse (Fig. 8.9) it is boat-shaped, with a keel formed by a ventral crest.

There are said to be 6–8 sternebrae in the domestic species (e.g. Barone, 1986, p. 433), but it is not always clear what is meant by 'sternebra'. The manubrium is sometimes said to be the first sternebra, and the xiphoid process the last sternebra (e.g. Evans and Christensen, 1979, p. 177). However, the intention of the NAV (1994) is evidently to consider the sternebrae to belong only to the body of the sternum. If so, there are eight sternebrae in the dog (Fig. 8.8) and six in the horse (Fig. 8.9), and the manubrium and xiphoid process are additional structures.

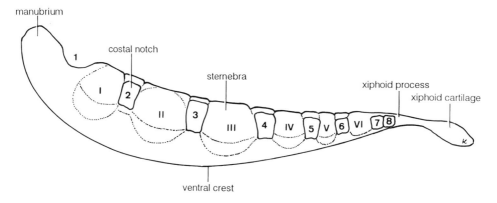

Fig. 8.9 Left lateral view of the sternum of a horse. The sternum is boat-shaped, the prominent ventral crest representing the keel. The body of the sternum has six sternebrae (I–VI). The manubrium is fused to the first sternebra. The xiphoid cartilage projects from the xiphoid process at the caudal end of the sixth sternebra. The costal cartilage of the first of the eight sternal ribs (1) articulates with the manubrium. The others (2–8) articulate with costal notches on the body of the sternum, the notches of 7 and 8 being confluent.

The points on the sternum where the costal cartilages articulate, i.e. the sternocostal articulations, are known as **costal notches** (incisurae costales) (Figs 8.8, 8.9). Being synovial, each joint is supported by a joint capsule and a **radiate sternocostal ligament** (lig. sternocostale radiatum) (Fig. 8.8) that spreads out between the distal end of the costal cartilage and the dorsal and ventral surfaces of the body of the sternum.

The dorsal surface of the sternum is almost completely covered by the **transverse thoracic muscle** (m. transversus thoracis). Its fibres are essentially transverse, passing from the sternum to the costochondral junction of the sternal ribs (Section 8.9.2).

8.7   Embryonic derivation of vertebrae, ribs, and sternum

These structures are all mesodermal derivatives. The vertebrae and ribs arise from somites, and the sternum from the lateral mesoderm.

8.7.1   *Formation of ectoderm, mesoderm, and endoderm*

The fertilized ovum divides repeatedly by mitosis to form a solid ball of cells (Latin: morula, mulberry). This soon becomes a hollow sphere (blastocyst), with a wall that is *one cell thick* (trophoblast cells) surrounding the central cavity (blastocoele). The trophoblast cells sustain the nutrition of the blastocyst by attaching it to the uterine wall (Greek: trophikos, nourishment). The blastocyst now elongates into a sausage-shaped sac. At one end of this sac a small cluster of cells (embryonic disc, or inner cell mass) proliferates beneath the trophoblast cells. Then the trophoblast cells that cover the embryonic disc degenerate, thus exposing the embryonic disc on the surface of the blastocyst. In principle, the embryonic disc forms the embryo, whereas the trophoblast cells extending beyond the rim of the embryonic disc contribute to the fetal membranes of the placenta.

The outermost cells of the embryonic disc are now the **ectoderm**. The innermost cells of the embryonic disc, i.e. those facing the cavity of the blastocyst, bud off a layer of cells. This is the **endoderm**. The wall of the blastocyst is now *two cells thick* (bilaminar). Between these two layers, the embryonic disc now produces a third layer of cells that spreads rapidly between ectoderm

and endoderm. This is the **mesoderm**. The mass of proliferating cells that form the endoderm and mesoderm lies in the *longitudinal axis* of the embryonic disc (primitive streak). The mesodermal **notochord** develops from what becomes the *cranial* end of the primitive streak. The disposition in the embryonic disc of the ectoderm, mesoderm, endoderm, primitive streak, and notochord, is seen in Fig. 8.10.

At its bilaminar stage, the deep layer of the **embryonic disc** (discus embryonicus) that forms the **endoderm** (endoderma) is known at the **hypoblast** (hypoblastus): the superficial layer is the **epiblast** (epiblastus), and forms the other two germ layers, namely the ectoderm and mesoderm (Latshaw, 1987, p. 38). At a point on the margin of the disc the epiblast becomes thicker by cellular proliferation, this thickening establishing the *caudal* end of the embryo. This thickening enlarges into the **primitive streak** (linea primitiva) (Fig. 8.10A,B) (Noden and de Lahunta, 1985, p. 32). The proliferating cells of the primitive streak are particularly active at its *cranial end*, forming an enlargement, the **embryonic node** (nodus embryonicus), also known by several synonyms (primitive node or knot, Hensen's node). Thus the primitive streak and embryonic node have established the long axis, and the head and tail ends, of the developing embryo.

Mesoderm proliferates from the deep surface of the primitive streak (Fig. 8.11) and extends caudally, laterally, and cranially between the ectoderm and endoderm (Fig. 8.10B). The embryonic disc is now trilaminar. Eventually the advancing mesoderm becomes interposed between the ectoderm and endoderm over almost the whole area of the embryonic disc, constituting the **intraembryonic mesoderm** (mesoderma embryonicum); it also extends beyond the edges of the embryonic disc as the **extraembryonic mesoderm** (mesoderma extraembryonicum) (Fig. 8.10B). Intraembryonic mesoderm is temporarily absent (Fig. 8.10B) from a small longitudinal strip in the midline where the notochord is about to form.

The **notochord** (notochorda) arises as a rod of tightly packed mesodermal cells from the *cranial* end of the primitive streak, growing towards the head end of the embryo (Fig. 8.10A). The rod enters the temporarily unoccupied midline zone between the cranially advancing lateral extensions of the mesoderm (Patten, 1958, p. 112) (Fig. 8.10B).

8.7.2   *Formation of paraxial, intermediate, and lateral mesoderm*

The mesodermal mass on each side of the notochord increases in amount, and because it lies

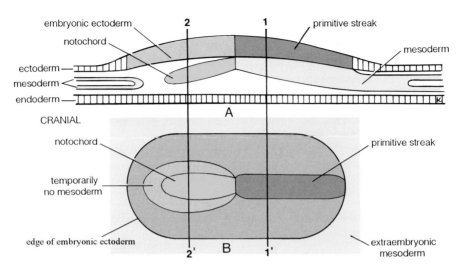

Fig. 8.10 Diagrams of the embryonic disc to show the formation of the notochord from the primitive streak. A. Diagrammatic median longitudinal section of the embryonic disc through the primitive streak. The three germ layers are present (ectoderm, mesoderm, and endoderm) so the disc has reached the trilaminar stage. B. Dorsal view of the same embryonic disc, the ectodermal covering of the disc being portrayed as though transparent so that the notochord and other mesoderm (grey-green) are visible. The rod-like notochord arises from the cranial end of the primitive streak, extending cranially between the ectoderm and the endoderm into a region temporarily unoccupied by the invading mesoderm. 1–1′ is the plane of the transverse section in Fig. 8.11; 2–2′ is the plane of the transverse section in Fig. 8.12.

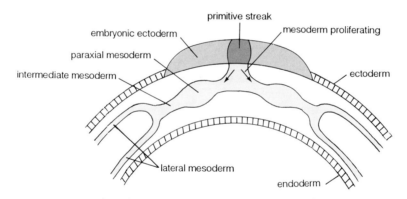

Fig. 8.11 Diagrammatic transverse section through the embryonic disc to show the origin of the mesoderm. The section is cut at 1–1′ in Fig. 8.10A,B. The mesoderm arises from the primitive streak (arrows). The three great divisions of the mesoderm, i.e. the paraxial, intermediate, and lateral mesoderm, have been formed.

on either side of the midline this enlargement of the mesoderm is named the **paraxial mesoderm** (or dorsal mesoderm) (Fig. 8.11). The mesoderm is continued laterally by a relatively thin sheet known as the **intermediate mesoderm** (Fig. 8.11), and this eventually contributes to the formation of the **urogenital system**. Beyond the intermediate mesoderm is the **lateral mesoderm** (or lateral plate mesoderm) (Fig. 8.11).

Clefts appear in the lateral mesoderm, splitting it into an outer layer of **somatic mesoderm** (somatic meaning 'body') and an inner layer of **splanchnic mesoderm** (splanchnic meaning 'visceral'). The clefts coalesce to become the **coelom** (Fig. 8.12).

The **somatic mesoderm** and the overlying ectoderm comprise the **somatopleure** (Fig. 8.12). The somatic mesoderm of the somatopleure con-

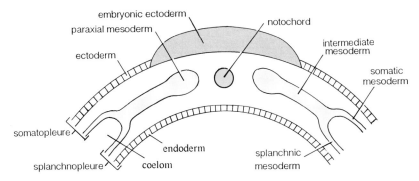

Fig. 8.12 Diagrammatic transverse section through the embryonic disc to show the notochord and the paraxial, intermediate, and lateral mesoderm. The section is cut at 2–2′ in Fig. 8.10A,B. The lateral mesoderm has split into the outer somatic mesoderm and the inner splanchnic mesoderm, with the coelom between them. The somatic mesoderm combines with the ectoderm to form the somatopleure, and the splanchnic mesoderm with the endoderm to form the splanchnopleure.

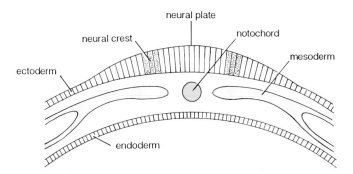

Fig. 8.13 Diagrammatic transverse section showing the origin of the neural plate. The neural plate arises as a thickening of the ectoderm dorsal to the notochord. The neural plate eventually becomes many cells thick. The cells of the neural crest first form in the lateral margins of the neural plate.

tributes to the **body wall**, including the formation of the sternum, parietal pleura, and parietal peritoneum; it also forms the parietal pericardium. Furthermore, it migrates into the limb buds where it forms the skeleton of the **limbs**.

The **splanchnic mesoderm** and the adjacent endoderm together constitute the **splanchnopleure** (Fig. 8.12). The splanchnic mesoderm becomes involved in the formation of visceral structures, including the **visceral pleura** and the **visceral peritoneum**, the **smooth muscle of the gut wall**, and the **myocardium** and **visceral pericardium**.

The ectoderm immediately dorsal to the notochord thickens to become the **neural plate** (Fig. 8.13). The lateral edges of the neural plate rise up to form the left and right **neural folds**, thus defining the **neural groove** (Fig. 8.14). The folds unite in the midline to establish the **neural tube**, from which the **central nervous system** will develop. As the neural tube becomes complete, the ectoderm closes over it dorsally (Fig. 8.15). Cells near the lateral edge of the neural plate form a pair of longitudinal aggregations known as the **neural crest** (Fig. 8.13). These come to lie at the apex of each neural fold (Fig. 8.14), as the folds close to form the neural tube, and detach themselves as a pair of masses on the dorsolateral aspect of the closed neural tube (Fig. 8.15).

Nomina Embryologica Veterinaria (1992) terms are as follows: paraxial mesoderm, mesoderma paraxiale; intermediate mesoderm, mesoderma intermedium; lateral mesoderm, mesoderma laterale; somatic mesoderm, mesoderma somaticum; splanchnic mesoderm, mesoderma splanchnica; somatopleure, somatopleura; splanchnopleure, splanchnopleura; neural plate, lamina neuralis; neural fold, plica neuralis; neural groove, sulcus neuralis; neural tube, tubus neuralis.

Cells of the **neural crest** (crista neuralis) migrate all over the body. In particular they form most of the neurons (and their accompanying **Schwann cells**) that have their cell bodies in the *peripheral* nervous system (e.g. **dorsal root ganglion cells**, and **postganglionic autonomic neurons**). They also contribute extensively to connective tissues in the head (Williams *et al.*, 1989, p. 137).

8.7.3 *Differentiation of somites*

The paraxial mesoderm becomes divided into a series of paired block-like segmental masses called **somites** (Fig. 8.16), starting at the cranial end of the embryo. As the embryo grows, further **segmentation** adds more somites to the caudal end of the series. Each somite differentiates into the **dermatome** forming the dermis of the skin, the sclerotome forming bone, and the myotome forming muscle (Fig. 8.17).

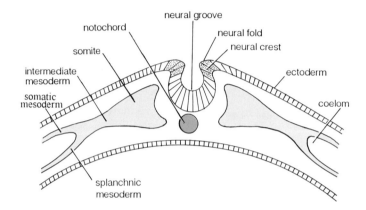

Fig. 8.14 Diagrammatic transverse section showing the neural groove. The neural groove is formed by the left and right neural folds that rise up from the neural plate. The folds are about to unite in the midline, thus closing the neural tube. The cells of the neural crest lie at the apex of each neural fold, where the folds will meet.

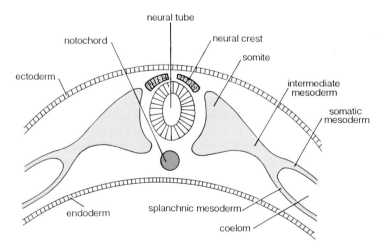

Fig. 8.15 Diagrammatic transverse section showing the neural tube and neural crest and their relationship to the ectoderm and mesoderm. The ectoderm has closed over the neural tube (which has become many cells thick). The cells of the neural crest have taken up a position dorsolateral to the neural tube. The neural tube is flanked laterally by the paraxial mesoderm, which has enlarged into somites.

8.7.4 *Formation of vertebrae*

The vertebrae are mesodermal structures formed from somites by the rearrangement of segmental sclerotomes into **intersegmental** vertebrae (Fig. 8.18).

Mesenchymal cells of the sclerotome sweep ventromedially to surround the notochord, separating it dorsally from the neural tube and ventrally from the gut. The mesenchyme of the caudal half of each sclerotome becomes condensed (Fig. 8.18A) and fuses with the more diffuse cranial half of the sclerotome immediately caudal to it (Fig. 8.18B,C); at the same time it separates itself from its own cranial component by the formation

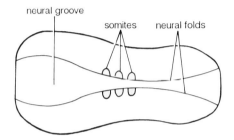

Fig. 8.16 Dorsal view diagram of an early embryo to show the first somites. At the cranial end of the embryo, the paraxial mesoderm has become divided into paired segmental blocks, the somites.

of a fissure (Fig. 8.18B). This new block of mesoderm, reconstituted from two of the original somites, now develops into a vertebra.

The dense cranial component of the rearranged vertebra forms the cranial part of the vertebral body, its arches, and its lateral processes, and in the thoracic region the associated ribs; the other parts of the vertebra develop from the diffuse caudal component that originally came from the next sclerotome (Fig. 8.18D). So in relation to the somites (which really are segmental), the definitive vertebra is **inter**segmental. Since the **spinal nerves** emerge between the vertebrae they are truly segmental.

The exact contribution of the cranial and caudal component of each sclerotome is controversial, but the rearrangement of the segmental sclerotome into an intersegmental vertebra still forms the basis of the description of vertebral development (e.g. see Noden and de Lahunta, 1985, p. 142; Williams *et al.*, 1989, p. 159).

The **anulus fibrosus** of the intervertebral disc probably arises from mesenchyme derived from the dense cranial component of each rearranged vertebra (Noden and de Lahunta, 1985, p. 142). As stated above, the notochord forms the **nucleus pulposus** (Fig. 8.18C), but atrophies and finally vanishes from within the vertebral bodies (Williams *et al.*, 1989, p. 161).

8.7.5 *Formation of ribs*

Like the vertebrae, the ribs are formed from sclerotomes. They arise as paired cartilaginous

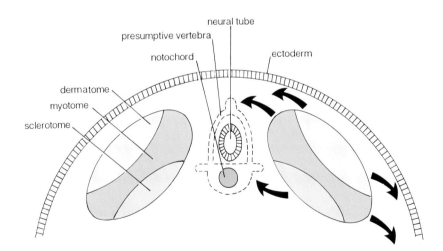

Fig. 8.17 Diagrammatic transverse section of an early embryo to show the differentiation of the somite into its three basic components. The dorsolateral part of the somite (light green) becomes the dermatome, and distributes its mesenchymal cells under the ectoderm (upper arrows) to form the dermis. The ventromedial part (medium green) becomes the sclerotome, and forms vertebrae and ribs (ventromedial arrow). The middle part of the somite (darker green) becomes the myotome, and forms the axial (medial arrow) and limb musculature (lateral arrow). The future position of the vertebra is shown in broken lines.

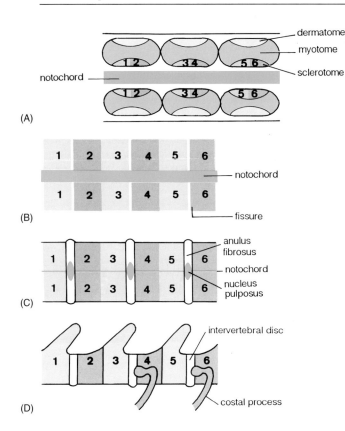

(A)

(B)

(C)

(D)

Fig. 8.18 Diagrams showing the contribution of the sclerotome to formation of vertebrae. A, B, and C are horizontal sections through the developing vertebrae, and D is a lateral view of the developing vertebrae. In A, the somites, including their sclerotomes, are **segmental**. The mesenchyme of each sclerotome, however, has differentiated into a dense caudal component (2, 4, 6) and a diffuse cranial component (1, 3, 5). In B and C, the dense and diffuse components of each sclerotome have been separated by a fissure. The two components become rearranged, the vertebrae now being formed by 2 combined with 3, 4 with 5, and so on. Each vertebra resulting from this fusion is **inter**segmental. In D, the dense component (2, 4, 6) has formed the cranial part of the definitive vertebral body, the arch, and the lateral processes, and also the ribs. The diffuse component (1, 3, 5) has formed the rest of the vertebra. In C, the notochord forms the nucleus pulposus of the intervertebral disc between each vertebral body, but within each vertebral body the notochord is reduced and finally disappears. The anulus fibrosus is formed by sclerotomal mesenchyme from the dense cranial component of each sclerotome, adjacent to the fissure.

costal processes from the developing vertebral arches. In the thoracic region, these costal processes extend laterally into the developing body wall and form definitive ribs (Fig. 8.18D).

The ribs are formed from the dense component of each sclerotome (Fig. 8.18D) (Williams *et al.*, 1989, p. 161). The ossification of the ribs starts dorsally and proceeds ventrally, stopping short of the sternum and thus creating the flexible costal cartilages (Krahl, 1964, p. 231).

Much reduced paired costal processes appear in all the other vertebral regions, except perhaps the coccygeal (Williams *et al.*, 1989, p. 161). However, the proximal end of each of these costal elements fuses with the cartilage of the vertebra to which it belongs, thus contributing to the transverse process of the vertebra (Section 8.2). The foramen transversarium, penetrating the root of the transverse process of cervical vertebrae, is homologous to the gap (Fig. 8.2) between the transverse process of the vertebra, and the articular head, neck and tubercle of a typical rib.

The first lumbar vertebra of the dog may have a rib in place of the transverse process, on one or both sides (Dennis, 1987). In man an extra rib may articulate with the seventh cervical vertebra, and this sometimes dam-

ages the brachial plexus or obstructs the subclavian vessels, giving nervous and vascular symptoms (Williams *et al.*, 1989, p. 336).

In the thoracic region, the costal processes become ossified, except at their distal ends which remain cartilaginous as the **costal cartilages**.

8.7.6 *Formation of the sternum*

The sternum is a mesodermal structure, but unlike the other components of the rib cage it is not derived from somites but from mesenchyme (Fig. 8.19A,B,C).

The sternum originates by the fusion of a pair of mesenchymal **sternal bars**, lying laterally in the developing body wall (Fig. 8.19A). The sternal bars arise from the somatic mesoderm (i.e. from the lateral mesoderm), and not from the sclerotome (Noden and de Lahunta, 1985, p. 144). After conversion to cartilage, the left and right sternal bars fuse together, starting at their cranial ends (Fig. 8.19B,C). Although they arise independently, the cartilaginous ribs of the first eight or so pairs unite with the cartilaginous sternal bars to form the sternal

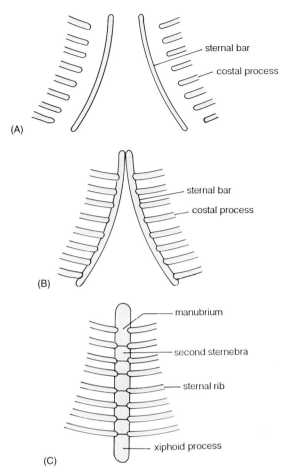

(A)

sternal bar

costal process

(B)

sternal bar

costal process

(C)

manubrium

second sternebra

sternal rib

xiphoid process

Fig. 8.19 Diagrams to show the development of the sternum. A. The sternum arises from the lateral mesoderm as a pair of mesenchymal sternal bars. The primordial costal processes (which will form the ribs) are not at first attached to the sternal bars. B. The sternal bars begin to fuse, starting at their cranial ends. The first eight pairs of ribs have joined the sternal bars. These are the sternal ribs. C. The paired sternal bars have fused to form the body of the sternum, which now becomes divided into segmental sternebrae.

ribs (Section 8.4). The body of the sternum becomes differentiated into segmental **sternebrae** (Fig. 8.19C). Cases of a cleft or perforated sternum in man reflect the paired derivation of this bone (Arey, 1958, p. 411).

8.8   Vertebral muscles

The muscles of the vertebral column are classified as **epaxial** or **hypaxial**. The epaxial muscles lie

dorsal to the transverse processes of the vertebrae, and get their nerve supply from the **dorsal rami** (dorsal divisions) of the spinal nerves (Fig. 2.1, Section 2.2). The hypaxial muscles lie *ventral* to the transverse processes and are innervated by **ventral rami**. The **epaxial vertebral muscles** consist of continuous and complex systems of short overlapping fascicles, extending from the ilium or sacrum all the way to the skull. Some of the fascicles are very short, passing between two adjacent vertebrae. Many others traverse one, two, three, four, or more vertebrae. Most of them attach to transverse processes, mamillary processes, and spines, and many of those in the thoracic region attach to the proximal ends of the ribs and therefore are potentially involved directly in respiration.

It is possible to identify and name quite numerous epaxial muscles that are associated with the **thoracic vertebrae**; a few of these (e.g. **longissimus thoracis** (Fig. 8.20) and **iliocostalis thoracis** (Fig. 8.21)) are conspicuous in the dissection room and recognizable radiographically (Fig. 24.8). Unquestionably these muscles play an important part in the life of the animal, particularly in carnivores where dorsal extension of the vertebral column by the epaxial muscles and ventral flexion by the hypaxial muscles are major factors in their bounding gait at full speed. They are all also potentially *inspiratory* muscles (Sections 8.9.2; 10.10.1), acting *indirectly* by dorsal extension of the thoracic vertebral column, and some of them *directly* (for example iliocostalis, as its name implies, and longissimus thoracis) because of their attachments to the ribs. However, the ability to name and identify the individual epaxial muscles in the thoracic region has little value physiologically or clinically.

The hypaxial muscles are not restricted to muscles that are directly attached to the vertebrae, but also include the muscles of the thoracic and abdominal walls (Sections 8.9–8.11).

The epaxial and hypaxial muscles all arise embryologically from the myotome (Section 8.7.3).

The main **epaxial vertebral muscles** can be subdivided into three longitudinal systems, lateral, intermediate, and medial, lying in a lateromedial, and at the same time ventrodorsal, series (Evans and Christensen, 1979,

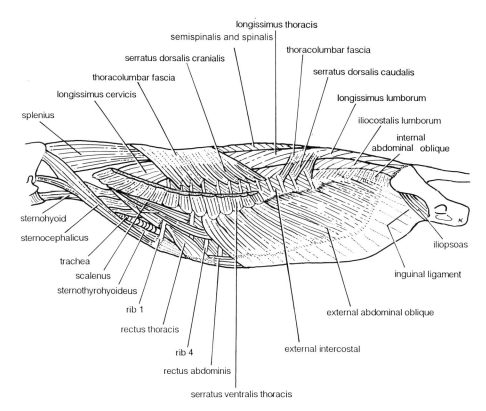

Fig. 8.20 Superficial muscles of the vertebral column, and of the lateral thoracic wall and abdominal wall of the dog. The serratus ventralis attaches to the medial surface of the scapula, and is transected when the limb is removed. The fibres of the external intercostal and external abdominal oblique muscles slope in the same direction, caudoventrally. The three great systems of epaxial muscles, i.e. the iliocostalis muscle, longissimus muscle, and the medial group of short segmental muscle bundles lying directly on the vertebrae (e.g. spinalis and semispinalis), are partly concealed by the serratus dorsalis muscles.

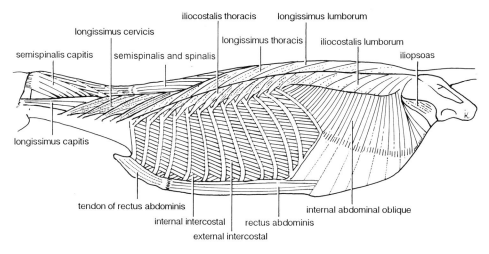

Fig. 8.21 Deeper muscles of the vertebral column, and of the lateral thoracic wall and abdominal wall of the dog. The external abdominal oblique and serratus muscles have been removed, exposing epaxial vertebral muscles and the external intercostal muscles. The main epaxial muscles are the iliocostalis (laterally placed), longissimus (intermediate in position), and the spinalis and semispinalis muscles (lying medially). The longissimus and iliocostalis muscles have lumbar, thoracic, and cervical components. The fibres of the external intercostal muscles slope caudoventrally. In most species, the external intercostal muscles are not present in the spaces between the costal cartilages, these spaces being occupied only by the internal intercostal muscles; in the dog the external intercostal muscles are present in the more caudal of the interchondral spaces.

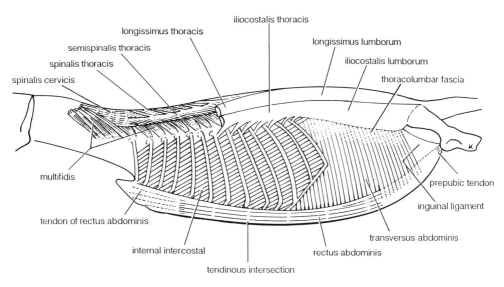

Fig. 8.22   Deepest muscles of the vertebral column and of the lateral thoracic wall and abdominal wall of the dog. The longissimus and iliocostalis muscles have been transected and their cranial parts removed, exposing some of the most medial epaxial muscles (semispinalis, spinalis, and multifidis). The external intercostal muscles have been removed to show the internal intercostals. The fibres of the internal intercostal muscles slope caudodorsally, at right angles to those of the external intercostals, and occupy the interchondral spaces as well as the bony intercostal spaces. Removal of the internal abdominal oblique reveals the transversus abdominis muscle. The rectus abdominis is subdivided by tendinous intersections.

p. 305). (Some smaller vertebral muscles, such as **serratus dorsalis**, may also be epaxial, but are considered below in Section 8.9.2). The lateral system is formed by the **iliocostalis muscle** (Figs 8.21, 24.8). The intermediate system is formed mainly by the powerful **longissimus muscle** (Fig. 8.20). (The iliocostalis and longissimus muscles are further divided regionally into cervical, thoracic, and lumbar components.) The medial system, which is largely covered by the longissimus system, consists of a complex group of short muscles that lie more or less directly on the vertebrae, including the **multifidis**, **spinalis**, and **semispinalis** muscles (Fig. 8.22), and the **rotatores**, **interspinales**, and **intertransversarii** muscles; these muscles are also known as the **transversospinalis system**.

In general, the fascicles in the iliocostalis and longissimus systems are directed cranioventrally (Dyce *et al.*, 1987, p. 45) (Fig. 8.21), whereas those in the complex medial system run craniodorsally (Dyce *et al.*, 1987, p. 395) (e.g. multifidis and semispinalis in Fig. 8.22).

The longitudinal muscle systems are classified by the NAV (1994) into the **erector spinae transversospinalis**, **interspinales**, and **intertransversarii systems** (Schaller *et al.*, 1992, pp. 108–111). The erector spinae system includes iliocostalis and longissimus. The transversospinalis system is as just mentioned above, except that in the NAV (1994) it excludes the interspinales and intertransversarii muscles, which now constitute their own systems.

When all the epaxial systems on both sides of the body

contract together they dorsally extend the vertebral column. When they contract on only one side they produce lateral movement of the vertebral column. As already stated, extension and flexion of the vertebral column are important in locomotion of **carnivores** at high speed. In the **horse**, however, contraction of the epaxial and hypaxial muscles maintains the thoracolumbar vertebral column relatively rigidly, with minimal extension and flexion. Extension and flexion do occur at the lumbosacral articulation of the horse, contributing to the length of the stride. **Injury** to the epaxial muscles in the horse can cause back pain, leading to stiff hind limb action, faulty backing and jumping, and resentment of palpation, grooming and saddling (de Lahunta and Habel, 1986, p. 210).

8.9   Muscles of the lateral and ventral thoracic walls

8.9.1   *Intercostal muscles*

The external and internal intercostal muscles occupy the intercostal spaces. The **external intercostal muscles** lie superficially in the intercostal spaces, covering the deeper internal intercostal muscles (Fig. 8.23). The fibres of the external intercostal muscles run caudoventrally between

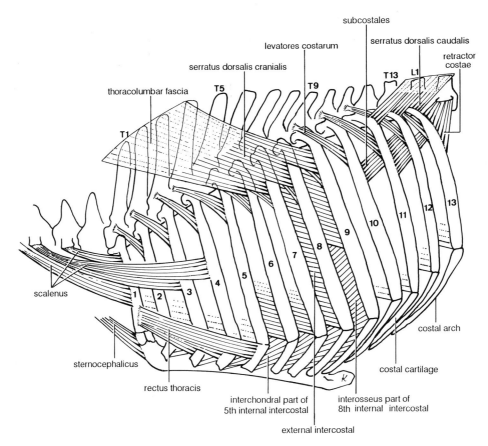

Fig. 8.23 Semi-diagrammatic view of the left thoracic wall of a standard mammal to show the principal accessory muscles of respiration. Muscles that can pull the ribs cranially (scalenus, serratus dorsalis cranialis, levatores costarum, rectus thoracis) or tilt the body of the sternum ventrally (sternocephalicus) are potentially inspiratory. Muscles that pull the ribs caudally (serratus dorsalis caudalis, retractor costae, subcostales) are potentially expiratory. The subcostal muscles occur in carnivores only. The external intercostal muscle is shown complete in the seventh intercostal space; typically, the external intercostal muscles do not continue into the interchondral space. In the eighth intercostal space the distal two thirds of the external intercostal have been removed, exposing the internal intercostal muscle which not only continues into the interchondral space but is best developed therein. Skeleton based on the ox: 1–13, ribs one to thirteen; T1, T5, T9, T13, thoracic vertebrae; L1, first lumbar vertebra.

the ribs (Fig. 8.21), but not between the costal cartilages (Fig. 8.23).

The **internal intercostal muscles** have two components. The **interosseous component** consists of fibres that run between the bony ribs, at right angles to the external intercostals and therefore sloping caudodorsally (Fig. 8.22). The **interchondral component** lies in the interchondral space. Its fibres run between the costal cartilages, still sloping caudodorsally (Fig. 8.23). The interchondral component of the internal intercostal is

thicker and more powerful than the interosseous component.

The forces of the **external intercostal muscles** give them an **inspiratory action** (Section 10.9). The forces of the *interosseous* part of the **internal intercostal muscle**, as the contrary direction of their fibres suggests, are opposite to those of the external intercostal, i.e. **expiratory**. On the other hand, the forces of the *interchondral* part of the **internal intercostals** are **inspiratory** (Section 10.9). Thus the respiratory action of the internal intercostal muscle is reversed at its costal cartilage.

In summary, the external intercostal muscles and the interchondral components of the internal intercostals are inspiratory; the interosseous components of the internal intercostals are expiratory.

The intercostal muscles arise in the embryo from the myotome.

There are species variations in the relative development of interosseous and interchondral components of the intercostal muscles. In general, however, the **external intercostal muscles** have strongly developed interosseous components, but limited or non-existent intercartilaginous components; the reverse applies to the **internal intercostal muscles**, which possess well-developed interchondral parts ventrally but weak interosseous parts, especially dorsally. Thus in the *horse* (Sisson, 1975, p. 402) and *ox* (Getty, 1975, p. 818) the **interchondral component** is absent from the external intercostal muscle, and is reduced to a membrane in *man* (Krahl, 1964, p. 236), but is strong in the internal intercostal muscle; the **interosseous component** of the internal intercostal muscle disappears or converts into a membrane near the vertebrae in the *ox* and *man*, and in the *ox* is generally thinner than the external intercostal but in the *horse* it extends over the entire intercostal space. In the *pig* (Sisson, 1975, p. 1260), the **interchondral part** of the internal intercostal is thick. In the *dog* (Evans and Christensen, 1979, p. 318) the external intercostal lacks an **interchondral part** in the most cranial intercostal spaces, but in the caudal intercostal spaces it occupies more and more of the interchondral space. The **interosseous part** of the internal intercostal muscle of the *dog* is weaker than the external intercostal; however, the **interchondral part** of the internal intercostal fills the interchondral space and is of notable thickness.

The **interchondral components** of the internal intercostal muscles may appear to be a rather insignificant anatomical detail. However, they turn out to be *the most important inspiratory part of the intercostal musculature* (Decramer, 1993) (Section 10.9). They are designated by some physiologists as the 'parasternal intercostal muscles'. The relatively great bulk of the parasternal intercostals, as described in the preceding paragraph, indicates their functional importance.

In the middle two quarters of the more caudal intercostal spaces in man (Williams *et al.*, 1989, p. 592) there is a third but indistinct intercostal muscle, deep to the other two intercostal muscles and therefore lying next to the parietal pleura. This is the **m. intercostalis intimus** of the human (NA, 1989). It can be identified by the intercostal artery vein and nerve, which, as they pass ventrally, come to lie between the third layer of intercostal muscle and the internal intercostal muscle (Krahl,

1964, p. 236). This muscle can be found in the dog, but seems to have been generally overlooked by veterinary anatomists, or interpreted as the m. subcostalis (as by Dyce *et al.*, 1987, p. 49); it is not listed in the NAV (1994). The third intercostal muscle is far too feeble to have any physiological significance, but what makes it interesting is not respiratory mechanics but the insight it gives into the anatomy of the lateral body wall. The development of the diaphragm in mammals appears superficially to divide the lateral wall of the body cavity into two very different regions, a thoracic region with ribs and an abdominal region without ribs.

However, it will be recalled (Section 8.4) that ancestral tetrapods had a pair of ribs in almost every segment of the body, a condition still retained in contemporary snakes. Therefore, on grounds of phylogeny, in a mammal the lateral thoracic and lateral abdominal walls ought to have basically the same structure. This prediction is confirmed by the presence of the third (deep) intercostal muscle. The three intercostal muscles (external, internal, and deep) in the lateral thoracic wall are homologous (Krahl, 1964, p. 236) to the three abdominal muscles in the lateral abdominal wall (i.e. the external oblique abdominal, the internal oblique abdominal, and the transverse abdominal muscles). In the thoracic wall these three layers of muscle are simply interrupted by ribs, thus creating intercostal muscles. The direction of the fibres of the **external** intercostal muscle (Fig. 8.21) is therefore the same as that of the **external** oblique abdominal muscle (Fig. 8.20), i.e. caudoventral; likewise, the direction of fibres in the **internal** intercostal muscle (Fig. 8.22) is necessarily the same as that of the **internal** oblique abdominal muscle (Fig. 8.21), i.e. caudodorsal. These homologies of the thoracic and abdominal walls are nicely completed by the **endothoracic fascia** (Section 9.8), which is homologous to the **transversalis fascia** of the abdominal wall (Williams *et al.*, 1989, p. 1268). All this is good news for the student: if he knows the anatomy of the abdominal wall he also knows the anatomy of the thoracic wall – two for the price of one.

8.9.2 Other muscles of the lateral and ventral thoracic walls

The muscles of the lateral thoracic wall include: (a) intrinsic thoracic muscles with all their attachments within the thoracic skeleton (e.g. the intercostal muscles); (b) thoracic vertebral muscles with attachments to the ribs (e.g. longissimus thoracis, Fig. 8.20); (c) limb muscles, with attachments to the ribs or sternum (e.g. serratus ventralis thoracis, Fig. 8.20); (d) neck muscles with attachments to the ribs or sternum (e.g. sternocephalicus, Fig. 8.20); and (e) abdominal muscles (Section 8.10). All of the muscles of the lateral thoracic wall develop from the myotome.

Virtually any muscle that is attached to the lateral or ventral thoracic wall, either to the ribs or the sternum, is potentially a respiratory muscle. However, most of these muscles are not significantly involved in **resting breathing** (eupnoea), which is performed by the diaphragm and intercostal muscles. But many of them do act as **accessory muscles of respiration** (Section 10.10) during the hyperventilation of exercise or the distressed breathing of respiratory disease.

Intrinsic thoracic muscles

The **transversus thoracis** muscle lies, essentially transversely, on the dorsal surface of the sternum (Fig. 8.8). In carnivores, its fibres pass craniolaterally (St. Clair, 1975, p. 1518) from the sternebrae to the costal cartilages of sternal ribs and are therefore *potentially expiratory*. In some species (horse, Sisson, 1975, p. 405; man, Williams *et al.*, 1989, p. 592) the most caudal bundles lack the cranial element in their direction and even tend to run caudolaterally. The **subcostal** muscles (Fig. 8.23) lie at the proximal ends of the most caudal ribs in carnivores, deep to the internal intercostal muscles (Schaller *et al.*, 1992, p. 110); their fibres pass obliquely between several ribs, sloping caudodorsally like the internal intercostal muscles, and are therefore *potentially expiratory*. The **rectus thoracis** muscle (Fig. 8.23) runs caudoventrally between the distal end of the first rib and the costal cartilages or distal ends or ribs 3, 4, or 5, and would seem to be *potentially inspiratory*.

Thoracic vertebral muscles

The **iliocostalis** and **longissimus systems** (Fig. 8.21, Section 8.8) attach to the vertebrae and ribs. Since their fibres run caudodorsally from the ribs they have expiratory possibilities. However, all the *epaxial* thoracic muscles are capable of contributing to *inspiration* by dorsally extending the thoracic vertebral column; this spreads the ribs, slightly increases the width of the intercostal spaces, and allows the ribs a greater range of movement (Williams *et al.*, 1989, p. 595) (Section 10.10.1). The **serratus dorsalis** muscles are a series of segmental muscles running between the thoracolumbar fascia (covering the longissimus and iliocostalis systems) and the proximal ends of the ribs. The fibres of the **serratus dorsalis cranialis** (Fig. 8.20) slope caudoventrally (like the external intercostal muscle) and are therefore *inspiratory*; the fibres of the **serratus dorsalis caudalis** muscle (Fig. 8.20) are directed caudodorsally (like the internal intercostal) and are therefore *expiratory*. The **levatores costarum** muscles (Fig. 8.23) are like a smaller, deeper, but more extensive version of the serratus dorsalis cranialis. Thus they are segmental muscles running from the thoracic vertebrae, caudoventrally, to the proximal ends of the ribs. Like the serratus dorsalis cranialis, they are *inspiratory*. The **retractor costae** muscle (Fig. 8.23) is a very small muscle running caudodorsally from the proximal end of the last rib to the thoracolumbar fascia; it thus resembles the serratus dorsalis caudalis, and is *potentially expiratory*.

Limb muscles with attachments to the ribs or sternum

The fibres of the **serratus ventralis thoracis** muscle run from the ribs of the cranial half of the thorax (Fig. 8.20) to the scapula. The more caudal of these fibres slope caudoventrally (like those of the external intercostal muscles) and are therefore *potentially inspiratory*, but since the scapula is lateral to the thorax the entire muscle is capable of expanding the thorax laterally. The **latissimus dorsi** muscle runs between the humerus and the thoracolumbar fascia and caudal ribs; most of its fibres run caudodorsally and are therefore *potentially inspiratory*. The **superficial** and **deep pectoral** muscles are attached to the humerus and to the sternum, and (deep pectoral) to the costal cartilages also. In the horse, pig, and ruminant, the **subclavius** muscle (previously called m. pectoralis cleidoscapularis in the pig and horse; Schaller *et al.*, 1992, p. 110) passes craniodorsally from the first few costal cartilages to the supraspinatus or brachiocephalic muscle and is *potentially inspiratory*.

Neck muscles with attachments to the ribs or sternum

The substantial **scalenus** muscles (Fig. 8.20) pass craniocaudally between the cervical vertebrae and the first ribs. In the horse (and sometimes in the sheep) they are limited to rib 1, and in man to ribs 1 and 2 (Williams *et al.*, 1989, p. 586); in other domestic species they attach (variably) to ribs 4–9 (Schaller *et al.*, 1992, p. 104) and therefore have greater *inspiratory* possibilities. The **sternocephalicus** muscle (Figs 5.1, 8.20) attaches caudally to the manubrium (and the first costal cartilage in the ox; Sisson, 1975, p. 804) and cranially to the skull (mastoid and occipital parts) in the dog, to the mastoid process only in the pig and sheep (Schaller *et al.*, 1992, p. 104), to the skull and mandible in the ox (Sisson, 1975, p. 804), and to the mandible only in the horse (Schaller *et al.*, 1992, p. 104). In man, this muscle (the **sternocleidomastoideus**) runs between the manubrium and clavicle caudally, and the mastoid process and occiput cranially. Any respiratory action of sternocephalicus (which appears to be substantial in man and dog, Section 10.10.1) depends on its ability to pivot the first rib about its articulation with the vertebral column, and to pivot the sternum about its articulation with the first rib, both of these movements causing the caudal end of the sternum to swing ventrally (*inspiratory*).

8.10 Abdominal muscles

The **abdominal muscles** play an essential role in posture and locomotion. They are also the most powerful muscles of *expiration*, although during resting breathing expiration is attained entirely passively. They are used mainly for expiration during hyperventilation of exercise or forced expiration in respiratory disease (Section 10.10.2). They are also important for expulsive efforts such as *defecation* and *coughing*.

The fibres of the **external abdominal oblique muscle** slope caudoventrally, from the ribs and thoracolumbar fascia to the linea alba, pubic brim, and the iliopsoas muscles (Fig. 8.20). The fibres of the **internal oblique abdominal muscle** (Fig. 8.21) run cranioventrally, at right angles to those of the external oblique, from the thoracolumbar fascia and tuber coxae to the last rib and linea alba. The **transversus abdominis muscle** is the deepest of the abdominal muscles. Its fibres are directed more or less dorsoventrally (Fig. 8.22), from the thoracolumbar fascia and the medial surface of the ribs to the linea alba. The **rectus abdominis muscle** (Fig. 8.22) is attached cranially to the sternum and costal cartilages by a flat tendon, and caudally to the pubis by the prepubic tendon.

The fibres of the oblique abdominal muscles are so orientated (Figs 8.20, 8.21) that their contraction will pull the ribs caudally, thus creating an *expiratory movement* of the rib cage. During forced expiration or expulsive efforts, all of the abdominal muscles participate in compressing the abdominal wall, thus raising the intra-abdominal pressure and forcing the cupola of the diaphragm cranially into the rib cage.

8.11 Diaphragm

The diaphragm is a musculotendinous dome, separating the thoracic and abdominal cavities. The dome projects cranially into the rib cage, and is therefore convex on its thoracic surface and concave on its abdominal surface. Its periphery is formed by a continuous rim of skeletal musculature (Fig. 8.24), consisting of a lumbar component, a costal component, and a sternal component. The muscle fibres of these three components converge onto the central tendon (Figs 8.24, 8.25).

8.11.1 Diaphragmatic cupola

The most cranial part of the dome is known as the **diaphragmatic cupola**. At the end of a resting expiration in most species the cupola reaches cranially to about the level of the sixth rib (Fig. 8.25), where typically it is in contact with the pericardium (Figs 23.3, 23.4). The cupola tends to be slightly asymmetrical, the right half tending to bulge somewhat further cranially than the left; this asymmetry is discernible in dorsoventral thoracic radiographs of the dog (Section 24.7.4; Fig. 24.3).

The right half of the diaphragmatic cupola (cupula diaphragmatis) often projects further cranially than the left not only in the dog (Grandage, 1974), but also in the horse (Sisson, 1975, p. 406) and man (Williams *et al.*, 1989, p. 592). When viewed from the ventral (or dorsal) aspect the profile of the cupola is then sinuous with a bulge on each side, the two bulges being separated by a *cardiac impression* (Fig. 24.1). In the carnivores and pig the left half of the diaphragmatic cupola is attached to the fibrous pericardium by the phrenicopericardiac ligament (Section 9.4). When viewed laterally, the cranioventral slope of the cupola and diaphragm as a whole is less marked in the horse (Fig. 23.3) than in the ox (Fig. 23.4) and the other domestic species, because of the greater length of the thorax in the horse.

The word 'cupola' is a perfectly respectable English word for a dome (*Oxford English Dictionary*), whereas the word 'cupula' is strictly the late Latin source of the English 'cupola'. As such, cupula is correct as the official Latin term, cupula diaphragmatica, adopted by the NAV (1994), but is not really appropriate in an anatomical text written in English. Nevertheless the Latin 'cupula' has been widely adopted in English textbooks on *veterinary anatomy*. However, the English 'cupola' is used in current leading works on *human anatomy* as in *Gray's Anatomy* (Williams *et al.*, 1995, p. 816), and is also preferred here.

8.11.2 Tendinous centre

The tendinous centre is more or less V-shaped (Fig. 9.5), this shape being caused by invasion into the *dorsal* periphery of the tendon by the ventrally directed muscle fibres of the crura. Most of the fibres of the tendon radiate from the centre and into the muscular periphery, but many of them interlace in various directions (Fig. 8.24).

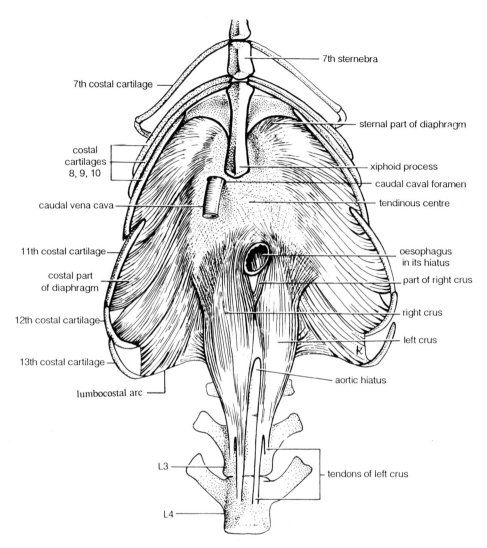

Fig. 8.24 Ventral view of the diaphragm of a cat. In this species and the dog the left and right crura arise by a bifid tendon from the third and fourth lumbar vertebrae. The aortic hiatus lies between the origins of the two crura. The fan-shaped muscle of the right crus is much broader than that of the left crus. The oesophageal hiatus is formed between two bundles of the right crus. The costal part of the diaphragm consists of muscle bundles arising from the costal cartilages and bodies of ribs 8–13, as in the dog. The tendinous centre is roughly heart-shaped, the heart image being upside-down in this view. The fibres of the tendon radiate from the musculature of the costal part towards the centre, but are also interlaced. The caval foramen lies in the tendinous centre, to the right of the midline.

The shape and relative size of the tendinous centre (centrum tendineum) vary in the species. In the *dog* the tendon is relatively small in area (Evans and Christensen, 1979, p. 321) and Y-shaped (Dyce *et al.,* 1987, p. 399). In the *pig* (Sisson, 1975, p. 1260) and *cat* (Fig. 8.24) the tendon is more circular in outline than in the *horse* where it is dorsoventrally elongated (Sisson, 1975, p. 406). In *man* it is V-shaped.

8.11.3 *Lumbar component of the diaphragm: the crura*

The left and right lumbar components of the diaphragm consist of a pair of fan-shaped skeletal muscles, the **left crus** and **right crus** of the diaphragm (Fig. 8.24). The two crura arise from the

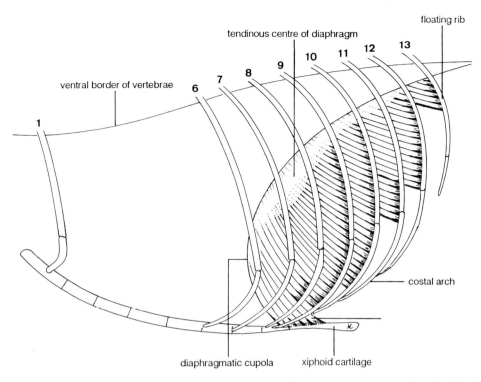

Fig. 8.25   Lateral view diagram of the costal part of the diaphragm of the dog. The dome-shaped cupola of the diaphragm reaches cranially to about the level of the sixth rib. The costal part of the diaphragm consists of bundles of skeletal muscle fibres that arise from costal cartilages and bodies of ribs 8–13, at the sites indicated by dense shading of fibres. The fibres slope craniodorsally and medially, converging on the tendinous centre. During inspiration these fibres pull the tendinous centre **caudally**, thus increasing the *craniocaudal* dimension of the rib cage; this is probably the main factor in inspiration. However, if the central tendon is fixed in position, the fibres pull their ribs and costal cartilages **cranially**, thereby expanding *transversely* the caudal part of the rib cage and aiding inspiration. The sternal component of the diaphragm arises from the xiphoid cartilage.

first three or four lumbar vertebrae as tendons, the tendon forming the handle of each fan. The muscle of the fan spreads out cranioventrally to insert onto the dorsal part of the tendinous centre of the diaphragm. The musculature of the left and right crura is not bilaterally symmetrical, that of the right crus being much larger and extending across the midline to the left side.

In veterinary anatomy, though not human anatomy (see Williams *et al.*, 1989, p. 592), it is customary to subdivide both the left crus (crus sinistrum) and the right crus (crus dextrum) into a lateral, intermediate, and medial component. The caudal edge of the lateral component forms the **lumbocostal arch** (arcus lumbocostalis) of the NAV (1994) (Fig. 8.24). However, some of these muscle masses are admitted to be 'only indistinctly separable' (Evans and Christensen, 1979, p. 322) or 'in part artificial' (Sisson and Grossman, 1969, p. 289), and the three

components are not recognized by the NAV (1983). Evans and Christensen (1979, p. 323) state that, in the dog, the tendon of origin of the right crus forms all three parts of the right crus plus the medial component of the left crus; the tendon of the left crus forms the intermediate and lateral components of the left crus. According to this method of description, the oesophageal hiatus lies between the right medial and left medial components.

8.11.4   *Costal component of the diaphragm*

The costal component of the diaphragm (pars costalis) is the rim of skeletal muscle forming the lateral border of the diaphragm. Its muscle fibres are attached to the medial surfaces of the more caudal ribs. The fibres diverge away from the thoracic wall at an acute angle, and converge radially on the central tendon (Fig. 8.25).

The site of attachment of these fibres is important clinically, since it determines the position of the **costodiaphragmatic line of pleural reflection** (Section 23.8, Fig. 23.2A–C). Basically, the zone of attachment of the fibres is parallel to the costal arch. However, the attachments to the ribs are not along a slender line, but quite a broad zone. In the **dog** (Fig. 23.2C) this zone follows the costal arch closely at its cranial end, but diverges cranially from the caudal part of the costal arch; in the **horse**, the zone of attachment lies well craniodorsal to the costal arch (Fig. 23.2A); in the **ox** it is even more craniodorsal to the costal arch (Fig. 23.2B). The parietal pleura is reflected from the lateral thoracic wall onto the diaphragm, and this has to happen along the craniodorsal border of the attachment zone of the costal musculature of the diaphragm. For all these reasons, the costodiaphragmatic line of pleural reflection is somewhat craniodorsal to the costal arch in the dog (Fig. 23.2C), about a hand's breadth craniodorsal in a small pony (Fig. 23.2A), and very far craniodorsal in the ox (Fig. 23.2B).

To understand the **actions of the diaphragm in breathing** it is essential to appreciate the *slope* of its costal muscle fibres, and this is only possible on a lateral view diagram such as Fig. 8.25. A glance at this diagram shows that these fibres can be regarded as running **craniodorsally** from the ribs to the tendinous centre; however, the fibres can equally well be visualized as running in the reverse direction, i.e. sloping **caudoventrally**, from the tendinous centre to the ribs (their orientation then being the same as the inspiratory external intercostal muscles). Figure 8.25 therefore shows that the costal muscles of the diaphragm **should** be able to pull the *tendinous centre caudally*, and thus cause inspiration. But **might** they be able to reverse their action? Perhaps they could then pull the more *caudal ribs* (i.e. the four asternal ribs, and the last two sternal ribs) *cranially*; this would expand the caudal part of the rib cage, causing inspiration. Both of these actions can actually happen. However, the centre of the diaphragm is, of course, mobile. The riddle, then, is to see how the centre of the diaphragm could be rendered *immobile*, i.e. fixed in position, so that the costal component of the diaphragm could contribute to inspiration by expanding the caudal part of the rib cage. The answer is that the tendinous centre can

be fixed in position by raising the intra-abdominal pressure (Section 10.8).

The attachments of the costal muscle fibres of the diaphragm are complex and vary with the species. In the *dog* (Fig. 8.25), they arise from part of the costal cartilage of rib 8, from the costal cartilages and bodies of ribs 9 and 10, and the bodies of ribs 11, 12 and 13 (Evans and Christensen, 1979, p. 323). Sisson (1975, p. 406) and Getty (1975, p. 820) stated that the origin extends along the ninth costal cartilage in the *horse* and the eighth in the *ox*, but from there to the last rib the attachments are from the bodies of the ribs at an increasing distance dorsal to their costochondral junctions.

8.11.5 *Sternal part of diaphragm*

The muscle of the sternal component of the diaphragm arises from the xiphoid cartilage (Fig. 8.25). It helps to pull the tendinous centre caudally during inspiration, but is presumably too small to make a major contribution to breathing.

8.11.6 *Diaphragmatic apertures*

Three openings in the diaphragm connect the thoracic and abdominal cavities, namely the aortic hiatus, the oesophageal hiatus, and the caval foramen.

The **aortic hiatus** lies between the tendons of origin of the left and right crura, and is completed dorsally by the lumbar vertebrae; the aorta, azygos vein, and thoracic duct pass through it.

The **oesophageal hiatus** is formed by a separation of muscle bundles of the medial part of the right crus (Fig. 8.24); the oesophagus and its blood vessels, and the dorsal and ventral vagal trunks (Section 3.11), pass through the oesophageal hiatus.

The **caval foramen** is an opening in the tendinous centre of the diaphragm and transmits the caudal vena cava; it lies to the right of the midline, somewhat caudodorsal to the most cranial part of the cupola of the diaphragm (Figs 8.24, 23.3, 23.4, 24.5).

The adventitia of the caudal vena cava is tightly attached to the tendinous rim of the caval foramen. However, the attachments of aorta and oesophagus within their hiati are rather more elastic; this allows some freedom of movement during breathing and, in the case of the oesophagus, swallowing.

Abdominal organs, usually the stomach, sometimes herniate through the diaphragm and into the thorax, constituting **diaphragmatic hernia** (Section 25.13).

8.12 Embryonic development of pleura and pericardium

8.12.1 Formation of intraembryonic and extraembryonic coelom

The first signs of the developmental origin of the **coelom** arise when clefts appear in the lateral mesoderm (Section 8.7.2). These clefts split the lateral mesoderm into an outer layer of **somatic mesoderm** and an inner layer of **splanchnic mesoderm**. The clefts coalesce to become the **coelom** (Fig. 8.14).

On each side of the embryo, **lateral body folds** (Fig. 8.26) undercut the body of the embryo along its whole length. The folds meet in the ventral midline thus completing the ventral body wall, except at the site of the **umbilicus** (Fig. 8.26) which remains as a stalk connecting the embryo to its extraembryonic structures.

At the early stage in Fig. 8.26, the intra-embryonic coelom connects to the extra-embryonic coelom by an umbilical part of the extraembryonic coelom. This continuity between the two components of the coelom is soon closed off in the primitive umbilical ring, although the yolk sac and the vitelline vessels, and the allantois with its umbilical vessels, still pass through the ring. The investment of the yolk sac and allantoic stalks by the amnion marks the formal conversion of the primitive umbilical ring into the **umbilical cord**.

In the early embryo the **intraembryonic coelom**, when first formed, consists of a pair of elongated cavities, one on each side of the body, extending through the whole length of the thoracic and abdominal regions. This cavity must now be divided into the pleural, pericardial, and peritoneal cavities.

8.12.2 Separation of pleural and pericardial cavities

On each side of the body, the **pleuropericardial coelom** is now divided into pleural and pericardial cavities. This process begins by the formation of the **pleuropericardial fold** from the somatic mesoderm of the lateral wall of the coelom; this is a

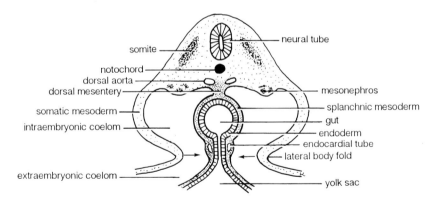

Fig. 8.26 Diagrammatic transverse section of an early embryo showing the separation of the intra- from the extraembryonic coelom. The left and right lateral body folds undercut the body of the embryo on each side, forming the ventral body wall, except at the level of the umbilicus. Here, the folds leave a stalk, connecting the embryo to its extraembryonic structures. At the very early stage of this diagram, the stalk constitutes a primitive umbilical ring. The extraembryonic coelom extends through this ring, forming direct continuity between the intra- and extraembryonic coelom. As the lateral body folds impinge on the ring, the umbilical part of the coelom is obliterated (arrows). The intra- and extraembryonic coeloms are then no longer continuous. The yolk sac and allantois, and their blood vessels, still pass through the ring which later becomes the umbilical cord. The endoderm forms the gut tube, which is suspended in splanchnic mesoderm (dense stipple). In the region of this transverse section, the gut tube is open ventrally to form the yolk sac; elsewhere throughout the thoracic and abdominal regions of the embryo, the gut tube is closed ventrally when the fusion of the lateral body folds completes the ventral body wall.

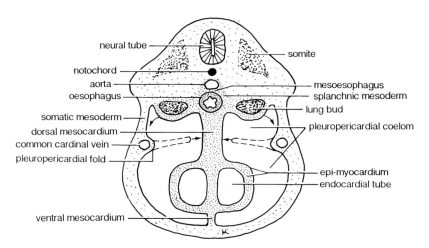

Fig. 8.27 Diagrammatic transverse section of an embryo to show the onset of separation of the pleural and pericardial cavities. The somatopleuric mesoderm of the lateral body wall forms a ridge, the pleuropericardial fold. This grows towards the midline (broken lines and medial arrows). The developing lung bud has grown caudally, and arrived in the splanchnopleuric mesoderm (dense stipple) in a position dorsal to the pleuropericardial fold. Here it now begins to bulge ventrolaterally (upper arrows). The paired endocardial tubes are suspended by the dorsal and ventral mesocardium.

longitudinal ridge housing the common cardinal vein (Fig. 8.27). This vein runs caudocranially to the sinus venosus.

The pleuropericardial fold grows medially (Fig. 8.27) and fuses with the dorsal mesocardium, thus forming the **pleuropericardial membrane**. This membrane now separates the pleural from the pericardial cavity (Figs 8.28, 8.30).

The left and right **lung buds** arose from the endoderm of the foregut (Section 5.1), and acquired a coat of splanchnic mesoderm forming smooth muscle, connective tissue, and blood vessels. The lung buds have now grown sufficiently far caudally to reach a position dorsal to the developing pleuropericardial fold (Fig. 8.27). As the lungs enlarge still more they bulge into the **pleural cavity** (Fig. 8.28). Clefts form in the somatic mesoderm of the lateral body wall (a process resembling the gradual splitting of the lateral mesoderm to form the original coelom; Section 8.7.2). The clefts coalesce (Fig. 8.28), allowing the lungs to invade the lateral body wall by extending the pleural cavity laterally and ventrally (Fig. 8.29).

The invasion of the lungs into the somatic mesoderm of the lateral body wall splits off the **parietal pericardium** (Figs 8.28, 8.29). The heart is now completely enclosed between the visceral

and parietal pericardium (in strict terms, as in Fig. 8.29, it is enclosed between the visceral serous pericardium and the parietal serous pericardium). The pericardium itself is flanked on each side by the pleural cavity and lungs (Fig. 8.29). Dorsally the pericardium is continuous with the mediastinum. In the ventral midline, the cleft-like splitting of the body wall is arrested, thus contributing to the **ventral mediastinum** (see 'site of ventral mediastinum' in Fig. 8.28). Once it is completed, the ventral mediastinum connects the parietal pericardium (parietal serous pericardium) to the ventral thoracic wall (Fig. 8.29). The heart within its pericardium is now incorporated in the mediastinum (Fig. 8.29).

8.12.3 *Embryonic derivation of the mediastinum*

The **mediastinum** in the fully developed thorax is a median partition between the left and right pleural sacs (Section 9.4, Fig. 9.1). It contains most of the thoracic organs, but not the lungs.

It arises as a broad mass of splanchnic mesoderm in the midline, extending from the ventral aspect of the vertebrae to the ventral body wall (dark stipple in Figs 8.28, 8.29). It contains the

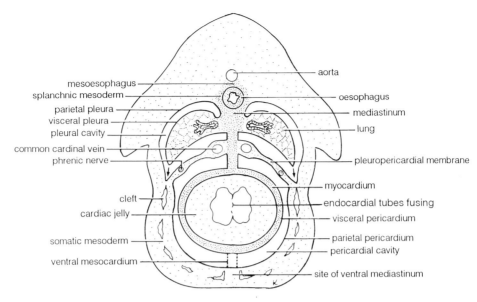

Fig. 8.28 **Diagrammatic transverse section of an embryo to show the completion of separation of the pleural and pericardial cavities.** The pleural cavity invades the somatic mesoderm of the lateral body wall (arrows) via the coalescence of clefts. Splanchnic mesoderm (dark stipple) forms the mediastinum, and the myocardium and visceral pericardium. The ventral mesocardium disappears (broken lines).

developing aorta, oesophagus, and heart. Contributions to it are made by the mesocardium (Fig. 8.27) and the mesoesophagus (Figs 8.27, 8.28).

The mediastinum is divided into regions, based on the pericardium (Section 9.4). The cranial mediastinum is derived from the dorsal mesocardium, and the caudal mediastinum comes from the mesoesophagus (Noden and de Lahunta, 1985, pp. 287–288). The ventral mesocardium (Fig. 8.27) originally suspends the tubular heart, but it degenerates (Fig. 8.28) except at the cranial and caudal ends of the tube, thus enabling the heart to bend into its sigmoid form during its subsequent development (Section 15.2) (Noden and de Lahunta, 1985, p. 235).

8.12.4 *Developmental sources of pleura and pericardium*

A grasp of the basic principle of the derivation of the coelom, i.e. that it arises between the somatic and splanchnic mesoderm, makes it possible to work out the developmental sources of the various parts of the pleura and pericardium.

The developing lung causes the splanchnic mesoderm

to bulge (Fig. 8.27). The outer surface of the bulge becomes the **visceral pleura** (pulmonary pleura); therefore the visceral pleura must of course be derived from the *splanchnic mesoderm* (Arey, 1958, p. 266). The lining of the pleural cavity, the **parietal pleura**, comes from the lateral body wall and the pleuropericardial membrane (Fig. 8.27); therefore the parietal pleura must be derived from the *somatic mesoderm* (Arey, 1958, p. 266).

Like the embryonic gut (Fig. 8.26), the **heart** is originally suspended by a dorsal and ventral mesentery consisting of splanchnic mesoderm; the splanchnic mesoderm suspending the heart takes the form of the dorsal and ventral **mesocardium** (dense stipple in Fig. 8.27). The outer surface of the heart is covered by the **visceral pericardium** (labelled according to the NAV (1994) as the 'visceral serous pericardium' in Fig. 8.29), and the interior is lined by the **endocardium**; between them is the muscle of the **myocardium** (Fig. 8.29). All of these components of the heart must necessarily come from the *splanchnic mesoderm*. On the other hand, the **parietal pericardium** (labelled 'parietal serous pericardium' in Fig. 8.29) is derived from *somatic mesoderm*, since it arises from the split in the *somatic mesoderm* of the lateral body wall (Fig. 8.28), and from the pleuropericardial membrane which is also somatic mesoderm.

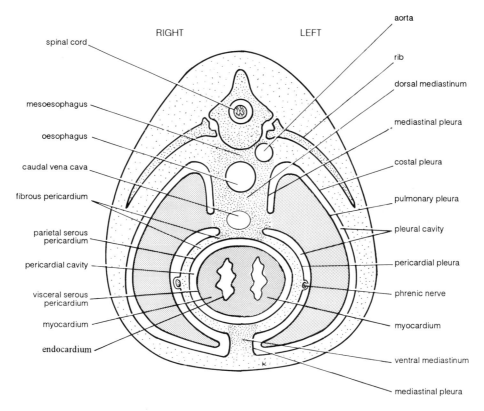

RIGHT   LEFT

aorta

spinal cord

rib

dorsal mediastinum

mesoesophagus

mediastinal pleura

oesophagus

costal pleura

caudal vena cava

fibrous pericardium

pulmonary pleura

parietal serous pericardium

pleural cavity

pericardial cavity

pericardial pleura

visceral serous pericardium

phrenic nerve

myocardium

myocardium

endocardium

ventral mediastinum

mediastinal pleura

Fig. 8.29 Diagrammatic transverse section of an embryo to show the final position of the pleural cavity and the formation of the pericardium. The lungs have pushed the pleural cavity right round the heart, to the ventral mediastinum. The splitting of the somatic mesoderm that made this possible has formed the pericardium, which therefore consists of somatic mesoderm. The mediastinum is composed of splanchnic mesoderm (dark stipple). The parietal pleura is known as costal, pericardial, and mediastinal pleura, according to the structures that it covers. The terms adopted here for the pericardium are those of the NAV (1994); see Section 20.2 for alternative terms.

8.13 Embryonic development of the diaphragm

During development the left and right pleuropericardial folds (Fig. 8.27) develop into the left and right pleuropericardial membranes (Fig. 8.28), and these now largely separate the pleural cavity from the pericardial cavity. However, the pleural cavity and peritoneal cavity still continue to form a single **pleuroperitoneal coelom** on each side of the embryo body, throughout the whole length of the thoracic and abdominal regions (Section 8.12.1). Therefore the next developmental step is to separate the pleural and peritoneal cavities.

The **septum transversum** arises during the early differentiation of the heart as a mesodermal plate lying transversely between the pericardial and peritoneal cavities (Fig. 8.30). It is, however, only an imperfect septum between the two cavities. This is because the original continuity of the pleuroperitoneal coelom on each side of the body still persists as a left and right **pleuroperitoneal canal** over the dorsal rim of the septum transversum (Figs 8.30, 8.31).

On each side of the body the pleuroperitoneal canal is finally closed by the **pleuroperitoneal fold** (plica pleuroperitonealis) (Fig. 8.31). This forms from the dorsolateral aspect of the wall of the pleuroperitoneal canal. It descends like a shutter, fusing with the septum transversum ventrally and

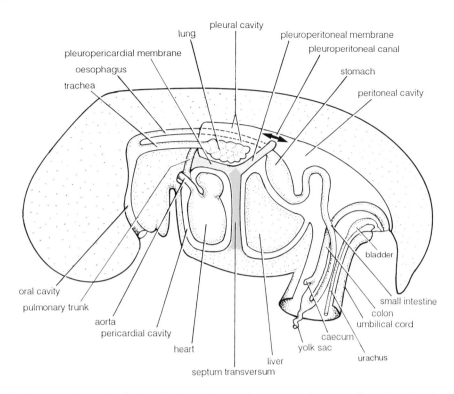

Fig. 8.30 Highly schematic longitudinal section through an embryo to show the separation of the pleural and peritoneal cavities. The section has passed through the body in a sagittal plane, just to the left of the midline. The thoracic oesophagus is shown in broken lines to indicate that it lies embedded in the mesoesophagus and has therefore escaped the cut. The septum transversum (dark green) is a transverse mesodermal plate between the pericardial and peritoneal cavities. The pleuroperitoneal fold (light green) grows ventrally from the dorsolateral wall of the peritoneal part of the coelom, forming the pleuroperitoneal membrane. The pleuroperitoneal membrane has fused ventrally with the dorsal rim of the septum transversum (Fig. 8.31). The pleuroperitoneal membrane also extends medially to blend with the caudal mediastinum (Fig. 8.32). In this diagram the medial extension of the membrane is not yet complete, leaving a last remnant (arrows) of the (closing) pleuroperitoneal canal (pleuroperitoneal hiatus). The abdominal cavity is at first too small to accommodate the rapid elongation of the developing loop of small intestine. Some of the intestinal loop is therefore temporarily pushed into the extraembryonic coelom within the umbilical cord. Adapted from Goodrich (1930), Fig. 649; Patten (1948), Fig. 111; Arey (1958), Fig. 252.

with the **mesoesophagus** (caudal mediastinum) medially, to form the **pleuroperitoneal membrane** (Fig. 8.32). At last, a complete partition separates the peritoneal cavity from the pleural cavity: this partition is the **diaphragm** (Fig. 8.32).

During the subsequent enlargement of the thoracic cavity, the **body wall** contributes mesoderm to the periphery of the diaphragm. By this means the diameter of the diaphragm is able to increase progressively as the diameter of the rib cage increases.

Initially the diaphragm is a connective tissue membrane. The muscle of the diaphragm, which is of course skeletal muscle, comes from myoblasts derived from cervical somites. The original source of these myoblasts is indicated by the cervical spinal nerves that form the **phrenic nerve**; the phrenic nerve innervates **all** the skeletal muscle of the diaphragm, i.e. both its costal and lumbar (crural) musculature. In the domestic mammals in general, the phrenic nerve arises from spinal nerves C5, C6, and C7, and from C3, C4, and C5 in man.

To sum up, the diaphragm develops from four main sources (Fig. 8.32): (i) the midline septum transversum, (ii) the left and right pleuroperitoneal membranes, (iii) the midline mesoesophagus, and (iv) the left and right lateral

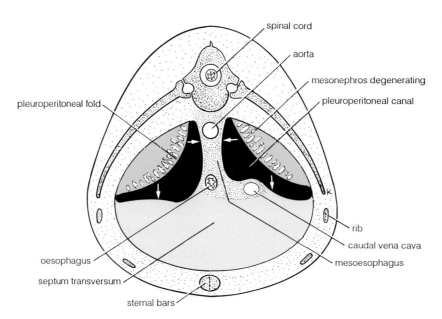

Fig. 8.31   Diagram of the caudal surface of the developing diaphragm. The septum transversum forms the ventral half of the partition between the pleural and peritoneal cavities. The pleuroperitoneal membrane grows down ventrally and medially (arrows) from the dorsolateral wall of the pleuroperitoneal coelom. It fuses ventrally with the dorsal edge of the septum transversum, and medially with the mesoesophagus (dorsal mediastinum). The enlargement of the mesonephros contributes to the ventromedial extension of the pleuroperitoneal fold, but at this stage the mesonephros is degenerating.

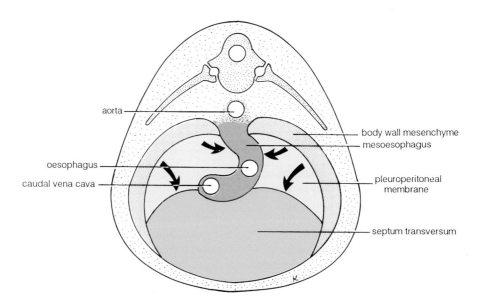

Fig. 8.32   Highly schematic cranial view of the diaphragm of a mammal to show the sources of its main components. The septum transversum (dark green) forms the tendinous centre. Much of the lateral and dorsal parts, including the costal and lumbar musculature, probably come from the lateral body wall (grey stipple). The pleuroperitoneal folds (light green) have grown ventrally to unite with the dorsal rim of the septum transversum (ventral arrows), and medially (medial arrows) to fuse with the caudal mediastinum (mesoesophagus) (grey). From Broman (1905).

body walls. The skeletal muscle cells of the diaphragm are seeded from the myotomes of cervical somites (5, 6, and 7 in the domestic mammals).

The exact developmental sources of the various components of the diaphragm are not known. On the basis of classical embryological studies (Goodrich, 1930, p. 650), it seems to be agreed that the septum transversum forms the tendinous centre, and that most of the lateral and dorsal parts of the diaphragm, including the costal and lumbar components, may come from the lateral body wall, although the exact contribution from this source is unknown (Noden and de Lahunta, 1985, pp. 288–289). If the latter suggestion is correct, the myoblasts must originally have migrated from the myotomes of somites C5, C6, and C7 into the lateral body wall, and subsequently continued their journey to end up in the costal and lumbar (crural) musculature.

It may seem astonishing that a thoracolumbar partition should be innervated by *cervical* segments of the spinal cord. The explanation (Arey, 1958, p. 287) is that the septum transversum forms along the pericardium at a very early stage, when the heart is developing between the head and the yolk sac, at a level somewhat **cranial** to the first cervical somites. The septum transversum then begins what, to use Arey's (1958, p. 285) words, is usually described as 'an extensive caudal migration'. However, this displacement is caused mainly by relatively fast growth in a **cranial** direction of the **dorsal** parts of the embryo, including the somites, thus leaving behind the more ventral parts including the septum transversum (relative to the somites). When opposite to the fifth cervical segment (in most mammals), the septum transversum picks up the phrenic nerve, by way of the pleuropericardial membrane (Fig. 8.28).

The pleuroperitoneal fold is associated with the **mesonephros** (Noden and de Lahunta, 1985, p. 289). As the mesonephros enlarges it extends the pleuroperitoneal fold. Subsequently the mesonephros degenerates (Fig. 8.31), but the fold persists and (as the now complete pleuroperitoneal membrane) closes the diaphragmatic partition.

The **liver bud** develops against the caudal surface of the septum transversum (Fig. 8.30), which it then invades. As the liver enlarges it pulls away from the septum transversum (Arey, 1958, p. 285), thus forming ventral mesentery that becomes the **falciform ligament** and the **coronary ligaments** (Langman, 1971, p. 281). (Section 16.5).

8.14   The body cavities in other vertebrates

The **pericardial sac**, enclosing the heart and thus isolating the heart from the peritoneal cavity, is the only component of the body cavities that is virtually constant in all vertebrates. The **peritoneal cavity** in vertebrates in general is divided as in mammals into a left and right side by a dorsal mesentery and sometimes also by a ventral mesentery (Fig. 8.33), but the arrival of lungs imposes great differences between mammals and all other vertebrates. In amphibians and reptiles the lungs are suspended in the peritoneal cavity (general coelom) by a pair of pulmonary folds. These folds form left and right **pulmonary recesses** (Fig. 8.33), which forecast the left and right pleural cavities of mammals but differ from the latter by opening freely into the peritoneal cavity. In birds each lung is totally enclosed within a **pleural cavity**, but each pleural cavity remains closely attached to the dorsal body wall. Reptiles and birds have no structure with anatomical characteristics or respiratory functions that even remotely resemble those of the mammalian **diaphragm**.

The details of the phylogenetic history of the mammalian diaphragm have been lost in the long line of extinct reptilian ancestors (Goodrich, 1930, p. 655). Nevertheless, there are indications (Romer, 1962, pp. 290–296) that the embryology of the mammalian body cavities and diaphragm recapitulates the phylogeny. The **caudal 'migration' of the heart** is always repeated in phylogeny (Goodrich, 1930, p. 614). The **pericardium** is situated far cranially in fishes; in tetrapods, it retreats further and further caudally, caudal to the gill (pharyngeal) arches. This change, which begins in Amphibia, accompanies the differentiation of a well-defined **neck** in amniotes and culminates in the withdrawal of the heart into the full protection of the sternum and rib cage in reptiles, birds, and mammals.

In the early embryo of all vertebrates the **pericardial cavity** opens widely at its caudal aspect into the general coelomic cavity (Romer, 1962, p. 290). A primitive vertebrate could therefore be postulated, in which the pericardial cavity lacked any separation from the peritoneal cavity, but such an animal remains hypothetical. According to Romer (1962, p. 290), in all vertebrate embryos, the **septum transversum** arises caudal to the heart and blocks off the ventral part of the pericardial cavity from the peritoneal cavity, but leaves a gap dorsally. In some cyclostomes as well as in elasmobranchs and a few lower actinopterygian fishes, the gap persists in the adult as a small opening between the pericardial and the general coelom. In most vertebrates, however, including typical fish, the gap is closed, thus sealing off the pericardial cavity from the rest of the coelom.

The remainder of the coelomic cavity is partly subdivided into left and right halves by the **dorsal and ventral mesentery**. The ventral mesentery persists in some fishes and salamanders, but usually disappears along most of its length. Cranially it persists in association with the stomach and liver as the lesser omentum and falciform ligament, and caudally with the bladder.

When **lungs** are present, as in some bony fishes and all

terrestrial vertebrates, they grow caudally on either side of the **mesoesophagus** and dorsal to the pericardium. In amphibians and most reptiles the lungs are typically suspended from the dorsal body wall by paired dorsal mesenteries, the left and right **pulmonary folds**, which continue ventrally onto the liver (Fig. 8.33). The pulmonary folds form a **pulmonary recess** on each side of the mesoesophagus at the cranial end of the general coelom, thus foreshadowing the left and right pleural cavities of higher tetrapods, but caudally each of these recesses opens freely into the general coelom. In some reptiles there is a partial closure of the pulmonary recesses, and in some lizards and snakes, and particularly in crocodilians (which of the extant reptiles are the most closely related to birds), the left and right **pleural cavities** are completely separated from the rest of the coelom, much as in mammals (Romer, 1962, p. 294). In birds the pleural cavities are totally separated, but the splitting of the lateral body wall that allows the pleural cavities and lungs of mammals to sweep ventrally around the heart (Fig. 8.28) does not occur in birds; as a result, the lungs of birds remain entirely *dorsal* in position, so much so that they can easily be overlooked in dissection. In marked distinction to mammals, the peritoneal cavity of birds is subdivided into five closed cavities (King and McLelland, 1984, p. 79).

Paired **nephric folds** support the mesonephros in vertebrates (Goodrich, 1930, p. 631). In the higher vertebrates they become involved in separating the pleural from the peritoneal cavity. Finally in the mammal they express themselves as the left and right **pleuroperitoneal folds** (Goodrich, 1930, p. 647), thus completing the formation of the diaphragm.

Although the term '**diaphragm**' has sometimes been applied to the horizontal and oblique septa of birds, there is no structure in the bird or reptile that is physiologically similar or embryologically homologous to the mammalian diaphragm (Goodrich, 1930, p. 655; King and McLelland, 1984, p. 136). The 'diaphragm' in the form that occurs in mammals is unique to mammals.

8.15   Anomalous development of the diaphragm

Diaphragmatic hernia in domestic mammals is usually caused by trauma (Section 25.13). Three varieties of congenital diaphragmatic hernia also occur in calves, dogs, and cats, though relatively rarely, namely pleuroperitoneal, hiatus, and pericardioperitoneal hernias. In pleuroperitoneal hernia abdominal viscera enter the pleural cavity through an aperture in the tendinous centre of the diaphragm. In hiatus hernia abdominal viscera pass into the pleural cavity through the oesophageal hiatus (Section 8.11.6).

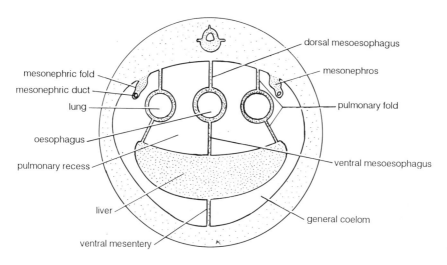

Fig. 8.33   Highly schematic transverse section through the body of a lizard, showing the partial separation of the pleural cavities. On each side of the body the tube-like lung is suspended from the dorsal body wall by a pulmonary fold which continues to the liver. A left and right pulmonary recess is formed between the mesoesophagus and the left and right pulmonary folds. The pulmonary recesses are, however, directly continuous caudally with the general coelom. Based on structural data from Goodrich (1930).

In pericardioperitoneal hernia, herniation of abdominal viscera into the pericardial cavity occurs through a defect in the ventral part of the diaphragm.

(1) Pleuroperitoneal hernia

This seems to be the best known congenital diaphragmatic hernia (Latshaw, 1987, p. 177), but is nevertheless rare in the domestic species (Noden and de Lahunta, 1985, p. 290). The defect is in the dorsal part of the tendinous centre of the diaphragm, and is probably caused by failure of the pleuroperitoneal membrane to fuse with the septum transversum (at the lateral arrows in Figure 8.31), leaving a permanent pleuroperitoneal canal (hiatus).

In man pleuroperitoneal hernia is one of the more common malformations in the newborn (Langman, 1971, p. 288). It usually occurs on the left side, and allows the stomach, spleen, and part of the liver to herniate into the pleural cavity, thus compressing the heart and lung and causing grave dyspnoea. Sometimes the diaphragm is in fact intact, but is weakened by being still in its original membranous form; the hernia is then contained in a membranous sac (Arey, 1958, p. 291).

(2) Hiatus hernia

In the domestic species congenital hiatus hernia is rare, but cases have been reported in the dog (Latshaw, 1987, p. 178). The hernia occurs at the oesophageal hiatus (Section 8.11.6), and is presumably due to incomplete fusion of the pleuroperitoneal membrane with the mesoesophagus (at the medial arrows in Figure 8.31).

(3) Pericardioperitoneal hernia

In this congenital condition there is an aperture, generally in the ventral part of the diaphragm (Latshaw, 1987, p. 178), thus connecting the peritoneal and pericardial cavities. Diaphragmatic defects of this kind are much less common than pleuroperitoneal anomalies. As Noden and de Lahunta (1985, p. 290) pointed out, there is no natural connexion between the pericardial and peritoneal cavities in the developing embryo. Therefore, in contrast to the other two diaphragmatic hernias, this condition is not caused by the failure of a normal aperture to close.

As stated in Section 8.13, the liver invades the caudal surface of the septum transversum. Later the huge enlargement of the liver forces it to withdraw caudally from the septum transversum, thus forming the falciform ligament (ventral mesentery). Evidently this retraction of the liver is sometimes faulty, causing an opening in the ventral part of the diaphragm, or else leaving a weak area where the tissue is so thin that it ruptures (Noden and de Lahunta, 1985, p. 290). Abdominal viscera may then enter the pericardial cavity as a pericardioperitoneal hernia, causing abnormal cardiac or digestive functions.

8.16 Blood supply of the thoracic walls

8.16.1 *Vertebral muscles and muscles attaching forelimb to trunk*

The epaxial vertebral muscles are supplied by the subclavian, intercostal, and lumbar segmental arteries. The venous drainage is by satellite veins of these arteries.

The epaxial vertebral muscles at the cranial end of the thorax receive their **arterial supply** from the **subclavian artery**, via the **costocervical trunk** and its **deep cervical artery** (Fig. 8.34). The remainder of the epaxial vertebral musculature is supplied by segmental **dorsal branches** arising from the **dorsal intercostal arteries** and from **lumbar arteries** (Fig. 8.34). The dorsal branches end in the skin as **dorsal cutaneous branches**.

In the dog (Evans and Christensen, 1979, pp. 682, 692), the **costocervical trunk** supplies the thoracic part of the serratus ventralis muscle by its **dorsal scapular artery** (Fig. 8.34). The superficial pectoral muscle is supplied by the **external thoracic artery**, and the deep pectoral muscle and latissimus dorsi are supplied by the **lateral thoracic artery**; these two arteries are branches of the **axillary artery** (Fig. 8.34).

The **venous drainage** by the dorsal intercostal veins empties into the **azygos system** (Section 17.5). The paired **costocervical veins** empty into the cranial vena cava.

8.16.2 *Blood supply of rib cage: intercostal vessels*

The intercostal muscles are supplied by **dorsal intercostal arteries** which arise from the thoracic aorta. The intercostal muscles are also supplied by **ventral intercostal arteries** (strictly, ventral intercostal **rami**) which are formed by the **internal thoracic artery** and its continuation, i.e. the **musculophrenic artery** (Fig. 8.34). The dorsal and ventral intercostal arteries anastomose end to end. The dorsal and ventral intercostal arteries lie along the *caudal* border of the rib, and therefore in **thoracocentesis** (Section 25.1) the needle is usually inserted at the cranial border of the rib (but not in the dog, see below).

The **internal thoracic artery** (Fig. 8.34) arises from the **subclavian artery**, and runs along the dorsal surface of the sternum, giving off the ventral intercostals. It also forms **perforating rami**

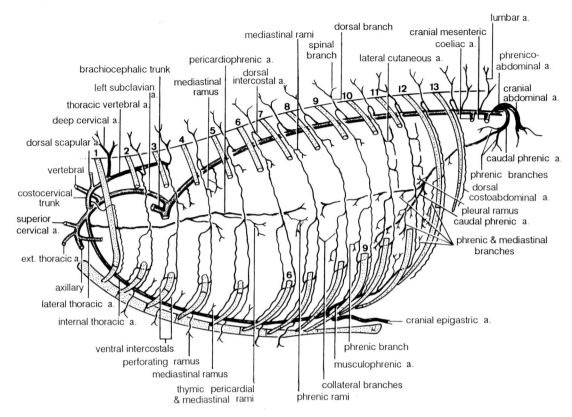

Fig. 8.34 Diagrammatic left lateral view of the arteries supplying the thoracic walls in the dog. The arterial pattern in this diagram applies to other domestic species, except in the following details. The cranial abdominal artery occurs only in the carnivores and pig. The caudal phrenic artery is absent in the horse, but cranial phrenic arteries arise from the aorta at the aortic hiatus in this species and supply the crura. The thoracic vertebral artery occurs only in the dog, and is replaced in the other species by the supreme intercostal artery. In the pig and ruminants phrenic rami from the first two lumbar segments of the aorta supply the crura.

that supply the pectoral muscles and skin, and **mammary branches** in species with thoracic mammary glands.

The **venous drainage** of the rib cage is by satellite veins of the above arteries.

In all the domestic species the first three or four dorsal intercostal arteries arise from a branch of the **costo-cervical trunk**. In the *horse, ox,* and *pig* this branch is the **supreme intercostal artery**, but in the *dog* it is the **thoracic vertebral artery** (Simoens, 1992, pp. 277, 279, 283).

The dorsal intercostal arteries form **collateral rami** (Fig. 8.34) in the dog, pig, and horse; these traverse the rib to its cranial border (dog, pig), or traverse the intercostal space to the cranial border of the following rib (horse) (Schummer *et al.*, 1981, p. 120). They then de-

scend ventrally in the intercostal space close to the cranial border of the rib, towards the ascending ventral intercostal rami. In the dog they anastomose distally with the ventral intercostal rami that ascend the cranial border of the rib (Fig. 8.34); during their course distally, they lie on the medial surface of the rib and are therefore protected from the needle during thoracocentesis in the middle level of the thoracic wall. The collateral rami supply the intercostal muscles adjoining the cranial border of the rib; the collateral rami of the last few intercostal arteries supply **phrenic rami** (Fig. 8.34) to the diaphragm (Evans and Christensen, 1979, p. 714).

Lateral cutaneous rami (Fig. 8.34) arise from the dorsal intercostal arteries and penetrate the intercostal muscles to supply the skin of the lateral thoracic wall (Simoens, 1992, p. 302). These accompany the dorsal and lateral cutaneous rami of the thoracic spinal nerves (Fig. 8.35) (Krahl, 1964, p. 237).

The **perforating rami** of the internal thoracic artery in the dog are restricted to the second to the seventh interchondral spaces (Evans and Christensen, 1979, p. 690).

Usually in the *dog* (Fig. 8.34), and sometimes in other species, including the horse (Schummer *et al.*, 1981, Fig. 88) and pig (Simoens, 1992, Fig. 279A), the **ventral intercostal rami** are double, both in each interchondral space and along the ventral end of the rib (Evans and Christensen, 1979, p. 690). Since these vessels may therefore accompany both the cranial and the caudal border of the rib (Fig. 8.34), a **thoracocentesis** is performed through the *middle* of the intercostal space (Section 25.1) rather than at the cranial border of the rib.

The **dorsal intercostal veins** empty into the **azygos system** (Section 17.5). The **ventral intercostal veins** drain by the (satellite) musculophrenic and internal thoracic veins into the cranial vena cava or brachiocephalic vein (Simoens, 1992, p. 344).

In the *horse* and *ox*, there is a **superficial thoracic vein**, which is not satellite to any artery. In the horse, this begins as a conspicuous subcutaneous vein on the ventral abdominal wall, the **cranial superficial epigastric vein** also known as the 'spur vein', which continues as the superficial thoracic vein along the ventrolateral thoracic wall at the ventral edge of the cutaneous muscle; it finally passes craniodorsally into the axillary space to enter the **thoracodorsal vein** which continues immediately into the axillary vein (Simoens, 1992, p. 364). It may be raised on the thoracic wall and used for intravenous injection or blood sampling. It can be lacerated in the horse by sharp spurs, and must be avoided during thoracotomy in the ox (Section 25.3). In the cow the superficial thoracic vein occasionally anastomoses with the cranial superficial epigastric vein ('milk vein'), thus forming a continuous **milk vein** from the udder to the axilla.

Because of their many anastomotic connections, the intercostal vessels provide important collateral circulatory pathways following surgical or pathologic interruption of normal major pathways (Krahl, 1964, p. 237).

8.16.3 *Blood supply of diaphragm*

The arterial supply to the diaphragm is from the aorta and the internal thoracic artery. The venous drainage is directly into the caudal vena cava where it goes through the diaphragm.

The main arterial supply comes from the caudal phrenic artery and the musculophrenic artery. The **caudal phrenic artery** arises essentially from the aorta, at about the level of the costal arch (Fig. 8.34). The **musculophrenic artery** is one of the two terminal branches of the **internal thoracic artery** (the other being the **cranial epigastric artery**. It runs dorsocaudally along the costal arch, supply-

ing the costal musculature of the diaphragm by **phrenic branches** (Fig. 8.34).

The arterial supply to the diaphragm comes from several arteries, which vary with the species.

The **caudal phrenic artery** may arise by a common root shared with some other large artery, e.g. the cranial abdominal (Fig. 8.34) in the dog (Evans and Christensen, 1979, p. 728) and the coeliac artery in the ox and pig (Schummer *et al.*, 1981, p. 72). In the dog it supplies the crus, continues over the tendinous centre, and finally ramifies in the costal musculature of the diaphragm; there it anastomoses with phrenic branches of intercostal arteries 10, 11, and 12, and with the pericardiophrenic artery (Fig. 8.34). The caudal phrenic artery is absent in the horse, but in this species a **cranial phrenic artery** arises from the aorta at the level of T16 and supplies the crura; this artery is said to occur only in the horse (Schummer *et al.*, 1981, p. 122), but according to Simoens (1992, p. 302) it has also been described in the ruminants and pig. The **pericardiophrenic artery** is a branch of the internal thoracic artery. It usually ends in the pericardium, but may accompany the phrenic nerve to the diaphragm and may anastomose with the caudal phrenic artery (Schummer *et al.*, 1981, p. 76) (Fig. 8.34). Smaller **phrenic rami** arise from various other sources; examples are the first few lumbar arteries in the ox and pig and in the dog (Fig. 8.34) the more caudal of the dorsal intercostal arteries. These various phrenic arteries supply the diaphragmatic part of the parietal pleura (Section 9.9).

The main **venous drainage** of the diaphragm is by the large paired **cranial phrenic vein** (Simoens, 1992, p. 372) which drains into the caudal vena cava as it passes through the tendinous centre of the diaphragm (Section 8.11.6); these vessels are not satellites of arteries. This drainage is augmented by **phrenic rami** of the **musculophrenic vein** (satellites of the artery); these vessels drain the costal musculature via the internal thoracic vein into the cranial vena cava (Simoens, 1992, p. 344). **Caudal phrenic veins** (satellite veins of the arteries) drain the crura into the caudal vena cava in carnivores, and into the azygos system in the pig. The **pericardiophrenic vein** is a satellite of the artery, and empties via the internal thoracic vein into the cranial vena cava (Nickel *et al.*, 1973, p. 195).

8.17 Nerve supply of thoracic walls

The number of **thoracic spinal nerves** is the same as the number of thoracic vertebrae (13 in the carnivores and ruminants, 14 or 15 in the pig, and 18 in the horse). In all the domestic mammals, and indeed in almost all mammals, there are eight pairs of **cervical spinal nerves** even though there are only seven cervical vertebrae. This is because the first pair of cervical spinal nerves emerges from the spinal cord between the skull and the first cervical vertebra (the atlas), whereas the last pair comes out between the last cervical vertebra (the seventh) and the first thoracic vertebra. Therefore the first **thoracic** spinal nerve must emerge *caudal* to vertebra T1. Consequently each thoracic spinal nerve (and all other spinal nerves) bears the same number as the vertebra that lies immediately *cranial* to it (e.g. vertebra T5 *precedes* nerve T5).

Each segment of the dorsal, lateral, and ventral **thoracic walls** receives a sensory (afferent) and a motor (efferent) innervation from its corresponding **thoracic spinal nerve**. On the other hand, the caudal thoracic wall is formed by the diaphragm, which obtains its myoblasts from cervical somites (Section 8.13) and is therefore innervated by cervical spinal nerves, via the **phrenic nerve**.

A typical spinal nerve is formed by the union of its dorsal and ventral roots (Section 2.2). Peripheral to the union of its two roots the spinal nerve leaves the vertebral canal through the **intervertebral foramen** and divides into a **dorsal primary ramus** (dorsal division) and a **ventral primary ramus** (ventral division) (Figs 2.1, 8.35). The spinal nerve connects to the sympathetic vertebral ganglion of the same segment (Fig. 2.3) by a white and a grey **ramus communicans** (Section 2.3). The ventral primary ramus of the first two thoracic spinal nerves contributes to the **brachial plexus**, but the connection of T2 to the plexus is slender.

A typical spinal nerve forms a **meningeal ramus** (ramus meningeus) that re-enters the vertebral canal and supplies the meninges.

8.17.1 *Dorsal thoracic wall*

The epaxial vertebral muscles in the thoracic region (Section 8.8), and the skin that covers them, are supplied by the thoracic spinal nerves (Fig. 8.35).

The **medial ramus** of the **dorsal** primary ramus supplies the epaxial muscles. The **lateral ramus** (Fig. 8.35) of the **dorsal** primary ramus forms a sensory **cutaneous ramus** to the skin over these muscles.

8.17.2 *Lateral and ventral thoracic walls: intercostal nerves*

The muscles of the rib cage and abdominal wall are included in the hypaxial musculature, and are therefore innervated by the **ventral primary rami** of the thoracic spinal nerves. The ventral primary ramus continues as the **intercostal nerve** (n. intercostalis) (Fig. 8.35), running along the caudal border of the rib.

The main trunk of the intercostal nerve innervates the **external** and **internal intercostal muscles**, and the **abdominal muscles** that are attached to the rib cage. Intercostal nerves also supply several other (though not all) of the **accessory muscles of respiration** (Section 10.10). Thus the intercostal nerves are responsible for the motor innervation of most of the muscles with respiratory actions, with the notable exception of the diaphragm.

The intercostal nerves supply somatic afferent fibres, in **cutaneous rami** (Fig. 8.35), to the skin of the lateral and ventral thoracic walls; these accompany the lateral cutaneous rami of the dorsal intercostal arteries (Fig. 8.34). The more caudal intercostal nerves send branches to the skin of the ventral abdominal wall.

The intercostal nerves also supply somatic afferent fibres to much of the **parietal pleura** (Section 9.11), i.e. to the costal pleura and to the peripheral part of the diaphragmatic pleura. These nerve pathways to the pleura have the same sensitivity to pain as the skin, as is predictable from the somatic origins of all of these structures.

In addition to those just mentioned, several other muscles of the lateral and ventral thoracic walls (Section 8.9.2) receive a motor innervation from intercostal nerves. Three of these are intrinsic thoracic muscles, namely the **transversus thoracis**, **rectus thoracis**, and **subcostalis muscles**; three more are vertebral muscles, i.e. **serratus dorsalis**, **levatores costarum**, and **retractor costae**; one other is a neck muscle, **scalenus**, though this is also innervated by cervical spinal nerves. Of the limb muscles that are attached to the thoracic wall, the **serratus ventralis thoracis** is innervated by the **long thoracic nerve** (nervus thoracicus longus), the **latissimus dorsi** by the **thoracodorsal** (n. thoracodorsalis) and **pectoral nerves** (nn. pectorales), and the **pectoral muscles** by the **pectoral nerves** and cervical spinal nerves. **Sternocephalicus** is innervated by the **spinal accessory**

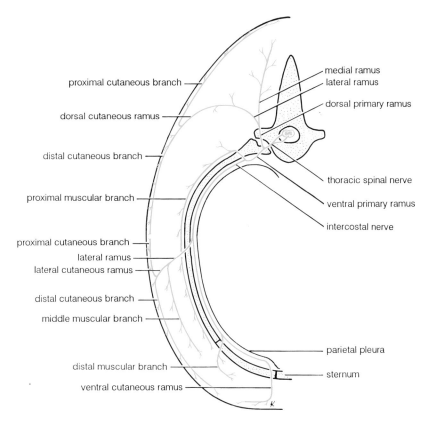

Fig. 8.35   Diagram of the innervation of the dorsal, lateral, and ventral walls of the thorax by a thoracic spinal nerve.
Immediately after emerging from the intervertebral foramen the spinal nerve divides into its dorsal primary ramus and ventral
primary ramus (Fig. 2.3). The **dorsal primary ramus** divides into a medial ramus and a lateral ramus. The medial ramus is purely
motor, innervating the epaxial musculature. The lateral ramus gives off a few motor branches, and continues to the skin as the
dorsal cutaneous ramus which ends in a proximal and a distal branch. The **ventral primary ramus** continues as the intercostal
nerve itself, supplying the intercostal muscles. The intercostal nerve immediately forms a proximal muscular branch which also
supplies the intercostal muscles. Half way along its course, the intercostal nerve gives off a lateral ramus; this forms a middle
muscular branch that supplies muscles attached to the thoracic wall, and ends as the lateral cutaneous ramus with a proximal
and a distal branch. Near the distal end of its course, the intercostal nerve gives rise to a distal muscular branch which innervates
the rectus thoracis and rectus abdominis muscles. The intercostal nerve itself ends as the ventral cutaneous ramus.

nerve (n. accessorius) and cervical spinal nerves. All
of these muscles have a *potential respiratory action*,
and several of them (transversus thoracis, levatores
costarum, and scalenus) are known to participate in
breathing in appropriate circumstances (Section 10.10).

The periphery of the costal part of the **diaphragm** does
receive some afferent fibres and vasomotor efferent
fibres from the more caudal intercostal nerves (Krahl,
1964, p. 237), this being consistent with the derivation
of the dorsolateral border of the diaphragm from the
mesenchyme of the body wall (Fig. 8.32). But no part of
the musculature of the diaphragm receives somatic effer-

ent fibres from intercostal nerves, since this function is
taken over entirely by the phrenic nerve.

The intercostal nerve is separated from the caudal
border of the rib by the intercostal artery and vein. In the
dog (Kitchell and Evans, 1993, p. 862), in most of the
intercostal spaces the intercostal nerve and vessels are
covered medially only by the **parietal pleura**. The parietal pleura receives a somatic afferent innervation from
the intercostal nerves.

The position of the intercostal nerve in the intercostal
space helps to identify the vestigial third intercostal muscle, the **intercostalis intimus** in man (Section 8.9.1). This

muscle lies adjacent to the parietal pleura, and is separated from the internal intercostal muscle by the intercostal artery, vein, and nerve.

The nomenclature of the branches of the intercostal nerve was criticized by Bailey *et al.* (1984), who suggested changes. The terms used here are based on those of Bailey *et al.* (1984), though with some minor simplifications (the terminal branches of the dorsal and lateral cutaneous rami are here named proximal and distal, instead of dorsal and ventral).

In the pig and carnivores, the distal branch of the lateral cutaneous ramus forms **lateral mammary rami**, and the ventral cutaneous ramus forms **medial mammary rami** (rami mammarii laterales, mediales) (Simoens, 1992, p. 490).

The second **intercostal nerve** forms an exceptionally large lateral cutaneous ramus, with a sensory field extending to the brachial region; hence the name **nervus intercostobrachialis** (Schaller *et al.*, 1992, p. 490) is appropriate. Electrophysiological studies by Bailey *et al.* (1984) showed that in the dog the third intercostal nerve sometimes forms a similar intercostobrachial nerve. These two nerves in the dog have then been named the **cranial** and **caudal intercostobrachial nerves** by Bailey *et al.* (1984). Of these two the **cranial** nerve forms a dorsal branch which innervates the skin over the deltoideus muscle and the origin of the long head of triceps, and a ventral branch which innervates the skin over the lateral surface of the long head of triceps as far distally as the lateral epicondyle of the humerus; the **caudal** nerve slightly augments the sensory cutaneous field of the cranial nerve. This extensive cutaneous field is of diagnostic significance in **avulsion of the roots of the brachial plexus** (usually occurring after a traffic accident). The connection of the second thoracic spinal nerve to the brachial plexus is so delicate that it usually escapes avulsion. Consequently the cutaneous sensory field of the intercostobrachial nerves usually remains sensitive (Kitchell and Evans, 1993, p. 864).

The ventral extension of the last thoracic nerve forms the **costoabdominal nerve**, supplying the abdominal wall ventral to the costal arch (Kitchell and Evans, 1993, p. 865).

Campbell (1964, p. 538) reviewed the roles of intra- and extrafusal (gamma and alpha) motor pathways to the respiratory muscles. There is histological evidence that the intercostal muscles contain numerous **muscle spindles**. There is also electrophysiological evidence of afferent activity in the dorsal roots of intercostal nerves in phase with breathing, some of this activity being consistent with the responses of **tendon receptor organs** as well as muscle spindles. As in the somatic motor control of skeletal musculature generally, the intercostal muscles may be driven by the **gamma (intrafusal) neuron**; the discharge of the gamma neuron stretches the **annulospiral receptor** within the muscle spindle, and this activates the well known monosynaptic reflex arc that is completed by the discharge of the **alpha (extrafusal) motor neuron**. Or the intercostal extrafusal muscle fibres may be driven directly by the alpha motor neuron. At the time of Campbell's review, however, there was little evidence of the functional linkage of the alpha and gamma systems, but Comroe (1975, p. 84) concluded that the gamma system does operate in the control of the respiratory muscles. Derenne *et al.* (1978, p. 378) confirmed this conclusion (Section 8.17.3). (See Vol. 1 of this series (King, 1987) for an account of the structure and function of the alpha and gamma neuron and the muscle spindle reflex.)

8.17.3 *Diaphragm: phrenic nerve*

The muscle of the diaphragm consists of striated muscle fibres, and therefore has a typical somatic motor innervation (Section 1.2). It generally acts without conscious control, but so do the intercostal muscles and many other skeletal muscles such as those controlling posture. It can also function under conscious control, during both breathing and expulsive efforts such as coughing and defecation.

The paired **phrenic nerve** innervates **all** the skeletal muscle of the diaphragm, i.e. both its costal and lumbar (crural) musculature, and is therefore the sole somatic motor supply to the diaphragm.

The phrenic nerve is a typical somatic nerve. It arises from somatic efferent neurons in the ventral horn of the *cervical* spinal cord (Fig. 11.1; Section 11.3). Its axons leave the spinal cord in several *cervical spinal nerves*, and then combine together in the neck to form the phrenic nerve. After entering the thoracic cavity at the thoracic inlet, the left and right phrenic nerves pass on either side of the heart to end in the diaphragm (Fig. 9.5). The phrenic nerve also supplies acutely sensitive pain fibres to the parietal pleura.

In the domestic mammals in general, the **phrenic nerve** (n. phrenicus) arises from spinal nerves C5, C6, and C7. Its three rootlets combine into the phrenic nerve just cranial to the thoracic inlet. The main trunk runs caudally within the **mediastinum**, along the pericardium covering the base of the heart. The **left nerve** passes across the pulmonary trunk, the left auricle, and left ventricle, and then goes via the caudal mediastinum to the cupola of the diaphragm (Figs 9.2, 9.5). The **right nerve** follows the great veins in its journey to the cupola of the diaphragm, running caudally on the cranial vena cava, across the right atrium, and finally along the caudal vena cava in the **plica vena cava** (Figs 9.2, 9.5). Since the nerve lies essentially within the mediastinum (as of course does the heart), it is therefore covered by a small fold (plica) of the mediastinal component of the parietal pleura.

The phrenic nerve supplies **somatic afferent** fibres to the mediastinal (parietal) pleura and to the parietal pericardium and fibrous pericardium (Section 20.2) (Williams *et al.*, 1989, p. 1129); all these structures are therefore sensitive to the usual broad range of painful stimuli (Section 9.12).

At the heart, the **phrenic nerve** lies between the pericardial pleura and the fibrous pericardium (Fig. 8.29). In its course across the heart it is accompanied by the **pericardiophrenic vessels** (Fig. 8.34). The caudal vena cava is contained within its own fold of mediastinal pleura, the **plica vena cava**, and the right phrenic nerve lies in a small sub-fold of the plica vena cava on the right surface of the vein (Fig. 9.2).

The left phrenic nerve supplies the left half of the diaphragm, and the right nerve supplies the right half. On reaching a point lateral to the tendinous centre (Kitchell and Evans, 1993, p. 841), each nerve forms three main branches, ventral, lateral, and dorsal. These branches supply the corresponding thirds of its half of the diaphragm. Cutting the phrenic nerve in the neck totally paralyses the appropriate half of the diaphragm, which then atrophies (Williams *et al.*, 1989, p. 1130).

The phrenic nerve (Derenne *et al.*, 1978, p. 376) consists essentially of myelinated fibres, the diameter having a unimodal peak of between 9 and 11 μm, the **conduction velocity** being about 80 m per second. The **motor units** are surprisingly small, from 25 to 80 depending on the species, such low values being typical of muscles performing precise and fine movements, for example the extrinsic muscles of the eyeball.

The phrenic nerve contains a substantial assortment of **somatic afferent fibres** (Williams *et al.*, 1989, p. 1128). Some of these are distributed to the mediastinal pleura and pericardium; at the diaphragm itself, others go to the central regions of the diaphragmatic pleura and to the peritoneum on the abdominal surface of the diaphragm (Hare, 1975, p. 132; Williams *et al.*, 1989, pp. 1129–1130). All of these afferent fibres supply *parietal* elements, i.e. the parietal pleura, fibrous and parietal pericardium, and parietal peritoneum; since these elements are all derived developmentally from the **somatic** mesoderm (Sections 8.12, 8.13), it is to be expected that they will be innervated by somatic afferent fibres, and will therefore be highly sensitive to painful stimuli (Section 9.12).

The phrenic nerve also contains another variety of somatic afferent fibres, namely **muscle proprioceptive afferent fibres** (Williams *et al.*, 1989, p. 1130). The review by Derenne *et al.* (1978, p. 376) showed that **muscle spindles** are present in the diaphragm, but are much less numerous than in the intercostal muscles; the stretch reflex plays a major role in the intercostal muscles, but has not been demonstrated in the diaphragm. Yet tendon organs are abundant in the diaphragm.

The phrenic nerve acquires **sympathetic motor axons**, presumably vasomotor, from connections with the **caudal cervical ganglion** or the adjacent **sympathetic trunk**, and with the **coeliac plexus** (Kitchell and Evans, 1993, p. 841).

The parietal pleura on the dorsolateral periphery of the diaphragm receives afferent fibres from the intercostal nerves (Section 8.17.2).

Chapter 9
Pleural Cavity

9.1 Pleural sac

During its early development, the growing lung bulges ventrally into the roof of the intra-embryonic coelom (arrows in Fig. 8.27), the bulge being covered by splanchnic mesoderm (Section 8.12.2). At a slightly later stage of development (Fig. 8.28), the growth of the **pleuropericardial membrane** separates a primitive pleural cavity, or **pleural sac**, from the pericardial cavity. Continuing enlargement of the lung causes it to protrude into the pleural sac by invaginating the dorsomedial wall of the sac.

The part of the sac that actually coats the surface of the lung becomes the **visceral pleura**. (Strictly, the visceral pleura is named the **pulmonary** pleura, since it is attached all over the lung, but in the embryological context the term *visceral* pleura is more meaningful, since it forms a logical partner to *parietal* pleura.) At the neck of the invaginated pleural sac the visceral pleura is directly continuous with the outer wall of the sac, which has now become the **parietal pleura**. The neck of the sac encloses the **root** of the lung (Figs 5.3, 9.1). The coating of the lung, i.e. the visceral pleura, is formed from the splanchnic mesoderm, but the parietal pleura has been derived from the somatic mesoderm. The space between the visceral and parietal pleura is the **pleural cavity**.

Since the lung has developed by *invaginating* the wall of the pleural sac, the mature lung cannot actually be inside the lumen of the sac (i.e. within the pleural cavity), yet it is surrounded by the pleural sac. In the same way, a fist pushed into the wall of a softly inflated rubber balloon is not inside the lumen of the balloon, but is nevertheless surrounded by the balloon. Moreover, just as the fingers of the fist are free to extend and retract within the invaginated balloon, so also are the lobes of the lung free to expand and contract within the invaginated pleural sac.

The left and right pleural sacs are separated by the **mediastinum** (Fig. 8.28).

9.2 Pulmonary pleura

The visceral pleura (**pulmonary pleura**) (Fig. 9.1) is attached to the surface of the lung, including the **fissures** that separate the lobes of the lung from each other (Fig. 9.3). To allow the great fluctuations in the volume of the lung during breathing, the visceral pleura contains abundant elastic fibres. These fibres are continuous with the elastic continuum of the lung (Section 6.9).

The fissures between the lobes are deepest in the domestic carnivores (Section 5.6). In the lung of the dog (Fig. 5.4) the pulmonary pleura (pleura pulmonalis) extends to the full depth of the fissures and reaches the lobar bronchi, except between the cranial and caudal parts of the left cranial lobe (Fig. 9.3) (Evans, 1993, p. 486).

The site where the visceral pleura becomes continuous with the parietal pleura (pleura parietalis) is the **root** of the lung (Section 5.5), where the airways, vessels, and nerves enter and leave the lung. At the root, the surface of the lung is not covered with pleura, forming a bare area known as the **hilus** of the lung (hilus pulmonis); the **pulmonary ligament** extends from the hilus, and the lung surface that this ligament encloses is also devoid of pleura (Fig. 5.3, Section 5.5).

The *thickness* of the pulmonary pleura varies with the species. It is relatively thick in the horse, ox, sheep, pig, and man, and relatively thin in the dog and cat (Section 9.7).

9.3 Parietal pleura

As just stated, the parietal pleura is derived from somatic mesoderm. It lines the wall of the pleural

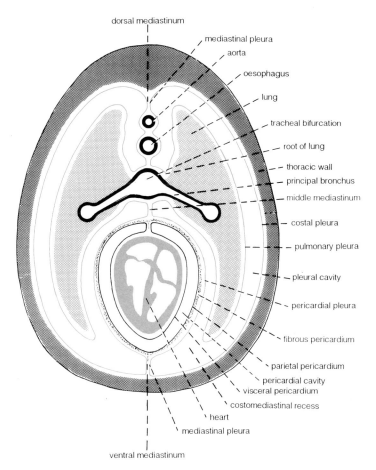

dorsal mediastinum

mediastinal pleura

aorta

oesophagus

lung

tracheal bifurcation

root of lung

thoracic wall

principal bronchus

middle mediastinum

costal pleura

pulmonary pleura

pleural cavity

pericardial pleura

fibrous pericardium

parietal pericardium

pericardial cavity

visceral pericardium

costomediastinal recess

heart

mediastinal pleura

ventral mediastinum

Fig. 9.1 Highly diagrammatic transverse section through the thorax to show the basic arrangement of the pleura and pericardium in the mature mammal. The pleura is green. The parietal pleura lines the thoracic walls and mediastinum as the costal and mediastinal pleura. The part of the mediastinal pleura that covers the pericardium is known as the pericardial pleura. The lung is covered by the pulmonary (visceral) pleura. The principal bronchus is the main element of the root of the lung. At the root, the parietal pleura is continuous with the visceral pleura. The pleural cavity lies between the parietal pleura and visceral pleura. The pleural cavity extends ventrally as the costomediastinal recess. The lung moves into this recess during inspiration. The pleural cavity is a potential space occupied in life by only a thin film of pleural fluid. The left and right pleural cavities are separated by the mediastinum. In the mediastinum, the heart is invaginated into the sac-like pericardium. The structure labelled parietal pericardium is conveniently known by that term, but is strictly the parietal layer of the serous pericardium. It is reinforced externally by the fibrous pericardium. The structure labelled visceral pericardium is again conveniently so named, but is strictly the visceral layer of the serous pericardium. It is so closely attached to the myocardium that it becomes an integral part of the heart wall, and is therefore known alternatively as the epicardium. The pericardial cavity lies between the parietal and visceral pericardium, and is a potential space containing only a small volume of pericardial fluid. For clarity, the volumes of the pleural and pericardial cavities are much exaggerated in the diagram.

cavity. Depending on the region of the wall that it covers, the parietal pleura is divided into three main components: the **costal pleura** lines the inside of the lateral wall of the rib cage (Fig. 9.1); the **mediastinal pleura** lines the mediastinum (Fig. 9.1); the **diaphragmatic pleura** lines the cranial surface of the diaphragm (Fig. 9.4). Like the visceral pleura, numerous elastic fibres are needed to enable the parietal pleura to adjust to the movements of the thoracic wall during breathing.

The **costal pleura** (pleura costalis) covers the ribs and intercostal muscles laterally, the sternum and transversus thoracis muscle ventrally, and the vertebral bodies dorsally. The strips covering the ribs themselves are thin but firmly attached, whereas those covering the intercostal muscles are thick but loosely attached (Evans, 1993, p. 485).

The **mediastinal pleura** (pleura mediastinalis) becomes continuous with the costal pleura ventrally along the dorsal surface of the sternum, and dorsally along the vertebral bodies (Fig. 9.1). The part of the mediastinal pleura that covers the pericardium is known as the **pericardiac pleura** (pleura pericardiaca).

The **diaphragmatic pleura** (pleura diaphragmatica) is reflected from the costal pleura along the line where the costal musculature of the diaphragm diverges cranially from the lateral thoracic wall (Fig. 8.25), thus forming the **costodiaphragmatic line of pleural reflection** (Fig. 23.2A; Sections 8.11.4 and 23.8). The acute angle of divergence of the diaphragmatic from the costal pleura (Fig. 9.3) forms the **costodiaphragmatic recess** (recessus costodiaphragmaticus) (Section 9.6.1).

9.4 Mediastinum

The mediastinum is the partition between the left and right pleural sacs. It is formed by the apposition of the mediastinal pleura of the left and right pleural sacs, with a connective tissue filling between these two sheets. Its developmental origin is described in Section 8.12.3. It contains most of the structures in the thoracic cavity, including the heart in its pericardial sac, the thoracic trachea,

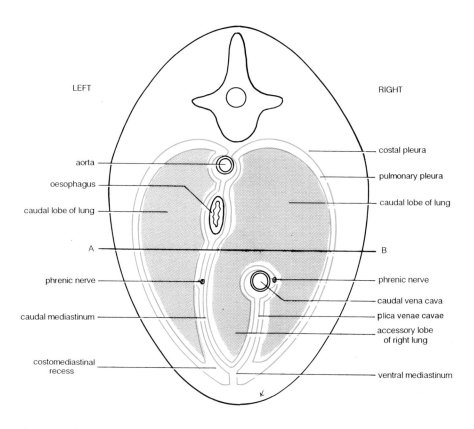

Fig. 9.2 Diagrammatic transverse section through the thorax of a mature mammal caudal to the heart to show the position of the mediastinum to the left of the midline and the plica venae cavae to the right of the midline. The pleura is green. The plica venae cavae is a fold from the ventral mediastinum, carrying the caudal vena cava. Between the plica venae cavae and the mediastinum is the mediastinal recess, containing the accessory lobe of the right lung. The volume of the right lung is so much greater than that of the left that the mediastinum is deflected to the left of the midline. A–B is the plane of the horizontal section in Fig. 9.3.

the thoracic oesophagus, the thymus, mediastinal lymph nodes, most of the great vessels going in and out of the heart, and nerves associated with the heart and lungs.

Major structures that are *not* in the mediastinum are the lungs, caudal vena cava, and the right phrenic nerve in the caudal part of its course. At the root of the lung, the mediastinal pleura is reflected onto the surface of the lung as the pulmonary pleura (Fig. 9.3). Caudal to the heart, the caudal vena cava and right phrenic nerve are contained in their own private fold of

parietal pleura, the **plica venae cavae** (Section 9.5).

If one pleural cavity is opened widely to the atmosphere in the live animal, there is an immediate unilateral **pneumothorax** (gas in the pleural cavity) on that side, causing the lung to collapse (Section 10.3). During each subsequent inspiration the pressure in the opened pleural cavity remains atmospheric, but the pressure in the closed pleural cavity falls well below atmospheric. Thus there is a substantial pressure gradient across the mediastinum during each inspiration, causing the

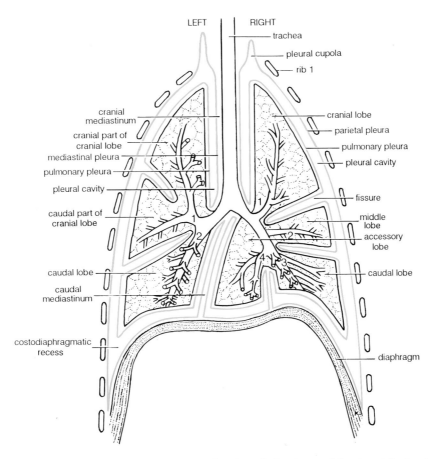

Fig. 9.3 Dorsal view of a diagrammatic horizontal section through the thorax of the dog at the level of the tracheal bifurcation, to show the lobes of the lung and their pleural coverings, and the lobar and segmental bronchi. The section is cut in the plane A–B of Fig. 9.2, i.e. dorsal to the heart. The pleura is green. In the domestic carnivores the fissures between the lobes of the lung are exceptionally deep, so that the pulmonary (visceral) pleura reaches the lobar bronchi. The left pleural cupola projects further into the neck than the right. 1–4 in the right lung, and 1 and 2 in the left lung, are the lobar bronchi of the dog, as shown in Fig. 5.4. The branches from each of these lobar bronchi are the segmental bronchi in this species, as recognized by Amis and McKiernan (1986, Fig. 10) from their bronchoscopic observations.

mediastinum to bulge into the unopened side of the thorax. If the mediastinum ruptures, there is an immediate bilateral pneumothorax and both lungs collapse. Whether or not the mediastinum ruptures after unilateral pneumothorax probably depends mainly on species differences in the thickness and structure of the mediastinum. The risk of rupture appears greatest in the horse and dog, since in both of these species the mediastinum is relatively thin and may have natural **fenestrations**.

The *pressures* in the pleural cavity are considered in Section 10.4.

In principle, the sheet of mediastinal pleura of the left pleural sac faces the sheet of mediastinal pleura of the right pleural sac; these two sheets, together with the connective tissue of **endothoracic fascia** (fascia endothoracica) that unites them, form the vertical partition between the two pleural cavities in the midline, as shown in Fig. 9.1. This partition is the **mediastinum** (Section 9.4). In reality, however, the right lung is so much greater in volume than the left (Section 5.5) that the caudal mediastinum is displaced to the left of the midline (Figs 9.3, 9.4).

Where it meets the diaphragm, the mediastinal pleura becomes continuous with the **diaphragmatic pleura** along a line of reflexion that curves over the left side of the cupola, between the aorta and oesophagus dorsally and the sternal region ventrally (Fig. 9.5); at the dorsal end of this line of reflexion, the caudal ends of the left and right **pulmonary ligaments** (Section 5.5) also become continuous with both the diaphragmatic pleura and the mediastinum (Fig. 9.5).

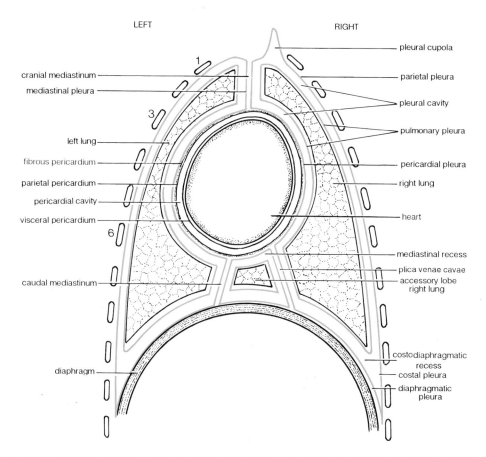

Fig. 9.4   Dorsal view of a diagrammatic horizontal section through the thorax of a horse at the level of the heart, to show the disposition of the pleura and pericardium. The pleura is green. The sac-like pericardium, containing the heart, lies within the mediastinum. The accessory lobe of the right lung occupies the mediastinal recess. In this species only the right pleural cupola enters the neck.

The mediastinum is divided into regional components, according to its relationships to the heart (Schaller *et al.*, 1992, p. 192). The **cranial mediastinum** (mediastinum craniale) lies cranial to the pericardium (Fig. 9.4), and the **caudal mediastinum** (mediastinum caudale) caudal to the pericardium (Fig. 9.4). The **dorsal mediastinum** (mediastinum dorsale) is the region between the vertebrae and the pericardium, whereas the **ventral mediastinum** (mediastinum ventrale) is between the pericardium and the sternum (Fig. 9.1). The **middle mediastinum** (mediastinum medium) contains the heart and pericardium (Fig. 9.1).

The **cranial mediastinum** contains the thoracic trachea, the thoracic oesophagus, the thymus, cranial mediastinal lymph nodes, the internal thoracic vessels, the cranial vena cava, the brachiocephalic vessels, thoracic duct, the phrenic nerves, cardiosympathetic nerves, vagus nerve, cardiovagal nerves, and recurrent laryngeal nerves (Schaller *et al.*, 1992, p. 192).

The **middle mediastinum** contains the pericardium and the heart, and the left and right phrenic and left and right vagus nerves as they pass caudally across the heart (Schaller *et al.*, 1992, p. 192; Evans, 1993, p. 485).

The **dorsal mediastinum** contains the thoracic trachea and its bifurcation, and the great arteries and veins associated with the base of the heart (Schaller *et al.*, 1992, p. 192).

In the immature animal, the cranial part of the **ventral mediastinum** contains the thoracic component of the thymus (Section 14.19.2). The ventral mediastinum also contains the paired **sternopericardiac ligaments** (ligamenta sternopericardiaca) in ruminants and the pig, at the levels of the fifth and sixth costal cartilages, respectively, and the single **sternopericardiac ligament** (ligamentum sternopericardiacum) in the horse at the fourth or fifth costal cartilage (Schummer *et al.*, 1981, p. 16). In man also, the ventral mediastinum contains an ill-defined superior and inferior sternopericardiac ligament (Williams *et al.*, 1989, p. 695). The sternopericardiac ligaments secure the heart in position, ventrally and caudally (Section 20.2).

The **caudal mediastinum** contains the oesophagus and aorta. In carnivores it contains the **phrenicopericardiac ligament** (ligamentum phrenicopericardiacum) (Fig. 9.5) (Nickel *et al.*, 1973, Fig. 8), and a similar ligament is present in the pig (Simoens, 1992, p. 234). In the dog, the caudal mediastinum (presumably reinforced by the phrenicopericardiac ligament) is commonly visible in dorsoventral thoracic radiographs (Section 24.7.4), projecting cranially from the left side of the diaphragmatic cupola (Figs 24.1, 24.3). Grandage (1974) concluded from lateral radiographs of the dog on its right side that the heart is suspended by the attachment of the phrenicopericardiac ligament to the *left* half of the diaphragmatic cupola (Section 24.9.5).

The standard reference works on veterinary anatomy are reticent about what, if any, relationship exists between these pericardiac ligaments and the mediastinum; it is usually left to the reader to conclude that the only route by which these ligaments can pass from the pericardium to the sternum or diaphragm must be between the two pleural sheets of the mediastinum. Fortunately Williams *et al.* (1989, p. 1272) state explicitly that that indeed is where these ligaments go, and this is more or less consistent with Fig. 8 of Nickel *et al.*, 1973).

There also appears to be uncertainty in the classical anatomical reference works about **fenestrations** and the **thickness** of the mediastinum in the domestic species, despite the clinical importance of these characteristics. Fenestrations or extreme thinness could indicate that a unilateral pneumothorax, pleural effusion, or infection might become bilateral and fatal. It seems to be generally agreed that in all **newborn** domestic mammals the mediastinum *does* form a perfect sagittal partition between the left and right pleural cavities, and that it remains a complete partition in the **adult ox**, **goat**, and **pig** (Nickel *et al.*, 1973, p. 6; de Lahunta and Habel, 1986, p. 200).

In the **horse**, however, the caudal mediastinum ventral to the oesophagus was reported by Sisson and Grossman (1969, p. 540) to be very delicate and usually fenestrated, thus giving communications between the two pleural cavities. However, some of the openings were presumed to be artefacts caused while examining the membrane, and the sheer transparency of the membrane may account for others; it was noted that apertures do not exist in the fetus, and are sometimes definitely absent in adults. Hare (1975, p. 517) reaffirmed these comments. Dyce *et al.* (1987, p. 156) maintained that the mediastinum of the *dead* horse always has many small openings, though there is doubt whether these fenestrations exist in the intact thorax. According to Nickel *et al.* (1973, p. 6), in the **horse** and **carnivores** openings appear *postnatally* in the ventral part of the caudal mediastinum through which the two pleural cavities can communicate; such openings also appear, though rarely, in the cranial mediastinum of lean **sheep**, and others have been observed in the middle mediastinum of **carnivores**. Hare (1975, p. 1569) considered the mediastinum in the **dog** to be complete, but so thin and delicate in its caudal ventral part that any marked pressure difference would rupture it. Evans (1993, p. 483) agreed that the tissue in the mediastinum of the dog is extremely scanty and that the pleura that covers it is not fenestrated. On the other hand, clinicians (Anon., 1993) hold that in the dog and cat fenestrations are normally present, so that pneumothorax and pleural effusions in these species are usually bilateral (Section 25.1).

The topic of mediastinal fenestrations was reviewed by de Lahunta and Habel (1986, p. 200). Such fenestrations have been observed in the **adult horse, dog, cat**, and some old **sheep**, but do *not* occur in the **ox, goat**, or **pig**, or in very young animals of any species. They are of **very small diameter**, less than 1 mm in the horse and **microscopic** in the dog. There is some clinical evidence that the openings may be a real danger in the **horse**, but nevertheless they can apparently become closed during inflammation. Acute unilateral pneumothorax is not fatal in the **dog**, provided that the mediastinum is not disturbed. **Cattle** tolerate unilateral pneumothorax during pericardial drainage. However, Fowler (1973) strongly advised intubation, and the immediate availability of positive pressure ventilation, before opening the thorax of the ox as well as the horse.

As stated in the preceding paragraphs, the **thinness of the mediastinum** has been noted in the **dog** and particularly emphasized in the **horse**. Fowler (1973) confirmed the thinness and fragility of the mediastinum in the **horse**. He also called attention explicitly to the relative **thickness** of the mediastinal pleura in the **ox** and **sheep**.

The loose fascia that covers the trachea and oesophagus in the neck continues into the cranial mediastinum and can act as a pathway for the spread of infection (Section 5.4.6).

9.5   Plica venae cavae

This is a fold of parietal pleura that contains the caudal vena cava. It arises from the right side of the ventral part of the caudal mediastinum (Fig. 9.5). It is continuous cranially with the pericardial pleura and caudally with the diaphragmatic pleura (Fig. 9.4). Since the **caval foramen** of the diaphragm (Section 8.11.6) lies to the right of the midline, the plica blends with the diaphragmatic pleura along the right side of the diaphragmatic cupola. In a sub-fold alongside the vena cava, the plica venae cavae carries the right phrenic nerve (Figs 9.2, 9.5).

Between the plica venae cavae and the caudal mediastinum there is a ventrally directed pocket of the pleural cavity, the **mediastinal recess**. This

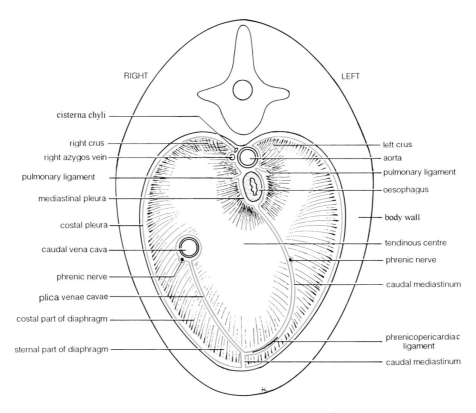

Fig. 9.5   Diagrammatic cranial view of the diaphragm of a dog, to show the attachment of the caudal mediastinum and plica venae cavae. The transected pleura is green. The mediastinum is deflected to the left by the relatively great volume of the left lung. On the surface of the diaphragm the pleura of the caudal mediastinum and plica venae cavae is continuous with the diaphragmatic pleura (not shown).

pocket contains the **accessory lobe** of the right lung (Fig. 9.2).

> In man, the accessory lobe of the right lung and the plica venae cavae are absent.

9.6 Anatomy of pleural cavity and pleural recesses

The pleural cavity (Fig. 9.1) is a potential space between the visceral and parietal pleura, occupied by nothing more than a thin film of **pleural fluid**. As already stated (Section 9.1), the lung is not in the pleural cavity, but invaginated into it. The pleural fluid has very important lubricating properties.

Because the volume of the lung becomes much smaller during each expiration, its lobes have to withdraw partially from their invaginated position within certain regions of the pleural cavity; at the next inspiration the lung expands and re-enters these regions. The most mobile parts of the lung during breathing (Section 5.7) are, (i) the basal border of its caudal lobe, and (ii) its ventral border (Fig. 5.3). These parts of the lung move in and out of regions of the pleural cavity that are known as the **costodiaphragmatic recess** and the **costomediastinal recess**. The lubricating qualities of the pleural fluid are essential to the movements of the lung in and out of these recesses.

> Presumably because of the difficulty of accurately measuring it, few authorities risk an estimate of the volume of the pleural fluid, but it has been put at 'only a few ml' (West, 1975, p. 92) or less than 15 ml in man and 1 ml in the rabbit (Wang, 1975).
>
> Since the pleura is permeable to gases and interstitial fluid (Agostoni and Mead, 1964, p. 401), it might be expected that the sub-atmospheric pressure of the pleural fluid would draw either gas or water **into** the pleural cavity until the lungs collapse (Fenn, 1964, p. 358). In fact gas and water are immediately absorbed **from** the cavity, leaving only the film of pleural fluid. Gas is absorbed because the sum of the gas tensions in venous blood is less than atmospheric pressure. Water is absorbed because the oncotic pressure (colloid osmotic pressure) of the plasma proteins in the capillaries of the visceral pleura is high, whereas the hydrostatic pressure in these capillaries is low (Section 17.25.2); this gives a strong pressure in favour of absorption (Fenn, 1964, p. 358), at a normal value of about 20 mmHg (2.7 kPa) (Guyton, 1986, p. 380).

In the normal animal, the pleural fluid enables the visceral pleura to slide smoothly over the parietal pleura, without sound or pain. When the pleura becomes inflamed, the movements of the lung may be painful and friction sounds can be auscultated. If pleural effusion then forms, it separates the visceral and parietal pleura and the sounds disappear (Section 21.5.2).

9.6.1 *Costodiaphragmatic recess*

The costodiaphragmatic recess is the most caudolateral region of the pleural cavity, where the diaphragm is in contact with the lateral thoracic wall (Fig. 9.3); the two surfaces of this cleft-like potential space are formed by the costal pleura and the diaphragmatic pleura. In the live animal at the end of expiration (and in the dead animal where the lung is collapsed, as in the dissection room) this recess is extensive. During inspiration, however, the diaphragm pulls away from the lateral thoracic wall (Fig. 10.3C), and the expanding basal border of the caudal lobe of the lung moves into the large space so created. This is a major factor in inflation of the lung (Section 10.6.3).

The **costodiaphragmatic line of pleural reflection** (Fig. 23.2) forms the peripheral (caudoventral) limit of the costodiaphragmatic recess (Section 23.8).

9.6.2 *Costomediastinal recess*

The costomediastinal recess is the ventral region of the pleural cavity. Here, at the end of expiration in the live animal (and in the dissection room cadaver), the parietal pleura covering the ventral region of the lateral thoracic wall is in contact with the parietal pleura covering the ventral mediastinum and the ventral region of the pericardium (Figs 9.1, 9.2). Dorsoventral and transverse expansion of the thoracic wall in inspiration opens up this recess (Sections 10.6.1, 10.6.2), and the expanding ventral border of the lung moves in. This, too, is a substantial factor in lung inflation.

> There are three other recesses of the pleural cavity, i.e. the **mediastinal recess** (recessus mediastini), the **lumbodiaphragmatic recess** (recessus lumbodiaphragmaticus), and the **pleural cupola**. Of these, the mediastinal recess is simply a regional subdivision of the main pleural cavity, and the other two are respectively a

caudal and a cranial extension of the pleural cavity beyond the thorax. None of these three has any physiological significance, but the cranial extension has clinical importance.

9.6.3   *Mediastinal recess*

This recess is the pocket of pleural cavity between the plica venae cavae and the caudal mediastinal pleura, occurring in the right pleural cavity only. It contains the **accessory lobe** of the right lung (Fig. 9.2).

9.6.4   *The lumbodiaphragmatic recess*

This paired recess extends over the dorsal surface of the left and right crura of the diaphragm, caudal to the last rib and reaching the first lumbar vertebra, in the carnivores, pig, sheep, and goat (Schaller *et al.*, 1992, p. 192).

9.6.5   *Pleural cupola*

The pleural cavity extends cranial to the first rib in the domestic mammals generally, as the dome-like pleural cupola (cupula pleurae). In the dog (Fig. 9.3) both the left and the right components of the cupola extend 1–2 cm beyond the first rib and enter the base of the neck; the left is the more extensive, and is more closely related to the oesophagus than the right. In the horse and ox the cupola enters the neck on the right side (extending about 2–3 cm). The pleural cupola may be entered accidentally during surgery at the thoracic inlet or by a penetrating wound, causing pneumothorax (Section 25.12). In the pig the pleural cupola does not extend cranial to the first rib (Hare, 1975, p. 1291).

9.7   Microscopic structure of the pleura

The pleura is a serous membrane. Like all such membranes lining closed body cavities (e.g. pericardium, peritoneum), its surface is formed by a simple squamous epithelium of plate-like **mesothelial cells** lying on a **submesothelial connective tissue layer**. This connective tissue layer consists of collagen bundles interlaced with elastic fibres, thus providing the strength and the elasticity needed by both the parietal and the visceral pleura to allow the movements of breathing.

The submesothelial connective tissue layer of both the parietal and the pulmonary pleura contains pleural blood vessels and lymphatics, but the visceral pleura is much more vascular and has far more abundant lymphatics than the parietal pleura. Therefore the visceral pleura is particularly well equipped for the absorption of fluid. In the normal thorax it very effectively keeps the volume of pleural fluid at the proper minimum, and is the main route by which excess pleural fluid (**pleural effusion**) is removed (Section 17.27.2).

In the visceral (pulmonary) pleura, the **collagen** and **elastic fibres** of the submesothelial connective tissue layer pass through the vascular stratum to become continuous with the **fibrous and elastic continuum** of the lung (Section 6.9). The tension transmitted from the visceral pleura to the fibrous and elastic continuum holds open the alveoli, conducting airways, and blood vessels in the substance of the lung.

The **mesothelial cells** (mesotheliocytus) (Krahl, 1964, p. 241; Williams *et al.*, 1989, p. 1270) interdigitate with each other and are held together by desmosomes. Between the cell borders there are intercellular clefts occupied by a homogeneous, perhaps semifluid, intercellular substance. Their luminal surfaces carry microvilli and (at least in man) numerous cilia. There are many micropinocytotic vesicles. These structural characteristics are consistent with a capacity for exchange of substances across the pleura. However, there are differences in the structure of the visceral and parietal pleura (Krahl, 1964, p. 242), which correlate with differences in uptake capability.

The **submesothelial connective tissue layer** of the **parietal pleura** is attached to the endothoracic fascia (Section 9.8). It contains the usual lymphatics and blood vessels. The **visceral pleura** differs in possessing a particularly well-developed **vascular stratum** beneath the submesothelial connective tissue layer, thus making the visceral pleura much more vascular than the parietal. This vascular stratum contains abundant lymph vessels, as well as veins, arteries, and rich capillary networks; it lies on the surface of the exchange tissue of the lung, but its fibres and vessels are continuous with those of the **interlobular septa** (Section 5.8).

The **lymphatic vessels** of the vascular stratum of the **visceral (pulmonary) pleura** are organized into a network of anastomosing channels, extending over the whole surface of the lung (Section 7.8.2).

The **arterial supply** to the visceral (pulmonary) pleura is provided by the **bronchial arteries** in most mammals (Section 9.9). The terminal arterioles break up into a loose network of capillaries of unusually large diameter (Krahl, 1964, p. 242). The diameter may reach 30 μm, leading to the name '**giant capillaries**', but the structure of the wall is the same as that of any other capillary. The meshes of this capillary network are about ten times wider than those of the alveolar capillaries.

It is generally agreed that the **pulmonary (visceral) pleura** is the main avenue for the *absorption of pleural fluid* from the pleural cavity (Agostoni and Mead, 1964, p. 402; Wang, 1975). However, these authors supposed that this absorption is by the *blood capillaries* of the pulmonary pleura; the lymphatics of the pulmonary pleura were thought not to be involved in draining the normal pleural cavity, but were assumed possibly to offer an important emergency mechanism. Drake and Gabel (1995) have now reversed this conclusion: according to their view, the *lymphatics* of the pulmonary pleura very effectively keep the volume of the pleural fluid at a minimum in the normal thorax, as well as removing excess fluid if **pleural effusion** occurs. Anyway, by means of either its blood vessels or its lymphatics, the **vascular stratum** of the pulmonary pleura is critically important, both in maintaining the normal film of **pleural fluid** (Section 9.6), and in removing excess pleural fluid as in **pleural effusion** (Sections 17.27.2, 17.27.4). Most investigators have also believed that little, if any, of *the fluid from the lung itself* is normally drained by the lymphatics of the pulmonary pleura via the pleural cavity. However, Drake and Gabel (1995) found that fluid from the lung is drained by this pathway, even when the lungs are not oedematous; when pulmonary oedema has formed, a large volume is cleared by this route.

On the other hand, *particulate matter* (e.g. Berlin blue, India ink), cells, and **large molecular proteins**, are removed from the pleural cavity by the **parietal pleura** (Krahl, 1964, p. 242; Wang, 1975). Various structures seem to be involved in the removal of such particles. Wang (1975) showed that carbon particles injected into the pleural cavity of the normal rabbit and mouse are picked up by the **mesothelial cells** of both the parietal and the visceral pleura. However, abundant particles are subsequently found in the lymphatic capillaries of the parietal pleural, but there are no particles in those of the visceral pleura; thus ultimate removal is solely by the parietal lymphatics.

Wang (1975) and a few other investigators have found small numbers of **stomata**, 2–6 μm or more in diameter, between the mesothelial cells of the parietal pleura in various mammals. Macrophages and other large particles were often associated with the stomata. The stomata open directly into dilated submesothelial lymphatic channels. It is not certain that the stomata are permanent structures. No stomata have been found in the visceral pleura; also the lymphatic capillaries of the visceral pleura are usually separated from the mesothelium by a layer of connective tissue fibres. The stomata may widen during inspiration, by stretching of the pleura. Stomata may perhaps be involved in the removal of particulate matter and cells by the parietal pleura, and possibly stomata might become more numerous under pathological conditions.

The **mesothelial cells** of the **visceral pleura** are very sensitive to mechanical and chemical **irritants** (Krahl, 1964, p. 241). When irritated they retract, but still retain contact with neighbouring cells by cellular bridges; retraction widens the intercellular clefts, and may thus promote the transmission of fluids and uptake of particles through the pleura. The cells may also become rounded, divide, and migrate to cover local defects in the pleural surface. They are also able to abandon their epithelial connections and differentiate into macrophages (Krstic, 1984, p. 257). There are islets of smaller mesothelial cells with widened intercellular clefts containing many lymphocytes, suggestive of immune defence.

There are **species variations** in the **pulmonary (visceral) pleura** (McLaughlin *et al.*, 1961; Tyler *et al.*, 1971). The connective tissue beneath the mesothelium is extremely thin in the dog, cat, and Rhesus monkey. Also the blood supply of the visceral pleura in these animals is from the pulmonary artery; the bronchial artery (Section 17.4) supplies no pleural blood, except for some small branches at the hilus of the lung. On the other hand, in the ox, sheep, pig, horse, and man, the pleura is thick and highly vascularized by the **bronchial artery** (Section 17.4), especially in the horse. On the basis, evidently, of extensive experience of thoracic surgery in the horse, Fowler (1973) took an opposite view of the thickness of the equine pulmonary pleura, describing it as frankly thin; he reported that the visceral pleura can be used as an anchor for sutures in the ox (as in man), but found it too thin in the horse to serve this function.

9.8 Endothoracic fascia

The endothoracic fascia is a distinct layer of fibroelastic connective tissue that is interposed between the parietal pleura and the thoracic walls. It therefore lines the thoracic cavity throughout. It also forms the connective tissue filling of the mediastinum. Its fibres mingle with those of the adjacent connective tissue layer of the pleura.

The texture of the endothoracic fascia (fascia endothoracica) is looser than that of the intrinsic connective tissue layer of the parietal pleura, at least in man, and this enables it to be utilized as a plane for surgical separation of the pleura from the thoracic wall (Krahl, 1964, p. 239).

Dorsally the endothoracic fascia covers the ventral surfaces of the vertebral bodies, including various structure that lie against the dorsal body wall such as the aorta, azygos venous trunks, and sympathetic chain. Laterally it covers the costal wall, and caudally it continues over the diaphragm. In the dorsal and ventral midlines it forms the more or less sagittal sheet of fascia that constitutes the connective tissue 'filling' of the **mediastinum** (Section 9.4). At the thoracic inlet it reinforces the **pleural cupola** and then becomes continuous with the cervical fascia enclosing the trachea and oesophagus; this connection makes it possible for a septic lesion in the region of the trachea or oesophagus to spread into the thoracic cavity (Section 5.4.7) (Hare, 1975, p. 130).

There are species and regional variations in the thickness of the fascia and the relative proportions of collagenous to elastic fibres (Hare, 1975, p. 130). It is thick and highly elastic on the lateral thoracic wall where it crosses the intercostal spaces, but less thick on the ribs themselves. It is thick where it reinforces the pleural cupola. On the diaphragm it is very thin.

As pointed out in Section 8.9.1, the endothoracic fascia is homologous to the **transversalis fascia**, and therefore completes the homologies between the thoracic wall and the abdominal wall.

9.9   Blood supply of the pleura

The **arterial supply** to the **parietal pleura** is by regional systemic arteries, notably the intercostal arteries. The **venous drainage** of the **parietal pleura** is by the intercostal and other regional satellite systemic veins.

The **pulmonary (visceral) pleura** is supplied by the **bronchial arteries** in most of the domestic mammals, and by the **pulmonary arteries** in the remaining species (Section 17.4). The **venous drainage** of the **pulmonary pleura** is the same in both of these two groups of mammals, i.e. into the **pulmonary veins** (Section 17.5).

The arterial supply to the costal part of the **parietal pleura** comes from many small twigs of the intercostal arteries (Fig. 8.34). The diaphragmatic pleura is supplied by the various **phrenic arteries** (Fig. 8.34) (Section 8.16.3) (Hare, 1975, p. 131). The mediastinal pleura obtains a supply from the arteries that are topographically in a position to reach it. One source is the **pericardiophrenic artery** (Fig. 8.34), which runs caudally across the pericardium and within the mediastinum on the left side and within the plica venae cavae on the right side, but this is a small or very small artery (Ghoshal, 1975a, p. 569; Evans, 1993, p. 631). Branches are supplied to the ventral mediastinum by the **internal thoracic artery** (Fig. 8.34), and to the caudal mediastinum by the various **phrenic arteries**. The dorsal mediastinum of the dog receives 'two or more' branches directly from the **aorta** (Fig. 8.34) (Evans, 1993, p. 648) In man, 'numerous' small aortic mediastinal arteries supply the dorsal mediastinum (Williams *et al.*, 1989, p. 764).

As already stated (Section 9.7), the **visceral (pulmonary) pleura** is more vascular than the parietal pleura. According to McLaughlin *et al.* (1961) and Tyler *et al.* (1971), the pulmonary pleura is vascularized profusely by the **bronchial arteries** in the ox, sheep, and pig, and even more profusely in the horse and man; the pathways are by both hilar and interlobular branches. Williams *et al.* (1989, p. 1271) reaffirmed that in man the vascular supply to the pulmonary pleura is from bronchial vessels. On the other hand, Krahl (1964, p. 242) maintained that in man the supply by the bronchial artery is restricted to most of the mediastinal and interlobar surfaces of the lung, and part of the diaphragmatic surface; the costal surface and most of the diaphragmatic surface are supplied by numerous twigs of the pulmonary artery.

In the Rhesus monkey, dog, and cat, vascularization of the pulmonary pleura is said by McLaughlin *et al.* (1961) to be solely by the pulmonary artery, with no flow from the bronchial artery except for a few short branches to the hilus.

9.10   Lymphatic pathways from the pleura

As stated in Section 9.7, the **pulmonary pleura** contains a rich network of lymphatic channels. These absorb pleural fluid, maintaining the total volume at its normal minimal level. They also drain off excess fluid of pleural oedema.

The lymphatic channels of the pulmonary pleura run all over the surface of the lung, and converge on the root of the lung (Section 7.8.2). Here they empty into bronchial lymphatics accompanying the principal bronchus. These drain mainly into the **tracheobronchial lymph nodes**, which also receive the lymphatic drainage of the lung itself (Section 7.9.1).

The various parts of the **parietal pleura** have a regional drainage into intercostal, mediastinal, and sternal lymph nodes, and also into the tracheobronchial nodes.

The lymphatic pathways from the thoracic cavity are surveyed in Section 14.32.4.

9.11   Innervation of the pleura

The parietal pleura receives a sensory innervation from the intercostal nerves (Section 8.17.2) and the phrenic nerve (Section 8.17.3). Like the afferent pathways from the other parietal serous membranes (e.g. the parietal peritoneum), this innervation consists of somatic afferent fibres. Such fibres are acutely sensitive to the painful stimuli that affect the outer structures of the body (Section 4.4.4), including those of cutting, crushing, and burning.

The visceral (pulmonary) pleura has an autonomic afferent innervation, which is insensitive to cutting, crushing, and burning, but responds to the adequate stimuli for visceral pain (Section 4.4.1). The pathways for these afferent fibres from the visceral pleura are not known, but they presumably follow the bronchial tree in the bronchial rami of the vagus.

The somatic afferent innervation of the **costal pleura** and of the peripheral rim of the **diaphragmatic pleura** is supplied by the **intercostal nerves**; that of the **mediastinal pleura** and the central zone of the **diaphragmatic pleura** comes from the **phrenic nerve** (Hare, 1975, p. 132; Williams *et al.*, 1989, p. 1171). The pain responses to noxious stimulation of the parietal pleura in man have been summarized by Hare (1975, p. 132): irritation of the costal pleura causes pain that is localized on the thoracic wall at the site of stimulation; irritation of the peripheral rim of the diaphragmatic pleura causes diffuse pain in the lumbar or abdominal areas; irritation of the parts of the diaphragmatic pleura supplied by the phrenic nerve cause referred pain (Section 4.7), usually in the neck or shoulder.

Chapter 10
Respiratory Mechanics

I PRESSURE GRADIENTS

10.1 General principles

Fluids, that is gases and liquids, can only flow from a higher to a lower pressure, i.e. down a pressure gradient. The movement of blood requires a higher pressure in the heart than in the capillaries, and the heart obviously provides the driving force. To move air into the lung also requires a pressure gradient, from mouth to alveoli. It is not quite so obvious that, in this case, the driving force is *atmospheric pressure*.

If the pressure in the alveoli is one atmosphere, and the larynx and mouth are open, no air flows. The pressure gradient required to create air flow in inspiration can only be produced *naturally* by reducing the pressure in the alveoli *below* the atmospheric value. *Artificially*, the necessary gradient can be created by raising the pressure at the mouth **above** one atmosphere; this is known as **'positive' pressure breathing**, and can be accomplished by means of a pump.

Mammals **inspire** during natural breathing by enlarging the volume of the thorax. (Birds do it by increasing the volume of the thorax and abdomen together.) The mammalian thoracic wall is coupled to the surface of the lung by means of the thin film of pleural fluid in the pleural cavity (Section 10.5). Therefore if the volume of the thorax increases, the volume of the lung increases. The increase in the volume of the lung then causes the alveolar pressure to become slightly sub-atmospheric. There is now a pressure gradient from the mouth to the alveoli, and therefore atmospheric pressure pushes air into the lungs.

10.2 Forces and pressure gradients in inspiration and expiration

10.2.1 *Inspiration*

The lungs have a continual tendency to contract inwards, away from the thoracic wall. About one third of this inward force is caused by the elastic fibres (force E, in Fig. 10.1A) in the elastic continuum of the lung (Section 6.9), and about two thirds is caused by surface tension (force ST, in Fig. 10.1A) within the alveoli (Section 6.25). Together, force E and force ST can be known as the **forces of lung recoil** (or the forces of elastic recoil of the lungs).

In contrast, the thoracic wall has the opposite tendency, i.e. to spring outwards. These outward forces are produced by the elasticity of the thoracic wall in general, and in particular by ligaments acting on the proximal ends of the rib at the costovertebral articulations (force L1 in Fig. 10.1A) and on the distal ends of the costal cartilages at the sternocostal articulation. Together they can be called the **forces of thoracic wall recoil** (or forces of elastic recoil of the thoracic wall).

At the **end of a resting expiration**, these inward and outward forces on the lung and thoracic wall respectively come into equilibrium, at the **resting volume of the thorax** (Fig. 10.1A). During this phase of equilibrium neither the lungs, nor the thoracic wall, nor the air inside the lungs, is moving. The pressure outside the thoracic wall is atmospheric: so also is the pressure in the alveoli. There is no pressure gradient within the airways.

At the **onset of inspiration** an additional out-

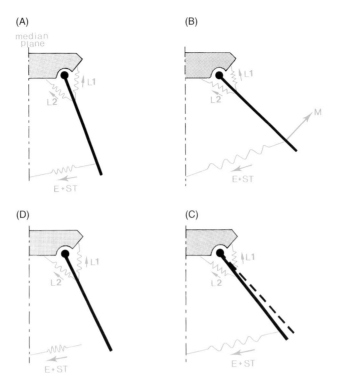

Fig. 10.1   Diagrams summarizing the main forces acting on the lateral thoracic wall during breathing. The thoracic wall is represented by a single rib, articulating with a vertebra and orientated as in a transverse section of the thorax. Movement of the rib to the left of the diagram is a medial movement; movement to the right is lateral. The median plane divides the thorax longitudinally into equal right and left halves. The forces are represented by springs. E, force of elastic tissue within lung. ST, force of surface tension within lung. L1, elastic force of ligamentous tissue acting on the proximal end of the rib at the vertebral articulation, and moving the rib laterally. L2, as L1 but moving the rib medially. M, force of inspiratory muscles acting on lateral thoracic wall. Ligamentous forces acting on the distal end of the rib and costal cartilage are ignored.

    A. At the end of a resting expiration. Forces E + ST + L2 are in equilibrium with force L1. Nothing is moving. The thoracic cage is at the resting volume of the thorax.

    B. At the end of a resting inspiration. Force M has moved the rib laterally. Forces E + ST + L2 are in equilibrium with M + L1. Nothing is moving.

    C. Shortly after the beginning of a resting expiration. Force M has ceased. Forces E + ST + L2 are moving the rib medially, overcoming the resistance of L1. Broken line, position of rib before expiration began.

    D. Pneumothorax. Air has been admitted to the pleural cavity. The lung collapses inwards through forces E + ST. The rib springs a substantial distance laterally (compare the position of the rib in A) because of force L1, but this movement stops when force L1 comes into equilibrium with force L2.

ward force (M in Fig. 10.1B) is applied to the thoracic walls by the muscles of inspiration. Forces M + L1 move the thoracic walls outward, and the volume of the thorax therefore increases. Because of the coupling of the thoracic walls to the lung surface, the surface of the lung is drawn outwards, and the volume of the lung simultaneously increases; this dilates the alveoli and thus causes a fall in the pressure within the alveoli.

    The fall in alveolar pressure in a **resting inspira-** **tion** is very small, at its peak being less than 1 mmHg (0.133 kPa) (slightly more than 1 cmH$_2$O (0.098 kPa)) below atmospheric pressure (Fig. 10.2). (mmHg can be converted to cmH$_2$O by dividing by 0.74; conventionally, these values below atmospheric pressure are written as '−1 mmHg' or '−1 cmH$_2$O', whereas pressures above atmospheric are preceded by a + sign.) In the **normal** animal this almost incredibly small pressure gradient from the mouth to the alveoli is enough to enable atmospheric pressure to push air into the airways.

Figure 10.2 shows that the fall in pressure in the alveoli reaches its peak of $-1\,cmH_2O$ ($-0.098\,kPa$) about half-way through inspiration; this peak coincides with the peak of airflow of about $0.51s^{-1}$. Thereafter, pressure and flow return simultaneously to zero at the turnover point between inspiration and expiration.

During **hyperventilation** as in **heavy exercise**, much greater pressure gradients are needed during inspiration to achieve the necessary flow rate of air. Respiratory diseases, such as **chronic obstructive pulmonary disease** (Section 7.17), may produce a severe increase in resistance to airflow (Section 6.14). A very large fall in alveolar pressure is now needed to achieve an adequate flow rate in inspiration, many times greater than the fall that is required during a normal resting inspiration.

The **forces of thoracic wall recoil** impart 'stiffness' to the rib cage, which can be expressed as the **compliance of the thoracic wall**. The compliance of the thoracic wall usually means the combined compliance of the lungs and rib cage together; the compliance of the lung is considered in Section 6.31. In man and the horse the stiffness of the rib cage is severe, i.e. the compliance of the thoracic wall is low. In small mammals such as the cat the thoracic wall is much more flexible, i.e. the compliance is high.

If the laryngeal glottis is firmly closed in *man*, vigorous inspiratory movements, at mid-capacity, may lower the **alveolar pressure** to -100 to $-140\,cmH_2O$ (-74 to $-103\,mmHg$) for 1–3 seconds (Agostoni and Mead, 1964, p. 404).

In the *galloping racehorse* the pressure in the oesophagus falls to about $-20\,mmHg$ ($-2.7\,kPa$) during inspiration, and it is likely that much of this fall in pressure will be transmitted to the alveoli (West and Mathieu-Costello, 1994).

Compliance is expressed as the relationship between volume and pressure (Section 6.31). The compliance of the thoracic wall alone can be measured directly if the lungs are removed, but it is possible to estimate thoracic wall compliance separately in the living animal. Crosfill and Widdicombe (1961) found thoracic wall compliance (expressed per unit lung volume) to be relatively high (about $0.5\,ml\,(cmH_2O)^{-1}\,ml^{-1}$) in the smaller laboratory mammals (mouse, rat, guinea pig, rabbit), and relatively low in the monkey, cat, dog, and man (about $0.1\,ml$

$(cmH_2O)^{-1}\,ml^{-1}$). Koterba *et al.* (1988) found data in the literature showing that, when normalized to body mass, the compliance of the equine thoracic wall is very low. The relatively high compliance of the thoracic wall in the cat as compared with that of man accounts for the occurrence of an inward ('expiratory') movement of the thoracic wall during inspiration in the cat but not in man (Sections 10.8, 10.11).

10.2.2   *Expiration*

At the **end of a resting inspiration** (Fig. 10.1C) the muscles of inspiration stop contracting, and the force M disappears. For a brief instant, when expiration is just about to begin, all forces are once again in equilibrium and neither the lungs, nor the thoracic wall, nor the air inside the lungs, is moving; the pressures outside the thoracic wall and inside the alveoli (Fig. 10.2) are once again atmospheric, and there is no pressure gradient in the airways.

However, **at the onset of a resting expiration**, the **forces of lung recoil** (E + ST in Fig. 10.1C) instantly cause the lung to get smaller; simultaneously, the elastic **forces of thoracic wall recoil** (represented by L2 in Fig. 10.C) contract the volume of the thorax. These elastic forces are all passive, their energy being stored during the stretching of the lung and thoracic wall throughout the previous inspiration. They compress the alveoli, and therefore the pressure within the alveoli rises above atmospheric pressure. A pressure gradient now exists from the alveoli to the mouth, and air flows out of the lung. The rib cage returns to the **resting volume of the thorax**. The elastic forces of thoracic wall recoil account for about one third of the energy needed for a resting expiration: the remaining two thirds are supplied by surface tension (ST).

The elasticity of the abdominal wall and abdominal contents adds a further, relatively small, force of **abdominal recoil** to the forces of expiration. These elastic forces arise from the compression of the abdominal contents and stretching of the abdominal wall when the diaphragm contracts during inspiration.

In resting breathing, the change in alveolar pressure during **expiration** is again very small, reaching only about $1\,cmH_2O$ (about $0.01\,kPa$) above atmospheric pressure (Fig. 10.2). The peak of the increase in alveolar pressure in a resting

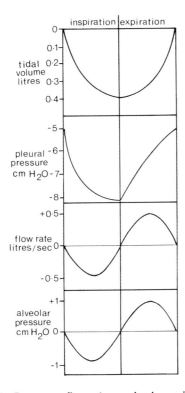

Fig. 10.2 Pressures, flow rates, and volumes in inspiration and expiration during resting breathing in a normal man. Before inspiration begins, pleural pressure is about $-5\,cmH_2O$, because the inward forces of the elastic tissue and surface tension of the lungs are balanced by the outward force of the costal articulations. Alveolar pressure is atmospheric, so there is no pressure gradient between the alveoli and the mouth, and therefore the volume and flow rate of inspired air are also zero. At the onset of inspiration, pleural pressure falls, establishing a small sub-atmospheric pressure in the alveoli. This sets up a pressure gradient from the mouth towards the alveoli, thus causing a flow of air to the alveoli giving a tidal volume of about 400 ml. At the onset of expiration, the pleural pressure rapidly becomes less sub-atmospheric, thus allowing the lungs immediately to collapse inwards. The alveolar pressure instantly rises above atmospheric. This creates a pressure gradient from the alveoli to the mouth, thus causing a flow of air from the lung. The inspiratory and expiratory pressure gradients are very small (only $1\,cmH_2O$ (0.098 kPa), respectively, below and above atmospheric), but this achieves a flow rate adequate for the resting healthy individual. The quantitative data are from West (1975).

expiration occurs about half way through expiration, coinciding with the peak of air flow (Fig. 10.2). Alveolar pressure and airflow then together return to zero at the end of expiration.

In **hyperventilation** as in **heavy exercise**, and in respiratory diseases such as **chronic obstructive pulmonary disease**, the alveolar pressure rises strongly above one atmosphere (Comroe, 1975, p. 128). This is because the **expiratory muscles** now apply active forces that compress the thoracic walls and thence the lungs. This creates a steep pressure gradient from alveoli to mouth, giving a much faster flow rate of expired gas (Section 10.12).

In **disease conditions** such as **chronic obstructive pulmonary disease** or **asthma** (Sections 7.17, 7.20), very steep gradients from alveoli to mouth may be needed in order to overcome airway resistance (Guyton, 1986, p. 477). In fact it is usually much more difficult for asthmatics to breathe out than in. This is because the high pressure within the thoracic cavity during expiration needed to overcome airway resistance also tends to compress the conducting airways and thus to increase still further the resistance to air flow (Section 10.12); in contrast, during inspiration, and particularly during forced inspiration, the sub-atmospheric pressure within the thorax tends to pull the conducting airways open, thus reducing airway resistance (Guyton, 1986, p. 476).

If the laryngeal glottis is closed, forceful expiratory efforts, in mid-capacity, can raise the alveolar pressure in man to $160-190\,cmH_2O$ (118–140 mmHg) above atmospheric pressure for 1–3 seconds (Agostoni and Mead, 1964, p. 404).

10.2.3 *Terms used to describe pulmonary volumes and capacities*

Various terms (Fig. 10.5) are used to describe the performance of the lungs (Guyton, 1986, p. 470). The *tidal volume* is the volume of air inspired or expired in one breath. The *inspiratory reserve volume* is the maximum volume that can be inspired in excess of a normal resting inspiration. The *expiratory reserve volume* is the maximum volume that can be expired in excess of a normal resting expiration. The *residual volume* is the volume remaining in the lungs after a maximum expiration.

The *inspiratory capacity* is the tidal volume plus the inspiratory reserve volume. The *functional residual capacity* is the expiratory reserve volume plus the residual volume, and is the volume of gas remaining in the lung after a normal resting expiration. The *vital capacity* is the maximum volume that can be expired after a maximal inspiration. The *total lung capacity* is the total volume contained by the lung after a maximal inspiration, and is therefore the vital capacity plus the residual volume.

10.3   **Pneumothorax**

Penetrating wounds of the thoracic wall (Section 9.4) or pleural cupola (Section 9.6.5) on one side of the body, or surgical interference with the surface of a lung (Section 20.11), may allow gas to enter the pleural cavity, resulting in unilateral pneumothorax. On the affected side, the lung now collapses inwards because of the forces of its elastic continuum and surface tension (E + ST in Fig. 10.1D). At the same time the thoracic wall springs outwards because of the elastic forces of the thoracic wall (L1 in Fig. 10.1D), until L1 is balanced by elastic force L2.

The increase of the thoracic volume above its resting value that occurs in pneumothorax is large. In man it is estimated at about 600 ml (Comroe, 1975, p. 116), i.e. about 30% more than a normal tidal volume. An estimate obtained by subtracting the functional residual capacity from the resting volume of the thoracic cavity (as given by Hildebrandt and Young, 1966, p. 749) suggests a smaller value of about 450 ml, i.e. about equivalent to tidal volume. According to Agostoni and Mead (1964, p. 392), if both of the pleural cavities were opened to the atmosphere in man, a volume of air equivalent to about 60% of the vital capacity (i.e. about 2700 ml) would be sucked into the yawning gap between the expanding thoracic wall and the collapsing lung.

The filling of one pleural cavity by air in severe unilateral pneumothorax displaces the mediastinum, and the organs that it contains, towards the other side of the thorax. This **mediastinal shift** (Blood and Studdert, 1988, p. 564) can compress the other lung, and can also cause kinking of one or more of the great blood vessels thus seriously impairing the flow of blood to and from the heart. The result is severe dyspnoea, congestion of cervical veins, and displacement of the trachea to one side.

10.4   Pleural pressure

At the end of expiration all forces on the thoracic wall are in equilibrium (Fig. 10.1A). But, since the lungs and thoracic wall are trying to pull apart, the pressure between them, i.e. within the pleural cavity, must be less than atmospheric. The actual value is about -4 mmHg (about -5 cmH$_2$O; Fig. 10.2)). The pressure within the pleural cavity is known as the pleural pressure or intrapleural pressure.

In strict physical terms, pleural 'pressure' is not a pressure but, for convenience, the term is nevertheless in general use (Hildebrandt and Young, 1966, p. 747). Pressure is a scalar quantity (i.e. it is sufficiently defined when the magnitude is given in appropriate units; Isaacs,

1971), and only exists in a homogeneous fluid (gas or liquid) phase. In the film of fluid that separates the parietal and visceral pleura, forces, shears, and stresses arise that are, in general, vector and tensor quantities (a vector quantity requires a direction to be stated in order to define it completely; Isaacs, 1971). To measure the pleural pressure directly it is necessary to **create** a homogeneous fluid phase by inserting a drop of liquid or a bubble of air on the end of a needle, between the parietal and visceral pleura.

The pressure in the pleural **fluid** is actually much lower than that in the pleural cavity, averaging about -10 cmH$_2$O (0.98 kPa) (Guyton, 1986, p. 380). This relatively low value is caused by the 'absorptive force' arising from the high oncotic pressure of the blood plasma in the capillaries of the richly vascular pulmonary pleura Section 9.7; see also Section 17.27, Pleural effusion).

10.4.1   Variations in pleural pressure during the breathing cycle

In normal resting breathing, the pleural pressure falls progressively during **inspiration** to a lowest value of about -8 cmH$_2$O (Fig. 10.2); the fall is progressive because the elastic forces within the lung increase progressively as the lung is stretched. In a **forced inspiration** the strong contraction of the inspiratory muscles reduces the pleural pressure to much lower values.

During **expiration** in **resting breathing**, the pleural pressure remains sub-atmospheric throughout (Fig. 10.2). But during a **forced expiration** it rises strongly above atmospheric pressure, because of the compression of the thoracic walls by the expiratory muscles. During the expulsive efforts of **defecation** and **parturition**, when the expiratory muscles contract powerfully against a closed laryngeal glottis, the pleural pressure reaches maximum values above atmospheric pressure corresponding to maximum alveolar pressures (160–190 cmH$_2$O, or 15.7–18.6 kPa, Section 10.2.2).

In the galloping Thoroughbred, the oesophageal pressure falls to -20 mmHg (-2.66 kPa) during inspiration (West and Mathieu-Costello, 1994).

10.4.2   Physiological and pathophysiological significance of pleural pressure

The pleural pressure is of general importance in thoracic physiology and pathophysiology. The left and right pleural cavities are separated by the **mediastinum**, and therefore the mediastinum and its contents are subjected to the pleural pressure. Thus the pleural pressure is exerted on the heart and its great vessels, the thoracic oesophagus, the thoracic trachea and its bifurcation into the left and right principal bronchi, and the thoracic duct. All of these structures are therefore affected by fluctuations in pleural pressure, some more importantly than others.

Since the great veins and the right side of the heart are thin-walled structures they are particularly affected by the variations in pleural pressure; for example, the venous return fluctuates during the normal respiratory cycle, and the heart rate and arterial pressure vary accordingly (Sections 13.3.5, 21.11).

As already mentioned, an animal suffering from an obstructive respiratory disease, e.g. an asthmatic human or a horse with chronic obstructive pulmonary disease, may have to raise the expiratory effort greatly in order to achieve an adequate flow rate of expired gas; the resulting increase in pleural pressure reduces the diameter of the principal bronchi, thus increasing the resistance to flow still further.

10.4.3 *Measurement of pleural pressure*

The pleural pressure can be measured directly by puncturing the thoracic wall with a large blunt needle. This drastic interventionist procedure can, however, be avoided clinically by taking advantage of the location of the thoracic oesophagus within the mediastinum. A small tubular balloon on the end of a tube can be swallowed and retained within the thoracic oesophagus (Fig. 24.8). The pressure in the thoracic oesophagus is generally taken to be equal to the pleural pressure. The thoracic oesophagus therefore gives the clinician a relatively non-interventionist way of recording the pressure changes within the thorax, and thence applying clinical tests for analysing breathing in disease conditions (Fenn, 1964, p. 360).

Hildebrandt and Young (1966, p. 748) remarked that swallowing a balloon is not only safer than intercostal puncture, but is also quite a memorable experience; thus, 'with a liberal supply of iced water, dedicated people are able to swallow and even to hold down a balloon with only slight flushing, sweating, eye-watering, gagging, choking, coughing, and occasional vomiting.'

Oesophageal pressure can closely approximate pleural pressure, particularly at small tidal volumes, but there are limitations and sources of error such as a regular cardiac artefact, spurious pressures generated by oesophageal peristalsis, quite substantial changes during flexion and extension of the neck (probably caused by compression of the oesophagus by the trachea), and variations at the apex and base of the lung (Mead and Milic-Emili, 1964, p. 373; Hildebrandt, 1974, p. 311).

10.4.4 *Transmural pressure*

The pressure events in the pleural cavity can be described in terms of transmural pressure (transpulmonary pressure). The transmural pressure (P_{tp}) is the pressure that distends the lung (Hildebrandt, 1974, p. 311). P_{tp} is the difference between the pleural pressure (P_{pl}) and the alveolar pressure (P_{alv}): $P_{tp} = P_{pl} - P_{alv}$. At the end of expiration, when nothing is moving, $P_{alv} = 0$ and P_{pl} is about $-5 \, cmH_2O$ ($-0.49 \, kPa$); therefore $P_{tp} = P_{pl}$, i.e. about $-5 \, cmH_2O$. About half way through a resting inspiration (Fig. 10.2), P_{alv} has fallen to its lowest value (about $-1 \, cmH_2O$ or $-0.1 \, kPa$); P_{pl} has fallen to about $-8 \, cmH_2O$ ($-0.78 \, kPa$). Therefore at this point during inspiration, $P_{tp} = -8 - -1, = -7 \, cmH_2O$ ($-0.68 \, kPa$).

10.4.5 *Effect of gravity on pleural pressure*

The lung is heavy, and the force of gravity drags the lung towards the ground. So long as the pleural cavity remains intact, the lung remains 'coupled' to the thoracic wall (Section 10.5), and cannot collapse downwards. However, the force of gravity gives the pleural pressure a gradient from top to bottom. Thus if breathing is arrested at the end of a resting expiration the pleural pressure everywhere is below atmospheric (negative), but the negativity is considerably greater at the 'top' than at the 'bottom' of the pleural cavity. For example, in a standing man the pressure in the cranial region of the pleural cavity is about 7.4 mmHg (0.99 kPa), but in the caudal region it is only about 1.8 mmHg (0.24 kPa) (Weibel, 1984, p. 307). It is known that in the horse the dorsal region of the pleural cavity is relatively negative, and indeed there is evidence that the most negative region is dorsocaudal – where lesions of **exercise-induced pulmonary haemorrhage** are most common (Section 17.28).

10.5 Coupling of lung to thoracic wall

In the normal thorax, the parietal pleura is separated from the pulmonary (visceral) pleura by only a thin film of **pleural fluid** (Section 9.6). The volume of this fluid is kept to a minimum by the absorptive qualities of the highly vascular pulmonary pleura (Section 9.7).

The film of pleural fluid provides a liquid coupling between the surface of the lung and the thoracic wall; it establishes complete and synchronous transmission of thoracic volume to lung volume, and at the same time allows the lung to slide freely over the thoracic wall. A good analogy is two glass slides held together by a film of water: one surface slides easily over the other, but it is very difficult to separate them by pulling one slide at right angles to the plane of the other.

In the living body the movements of the thoracic wall and the surface of the lung follow each other instantly, and yet the lobes of the lung are able to slide in and out of the **costodiaphragmatic** and **costomediastinal recesses** at a minimal energetic cost.

The forces that actually hold the lung against the thoracic wall, crucial though they are in the mechanics of breathing, seem nevertheless to be somewhat obscure (Agostoni and Mead, 1964, pp. 402–404). It has often been suggested that these forces depend on surface tension (forces of attraction between the molecules of a liquid at its *open* surface), or adhesion (forces between molecules), or cohesion (the force holding a solid or liquid together by attraction between its molecules). However, there are objections to all these propositions. There is normally no gas in the pleural cavity, and therefore no gas–liquid tension holding the parietal and visceral pleura together. Forces of adhesion and cohesion of the pleural liquid, and between the pleural liquid and the pleural membranes, could only act if the pleural layers were impermeable to liquids and gases, but they are not. Therefore the essential mechanisms that hold the lung and chest wall together appear to be those that keep the pleural cavity free of gas and nearly free of fluid (Section 17.27.2). A mechanism preventing the total removal of the pleural fluid provides the lubrication of the coupling system.

This raises the question, why is there any fluid at all in the pleural cavity? Evidently an additional elastic force, besides that of the lung, is needed to prevent the *complete* removal of pleural fluid. It has been suggested that this force is supplied by the local stretching of the pleural membranes when the amount of fluid has been reduced to the minimum. By lowering the pressure in the pleural fluid, such stretching would oppose the further removal of pleural fluid (Agostoni and Mead, 1964, p. 402).

10.6 Changes in the thoracic diameters during inspiration

The transverse, dorsoventral, and longitudinal diameters of the thoracic cavity are increased by the inspiratory movements of the ribs and diaphragm. The volume of the thoracic cavity will thus be increased, and the lungs will be correspondingly expanded.

10.6.1 *Transverse diameter*

Most of the ribs slope caudolaterally in the resting position, if viewed from a dorsal position (Fig. 10.3B). Therefore a cranial movement of the midpoint of the body of the rib increases the transverse diameter of the thoracic cavity. This widening by swinging the ribs cranially can be simply demonstrated by a bucket with two han-

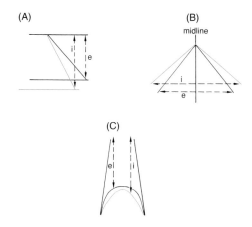

Fig. 10.3 Diagrams summarizing the changing dimensions of the thorax during breathing.

A. Left lateral view of the vertebral column (above) and sternum (below) joined by a rib. During inspiration, inspiratory muscles move the rib cranially to the position shown in green. The distance i exceeds e, showing that the dorsoventral measurement of the thorax increases during inspiration. This is known as the 'pump handle' action of a rib during inspiration.

B. Dorsal view of the vertebral column and one pair of ribs. During inspiration, inspiratory muscles move the ribs cranially to the position shown in green. Distance i exceeds e, showing that the transverse measurement of the thorax increases during inspiration. These widening movements of the two ribs resemble the widening movements of the handles of a two-handled bucket.

C. Dorsal view of the diaphragm in a horizontal section through the thorax. During inspiration, both the tendinous centre and the costal periphery of the diaphragm move caudally to the position shown in green. Distance i exceeds e, showing that the craniocaudal measurement of the thorax increases during inspiration.

dles. The two handles represent a pair of ribs, the two attachments of each handle being the costovertebral and sternocostal articulations. When the bucket is picked up by both handles, the handles come together; when the handles are put down, the distance between them widens.

The increase in the transverse diameter of the thorax opens the costomediastinal recess (Section 9.6.2), allowing the ventral border of the lung to move in.

10.6.2 *Dorsoventral diameter*

The dorsoventral diameter of the thoracic cavity increases during inspiration because of the 'pump handle' movement of the ribs. The essential point is that in the resting position most of the ribs slope caudoventrally, if viewed from a lateral position (Fig. 10.3A). Consequently a cranial movement of the distal end of the rib (the handle of the pump) depresses the sternum ventrally and increases the dorsoventral diameter of the chest (Fig. 10.3A). This ventral movement of the ventral end of the rib during inspiration, and hence of the sternum, can be felt in one's own thorax and is visible, for example, in a dog lying on its side.

The increase in the dorsoventral diameter of the thorax helps the opening of the costomediastinal recess (Section 9.6.2), allowing the ventral border of the lung to move in.

10.6.3 *Craniocaudal diameter*

Straightening of the diaphragm increases the craniocaudal dimension of the thoracic cavity (Fig. 10.3C). This increase is easy to visualize at the tendinous centre of the diaphragm, which moves caudally like a piston. The straightening of the diaphragm also increases the craniocaudal dimension by moving the costal component of the diaphragm caudally, thus opening the costodiaphragmatic recess (Section 9.6.1, Fig. 9.3). At the end of expiration the recess is only a potential space; but when the diaphragm contracts and moves caudally, the recess opens and the basal border of the caudal lobe of the lung pushes in (Section 5.7).

Extensive radiological studies have shown that the tendinous centre of the cupola of man moves caudally

about 1.5 cm in resting breathing and between 7 and 13 cm in deep breathing (Agostoni, 1964, p. 378).

II ACTIONS OF RESPIRATORY MUSCLES

10.7 Evolution of breathing mechanisms

Although the basic mechanics of air flow according to pressure gradients are simple, the expansion of the thorax by the inspiratory muscles was described by Fenn (1964, p. 359) as 'an ingenious engineering feat that only nature could accomplish'. The ribs form the bony framework of the barrel-like thorax, but they lie essentially parallel to the circumference of the barrel. It would seem scarcely possible to expand the circumference of the barrel by the shortening of muscles (such as the intercostal muscles and the costal component of the diaphragm) that more or less encircle its circumference.

One has to resist the anthropocentric temptation to regard the rib cage as 'custom-built' to suit the respiratory requirements of contemporary mammals, including man. On the contrary, the higher vertebrates (mammals, birds, and reptiles) have inherited this bony equipment from fishes which used it to support the body wall and only very rarely sought to use it for breathing. On abandoning the water for a terrestrial habitat, the higher vertebrates had to adapt the ribs as best they could for this new function. Therefore we should not be too surprised at finding the bony attachments and movements of the individual respiratory muscles of mammals to be so complex that their mechanical action cannot, even now, be precisely explained.

The inspiratory muscles are unique in being the only skeletal muscles on which life directly and continuously depends. They have to contract throughout a lifetime, during sleep as well as wakefulness. They are the skeletal muscles that we use the most.

At all times, breathing requires the coordinated contraction of several, and in hyperventilation many, respiratory muscles. The muscles that maintain resting breathing can be called the

principal muscles of respiration. The additional muscles that may come into action during resting breathing in some species, or particularly during hyperventilation, can be known as the accessory muscles of respiration.

The principal muscles of respiration are the **diaphragm** and the **interchondral component of the internal intercostal muscles**. These maintain inspiration in resting breathing in mammals generally. No muscles are used to contract the thoracic cage during expiration in resting breathing (Section 10.12), and therefore *no expiratory muscles are included in the category of principal muscles of respiration*.

The **external intercostal muscles** may contribute to *inspiration* during resting breathing in some mammalian species, and could therefore be classed as principal respiratory muscles, but their main role is probably to contribute during hyperventilation (Section 10.12). In some species other muscles, e.g. **scalenus** in man, participate consistently in resting *inspiration*. The **transverse thoracis** muscle (Section 8.9.2) and **transversus abdominis** muscle are active in resting *expiration* in the dog. These muscles could be classed as principal muscles of respiration, but because they are not active in mammals generally they are considered to be *accessory muscles* (Section 10.10.2).

Difficulties in relating studies on laboratory mammals to those on man were discussed by Decramer (1993). Much of the current knowledge of the mechanics of the respiratory muscles is based on observations on anaesthetized laboratory mammals and on human volunteers, supplemented by pathophysiological observations, particularly on human patients. However, there are rather elemental differences between the thoracic anatomy of man and that of quadrupedal mammals (Section 8.1). These include: dorsoventral flattening of the thorax in man, as opposed to lateral flattening in quadrupeds, and consequent differences in the curvatures and angles of the ribs and therefore of the geometry of the ribs; upright as opposed to horizontal posture; and varying stiffness, i.e. compliance, of the rib cage (the rib cage of man is more rigid, i.e. has lower compliance, than that of laboratory mammals; Section 10.11). Therefore it is doubtful whether these findings can be fully transposed from dog to man (Agostoni, 1964, p. 382) or vice versa. Nevertheless, Decramer (1993) concluded that 'the general pattern of motion of the chest wall is similar between upright humans and supine anaesthetized dogs'.

Electromyography has revealed the respiratory role of muscles attached to the thorax (Hildebrandt, 1974, p. 299). However, electromyographic activity in a particular muscle during, for example, inspiration does not prove that this muscle directly enlarges the thorax, i.e.

that it is an agonistic inspiratory muscle; its action may be only to regulate the action of other, truly agonistic, inspiratory muscles. Thus muscular activity synchronous with breathing may be a **consequence** of breathing rather than a cause (Agostoni, 1964, pp. 379, 382).

The evolution of **breathing mechanisms in vertebrates** was reviewed by Randall *et al.* (1981, p. 104). The earliest vertebrates were **fish**, using a buccal pump to force water by positive pressure from the buccal cavity and through the gills. Hypoxic water caused some fish to move to the air–water interface, where the buccal pump could also be used to force air into a gas bladder (*Lepidosteus*) or a primitive lung (Dipnoi, lungfish). At about the same time (pre-Devonian), some fish experimented with negative pressure breathing (aspiratory breathing). In this mechanism, the fish sucks air into the gas bladder by arching its back dorsally as it pokes its mouth through the surface of the water; this movement spreads the ribs and thus enlarges the body cavity – an inspiratory mechanism used to this day by man when making a maximal inspiration (Section 10.10.1). The buccal pump is still retained in such fish to force water through the gills. A modern example is found in the pirarucu (*Arapaima gigas*), which cannot survive if denied access to air.

The buccal pump is retained in **anuran** (tail-less) **amphibians** (frogs and toads). Some early amphibians may have ventilated their lungs by negative pressure. **Early reptiles** adopted aspiration breathing, thus increasing their ventilation rate and opening the way to a higher metabolism. Modern **chelonian reptiles** (turtles and tortoises) use negative pressure, but being enclosed in a carapace have abandoned movable ribs and inflate the lungs by enlarging the body cavity through extruding their limbs. **Crocodiles** have well-developed ribs and intercostal muscles, but inflate the lungs by pulling the liver caudally, a piston-like movement foreshadowing the caudal movement of the mammalian diaphragm; doubtless their intercostal muscles are used in the swift writhing movements of the trunk. **Lizards** do use their intercostal muscles for inspiration and expiration. In **snakes** a pair of ribs articulates with every vertebra (except the first three, in some species), though there is no sternum; the intercostal muscles can generate regional expansion of the body wall and thus inflate the lung or lungs within. **Birds** inflate their airsacs by expanding the rib cage through the action of intercostal muscles and accessory respiratory muscles. No sub-mammalian vertebrate has a structure homologous to the mammalian diaphragm (King and McLelland, 1984, pp. 136–137).

10.8 Inspiratory actions of the diaphragm

The diaphragm is much the most important inspiratory muscle in mammals. It is innervated by the phrenic nerve (Section 8.17.3). During **resting breathing** it generates almost all of the tidal volume. In the **hyperventilation of exercise**, it accounts for about 70% of the tidal volume (Section 10.11).

Nevertheless, although it is very much the dominant inspiratory muscle, the diaphragm is not essential for inspiration. If the diaphragm is paralysed the **vital capacity** (Fig. 10.5) is greatly reduced (Section 10.11), but the inspiratory intercostal muscles (Section 10.9) and accessory inspiratory muscles (Section 10.10.1) maintain **resting breathing** without signs of hypoventilation; the maximum **hyperventilation** in response to **exercise** will, however, be substantially reduced.

The diaphragm works through the integrated contraction of its two muscular components, i.e. its lumbar and costal components (Section 8.11). This integrated contraction has two inspiratory actions. Firstly, it moves the tendinous centre of the cupola caudally in a piston-like action. This increases the **craniocaudal** dimension of the thorax (Fig. 10.3C), including opening the costodiaphragmatic recess (Section 10.6.3).

Secondly, contraction of the diaphragm increases the **transverse** and **dorsoventral** diameters (Fig. 10.3A,B) of the **caudal part** of the thoracic cage. This second action depends on firmly fixing the position of the cupola, so that it cannot continue to move caudally. Such fixation is achieved by increasing the **intra-abdominal pressure**, to the point where it prevents any further movement of the cupola caudally.

Caudal movement of the cupola in itself compresses the abdominal viscera and raises the intra-abdominal pressure. On the other hand, active **contraction of the abdominal muscles** (Section 10.10) can achieve and maintain a large rise in intra-abdominal pressure in the normal animal.

Once the cupola is fixed by a sustained increase in intra-abdominal pressure, the muscle fibres of the costal component of the diaphragm can reverse their action. Figure 8.25 shows that the *functional direction* of the fibres of the costal component is **craniodorsal**, from the caudal ribs to the tendinous centre, if the attachment of the costal component to the ribs is fixed and the tendinous centre is free to move; the craniodorsal direction of the fibres causes the tendinous centre

to move *caudally*. However, if the central tendon is fixed (by intra-abdominal pressure) and the ribs are free to move, the *functional* direction of the fibres changes to **caudoventral**; the costal component then reverses its action and pulls the caudal ribs *craniolaterally* (Section 8.11.4). This craniolateral movement of the ribs has a strong inspiratory action by increasing the transverse and dorsoventral diameters of the caudal half of the thorax.

The mechanisms by which diaphragmatic contraction might expand the thoracic wall, and how diaphragmatic contraction interacts with the inspiratory intercostal muscles, are complex and still debated (Agostoni, 1964, p. 380; Derenne *et al.*, 1978, p. 382). The craniodorsal slope of the costal component of the diaphragmatic musculature (Fig. 8.25), and the certainty that these fibres must therefore produce a force *capable* of expanding the *caudal part* of the rib cage (Section 8.11.4), have been recognized for centuries. Galen (AD 130–200) experimentally eliminated all other inspiratory muscles and found that isolated contraction of the diaphragm does indeed expand the caudal part of the thorax; Vesalius (1514–1564) explicitly reached the same conclusion from anatomical reasoning (Derenne *et al.*, 1978, p. 122). Only in the last two centuries, however, has the significance of *intra-abdominal pressure* in the expansion of the rib cage been appreciated.

The extent to which the inspiratory contraction of the diaphragm **expands the rib cage** in **resting breathing** and **hyperventilation** varies between the species, within individuals of the same species as in man (Williams *et al.*, 1989, p. 595), and with posture. In resting breathing, such expansion should be most obvious along the costal arch. In **man** some expansion is indeed normally apparent in the region of the costal arch, and even in the cranial part of the lateral thoracic wall as well. (Decramer, 1993).

On the other hand, in the **cat** asleep on its side, the *whole* of the lateral thoracic wall, as far caudally as the costal arch, tends to move *medially* (i.e. in the *expiratory* direction) during each **inspiration** at the same time as the abdominal wall bulges *outwards*; however, this rather puzzling expiratory (medially directed) movement is explicable by the fall in pleural pressure caused by the caudal movement of the diaphragmatic cupola, which sucks the lateral thoracic wall inwards. It is presumed to occur mainly in species with a particularly flexible thorax, i.e. *with high thoracic wall compliance*, such as the cat and rabbit (Section 10.2.1) (Derenne *et al.*, 1978a,b, pp. 123, 383).

Any such *expiratory* movement of the thoracic wall caused by the diaphragm during each *inspiration*, must be inefficient and is therefore essentially unwanted. In resting breathing, it appears to be minimized or prevented, depending on the species, by activity of the *in-*

spiratory intercostal muscles (i.e. the external intercostal and interchondral component of the internal intercostal muscles; Section 10.11). In hyperventilation it ought to be eliminated altogether, presumably by powerful contraction of the inspiratory intercostal muscles, but the details of such a mechanism are uncertain.

The caudal movement of the cupola is believed to achieve **expansion** of the **caudal** part of the rib cage by two independent mechanisms (Decramer, 1993). Firstly, the *craniodorsal slope* of the *costal* component of the diaphragmatic musculature causes active expansion of the caudal part of the rib cage (as already described). Secondly, the rise in *intra-abdominal pressure* caused by the caudal movement of the cupola pushes the costal part of the diaphragm against the caudal part of the rib cage, and thus passively expands it. Thus the more the diaphragm is prevented by intra-abdominal pressure from moving caudally, the greater is the tendency for it to displace the caudal ribs craniolaterally and thus expand the caudal half of the rib cage. Intra-abdominal pressure is the effective agent (Derenne *et al.*, 1978, p. 123).

In the normal human subject, expansion of the rib cage in resting breathing is achieved not by the diaphragm alone, but by the co-ordinated action (Section 10.11) of the diaphragm and the **inspiratory intercostal muscles** (Decramer, 1993).

The diaphragm can inspire more air when it both moves the tendinous centre of the diaphragm caudally *and* expands the rib cage by means of its costal component, than when it only moves its centre caudally into the abdomen, at least in man. Thus when the greatest possible effort is made to obtain a **single maximal inspiration**, the ventrodorsal dimension of the abdomen is sharply *reduced* (as can be observed on oneself); the tendinous centre of the diaphragm must then move *cranially* to compensate for the decreased ventrodorsal depth of the abdomen – yet the further expansion of the thorax resulting from this cranial movement of the diaphragm brings in the greatest possible volume of air (Fenn, 1964, p. 359). It is virtually impossible to check observations of this kind on quadrupedal animals, since it is unrewarding to ask a dog, let alone a rabbit, to make a single maximal inspiration.

Fenn finally re-emphasized that, during '*normal*' (i.e. resting) breathing, the caudal movement of the diaphragm *does* cause protrusion of the abdomen in man, and it *does* account 'for a large fraction of the inspired air'. Decramer (1993) confirmed that there is evidence that in man 'downward (caudal) diaphragmatic displacement accommodates considerably more volume than lower rib cage expansion', although 'it is difficult to estimate their relative contributions'.

Incidentally, the old idea that men breathe with the abdomen and women with the thorax – doubtless a profitable theory for the corset industry – is incorrect: the mechanisms are the same in both sexes (Derenne *et al.*, 1978, p. 122).

Pathological changes in the abdomen, such as peritoneal effusion or a large tumour, raise the intra-abdominal pressure or directly obstruct the caudal movement of the tendinous centre of the diaphragm during inspiration. The result is that increased expansion of the lateral thoracic wall during inspiration then becomes a diagnostic sign (Section 23.4.1). A similar change in the respiratory movements occurs in pregnancy and excessive obesity.

Posture can be an important factor in breathing (Section 6.30.2). At the 1998 Conference of the Horse Race Betting Levy Board, Dr. Lesley Young pointed out that general anaesthesia is a dangerous procedure for horses since they are heavy animals not designed to lie down for long periods, especially on their backs. In this position the lungs are compressed, thus compromising the ability to breathe. This is believed to contribute to the relatively high perioperative mortality in horses compared to that of other domestic species.

To summarize, in mammals generally the diaphragm is the main factor in the expansion of the lung during resting breathing and hyperventilation. Its contraction causes (1) a caudal movement of the cupola, (2) an increase in intra-abdominal pressure, (3) an inspiratory expansion of the caudal region of the thoracic cage, (4) a decrease in pleural pressure, and (5) if the thoracic cage is compliant, an expiratory contraction of the cranial part of the cage though this may be largely cancelled by the action of inspiratory intercostal muscles.

10.9   Inspiratory actions of intercostal muscles

The **external intercostal muscles** lie between successive ribs, but not between the costal cartilages. The **internal intercostal muscles** have an **interosseous** component that lies between successive ribs, *and* an **interchondral** component situated between the costal cartilages (Section 8.9.1, Fig. 8.23). The intercostal muscles are innervated by the intercostal nerves (Section 8.17.2).

The fibres of the **external intercostal muscles** slope *caudoventrally* (Fig. 8.23). Theoretically each external intercostal muscle should exert a greater **torque** (or moment of force) on the more *caudal* of the two ribs on which it acts (Fig. 10.4B). (For a definition of torque, see Fig. 10.4A.) Therefore it should pull the *caudal* rib *cranially*. Consequently the **external** intercostal muscles are **inspiratory** muscles (Fig. 10.3A,B).

The slope of the **internal intercostal** fibres is *caudodorsal*. The *torque* of the **interosseous** com-

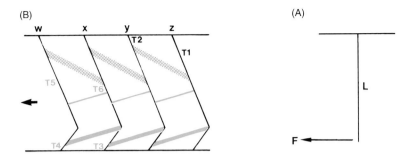

Fig. 10.4   Torque from action of intercostal muscles on ribs. A. A rod is hinged at its upper end on a body represented by the upper horizontal line. The torque, T, is a measure of the tendency of a force to rotate the body to which it is applied. The torque on the rod, $T = F \times L$, where F is the magnitude of the force and L is the perpendicular distance from the line of action of the force to the axis of rotation.

B. Highly schematic left lateral view diagram of four ribs, w, x, y, z, articulating dorsally with the vertebral column (upper horizontal line) and ventrally, via intercostal cartilages, with the sternum (lower horizontal line). The ribs are acted on by external intercostal muscles (black stipple) and internal intercostal muscles (green). An internal intercostal muscle comprises a feeble interosseous component (thin green line) and a strong interchondral component (thick green line). An intercostal muscle applies its force to two ribs, one cranial to it and the other caudal to it. Which of the two ribs will move depends on the torque exerted on each rib. The torque (T1) exerted by an external intercostal muscle on its **caudal** rib is greater than the torque (T2) exerted on its cranial rib; thus T1 moves rib z **cranially**. Moving the rib cranially increases the diameters of the rib cage (Fig. 10.3A), and therefore the external intercostal muscle is an **inspiratory** muscle. The torque (T3) exerted by the *interchondral* component of an internal intercostal muscle on its **caudal** rib is again greater than that exerted on its cranial rib (T4), and thus T3 moves rib X **cranially**. Therefore the *interchondral* component of an internal intercostal muscle is again **inspiratory**. The torque (T5) exerted by the *interosseous* component of an internal intercostal muscle on its **cranial** rib is greater than that exerted on its caudal rib (T6); thus T5 moves rib w caudally. Moving the rib caudally decreases the diameters of the rib cage, and therefore the *interosseous* component of an internal intercostal muscle is **expiratory**. The arrow points cranially.

ponent of the internal intercostal muscle is greater on the more *cranial* of the two ribs on which the muscle acts (Fig. 10.4B), and therefore it should pull this rib *caudally*. Consequently the **interosseous component** of the **internal intercostal** muscle is **expiratory**. Since the slope of the fibres in the interosseous part of the internal intercostal muscles is the opposite to that of the external intercostal muscles, it is to be expected that the action of these two muscles would be antagonistic.

The fibres of the **interchondral** component of the internal intercostal muscle also slope caudodorsally. Their *torque* is greater on the more *caudal* of the two costal cartilages on which they act (Fig. 10.4B). Therefore they should pull this cartilage *cranially*. Consequently the **interchondral** components of the internal intercostal muscles are **inspiratory**.

The analysis of torque explains how the **interosseous** and **interchondral** components of the

internal intercostal muscle can have the same slope and yet diametrically opposite actions. This surprising contrast can be examined in another way, i.e. by considering whether each muscle relates to the vertebral column or to the sternum. The fibres of the interchondral muscle may have the same direction as those of the interosseous component, but the action of the interchondral part has to be referred to the sternum and not to the vertebral column. The geometric relationship between the interchondral component and the sternum is similar to that between the external intercostal fibres and the vertebral column; consequently, both of them are inspiratory.

The **interchondral components** of the internal intercostal muscle ('parasternal intercostals', p. 197) are, in fact, the most important inspiratory element of the intercostal muscles. They are active during **resting breathing**, but account for only a small fraction of the inspired air. On the other hand, in **hyperventilation** as in **exercise** they are recruited and make a more substantial contribution to inspiration. The integration of the intercostal muscles into the overall muscular activities of inspiration is considered in Section 10.11.

If the intercostal muscles are paralysed, the **diaphragm** maintains **resting breathing** without difficulty; and in **hyperventilation** there is little decrease in exercise tolerance.

Terms used to describe the changes in lung volume during breathing are shown in Fig. 10.5.

For nearly 2000 years, since the time of Galen to the present day, the respiratory actions of the intercostal muscles have been the subject of lively controversy (Agostoni, 1964, p. 381). Participation in either expiration or inspiration was argued by some authorities, but others maintained that these muscles make no important contributions at all to respiratory movements, and merely prevent the intercostal spaces from being sucked in and out during breathing. As an anatomist, Krahl (1964, p. 237) pointed out that the latter action could be carried out adequately and at less energetic cost by fibrous membranes. He also noted that the combined length of the strips of external and internal intercostal muscles in man is nearly 20 metres, with a total mass greater than that of the gluteal muscles, and pointed out that such muscles would be an intolerable energetic extravagance if they did not do what other muscles do – control movement.

The complexity of rib movements defies the precise anatomical and geometrical analysis of the mechanical action of the intercostal muscles (Agostoni, 1964, p. 381). The analysis on the basis of torque (as in this section) is known as **Hamberger's theory** (published in Latin in 1748). It is plainly a simplification: for instance, according to such simple geometrical considerations the same group of muscles, for example the external intercostals, should have an opposing action at various points along the rib (Fenn, 1964, p. 359); thus it may be inspiratory along the proximal half of the rib where its action clearly relates to the vertebral column, but expiratory along the distal half of the rib where its action may relate to the sternum. This suggests that the intercostal muscles may work against themselves. Actually, this is not as improbable as it sounds. Calculations of the work of the external and internal intercostals on both sides of the body give a value similar to the total work of the respiratory apparatus; since the movements of the rib cage account for only a minor part of the vital capacity, the force of the intercostals must be applied very inefficiently.

Nevertheless, Hamberger's theory is in **general** agreement with most of the experimental work, and especially with electromyographic findings in man (Agostoni, 1964, p. 381).

10.10 Accessory muscles of respiration

The **accessory muscles** of respiration are those that do not consistently contribute to resting breathing, but become active during hyperventilation or disease. Some of these muscles are **accessory inspiratory muscles** and others are **expiratory muscles**.

10.10.1 Accessory inspiratory muscles

The **external intercostal muscles** are inspiratory, but are probably only intermittently active in **resting breathing**, and are therefore regarded as accessory inspiratory muscles.

In the **hyperventilation** of exercise, the external intercostal and parasternal intercostal muscles become strongly active. Several muscles that run from the neck or vertebral column to the thoracic wall also act as accessory inspiratory muscles (Section 8.8).

Any inspiratory intercostal activity in resting breathing, including that in the **interchondral components** of the **internal intercostal muscles** (the parasternal muscles), is probably not designed to expand the rib cage; its function is probably to resist unwanted expiratory movement resulting from the fall in pleural pressure created by the inspiratory action of the diaphragm (Section 10.8) (Derenne *et al.*, 1978, p. 382).

In distressed breathing (dyspnoea) in **respiratory disease**, yet other muscles that run from the forelimbs to the thoracic wall are also recruited. To achieve this an unusual posture may be adopted (Section 23.4.1).

Almost any muscle of the many that are attached to the lateral or ventral thoracic wall is potentially a respiratory muscle (Section 8.9.2), but only five are known to contribute substantially to inspiration. These are the external intercostal (Section 8.9.1), scalenus, sternocleidomastoid, levatores costarum muscles (Section 8.9.2), and the epaxial vertebral muscles (Section 8.8).

The **external intercostal muscles** (Section 8.9.1) are generally agreed to be inspiratory in action (Section 10.9), but there are differences of opinion as to whether they are consistently or only intermittently active during resting inspiration. They may therefore be regarded as accessory inspiratory muscles (Decramer, 1993). See also Section 10.11.

The **scalenus muscles** (Section 8.9.2) are invariably active in resting inspiration in man, and are likely to contribute to expansion of the thorax, but since they only attach to the first two ribs their contribution to inspiration would presumably be less than that of the parasternal intercostal muscles; they are not active in inspiration in the supine anaesthetized dog (Decramer, 1993).

The **sternocleidomastoid muscle** (Section 8.9.2) is not active in resting inspiration in normal persons, but in moderate inspiratory efforts and hyperventilation it does contract (Agostoni, 1964, p. 383; Decramer, 1993). In hyperventilation in man, the pivotal movement of the first rib (Section 8.9.2) allows the sternocleidomastoid muscle to swing the sternum cranioventrally, thus increasing the dorsoventral diameter of the thorax (Williams *et al.*, 1989, p. 498). In tetraplegic patients it is active and becomes greatly hypertrophied, and may even be able to sustain breathing alone for a time. This is probably the most important accessory muscle of inspiration, at least in man. There is some evidence that ventilation in the dog can be maintained by neck and shoulder muscles only (Agostoni, 1964, p. 383).

The **levatores costarum muscles** (Section 8.9.2) are active during resting inspiration in the dog and cat, and may be active in the caudal segments of the thoracic wall during resting inspiration in man (Decramer, 1993).

The **epaxial vertebral muscles**, e.g. longissimus thoracis (Section 8.8), contribute significantly to a very deep inspiration in man by dorsally arching the back, thus spreading the ribs and hence increasing the craniocaudal dimensions of the thorax (Krahl, 1964, p. 234). This is probably the most primitive inspiratory mechanism of all, since it is shared with air-breathing fish where it represents the first attempt at the evolution of mechanisms for breathing air instead of water (see Section 10.7).

The remaining accessory respiratory muscles with possible inspiratory actions include the **serratus dorsalis cranialis**, **serratus ventralis thoracis**, **latissimus dorsi**, **pectorales**, and **subclavius muscles** (Section 8.9.2). These sometimes show inspiratory activity, but normally their contribution to inspiration is probably negligible (Agostoni, 1964, p. 384). However, in respiratory distress (**dyspnoea**) from pulmonary disease, man and quadrupedal mammals can bring these accessory muscles into play by adopting an unusual posture (Section 23.4). By planting its front feet firmly apart and abducting its elbows, a quadrupedal animal can employ the pectoral muscles for inspiration. The human patient can grasp the arms of a chair or the sides of a bed, and then use the serratus ventralis thoracis (m. serratus anterior) to expand the rib cage (Krahl, 1964, p. 234). A dyspnoeic man or quadrupedal mammal may also extend its neck so that neck muscles (scalenus and sternocleidomastoid) can exert greater forces on the rib cage. Arching the back dorsally by the epaxial vertebral muscles spreads the ribs. Sitting upright shifts the abdominal viscera caudally, thus enhancing the caudal movement of the diaphragm in dyspnoeic man and domestic mammals.

10.10.2 *Expiratory muscles*

In principle, during **resting breathing** the expiratory muscles make no contribution to expiration, which is performed entirely passively by the combined forces of **lung recoil**, **thoracic wall recoil**, and **abdominal recoil** (Section 10.2.2).

During **hyperventilation** in **exercise** the expiratory muscles cause a substantial increase in ventilation. The **abdominal muscles** (Section 8.10) are by far the most powerful and important of the expiratory muscles (Section 10.12). Their contraction raises the intra-abdominal pressure and forces the cupola of the diaphragm cranially. Also the fibres of the oblique abdominal muscles are so orientated (Figs 8.20, 8.21, 8.22) that they pull the ribs *caudally* in a strongly expiratory movement.

The **interosseous component** of the **internal intercostal muscles** is another expiratory muscle, but it has relatively little functional importance.

When ventilation increases, as in exercise, muscles of expiration are progressively recruited. The **abdominal muscles** (Agostoni, 1964, p. 382) then become powerfully active in expiration. It is not clear what each individual muscle contributes (Decramer, 1993), but the **transversus abdominis** is probably the most important; indeed there is evidence that this muscle may even be regularly active during resting breathing in the anaesthetized and conscious dog (Decramer, 1993). Contraction of the abdominal muscles raises the intra-abdominal pressure, thus forcing the cupola of the diaphragm cranially, and simultaneously draws the more caudal ribs dorsocaudally (Agostoni, 1964, p. 382) thus reducing the transverse and dorsoventral dimensions of the thorax. The **rectus abdominis** compresses the abdomen, and draws the sternum caudally (Agostoni, 1964, p. 382), countering the inspiratory action of the sternocleidomastoid or sternomastoid muscle.

The **interosseous component** of the **internal intercostal muscle** becomes active during hyperventilation, during the later half of expiration (Agostoni, 1964, p. 382).

Although the **transversus thoracis muscle** (Section 8.9) is active in conscious and anaesthetized dogs during resting breathing, in man it only becomes active during forced expiration (Decramer, 1993).

10.11 Coordination of muscle actions during inspiration

The expansion of the lung during normal **resting breathing** is accomplished almost entirely by contraction of the diaphragm (Section 10.8).

In the **hyperventilation** of exercise, and in obstructive respiratory disease (Section 7.17) or bronchoconstriction (Section 7.20), the diaphragm and parasternal muscles progressively increase their activity, and the external intercostal muscles are recruited as well. In maximal ventilation a whole array of accessory inspiratory muscles may contribute (Section 10.10.1).

The coordination of **intercostal inspiratory activity** during resting breathing with the inspiratory action of the diaphragm is controversial even in man, despite intensive studies (Derenne *et al.*, 1978, p. 382). It is suggested that the diaphragm is the only important *contracting* (shortening) muscle. There is regular inspiratory activity in the **interchondral** components of the **internal intercostal muscles** (the **parasternal muscles**), and there may be some inspiratory activity in the **external intercostal muscles**. However, these inspiratory intercostal muscles are not primarily agonistic (shortening) but are mainly *fixating* in function, the purpose of their fixating action being to prevent unwanted motion. The unwanted motion is the inward, i.e. *expiratory*, distortion of the *cranial* part of the thoracic cage during the inspiratory movement of the diaphragm (Section 10.8). As already stated, this inward movement is caused by the fall in pleural pressure that is generated by the inspiratory movement of the diaphragm.

The fixating action of the parasternal and external intercostal muscles is believed to act on the *cranial* part of the thoracic cage in resting breathing, and this is supported by several lines of evidence. Firstly, the inspiratory activity of the parasternal muscles is confined to the *first four* intercostal segments (in man) (Derenne *et al.*, 1978, p. 382); and that of the external intercostals (in the dog) also occurs mainly in the more *cranial* intercostal spaces (Decramer, 1993). Secondly, supporting evidence comes from clinical observations. During most respiratory manoeuvres in a normal conscious human subject, the caudal part of the thoracic cage expands and the cranial part is **not** displaced inwards but clearly expands (Decramer, 1993). However, in human subjects under spinal anaesthesia up to T1, and in tetraplegic patients in which the function of the diaphragm has survived, the *cranial* part of the rib cage *does* move inwards during diaphragmatic contraction while the *caudal* part moves outwards: this shows that, in the normal human subject, expansion of the rib cage is achieved not by the diaphragm alone but by the coordination of the agonistic action of the diaphragm and the fixating action of other primary inspiratory muscles, especially the **interchondral component** of the **internal intercostal muscles** (Decramer, 1993).

Evidently the fixating action of the inspiratory intercostal muscles in man is effective. But thoracic wall compliance (Section 10.2.1) is relatively low in man (Crosfill

and Widdicombe, 1961; Derenne *et al.*, 1978, p. 123) and very low in the horse (Koterba *et al.*, 1988) so in these species thoracic distortion may be quite readily prevented by the fixating action of accessory inspiratory muscles. In the small laboratory mammals, and to a lesser extent in the cat and dog, thoracic wall compliance is relatively high (Crosfill and Widdicombe, 1961); the fixating action of the inspiratory intercostal muscles during resting breathing is apparently less effective in these species, since thoracic distortion does occur in resting breathing.

In the hyperventilation of **exercise** in man, the diaphragmatic electromyogram increases linearly as the minute volume rises to 50–60 litres min^{-1} (Derenne *et al.*, 1978, p. 383), with the increased activity and synchronization of **motor units** (Williams *et al.*, 1989, p. 595); the motor units of the diaphragm are small, as in muscles of precision (Section 8.17.3). (For definition of motor units see Vol. 1 in this series on the CNS; King, 1987.) Active **external intercostal muscles** are progressively recruited in the more caudal intercostal spaces as ventilation increases (Agostoni, 1964, p. 382), and presumably the **parasternal intercostals** increase their activity too (Derenne *et al.*, 1978, p. 383). Thus, as hyperventilation advances with the onset of moderate to heavy exercise, the inspiratory intercostal muscles not only continue their fixating function, but also extend their activity into strong agonistic inspiratory actions on the rib cage; in all probability, inspiratory movements of the **costal component** of the diaphragm augment this action on the rib cage, though this seems to be speculative. At a minute volume of 30 litres min^{-1}, the **scalene** and **sternocleidomastoid muscles** become consistently active (Derenne *et al.*, 1978, p. 383). In maximal hyperventilation the whole array of accessory inspiratory muscles may come into action (Section 10.10.1).

A minute volume of less than 50 litres min^{-1} (i.e. about eight times the resting minute volume) is regarded as characteristic of mild to moderate exercise in man, and more than 50 litres min^{-1} as moderate to severe exercise (Hildebrandt, 1974, p. 299).

In man the maximal ventilation is reduced by only 20–30% when the thorax is enclosed in a plaster cast (Comroe, 1975, p. 96). This appears to indicate very roughly the maximum contribution to inspiration by the combined efforts of the intercostal muscles and accessory respiratory muscles, the diaphragm contributing the remaining 70–80%. Calculations based on thoracic circumference and diaphragmatic excursion give a similar value for the diaphragmatic contribution to breathing, i.e. about 70% of the vital capacity (Agostoni, 1964, p. 378).

Although the diaphragm is very much the dominant inspiratory muscle, it is not essential for inspiration (Comroe, 1975, p. 95). If the diaphragm is paralysed the other inspiratory muscles take over, both the **interchondral component** of the **internal intercostal muscle** and the **external intercostal muscles** presumably playing a major role. A man with bilateral paralysis of the diaphragm but otherwise normal respiratory musculature has a vital capacity, when lying down, of about 33% of the normal value, confirming the rough estimate that the diaphragm normally contributes about 70%; in the standing position, with gravity to promote a caudal displacement of the diaphragm, the vital capacity is about 50% of normal (Hildebrandt, 1974, p. 298). Despite these reductions of vital capacity in the presence of diaphragmatic paralysis, hypoventilation does not occur during resting breathing provided that the thorax is otherwise normal (Comroe, 1975, p. 95).

If the intercostal muscles alone are paralysed, the diaphragm copes well, with little decrease in **exercise** tolerance (Comroe, 1975, p. 96).

10.12   Coordination of expiratory forces

During **resting breathing** the main forces that cause expiration (Section 10.2.2) are those of, (i) lung recoil (E + ST in Fig. 10.1C), (ii) thoracic wall recoil (L2 in Fig. 10.1), and (iii) a further small force of abdominal recoil.

These are all energy storing systems. Muscular work, done on the thoracic walls during inspiration, stores energy in the elastic fibres of the elastic continuum and surface tension of the lung (Section 6.9), and in the costal articulations. When the force of the inspiratory muscles ceases at the end of inspiration, this stored energy is released as expiration. The diaphragm compresses the gases and tissues in the gastrointestinal tract and stretches the abdominal wall; when inspiration ends, this stored energy drives the diaphragm back into the thorax, enhancing expiration. Thus the energetics of resting breathing are principally inspiratory.

Expiratory muscles make no contribution to expiration during resting breathing, but at **moderate exercise** they begin to participate. During the **hyperventilation** of **heavy exercise**, and in **obstructive respiratory disease**, the expiratory muscles, notably the abdominal muscles, play a major role in expiration. The abdominal muscles achieve this by forcing the diaphragm into the thorax and pulling the caudal part of the rib cage dorso-caudally (Section 10.10.2).

The strong action of the expiratory muscles during **hyperventilation** in **heavy exercise** compresses the conducting airways, and thus increases the resistance to airflow. A critical point may be reached where compression of the airways makes expiratory flow slower instead of faster, thus limiting the ventilatory capacity during maximal exercise.

In severe **obstructive respiratory disease** (Sections 7.17, 7.20), compression of the airways during forced expiration by means of the expiratory muscles may set fatal limits on the efforts to maintain adequate ventilation during resting respiration.

The volume of gas in the abdomen is regarded as normally negligible compared with the total volume of the abdomen in man (Agostoni and Mead, 1964, p. 394), but in herbivores it may be relatively greater and might therefore contribute to the force of abdominal recoil.

In resting breathing, the diaphragm and interchondral intercostal muscles continue to be active during the first two thirds of the expiratory phase, thus serving as a brake on expiratory flow (Derenne *et al.*, 1978, p. 383). In this way the inspiratory muscles 'let the system down gently', including in moderate exercise where the inspiratory muscles still act well into the expiratory phase (Mead and Agostoni, 1964, p. 422).

Mead and Agostoni (1964, pp. 421–423) reviewed breathing in man at **exercise**. The participation of the expiratory muscles during **hyperventilation** begins in **moderate exercise** at a minute volume of about 40 litres min^{-1}, appearing first in the last part of expiration. At a minute volume of about 45 litres min^{-1}, the tidal volume is increased to about 1500 ml (about three times the resting value of about 450–500 ml); but this increase takes place entirely in the **inspiratory phase**, and the lung volume at the end of expiration (i.e. the functional residual capacity, Fig. 10.5) remains near the resting value. Therefore the contribution of the expiratory muscles to the increase in minute volume is presumably to accelerate flow rate during expiration. The interosseous components of the internal intercostal muscles probably contribute to this supplementation of expiration.

In **heavy exercise** a fit young man can achieve a minute volume of up to 120 litres min^{-1} (West, 1975, p. 127). At a minute volume of 113 litres min^{-1} (Mead and Agostoni, 1964, p. 422), the tidal volume is increased to about 2300 ml (i.e. about four times the resting value, and one half of the vital capacity), but now the increase occurs in the **expiratory phase** as well as the inspiratory phase; moreover the pleural pressure rises above atmospheric during expiration, and is presumed to be close to levels where compression of the airways would become appreciable (Mead and Agostoni, 1964, p. 422). These are clear indications that the expiratory muscles are now participating in the expiratory effort, i.e. the **abdominal muscles** in particular (Section 8.10) and in some species the **transversus thoracis** (Section 10.10.2). The expiratory muscles are therefore important reserves that are brought into action during strong hyperventilation (Decramer, 1993).

The rise of pleural pressure above atmospheric is the key to the **critical upper limit** of ventilation during **extreme exercise**. An increase of the expiratory driving pressure above atmospheric compresses the conducting airways, and thus increases the resistance to airflow. Since the resistance is inversely proportional to the fourth power of the internal radius of the airway, a small reduction in airway diameter induces a large rise in resistance (Section 6.14). A critical point is reached in hyperventilation, where a rising pleural pressure, caused by extreme muscular expiratory effort to achieve yet faster flow during expiration, eventually has the opposite effect to that desired, i.e. it makes expiratory flow slower not faster. Thus dynamic compression of the conducting airways, and not muscular effort, sets the single most important limit on ventilatory capacity during maximum exercise (Mead and Agostoni, 1964, p. 418).

In **respiratory disease**, the *expiratory* flow is again the weakest link. Forced inspiration tends to *dilate* the conducting airways. But, in severe obstructive respiratory disease (Sections 7.17, 7.20), the *resistance* to airflow during strong expiratory efforts is *increased* by compression of the airways; the resistance to airflow may then reach the critical limit where it prevents any further increase in ventilation needed to maintain an adequate resting ventilation.

10.13   The energetic cost of breathing

The total energetic cost of breathing is the oxygen consumption of the respiratory muscles, but it is impossible to measure this directly. Therefore the total oxygen consumption of the body is measured during progressively increasing levels of ventilation (minute volume), and it is assumed that the corresponding step-like increases in oxygen consumption represent the energetic cost of each increment in ventilation.

The muscles of breathing perform work against two main forces: (i) the combined forces of lung recoil, thoracic recoil, and abdominal recoil, and (ii) the forces of airway resistance to gas flow (Section 6.14).

During **resting breathing** in the normal healthy subject, far more energy is expended on the first

of these two forces than on the second. The total energetic cost of the respiratory muscles during resting breathing is very low (only about 2–3% of the total resting metabolism).

In the **hyperventilation** of heavy **exercise**, the energetic cost may rise to 10% of the total metabolism. Large volumes of air must be shifted at very high velocity, and consequently most of the energy is expended on overcoming airway resistance. Furthermore, the powerful action of the expiratory muscles (particularly the abdominal muscles) raises the pleural pressure, and this *compresses* the conducting airways thus increasing the airway resistance still further (Section 10.12). Theoretically, there should be a critical limit in extreme muscular exercise beyond which any further effort to increase oxygen uptake will be offset by the increased oxygen consumption of the respiratory muscles (as may happen in very severe pulmonary disease). Normally, however, the limiting factor in exercise is likely to be oxygen transport, i.e. cardiac output, not oxygen uptake.

In **lung diseases** causing severe obstruction of the airways (Sections 7.17, 7.20), or extensive collagenous replacement of the elastic fibres of the lung (Section 7.19), or worse still both of these conditions together, the energetic cost of breathing may rise to one third of the total metabolism. Compression of the airways during forced expiration adds greatly to the problem. Eventually the respiratory muscles may use more oxygen than they bring in: this leads to death.

In addition to the forces of elastic recoil and airway resistance, the muscles of breathing work against two other forces. The first is variously described as 'the non-elastic deformation of tissue' (Otis, 1964, p. 465), 'the frictional resistance to motion of the lung tissues' (Tenney, 1977, p. 179), and 'the viscosity of the lung and chest wall structures' or 'tissue resistance' (Guyton, 1986, p. 469). The first of these expressions seems the most meaningful since its essential word is '**non-elastic**'. As noted in Section 6.9, elasticity in the strict physical sense is the property of a material to resume its original dimensions when the forces acting on it are removed: compliance is the property of being deformed under stress. The elastic fibres in the lung and thoracic walls meet the criterion of elasticity, but other tissues do not, yet are compliant. For example, the muscles on the outside of the thoracic wall, such as the pectoralis muscles, are required to be compliant when the thorax changes its shape during inspiration and expiration, but have low elasticity. Work is expended in deforming a ball of plasticine, and so it is when changing the shape of a muscle or a zone of loose connective tissue or fat.

The second additional force comprises **inertial forces**. Work is required to overcome the inertia of the thoracic tissues, and to accelerate gas flow from zero velocity. Both of these additional forces (non-elastic deformation of tissue, and inertia) are small, or negligible (in the case of inertia).

The muscular work during **resting breathing** in the normal subject accounts for only about 2–3% of the total resting metabolism in man (Guyton, 1986, p. 469), and a similar small value in small laboratory mammals including the cat and dog (Crosfill and Widdicombe, 1961). This amount is so small as to be of almost negligible functional significance in a *normal* animal, but in *respiratory disease* the muscular work of breathing can become a very serious burden (Otis, 1964, p. 463).

With increasing ventilation in **exercise**, the energetic cost per breath becomes progressively greater. Severe hyperventilation, as in very heavy exercise, does require substantial energetic expenditure. In one estimate (Guyton, 1986, p. 469) the amount of energy required for the faster respiratory rate during very heavy exercise can increase about 25-fold, but, since the total expenditure of body energy also goes up by 15–20 times, only about 3–5% of it is still used for breathing. Other estimates suggest that the energetic cost of breathing at high levels of exercise amount to about 10% of the total oxygen consumption of the body (Otis, 1964, p. 474). In theory, the critical limit in muscular exercise beyond which any further effort to increase oxygen uptake will be offset by the increased oxygen consumption of the respiratory muscles (as may happen in very severe pulmonary disease) might be encountered in exercise at a ventilation of about 150 litres min^{-1}, but is seldom if ever reached in normal individuals (Otis, 1964, p. 474). Cardiac output is usually the limiting factor in extreme exercise (Hildebrandt, 1974, p. 319).

In **obstructive respiratory disease** (Section 7.17) or **bronchoconstriction** (for example, asthma; Section 7.20) airway resistance can become so great that a very large energetic cost has to be paid to maintain a level of ventilation only just adequate for resting needs. This difficulty is compounded by compression of the conducting airways during the forced expiration needed to maintain an adequate tidal volume (Section 10.12). In **alveolar emphysema**, destruction of the alveolar walls and the subsequent replacement of the elastic tissue by collagenous tissue (Section 7.19) greatly reduces the lung compliance and correspondingly increases the energetic cost of breathing.

In any of these respiratory diseases, a third or more of the total energy expended by the body may be utilized by the respiratory muscles (Guyton, 1986, p. 469). A critical limit may be reached when the oxygen consumption of the respiratory muscles outruns the oxygen gained by breathing (Section 10.12): the excess energetic cost of breathing alone is then the cause of death (Guyton, 1984, p. 469).

10.14 Breathing strategies

It is possible to achieve a given total ventilation by various combinations of tidal frequency and volume of breathing. Work against the forces of elastic recoil (Section 10.13) increases progressively as tidal volume increases. On the other hand, the work against resistance to air flow increases progressively as the frequency increases.

In theory, however, each species evolves an optimal combination of frequency and volume that minimizes the total energetic cost of breathing whilst providing a proper volume of alveolar ventilation.

Values assembled by Comroe (1975) show the energetic cost (in g cm min^{-1}) of overcoming recoil and airway resistance in a man achieving a constant alveolar ventilation of 4000 ml min^{-1}. When the frequency is five breaths per minute and tidal volume 1000 ml, the cost of recoil is 25 000 and the cost of airway resistance is 3750, giving a combined cost of 28 750. If the frequency rises to 15 breaths per minute and the tidal volume falls to 411 ml, the cost of recoil is halved to 12 667 and that of airway resistance is increased by about 50% to 5720, so that the combined cost is reduced by more than one third to 18 387. When frequency is 40 breaths per minute and tidal volume 228 ml, the cost of recoil is further reduced by almost one fifth to 10 400 but that of airway resistance is increased by more than 100% to 12 476, giving almost a 25% increase in the combined cost to 22 876. Thus in man, employing a breathing frequency of 15 breaths per minute and a tidal volume of 411 ml is much more economical than the other two strategies.

The rate normally recorded in resting breathing in man is about 12 breaths per minute with a tidal volume of about 500 ml (Guyton, 1986, p. 472), but these values are presumably those obtained from test subjects. Individuals unaware of breathing commonly breathe at rest at between 15 and 20 per minute (Mead and Agostoni, 1964, p. 421), giving values for man more like those in Table 10.1.

Observations on a variety of laboratory mammals (e.g. by Crosfill and Widdicombe, 1961) have shown that the frequency adopted by each species does correspond quite closely with the estimated optimal frequency, but the physiological mechanism for achieving this relationship is uncertain (Otis, 1964, p. 473).

Table 10.1 Respiratory frequencies, tidal volumes, and work of breathing

	Body mass (kg)	Resp. frequency (breath min^{-1})	Tidal volume (ml)	Power per g body mass	
				(g cm min^{-1})	μW
Mouse[a]	0.032	109	0.18	4.25	6.94
Rat[a]	0.25	97	1.55	1.9	3.10
Guinea pig[a]	0.69	42	3.7	0.52	0.85
Rabbit[a]	2.4	39	15.8	0.62	1.01
Cat[a]	3.7	30	34	0.63	1.03
Dog[a]	12.6	21	144	0.55	0.90
Man[b]	70	16	400	0.43	0.70
Cow[c]	514	30	3800		
Horse[d]	474	12	6700		

[a] Values obtained from Table 3 of Crosfill and Widdicombe (1961).
[b] Values obtained by Crosfill and Widdicombe (1961) from Altman *et al.* (1958) *Handbook of Respiration*, Saunders, Philadelphia.
[c] Values obtained from Tenney (1977, Tables 15.2, 15.4).
[d] Values obtained from Koterba *et al.* (1988).

10.14.1 *Mammals in general*

As has been said many times in this chapter, during **resting breathing** inspiration takes place actively, by means of the muscles of inspiration: expiration occurs passively, powered by energy stored in the expanded lungs and thoracic wall during the previous inspiration. Thus the muscles of inspiration do all the work, not only for inspiration but also for expiration.

The forces acting on the thorax come into equilibrium at the end of expiration (Fig. 10.1A, Section 10.2.1). The volume of the thorax at this point is the **resting volume of the thorax**. The next inspiration starts **from** the resting volume of the thorax.

During **moderate exercise** the expiratory muscles begin to contribute actively to expiration. Even then, however, expiration still ends at the resting volume of the thorax, thus leaving the lung volume the same as it was at the end of expiration during resting breathing (Section 10.12). Only during hyperventilation as in **heavy exercise** do the expiratory muscles drive expiration beyond the resting volume of the thorax and into the expiratory reserve volume (Fig. 10.5).

10.14.2 *The horse: biphasic breathing*

It is more economical in energy to breathe **around** rather than **from** the resting volume of the thorax,

as is shown in Fig. 10.6. This strategy of breathing, which has been christened **biphasic breathing**, has been found in the horse. The reason for calling it biphasic is that both inspiration and expiration have a biphasic pattern, *initially passive* and *finally active*.

In the horse, the *first* phase of **expiration** is **passive**, as in other species; however, when the resting volume of the thorax is reached there is a *second* phase, of **active expiration** caused by contraction of the abdominal muscles, and this causes the end-expiratory volume to be less than the lung volume at the resting volume of the thorax. Starting from the end-expiratory volume, the *first* phase of **inspiration** is a **passive inflation** to the resting volume of the thorax, using energy stored by the previous expiration. Inspiration then continues by a *second* phase of **active inflation**, by means of the diaphragm and (probably, in the horse) the external intercostal muscles. Thus in the horse both inspiration and expiration have a biphasic pattern, initially passive and finally active.

Observations on **horses** by Koterba *et al.* (1988) have shown that this species has adopted a biphasic strategy of breathing. **Biphasic breathing** is an economical strategy. Figure 10.6 compares two identical tidal volumes, A to B being the typical mammalian cycle and G to D being a biphasic breathing cycle. The oblique line represents the relaxation-pressure 'curve'. In the cycle A to B, inspira-

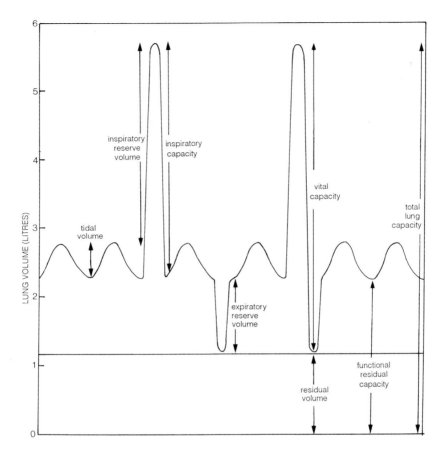

Fig. 10.5   Diagram of pulmonary volumes and capacities in man during resting breathing and maximal inspiration and maximal expiration. The diagram begins on the left with two breaths during resting breathing; the tidal volume is about 500 ml (at a frequency of about 12 per minute, giving a minute volume of about 6 litres min^{-1}). Expiration occupies more than half the cycle, the inspiratory rise being more abrupt than the expiratory fall. Next comes a single maximal inspiration. In maximal breathing, inspiration and expiration are about equal in duration. The inspiratory reserve volume is the volume that can be inspired in excess of a normal tidal volume (about 3 litres). The inspiratory capacity is the tidal volume plus the inspiratory reserve volume (about 3.5 litres). The expiratory reserve volume is the volume that can be expired forcefully at the end of a resting expiration (about 1.1 litres). The vital capacity is the maximum amount of air that can be expired after a maximal inspiration (about 4.5 litres). The residual volume is the volume still in the lungs after a maximal expiration (about 1.2 litres). The functional residual capacity is the expiratory reserve volume plus the residual volume, and is the volume of gas remaining in the lung after a normal expiration (about 2.3 litres). The total lung capacity is nearly 6 litres. The quantitative data are from Guyton (1986, pp. 470–471).

tion starts at the resting volume of the thorax, A, and ends at B. It requires a pressure change of BC, which has to be developed across the system by the muscles of inspiration. The total work needed to overcome recoil forces during inspiration would then be equal to the area ABC.

The cycle G to D is biphasic. The first part of inspiration, G to A, is passive because work equivalent to the area AFG is recovered from elastic energy stored during the last half of the previous expiration; in the second half of inspiration, A to D, work is required from the inspira-

tory muscles, and is equivalent to the area ADE. The first half of expiration, D to A, is passive by recovering the energy stored as ADE in the previous inspiration; the second half of expiration, A to G, requires work from the expiratory muscles, equivalent to the area AFG. The work required to overcome recoil forces during the whole G to D cycle would be ADE plus AFG. But the area of ABC, the work required to overcome recoil forces during the whole of the monophasic A to B cycle, is twice as great as that of ADE + AFG.

Otis (1964, pp. 465–466) envisaged a biphasic cycle as

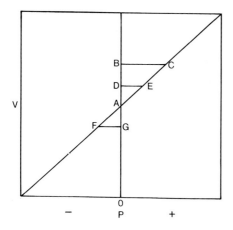

Fig. 10.6 Highly schematic diagram of pressure–volume relationships for the total respiratory system. The oblique line represents the relaxation–pressure relationships. In mammals in general, an inspiration involving a volume change from A to B would start at the resting volume of the thorax, A, and require a pressure change represented by BC; the work by the inspiratory muscles against recoil forces would be represented by the area of ABC. Biphasic breathing would occur on either side of the resting volume of the thorax at A. The same volume change, but from G to D, would then require muscular work against recoil; this work is represented by the area ADE for the inspiratory muscles and AFG for the expiratory muscles. The area of ABC is twice that of ADE plus AFG. Thus the work required to overcome recoil forces is reduced by half in the biphasic strategy of breathing. The horse adopts a biphasic strategy. V, tidal volume; P, pleural pressure.

one that theoretically may be encountered, but there appears to be no clear evidence that it occurs in any species other than the horse. The cow is similar to the horse in size, but has not adopted a biphasic strategy of

breathing; compared with the horse (Table 10.1), it has retained a relatively fast rate of breathing and low tidal volume.

Thus it appears that the horse has invented an economic strategy of breathing. Probably the volume of the active phase of inspiration in the horse is not equal to that of the active phase of expiration. Even so, it should be an energetic improvement on the 'monophasic' strategy of other mammals.

Birds, as represented by the domestic fowl, have evolved a balanced biphasic breathing strategy: if all muscular forces are eliminated, the thorax comes to rest **midway** between full inspiration and full expiration (King and McLelland, 1984, p. 137). They breathe equally above and below the resting volume of the thorax as in Fig. 10.6, and thus take full advantage of the biphasic strategy. The energetic demands of flight are severe. The humble house sparrow must increase its oxygen consumption by about 13 times in order to achieve sustained powered flight, and this is equivalent to the energetic performance of an Olympic athlete. Selection pressures for energetic economy must have been intense in birds.

Koterba *et al.* (1988) suggested various factors that seem to favour the evolution of a **biphasic equine breathing strategy**. Although the **lung compliance** of the horse is similar to that of other mammals (Section 6.31), its **thoracic wall compliance** (Section 10.2.1) is very low. In a large animal, such a stiff thoracic wall is presumably an advantage for supporting locomotor functions and stabilizing end-expiratory lung volume during changes in posture. However, the energetic cost of overcoming the thoracic recoil forces during inspiration will be high if thoracic wall compliance is so low, especially in the slow deep breathing that characterizes the horse. The biphasic strategy adopted by the horse minimizes this elastic work. Furthermore, a low frequency during resting breathing gives the horse a maximal respiratory reserve, since the maximum frequency of its breathing is limited by the maximum frequency of its stride.

Chapter 11
Control of Breathing

Breathing is truly a strange phenomenon of life, caught midway between the conscious and the unconscious, and peculiarly sensitive to both.

Richards (1953)

11.1 Respiratory 'centres'

Autonomic activities are generally controlled within the brain by so-called 'centres', that co-ordinate the afferent and efferent neuronal pathways involved in a particular function (Section 1.5). As a general rule, such autonomic 'centres' are components of the **reticular formation**, which is an ascending (afferent) and descending (efferent) network of neurons forming the most extensive and the most primitive part of the brain and spinal cord. An example is the 'cardiovascular centre' (Section 19.12), controlling circulation.

Breathing is controlled by four respiratory 'centres' in the hindbrain, (1) the medullary respiratory 'centre' (2) the pneumotaxic 'centre' (3) the apneustic 'centre', and (4) the central chemoreceptor area. These 'centres' interact with their afferent neuronal input, and with each other. Their efferent (motor) output to the respiratory musculature produces automatic rhythmic breathing, which involuntarily maintains the O_2 and CO_2 tensions of alveolar gas and arterial blood at optimum levels regardless of whether the body is at rest or exercise.

Breathing is also under voluntary control. This enables the automatic neuronal rhythm to be consciously overruled as in phonation, coughing, sighing, yawning, and sniffing, and for expulsive efforts such as defecation, parturition, and practising the trombone. The voluntary control system lies in the forebrain.

Furthermore the respiratory 'centres' are subordinate to several other 'centres' such as those that regulate body temperature and control vomiting, since these functions require an adjustment of breathing.

None of the respiratory 'centres' is visible histologically as a circumscribed group of neurons, so the term 'centre' is somewhat misleading. However, it forms a useful basis for discussion.

The first three of the four respiratory 'centres' listed above are a part of the reticular formation (Section 1.5) of the pons and medulla oblongata (Wang and Ngai, 1964, p. 488; Brodal, 1981, p. 423; Williams *et al.*, 1989, p. 995). The fourth, the central chemoreceptor area, is of unknown neuronal structure (Section 11.10).

The ascending and descending respiratory neuronal pathways within the reticular formation intermingle intimately and exchange many synaptic contacts. It is a general characteristic of individual neurons of the reticular formation that they form synaptic contacts with many other widely separated neurons. Therefore it is predictable that the respiratory 'centres', far from being well-defined compact clusters of specifically inspiratory or expiratory neurons, actually overlap each other and even overlap other autonomic control 'centres' in the hindbrain. In short, the neuroanatomical basis of control of respiration by the reticular formation is recognized to be a complex problem (Brodal, 1981, p. 421).

11.2 Medullary respiratory 'centre'

The medullary respiratory 'centre' is a bilateral longitudinal column of nerve cells (Fig. 11.1), extending through virtually the whole length of the reticular formation of the medulla oblongata.

A **peripheral** sensory (afferent) input projects into the medullary respiratory 'centre' through three main neuronal pathways. These pathways arise from (a) mechanoreceptor endings in the bronchi and trachea (Fig. 11.1), (b) arterial

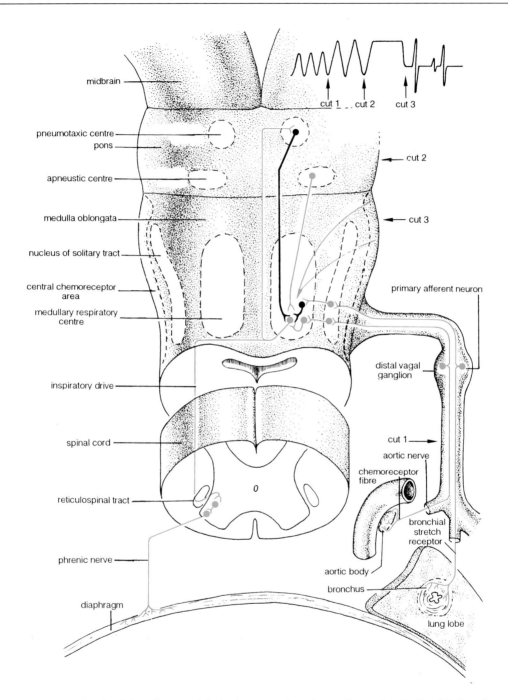

Fig. 11.1 Schematic dorsal view diagram of the brainstem to show the respiratory 'centres' and their main neuronal connections. The pneumotaxic, apneustic, and medullary respiratory centres belong to the reticular formation. The inspiratory drive pathway is represented by a neuron with its cell station in the medullary respiratory centre. Its axon descends the spinal cord in the reticulospinal tract, synapsing with the neurons of the phrenic nerve. The bronchial stretch receptor pathway ascends by the vagus nerve to the nucleus of the solitary tract. It ends by an inhibitory neuron (black) in the medullary respiratory centre, which reflexly inhibits the inspiratory drive. The peripheral arterial chemoreceptors in the aortic body ascend via the vagus nerve and nucleus of the solitary tract, and reflexly excite the inspiratory drive. The pneumotaxic 'centre' is activated by a collateral

chemoreceptor endings in the aortic bodies (Fig. 11.1) and carotid body (Fig. 19.8), and (c) mechanoreceptor endings in joints.

A **central** afferent input projects into the medullary respiratory 'centre' from slightly higher levels of the brainstem, again from three main sources (Fig. 11.1). These are (i) the pneumotaxic 'centre' in the pons, (ii) the apneustic 'centre' also in the pons, and (iii) the central chemoreceptor area in the medulla oblongata.

The **efferent** (motor) drive (**the inspiratory drive pathway**) that actually induces the muscular activity of inspiration arises in the medullary respiratory 'centre' (Section 11.3).

The structure and function of the **medullary respiratory 'centre'** have been studied by a wide range of experimental techniques, including ablation, stimulation, microelectrode recording, and labelling, all of which have technical limitations. Attempts have been made to divide it into an **inspiratory** and an **expiratory 'centre'**. Some accounts (Wang and Ngai, 1964, p. 493–494) localized the **inspiratory** neurons in the *ventral* part of the medullary reticular formation and the **expiratory** neurons in the *dorsal* part. Brodal (1981, p. 423) agreed that an **inspiratory** area or inspiratory 'centre' lies in the *ventromedial* part of the medullary reticular formation, but regarded the **expiratory** region as essentially *rostral* and *lateral* in position. Bowsher (1988, p. 81) placed the **inspiratory** component in the *lateral* and *rostral* site, and the **expiratory** component in the *ventromedial position*. Barr and Kiernan (1983, p. 153) located the **inspiratory** zone in a *medial* position (gigantocellular reticular nucleus) and the **expiratory** zone in a *lateral* position (parvocellular reticular nucleus). Guyton (1986, p. 504) concluded that the **inspiratory** neurons are sited mainly in a *dorsal* respiratory group, whereas both **expiratory** and **inspiratory** neurons lie in a *ventral* group. Observations based on microelectrode recordings (Young, 1974, p. 365), which have the advantage of revealing the activity of cells or axons after only minimal damage, show the

inspiratory neurons in an essentially *rostral* position (rostral to the obex) and the **expiratory** neurons *caudal* (relative to the obex). All of these studies are based mainly on the cat and to lesser extent on the rabbit. In the rat (Ezure *et al.*, 1988), almost all of the respiratory neurons were in a *ventral* column, **expiratory** neurons being concentrated at both the *rostral* and the *caudal* end of the column and **inspiratory** neurons grouped in the *middle*; a dorsal column was virtually non-existent. Thus, on the basis of differing techniques and species, the site of the **inspiratory group** of neurons in the longitudinal column formed by the medullary respiratory 'centre' has been variously judged to be: ventral, ventromedial, medial, lateral–dorsal, rostral, and in the middle; and the **expiratory group** dorsal, ventral, ventromedial, lateral, rostral–lateral, and both rostral and caudal.

Readers who have got this far will probably have concluded that the case for a localized **inspiratory** and a localized **expiratory medullary 'centre'** has not yet been made out; if so, they will be in good company, since Brodal (1992, p. 294) came to the same conclusion. The inherent neuroanatomical complexity of the reticular formation makes this likely, anyway.

11.3   Inspiratory drive pathway to the respiratory muscles

The motor axons of the medullary respiratory 'centre' project down the spinal cord (Fig. 11.1) in the **medullary reticulospinal tract** (see Vol. 1 of this series on the CNS; King, 1987). Many of these efferent projections end by making synapses with interneurons in the ventral horn of cervical segments C5, C6, and C7; these interneurons in turn project on somatic motor neurons (motoneurons) which send their axons (Figs 11.1, 19.8) through the **phrenic nerve** to the skeletal muscle fibres of the diaphragm (Section 8.16.3).

Other efferent axons in the medullary

Fig. 11.1 (Continued)   branch from the inspiratory drive pathway. This centre also reflexly inhibits the inspiratory drive by an inhibitory neuron (black). The apneustic 'centre' is tonically excitatory to the inspiratory drive. The central chemoreceptor area forms the ventrolateral surface of the medulla oblongata. It is excitatory to the inspiratory drive pathway. Its neuronal connections are not known.

The respiratory tracing in the top right corner of the diagram reads from left to right, inspiration being up. It shows the effects on breathing of three successive cuts. Cut 1, through the left and right vagus nerves, eliminates the bronchial stretch receptor and causes deeper slower breathing. Cut 2, transecting the middle of the pons and made after cut 1, eliminates the pneumotaxic 'centre' and causes apneusis (arrest in inspiration). Cut 3, transecting the rostral part of the medulla oblongata and made after cuts 1 and 2, eliminates the apneustic 'centre', but leaves most of the central chemoreceptor area intact and causes expiration followed by irregular gasping.

Neuronal pathways green (except inhibitory neurons, black).

reticulospinal tract continue into the thoracic spinal cord. There, via interneurons, they activate motoneurons in the ventral horn of each thoracic spinal nerve. The axons of these motoneurons are distributed through the **intercostal nerves** to the inspiratory intercostal muscles (i.e. to the **interchondral component** of the internal intercostal muscles, and to the **external intercostal muscles**; Section 8.9.1).

The chain of neuronal projections, from the medullary respiratory 'centre' to the effector endings of motoneuron axons on the muscle fibres of the diaphragm and inspiratory intercostal muscles, is the **pathway of the inspiratory drive**.

Impairment of the pathway of the inspiratory drive may lead to **respiratory insufficiency** (Section 17.29). Lesions in the reticular formation of the medulla oblongata may damage the respiratory centres, causing depressed and irregular breathing. Paralysis of the diaphragm and intercostal muscles follows severance of the spinal cord between segments C1 and C4. Severance caudal to C7 leaves the diaphragm unimpaired but paralyses the intercostal muscles.

The fibres in the medullary reticulospinal tract mostly or entirely cross over in the cat, as in Fig. 11.1, whereas in the rat the projections are mainly bilateral; there is growing evidence that in both the cat and rat the fibres make **monosynaptic connections** directly with the motoneurons of the phrenic nerve (Ellenberger and Feldman, 1988; Yamada *et al.*, 1988). In Fig. 11.1 the terminal relay is made, much more typically though perhaps incorrectly, via an interneuron.

The inspiratory muscles are evidently activated by the classical gamma neuron linkage, via the annulospiral receptor through the dorsal root, to the alpha neuron (King, 1987). This alpha–gamma linkage can be demonstrated experimentally by cutting the dorsal roots of the thoracic spinal nerves, which results in intercostal paralysis (Campbell, 1964, p. 538).

11.4   Mechanoreceptor projections from airways to medullary respiratory 'centre'

Stretch receptors (mechanoreceptors) lie in the walls of the trachea and larger bronchi (Section 4.16). These can be known as **bronchial stretch receptors**. Their autonomic afferent axons travel at first in the **bronchial rami** of the vagus (Figs 3.3, 11.1), and then ascend the main trunk of the vagus

(Section 4.3.3) to project into the **nucleus of the solitary tract**. There, they synapse with a short connecting neuron that makes a relay into the medullary respiratory 'centre'. In the medullary respiratory 'centre', the connecting neuron synapses with a short *inhibitory* neuron (black, in Fig. 11.1). The inhibitory neuron projects on the neuron at the top of the inspiratory drive pathway.

This sequence of neurons is activated by the stretching of the mechanoreceptor in the airway wall during inspiration. The frequency of discharge by the receptor increases more or less linearly with tension (Fig. 11.2A,B). It tires very little during sustained inflation (Fig. 11.2C), and is therefore an example of a slowly-adapting receptor (King, 1987). The physiological characteristics of these respiratory mechanoreceptor neurons resemble those of the baroreceptors in the wall of the carotid sinus (Section 19.4, Fig. 19.4).

The activity of the bronchial stretch receptor reflexly *inhibits* the inspiratory drive, and therefore *arrests inspiration*, allowing expiration to follow immediately. This is the **inflation reflex** or **Hering–Breuer reflex**. By curtailing the inspiratory phase of each breath, this reflex accelerates the rate of breathing.

Irritant receptors in the epithelium of the upper and lower airways induce various protective reflexes such as coughing, laryngeal and bronchial constriction, and mucous secretion, thus defending the lungs against irritant gases and particles (Section 4.16). Their afferent pathways travel in the vagus nerve to the nucleus of the solitary tract, and thence to the medullary respiratory centre.

The Hering-Breuer reflex has been found in many mammals, including the dog and cat among the domestic mammals. The strength of the reflex varies with the species, being strongest in the guinea pig or rabbit and exceptionally weak in man (Widdicombe, 1964, p. 590). In man, it only comes into play in large tidal volumes, starting when the tidal volume is about three times its resting value (Guyton, 1986, p. 505). It therefore appears to be mainly a protective mechanism in man, for preventing over-inflation of the lungs.

There are two groups of *irritant receptors*. Rapidly adapting irritant stretch receptors (Section 4.16.2) occur throughout the trachea and larger bronchi. C-fibre receptors (also named J-fibre receptors) (Section 4.16.3) comprise a pulmonary group at the alveolar level, and a bronchial group (probably) in the smaller bronchi.

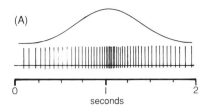

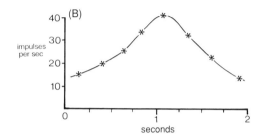

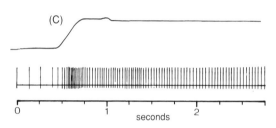

Fig. 11.2 A. **Discharges of a single bronchial stretch receptor axon in the vagus nerve during the course of one breath.** The upper record is a trace of resting breathing, inspiration up. The frequency of discharge is directly proportional to the degree of inflation. After Adrian (1933).

B. **Frequency of discharge of the axon in A.** The frequency rises and falls along a smooth curve as the volume of the lung increases and decreases. After Adrian (1933).

C. **Discharge of a single bronchial stretch receptor axon in the vagus nerve during sustained inflation.** The upper record is intratracheal pressure. The receptor fires at a frequency of about $40\,s^{-1}$ during the first second of inflation. Then the frequency falls to about $30\,s^{-1}$, but is maintained at that level. This is a slowly adapting receptor. After Knowlton and Larrabee (1946).

11.5 Arterial chemoreceptor projections to the medullary respiratory 'centre'

Other afferent neuronal pathways affecting breathing arise from peripheral *arterial chemoreceptors* in the **aortic bodies** and **carotid**

body (Section 4.17.2). Those arising in the **aortic bodies** project via the **aortic nerve** and then in the main trunk of the **vagus nerve** (Section 4.3.3), to end in the nucleus of the solitary tract (Figs 11.1, 19.8). The chemoreceptors in the **carotid body** project via the **carotid sinus nerve** and **glossopharyngeal nerve** (Section 4.3.2), to end in the nucleus of the solitary tract (Fig. 19.8). The identity of the actual chemoreceptor, i.e. whether it is a nerve ending or a receptor cell, is considered in Section 19.9.3.

On reaching the **nucleus of the solitary tract**, the afferent fibres synapse with short neurons that project the chemoreceptor signals into the **medullary respiratory 'centre'** (Figs 11.1, 19.8). Here they excite the neurons at the top of the inspiratory drive pathway (Section 11.2), which activates the diaphragm and the inspiratory components of the intercostal muscles.

The arterial chemoreceptors in the aortic bodies (Section 19.11) and carotid body (Section 19.9) are excited by an *increase* in either the *carbon dioxide* concentration or the *hydrogen ion* concentration of the blood. They are also stimulated by a *fall* in the arterial *oxygen concentration* – this is the only mechanism by which breathing responds to a *fall* in the P_{O_2} of arterial blood. They induce a reflex **increase in breathing**.

11.6 Mechanoreceptor projections from joints to the medullary respiratory 'centre'

Somatic mechanoreceptor endings in the joints of the limbs and ribs project into the medullary respiratory 'centre'. Movements of the joints stimulate these receptors, causing them to project **excitatory** impulses to the 'centre' and thus reflexly **increase breathing**. This may be one mechanism by which **exercise** stimulates breathing (Section 11.14).

Passive movements of the limbs about a joint stimulate breathing reflexly in unanaesthetized and anaesthetized animals (Comroe, 1975, pp. 91, 239). This could help to explain the instant increase in breathing that occurs with the immediate onset of movement. The pathway begins with joint proprioceptors, and probably projects to the medullary respiratory 'centre' via the spinoreticular tract.

Also, there are (seemingly inconclusive) indications

that signals are projected from intercostal muscle spindles to the medullary respiratory 'centre', and thus influence the inspiratory drive (Derenne *et al.*, 1978, p. 379).

11.7   Nucleus of the solitary tract

The nucleus of the solitary tract is one of the nuclei of the cranial nerves. These nuclei form a series of fundamental landmarks in the architecture of the brain stem that merit full consideration in their own right (King, 1987). The nucleus of the solitary tract is of interest here, because it is a basic relay station in the important respiratory reflexes that arise from afferent receptor endings in the airways.

All autonomic (visceral) afferent pathways from the head, and many from the trunk, end by projecting into this elongated (bilateral) nucleus in the medulla oblongata (Section 4.2.4). These autonomic afferent pathways necessarily convey a wide range of visceral signals, including all those from the alimentary tract and the cardiovascular system. Therefore the nucleus of the solitary tract is far from being an exclusive component of respiratory pathways.

However, some of its incoming afferent pathways do profoundly affect breathing. Among these are the mechanoreceptor pathways of the **Hering-Breuer inflation reflex** from the lower airways, and the **arterial chemoreceptor pathways** from the aortic and carotid bodies; as already stated, these pathways make synapses in the nucleus of the solitary tract with short connecting neurons that then project into the **medullary respiratory 'centre'** (Fig. 11.1).

11.8   Pneumotaxic 'centre'

The pneumotaxic 'centre' is an ill-defined bilateral area of the reticular formation, in the rostral part of the pons. The pneumotaxic 'centre' receives projections from the medullary respiratory 'centre'. In Fig. 11.1, these projections are represented schematically by a collateral branch from a neuron of the inspiratory drive. In the pneumotaxic 'centre', this collateral branch synapses with an **inhibitory neuron** (black, in Fig. 11.1), which projects back to the medullary respiratory 'centre'.

The inhibitory neuron transmits impulses to the neurons at the top of the medullary reticulospinal tract, and thus inhibits the discharge of the **inspiratory drive pathway**. The effect of this is to *arrest inspiration* and thus induce expiration; by curtailing the duration of inspiration it increases the rate of breathing. The action of the pneumotaxic 'centre' on breathing is therefore the same as that of the Hering–Breuer inflation reflex.

The pneumotaxic 'centre' lies in the rostral few millimetres of the pons (Wang and Ngai, 1964, p. 490). In the cat, and probably also in the rat, it is within the **medial parabrachial nucleus** (St. John, 1986; Yamada *et al.*, 1988), which is a part of the lateral column of the pontine reticular formation (Williams *et al.*, 1989, p. 990).

The projections from the medullary respiratory nucleus to the pneumotaxic 'centre' are likely to be multineuronal rather than collateral branches of the type shown in Fig. 11.1.

The projections of the pneumotaxic 'centre' to the medullary respiratory 'centre' appear to be diffuse and multiple, with some fibres crossing over (decussating) and others remaining ipsilateral (St. John, 1986).

11.9   Apneustic 'centre'

The apneustic 'centre' lies in the reticular formation in the caudal part of the pons (Fig. 11.1). Its neurons project *excitatory* impulses to the neurons at the top of the **inspiratory drive pathway** in the medullary respiratory 'centre'.

Its stimulatory impulses seem to be delivered in a continuous (tonic) stream, exerting a strong inspiratory drive. If these are the only signals reaching the medullary respiratory 'centre' (that is, if all *inhibitory* signals to that 'centre' are eliminated), breathing is arrested and held in full inspiration. This condition is known as **apneusis**, hence the name of the centre.

11.10   Central chemoreceptor area

The central chemoreceptor area is a thin shell of nervous tissue, forming the ventrolateral surface of the medulla oblongata and bathed by cerebrospinal fluid. Neurons within the area are highly sensitive to CO_2. They respond by projecting strong excitatory signals to the neurons at the top of the **inspiratory drive pathway** in the medullary respiratory 'centre'. Thus they cause a large **increase in breathing**.

In view of the extreme sensitivity of the body to carbon dioxide (Section 11.11), it might be expected that in the medullary respiratory 'centre' itself there would be neurons that are directly stimulated by CO_2. Actually, the neurons in the medullary respiratory 'centre' (and those in the pneumotaxic 'centre') are not excited by increased concentrations in the blood of CO_2 or hydrogen ions (Guyton, 1986, p. 506). On the contrary, the neurons at the top of the inspiratory drive, and those that form the phrenic nerve in the ventral horn, are directly *depressed* by CO_2 (Derenne *et al.*, 1978, p. 380). Furthermore, after their initial phase of responsiveness, the neurons of the central chemoreceptor area themselves are depressed by increased P_{CO_2} even more readily than the neurons in the medullary respiratory 'centre' (Comroe, 1975, p. 65). Moreover, most **general anaesthetic** agents diminish the response of the neurons in the central chemoreceptor area to CO_2 (Comroe, 1975, p. 65). Therefore it is important in general anaesthesia not to allow a build-up of CO_2 in the blood. Likewise, inhalation of carbon dioxide is seldom used therapeutically to increase ventilation (Comroe, 1975, p. 64).

The structure and function of the central chemoreceptor area have been reviewed by Bruce and Cherniak (1987). It is about 1 mm thick, and being no more than a thin, essentially *superficial*, layer of nervous tissue it cannot be a part of the core of the brainstem, i.e. the reticular formation. Indeed it differs from all the other respiratory 'centres' in that its neuronal pathways are still entirely unknown, despite intense investigation.

After all known **peripheral arterial chemoreceptors** (those in the carotid and aortic bodies) have been eliminated, breathing CO_2 causes a powerful increase in ventilation; therefore there must be **central chemoreceptors** somewhere in the brain that are stimulated by acidity or an increase in CO_2. Indeed the drive arising from the stimulation of these chemoreceptors by CO_2 and/or acid is thought to be the major source of the tonic input into the central respiratory rhythm generator.

It was at first believed that CO_2 would directly stimulate neurons in the central chemoreceptor area. However, it is now generally recognized that molecular CO_2 would have no direct action, and that the concentration of **hydrogen ions** is crucial. However, CO_2 would have a strong *indirect* effect. This is because carbon dioxide in the blood passes very easily through the blood–brain and blood–cerebrospinal fluid barrier. As soon as it gains the **interstitial fluid**, it reacts with water to form

carbonic acid, and this dissociates into hydrogen and bicarbonate ions; it is mainly the hydrogen ions that stimulate the chemoreceptors in the brain. On the other hand, hydrogen ions in the blood do not pass so easily through the blood–brain and cerebrospinal fluid barriers, and therefore would have less effect.

Although the stimulation of breathing is probably caused mainly by the hydrogen ions in the interstitial fluid of the chemoreceptor area, it is possible that an increase in the concentration of CO_2 in the **cerebrospinal fluid** may also strongly stimulate the cells of the central chemoreceptor area.

No cells have yet been identified in the central chemoreceptor area that are indisputably chemoreceptors responding to these stimuli. Nevertheless there is abundant evidence that the direct application of chemical, electrical, and thermal stimuli to the ventrolateral surface of the medulla oblongata evokes respiratory responses; for example, the application of acetylcholine to this surface excites breathing, whereas local anaesthetic depresses breathing and may even lead to apnoea.

It is therefore proposed, albeit with due caution, that the central responses to CO_2 and to blood acid–base changes arise from chemoreceptors in the shell of nervous tissue that forms the ventrolateral surface of the medulla oblongata, i.e. the central chemoreceptor area.

11.11 Main stimuli to breathing

The levels of oxygen and carbon dioxide in the blood regulate the pattern of breathing. Rather unexpectedly, carbon dioxide is a much stronger regulator than oxygen. This is because the concentration of **carbon dioxide** acutely affects the acidity of the body.

The rates of reactions catalysed by enzymes are usually strongly influenced by changes in the acidity of the body fluids. Extreme acidity and extreme alkalinity can also dangerously disturb the excitability of the nerve cells. Clearly, the body needs mechanisms that monitor and adjust the concentration of CO_2 accurately and rapidly.

Even so, readers may be unimpressed by this argument – after all, disorganized enzymes and action potentials may well be inconvenient, but without oxygen they die. Be reassured. The body has evolved safety margins (Section 14.3.1) that enable it to maintain adequate oxygen concentrations at its cells, even when the gaseous oxygen supply is grossly defective. For example, if the P_{O_2} of alveolar gas falls to only half its normal value, the haemoglobin of arterial blood will still be about 80% saturated (Fig. 14.1).

To illustrate the powerful influence of carbon dioxide over pH (Attwell, 1986, p. 24), assume that the metabolic production of CO_2 is constant and consider the effect of varying the alveolar ventilation from the value required to maintain pH at 7.4. The CO_2 concentration in arterial blood is roughly inversely proportional to alveolar ventilation, so halving the alveolar ventilation doubles the concentration of CO_2 and this lowers the extracellular pH by about 0.2 of a unit; changing the pH from 7.1 to 7.2 increases almost 20-fold the activity of phosphofructokinase, the enzyme that regulates the rate of glycolysis. However, the ventilation can be diminished to nearly zero, or increased by a factor of more than 10; ventilation changes of this magnitude can shift the pH towards dangerous levels. Extreme acidity can depress the nervous system so severely that death from coma results. Extreme alkalinity leads to spontaneous action potentials in peripheral nerves which can result in death through spasm (tetany) of the muscles of respiration.

11.11.1 *Increased carbon dioxide as a stimulus to breathing*

Metabolism of oxygen in the cells generates carbon dioxide, which diffuses through the tissue fluid and capillary endothelium, and then into the blood plasma and the erythrocytes.

When dissolved in blood, the CO_2 reacts with water to form **carbonic acid** (H_2CO_3); the carbonic acid ionizes (at blood pH) into **hydrogen ions** and **bicarbonate ions** (HCO_3):

$$CO_2 + H_2O \leftrightarrow H_2CO_3 \leftrightarrow H^+ + HCO_3^-$$

Thus the uptake of carbon dioxide by the blood increases the hydrogen ion concentration and lowers the pH of the blood.

The cells of the body cannot tolerate an acid pH. In man and the domestic animals, the average pH is normally close to 7.4 and must remain between about 7.0 and 7.8. It is therefore essential that the P_{CO_2} of the blood and tissues is regulated continuously, swiftly, and exactly; adjustment of respiration is the only effective means available to the body for doing so. Therefore the key stimulus in the regulation of breathing is the concentration of carbon dioxide in the blood.

It is the role of the neurons in the **central chemoreceptor area** to monitor this stimulus closely and respond to it instantly; a *single* breath of air containing 7% CO_2 causes the next *several*

breaths to have a greater tidal volume. The sensitivity of the central chemoreceptor area to carbon dioxide enables it to play a major part in maintaining the pH of the blood within an acceptable range. This it does, as follows: (i) it causes an increase in breathing (minute volume) if the hydrogen ion concentration rises (acidity), thus promptly removing excess CO_2 and therefore raising the pH towards normal; and (ii) it causes a decrease in breathing if the hydrogen ion concentration falls (alkalinity), thus allowing carbon dioxide to accumulate and the pH to fall towards normal.

Respiration is not, of course, the only mechanism in the body for **regulating pH**. All the body fluids contain **acid–base buffers** that act instantly to rectify excessive changes in pH, and the **kidneys** readjust pH by excreting an acid or alkaline urine. The renal mechanism is the most powerful, but takes many minutes or even days to act. The respiratory control mechanism is much faster, taking only a few minutes to correct the pH after a sudden change; but its responsiveness fades within a few days.

If the lungs fail to remove sufficient carbon dioxide from the blood, the hydrogen ion concentration may rise and the pH fall. This can occur in **respiratory diseases** involving a venous-to-arterial shunt (Section 6.30), or airway obstruction (Section 7.17), or excessive dead space as in alveolar emphysema (Section 7.19). The condition is then known as **respiratory acidaemia**.

The respiratory response to an **increase in arterial P_{CO_2}** is immediate and roughly proportional (Weibel, 1984, p. 390). For example, as just stated, a single breath of air containing 7% CO_2 causes the next several breaths to have a greater tidal volume. Increasing the arterial P_{CO_2} from 40 to about 43 mmHg (5.3 to 5.7 kPa) (an increase of about 8%) will lead to a rapid increase in ventilation from about 5 litres min^{-1} to about 8 litres min^{-1} (an increase of about 60%); a similar further increase of arterial P_{CO_2} to about 46 mmHg (6.1 kPa) could at once increase the minute volume to about 15 litres min^{-1} minute (an additional 90%, approximately); yet another similar increase in arterial P_{CO_2} to 50 mmHg (6.7 kPa) could increase the minute volume to about 30 litres min^{-1} (a further 100% increase). When such changes are expressed in terms of pH, a fall from the normal value of 7.4 to 7.0 increases the rate of alveolar ventilation four- or fivefold (Guyton, 1986, p. 443).

As already stated, when dissolved in blood, the CO_2 reacts with the water in the **plasma** to form carbonic acid, and then bicarbonate, but the formation of bicarbonate in the plasma is too slow (needing many seconds or minutes to occur) to be important for **transport** by the blood plasma (Guyton, 1986, p. 501). However, the CO_2 also diffuses into the **erythrocytes**. Here it encounters an enzyme, **carbonic anhydrase**, that accelerates the formation of carbonic acid so much that the reaction to form bicarbonate is completed within a small fraction of a second. Almost instantly, the carbonic acid thus formed in the erythrocytes dissociates into hydrogen and bicarbonate ions. Many of the bicarbonate ions diffuse into the plasma, and most of the hydrogen ions combine with haemoglobin. About 70% of the carbon dioxide transported from the tissues to the lungs is accounted for by the (reversible) combination of carbon dioxide with water in the erythrocytes under the influence of carbonic anhydrase (Guyton, 1986, p. 501).

Some carbon dioxide combines with haemoglobin to form **carbaminohaemoglobin**. A much smaller amount reacts similarly with plasma proteins. About 20% of the total quantity of carbon dioxide is transported as **carbamino compounds**. About 10% is transported to the lungs in simple solution in the plasma as dissolved CO_2.

The reactions forming bicarbonate and carbamino compounds are reversible, and when reversed they **release carbon dioxide in the lungs**. The key to these reversals is the binding of oxygen to haemoglobin in the alveolar capillaries, since this displaces carbon dioxide from the blood (the **Haldane effect**). The combination of oxygen with haemoglobin makes the haemoglobin into a stronger acid. This causes the haemoglobin to release hydrogen ions, and these bind with bicarbonate ions thus reforming carbonic acid. The carbonic acid in turn dissociates into water and carbon dioxide (accelerated by carbonic anhydrase), allowing the carbon dioxide to escape from the blood into the alveolar gas. Thus the reaction that enables the bulk of the carbon dioxide to be transported from the tissues to the lung, is now reversed to release the carbon dioxide into the alveoli.

The concentration of CO_2 in the blood affects the cerebral circulation. Thus **hypercapnia** (an increased CO_2 concentration in arterial blood) dilates the cerebral blood vessels and increases cerebral blood flow (Comroe, 1975, p. 257). **Hypocapnia** (a decreased concentration in arterial blood) causes cerebral ischaemia. Hypocapnia (with respiratory alkalosis) occurs in hyperventilation by an animal at **high altitude**. Incapacitation of man at high altitude (light-headedness, for example) may be due in part to cerebral ischaemia (Comroe, 1975, p. 259).

11.11.2 *Oxygen lack as a stimulus to breathing*

As already stated, the level of the oxygen in the blood plays a much smaller role than CO_2 in the regulation of breathing. The P_{O_2} **of inspired air** can be decreased to about half of its normal value before ventilation becomes noticeably increased. The reason for this is that normal breathing maintains the **alveolar** P_{O_2} at a substantially higher level than that needed to saturate the haemoglobin of arterial blood (Section 14.3.1) – a major **safety factor**. However, if ventilation is progressively reduced, or if the P_{O_2} of the inspired air is progressively reduced, the P_{O_2} of arterial blood eventually falls sharply with potentially fatal consequences. The P_{O_2} **of arterial blood** leaving the heart is normally about 95 mmHg (12.7 kPa), and can fall to about 60 mmHg (7.9 kPa) without any clear effect on breathing. If it falls further to 40–20 mmHg (5.3–2.7 kPa), this is incompatible with life for more than a few minutes.

None of the respiratory 'centres' in the brain stem is directly affected by changes in arterial P_{O_2}. But throughout the whole of such a fall in arterial P_{O_2}, and particularly between 60 and 30 mmHg (7.9 and 3.9 kPa), the **peripheral arterial chemoreceptors** (Section 19.9) discharge progressively faster to the nucleus of the solitary tract, and thence to the medullary respiratory 'centre'. In response, the minute volume of breathing also increases progressively, but only by the relatively small factor of 1.5–1.7 at the most, even when death may be imminent. In contrast, a great increase in blood P_{CO_2} can increase breathing 10- to 20-fold.

The reason for such a small increase in breathing when arterial P_{O_2} falls, even to such dangerously low levels, is that the resulting increase in ventilation washes CO_2 from the blood, thus eliminating the most powerful stimulus to breathing. Hence the respiratory stimulus of falling oxygen levels is largely cancelled out by the depressor effect on the central chemoreceptor area of a fall in the concentration of carbon dioxide.

Normally, regulation of breathing by the peripheral arterial chemoreceptors, in response to falling oxygen levels in the blood, is therefore of virtually no significance. However, if abnormal conditions arise in which the carbon dioxide content of the blood increases at the same time as the oxygen content decreases, then the two receptor mechanisms reinforce each other. The response of the peripheral arterial chemoreceptors to O_2 can now have a more powerful effect on breathing than the response of the central chemoreceptor area to CO_2.

Decreasing the P_{O_2} **of inspired air** from the normal level of 159 mmHg (21.2 kPa) by decrements of 10% has little effect on ventilation until the level has fallen to about half the normal value or less (about 60 mmHg) (7.9 kPa) (Weibel, 1984, p. 390). Even when alveolar ventilation has decreased to about half its normal value, the blood is still within 10% of complete saturation (Guyton, 1986, p. 510). Thus when the P_{O_2} of inspired air is within the upper range (159 to about 60 mmHg), blood has a very wide margin of safety (Weibel, 1984, p. 391). But below 60 mmHg the oxygen–haemoglobin equilibrium curve falls rapidly, and the capacity of the blood for the transport of oxygen is dangerously diminished.

The principal reason for the low sensitivity of the body's responses to a fall in arterial P_{O_2} is that the **normal alveolar P_{O_2}** is higher than the minimal level required to saturate the haemoglobin of arterial blood almost completely (Section 14.3.1) (Guyton, 1986, p. 510). This gives the mechanism for the uptake of gaseous oxygen a large **safety factor**, whereas the mechanism for the removal of carbon dioxide has no such margin of safety. Also, in normal pulmonary flow, the blood is almost saturated with oxygen when it has traversed only the first third of the **pulmonary capillary** (Guyton, 1986, p. 494) giving a second **safety factor** in oxygen transport (the removal of carbon dioxide from the pulmonary capillary enjoys similar efficiency). There is a third substantial **safety factor**, since the intracellular P_{O_2} is normally about 23 mmHg (3.1 kPa) but only 3 mmHg (0.4 kPa) are needed to provide fully for cell metabolism.

11.12 Rhythm of breathing

In the normal animal breathing proceeds rhythmically and unconsciously, with automatic adjustments which maintain homeostasis generally. What controls this rhythm?

11.12.1 *Role of bronchial stretch receptors*

Since the bronchial stretch receptors in the lung discharge in direct proportion to the degree of inflation, the medullary respiratory 'centre' is being continuously informed of the degree of lung inflation.

As stated in Section 11.4, the stretch receptor axon synapses in the **nucleus of the solitary tract** with a short connecting neuron that projects into the **medullary respiratory 'centre'**. Here, the connecting neuron synapses with an **inhibitory neuron** (black, in Fig. 11.1). This inhibitory neuron, in turn, synapses with the neuron at the top of the inspiratory drive pathway.

As the lung inflates during inspiration, the neurons at the top of the inspiratory drive pathway are bombarded by progressively increasing numbers of inhibitory impulses. These impulses eventually inhibit the inspiratory drive neuron, so inspiration stops and expiration begins. This gives the medullary respiratory 'centre' an automatic cut-out device or, in engineering parlance, a *negative feedback* system.

Could inhibition by the stretch receptors of the lung be the cause of the rhythm of breathing? If so, cutting both vagi (cut 1 in Fig. 11.1) should break the rhythm entirely. But this is not what happens: certainly breathing is much *slower* and *deeper* after **bilateral vagotomy** (as could be predicted from the loss of the inhibitory stretch receptor impulses), but the rhythm persists (see the respiratory tracing in the top right corner of Fig. 11.1).

11.12.2 *Role of the pneumotaxic 'centre'*

As shown in Fig. 11.1, the axon descending from the top of the inspiratory drive pathway forms a collateral which projects rostrally to the pneumotaxic 'centre' (Section 11.8). In the pneumotaxic 'centre' it makes a synapse with an **inhibitory neuron** (black in Fig. 11.1), which projects back to the medullary respiratory 'centre'. Here, the inhibitory neuron synapses with the motor neuron at the top of the inspiratory drive pathway. This is therefore another negative feedback circuit, which tends rhythmically to curtail the firing of the inspiratory drive pathway, and thus arrests inspiration and initiates expiration.

If the left and right pneumotaxic 'centres' are severed from the medullary respiratory 'centres' on both sides of the brainstem (cut 2 in Fig. 11.1), breathing becomes deeper and slower, but is still rhythmic. The function of the pneumotaxic 'centre' is therefore essentially the same as that of the Hering–Breuer inflation reflex.

If both vagi are cut first, and then the left and right pneumotaxic 'centres' are also eliminated (that is, if cut 1 is followed by cut 2 in Fig. 11.1), rhythmic breathing stops. The animal inspires and breathing then remains arrested in full inspiration, a state known as **apneusis** (see the respiratory tracing between cuts 2 and 3 in Fig. 11.1). The animal will suffocate. The reason for apneusis appears to be the continued activity of the apneustic 'centre'.

11.12.3 *Role of the apneustic 'centre'*

The apneustic 'centre' (Section 11.9) seems to exert a steady (tonic) stimulation of the neurons at the top of the pathway of the inspiratory drive. Therefore as long as the apneustic 'centre' remains intact, after the vagi and pneumotaxic 'centres' have been eliminated, the pathway of the inspiratory drive is maintained in a state of constant stimulation giving apneusis.

If the left and right apneustic 'centres' are also now eliminated (cut 3 in Fig. 11.1) the apneusis ends. Expiration occurs, and is followed by irregular gasping, each breath being nearly always maximal (see the respiratory tracing in Fig. 11.1, after cut 3). This may be due to the activity of the central chemoreceptor area, which will still be partly intact.

If the vagus nerves and left and right pneumotaxic 'centre' are preserved intact, they rhythmically regulate the influence of the apneustic 'centre' (Wang and Ngai, 1964, p. 497).

11.12.4 *Role of the central chemoreceptor area*

The neurons in the central chemoreceptor area are excited by an increase in CO_2. When excited they apparently stimulate the inspiratory drive pathway. The stimulation which they apply to the pathway of the inspiratory drive would fluctuate irregularly as the concentration of CO_2 in the body rises and falls; this is shown by the irregular gasping that follows cuts 1, 2, and 3 in Fig. 11.1. A gasp eliminates some CO_2 and reduces the central chemoreceptor drive. After the gasp is over CO_2 accumulates again, and thus restimulates the chemoreceptors. Consequently the central chemoreceptors may be able to impart a very primitive and irregular rhythm to the pathway of the inspiratory drive, and hence to breathing.

11.12.5 *Role of the medullary respiratory 'centre'*

The medullary respiratory 'centre' is the **central respiratory rhythm generator**. It acts as a central respiratory computer, where all incoming information affecting breathing, from all over the body, is assembled and analysed. On the basis of these data, it decides on the best adjustments of the depth and rate of breathing for maintaining homeostasis. It then executes these decisions by means of its motor output through the reticulospinal tract, especially through its inspiratory drive pathway (Fig. 11.1) but also (if necessary) through pathways to the muscles of expiration. Its commands through these motor pathways can, however, be overruled by conscious decisions in the highest 'centres' of the brain (Section 11.13).

Feedback from vagal stretch receptors and feedback from the pneumotaxic 'centre' are certainly important mechanisms in maintaining the respiratory rhythm. Nevertheless, it seems unlikely that these negative feedback mechanisms alone could be the basis of the rhythm generator, although this was what the discoverers of the respiratory 'centres' in the 1920s and 1930s had hoped (hence their coining of the term 'pneumotaxic centre'). For example, it is difficult to reconcile the duration of the inspiratory phase of breathing with the hypothetical circuit between the medullary and pneumotaxic 'centres'.

There is a general consensus that there must somewhere be a central generator of the rhythm, emitting repetitive bursts of inspiratory action potentials (Guyton, 1986, p. 504). Evidence for this includes the claim by some workers that a respiratory rhythm can be maintained by the medullary 'centre', even when the 'centre' is completely isolated from 'any neural input whatsoever' (Young, 1974, p. 366) – an ambitious proposition experimentally.

One view is that this rhythm generator resides entirely within the **medullary respiratory 'centre'** itself, through the interaction of tonically active, inspiratory and expiratory neurons; the inspiratory neurons in the 'centre' would inhibit the expiratory neurons, and vice versa, producing an **oscillatory system**. The input into this system from the pulmonary stretch receptors and the pneumotaxic 'centre' would do no more than modify the rhythm. Many industrial mechanical and electrical systems are capable of such oscillation, and neural oscillatory systems may well turn out to resemble these non-neural oscillatory systems; consequently much recent research into the neural control of breathing has concentrated on control system engineering and mathematical models (Young, 1974, p. 367).

Another view suggested that control of the rhythm resides in some intermediary pool of neurons called the **'off-switch' pool**; all respiratory input (including that of the bronchial stretch receptors and the pneumotaxic 'centre') would go into this pool, which must reach a threshold before its inhibitory output to the top of the pathway of the inspiratory drive can terminate inspiration (Petersen, 1987, p. 18).

Recently Duffin *et al.* (1995) concluded that we are nearer to the solution of this problem than ever before, and that the key mechanisms governing the rhythm-generating process lie in the reticular formation of the **rostral ventrolateral medulla**. This region of the reticular formation lies immediately dorsal to, and in contact with, the central chemoreceptor area (Kuwaki *et al.*, 1995). However, the neuronal connections, neurotransmitters, and neuromodulators forming a network oscillator in this rostral–ventrolateral region have still to be identified (Duffin *et al.*, 1995).

11.13   Control of breathing by higher 'centres'

In the course of an ordinary day there are countless occasions when any mammal overrules the respiratory rhythm generator in order to execute respiratory actions under conscious control (Section 11.1). These actions are particularly important in man, since many of them relate to vocalization (talking, shouting), but dogs bark, cats mew, horses neigh, and cows moo. Other actions demanding conscious regulation of breathing include expulsive efforts such as **defecation** and **coughing**, which begin with a deep inspiration, continue with closure of the laryngeal glottis, and end with forcible and sustained contraction of the muscles of expiration. All of these are essentially *expiratory* actions, but non-rhythmic *inspiratory* actions also occur under conscious control, for example **sniffing**, **sighing**, and **taking a deep breath** before shouting a message or singing a long passage.

Not much is known about the neuronal basis for these actions, but three things seem clear. Firstly, they originate in the cerebral cortex of the forebrain. Secondly, they bypass the respiratory 'centres', including the medullary respiratory 'centre'. Thirdly, the final neuron in the chain is the motoneuron (somatic efferent neuron) in the ventral horn of the spinal cord.

Because of the obvious interest in speech and emotional expression in man, the **respiratory areas of the cerebral cortex** have been extensively explored in man and lower mammals (Young, 1974, p. 361). Respiratory motor activity, excitatory or more commonly inhibitory, is associated with parts of the primary and secondary motor areas of the cortex. The excitatory responses in the cat and dog are acceleration in the rate of breathing with or without changes in amplitude; inhibitory responses are reductions in both rate and amplitude (Wang and Ngai, 1964, p. 499). Stimulation of these respiratory regions also produces various forms of vocalization, accompanied by licking, chewing, and swallowing movements, involving the skeletal musculatures as would be expected from stimulation of the motor cortex. Respiratory responses can also be evoked from the cortical components of the limbic system (Young, 1974, p. 362; King, 1987, p. 112).

According to Comroe (1975, p. 22) the motor output from these cortical areas descends partly directly through the **corticospinal (pyramidal) tracts** to the phrenic and intercostal motoneurons, and partly indirectly through the **descending reticular formation**. According to Guyton (1986, p. 513) the descending pathway is corticospinal. Young (1974, p. 362) observed that, since (a) these cortical respiratory areas generate essentially voluntary respiratory actions and (b) are associated with the motor areas that form the pyramidal tracts and execute voluntary muscular activities, one would indeed expect conscious respiratory actions to be projected through the pyramidal system. However, section of the pyramidal tract in the cat does not affect the respiratory responses to cortical stimulation. It is therefore concluded that the pathways are not pyramidal but extrapyramidal. The **extrapyramidal pathways** would presumably be reticulospinal, but without in any way involving the pontine and medullary respiratory 'centres'. In principle, the cerebral cortex does project extrapyramidal motor activities through the **basal nuclei** (especially the globus pallidus) to the **descending reticular formation** of the brainstem, and on down the spinal cord in the reticulospinal tracts (King, 1987, p. 151). Respiratory cortical projections descending through this extrapyramidal system have been traced as far as the medullary reticular formation (Wang and Ngai, 1964, p. 500).

11.14   Control of breathing during exercise

During exercise, even when very strenuous, the arterial P_{CO_2} and P_{O_2} in a healthy individual remain close to normal resting values, despite the huge increase in the production of carbon dioxide and the strong demand for oxygen by the contracting musculature – a tribute to the body's amazing powers of homeostasis. Breathing during such heavy exercise is accurately regulated so that the blood gases, and therefore also pH, remain constantly at optimal levels.

It might be argued that surely all this could be achieved by the **central chemoreceptor area** with its capacity for responding to increases in acidity in exercise as the blood levels of CO_2 rapidly rise, and by the **peripheral arterial chemoreceptors** with their responsiveness to hypoxaemia as the muscles burn up oxygen. However, two surprising changes in breathing during exercise show beyond doubt that the regulation of breathing is not controlled by the central chemoreceptors alone. Although it might be expected that the minute volume would simply increase progressively as the work of exercise increased, there is, first, an *instant* abrupt *increase* in ventilation; this may even start *before* muscular activity begins, and certainly happens during the first few seconds after the onset of exercise, while the P_{CO_2} still remains at its pre-exercise level. Secondly, there is an equally *instant* and *abrupt fall* in minute volume immediately exercise stops, despite the high arterial P_{CO_2} that then exists.

These two events in ventilation, one at the beginning of exercise and one at the end, must be regulated by some factor other than the levels of the blood gases. This additional factor is believed to be neuronal. It is proposed that the **motor area of the cerebral cortex** not only activates muscular activity in exercise but also projects excitatory impulses to the **medullary respiratory 'centre'**. It is possible that, during exercise, **proprioceptors** in the joints also transmit excitatory impulses to the medullary respiratory 'centre' (Section 11.6).

Breathing during exercise is therefore regulated mainly by excitatory pathways from the cerebral cortex and possibly also from joints. The role of the central chemoreceptor area is probably limited to minor adjustments in response to arterial P_{CO_2}.

During maximum exercise (Young, 1974, p. 389), a trained athlete may achieve a sustained minute volume of about 120 litres min^{-1} (about 20 times the resting value of approximately 6 litres min^{-1}), thus quite closely approaching his maximum (transitory) voluntary ventilation of about 160 litres min^{-1}. The ventilation during exercise increases linearly with increasing oxygen consumption. On the other hand the arterial P_{O_2} and P_{CO_2} change scarcely at all, even though the oxygen consump-

tion and carbon dioxide production can increase by as much as twenty times (Guyton, 1986, p. 511).

At the onset of exercise, ventilation increases abruptly during the first few seconds; sometimes it even increases *before* exercise begins. During this very brief initial phase the arterial P_{CO_2} often even falls briefly below normal, although the contracting muscles have started to produce large amounts of carbon dioxide, so clearly a rising concentration of CO_2 is not the stimulus. Probably the **cortical motor pathways** that control the active musculature also project excitatory connections to the medullary respiratory 'centre', conveying an **anticipatory signal** (Section 22.16.1(d). (An anticipatory vasodilation also occurs in skeletal muscle that is about to become active, Sections 13.3.4 and 22.16.1(b).) Immediately movement has started, **joint proprioceptors** (Section 11.6), and perhaps **muscle spindles** (Section 11.6) (though the evidence for this is not strong; Hornbein and Sørensen, 1974, p. 389), are assumed to project **reinforcing excitatory impulses** into the medullary respiratory 'centre'.

After this very short 'onset' (first) phase of exercise, ventilation in a second phase rises rapidly within a few seconds and then increases more slowly over several minutes until it reaches a relatively constant steady state. Within the first half minute or so of this second phase the arterial P_{CO_2} returns to its normal value, and it then remains at that level. The amount of carbon dioxide released into the blood from the contracting muscles now roughly matches the increased rate of ventilation. During this second phase, the **central chemoreceptor area** makes upward or downward adjustments in ventilation, in order to balance alveolar ventilation against the rate of metabolism.

In a third phase, ventilation and arterial P_{CO_2} and P_{O_2} are in steady state. The constancy of arterial P_{CO_2} and P_{O_2} appears to eliminate these factors as possible stimuli for regulating exercise hyperpnoea, since it seems unlikely that arterial gas tensions could account for such delicate control (Young, 1974, p. 390). Moreover, a very high alveolar P_{CO_2} in exercise could only account for about two thirds of the increase in ventilation, since the maximum minute volume achieved by breathing CO_2 is only two thirds of that occurring in heavy exercise (Guyton, 1986, p. 511). The conclusion seems inescapable that, throughout the steady state phase, ventilation is regulated by neuronal control from the forebrain and possibly from joint proprioceptors (Guyton, 1986, p. 513). Doubtless, however, the central chemoreceptor area and peripheral arterial chemoreceptors monitor the arterial P_{CO_2} and P_{O_2}, and supervene if errors occur in the forebrain and proprioceptor control.

A fourth phase occurs when exercise stops. Ventilation instantly falls precipitously, in a few seconds, about half-way towards its pre-exercise level, and then diminishes slowly and progressively towards normal in the following minutes (Young, 1974, p. 389). The abrupt fall must presumably be due to sudden cessation of cortical and proprioceptive signals to the medullary respiratory 'centre', coincident with the cessation of cortical signals to the now inactive musculature. The final gradual recovery to normal is presumably governed by the central chemoreceptor area.

On experimental grounds, it is suggested (astonishing though it may seem) that neuronal control by the forebrain of breathing during exercise appears to be partly, if not entirely, a *learned response* (Guyton, 1986, p. 513). After repeated periods of exercise the forebrain seems to improve its ability to maintain the blood gases at normal levels.

Part 3
Circulatory System

Chapter 12
Blood Vessels

I GENERAL PROPERTIES OF THE CIRCULATORY SYSTEM

12.1 Fluid compartments

Water accounts for about 70% of the body weight – so even our greatest heroes are only 70% water. The two main fluid compartments are the intracellular and extracellular fluid. Separating these two compartments is the cell membrane (**plasmalemma**). The **intracellular fluid** is the site of all the metabolic processes of the body. The **extracellular fluid** consists of two main subcompartments, the **blood plasma** and the **interstitial fluid** (tissue fluid). In these body fluids, water is the solvent. Dissolved in the water are numerous inorganic and organic solutes. Together, the blood plasma and the interstitial fluid form the **internal environment**. The functions of the cardiovascular system are directed towards maintaining the **homeostasis** of the internal environment.

> **Transcellular fluids** constitute a further subcompartment of the extracellular compartment. These are the products of secretory cells in the alimentary and respiratory tracts, and also include the pleural, pericardial, peritoneal, and cerebrospinal fluids (Woodbury, 1974, p. 451).

12.2 Interstitial fluid and ground substance

The **interstitial fluid** (tissue fluid) is the lifeline between the cell and the blood plasma. It transports the fuel supply of the cell from the blood plasma, and the exhaust products of metabolism in the other direction. How do these transport systems through the interstitial fluid actually manage to move? Are they streams of fluid transferred in bulk (i.e. mass flow, also known sometimes as transport by convection), or are they diffusion pathways? The answers to these questions are influenced by the structure of the **intercellular substance** or 'interstitium', in which the cells are held. The term **interstitium** (Latin: inter, between; sistere, to place) is preferred to interstitial substance because it is shorter and matches 'interstitial fluid'. The **interstitium** is the filling between the cells of the body. It has two components, ground substance and fibres embedded in the ground substance. The fibres are collagen, elastic, and reticular fibres.

The **ground substance** holds the key to the transport of water and solutes between the cell and the blood plasma. It is founded on very large molecules formed by combinations of carbohydrate and protein complexes. The filaments of these huge molecules branch and coil in three dimensions, extending throughout the spaces between the fibres and the cells. The **water** in the interstitium, i.e. the **interstitial fluid**, binds to the molecular filaments by hydrogen bonding. The combination of the carbohydrate–protein filaments with water produces the characteristics of a viscous gel, and is commonly known as the **tissue gel**.

The proportion of water in the tissue gel is high. Almost all of it is **bound water**, but there is also a very small amount of **free water**. The free water normally takes the form of minute vesicles, or tiny channels running alongside collagen fibres or following the surfaces of cells; such channels were noted in the alveolar wall of the lung (Section 6.20). If **oedema** develops (Section 14.9), these vesicles and channels enlarge greatly.

The interstitial fluid comes from the arterial ends of the capillaries (arterial capillaries) as a filtrate of blood plasma (Section 14.1) (strictly an ultrafiltrate, since colloidal material is retained). It enters the interstitium in the form of free fluid, but nearly all of it immediately becomes bound. Of the fluid that is continually leaving the interstitium, about 90% is reabsorbed into the venous ends of the blood capillaries (Section 14.4); the remaining 10% escapes via the lymphatics as free fluid (Section 14.6.1).

Diffusion through the tissue gel is rapid, almost as rapid as through free fluid. Water, electrolytes, nutrients, metabolites, oxygen, and carbon dioxide are transported through the tissue gel by diffusion. Thus the tissue gel is the all-important roadway between the cell and the blood plasma.

Where the amorphous intercellular ground substance is a more rigid gel as in cartilage, it nevertheless contains a large amount of bound water which still allows diffusion. When the intercellular substance is impregnated with calcium and other salts, as in bone matrix, it finally becomes impermeable. Minute channels in the matrix (the bone canaliculi) are then required for diffusion.

The viscosity of the tissue gel has several functional advantages. It supports the cells and fibres, holding them apart and leaving space for diffusion between the blood capillaries and cells. It acts as a barrier, preventing bacteria from penetrating the tissues. It prevents interstitial fluid (tissue fluid) from percolating from the dorsal to the ventral parts of the body and piling up in the legs and feet.

It is estimated that the spaces between cells, i.e. the **interstitium** (substantia intercellularis), form about one sixth of the body (Guyton, 1986, p. 351).

The structure of the **ground substance** (substantia fundamentalis) was reviewed by Williams *et al.* (1989, p. 67). Two types of molecule predominate, **proteoglycans** and **structural glycoproteins**, both of which are combinations of carbohydrate and protein.

In **proteoglycans**, the carbohydrate component consists mainly of **glycosaminoglycans** (GAGs), previously called mucopolysaccharides. These are polysaccharide molecules made up of repeating disaccharides. In tissues they are nearly always combined with long filamentous proteins, and the combined molecules are then known as glycoproteins or proteoglycans depending on the relative proportions of the two constituents. The protein acts as a central core, from which the molecular filaments of the glycosaminoglycan radiate like the bristles of a brush. Some glycosaminoglycan–protein units may form even more immense, three dimensional, molecular com-

plexes by joining with hyaluronic acid (which is also a GAG) through another link protein. Glycosaminoglycans are very hydrophilic, and combine with many molecules of water by hydrogen bonding. This is the **bound water** that forms the **diffusion pathway** of the ground substance.

Structural glycoproteins generally provide adhesion between the cells and fibres in the ground substance. They consist of a protein and a carbohydrate component, but unlike proteoglycans the protein element predominates. **Fibronectin** has an affinity for collagen fibres and anchors fibroblasts to their supporting collagen fibrils. **Chondronectin** and **osteonectin** have similar functions in cartilage and bone. **Laminin** is a constituent of the basal lamina.

The **ground substance** is synthesized by fibroblasts in general connective tissue, and by chondroblasts and osteoblasts in cartilage and bone. In some sites it can be synthesized also by smooth muscle cells.

Some bacteria synthesize the enzyme **hyaluronidase**. This hydrolyses hyaluronic acid and other glycosaminoglycans, thus decreasing the viscosity of the ground substance and promoting the spread of infection.

Before the evolution of multicellular organisms, unicellular organisms depended on the homeostasis of the vast volume of sea water of the pre-Cambrian ocean. When the association of unicellular organisms first led to the formation of primitive multicellular animals, some of the surrounding sea water was supposedly incorporated to become the intercellular fluid (Woodbury, 1974, p. 451).

12.3 Diffusion

The cells of the body live by diffusion through the interstitial fluid, which delivers oxygen and nutrients from the blood plasma to the cell, and removes metabolic waste products such as carbon dioxide from the cell to the blood plasma.

Diffusion depends on the movement of solutes from regions of high concentration into regions of low concentration. For example, when a cell respires, the concentration of oxygen within its cytoplasm is reduced. The concentration within the cell falls below that of the interstitial fluid, thus establishing a concentration gradient, and oxygen then diffuses from the interstitial fluid into the cell. Metabolic waste products diffuse in the opposite direction. The rate of diffusion of a substance depends on the slope of its concentration gradient. The *steepness* of this slope is determined by the difference in concentration outside and inside the cell, and on the distance travelled. Diffusion is very slow over distances as great as 1 cm, but very fast over short distances of about 7 μm (approximately the diameter of a red blood cell).

The basic design requirement of the circulatory system is therefore to deliver blood in a very thin-walled tube as close as possible to every cell, thus creating the steepest possible concentration gradient at each cell. The *distance factor* of diffusion is so critical that even the one or two layers of smooth muscle in the wall of an arteriole (Fig. 12.2) form an effective barrier to diffusion. Therefore virtually all the exchange between blood and cells takes place across **capillary** walls, where the only tissue barrier is a single endothelial cell about 1 μm thick (Fig. 12.4).

Very active tissues such as the grey matter of the brain, skeletal muscle, and the myocardium have a capillary in the immediate proximity of every cell (Fig. 18.3, Section 18.3). On the other hand, cells with lower metabolic requirements, such as those in hyaline cartilage, can survive at much greater distances from their blood supply. Nevertheless, it is believed that, with rare exceptions, no functional cell in the body is more than 30 μm from a capillary.

> **Diffusion** is restricted to transport over short distances (Schmidt-Nielsen, 1990, p. 571). This is because diffusion time increases with the square of the diffusion distance, so that diffusion over 10 μm takes 100 times longer than diffusion over 1 μm. Thus if diffusion of oxygen over 1 μm takes 0.0001 s, it takes 0.01 s to diffuse over 10 μm, 100 s to diffuse over 1 mm, nearly 3 h for 10 mm, and over 3 years for 1 m, which is about the distance from the lungs to the limbs in a large mammal.
>
> A cylinder of protoplasm 1 cm in diameter and devoid of oxygen would take 3 h to become 90% saturated if suddenly plunged in pure oxygen. But a cylinder 7 μm in diameter would take only 0.0054 s to reach 90% saturation (Rushmer, 1966, p. 544).
>
> Diffusion over long distances is plainly ineffective, and transport by mass movement (i.e. convection) must then take over (Schmidt-Nielsen, 1990, p. 571).
>
> Diffusion (i.e. random molecular diffusion) results from the thermal kinetic energy possessed by individual particles.

12.4 Characteristics of the systemic and pulmonary circulations

The following survey applies mainly to the circulatory system after the animal is born, i.e. to the postnatal circulation. The fetal circulation is considered in Chapter 16.

12.4.1 *The systemic circulation*

The systemic circulation has the **left ventricle** as its pump, and serves the central and peripheral nervous systems, myocardium, skeletomuscular system, alimentary tract, urogenital system, and endocrine system.

Some of these systems have large and continuous metabolic demands. This is especially true of the central nervous system and myocardium. The metabolic requirements of some of the other systems fluctuate extremely, and sometimes at very short notice. For example, the skeletal musculature increases its oxygen demand about 20-fold during severe exercise, and needs an appropriate increase in blood supply. Blood flow through the skin is substantially increased by a rise in external temperature. Gastrointestinal activity and blood flow go up after a meal. There is not enough blood in one body to meet the maximum demands of all these systems simultaneously. Consequently blood flow has to be redistributed from one part of the body to another to satisfy their changing metabolic requirements.

Moreover, distances from the pump to the outlying regions like the muscles of the lower part of the hind limb are often great, and therefore some very long columns of fluid have to be moved.

> In the horse at rest about 80% of the blood volume is in the systemic circulation; of this volume, 60% is in the veins and venules and only 15% in the arteries (Evans, 1994, p. 138).

12.4.2 *The pulmonary circulation*

The pulmonary circulation has the **right ventricle** as its pump, and supplies the lungs alone. Since the structure and activity of all parts of the lung are essentially the same, only relatively minor adjustments in the distribution of blood are needed. Moreover, only comparatively short columns of blood need be moved.

> In the resting horse, about 20% of the blood volume is in the pulmonary circulation (Evans, 1994, p. 138).

12.4.3 General design requirements of the systemic and pulmonary circulations

The functional characteristics of these two great divisions of the cardiovascular system dictate the following basic design requirements. The **systemic circulation** will be a high pressure, high resistance system. The **high head of pressure** has two immediate objectives. Firstly, it provides an instantly accessible store of potential energy which can enable blood to be driven continuously to the central nervous system and myocardium. Refined mechanisms are available for rapidly and selectively opening or closing arterial channels, thus regulating the distribution of flow to different parts of the body. For example, in **exercise** the immediate opening of arterioles in skeletal muscles that suddenly become strongly active results in an instant increase in blood flow in those muscles: conversely, during exercise the gastrointestinal tract will usually be inactive, so the arterial vasculature supplying the gut is strongly constricted in order to decrease its blood flow to the minimum. Secondly, the high head of pressure provides the hydrostatic forces required (a) to reach the outlying parts of the body, and then (b) to drive fluid and dissolved substances through the capillary walls and into the interstitial fluid.

The **pulmonary circulation**, in contrast, will be a low pressure, low resistance system, with relatively little capacity for altering the distribution of flow (Section 17.12).

12.4.4 Arterial pressure

Arterial pressure (P) is directly proportional to the cardiac output (V) (the volume ejected by the left ventricle per minute) and to the total peripheral resistance (R); i.e. $P = V \times R$. This means that if the cardiac output remains constant, the pressure will rise or fall as the resistance increases or decreases. Thus regulation of resistance can regulate pressure.

12.4.5 Resistance

The resistance of a vessel depends on its length, and especially on its internal radius. Flow in blood vessels is typically laminar, not turbulent. During laminar flow of a fluid (i.e. a liquid or a gas) in a tube, the resistance is directly proportional to the length; therefore doubling the length doubles the resistance. The resistance of the tube is also inversely proportional to the internal radius to the fourth power; therefore halving the radius increases the resistance 16 fold (**Poiseuille's law**). In terms of flow, this means that if the pressure remains constant, halving the internal radius decreases the flow to one sixteenth of its original value.

The reason why narrowing the internal calibre affects resistance and flow so drastically is that, in laminar flow, the innermost laminae of fluid are restrained by shearing stress against the vascular wall, whereas the axial laminae flow rapidly; in a very narrow tube *all* the fluid is near the wall, and there are no fast flowing axial laminae (Section 6.14).

Since arterial pressure is directly proportional to vascular resistance, varying the internal radius of arteries and arterioles is a potent method of maintaining arterial pressure. Furthermore, varying the internal radius (and hence the resistance to flow) is the principal mechanism for diverting the arterial flow from one part of the circulation to another.

12.4.6 Conductance

The conductance of a vessel is the rate of flow relative to the difference in pressure at each end of the tube. It is inversely related to the resistance of the tube; as the resistance goes up, conductance goes down. Conductance (C) is therefore the reciprocal of resistance (R), or $C = 1/R$. Conductance is usually expressed as $mls^{-1}/mmHg^{-1}$.

12.4.7 Tension

The pressure inside a blood vessel puts the wall of the vessel under tension. Tension (T) is directly proportional to pressure (P); the greater the pressure the greater the tension. The tension is also directly proportional to the internal radius (r); as the radius goes up so the tension goes up. Thus $T = P \times r$ (the Laplace law). It therefore follows that, for a given pressure, the tension that develops in the walls of vessels of large calibre will be much greater than the tension in the walls of small vessels. The Laplace equation shows how the very small radius of a capillary (about 3.5 μm) could enable it to withstand pressures up to 30 mmHg (3.9 kPa) (at the arterial end of the capillary bed), even though its wall consists of only a single cell (endothelial cell) less than 1 μm thick (Section 12.12).

Strictly the tension is proportional to the transmural pressure, that is the difference between the pressure *inside* the vessel and the pressure *outside*. If a high pressure inside is balanced by an equally high pressure outside, there will be no tension in the wall.

II MICROSCOPIC ANATOMY OF BLOOD VESSELS

12.5 Types of blood vessel

12.5.1 Anatomical classification

The anatomical classification of blood vessels recognizes at least nine main varieties, namely elastic arteries, muscular arteries, arterioles, metarterioles, capillaries, sinusoids, postcapillary venules, muscular venules, and veins. The structure of these vessels is considered in Sections 12.8–12.16.

In histological sections there are intermediate vessels which cannot be classified firmly into one group or another. The diameters of blood vessels in histological sections vary greatly, depending on vasoconstrictor and vasodilator influences, including fixation.

12.5.2 Functional classification

The functional classification of blood vessels distinguishes conducting, distributing, resistance, exchange, and capacitance vessels.

Conducting arteries are low-volume, high-pressure, **elastic arteries** *arising from the heart*. They include the aorta, pulmonary arteries, brachiocephalic, subclavian, and common carotid arteries.

Distributing arteries include large and small **muscular arteries**, with a contractile capability enabling them to distribute blood selectively to the various components of the body. Most of the arteries of the body (excluding elastic arteries) belong to this category. For example, they include the femoral artery and its branches to individual skeletal muscles such as gracilis, the cranial mesenteric artery and its branches to the caecum, and the branches of the pulmonary arteries within the lobes of the lung.

Resistance vessels include all **arterioles** (large, medium, and small) and **metarterioles**. They are the main source of peripheral resistance in the circulatory system; it is across these vessels that the main fall in arterial pressure occurs in the live animal. They therefore control arterial pressure in general (Section 12.10). They also control the microcirculation of the various tissues. The **total peripheral resistance** is the resistance of the entire systemic circulation. About half of the total peripheral resistance resides in the arterioles.

Exchange vessels are capillaries, sinusoids, and postcapillary venules. Exchanges between the blood plasma and the interstitial fluid take place through the walls of these vessels. Materials so exchanged include oxygen, carbon dioxide, nutrients, water and inorganic ions, vitamins, products of metabolism, hormones, antibodies, and defensive cells.

Capacitance (reservoir) **vessels** are muscular venules and veins, with large volume and low pressure, that return the blood to the heart.

Mellander and Björnberg (1992) distinguished two groups of resistance vessels, namely 'large-bore' arterial resistance vessels greater than 25 μm in diameter (i.e. large and medium sized arterioles), and 'small arterioles' less than 25 μm.

Kuo *et al.* (1992) noted that 50–80% of vascular resistance resides in arterioles 10–100 μm in diameter.

12.6 Structural components of blood vessels

12.6.1 Endothelium

All blood vessels, lymphatic channels, and the chambers of the heart, are lined internally by **endothelial cells**. The smoothness of endothelial cells confers low frictional resistance to blood flow. The walls of **blood capillaries** (Fig. 12.5) are formed by endothelial cells, supported only by a **basal lamina** (Section 12.12). The walls of sinusoids (Section 12.13) and lymphatic capillaries (Section 14.6.1) are also formed by endothelial cells, but lack a basal lamina.

It is of imperative importance that the blood should not clot on the luminal surface of normal endothelium. To avoid coagulation, the endothelial cell must be completely intact as well as perfectly smooth. Roughened imperfections in the endothelial surface damage blood cells in general and **platelets** in particular. Injured platelets, and platelets in contact with the collagen of a disrupted vascular wall, become activated and release substances (phospholipids) which are involved in initiating **extrinsic** and **intrinsic clotting reactions** (Section 12.21.2). Endothelial cells in perfect condition have a monomolecular layer of protein adsorbed to their luminal surface, and this repels both platelets and **clotting factors**: damaged endothelial cells lose this vital protective layer against coagulation.

12.6.2 *Intima, media, and adventitia*

The walls of all blood vessels except the very smallest have three layers, the (tunica) intima (interna), (tunica) media, and (tunica) adventitia (externa). In **arteries** (Figs 12.1, 12.2), the **intima** comprises a lining of endothelial cells, a thin layer of subendothelial connective tissue, and an **internal elastic membrane** (membrana elastica interna). The **media** is composed of concentric layers of smooth muscle cells and elastic fibres, each in varying proportions depending on the type of artery; an **external elastic membrane** (membrana elastica externa) lies in the media, at the boundary with the adventitia. The **tunica adventitia** consists of collagen and elastic fibres, which blend imperceptibly with the surrounding connective tissue. In large arteries the adventitia contains **vasa vasorum**, small blood vessels supplying the vascular wall, and lymphatics. **Axons** may be found in any of the three tunics.

In the walls of **veins** (Fig. 12.8), the internal and external elastic membranes are ill-defined or absent. The amount of smooth muscle and elastic fibres in the media is relatively small, but collagen fibres are relatively abundant. There are also many collagen fibres in the adventitia, which is often the thickest layer of the wall.

The **endothelium** of the tunica intima confers low frictional resistance to blood flow. The **elastic membranes** and **elastic fibres** in the tunica media provide elasticity during pulsatile pressure changes or distension. The **smooth muscle cells** in the tunica media make it possible to regulate the internal calibre. The **collagen fibres** in the adventitia and the collagenous connective tissue in the intima provide protection against longitudinal and circumferential stresses.

The walls of the smallest vessels, i.e. **metarterioles**, **capillaries**, and **postcapillary venules** (and **sinusoids** may also be included in this group), are so thin (only one or two cells thick) that the terms intima, media, and adventitia are no longer meaningful. For example, it is difficult to visualize a 'middle' tunic in a vessel such as a metarteriole that is only two cells thick.

12.6.3 *Distensibility of vascular walls*

According to the **Laplace equation** (Section 12.4.7), the tension in the walls of blood vessels increases as the radius increases, and this explains the presence of **elastic fibres** in ever greater numbers as vessels get larger: for example, elastic elements are negligible in metarterioles, but ordinary arterioles have an inner elastic lamina, and small muscular arteries have an inner and outer elastic lamina as well as elastic fibres scattered throughout the smooth muscle cells of the media. Similarly, variable numbers of elastic fibres first appear in small muscular venules, between the endothelium and the smooth muscle cells.

The elastic tissue in these various vessels applies enough restraining force in the wall to balance, passively, the distending force of the blood pressure, and does so at a minimal cost of energy. The highly elastic walls of the great arteries near the heart act as shock absorbers withstanding the full impact of ventricular contraction.

Despite the presence of so much elastic tissue and the familiar pulsatile bulging with each heart beat, the walls of blood vessels do not follow the laws of simple elastic systems as exemplified by a rubber band. A piece of elastic obeys **Hooke's law**: it lengthens in direct proportion to increasing tension, until it finally yields completely; in other words, a plot of tension against length gives a straight line, until the point of yield. In blood vessels, when the wall is stretched its resistance is not proportional to each additional stretch; its resistance becomes relatively stronger and stronger at each additional stretch. Thus blood vessels have non-linear elastic properties, becoming disproportionately stiffer with increasing tension.

This peculiar elastic behaviour of blood vessels is caused by the **combination of elastic and collagen fibres** in the wall. The elastic fibres are first brought into play by only a very slight stretching of the wall, and subsequently show a more or less linear elastic response to further stretching. On the other hand, the collagen fibres have a certain amount of 'give' as they become straightened out, but reach their limit of extension rather abruptly; their main function is therefore to prevent overdistension.

Thus the elastic fibres in the wall of a blood vessel resemble the rubber wall of a fire hose: the collagen fibres are like the canvas coat enclosing the outside of the hose as a protective limiting jacket. Compare the similar protective role of collagen fibres in preventing overdistension of the wall of pulmonary alveoli (Section 6.9). When a fire hose is not carrying water it can be flattened and rolled up. Veins, with a thick collagenous adventitia, are also flattened when more or less empty and this, indeed, is the secret of their ability to accommodate large quantities of blood (Section 12.16.3); filling a vein entails little more than changing its shape from flat to cylindrical.

12.7 The microcirculation

The smallest blood vessels are grouped together as the '**microcirculation**'. No rules decide exactly which vessels should be included in the microcirculation, but as a working guide it usually includes all blood vessels that are too small to be visible to the naked eye. Since the limit of resolution of the naked eye is about $100\,\mu m$, vessels with a diameter less than this belong to the microcirculation. Many arterioles and muscular venules have diameters between 100 and $50\,\mu m$, and are therefore included in the microcirculation. But the main components are the vast numbers of vessels which are even smaller, i.e. the **metarterioles**, the **capillaries**, and the **post-**

capillary venules. Also included are arteriovenous shunts (Section 12.17).

12.8 Elastic arteries

Elastic arteries are **conducting arteries** (Section 12.5). Their principal role is simply to act as channels for conveying blood. They are always of large calibre, and most of them are near the heart. Examples are the aorta and its main branches (the brachiocephalic, common carotid, and subclavian arteries), and the pulmonary arteries.

The **intima** is lined by endothelial cells, with subendothelial connective tissue. The intima possesses a fenestrated **internal elastic membrane** or lamina, but this is inconspicuous because there are similar elastic laminae in the media.

The **media** is the most distinctive structural feature of an elastic artery. It consists of a series of concentric fenestrated **elastic lamellae** (about 40 in man). 'Fenestrated' means that these lamellae are not continuous sheets but are perforated by many apertures. Between the elastic lamellae lie scattered smooth muscle cells. The **external elastic membrane** (or lamina) of the media is more or less indistinguishable from the outermost elastic lamella of the media.

The **adventitia** possesses yet more elastic fibres reinforced by collagen fibres. These merge with the surrounding connective tissue.

The powerful elastic components in the walls of elastic arteries (and large muscular arteries) are a device for storing potential energy and releasing it to drive blood through the smaller vessels. Where does this potential energy come from?

The source is the muscular work done by the left ventricle in the systemic circulation and the right ventricle in the pulmonary circulation. A similar form of **stored energy** occurs during resting breathing, when some of the energy released by contraction of the inspiratory muscles is stored by the elastic continuum of the lung, and then used for expiration (Section 10.2.2). The elastic recoil of the arterial walls thus creates a reservoir of arterial pressure. This smoothes out the steep fluctuations in pressure and flow which arise from the repetitive ventricular contraction and relaxation, so maintaining the continuity of blood flow required by metabolically very active tissues such as the nervous tissues of the brain. The reservoir of pressure also gives the ventricle time to relax and refill in preparation for its next contraction.

The great elastic arteries such as the aorta make a major contribution to the reservoir of pressure in the systemic circulation. In addition, their highly elastic walls act as shock absorbers withstanding the full impact of ventricular contraction.

> The elastic artery is known in the *Nomina Histologica* (1994) as arteria elastotypica.
>
> As would be expected from the current interest in human cardiovascular disease, changes in the structure of the aortic wall in man with advancing age and disease have been extensively studied (Krstic, 1984, p. 24; Williams *et al*., 1989, p. 685). In children the intima may be almost insignificant, but in young adults it thickens because of lipid deposits and fibromuscular proliferation, and after middle age the intima may become grossly thickened (Fig. 18.4) (arteriosclerosis and atherosclerosis, Section 18.9). These changes affect the large arteries of man, and particularly the aorta, coronary, and cerebral arteries.

12.9 Muscular arteries

Muscular arteries, large and small, are **distributing arteries** (Section 12.5, ii). Their principal role is to control the distribution of blood according to the metabolic needs of the various components of the body. They include most of the arteries of the body, except the elastic arteries.

> The terms 'large' and 'small' as applied to muscular arteries (arteria myotypica) are arbitrary, and there is no agreement about their measurements. The axillary or femoral arteries would generally be accepted as 'large', and if a branch of such an artery were not much thicker than a hair it could be reasonably described as 'small'. This leaves the boundary between large and small undefined, although the functions of the vessel might well change in this intermediate form. More difficult is the point which distinguishes a small muscular artery from a large arteriole, a transition where functional changes become quite probable. The contractility of arterial and arteriolar walls creates further difficulties in distinguishing large from small, since contraction varies with the functional state of a vessel in the live animal and with the effects of fixation after death (Section 12.5.1).

12.9.1 *Structure of muscular arteries*

In a muscular artery (Fig. 12.1), the **intima** is lined by endothelial cells backed by a greater or lesser amount of connective tissue depending on the size of the vessel. The **internal elastic membrane** is a conspicuous refractile line, which is usually wavy because of the contraction of the smooth muscle cells in the media during fixation. In a transverse histological section it forms a reliable landmark for identifying the outer limit of the intima. **Fenestrations** of the inner elastic membrane allow diffusion of metabolites between the media and the lumen. The **media** consists of layer upon layer of circular or spiral **smooth muscle cells**, with a relatively weak **external elastic membrane** (Fig. 12.1). The **adventitia** consists of connective tissue with collagen and elastic fibres, which blends with the surrounding connective tissue. **Sympathetic vasomotor fibres** in the adventitia innervate smooth muscle cells in the media (13.3.1).

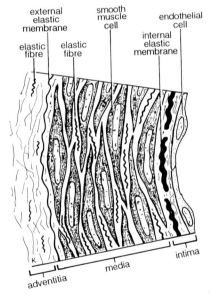

Fig. 12.1 Semidiagrammatic transverse section of a segment of the wall of a small muscular artery. The tunica intima consists of a lining of endothelial cells with a thin layer of connective tissue, and a fenestrated though strong internal elastic membrane. The tunica media has concentric layers of circular or spiral smooth muscle cells, with some elastic fibres and a relatively weak external elastic membrane. The tunica adventitia is formed by connective tissue with collagen and elastic fibres, blending with surrounding connective tissues.

12.9.2 *Contractile elements of muscular arteries*

By varying the internal radius of its vessels, the smooth muscle in the media controls the appropriate distribution of blood to the various parts of the body. For example, at the **onset of exercise** the distributing arteries to the musculature of the limbs (the axillary and femoral arteries) dilate, and the distributing arteries to the gastrointestinal tract (the coeliac, and cranial and caudal mesenteric arteries) constrict.

Smaller distributing arteries can provide fine-tuning of the blood flow in the limbs. For example, if the exercise were to make particularly heavy demands on the extensor muscles of the elbow (triceps brachii), the smaller muscular arteries supplying these muscles would be especially dilated.

These vasodilator and vasoconstrictor adjustments of the smooth muscle in the tunica media are achieved through the modification of the **basal tone** of the vascular smooth muscle (Section 13.1) by the metabolic, neural, hormonal, myogenic, and endothelial factors considered in Sections 13.2–13.6.

Regulation of the smooth muscle of distributing arteries also contributes to the adjustment of the **total peripheral resistance** and hence the maintenance of arterial pressure at appropriate levels.

> The smooth muscle cells (Williams *et al.*, 1989, p. 686) are mainly *spiral* in orientation, except in small arteries where they are mostly circular. In arteries that undergo repeated bending, such as the carotid and axillary arteries, there are longitudinal muscle cells in both the intima and the media. Adjacent myocytes communicate by gap junctions, thus allowing the transmission of the contractile impulse from cell to cell.

12.9.3 *Elastic elements of muscular arteries*

Although the characteristic feature of distributing (muscular) arteries is smooth muscle, there are also powerful elastic components in the walls of these vessels. In addition to the strong **internal elastic membrane** in the intima, there is generally a less powerful **external elastic membrane** in the outer border of the media. **Elastic fibres** are also dispersed throughout the media, between the layers of smooth muscle, and there are some in the adventitia.

These elastic elements contribute an elastic recoil to the walls of distributing arteries, detectable when **taking the pulse**, for example, at the femoral artery of a dog. This capacity for elastic recoil enables the distributing arteries to aid the conducting (elastic) arteries in creating a reservoir of arterial pressure and smoothing out the pulsatile fluctuations in pressure and flow that arise from ventricular contraction.

12.10 Arterioles

Arterioles (arteriolae) are **resistance vessels** (Section 12.5). Their principal role is to regulate the total peripheral resistance and hence arterial pressure. The **smallest arterioles** also collaborate with **metarterioles** to regulate the **microcirculation**, by controlling the flow of blood through the capillary beds.

The structural transition from artery to arteriole is not abrupt but gradual. There is no agreement about the external diameter that distinguishes an artery from an arteriole, both of which are variably contractile anyway, although it is sometimes assumed that an arteriole will be not more than 100 μm in external diameter (see the advanced text below). The best criterion for identifying an arteriole is the presence of only one or two layers of smooth muscle cells in its **tunica media** (Fig. 12.2), the muscle cells being circular or spiral in orientation. The smooth muscle layers are **continuous**, rather than intermittent as in a metarteriole (Section 12.11). The **intima** of an arteriole usually has a thin fenestrated **internal elastic membrane** (Fig. 12.2), but the smallest arterioles lack elastic elements altogether. The internal lining of the intima is formed by the usual single layer of endothelial cells, supported by a few connective tissue fibres. There is a **tunica adventitia** of loose connective tissue carrying unmyelinated axons that innervate the smooth muscle.

As the arterioles branch into metarterioles, and the metarterioles into capillaries, the **total cross-sectional area** of each pair of vessels so produced exceeds the area of the parent vessel (as in the conducting division of the pulmonary airways, Section 6.8); this slows the velocity of blood flow in these small-bore vessels (Section 12.12.6) and *passively* decreases the total peripheral resistance to blood flow.

However, *active* contraction and relaxation of the smooth muscle in the walls of arterioles is the main factor in the regulation of the **total peripheral resistance** (Section 12.4.5); and (since arterial pressure = cardiac output × total peripheral resistance) the arterioles have a profound influence on **arterial pressure** in general. Arterioles account for at least half of the resistance in the entire systemic circulation, and it is for this reason that they belong to the group of vessels known as **resistance vessels** (Section 12.5). Like the smooth muscle of muscular arteries, that of arterioles has an inherent **basal tone** (Section 13.1) which can be modulated by metabolic, neural, hormonal,

myogenic, and endothelial factors (Sections 13.2–13.6).

Arterioles also regulate the flow through the microcirculation in response to changes in the metabolic activity of the tissues. As an example, consider the adjustments of the blood supply in the skeletal musculature at the sudden **onset of exercise**. The smooth muscle cells of the arterioles have a sympathetic adrenergic innervation. This acts on alpha receptors and is therefore vasoconstrictor in effect (Sections 13.3.1 and 13.3.2). The sudden onset of exercise induces immediate sympathetic activity throughout the body. This at once causes a generalized/vasoconstriction, including the arterioles in the active muscle.

The vasoconstriction in the active tissue is now overruled by an **ascending vasodilation** (Section 13.8), which starts at the smallest arterioles and the metarterioles. The vasodilation is initiated by metabolic factors (Section 13.2), for instance by a fall in the oxygen concentration in the active tissue; this is predictable, since these small vessels are in intimate contact with the now highly active tissue. The vasodilation is augmented by the effects of shear stress on the endothelium (Section 13.6), and finally reaches the distributing (muscular) arteries (Section 13.8). It is also possible that, *at the very onset of exercise*, the sympathetic vasoconstriction in skeletal muscle may be modulated by the **vasodilator** action of sympathetic **cholinergic** fibres (Section 13.3.4).

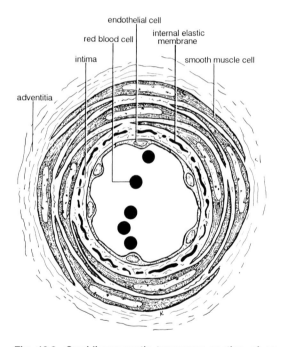

Fig. 12.2 Semidiagrammatic transverse section of an arteriole. The tunica intima has a lining of endothelial cells. The nuclei tend to bulge into the lumen. The endothelium is supported by a small amount of connective tissue and a thin fenestrated internal elastic membrane. The tunica media comprises two overlapping layers of circular or spiral smooth muscle cells. There is no external elastic membrane. The tunica adventitia consists of connective tissue, blending with surrounding tissues. The red blood cells, about 7 μm in diameter, provide a scale of measurement.

The internal lumen of arterioles is lined by non-fenestrated endothelial cells. In small arterioles the **internal elastic membrane** (membrana elastic interna) is missing. The internal elastic membrane of medium-sized arterioles may be reduced to patches of elastic tissue, allowing processes of endothelial cells to pass through and attach to smooth muscle cells in the media by **myoendothelial junctions** (gap junctions) (Krstic, 1984, p. 25); it has been suggested (Smiesko and Johnson, 1993) that these junctions may transmit vasodilator signals, stimulated by shear stress on the endothelial surface (thus supporting the release of vasodilator substances such as nitric oxide from the endothelial cells when the flow rate of blood increases, Section 13.6).

Rhodin (1974, p. 346) pointed out that, since the structural transition of artery into arteriole is gradual, no exact point in the change can be identified anatomically. The highest estimate of the **maximum external diameter** of an arteriole is 'generally less than 500 microns' (Junqueira and Carneiro, 1983, p. 251). Rhodin (1974, p.

348), himself an authority on the structure of the microcirculation, considered it to be 'generally agreed that arterioles are microvessels with a diameter of less than 300 microns'. Other estimates are much lower, for example 100 μm being the largest size according to Krstic (1984, p. 25) and Williams *et al.* (1989, p. 686). Estimates of the **minimum** external diameter of an arteriole are also erratic. If it be granted that an arteriole eventually dwindles into a metarteriole, then the **maximum** external diameter of a metarteriole is presumably the same as the **minimum** external diameter of an arteriole. Williams *et al.* (1989, p. 686) give the diameter range of metarterioles as 10–15 μm at their beginning and as little as 5 μm at their end; this yields a minimum arteriolar external diameter of 10–15 μm. Krstic (1984, p. 259) gives no estimate of the external diameter of a metarteriole, but draws one about 15 μm in diameter and agrees with Williams *et al.* (1989, p. 686) that metarterioles gradually diminish down to 5 μm.

The patient reader can see that there are almost as many estimates of these parameters as there are experts. For the teacher and students this creates difficulties, since students in the practical laboratory are apt to ask, 'is this an arteriole?' As already pointed out (Section 12.5.1), diameter has little meaning as a criterion for distinguishing between blood vessels. The number of muscle layers is a better criterion, but there is little agreement about that, too. Rhodin (1974, p. 344) estimated the number of layers in muscular arteries as commonly 40 down to 10, with a minimum of 3–4 in small muscular arteries. Krstic (1984, p. 274) gave the range of layers in large to small muscular arteries as 60 to a minimum of three. These views would allocate the arteriole just one or two muscle layers. Williams *et al.* (1989, p. 686) gave no estimate for muscular arteries, but mentioned 'one or two' layers of muscle in arterioles.

To summarize, in view of the effects of fixation it is probably best not to tie the boundary between muscular artery and large arteriole to any particular measurement, but to put it from 300 μm down to 100 μm in external diameter. On the other hand, the number of muscle layers can be stated somewhat more precisely, the smallest muscular artery having three or four layers and the arteriole one or two layers.

In the histology laboratory, the perplexed student can use a simple test when searching with a microscope for an arteriole under a beady professorial eye: if the muscle layers can be counted, the vessel is an arteriole. This is because in histological sections the more numerous muscle layers in even a very small muscular artery lose their definition.

Guyton (1986, p. 348) reported some interesting observations on the hierarchy of branches within the microcirculation. Having entered an organ, an 'artery' then divides six to eight times before the diameter falls as low as 40 μm. (At this point, Guyton regards the vessel as an 'arteriole'.) It then branches 2–5 more times to reach a diameter of about 9 μm. Its subsequent progeny are then capillaries. Unfortunately the authority for this information is not stated.

12.11   Metarterioles

Metarterioles are included among **resistance vessels** (Section 12.5), since they contribute substantially to total peripheral resistance. However, in collaboration with the smallest arterioles, metarterioles are also the main factor controlling the perfusion of the microcirculation.

The metarteriole (Fig. 12.3) comes after the arteriole, as its name implies (Greek: meta, after), and gives rise to the capillaries. For this reason it is also known as a **precapillary arteriole** or as a **terminal arteriole**.

A metarteriole is lined internally, as usual, by endothelial cells. There are also a few collagen fibres in the **tunica intima**, but the internal elastic membrane is lost. At the *proximal* end there is a single layer of smooth muscle cells, circular or spiral in orientation (Figs 12.3, 12.9); these are intermittent so that substantial lengths of the vessel, particularly towards its distal end, have no

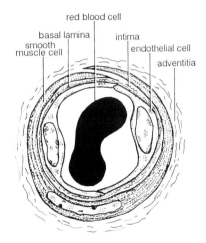

Fig. 12.3 Semidiagrammatic transverse section of a metarteriole. The tunica intima comprises endothelium and a few collagen fibres. There is a single layer of circular or spiral smooth muscle cells. External connective tissue blends with the surrounding tissues. The internal lumen is large enough to admit one red blood cell, but relaxation of the muscle may allow several to enter. Contraction may close the lumen.

muscle cells (Fig. 12.9). (Where there are no muscle cells, there cannot be a tunica media.) The internal diameter is capable of allowing a single red blood cell to go through as in Fig. 12.3, but in histological sections the action of the fixative on the smooth muscle may virtually close the internal lumen; on the other hand, if a vascular bed is well perfused with blood at the moment of death, the lumen of a metarteriole may be distended enough to accommodate several red cells.

The smooth muscle cells of metarterioles, like all other vascular smooth muscle, have **basic tone** (Section 13.1). By the modulation of their tone, they play a major role in regulating **recruitment of capillaries** (Section 12.12.7) and hence in controlling the volume of flow through the capillary beds of a tissue, according to the changing metabolic activity of different parts of that tissue. Because of this regulation of the capillary bed, the metarteriole and its strategically placed smooth muscle cells constitute what is known as the **precapillary sphincter**.

Unlike arterioles, the smooth muscle of metarterioles usually if not always **lacks a nerve supply**, and must therefore depend totally on non-neuronal factors for control of its basic tone; these include metabolic (Section 13.2.1), hormonal (Section 13.4), myogenic (Section 13.5), and endothelial factors (Section 13.6). Of these, the **metabolic factors** dominate, since metarterioles (like the smallest arterioles) are in particularly close contact with the tissues and their metabolites. Thus dilation of the metarterioles, in tissue like skeletal muscle that suddenly becomes metabolically active, begins the process of **ascending vasodilation**. Once started by metabolic factors from active tissue such as skeletal muscle at the onset of **exercise**, the vasodilation ascends the various grades of arterioles and muscular arteries by means of the effects of shear stress on the endothelium (Section 13.8).

Metarterioles contribute substantially to the **peripheral resistance** in the systemic arterial system. Nevertheless, their lack of innervation presumably restricts their participation with arterioles in *regulating* the total peripheral resistance, and hence in regulating the arterial pressure. Together, arterioles and metarterioles account for about half of the resistance in the systemic circulation.

The metarteriole (metarteriola) is the structural basis for the so-called '**precapillary sphincter**'. The classical concept of a precapillary sphincter (e.g. Williams *et al.*, 1989, p. 686) assumed that one or two smooth muscle cells surround each capillary **at the point where it comes off the metarteriole**. Rhodin (1974, p. 350), who had made a study of the subject, took a simpler view and regarded the whole length of the metarteriole as the precapillary sphincter, an interpretation apparently shared by Krstic (1984, p. 342). A metarteriole could vary the blood flow through its capillary bed by increasing, reducing, or completely closing part or all of its lumen, thus shunting the blood to other parts of the microvascular bed or bypassing it altogether (Fig. 12.9); the regulation of such changes is believed to be dominated by metabolic factors (Section 13.2.1). The precapillary sphincter, then, **is** the metarteriole.

A metarteriole (Rhodin, 1974, p. 350) varies in length from about 5 to 100 μm or more, and has an unpredictable lumen ranging from a maximum of perhaps 30 μm to a minimum of 5 μm or less, depending on the state of its smooth muscle cells and the pressure inside the lumen. Along the metarteriole, an increasing number of endothelial cell processes establish **cell junctions** with the smooth muscle cells, especially with the last muscle cells along the vessel; by these connections vasomotor factors derived from the endothelium (Section 13.6) may contribute to the regulation. Sparse connective tissue at the rim of the vessel blends with the connective tissue of the surrounding tissue.

Physiological arguments *against* the possibility that metarterioles participate in the regulation of peripheral systemic resistance were summarized by Wiedeman *et al.* (1976), though it was agreed that they do regulate the distribution and rate of flow of blood in the microcirculation. These authors also reviewed the evidence for the motor innervation of these vessels, and concluded that such innervation is indeed lacking.

12.12   Capillaries: endothelial cells

The **blood capillary** is the principal example of an **exchange vessel** (Section 12.5.2). All blood capillaries have one essential feature in common: their wall is only one cell thick, that cell being an endothelial cell.

They can be classified into different types, but these relate only to minor details such as site (arterial or venous end of the capillary bed) and the nature of the endothelial lining (thick, thin, fenestrated).

It is estimated that the body contains about 10 000 million capillaries (vas capillare), with a total surface area of about 500–700 m² (Guyton, 1986, p. 348). The length of an individual capillary ranges between 200 and 1000 μm (Krstic, 1984, p. 61). Zweifach (1959) calculated that their total length is nearly 60 000 miles (96 000 km), and that together they comprise the largest organ in the body, their total bulk being more than twice that of the liver. If all were open simultaneously they would contain all the blood in the body.

Classifications of capillaries (Rhodin, 1974, p. 352; Krstic, 1984, p. 61) recognize continuous capillaries with thick endothelium, continuous capillaries with thin endothelium, fenestrated capillaries, glomerular capillaries, arterial capillaries, true capillaries, and venous capillaries. **Continuous capillaries with thick endothelium** have a relatively thick endothelial cell (300–800 nm thick), many pinocytotic vesicles, and no fenestrations; these occur in skeletal, cardiac, and smooth muscle, ovary and testis, and brown adipose tissue. **Continuous capillaries with thin endothelium** have a relatively thin endothelial cell (100–200 nm) and few pinocytotic vesicles; these occur in the lung, central nervous system, spleen, thymus, lymph nodes, bone, and connective tissue. **Fenestrated capillaries** have even thinner endothelial cells (average 80 nm) with fenestrations (Section 12.12.5). Sinusoids (Section 12.13) are sometimes known as **discontinuous capillaries**.

Arterial capillaries (vas capillare arteriale) have essentially the same structure as **venous capillaries** (vas capillare venosum) (Krstic, 1984, p. 61), yet venous capillaries are believed to be several times more permeable (Guyton, 1986, p. 354). Arterial capillaries arise directly from a metarteriole, and venous capillaries drain into a **postcapillary venule**; the so-called **true capillary** separates an arterial from a venous capillary. According to Krstic (1984, p. 62) two or three true capillaries are confluent into a single venous capillary. For 'sinusoidal capillaries' see Section 12.13.

Besides being more permeable, venous capillaries are more numerous than arterial capillaries, and therefore the total surface area of venous capillaries is several times greater than that of arterial capillaries (Guyton, 1986, pp. 354, 358).

12.12.1   *Calibre of capillaries*

The calibre of an average capillary is wide enough to allow erythrocytes to pass through one at a time (Fig. 12.4). An erythrocyte is a biconcave disc about 7 μm in diameter, but being very pliant it often becomes bell-shaped and, by presenting its

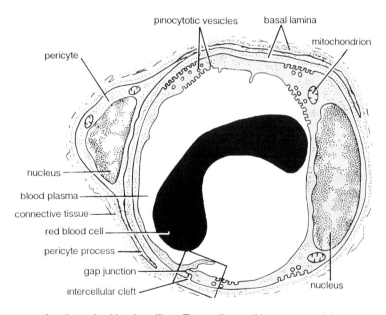

Fig. 12.4   Transverse section through a blood capillary. The capillary wall has two essential components, an endothelial cell (green) and the basal lamina of an endothelial cell. In some capillaries two or more endothelial cells may be present in a transverse section. The overlapping edges of the endothelial cell interlock at the intercellular cleft (inside the square, see Fig. 12.5). The cleft is sealed in one or more places by spot-like gap junctions. The endothelial cell has many pinocytotic vesicles about 60 nm in diameter. The slender cell processes of a pericyte surround most of the endothelial cell. The pericyte has a basal lamina, which blends with that of the endothelial cell.

convex surface forwards, it squeezes through capillaries with an internal diameter of only 3–4 μm. In histological sections a capillary in transverse section appears as a minute thin-walled ring, sometimes containing a single tight-fitting red blood cell. Occasionally a section passes through the nucleus of the endothelial cell, and this then appears as a basophilic crescent partly encircling the lumen.

> The internal **diameter** of a typical capillary is about 7–9 μm (Ham, 1974, p. 573), 20 μm when distended (Catchpole, 1966, p. 619), and about 3 μm when almost collapsed (Krstic, 1984, p. 60).

12.12.2 Structure of capillary wall

The essential structural difference between a capillary and a metarteriole is that the capillary has no smooth muscle. The wall of a capillary is therefore reduced to two essential components, a thin **endothelial cell** and a **basal lamina** (Fig. 12.4). Externally there is a sparse network of connective tissue fibrils. Largely enclosing the outer surface of a capillary with its slender cell processes there is often an elongated cell called a **pericyte** (Fig. 12.4), of unknown function.

12.12.3 The endothelial cell of capillaries

The endothelial lining of a capillary sometimes consists of a single endothelial cell rolled up, with its adjoining edges overlapping each other (Fig. 12.4). In other capillaries, segments of two or more endothelial cells may be visible in a transverse section.

The overlapping edges of endothelial cells are usually interlocked, as in Fig. 12.4 and the enlarged view in the top diagram of Fig. 12.5. Between the overlapping edges there is a gap, the **intercellular cleft**. The cleft is completely sealed in various places by spot-like gap junctions; elsewhere the cleft is held open by very large protein–carbohydrate macromolecular complexes, similar to those that form the **ground substance** of the **interstitium** (Section 12.2). (In physiological texts the intercellular clefts, together with pinocytotic vesicles and fenestrations, are often referred to as 'pores'.) The cleft is the principal pathway between the blood plasma and the interstitial fluid

for the **transport** of water and its small molecule solutes. Thus it provides both for **diffusion**, and for **filtration** and **reabsorption**. It is also used by leucocytes to migrate from the blood to the interstitium during **inflammation** (diapedesis; Section 12.14). **Postcapillary venules** participate extensively in all of these functions. Thus both capillaries and postcapillary venules are the principal **exchange vessels** of the circulatory system (Section 12.5.2).

In a typical capillary (Ham, 1974, p. 574), most of the **intercellular cleft** is about 20 nm wide, but it is narrowed to about 2 nm at **gap junctions** of the macula type (Fig. 12.5, top diagram). These gap junctions form minute spot-like areas of close adhesion between the overlapping edges of the endothelial cells; their function is to anchor the endothelial cells to each other. Apart from the scattered gap junctions, however, the cleft remains about 20 nm wide. It is occupied by proteoglycans, mainly hyaluronic acid (Guyton, 1986, p. 349). It is through the cleft that the water and its small molecule solutes are transported, both by diffusion and filtration (Wiederhielm, 1974, p. 132; Navaratnam, 1975, p. 137).

In the capillaries of the **brain**, however, the overlapping edges of the endothelial cells are attached by **tight junctions**, of the zonula occludens type (Krstic, 1984, p. 42). These form a continuous seal, leaving no gap anywhere between the overlapping edges, and thus contributing to the **blood–brain barrier** which blocks the movement of large molecules. A similar blood–tissue barrier occurs in some other organs, for example the testis (Williams *et al.*, 1989, p. 691).

Since **endothelial cells** are thin squamous cells, the nucleus tends to bulge into the lumen of a blood vessel (Figs 12.2, 12.6). The **organelles** (Krstic, 1984, p. 140) are not very abundant, as might be expected from the thinness of the cytoplasm. Among them are a centriole, a small Golgi apparatus, a few lysosomes, some free ribosomes, some bundles of microfibrils, a few large granular vesicles of unknown function (Rhodin, 1974, p. 340), and – the most conspicuous feature – a large number of pinocytotic vesicles. The plasmalemma has microvilli, which are less numerous in blood vessels with higher flow rates.

On the whole, **endothelial cells** do not look particularly active, though they are very rich in certain enzymes including **ATPase** and **adenylcyclase** (Krstic, 1984, p. 140). Nevertheless, researches in the last decade have shown that endothelial cells in metarterioles, arterioles, and muscular arteries continuously release extremely potent vasoactive agents that diffuse into the adjoining vascular wall, causing local vasodilation (e.g. nitric acid) or vasoconstriction (e.g. endothelin-1); these **endothelium-derived vasomotor agents** are produced

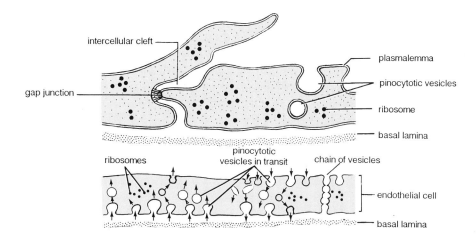

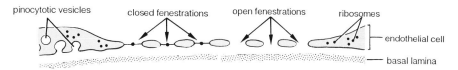

Fig. 12.5 **Semischematic sections through endothelial cells of blood capillaries at high magnification. Top diagram: The intercellular cleft in the square in Fig. 12.4.** In the cleft, the edges of the endothelial cell (green) are firmly attached by scattered gap junctions of the spot variety, one such junction being shown. At these points, the cleft is narrowed to about 2 nm. The rest of the cleft is held open by protein–carbohydrate macromolecules similar to those forming the interstitial ground substance, the gap being up to 20 nm wide. The clefts account for the great majority of diffusion, and filtration and reabsorption, across the capillary wall.

Middle diagram: pinocytotic vesicles. On the left, pinocytotic vesicles are detaching themselves from the plasmalemma of the endothelial cell (green), crossing the cytoplasm, and blending with the plasmalemma on the other side of the cell to discharge their contents into the blood plasma (upward arrows). In the right centre, vesicles are filling from the blood plasma, detaching themselves, crossing the cytoplasm, and emptying into the interstitial fluid (downward arrows). At the right, vesicles are blending into a continuous channel.

Bottom diagram: fenestrations. A fenestration is a circular area about 70 nm in diameter. Fenestrations occur in specialized endothelial cells. Usually there is a delicate closing membrane with a central knob, the membrane probably being formed by fusion of the inner and outer plasmalemma. Fenestrations of this type occur, for example, in the capillaries of endocrine organs. In glomeruli, there are no closing membranes. Redrawn and modified from Renkin (1978).

particularly by the endothelium of **resistance vessels**, i.e. arterioles and metarterioles, and are therefore of the greatest importance in the automatic regulation of systemic arterial pressure and the blood flow in individual organs (Section 13.6).

12.12.4 *Pinocytotic vesicles of endothelial cells*

Endothelial cells have many **pinocytotic vesicles** (Figs 12.4, 12.5). They lie along both the luminal and the peripheral surface of the endothelial cell,

and within its cytoplasm as well. Sometimes they coalesce, forming a more or less continuous channel across the cell (Fig. 12.5, middle diagram). It is generally accepted that pinocytotic vesicles transport large molecular proteins across the capillary wall. They appear to arise as invaginations or evaginations of the endothelial plasmalemma.

The **pinocytotic vesicles** (vesiculae pinocytoticae) of endothelial cells are about 60 nm in diameter (Krstic, 1984, p. 261), i.e. about two to three times greater in diameter than the wider parts of the intercellular cleft.

12.12.5 *Fenestrated endothelial cells*

In a few special tissues such as the endocrine organs and the kidney, where the transfer of substances from the blood is particularly active, there are pore-like fenestrations in the endothelial cells of the capillaries. A fenestration is a circular area where the endothelial cell is reduced to a delicate closing membrane (Fig. 12.5, bottom centre), by the apparent fusion of the inner and outer plasmalemma of the endothelial cell.

In an endotheliocytus fenestratus, a typical fenestration is a circular area about 70 nm in diameter (Rhodin, 1974, p. 356). The closing membrane, which has a central thickening (Fig. 12.5, bottom, left central), is derived from the plasmalemma (Krstic, 1984, p. 62), and not from the basal lamina as stated by Williams *et al.* (1989, p. 689). Capillaries of this type are found in endocrine organs, dermis, the kidney, and also in the choroid plexus, ciliary body, and intestinal mucosa (Rhodin, 1974, p. 354). However, the fenestrations in the **glomerular capillaries** are open and have no closing membrane (Rhodin, 1974, p. 356), so that the only barrier between the plasma and the filtrate is the basal lamina; however, the basal lamina is unusually thick, and therefore forms an effective barrier to all plasma proteins (Wiederhielm, 1974, p. 131).

12.12.6 *Velocity of capillary blood flow*

Because the combined cross-sectional area of the two tubes produced by each branching of an arteriole and metarteriole is greater than the cross-sectional area of the parent vessel (Section 12.10), the total cross-sectional area of all the capillaries together exceeds that of the aorta by a factor of several hundred. Since the total volume of blood flowing through all the capillaries roughly equals that flowing through the aorta, the velocity of flow in the capillaries is therefore very much slower than in the aorta (a few millimetres per second). The reduced velocity in the capillaries gives time for the exchange of substances between the blood and interstitial fluid, yet the rate of flow is not so slow that the cells in the tissues outrun their fuel supplies.

Estimates of the velocity of flow in capillaries vary: 0.07 mm per second (Rushmer, 1966, p. 546); 0.8–2.0 mm per second (Catchpole, 1966, p. 619); 1–10 mm per second (Wiederhielm, 1974, p. 132). The velocity in the aorta is about 50 cm per second (Rushmer, 1966, p. 545).

12.12.7 *Capillary recruitment*

In resting tissues (for example quiescent glands or inactive skeletal musculature) considerable numbers of capillaries are closed at any particular moment. There tends to be a phasic opening of capillaries in one area of a tissue as those in another area close. When a large region of such a tissue is becoming progressively active, more and more of its capillaries open and are perfused. This is known as capillary recruitment, as in the lung (Section 6.29). Eventually almost the entire capillary bed may be opened, and blood flow in the tissue can then increase to its maximum.

The **control of recruitment** lies in the **metarterioles** and the **smallest arterioles**. The smallest arterioles are probably innervated (Section 13.3.1), but the metarterioles are not. However, lying as they do in the closest possible contact with the active tissues, both the metarterioles and the smallest arterioles are believed to be regulated mainly by **metabolic factors** (Section 13.2.1). For example, their smooth muscle cells respond directly to a fall in oxygen concentration by relaxing, i.e. by vasodilation.

The concept that an individual capillary has an autonomous capacity to **change its diameter**, independently of the contraction of arterioles or metarterioles, has attracted the attention of researchers from the end of the nineteenth century onwards (Hammersen, 1976). There is, of course, no doubt that the diameter of blood capillaries does change from moment to moment in living tissues, but are such changes due to active contraction and relaxation of the capillary wall or are they simply passive changes caused by variations in pressure across the capillary wall?

The discovery of numerous **microfilaments** in endothelial cells appeared to confirm the idea of active contraction. However, such microfilaments are now known to predominate in endothelial cells which are subjected to particularly severe stresses, such as the endothelial cells that line **venous valves**; they also increase significantly in number in hypertension. Microfilaments are therefore now interpreted as a source of tensile strength, not contractility (Hammersen, 1976).

It was also suggested that **pericytes** might be contractile, endowing their capillaries with contractility, but Rhodin (1974, p. 358) concluded that experimental investigations had failed to demonstrate contractility. More recent observations (Shepro, 1988) did show pericyte contractility in response to vasoactive agents (e.g. histamine and serotonin), but only with the action of regulating the closeness of endothelial cells to one another. The enquiry now seems to be in abeyance.

12.13   Sinusoids

A **sinusoid**, like a capillary, is an endothelial channel connecting the arterial to the venous side of the circulation. However, its structure differs from that of a capillary: (1) instead of being a slender tube, the sinusoid is an irregular bulging vessel of much greater capacity than a capillary; (2) its endothelial lining is discontinuous, with spaces between the individual endothelial cells; (3) the endothelial cells have multiple fenestrations; (4) the basal lamina is almost entirely absent.

These structural features promote the interchange of fluids and macromolecules between plasma and interstitial fluid, and therefore sinusoids are included among the **exchange vessels** (Section 12.5). In particular, they allow the relatively easy **movement of cells** across the endothelium. Sinusoids are therefore characteristic of haemopoietic organs such as the spleen and bone marrow in which there is much movement of cells, and also of the liver. In the **spleen** the gaps between the endothelial cells are wide enough to allow the exchange of erythrocytes and lymphocytes between the blood plasma and the reticular tissue of the red pulp. In the **bone marrow** similar wide spaces enable newly formed blood cells to pass into the circulation. In the **liver**, the openings in the sinusoidal walls allow blood plasma to fill the **perisinusoidal space** (of Disse) and thus make a particularly intimate contact with the surfaces of the liver parenchymal cells.

Sinusoids tend also to be associated with **phagocytic activity**. In the liver, **stellate macrophages** (macrophagocytus stellatus, or von Kupffer cells) are interposed between endothelial cells, projecting into and even across the lumen of the sinusoid. In the spleen, the **cords of the red pulp**, which lie between the sinusoids, contain many splenic macrophages (Section 14.18.2). In the bone marrow, there are free macrophages and **phagocytic reticular cells** in the supporting fibrillar network. However, sinusoids are also found in the **adrenal gland** and **hypophysis**, and here they are not associated with phagocytosis.

Almost all authorities regard the sinusoid (vas sinusoideum) as a type of capillary (vas capillare sinusoideum; NH, 1983). They are sometimes known as 'discontinuous capillaries' (Krstic, 1984, p. 61), because of the spaces between their endothelial cells. However, their structure and function are so different from those of capillaries that it is more logical to regard them as a discrete class of blood vessel.

12.14   Postcapillary venules

Several capillaries drain into one **postcapillary venule** (Fig. 12.9). The postcapillary venule resembles an outsize capillary, although its calibre may be only slightly larger than that of a capillary. Its wall consists of an endothelial lining, basal lamina, and numbers of pericytes, with some connective tissue externally (Fig. 12.6). There are no smooth muscle cells. The edges of adjoining endothelial cells frequently overlap like those of capillaries. Unlike capillaries, however, junctional specializations are often missing and therefore the intercellular cleft is particularly accessible for exchange functions.

Postcapillary venules are **exchange vessels** (Section 12.5). They associate themselves with capillaries in forming a vast area for the exchange of gases, water, nutrients, and metabolites between the blood plasma and the interstitial fluid. Also the scarcity of specialized intercellular

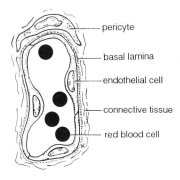

Fig. 12.6 Semischematic transverse section through a postcapillary venule. The wall consists of endothelial cells, basal lamina, and pericytes, and some outer connective tissue blending with the surrounding tissue. There are no smooth muscle cells. The red blood cells (about 7 μm in diameter) give a measuring scale.

junctions in postcapillary venules particularly promotes the migration (**diapedesis**) of blood cells through the vascular wall. The postcapillary venule is a specially important site for the diapedesis of granular leucocytes and the formation of **oedema** during the **inflammatory response** of tissues (Section 14.9.2).

The typical postcapillary venule (venula postcapillaris) is about 10–50 µm in diameter, and about 50–700 µm in length (Krstic, 1984, p. 341). Its endothelial cells are about 200–400 nm thick, roughly intermediate between the endothelial cells of thick and thin continuous capillaries (Section 12.12).

Postcapillary venules in the inner cortex (thymus-dependent zone) of **lymph nodes** (Section 14.17) (Krstic, 1984, p. 341) are a specialized variant. Their endothelial cells are cuboidal or even columnar, and therefore much thicker than the endothelial cells of any other blood vessels. They appear to provide a migratory pathway for T-lymphocytes entering lymph nodes from the blood stream (Section 14.12.3). Since the endothelial cells here are so tall, the contact between the two endothelial cells is closed on one side before the lymphocyte has forced them apart on the other side.

12.15 Muscular venules

Muscular venules form the small venous channels that are commonly called '**venules**'. When empty (and seen in histological sections) they appear as thin-walled *irregular ovals*, or partly collapsed vessels, in contrast to their satellite arterioles which have a much thicker muscular wall and a more consistently *circular* shape (Fig. 12.7).

The luminal surface of the **intima** is lined by endothelial cells. The **media** is weakly developed, with only one or two layers of innervated smooth muscle cells (compare the several muscle layers in the arteriole in Fig. 12.2). The **adventitia** consists of a relatively thick layer of collagenous connective tissue, with sympathetic vasomotor axons.

The general tendency for muscular venules in resting tissues to be semi-collapsed, and their relatively well developed tunica adventitia, show them to be **capacitance vessels** (Section 12.5.2), contributing to the venous reservoir (Section 12.16.3).

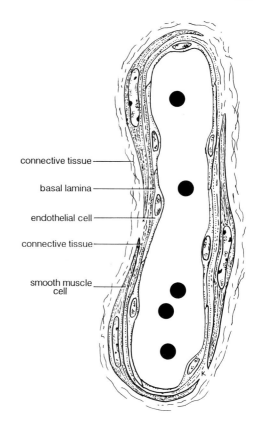

connective tissue
basal lamina
endothelial cell
connective tissue
smooth muscle cell

Fig. 12.7 Semischematic transverse section through a muscular venule. The partly collapsed profile is typical. The tunica intima is formed by endothelial cells, basal lamina, and some connective tissue. The media consists of one or two layers of smooth muscle cells. There is never an internal or external elastic membrane.

The external diameter of muscular venules (venulae musculares) ranges from 50 µm to 1 mm. The structure (Rhodin, 1974, p. 360) is characterized by an internal lining of relatively thick, continuous, endothelial cells joined together (Krstic, 1984, p. 274) by zonulae occludentes and gap junctions. The endothelial cells are backed by a basal lamina. An elastic membrane is never present, but scattered elastic and collagen fibres lie between the endothelium and the layer of smooth muscle cells (Rhodin, 1974, p. 360).

The structure of the endothelial cells, their close attachments to one another, and their fibrillar support, indicate **capacitance** but little exchange. In contrast to postcapillary venules, they therefore play little or no part in normal diffusion, or in the movements of cells and the formation of oedema during inflammation.

12.16   Veins

12.16.1   *Basic structure*

Veins (venae) (Fig. 12.8) have thinner walls than their satellite arteries, but the intima, media, and adventitia are recognizable. The **intima** is formed from non-fenestrated endothelial cells, supported by a basal lamina and a thin layer of collagen fibrils. Depending on the size of the vein, the **media** often consists of two or three, or several, layers of innervated circular smooth muscle cells, with some elastic and collagen fibres. The smooth muscle endows veins with **basal tone** (Section 13.1). Compared with arteries of similar size (i.e. their satellite arteries), veins have much less smooth muscle and elastic tissue. On the other hand, collagen fibres are relatively far more abundant than in arteries; the **adventitia** is often the thickest layer, consisting of many collagen fibres and a few elastic fibres.

Veins are categorized by size (Krstic, 1984, pp. 441–442). The range of **diameters** of small veins is 0.2–1 mm, medium-sized veins 1–10 mm, and large veins 10 mm and more.

In **medium-sized** and **large veins** (Rhodin, 1974, p. 364), a widely fenestrated **internal elastic membrane** sometimes occurs. The tunica media is very thin, with only a limited number of smooth muscle cells, but the adventitia is very thick, consisting of collagen and elastic fibres and some smooth muscle cells. In the largest veins (Williams *et al.*, 1989, p. 691) the adventitia is much thicker than the media, and contains abundant **longitudinal smooth muscle fibres**. In the **caudal vena cava**, collagen bundles interwoven with elastic fibres form a spiral meshwork around the vessel, which allows it to shorten and lengthen with the movements of the diaphragm. The great veins that enter the heart (venae cavae, pulmonary veins, and coronary sinus) acquire **cardiac muscle fibres** in the media. In some of the largest veins (e.g. caudal vena cava, azygos, hepatic, hepatic portal, cranial mesenteric, splenic, renal, external iliac) the smooth muscle in the adventitia actively propels blood towards the heart (Krstic, 1984, p. 442).

12.16.2   *Valves: muscle pump*

Valves first appear in medium-sized veins, and especially in limbs which support the body against the force of gravity. The largest veins, such as the great veins in the abdomen and thorax, have no valves.

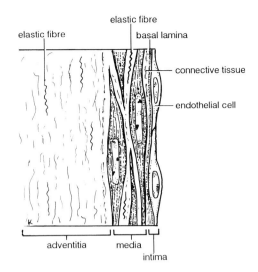

Fig. 12.8   Semischematic transverse section through a segment of the wall of a small vein. The tunica intima consists of endothelial cells, basal lamina, and a small amount of connective tissue. In small veins there is no internal elastic membrane. The tunica media contains two or three layers of circular smooth muscle cells. The adventitia is the thickest layer, consisting of collagenous connective tissue with a few elastic fibres.

Each valve is a pocket-like **semilunar cusp** attached to the interior of the vein, with the opening of the pocket directed towards the heart. The pocket is therefore flattened when the blood streams over it on its way towards the heart. If the blood flow is reversed (i.e. *away* from the heart), it catches the crescentic free border of the valve so that the pocket fills. Usually the pockets occur in pairs on opposite sides of the lumen; when both of them fill, their free borders touch and seal the lumen of the vein against reflux.

In the standing quadrupedal animal and in man, the weight-bearing limbs extend well below the level of the heart. Therefore the limb veins contain long vertical columns of blood. The hydrostatic pressure in the bottom of a *continuous* vertical column of liquid exceeds that at the top by the length of the column multiplied by the density of the fluid. The pressure at the bottom of a *continuous* column of blood in a long vein in the limb of a large animal such as a man or a horse will be high, and this would lead to excessive filtration across the capillary beds drained by such a vein. However, the valves of the vein convert its

column of blood into a series of *short segments.*
The hydrostatic pressure is greatly reduced in
each individual segment, in proportion to its reduction in length.

Contraction of the muscles in the limb, as in
walking, applies pressure to the veins. This causes
the blood to move towards the heart, since the
valves prevent movement towards the foot. This
action of the muscles of the limb is known as the
muscle pump. In the horse, the muscle pump is
reinforced by compression of the venous plexuses
on either side of the cartilages of the hoof.

If an animal stands still for a long time, there is
no muscle pump and blood accumulates in the
veins of the limbs. The valves are then kept open,
and the blood becomes a continuous column.
Oedema then tends to form in the distal part of
the limb (Section 14.9.1).

The muscle pump contributes substantially to
the **venous return to the heart** (Section 13.3.5).

When a large animal such as a horse or man stands still,
the flow of blood through the capillary beds fills the veins
of the limbs, the valves are held open, and the pressure at
the bottom of the now *continuous* column of blood is
about 80 mmHg (10.7 kPa). This pressure will be transmitted to the blood capillaries in the foot and other distal
parts of the limb. (The normal hydrostatic pressure at
the arterial end of a capillary is about 32 mmHg
(4.3 kPa); see Section 14.3.) When the animal walks, the
tissue pressure in the contracting muscles may reach
about 85 mmHg (11.3 kPa) (Wiederhielm, 1974, p. 143),
and this provides the force of the **muscle pump**. Since
the valves prevent regurgitation, the blood is forced
onwards towards the heart.

If an animal stands still for a long time, the high
capillary pressure in the distal part of the limb leads to
excessive filtration through the capillary wall, and this
may result in **oedema** (Section 14.9.1). The muscle pump
is also one of the main forces that move **lymph** towards
the heart (Section 14.8). Therefore, if the muscle pump
is not exercised, not only is there excessive filtration
but there is also decreased lymphatic drainage (Section
14.9.4) and this accentuates the oedema in the distal
part of the limb. In horses, oedema from this cause is
known as '*stocking-up*' or '*filling of the limb*' (Section
14.9.4).

In man, excessively large volumes of blood can be
retained in the legs during prolonged standing. It is well
known that soldiers standing to attention during protracted parades sometimes faint. As much as 10% of the
total blood volume can be sequestered in the legs during
such prolonged standing. This can impair the venous
return to the heart enough to diminish cardiac output,

reduce arterial pressure, and induce unconsciousness
(Wiederhielm, 1974, p. 143).

Structurally, a **venous valve** (Williams *et al.*, 1989,
p. 169) is a pocket-like reflection of the intima, reinforced by collagen and elastic fibres. The wall of the vein
facing each cup is slightly dilated, so that when the
paired valves close the adjoining wall bulges giving the
external surface of the vein a beaded appearance.

12.16.3 *Venous blood flow: venous reservoirs*

The flow of blood in systemic veins depends fundamentally on the pressure head in the aorta.
However, the **systemic venous pressure** has fallen
to about 15 mmHg (2.0 kPa) at the venous end of
a capillary bed, if the bed is at the level of the
heart. The **right atrial diastolic pressure** (Section
22.2) fluctuates around atmospheric pressure;
right atrial systolic pressure reaches maxima of
about 5 mmHg (0.7 kPa). Small though it is, this
basic pressure gradient from the capillaries to
the heart (from about 15 mmHg (2.0 kPa) at the
venous end of the capillaries, down to 5 mmHg
(0.7 kPa) at the right atrium) is nevertheless great
enough to move blood back to the heart, the veins
being low resistance vessels. The pressure in the
right atrium is known as the **central venous pressure**. Superimposed on the basic venous pressure
gradient are fluctuations in intrathoracic and
intra-abdominal pressures caused by breathing
(Section 13.3.5); these fluctuations are sometimes
very large, as in forced expiration when contraction of the abdominal muscles steeply raises the
intra-abdominal pressure, compressing the great
abdominal veins accordingly. Thus breathing augments the venous return to the right atrium.

The **systemic veins** (muscular venules and
veins) are a major **venous reservoir** for the storage
of blood. In the **resting animal**, they contain over
60% of all the blood in the body. The **splanchnic**
and **cutaneous veins** form the major components
of this systemic venous reservoir. The **liver** and
spleen also serve as venous reservoirs, since they
contain mobile reserves of blood amounting to
about another 5% (or more) of the total blood
volume. A further 10% of the total blood volume
is in the **pulmonary vasculature** (Section 17.17).
Together, all of these sites constitute the **blood
reservoir** of the body, and contain about 75% of
the total blood volume. From the systemic com-

ponents of this reservoir, blood is fed to the right side of the heart and then to the lungs.

At first sight, the walls of veins have a structure that seems not too well-adapted for the function of **storage**. Their soft, flexible walls are thinner than the walls of their companion arteries, and contain fewer elastic fibres and smooth muscle cells; their collagen, on the other hand, is relatively more abundant, especially in the adventitia which is typically the thickest layer. These structural features might seem to limit the ability of such vessels to accommodate large variations in volume. However, like venules, veins tend to be flattened or elliptical in cross-section. It is the ability to **change shape** (rather than undergo elastic stretching) that enables veins to vary their capacity, and thus to play such an important role as **capacitance vessels** for storing blood.

A simple conversion of a vein from a flattened oval to a **circular** cross section greatly increases its capacity, and yet the increase in pressure (and hence the energetic cost) needed to accomplish this is very small. Strictly the pressure should be referred to as the **transmural pressure**, since it is the pressure across the wall (from the inside to the outside of the vessel) that changes the shape. It follows that veins have a high **compliance** (change in volume per unit change in transmural pressure; Section 6.31). The abundant collagen fibres prevent over-distension (Section 12.6.2).

At the sudden onset of **severe exercise**, as in **fight and flight**, there is a mass discharge of the **sympathetic system** (Section 22.16). The strong vasoconstrictor action of this discharge has two immediate circulatory effects. (1) By causing contraction of the smooth muscle in the venous walls it instantly releases from the blood reservoir of the body a very great additional volume of blood for utilization by the skeletal musculature; much of this blood comes from the splanchnic and cutaneous veins. (2) It simultaneously closes, for a short period, the arterial input to tissues which are not required in the emergency; for example, the splanchnic arterial circulation would be temporarily shut down. The coronary and cerebral arterial systems are exempted from closure, even temporarily, since the brain and heart must be fully active during exercise; these vessels have a very weak vasoconstrictor innervation (Section 13.3.2). The result is that (in man) about 2 litres of

blood (the total blood volume being about 5 litres) immediately become available to the active skeletal musculature. The blood flow to the musculature thus suddenly increases more than 20 times above the resting values, and its metabolic activity goes up about 50-fold. These circulatory and metabolic changes are splendid for the Olympic athlete, but for the predator and prey they are a matter of life and death.

The shunting of blood from the systemic veins in fight and flight is activated by the sympathetic vasoconstrictor innervation of the smooth muscle in the venous walls. Such vasoconstrictor innervation is particularly well developed in the splanchnic and cutaneous veins (Section 13.3.5), which are the principal systemic venous reservoirs. Severe **haemorrhage** is followed by a similar shunting of blood from the venous reservoirs of the splanchnic and cutaneous systemic veins, liver, and spleen, by means of sympathetic venoconstriction. This maintains an adequate venous return to the heart, and hence cardiac output, despite the reduction in blood volume.

Wiederhielm (1974, p. 141) indicated that a rise of only 1 mmHg (0.13 kPa) is enough to convert the elliptical profile of a vein into a circular cross section, and this simple change increases the capacity of the vein three-fold. A further small rise of pressure (to about 10 mmHg, 1.3 kPa) stretches the elastic fibres in the wall, readily allowing an additional increase in capacity (about sixfold, in all). After this, more and more of the collagen fibres approach their limit of extension; the wall then becomes progressively much stiffer, requiring a large increase in pressure to achieve a further small increase in capacity.

12.17   Arteriovenous shunts

An **arteriovenous shunt** is a communication between the arterial and venous side of the circulation, thus bypassing the capillary network. There are several varieties, but the main one is a simple arteriovenous anastomosis.

A **simple arteriovenous anastomosis** connects an arteriole with a muscular venule (Fig. 12.9). It often has a thick muscular wall of smooth muscle cells, with a sphincter-like action. The smooth muscle cells are innervated by excitatory sympathetic postganglionic efferent axons, which can

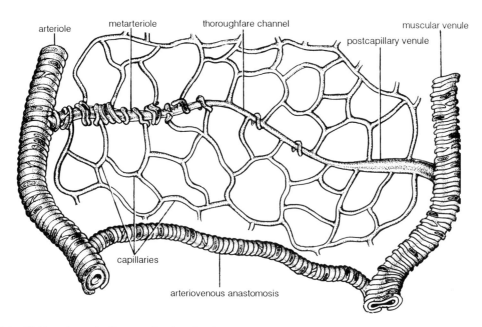

Fig. 12.9 Highly schematic diagram showing the elements of the microcirculation. The microcirculation consists of all blood vessels under 100 μm in diameter. It includes small arterioles, muscular venules, and arteriovenous shunts, but is formed mainly by metarterioles, capillaries, and postcapillary venules. A metarteriole has a single layer of intermittent circular or spiral smooth muscle cells. Some of these muscle cells are entwined around the root of a capillary as it arises from the metarteriole. This led to the concept of the 'precapillary sphincter', but the whole length of the metarteriole acts as a precapillary sphincter. The metarteriole often leads directly into a thoroughfare channel, which has a slightly larger calibre than a capillary and possesses a few circular smooth muscle cells. The arteriovenous anastomosis shown in the diagram is of the simple type, directly connecting the arteriole to the muscular venule. It has a thick wall comprising innervated circular smooth muscle cells which can close the anastomosis.

close the anastomosis. The muscle cells are also influenced by metabolic, humoral, myogenic, and endothelial factors (see advanced text).

At first sight it may appear likely that an arteriovenous anastomosis, when open, will **de-crease** the volume of blood flowing through the tissues that it serves, simply because it short circuits the arteriole to the venule and thereby cuts out the capillary bed. Some anastomoses do indeed have this function, the physiological objective being to divert blood **away** from tissue that is functionally inactive. For example, this is the action of the arteriovenous anastomosis in a villus of the gastrointestinal tract; it diverts blood away from the capillary beds of the villus when no intestinal absorption is in progress.

Many other arteriovenous anastomoses have the opposite effect: when one of these is open, it **increases** blood flow through its territory. Examples of these occur in the skin, where they

play an important part in **thermoregulation**. They open when the body temperature rises. There are so many of them in the skin of regions like the ears and feet that, when the anastomoses open, the total volume of blood flowing through the skin greatly **increases**. This enables heat to be lost: conversely, they close when the body temperature falls, thus conserving heat. The smooth muscle in their walls has a dense innervation by sympathetic vasoconstrictor fibres; a small increase or decrease in the discharge of these axons greatly decreases or increases respectively the blood flow through these anastomoses.

Another common type of arteriovenous anastomosis is the **thoroughfare channel**. This connects the end of a metarteriole to the beginning of a postcapillary venule (Fig. 12.9). It has a slightly larger calibre than a capillary and possesses an occasional circular smooth muscle cell, but otherwise has the same structure as a capillary.

A third variety of arteriovenous anastomosis is a **glomeriform arteriovenous anastomosis** (anastomosis arteriovenosa glomeriformis). Like the simple arteriovenous anastomosis (anastomosis arteriovenosa simplex), this has an innervated contractile wall. It differs from the simple type in that the contractile part is limited to a short segment which is highly convoluted. This convoluted contractile segment is enclosed by a dense connective tissue capsule, thus forming a small compact spherical 'glomus' (Latin: glomus, a ball of thread).

The structure, distribution, and function of arteriovenous anastomoses were reviewed by Sherman (1963). Five anatomical variants have been identified, but these include some that appear to be no more than intermediate types between simple and glomeriform anastomoses. Arteriovenous anastomoses in one form or another have been found in all the important organs of the body, including the heart, lungs, gastrointestinal tract, urogenital organs, endocrine organs, and central nervous system.

Both the simple (Krstic, 1984, p. 18) and the glomeriform types (Krstic, 1984, p. 174) are common in exposed regions of the **dermis**, especially in the external ear, lips, nose, and digits (Le Gros Clark, 1965, p. 205). Also large numbers of the simple type of shunt are found all over the dorsal mucosal surface of the dog's **tongue** (Chibuzo, 1993, p. 411). All these parts of the body are involved in **thermoregulation**. Le Gros Clark (1965, p. 204) proposed that the anastomoses are so numerous and of such large calibre that, when *open*, they *increase* the total volume of blood flow through the region much more than is possible through the capillary beds alone. An alternative explanation (Scott, 1986, p. 81) of the thermoregulatory function of these dermal anastomoses is that, when opened, they fill the deep venous plexi in the dermis with warm blood, enabling heat to be lost from the plexi to the environment. Likewise the arteriovenous anastomoses in the surface of the dog's tongue dilate if the body temperature rises, in order to increase *evaporative cooling by panting* (Le Gros Clark, 1965, p. 205).

Dermal arteriovenous anastomoses appear also to control the *local*, as opposed to the *general*, body temperature. For example (Sherman, 1963, p. 260), if a finger is immersed in iced water the temperature of its skin falls, but while the finger is still immersed a sudden rise in its skin temperature occurs. This rise coincides with an increase in the total blood flow through the skin of the finger and marked decrease in capillary flow. Here, the function of the arteriovenous anastomosis is rewarming of the exposed part (Williams *et al.*, 1989, p. 694). In principle, therefore, the function of arteriovenous anastomoses in these tissues is to *increase* the blood flow by *opening*.

In certain other tissues, arteriovenous anastomoses *increase* the blood flow by *closing* (Williams *et al.*, 1989,

p. 694). One or two arteries run to the tip of an **intestinal villus** without branching, and there form a capillary network (Krstic, 1984, p. 210); one or two veins collect the blood from the capillaries, and convey it to veins in the submucosa. At the tip of the villus there is a simple arteriovenous anastomosis connecting the arteries to the veins. When alimentary absorption is active the anastomosis is closed and the capillary bed is perfused. In the absence of absorption the anastomosis opens and blood is diverted from the capillaries.

The **control of blood flow through arteriovenous anastomoses** seems to be multifactorial (Sherman, 1963, p. 259). There is an inherent **basal tone** but it is unusually weak. What tone there is, is modulated by a profuse autonomic innervation, humoral substances, oxygen tension and pH (metabolic factors), intravascular pressure (myogenic factors), and presumably also by factors derived from the endothelium in response to shear stress. No clear cut patterns of regulation have emerged, except that arteriovenous anastomoses are highly responsive vessels, and that they often react differently from neighbouring arteries or arterioles to the same stimuli.

The contractile cells of a **glomeriform anastomosis** are modified smooth muscle cells (Kristic, 1984, p. 174). They are pale and swollen, resembling epithelial cells, and are therefore called '**epithelioid cells**' (Williams *et al.*, 1989, p. 694). These peculiar cells have been found, in variable numbers, in nearly all arteriovenous anastomoses (Sherman, 1963).

The *mechanisms* by which arteriovenous anastomoses *open and close* are not entirely clear (Williams *et al.*, 1989, p. 694). When circular smooth muscle cells are present they presumably close the lumen, perhaps aided by the epithelioid cells. If there are no smooth muscle cells, the lumen may be closed by *swelling* of the epithelioid cells.

Thoroughfare channels are also known as **preferential channels**. The muscle cells are placed so far apart (Fig. 12.9) that the channel is almost indistinguishable from a true capillary (Zweifach, 1959). Direct flow through the thoroughfare channel is presumably controlled by the last muscle cells of the metarteriole. The physiology of thoroughfare channels is not known.

12.18 Artery-to-artery anastomoses: collateral circulation

It is quite common for a small artery to form a branch that anastomoses directly with another similar artery, before either of them forms its capillary bed. Arterial anastomosis between major arteries may even occur **end-to-end**. A notable example of arterial anastomosis is the **cerebral arterial circle** on the ventral surface of the forebrain, which acts as an arterial Piccadilly Circus receiving several incoming arteries and giving off various outgoing arteries (see King, 1987).

Although perhaps not quite on the grand scale of the cerebral arterial circle, anastomoses of substantial arteries occur in many other parts of the body. End-to-end anastomoses between the cranial and caudal **mesenteric arteries** and their branches are found along the mesenteric border of the intestines. The dorsal and ventral **intercostal arteries** are another example of end-to-end anastomosis (Section 8.16.2). If such arteries are cut surgically, they bleed from both of the cut ends; both ends must be ligated, and such ligation may be carried out with impunity. In the limbs, the arteries proximal to a joint tend to anastomose with arteries distal to the **joint**; the movement of a joint may obstruct one set of its arteries, but the flow may be restored by the anastomosing vessels. Anastomoses between arteries become progressively more numerous as the branching of the arterial tree proceeds; in other words small arteries anastomose more often than large arteries. The direction of blood flow in any such anastomosing network of arteries, or veins, is determined solely by the **pressure gradients** in the various vessels, since a fluid will only flow from a greater to a lesser pressure.

The many anastomoses that occur between small arteries form the basis for the development of a **collateral circulation**, if an artery is closed by disease or trauma. This is a matter of great clinical importance. Although the collateral vessels may at first be of small diameter, they tend to dilate quite rapidly and can often form a perfectly adequate alternative pathway. However, much depends on the metabolic demands of the affected tissue. The more active the tissue, the more time it requires to form a viable collateral circulation. The rate of occlusion is also important: a sudden total occlusion may kill the tissues in its territory, whereas a gradual occlusion may allow the development of an adequate collateral pathway. See also Section 12.19.

If the **femoral artery** is suddenly occluded (Guyton, 1986, p. 236), the blood flow to the distal leg falls within a few seconds to about one eighth of its normal flow. During the next 1 or 2 minutes, the collateral circulation dilates and the blood flow returns to about 50% of normal. During the next week or longer, the blood flow

reaches nearly normal values. The initial opening of the collateral vessels seems to be started by metabolic factors.

The subsequent gradual improvement of a collateral circulation is believed to be controlled by the progressive increase in the release of **nitric oxide** (or some other **endothelium-derived vasorelaxant**). This release occurs in response to the increasing blood flow and the resulting increase in the shear stress on the endothelium of the collateral vessels (Section 13.6).

12.19   End-arteries

Some organs contain arteries that make no direct arterial anastomotic connections with any other arteries, and may even lack anastomoses via their capillary beds. If such an artery be closed, the territory that it supplies must die. Such vessels are known as **end-arteries**. An extreme example is the **central artery of the retina**. In man, and probably in the domestic mammals, this is a true end-artery. Blocking it by a clot or embolus results in permanent blindness in that eye, since there is no alternative route by which the retina can obtain a blood supply.

True end-arteries are scarce, but **functional end-arteries** are quite common and are particularly important in the brain and heart. A functional end-artery is one that does anastomose with neighbouring arteries, but the anastomoses are too small to be functionally effective and therefore the artery **functions** as though it were an end-artery. For example, in the white and grey matter of the brain there are no end-arteries in the strict anatomical sense, since the small arteries do anastomose through their capillary beds and to some extent by direct arteriolar connections. But these anastomoses do not provide an adequate collateral circulation, and if a small artery is blocked by a thrombus or embolus the territory that it supplies will die. The reason for this is the metabolic activity of neurons in the brain, which is so extreme that pyramidal cells in the motor cortex are fatally injured 8 minutes after occlusion of the main arterial supply to the brain.

Functional end-arteries also occur in the **myocardium** (Section 18.9). Anastomoses are found in the coronary arterial vasculature, but only between one arteriole and another arteriole, and across their capillary beds. Since the cardiac muscle cells are constantly active and cannot rest, they demand a continuous and generous oxygen supply. The first few days after the sudden occlusion of a branch of a coronary artery are critical. During this period, the collateral circulation is often insufficient and the myocardial cells in its territory may die, and this can result in fatal **fibrillation** of the heart (Section 21.23.2). If that period is survived, the collateral circulation builds up and may eventually restore normal levels of myocardial blood flow.

The penicillar arteries of the spleen are said to be true end arterioles (Section 14.18).

12.20 Angiogenesis

Remodelling of arterioles, capillaries, and venules occurs not only during embryonic development but also throughout adult life, resorbing ineffective pathways and adding new ones. Such remodelling is the basis for the **long-term adjustment** of the vascular bed in a tissue that is experiencing a sustained change in its metabolic activity (Section 13.2.2). An example is the increase in the capillary beds of muscle that occurs during athletic training.

Angiogenesis is particularly important in **repair** of damaged tissues. The injured area is invaded by solid cords of cells; these proliferate from surviving endothelium, smooth muscle cells, and fibrocytes, or by the differentiation of primitive mesenchyme cells in the connective tissue. The cords become canalized and anastomose, forming vascular beds. Some of the vessels acquire a fibromuscular coat and innervation, thus converting to arterioles and venules.

The **bronchial circulation** in the lung is a productive site of angiogenesis in adult tissues (Section 17.9).

Another site of potential angiogenesis is the coronary circulation in man (Section 18.9.3).

The stimuli for these remarkable adaptive and defensive responses appear to be various polypeptide **growth factors (mitogens)**, for example **platelet-derived growth factor** (PDGF). These are released by macrophages, activated T-lymphocytes, and platelets (Section 12.21.2); at least in the myocardium (Section 18.9.3) they may also be produced by endothelial cells, and appear to be potentiated by heparin released by local mast cells (Schaper *et al.*, 1988). After release, the growth factors interact with molecular receptor sites on the endothelial and smooth muscle cells of adjacent microvasculature, and angiogenesis begins. The chemotactic gradients established by such factors presumably control the orientation of the new vessels (Williams *et al.*, 1989, p. 684).

III PHYSIOLOGICAL HAEMOSTASIS

Haemostasis means prevention of blood loss.

12.21 Injuries to blood vessels

12.21.1 *Injuries to large arteries*

Arteries rely mainly on contraction of the smooth muscle in their walls to seal substantial injuries. A blood clot alone is too slow, and may not be strong enough to arrest bleeding.

The smooth muscle in an arterial wall instantly contracts vigorously in response to **mechanical stimuli** such as pricking, traction, cutting, and crushing. This response can be powerful enough to prevent fatal haemorrhage, even after loss of a whole limb through crushing trauma. Electrical coupling between smooth muscle cells (Section 3.17) enables contraction of the smooth muscle in an arterial wall to spread circumferentially around the site of injury. The clot helps by releasing **serotonin** from **platelets** that aggregate during clotting. Serotonin has a powerful vasoconstrictor action on the smooth muscle cells nearest to the arterial lumen.

A localized injury to an artery (Keatinge, 1979), such as a needle puncture through its wall, produces a ring contraction. This response still occurs after blocking the innervation of the smooth muscle in the tunica media, and is therefore a direct response of the smooth muscle cells to **mechanical stimulation**. At the point of injury, the smooth muscle cells undergo depolarization, which is then transmitted from cell to cell at points of low electrical resistance (via gap junctions or, more simply, across the closely apposed cell membranes). The conduction extends round the wall of the artery, but is not conducted very far along the vessel longitudinally.

This mechanical stimulation is reinforced by powerful **vasomotor agents** released by platelets in the clot, notably **serotonin**. The smooth muscle in the innermost part of the tunica media of arteries (i.e. the part of the media that adjoins the intima) is not innervated, but is much more sensitive than the outer muscle to all the common vasoconstrictor agents (Keatinge, 1979). Consequently a thrombus on the inside of an artery produces much more effective vasoconstriction than a clot on the outside.

In **surgical haemostasis**, the surgeon utilizes the mechanical responsiveness of the arterial wall, and its sensitivity to the vasoconstrictor effect of an internal blood clot, when crushing an artery with a haemostat.

12.21.2 *Injuries to small blood vessels: platelet plugs*

Hundreds of minute breaks in the walls of the very small blood vessels of the **microvasculature** are caused by the bangs and knocks of everyday life. Such breaks are closed by a platelet plug. The process of plugging occurs in two stages: (1) adhesion of platelets to the injured vascular wall, and (2) aggregation of platelets by sticking to each other (Fig. 12.10D).

Platelets are small discs, like flying saucers (Fig. 12.10A). They are budded off from the giant **megakaryocytes** in the bone marrow. Although a platelet has no nucleus and cannot reproduce itself, it contains remnants of the endoplasmic

reticulum and Golgi apparatus of the parent megakaryocyte; these remnants synthesize various enzymes, including the **serotonin** that causes the vasoconstriction of damaged arteries (Section 12.21.1), and various agents involved in blood-clotting (see Section 12.21.3).

Platelets become activated when they contact the injured luminal surface of a blood vessel, by touching either damaged endothelium that has lost its smoothness, or the collagen fibres beneath the endothelium. Activation of platelets by contact with roughened endothelium is known as **contact activation**. The activated platelets swell, become lumpy, and throw out slender radiating cell processes (Fig. 12.10B).

The surface of the platelet is lined by molecular receptors that bind it to the damaged vascular wall, thus causing the initial **adhesion** of platelets. The adhering platelet is now thoroughly sticky, and its cell processes bind to those of other platelets (Fig. 12.10C). This causes platelets to clump into amorphous masses (Fig. 12.10D), i.e. **aggregation**. If the wound in the vessel wall is small, the clump of aggregated platelets completely plugs the wound and stops the escape of blood; yet it allows blood to go on flowing within the vessel. But the plug of platelets is fairly loose, and to close larger wounds the plug has to be reinforced by the formation of a **blood clot**; this often stops the flow of blood within the vessel.

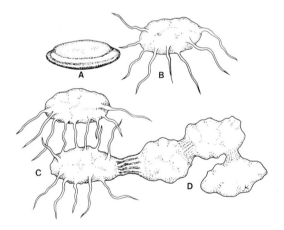

Fig. 12.10 Diagram showing the formation of a platelet plug. A. **Normal platelet.** It is disc shaped. B. **Activated platelet.** The platelet has thrown out long irregular radiating cell processes. C. **Beginning of aggregation.** The cell processes of two platelets have made contact. D. **Aggregation.** Three platelets have fused into an amorphous mass. Redrawn and modified from Booyse and Rafelson (1972).

Platelets (thrombocyti) are oval or circular biconvex corpuscles, about 2–4 µm in diameter. They are released into the blood sinuses of the bone marrow by the fragmentation of megakaryocytes (megakaryocyti) (Krstic, 1984, p. 337). The megakaryocyte degenerates after forming about 2000 platelets. There are about 250 000 to 300 000 platelets per mm^3 of blood. After a life span of about 10 days they are destroyed in the spleen and lungs.

Factors possessed by platelets, and the functions of these factors, are as follows: (1) Molecules of **actin** and **myosin**. These cause strong contraction of platelet cell processes that radiate from the platelet, and thus contribute to **clot retraction** during the hour or so after a clot is formed. (2) **Calcium ions**. These are involved in the activation of platelets for aggregation, and in nearly all the steps in blood clotting. If calcium ions are absent clotting does not occur. (3) **Phospholipids**. These activate intrinsic blood clotting. (4) **Fibrin-stabilizing factor**. This reinforces the linkage between fibrin molecules, thus greatly increasing the strength of a blood clot. (5) **Glycoprotein receptor molecules on the platelet surface.**

These are utilized in the adhesion of platelets to damaged vascular walls. (6) **ADP** and **thromboxane**. Together these are responsible for activation of platelets for aggregation. (7) **Serotonin**. This causes vasoconstriction of injured arteries. (8) **Platelet-derived growth factor**. PDGF stimulates proliferation of vascular smooth muscle cells and fibroblasts in angiogenesis for vascular repair.

The mechanisms of **adhesion** and **aggregation of platelets** at the damaged vascular wall were reviewed by Ross and McIntire (1995). Both the endothelial cells and the platelets contain a multimeric protein molecule, vWF (the von Willebrand factor), and can release it into the blood plasma and into the collagen matrix that underlies damaged endothelium. The glycoprotein coat on the cell membrane of platelets is equipped with an adhesive molecular receptor (glycoprotein Ib-IX, known as GPIb because the Ib component does the binding). GPIb binds with vWF, thus causing adhesion of platelets to the collagen beneath eroded endothelium. Another adhesive glycoprotein receptor (GPIIb-IIIa) is abundant on the platelet surface, but in unactivated platelets it has no ligand-binding capability. Activated adherent platelets release large quantities of **ADP**, and they also synthesize the enzyme **thromboxane** (a type of prostaglandin). Neighbouring unactivated platelets become activated by the combined action of ADP and thromboxane (Guyton, 1986, p. 77), extracellular **calcium ions** also being required. The GPIIb-IIIa on the surface of the activated platelets can now bind to vWF of platelets that are adhering to the vessel wall; thus the platelets can now stick to each other, and this results in platelet aggregation (Ross and McIntire, 1995). Glycoproteins Ib and IIb-IIIa are the most studied, and apparently the most important, platelet receptors.

12.21.3   *Mechanisms by which a blood clot forms*

A blood clot forms in three steps. (1) Damage to the vascular wall or to the blood itself causes the formation of **prothrombin activator**. (2) The prothrombin activator converts **prothrombin** into **thrombin**. (3) Thrombin converts **fibrinogen** into threads of **fibrin** which trap platelets and blood cells to form a clot.

A few minutes after a clot has formed, the **actin** and **myosin molecules** in the radiating cell processes of the trapped platelets begin to contract, causing **clot retraction**. This pulls together the ruptured edges of the blood vessel, thus contributing to haemostasis. It also makes the clot much smaller, and may then diminish the obstruction to blood flow within the vessel.

The formation of **prothrombin activator**, the *first stage* in the formation of a blood clot, is initiated by either an extrinsic or an intrinsic pathway (Guyton, 1986, p. 77). The **extrinsic pathway** starts from trauma to the vascular wall or contact with tissues outside the vascular wall; traumatized tissues release several factors involved in clotting, notably phospholipids, known collectively as **tissue thromboplastin**. The **intrinsic pathway** starts from trauma to the blood itself; this includes the **contact activation** of platelets that strike roughened endothelial cells and then release phospholipids.

Both the extrinsic and the intrinsic pathways now proceed through a cascade of reactions with 'blood-clotting factors'; these factors are plasma proteins (factors VII, X, and V for the extrinsic pathway, and factors XII, XI, IX, VIII, X, V for the intrinsic pathway). In both pathways, these reactions culminate in the formation of the complex called **prothrombin activator**.

The *second stage* in the formation of a blood clot is the conversion of **prothrombin** into **thrombin**. Prothrombin is a plasma protein present in normal blood plasma. In a matter of seconds the prothrombin activator converts prothrombin into thrombin.

In the *third and final stage* in the formation of a blood clot, thrombin polymerizes **fibrinogen** molecules into **fibrin** threads, again in seconds. Fibrinogen is a high molecular weight plasma protein, formed in the liver. Being of high molecular weight, fibrinogen normally diffuses into the interstitial fluid in only small quantities, and therefore interstitial fluid clots only weakly. However, a pathological increase in capillary permeability does allow interstitial fluid to clot like blood. Thrombin also activates a **fibrin-stabilizing factor** released from platelets caught in the clot; this stabilizing factor increases the linkages between the threads of fibrin and thus greatly strengthens the clot.

Calcium ions are required for all the reactions in the extrinsic pathway of blood clotting, and nearly all of those in the intrinsic pathway.

12.22   Natural removal of blood clots

A small blood clot in the wall of a vessel is typically invaded by fibroblasts and converted into fibrous tissue within a few days. A large blood clot is lysed (disintegrated) by enzymes that are already in the clot but have to be activated before they can work; the process of **enzymal lysis** takes several days. Vast numbers of minute clots in the microvasculature are also removed by enzymal lysis. Unfortunately, these lytic mechanisms are seldom able to reopen large vessels, and therefore a major blood clot, such as a massive pulmonary embolus (Section 17.9.4), is a life-threatening emergency.

A newly formed clot (Guyton, 1986, p. 82) contains a large quantity of a plasma protein called **plasminogen** or **profibrinolysin**. After activation by thrombin, or by any of several factors derived from endothelium or damaged tissues, plasminogen becomes **plasmin** or **fibrinolysin**, a proteolytic enzyme like trypsin. Plasmin digests the fibrin threads of a clot.

12.23 Mechanisms preventing unwanted clotting

12.23.1 *The luminal surface of the endothelial cell*

The endothelial cell itself (Section 12.6.1) probably provides the main protection against clotting inside a normal blood vessel. The luminal surface of the endothelial cell has an inherent *smoothness* that enables platelets to bounce off without being damaged, thus avoiding **contact activation**. A monomolecular protein layer that is adsorbed to the luminal surface of the endothelial cell *repels* clotting factors and platelets (Section 12.6.1).

12.23.2 *Velocity of blood flow*

Small quantities of **thrombin** are continually formed in normal blood, but are normally removed by macrophages, especially by the **stellate macrophages** (von Kupffer cells) in the liver. However, if the blood flow is slow, as in veins, the concentration of coagulation factors may increase to the level where clotting begins. If the blood flow stops altogether for hours, for instance in the leg veins of human patients immobilized in bed, clotting is very probable. Such patients should twiddle their toes, thus keeping the flow going by means of the **muscle pump** (Section 12.16.2).

12.23.3 *Heparin*

Heparin is contained in the basophilic granules of the **basophilic granulocyte** and the **mast cell**. It is a potent anticoagulant.

Mast cells are large (20–30 µm diameter) oval or spherical wandering cells, with a round or oval nucleus. In standard histological sections they can be recognized by their content of large purple granules (metachromasia). They accompany the blood vessels of connective tissue generally. They are particularly numerous around the capillaries of the lungs; here, they presumably prevent the enlargement of the many small embolic blood clots that are filtered out daily by the pulmonary microvasculature (Section 17.24).

The contents of the metachromatic granules include not only **heparin** but also **histamine**, and in some species **serotonin**; around the granules are **leukotrienes**, **prostaglandins**, **platelet-activating factor**, **eosinophilic chemotactic factor**, and **hydrogen peroxide** (Krstic, 1984, p. 246), and also bradykinin (Guyton, 1986, p. 521). Several of these substances are released from mast cells during **allergic reactions** (Section 14.27.6).

Heparin is an acid mucopolysaccharide, its concentration in the blood being normally very low. In itself it has a negligible anticoagulant action, but by combining with **antithrombin III** (Section 12.23.4) it potentiates about 1000-fold the ability of the latter to remove thrombin, thus creating an extremely powerful anticoagulant (Guyton, 1986, p. 82). Heparin is therefore extensively used in veterinary and medical practice in the prevention and treatment of undesirable clotting.

According to the *Nomina Histologica* (1994, p. 36), 'it is generally accepted that the **basophilic granulocyte** (granulocytus basophilicus) enters the tissue and becomes the "mastocytus"'. However, Krstic (1984, p. 180) concluded that, despite some similarities, mast cells and basophilic granulocytes probably do not belong to the same class of cells, since mast cells have no peroxidase-positive granules. Incidentally the basophil granulocyte is only about half the size of a mast cell.

12.23.4 *Antithrombin III*

Most of the thrombin formed from prothrombin is adsorbed to the fibrin threads as a clot develops. The remainder is inactivated by antithrombin III, an α-globulin. When activated by combining with **heparin**, antithrombin III becomes one of the most powerful anticoagulants in the blood itself (Guyton, 1986, p. 82).

12.23.5 *Plasmin*

The proteolytic enzyme **plasmin** (Guyton, 1986, p. 82) not only digests the fibrin threads of a blood clot (Section 12.22), but it also destroys many of the clotting factors in the surrounding blood, including factors V, VIII, XII, and prothrombin and fibrinogen. Plasmin thus lowers the clotting capability of the blood. Its tendency to do this is kept in balance by another factor in the blood, **α$_2$-antiplasmin**, that inhibits plasmin.

12.24 Disorders of blood clotting

The prothrombin and fibrinogen that play a major role in the formation of a blood clot (Section 12.21.3) are formed by the liver. The prothrombin activator (responsible for converting prothrombin into thrombin) is formed through a cascade of reactions with 'blood clotting factors'. The blood-clotting factors are plasma proteins that are also mostly formed by the liver. Thus the liver is extensively involved in the blood clotting mechanisms, and therefore severe **diseases of the liver** can produce a serious tendency to bleeding.

Vitamin K deficiency impairs the formation of blood clotting factors. **Warfarin** blocks the action of vitamin K. Several forms of **haemophilia** occur in domestic mammals; they are characterized by deficiencies of various blood clotting factors.

Disorders of clotting were reviewed by Gentry and Downie (1977, p. 44).

12.24.1 *Diseases of the liver*

Nearly all of the blood clotting factors are synthesized in the liver, and therefore malfunction of the liver can lead to bleeding problems.

12.24.2 *Vitamin K deficiency*

Vitamin K is essential for the synthesis of **prothrombin** and the three other clotting factors of greatest importance (**VII**, **IX**, and **X**). The group of fat-soluble compounds that constitute vitamin K are adequate in green feeds, but defects in fat digestion and absorption can lead to vitamin K deficiency.

12.24.3 *Dicoumarol*

Dicoumarol inhibits the synthesis of the clotting factors that are dependent on vitamin K. It is formed in mouldy sweet hay from the conversion of non-toxic **coumarin**, but is the active constituent (**warfarin**) of rodenticides and as such is a potential poison, highly toxic to all species and causing fatal haemorrhage.

12.24.4 *Thrombocytopenia*

Thrombocytopenia is a decrease in the number of platelets in the blood. In man and domestic animals this can arise from autoimmune conditions, resulting in multiple small haemorrhages in the microvasculature.

12.24.5 *Haemophilia*

Haemophilia is a congenital anomaly of the blood clotting mechanism. There are three variants (Blood and Studdert, 1988, p. 426). **Haemophilia A** and **haemophilia B** are transmitted by the female to the male as a sex-linked recessive gene. They therefore affect males predominantly, and only affect females in the rare instances when they are homozygous for the character. **Haemophilia A**, classical haemophilia, is caused by defective synthesis of **clotting factor VIII**. It occurs in dogs, horses, and cats. **Haemophilia B** is similar to haemophilia A, but is caused by a deficiency of **factor IX**. It occurs in dogs and cats. **Haemophilia C** is an autosomal dominant form, inherited as a recessive character (Blood and Studdert, 1988, p. 426). It is caused by a deficiency of **factor XI**, and is a minor disease in cattle.

IV HAEMOPOIESIS

12.25 Sites of haemopoiesis

Haemopoiesis begins in the mesenchyme of the **yolk sac** of the early embryo. It starts with a **totipotent haemopoietic stem cell**, that produces *all types of blood cell*. It does this by means of two subsidiary types of stem cell: (1) a **pluripotent haemopoietic stem cell** for producing all lineages of blood cells except lymphocytes (i.e. the erythrocyte lineage, granulocyte lineage, monocyte and macrophage lineage, and megakaryocyte and platelet lineage); and (2) a **pluripotent lymphopoietic stem cell** solely for lymphopoiesis. Since each of these two subsidiary stem cells produces *several* lineages of blood cells, it is known as a **pluripotent** stem cell, 'pluri-' meaning many: thus 'pluri-' describes its *multiple* productivity, and distinguishes it from the 'toti'-potent stem cell that alone can produce *all* types of blood cell.

Each lineage is headed by its own stem cell. Such a stem cell is committed to forming cells of its own lineage. Thus the stem cell of the erythrocyte lineage can form erythrocytes *only*, and therefore is not pluripotent. To distinguish it from the toti- and pluripotent stem cells, it is called a **committed stem cell**.

As pregnancy advances, the **totipotent haemopoietic stem cell** appears in the **liver**, which then becomes the main site of haemopoiesis, and in the **spleen**. Late in pregnancy the **bone marrow** acquires the **totipotent haemopoietic stem cell**. This forms (1) the **pluripotent haemopoietic stem cell**, that produces the erythrocyte lineage, granulocyte lineage, monocyte and macrophage lineage, and the megakaryocyte and platelet lineage; and (2) the **pluripotent lymphopoietic stem cell** that produces the B-lymphocyte and T-lymphocyte lineages. The other totipotent sites of blood cell formation, the liver and spleen, which for a period during pregnancy were capable of forming all of the blood cell lineages, now regress. From this stage onwards, the bone marrow is the *only* source of the totipotent stem cell.

The **pluripotent haemopoietic stem cell** in the bone marrow forms **committed stem cells** for each of its four lineages, i.e. for the erythrocyte lineage, granulocyte lineage, monocyte/macrophage lineage, and megakaryocyte/platelet lineage.

Towards the end of pregnancy **the pluripotent lymphopoietic stem cell** establishes itself not only in the bone marrow but also in the **thymus**. In the bone marrow it forms a **committed B stem cell**, which produces the **B-lymphocyte lineage** (Section 14.12.4); in the thymus it forms a **committed T stem cell** that produces the **T-lymphocyte lineage** (Section 14.12.5). From these committed B and T stem cells in the bone marrow and thymus, B- and T-lymphocytes are then seeded into the **peripheral lymphoid tissues**, i.e. into diffuse accumulations of lymphocytes in many mucous membranes (Section 14.15), into lymphonodules (Section 14.15), into lymph nodes (Section 14.17), and into the spleen (Section 14.18).

By the end of pregnancy the bone marrow and the peripheral lymphoid tissues (which include the spleen) are the only sites of haemopoiesis in the normal body.

The terms 'lymphoid' tissue and 'lymphatic' tissue are synonymous (Krstic, 1984, p. 238).

The mesodermal or endodermal origin of the totipotent haemopoietic stem cell is still controversial, but the cell itself is 'unquestionably mesenchymal in character' (Bannister, 1996, p. 1407). Current opinion supports the 'monophyletic' theory of haemopoiesis, in which all blood cells arise from a totipotent haemopoietic stem cell, as outlined above (Krstic, 1984, p. 188). Other authors have proposed polyphyletic theories. The topic is still being intensively researched, because of the potential role of marrow transplantation in treating genetic disorders and neoplasia in man (Bannister, 1996, p. 1412).

The **totipotent haemopoietic stem cell** seems to be structurally similar to the **pluripotent stem cells** (Bannister, 1996, p. 1412). The cells tend to be initially large, relatively undifferentiated, and rapidly dividing.

The nucleus is large and euchromatic and the cytoplasm somewhat basophilic. The cells get smaller as they proliferate, ribosomes become numerous, cytoplasmic basophilia increases, and the nucleus becomes more heterochromatic, smaller, and multilobar.

Haemopoiesis forms **cords** and **islands of cells** in the bone marrow, in various stages of development (Bannister, 1996, p. 1409). Several different cell lineages share one cord or island. One or more macrophages, dendritic in shape, lie at the core of each such cluster of cells. They appear to provide iron to developing erythrocytes and may regulate the rate of proliferation and maturation; no doubt they also participate in the removal of the cell debris (extruded nuclei, for instance) of haemopoiesis.

The main lineages of differentiating blood cells are referred to as '**colony-forming units**' (CFUs) (Krstic, 1984, p. 188). Thus **CFU-E** is the erythropoietic lineage, **CFU-G** is the granulopoietic lineage, and **CFU-M** is the megakaryopoietic lineage. Each of these lineages is headed by its own committed stem cell.

12.26   Bone marrow

Bone marrow occurs in the marrow cavities of bones. It has the same three basic structural components as lymphatic tissue (Section 14.11), i.e. (1) a network of fixed cells (**reticular cells**), suspended in (2) a framework of **reticular fibres**, and (3) **free cells** (haemopoietic in the red marrow) lodged in the meshes of the fixed cells and reticular fibres.

There are two types of bone marrow, red and yellow. In the fetus the bones contain **red marrow**. The **haemopoietic** free cells in red marrow consist of the *erythrocyte lineage*, the *granulocyte lineage*, the *monocyte–macrophage lineage*, the *megakaryocyte–platelet lineage*, and the *lymphocyte lineage*.

Between the islands of proliferating cells in the red bone marrow are large prominent **venous sinuses**, supplied by arterial capillaries. The sinuses are lined by thin **endothelial cells** that allow newly-formed blood cells to escape into the blood stream. Many macrophages are strung out on the reticular fibre meshwork; their job is to clear up the debris of haemopoiesis, such as the extruded nuclei of erythroblasts and fragments of megakaryocytes.

After birth, much of the red marrow is gradually converted into **yellow marrow**. This is achieved by the **reticular cells** (the fixed cells of the marrow), which become distended with fat globules and thus fill the marrow with fatty tissue yellow in colour.

In the growing animal, haemopoiesis is highly active in order to build up the required number of blood cells. Therefore the marrow cavities of the skeleton are almost entirely filled with **red marrow** (Schummer *et al.*, 1981, p. 6). In the adult, however, haemopoiesis simply maintains the normal quantity and quality of blood cells, and therefore the red marrow is less bulky and restricted to the spongy bone at the ends of long bones and within short, flat, and irregular bones. The spongy bone of ribs, vertebrae, and many short and flat bones, is filled with red marrow throughout life (Evans, 1993, p. 126).

The **endothelial cells** that line the venous sinuses are attached to each other by tight junctions that appear to form effective barriers between the newly-formed blood cells and the bloodstream. However, temporary **fenestrations** allow migrating cells to penetrate the endothelium. The fenestration fits the migrating cell tightly, and then closes behind it (Bannister, 1996, p. 1409).

In general, **yellow bone marrow** has little haemopoietic function. Nevertheless it can transform itself into red marrow in response to functional demands (Krstik, 1984, p. 50).

12.27   The erythrocyte lineage

By repeated mitosis in the red bone marrow, the **committed erythropoietic stem cell** at the head of this lineage produces a sequence of immature red blood cells. The first cells in the series are large, but subsequent cells get progressively smaller. The large cells divide rapidly and are therefore known as 'erythroblasts'. When cell division has finished, the nucleus is extruded and the cell enters the circulation. Finally all organelles are rapidly lost, the filling of the cytoplasm with haemoglobin is completed, and a fully qualified erythrocyte has been launched. The process of forming erythrocytes is known as **erythropoiesis**.

The first cell in the lineage (Bannister, 1996, p. 1413) is the large sized (14–20 μm) **proerythroblast** (proerythroblastus). Its cytoplasm is moderately basophilic, and already contains some ferritin. The next cell is the **basophilic erythroblast**. Haemoglobin synthesis begins, giving the subsequent cell in the series an acidophilic tinge to its otherwise basophilic cytoplasm, thus giving it the name **polychromatophilic erythroblast** (erythroblastus polychromatophilicus). The next generation is

frankly acidophilic, hence **acidophilic erythroblast** (erythroblastus acidophilicus). These cells stop dividing and extrude the nucleus, and thus become a **reticulocyte** (reticulocytus). (Unfortunately, the *Nomina Histologica* (1994) failed to distinguish this reticulocyte from the reticulocyte of connective tissue.) The reticulocyte of erythropoiesis retains a few fragments of organelles, which stain as a web-like basophilic reticulum, hence the name; for the next 24 hours these cells still take up ferritin and synthesize haemoglobin, but after that they lose their reticulum and are then **mature erythrocytes** (erythrocytus) (Krstic, 1984, p. 359).

The hormone **erythropoietin** arises from the kidney via a precursor, erythrogenin (Krstic, 1984, p. 151). Its formation is stimulated by hypoxia. It acts on the cells which differentiate into proerythroblasts. Erythropoietin is likely to be the main factor controlling the differentiation of erythrocytes, but its mode of operation is uncertain.

12.28   The granulocyte lineage

The granulocyte (granular leucocyte) lineage arises in the red bone marrow through mitotic division of the **committed granulocyte stem cell**. It culminates in the differentiation of neutrophils, basophils, and acidophils (neutrophilic, basophilic, and eosinophilic granulocytes).

Granules characteristic of the types of granulocyte form during the series of divisions. The nucleus becomes flattened on one side, horseshoe shaped, and finally divides into a greater or lesser number of lobes depending on the type of granulocyte.

The process of forming granulocytes is known as **granulopoiesis**. The first cell in the lineage is the **myeloblast**. This is a large cell (10–20 μm), similar in external appearance to the proerythroblast (Bannister, 1996, p. 1413). It differentiates into even larger **promyelocytes**. These synthesize specific proteins in the rough endoplasmic reticulum and Golgi apparatus, and store them in *non-specific* (primary) *granules*. Promyelocytes differentiate into smaller **myelocytes**, which are the last stage of proliferation. *Specific* (secondary) *granules* are now formed, distinguishing **neutrophilic**, **basophilic**, and **eosinophilic** myelocytes.

Eosinophils synthesize only one set of granules. It is not known whether the eosinophil differentiates from the same myeloblast or promyelocyte as the neutrophil, or whether it has a lineage of its own. The derivation of basophils seems even more uncertain (Bannister, 1996, p. 414).

In the **mature neutrophil** the nucleus has three to five lobes joined by thin strands of chromatin. The many specific granules are stainable with basic and acid dyes; hence the term neutrophil. Neutrophils are very mobile. Because of their phagocytic capabilities they are known as microphages. These and other functional characteristics are mentioned in Section 7.7.4. Immature forms, known as 'stab' neutrophils, can be identified by their heavily indented but unsegmented nucleus. Changes in the relative numbers of 'stab' neutrophils indicate the progress of some diseases (Schummer *et al.*, 1981, p. 4).

The **mature eosinophil** usually has a nucleus with two lobes connected by a thread of chromatin. The specific granules are coarse, round, eosinophilic, and of uniform size. The functional attributes of eosinophils are considered in Section 14.27.4.

In the **mature basophil** the nucleus is partly constricted into two lobes. The specific granules in the cytoplasm are much larger than those of neutrophils and eosinophils, vary in shape and size, and stain with basic and metachromatic dyes (Krstic, 1984, p. 180). According to the *Nomina Histologica* (1994, p. 29), it is generally accepted that the basophilic granulocyte enters the tissues and becomes the mast cell: Krstic (1984, p. 180) conceded some similarities between mast cells and basophils, but concluded that they do not belong to the same class of cells because basophils give a positive peroxidase reaction whereas mast cells do not. Basophil and mast cell functions are discussed in Sections 14.9.2, 14.27.4, 14.27.6, and 14.28.3.

12.29   The monocyte–macrophage lineage

Monocytes (Section 14.10) are formed in the red bone marrow.

The process is known as **monopoiesis**. The steps in monopoiesis are not yet clear. There is evidence that monocytes arise from the same committed stem cell as the neutrophil granulocyte. After a stage of proliferation as **monoblasts** they differentiate as **promonocytes**, forming lysosomes. They then enter the circulation and finally populate various tissues as macrophages of the **mononuclear phagocyte system** (Section 14.10). The definitive monocyte is a large cell (20 μm) with a large, kidney-shaped, euchromatic nucleus, well-developed Golgi apparatus, and many lysosomes and mitochondria (Section 14.10, Fig. 14.4).

12.30   The megakaryocyte–platelet lineage

Megakaryocytes are giant cells formed in the red bone marrow. They create platelets within their cytoplasm, and then extrude them by long narrow cytoplasmic protrusions and finally by disintegrating altogether (Section 12.21.2).

The formation of platelets is known as **thrombocytopoiesis**. The committed megakaryocyte stem cell gives rise to proliferative **megakaryoblasts**, from which the megakaryocytes arise. Successive mitoses then occur, *but without cytoplasmic division* (Bannister, 1996, p. 1414). Invaginations of the plasmalemma cut off regions of cytoplasm, which then break off the parent cell forming platelets. The nucleus, and finally the entire megakaryocyte, disintegrates.

12.31   The lymphocyte lineage

The B-lymphocyte and T-lymphocyte lineages are considered in Sections 14.12.2, 14.12.4, and 14.12.5.

Chapter 13
Regulation of Blood Vessels

13.1 Basal tone of blood vessels

Like cardiac muscle cells (Section 21.17), smooth muscle cells typically have an inherent capacity for spontaneous contractions, which are entirely independent of nerves or any other extraneous factor. Cardiac muscle cells contract and relax very rapidly: smooth muscle cells do so much more slowly, and the resulting sustained contractions endow smooth muscle with basal tone.

Such **basal tone** occurs in smooth muscle cells in the walls of **arteries** and **arterioles**, and almost certainly in **metarterioles**. There is also evidence that it occurs in **veins**. It sets a baseline of vascular calibre, on which all other regulatory mechanisms exert their excitatory (i.e. vasoconstrictor) or inhibitory (i.e. vasodilator) functions; in other words, blood vessels in their resting state, and in resting tissues, are already partly constricted, but can be relaxed or made even more constricted by other influences. These other influences are metabolic, neural, hormonal, myogenic, or endothelial.

Arterioles are maintained in a state of spontaneous tonic contraction through virtually an entire lifetime (Guyton, 1986, p. 146). Spontaneous rhythmical contractions also occur in the smooth muscle of the walls of the gastro-intestinal and urinary tracts (Creed, 1979); spontaneous myogenic activity of 'pacemaker cells' in the circular smooth muscle of the gut wall is a feature of the control mechanism of the enteric nervous system (Section 3.22). However, spontaneous activity is not a characteristic of all smooth muscle. In some arteries, including the carotid artery, the main pulmonary arteries, and ear arteries, the smooth muscle has been shown in the rabbit to be quiescent and devoid of spontaneous activity, as are the smooth muscle cells of the trachea, gall bladder, and ductus deferens; in these tissues, activity is normally initiated by nerves (Creed, 1979).

Systemic **venous tone** of intrinsic myogenic origin is also recognized, but its mechanisms and physiological significance are not yet fully understood (Monos, 1993).

Included among the arterioles with substantial basal tone are those of the **skin**. However, the contractile cells of **arteriovenous anastomoses** in the skin have little basal tone; they are highly responsive to the tonic discharge of the sympathetic vasomotor fibres that supply them, so inhibition of these fibres produces maximum dilation of the anastomosis (Rowell, 1974, p. 188). They are also regulated by humoral, metabolic, myogenic, and endothelial factors (Section 12.17).

The variation in vascular resistance (and hence in flow) that can be attained in an organ depends on the level of its basal arterial tone. For example, the arterioles in resting **skeletal muscle** have a high basal tone, and therefore the vascular bed can undergo very great vasodilation in **exercise**; blood flow increases more than 20-fold during maximal dilation so obtained (Hudlicka, 1985). The basal tone of the vascular smooth muscle of the **intestinal tract** also seems to be very high; if the basal tone is eliminated by drug action, the flow rate increases about 8-fold (Rowell, 1974, p. 218). On the other hand, kidney function is virtually maximal in the basal state, so an increase in blood flow over the resting value may be unobtainable (Feigl, 1974, p. 125).

13.2 Metabolic regulation of vascular tone

In most of the vascular beds of the body, the rate of blood flow is closely related to the metabolic activity of the tissues. If the activity increases, the blood flow increases: if the activity decreases, the blood flow decreases. These are **short-term adjustments**, occurring within seconds or minutes. There are also **long-term adjustments** that take days, weeks, or months.

13.2.1 Short-term adjustments

How do the tissues of the body achieve the homeostatic feat of a short-term **autoregulation** of blood flow? The main controlling factor is the **local concentration of oxygen in the tissues**. The oxygen supply to the cells in a tissue is critical, since cells die if their oxygen supply falls below minimal levels: such a crisis has to be dealt with locally. In virtually all the tissues of the body a short-term **local vasodilation** occurs *immediately*, if the oxygen delivered by the microcirculation falls below the minimal demands of the tissue. This acts by decreasing the **basal tone** of the smooth muscle in the arterioles and metarterioles of the microcirculation. The outstanding exception to this rule is the lung, in which the branches of the pulmonary arteries *constrict* in response to local hypoxia (Section 17.21.1).

This response by the smooth muscle cells of arterioles and metarterioles to a change in their metabolic environment may be direct, indirect, or a combination of direct and indirect.

In the **direct response**, the smooth muscle cells themselves react to the changing levels of oxygen within the vessel. The smooth muscle cells in the walls of arterioles and metarterioles require oxygen (and other nutrients) to maintain their contraction. If the supply of these substances decreases, the smooth muscle cells contract less strongly, resulting in local vasodilation and increased flow. Alternatively, if the tissue becomes more active metabolically, the availability of oxygen to the smooth muscle cells would decrease, again causing local vasodilation and increased flow. Conversely, if the supply of oxygen increases or the tissue becomes less active, the smooth muscle cells contract more strongly and vasoconstriction results, resulting in decreased flow. The essential point is that a fall in the oxygen supply weakens their basal tone, and therefore allows passive vasodilation.

The **indirect response** requires the participation of a **mediator**, i.e. a **vasodilator substance** released by the tissues. Thus a fall in the oxygen supply induces an increased release of the vasodilator substance, causing active vasodilation and increased blood flow. The nature of any such vasodilator substance – indeed its very existence – has been very elusive. However, in the last decade it has been discovered that **endothelial cells** produce vasomotor substances. One of them, **nitric oxide**, is a potent *vasodilator*; others are vasoconstrictors. Their mode of action in regulat-

ing vascular tone is discussed in Sections 13.6 and 13.8.

It should be re-emphasized that, for these mechanisms to work, the smooth muscle in the vascular walls must normally be maintained in a state of intermediate contraction, which can be increased or decreased as the metabolic need arises: this state of contraction is the **basal tone** of blood vessels (Section 13.1).

Another **mediator** of probable importance in inducing *vasodilation* during systemic or local hypoxia is **adenosine**. If the oxygen supply to cardiac muscle cells is lowered, ATP in the cell is degraded into adenosine. This is released into the myocardial interstitial fluid and causes local vasodilation (Section 18.5). During hypoxia, adenosine is also released from **skeletal muscle fibres** (Marshall, 1995), causing vasodilation by opening K^+ channels of, and hence hyperpolarizing, adjacent vascular smooth muscle cells.

The above account is based on **local autoregulation** in response to changes in the local availability of **oxygen**. As was emphasized in Section 11.11.1, an increase in the **carbon dioxide** concentration of the blood is life-threatening to the body as a whole, because it may lower the pH of the body fluids everywhere to levels of acidity at which cells in many tissues die: this crisis must be dealt with **systemically**, by adjustments in breathing.

However, changes in the pH of the body fluids can dangerously disturb the excitability of all **nervous tissue** in particular. Extreme acidity depresses the central nervous system so severely that coma and death can result; extreme alkalinity excites nervous tissue, inducing action potentials in peripheral nerves which can result in death from spasm of the muscles of respiration (Attwell, 1986, p. 1). The **cerebral circulation** therefore has a **local** mechanism for regulating blood flow in response to carbon dioxide and hydrogen ions (Guyton, 1986, p. 235). An increase in the concentrations of these substances dilates the arterioles of the brain, thus enabling the increased blood flow to wash out carbon dioxide from the tissues. The removal of carbon dioxide also removes carbonic acid and hence hydrogen ions. Conversely, a fall in the concentration of carbon dioxide and hydrogen ions below normal values induces vasoconstriction, thus allowing these substances to accumulate in the tissues until near normal levels are re-attained.

13.2.2 *Long-term adjustments*

The long-term adjustment of blood flow within a tissue requires the reconstruction of the vasculature of that tissue. Again, the mechanism for this probably depends on the tissue's requirement for oxygen. If a tissue becomes continuously more active, the constant demand for a sustained increase in the supply of oxygen stimulates **angiogenesis** (Section 12.20); this new vascular growth goes on until the increasing vasculature meets the oxygen demands of the tissues. For example, vascular augmentation occurs in animals adapted to life at high altitude. If a tissue becomes continuously *less* active, its oxygen demand decreases and its vascular tissue is remodelled to provide a lower blood flow.

13.3   Neural regulation of vascular tone

13.3.1   *Innervated and non-innervated blood vessels*

The smooth muscle in the media of **arteries** and **arterioles**, and usually also their satellite **veins** and **muscular venules**, is innervated by sympathetic vasomotor fibres. **Arteriovenous anastomoses** are particularly richly innervated.

In contrast, the **metarterioles** (i.e. the so-called precapillary sphincters) and presumably also the capillaries themselves are believed to have no nerve supply at all (Section 12.11).

The **sympathetic vasomotor fibres** of **muscular arteries** do not penetrate the whole depth of the smooth muscle in the tunica media (Keatinge, 1979). In **small muscular arteries** these fibres are generally confined to the adventitia and the outer surface of the tunica media. In **larger muscular arteries** they do penetrate the outer part of the tunica media, but not the inner quarter or half of the muscle layer. It is suggested that this inner part of the media remains nerve free because the axons are unable to withstand the pressures therein. Noradrenaline released by the effector terminals of the axons in the periphery of the tunica media diffuses into the inner, non-innervated, parts of the media and stimulates its smooth muscle. In small arteries excitation also passes from the outer to the inner layers of muscle cells by electrical transmission from cell to cell. Furthermore, the inner, non-innervated, layers of muscle cells are much more sensitive than the outer, innervated, layers to **circulating adrenaline** and **noradrenaline** (Section 13.4.1).

The innervation, or lack of innervation, of **metarterioles** (precapillary sphincter) is still controversial. However, there is increasing anatomical and physiological evidence that nervous control does not extend to these vessels (Wiedeman *et al.*, 1976). The current

view, therefore, is that metarterioles (and therefore the '**precapillary sphincter**'; Section 12.11) are either very sparsely innervated or, more typically, not innervated at all (Guyton, 1986, p. 231).

13.3.2   *Alpha- and beta-receptors*

As indicated in Section 13.3.1, the sympathetic motor system innervates the smooth muscle of the **arterial tree** with adrenergic vasomotor fibres throughout the body. In most organs, the **dominant** effect on the arterial tree of sympathetic nerve stimulation is **vasoconstriction**, acting through α-**adrenoreceptors** on the smooth muscle cells (Section 2.33.1). It is believed that *all* smooth muscle cells in **arteries** possess α-receptors. The smooth muscle in the wall of **veins** also is innervated by sympathetic vasomotor fibres in most tissues; the receptors are again mainly of the alpha type.

Beta-adrenoreceptors are of two types, β_1 being excitatory to the myocardium and β_2 being inhibitory to vascular (and other) smooth muscle (Section 2.33.1). **Beta$_2$-receptors** in **arteries** appear to be much fewer in number than α-receptors, and largely restricted to the vascular beds of skeletal muscle and the heart. Excitation of β_2-receptors by sympathetic nerve stimulation causes relaxation of vascular smooth muscle cells (Section 2.33.1), and hence **vasodilation** (see Section 13.3.4).

If stimulation of a sympathetic nerve excites both α- and β_2-receptors simultaneously in the smooth muscle in the arterial vasculature, the α-receptors generally dominate and vasoconstriction results.

Two of the major organ systems, the **heart** and **brain**, have a very weak arterial vasoconstrictor mechanism. This becomes important in the circulatory adjustments at the **onset of exercise**. Exercise begins with a massive discharge of the sympathetic nervous system. This has the effect (Section 13.8) of closing down the arterial supply to tissues (for example those of the gastrointestinal tract) that are not needed in exercise. However, the arterial supply to the heart and brain cannot be allowed to diminish, and therefore the **coronary** and **cerebral circulations** are exempted from a powerful vasoconstrictor adjustment.

Any *vasodilator* effects in skeletal muscle that may result from neuronal stimulation of **β-receptors** are normally completely masked by the altogether dominant *vasoconstrictor* effect of the more numerous **α-receptors** (Feigl, 1974, p. 124).

The domination of **α-receptors** is less clear in the **coronary arteries** than in the arteries of skeletal muscle (Guyton, 1986, p. 298). This is because α-receptors predominate in the coronary arteries in the **epicardium**, whereas **β₂-receptors** predominate in the **myocardial arteries**. Therefore stimulation of sympathetic cardiac nerves can cause either vasoconstriction or vasodilation, but usually constriction is slightly more obvious.

The **cerebral arteries** have an abundant sympathetic innervation (Section 2.23.5). Substantial species differences have been found in the vasoconstrictor influence of the sympathetic vasomotor innervation of the cerebral circulation (D'Alecy, 1974, p. 270). In man, sympathectomy or sympathetic blockade has little or no augmentative effect on cerebral flow, and therefore it was argued that the sympathetic innervation plays very little part in regulating cerebral blood flow; also this conclusion seems to be consistent with the enclosure of the brain within the rigid skull. However, in lower mammals electrical stimulation of the stellate ganglion produces a marked vasoconstriction and decrease in cerebral blood flow, acting through α-receptors. The probable explanation is that this vasoconstrictor effect is usually masked by the more powerful vasodilator action of carbon dioxide. However, it is now believed that in man a sudden increase in arterial pressure (as at the abrupt onset of severe exercise) induces a vasoconstriction of the **large** and **medium sized** cerebral arteries; this prevents a very high pressure from reaching the smaller cerebral arteries, and thus gives the brain some protection from haemorrhages (strokes) (Guyton, 1986, p. 340). The existence of adrenergic **β-receptors** in the cerebral circulation seems not to be established with certainty (D'Alecy, 1974, p. 270).

The **cutaneous arterial circulation** has only **α-receptors** (Rowell, 1974, p. 192). These can exert a powerful vasoconstrictor control, as in thermoregulation to prevent heat loss, or in the blanching of the human face in fear.

The smooth muscle in **cutaneous veins** and **splanchnic veins** is richly supplied by noradrenergic endings; the **veins in skeletal muscle** are virtually devoid of any adrenergic nerve endings (Rowell, 1974, p. 211).

For further discussion of the coronary, cerebral, and cutaneous vasculature see Section 13.4.1.

13.3.3   *Resting sympathetic tone*

In resting tissues, a steady tonic discharge of sympathetic vasomotor fibres maintains a continuous vasoconstrictor stimulus to the smooth muscle cells of most vascular beds. The resulting vasoconstriction is known as resting sympathetic tone. This **neural tone** is superimposed on the myogenic **basal tone** that is already inherent in vascular smooth muscle (Section 13.1).

Resting sympathetic tone is an important factor in the adjustment of blood flow in many tissues. For example, the splanchnic vasculature and the vasculature in skeletal muscle, and some parts of the cutaneous circulation, are subjected to resting sympathetic tone. In all of these vascular beds, a decrease in sympathetic tone can induce *passive vasodilation*; conversely, an increase in sympathetic tone can induce *active vasoconstriction*. Such variations in the degree of vasoconstriction, with corresponding variations in vascular resistance and hence in the rate of blood flow, can be achieved over wide ranges simply by increasing or decreasing the discharge rate of the sympathetic vasomotor fibres. In summary, the inherent myogenic basal tone of the smooth muscle cells themselves, and the superimposed sympathetic vasoconstrictor tone, combine together to provide a basis for the neuronal adjustment of blood flow within the various organs.

13.3.4   *Neuronal vasodilator systems*

Some tissues have **neuronal vasodilator systems**. These include the sympathetic vasomotor fibres acting on **β-receptors**, that have already been mentioned (Section 13.3.2); these occur in the vascular beds of skeletal muscle and the heart. In both of these tissues, the β-receptors are less numerous than the α-receptors, and therefore the *dominant* response to sympathetic nerve stimulation is *vasoconstriction*, even though the vasoconstrictor mechanism is very weak in the heart.

The arterial tree of skeletal muscle is also innervated by **sympathetic cholinergic vasodilator fibres** (Section 2.33.2). It is doubtful whether these play a major part in vasomotor control, with the exception of vasodilation in skeletal musculature at the **onset of exercise** (see advanced text).

A third variety of neuronal vasodilator mechanism occurs in the coronary and cerebral circulations. This consists of **parasympathetic (cholinergic) vasodilator neurons**. However, these vasodilator fibres have an almost negligible effect on the coronary circulation, metabolic factors, especially the oxygen consumption of the myocardium, being so highly dominant.

There are varying numbers of **β-receptor sites** on some vascular smooth muscle cells, and these are potential sources of vasodilation. They are innervated in the vasculature of **skeletal muscle** and the **heart**, and with the aid of appropriate agents to block the vasoconstrictor α-receptors that are considered in Section 13.3.2, can be shown to have a vasodilator function during sympathetic nerve stimulation.

Cholinergic sympathetic vasodilator nerve fibres (Section 2.33.2) have been found in **skeletal muscle** (but in **no** other tissue) in the cat and other lower mammals, but not in man (Guyton, 1986, p. 337). They probably play a significant role in the vasodilation of skeletal muscle at the very **onset of exercise** (Guyton, 1986, pp. 272, 337). Their motor pathway begins in the **motor area** of the **cerebral cortex**, and projects down through the hypothalamus to the **cardiovascular centres** in the medullary reticular formation (Section 19.12; Fig. 19.8). Thus at the instant when the predator launches its pursuit, or when the prey speeds away, a preliminary surge of blood pours through the vasculature of the skeletal musculature. This anticipatory circulatory adaptation forms an elegant companion to the anticipatory **increase in breathing** that occurs at, or even before, the onset of exercise (Section 11.14). In man a similar anticipatory vasodilation in skeletal muscle at the **onset of exercise** may be achieved by the action of circulating adrenaline on the **β-receptors** of vascular smooth muscle (Section 13.3.2). Once exercise is established, the control of vasodilation in the vascular beds of skeletal muscle is taken over completely by non-neuronal factors, i.e. local metabolic factors (Section 13.2) and endothelial agents (Section 13.6).

In the **coronary circulation** (Section 18.6) there is no evidence for cholinergic sympathetic vasodilator fibres. However, the coronary arterial tree does have **parasympathetic cholinergic vasodilator fibres**. These neuronal pathways reach the heart in the **cardiac rami** of the vagus nerve, being distributed along the branches of the coronary arteries (Rowell, 1974, p. 256) (Section 3.11.3). The postganglionic fibres in this pathway are cholinergic. Their functional role in controlling the coronary circulation is almost negligible, since metabolic factors dominate the flow of blood through the myocardium (Guyton, 1986, p. 298). The physiological role of these fibres is therefore uncertain, but they may have reflex functions in cardiac pathology such as myocardial infarction (Scott, 1986, pp. 64, 76) (Section 18.7).

The **parasympathetic vasodilator fibres** that supply the **cerebral circulation** (D'Alecy, 1974, p. 271) appear to arise from the **major petrosal nerve** (Section 3.9.1). If all other factors influencing cerebral blood flow are eliminated, stimulation of this pathway produces a substantial increase in cerebral blood flow.

Parasympathetic vasodilator fibres in the **pelvic nerve** (Section 3.12) supply the **erectile tissue** of the penis and clitoris.

There also appear to be purinergic and peptidergic vasodilator nerves, though their functional role is speculative (Scott, 1986, p. 66). **Purinergic neurons** may mediate the arteriolar dilation of the cutaneous **axon reflex**: if the skin is scratched, afferent receptors project sensory signals to the spinal cord; it is suggested that the afferent axons also project action potentials antidromically down collateral branches, and at their endings these release purines either directly or via an interneuron. Various **peptides** have been found in nerve endings associated with blood vessels in the brain, gastrointestinal tract, and heart. They may have a direct vasodilatory action, but they are often associated with other neurotransmitters and therefore may have an indirect modulating action.

The elder statesmen, noradrenaline and acetylcholine, are still prominent among vascular neurotransmitters. However, there is a whole array of young pretenders, some of which have been mentioned, that are clamouring for notice. These include: (1) various **neuropeptides**, among them being the recently discovered pituitary adenyl-cyclase-activating peptide (PACAP); (2) **ATP**, as a primary transmitter at sympathetic neurovascular junctions and as a cotransmitter with noradrenaline in vasoconstrictor neurons; (3) various transmitters released peripherally from *afferent* endings, including **calcitonin gene-related peptide** (**CGRP**), with its action in dilating gastric blood vessels and protecting the gastric mucosa from ulceration; and (4) **neural nitric oxide** (Section 2.34). These mechanisms of vascular innervation have been reviewed by Edvinson and Uddman (1993).

13.3.5 *Neural tone in veins: venous return to the heart*

In general veins are less well innervated than arteries. Nevertheless, veins and muscular venules (especially cutaneous and splanchnic veins) are strongly innervated by **vasomotor sympathetic fibres**. These vasomotor fibres act mainly by α-receptors and are therefore vasoconstrictors (Section 13.3.2). What is the overall function of these vasoconstrictor venous elements?

The systemic part of the venous system is a **venous reservoir** holding about two thirds of the total blood volume (Section 12.16.3). It would be functionally advantageous if this could be exploited as a mobile reserve of blood volume, since displacement of blood from the veins will increase the **venous return to the heart** and, by activating the Frank–Starling mechanism (Section 21.11), would then promote an increase in cardiac output. The pressure in the right atrium is known as the **central venous pressure**.

Various mechanisms contribute to the venous return to the heart in the standing animal, notably sympathetic venoconstriction, the muscle pump, and breathing.

Venoconstriction under the control of sympathetic vasomotor fibres contributes importantly to the venous return to the heart during sudden stress. It can rapidly mobilize substantial volumes of blood from the venous reservoirs (Section 12.16.3), notably from the splanchnic and cutaneous venous beds. This mobilization can form the motor part of a **baroreceptor reflex** from the **carotid sinus** (Section 19.12) in response to a fall in arterial pressure, especially after **haemorrhage**. Splanchnic and cutaneous venoconstriction also occurs at the sudden onset of severe **exercise**. Such immediate and widespread venoconstriction is consistent with the generalized increase in sympathetic activity in **fight and flight**, and meets the need to transfer blood at once to the active skeletal musculature. Splanchnic venoconstriction also occurs during **heat stress**, when large volumes of blood are transferred to the **cutaneous vessels** for cooling.

The **muscle pump** in the limbs utilizes contraction of the limb musculature during exercise, aided by control of the direction of flow by valves in the limb veins, to force venous blood from the limbs towards the heart (Section 12.16.2). In the horse, compression of the venous plexuses on either side of the cartilages of the hoof further augments the venous return at each step.

Changes in the intra-abdominal and intrathoracic pressure during breathing (Section 10.4.2) contribute to the venous return to the heart. During **inspiration**, the diaphragm raises the **intra-abdominal pressure** (Section 10.8), thus compressing the abdominal caudal vena cava and hepatic portal veins, and creating a pressure gradient from the abdomen towards the heart. Furthermore, the fall in **intrathoracic pressure** during inspiration is transmitted to the great veins in the mediastinum and to the thoracic caudal vena cava in the plica vena cava. These respiratory pressure changes augment the pressure gra-

dient towards the heart, and thus increase the venous return to the right atrium.

The **splanchnic veins** and **cutaneous veins**, unlike the veins in skeletal musculature (Rowell, 1974, p. 227) are richly innervated by sympathetic adrenergic fibres (Section 13.3.2). Direct electrical stimulation of the splanchnic nerves can expel 20–25% of the total blood volume from the intestines, liver, and spleen. However, it seems likely that somewhat more than half of this shift in blood volume is due to passive elastic recoil of the venous walls caused by vasoconstriction of the splanchnic arterial bed, and that only the remainder is accountable to active venoconstriction. Maximum sympathetic stimulation can expel 35–50% of the total blood content of the hindlimb into the central circulation (Rowell, 1974, p. 194), as might occur in heat stress in a resting animal.

Veins, in general, receive no sympathetic cholinergic innervation (Rowell, 1974, p. 211). Indeed, veins are believed to receive no specific vasodilator innervation of any kind (Smith and Hamlin, 1977, p. 112).

The increase in venous return to the right atrium that is induced by inspiration (Scott, 1986, p. 49) is quickly passed on to the pulmonary circulation, so that within a heart beat or two of the onset of inspiration, the right ventricle ejects a larger volume per beat. Each cycle of inspiration and expiration also promotes the filling of the pulmonary veins and their emptying into the left side of the heart (Section 17.15). These mechanical interactions between breathing and circulation have been a controversial field for over a century (Mead and Whittenberger, 1964, p. 18).

13.4   Hormonal regulation of vascular tone

13.4.1   *Adrenaline and noradrenaline*

Adrenaline and noradrenaline are released into the blood stream from the adrenal medulla when the sympathetic nerves to the adrenal medulla are stimulated. These two hormones circulate in the blood stream, and act on blood vessels in all parts of the body. Usually both of them cause vasoconstriction because of the general predominance of α-**receptors** in the smooth muscle cells of blood vessels (Section 13.3.2).

Circulating noradrenaline acts specifically via α-**receptors**, and therefore quite consistently causes vasoconstriction in almost all vascular beds. Circulating adrenaline can act via α-receptors to produce vasoconstriction, and as just stated this is its usual effect; however, in some tissues the blood vessels also have **β-receptors**, and then circulating adrenaline can also act via these receptors to produce vasodilation.

Hormones that induce contraction of smooth muscle cells usually do it by inducing an initial increase in the concentration of **calcium ions** inside the muscle cell, as happens when the cell is excited by an action potential (Guyton, 1986, p. 145). The hormone usually binds to a specific receptor protein lodged in the plasmalemma (cell membrane). This opens calcium ion channels and thus decreases (depolarizes) the membrane potential, but usually without causing an action potential. The flow of calcium ions into the cell causes it to contract. Some hormones, however, act without causing any change in the membrane potential. Such a hormone binds to a receptor protein in the cell membrane, forming **cyclic adenosine monophosphate (cAMP)**, which can alter the release of calcium ions from **intra**cellular organelles and change the degree of smooth muscle contraction (Section 2.36).

It is believed that the smooth muscle cells of all arteries and most veins possess **α-receptors** (Section 13.3.2). **Beta-receptors** seem to be confined mainly to the vascular beds of **skeletal muscle** and the **heart**, and even there are less numerous than α-receptors. In vascular beds that do possess β-receptors, the vasomotor responses to circulating **adrenaline** depend on the relative numbers of α- and β-receptors. However, the responses also depend on the size of the dose. It is suggested that this is because α-receptors have a higher threshold than β-receptors (Rowell, 1974, p. 210). Therefore high concentrations of circulating adrenaline stimulate α-receptors and cause vasoconstriction: low concentrations stimulate β-receptors and cause vasodilation.

The **arterial vasculature** of **skeletal muscle** possesses both α- and β-receptors. Circulating **noradrenaline** causes vasoconstriction via the α-receptors, and this is the dominant effect. However, circulating noradrenaline also appears to have a small effect on β-receptors, since blockade of β-receptors increases the vasoconstrictor action of noradrenaline (Rowell, 1974, p. 210). Presumably the overall vasoconstrictor action of noradrenaline due to α-receptors is normally somewhat weakened by a slight concurrent vasodilator effect due to the stimulation of β-receptors. **Adrenaline** produces vasodilation at low doses and vasoconstriction at high doses (Scott, 1986, p. 66), presumably in accord with the low threshold of β-receptors and the high threshold of α-receptors. The **veins** in skeletal muscle show negligible responses to circulating adrenaline and noradrenaline, or other vasoconstrictor drugs except vasopressin (Rowell, 1974, p. 211).

Both circulating adrenaline and circulating noradrenaline have potent effects on **splanchnic blood flow** (Rowell, 1974, p. 226). Circulating **noradrenaline** has, as usual, a strong vasoconstriction via α-receptors. Circulating **adrenaline** acts on β-receptors at least in man, giving marked vasodilation when infused in physiological concentration: some observers have obtained the same result in the dog, but others have found that in this species circulating adrenaline causes the opposite effect, i.e. splanchnic vasoconstriction.

In the **coronary circulation**, circulating **noradrenaline** once again acts through α-receptors and is vasoconstrictor in effect (Scott, 1986, p. 66). Circulating **adrenaline** acts on β-receptors, producing coronary vasodilation in response to high doses as well as low doses (Scott, 1986, p. 67).

Alpha-receptors are present in the **cerebral arterial vasculature**, but the presence of β-receptors is doubtful (Section 13.3.2). Intra-arterial injections of catecholamines have very little effect on cerebral blood flow. Yet, in a tissue bath, high doses of adrenaline and noradrenaline do cause constriction of isolated cerebral vessels; the reasons for this discrepancy between *in vivo* and *in vitro* observations are not known (D'Alecy, 1974, p. 270).

The **cutaneous vasculature** has no β-receptors, and therefore both circulating **adrenaline** and circulating **noradrenaline** are potent vasoconstrictors acting through α-receptors (Rowell, 1974, p. 192). However, this vasoconstrictor response to circulating catecholamines is weak compared with the effects of sympathetic vasoconstrictor action. Unlike the veins of skeletal muscle which show very small responses to circulating adrenaline and noradrenaline, **cutaneous veins** respond to both of these hormones by strong vasoconstriction (Rowell, 1974, p. 195).

The **sympathetic vasoconstrictor axons** that innervate the smooth muscle cells of arteries are restricted to the outer parts of the tunica media. The smooth muscle cells in the inner, non-innervated, part of the media are particularly sensitive to circulating adrenaline, noradrenaline, and other vasomotor agents such as angiotensin and vasopressin; circulating vasomotor substances reach these inner layers of smooth muscle by *diffusion* through the tunica intima.

13.4.2 *Other vasomotor agents*

Angiotensin II and vasopressin are particularly powerful **vasoconstrictor substances**. Angiotensin II constricts blood vessels in all parts of the body. Vasopressin is also known as antidiuretic hormone.

Vasodilator substances include kinins, notably bradykinin, and histamine. Serotonin and prostaglandins can be either vasodilator or vasoconstrictor in action, but most of the prostaglandins are vasodilators. Serotonin released from a blood clot has a powerful vasoconstrictor action on smooth muscle cells nearest to the lumen of large arteries, and thus helps to restrict haemorrhage if the arterial wall is damaged (Section 12.21).

13.5   Mechanical regulation of vascular tone: autoregulation

A sudden rise in arterial pressure causes an immediate increase in blood flow in most of the tissues of the body, but within a minute or so the blood flow in the tissues is somehow automatically restored to its normal value; likewise a fall in arterial pressure decreases blood flow, but this is quickly followed by a return to normal flow. The automatic maintenance of a normal rate of blood flow despite fluctuations in arterial pressure is known as **autoregulation**. The mechanism controlling it is often referred to as '**myogenic**', because it arises from the direct response of smooth muscle cells to stretching and relaxation.

The sudden stretching of the smooth muscle in the walls of small arteries and arterioles is a mechanical stimulus that causes the smooth muscle to contract, thus adjusting their tone. Therefore, when a rise in intravascular pressure dilates a vessel, the muscle in that vessel responds by contracting: conversely, when the intravascular pressure falls the muscle relaxes. Lymphatic vessels show similar responses to distension (Section 14.8). The urinary bladder also illustrates the contractile responses of smooth muscle to **mechanical stimulation** (Section 3.16.2).

Automatic regulation of local blood flow can also be explained by metabolic factors (Section 13.2.1). However, the review by Kuo *et al.* (1992) concluded that only **metarterioles** and the **smallest arterioles** (less than 20 μm) are dominated by **metabolic** factors; this is predictable, since these very small vessels are the ones that are in really close contact with the tissues and their metabolites (Smiesko and Johnson, 1993). **Myogenic regulation** dominates in **medium-sized arterioles** (20–100 μm), in which it induces substantial changes in vascular diameter. **Endothelial regulation** (Section 13.6) dominates in large arterioles (100–200 μm); the largest of these will be outside the organ, and therefore outside the range of metabolic factors (Smiesko and Johnson, 1993).

Neurogenic mechanisms are not involved in autoregulation (Mellander and Björnberg, 1992, p. 117).

Myogenic control in autoregulation interacts additively or negatively with the metabolic and endothelial control of arterioles. However, myogenic regulation appears to be critically important in the establishment of systemic arterial resistance, since at least 50% and perhaps up to 80% of vascular resistance resides in arterioles 10–100 μm in diameter (Kuo *et al.*, 1992) (Section 12.5). It is also postulated that myogenic regulation of small arteries and arterioles contributes importantly by maintaining the **stability of capillary pressure** during fluctuations in systemic arterial pressure (Guyton, 1986, p. 235). Mellander and Björnberg (1992) showed that, in the normal circulation, the capillary pressure remains virtually constant between 15 and 17 mmHg (2.0 and 2.3 kPa) even though the mean systemic arterial pressure is raised progressively from 50 to 180 mmHg (6.7 to 24.0 kPa). Mellander and Björnberg (1992) emphasized the imperative need to keep capillary pressure stable and not allow it to rise as mean arterial pressure rises; they estimated that, if myogenic autoregulation failed and at the same time aortic pressure increased to 125 mmHg (16.7 kPa) for 15 minutes, the net transcapillary filtration would cause the loss of about 50% of the total plasma volume – which, *in vivo*, would certainly lead to a catastrophic circulatory collapse.

It was at first suggested that the response to mechanical stimulation of the vascular wall was actually executed by a vasomotor *mediator* (e.g. nitric oxide for vasodilation, endothelin-1 for vasoconstriction) released by the endothelium in response to shear stress (Section 13.6). Endothelial regulation and myogenic regulation of blood vessels have mechanical stimulation in common. However, careful experimental removal of the endothelium, without compromising the adjacent smooth muscle, has shown that the endothelium is not required for the normal myogenic responsiveness of blood vessels of many different tissues (Kuo *et al.*, 1992, p. 6).

13.6   Endothelial regulation of vascular tone

The **endothelial cells** that line **small muscular arteries** and **large arterioles** continuously release a potent vasodilator agent, **nitric oxide** (NO). The stimulus is mechanical, namely the shearing stress (drag) caused by the flow of blood over the endothelium (Section 13.8). An increase in flow rate increases the drag, inducing the endothelial cells to increase the release of nitric oxide. The very short half-life of nitric oxide ensures that it has little effect downstream in the vasculature, but it does diffuse directly to the adjacent smooth muscle cells and causes them to relax. The resulting dilation of the vessel reduces the velocity of the stream and lowers the drag towards its original level. Conversely, a decrease in flow rate diminishes the release of nitric oxide, vasoconstriction results, and flow rate increases back to the original level.

This endothelium-dependent mechanism is another form of automatic regulation of blood flow. It has to be integrated physiologically into metabolic (Section 13.2) and myogenic (Section 13.3) regulation.

The **nitric oxide** produced by endothelial cells is commonly known as **endothelium-derived relaxing factor** (EDRF) or **endogenous nitrovasodilator**; it is synthesized in vascular endothelial cells from L-arginine (Lüscher and Dohi, 1992) by a constitutive Ca^{2+}-dependent enzyme named nitric oxide synthase (see Dikranien *et al.*, 1994). It had long been known that vascular perfusion of acetylcholine *in vivo* causes vasodilation, but this observation apparently could not be linked to current knowledge of the physiology of acetylcholine since it received little or no mention in leading reference works. However, in 1980 it was discovered that the vascular relaxations evoked by acetylcholine are fully dependent on the presence of endothelial cells, and are due to the release of nitric oxide from those cells (Kovách and Lefer, 1993). At that time, nitric oxide was known only as an environmental contaminant, for example in cigarette smoke and smog (Kovách and Lefer, 1993), and silo gas on farms, with dangerous toxic effects on the pulmonary alveoli (Blood and Studdert, 1988, p. 625).

In 1980 the discovery by R. Furchgott and his co-workers of endothelium-derived nitric oxide and its vasodilator action introduced a whole new dimension of research into cardiovascular physiology and pathophysiology (Kovách and Lefer, 1993). Moreover, as has happened before in the history of science, this discovery suddenly converged on two other totally different fields of biology, namely (1) neurotransmission by nitric oxide in many parts of the brain and in the enteric nervous system (Section 2.34), and (2) host defence mechanisms wherein nitric oxide is now found to be a powerful agent produced by macrophages and neutrophils, **cytotoxic** to bacteria and tumour cells; its production by defence cells is activated by **endotoxins** (lipopolysaccharide, LPS), and by **interferon-γ** (a **lymphokine**, Section 14.31.2) produced by cytotoxic T-lymphocytes. This tiny radical (NO) has the lowest molecular weight of any known bioactive agent secreted by a cell and an extremely short half-life. Yet it has these extraordinarily versatile functions, ranging from circulatory control and neuronal transmission to potent cytotoxity, depending on the amount present and the site of release (Kovách and Lefer, 1993).

Subsequently, several other extremely powerful **vasoactive agents** were found to be derived from endothelial cells, of which some are **vasodilators** and others are **vasoconstrictors** (Kovách and Lefer, 1993). The latter include peptides, e.g. **endothelin-1** which is strongly vasoconstrictor, and a cyclooxygenase-dependent factor (EDCF2), probably **prostaglandin H2** (Lüscher and Dohi, 1992). Endothelin-1, incidentally, turns out to be the mammalian homologue of the venomous safrotoxins of the asp (*Atractaspis engaddensis*) that killed Cleopatra (Brooks, 1997). Suddenly the humble endothelial cell with its slender cytoplasm and meagre organelles (Section 12.12) has emerged as a veritable power-pack of biogenic agents.

It has also been shown that endothelial cells release these vasoactive agents in response to a wide range of stimuli (Miller, 1992): (1) **metabolic stimuli**, e.g. partial pressure of oxygen; (2) **hormonal stimuli**, e.g. circulating catecholamines and acetylcholine; (3) **mechanical stimuli**, e.g. stretch of the vessel wall caused by pressure change, and shear stress of the blood flowing over the endothelial surface; and (4) **cellular stimuli** in the form of substances released from blood elements such as activated macrophages and aggregated platelets.

It seems likely that the **pathways of the vasoactive agent** to the nearby smooth muscle cells (Smiesko and Johnson, 1993) is by diffusion, but another possible pathway is offered by **myoendothelial junctions** (Section 12.10). Alternatively there may be electrical coupling via gap junctions, allowing hyperpolarization of the endothelial cell to spread to the smooth muscle cells (although there seems to be no evidence that endothelial cells are excitable cells).

As a result of these intensive researches during the last ten years, **endothelium-dependent contraction and relaxation** of the **arterial side** of the vascular system have now emerged as a whole complex of key mechanisms, subtly integrated, regulating vascular functions (Kovách and Lefer, 1993). (The endothelium of the venous side of the circulatory system awaits investigation (Smiesko and Johnson, 1993).

For example, the continuous formation of *vasorelaxant* **nitric oxide** in the endothelium of resistance arteries plays a particularly important part in regulating both mean arterial pressure, and tissue blood flow in individual organs, by controlling vascular resistance under physiological and pathophysiological conditions (Kovách and Lefer, 1993). As stated in Section 13.5, endothelial regulation (as opposed to myogenic and metabolic regulation) dominates in **large arterioles** of 100–200 μm (Kuo *et al.*, 1992), and these are vessels that contribute greatly to the peripheral vascular resistance (Section 12.5.2); this is one reason why nitric oxide contributes so importantly to the regulation of mean arterial pressure. Another reason is that a *vasodilator mecha-*

nism is also activated by the endothelial cells of **small muscular arteries** (Segal, 1992). Such arteries are indeed often called 'resistance arteries' (Smiesko and Johnson, 1993). The dilation of small muscular arteries is attained by a diffusible endothelial factor that is released by the endothelium in response to increased shear stress on the wall, or the dilation may be mediated by hyperpolarization of the endothelial cells (Segal, 1992). The release of **catecholamines** from sympathetic axon terminals can also be *inhibited* by an endothelium-derived factor (Kuo *et al.*, 1992); this is presumed to act presynaptically (Miller, 1992), and could thus block the sympathetic vasoconstrictor axon terminals at α_2-adrenoreceptor sites.

The graduated release of nitric oxide (or one of the other endothelium-derived vasorelaxants) in response to increasing blood flow is also thought to play a major role in the progressive opening of effective **collateral circulation** (Smiesko and Johnson, 1993) (Section 12.18).

Dysfunction of endothelial cells has now emerged as a major factor in **hypertension**, evinced as *decreased release of nitric oxide* from the endothelium and marked *reductions in endothelium-dependent relaxation* (Lüscher and Dohi, 1992). **Essential hypertension** in man accounts for many cerebrovascular strokes, myocardial infarctions, and sudden deaths. Hypertension is detected only sporadically in domestic mammals, partly because of technical difficulties in diagnosis, but it is recognized in dogs in a form resembling essential hypertension in man, and temporary episodes of hypertension occur in all species when suffering severe pain, and in horses with acute laminitis (Blood and Studdert, 1988, p. 465). There is evidence for a deficiency in the production or release of relaxing (i.e. vasodilator) factors from the endothelial cells, both in the natural process of ageing and also in essential hypertension in man and experimental rats.

Furthermore, **prostanoids** such as **prostacyclin (PGI$_2$)** that are normally released by endothelial cells, exert an excitatory influence on **baroreceptors** (Section 19.5.7) during increases in arterial pressure (Chapleau *et al.*, 1991). Baroreceptor activity is decreased in **chronic hypertension**, and this may be caused by endothelial dysfunction and hence impaired production of PGI$_2$.

Endothelial cell dysfunction is also a prominent, sensitive, and widespread vascular occurrence in **circulatory shock** (Kovách and Lefer, 1993, p. 147). Circulatory shock can be induced by various stimuli, including severe haemorrhage, endotoxaemia, mesenteric ischaemia and reperfusion, myocardial ischaemia and reperfusion, and trauma. According to Kovách and Lefer (1993, pp. 146–147) these types of shock are characterized by increased peripheral vascular resistance, hypoperfusion, and low blood flow. They share a period of **hypoperfusion** of certain organs; the hypoperfusion may be followed by reperfusion, but this improvement tends to be transient. Thus in haemorrhagic shock, the transient recovery is lost and hypotension again takes over (i.e. **postoligaemic shock**). It has been found that, in **postoligaemic shock**, there is a deficiency of endothelium-derived nitric oxide, and hence a failure permanently to relax the vessels that are suffering from hypoperfusion. The shock state can be successfully treated by any of an array of pharmacological agents that protect or restore the production of nitric oxide by the endothelium, including the semi-essential amino acid L-arginine which acts a substrate for nitric oxide.

In 1867 a young Edinburgh resident physician, T.L. Brunton, reported in the *Lancet* that inhalation of **amyl nitrite** relieved the pain of angina pectoris (Reeves, 1995). Brunton had graduated only one year earlier, but as a third year student had completed a thesis on digitalis, based mainly on experiments on himself. In the same year, Brunton moved to Leipzig where he published several more papers on the hypotensive action of amyl nitrite. His appointment at Leipzig almost exactly coincided with the sensational discovery there, in 1866, of the hypotensive action of the 'depressor nerve' by another young graduate, E. Cyon (Section 19.10.4). Amyl nitrite probably works by releasing nitric oxide, resulting in coronary vasodilation and hence the restoration of myocardial oxygen supply. Brunton came close to discovering the vasodilator activity of nitric oxide. He was well aware that the vasoreactivity of amyl nitrite and allied substances lay in their nitrite/nitrate moiety. However, biomedical science had to wait for more than a century for elucidation of the endothelial source and powerful vasodilator action of nitric oxide.

13.7   Central and peripheral regulation of arterial tone

As stated in Section 13.1, all vascular smooth muscle is in a state of **basal tone**. This basal tone sets a baseline on which all other factors regulating vascular tone are superimposed. These other regulatory factors are metabolic (Section 13.2), neural (Section 13.3), hormonal (Section 13.4), mechanical (myogenic) (Section 13.5), and endothelial (Section 13.6).

This complex array of factors regulates the tone of the smooth muscle of muscular arteries and arterioles by means of two control systems, one central and the other peripheral.

The **central control system** is responsible for the vascular requirements of the whole animal. It is based on the 'cardiovascular centre' in the brain stem (Section 19.12). It acts **indirectly** on the smooth muscle cells of muscular arteries and arterioles through baro- and chemoreceptor reflex arcs (Section 19.12). The effector (motor) components of these arcs are the sympathetic nervous system and circulating catecholamines (i.e. neural and hormonal regulatory factors).

The **peripheral control system** for regulating the vascular tone of muscular arteries and arterioles is responsible for the fine tuning of local vascular beds in particular organs, in order to meet their individual requirements. It works **directly** on the smooth muscle cells, (mainly) through metabolic and mechanical stimuli. The peripheral control system also works **indirectly** on the smooth muscle cells via the **endothelial cells**, again (mainly) through metabolic and mechanical stimuli. The direct and indirect mechanisms of peripheral control have to be integrated together.

Miller (1992) reviewed the interaction between the central and peripheral regulatory systems that control vascular tone, with particular reference to the role of the endothelial cell.

The effects of **mechanical stimuli** illustrate the complex integration that must take place between the **indirect** mechanisms of the endothelial system, and the more simple mechanisms of the **direct** myogenic responses of smooth muscle cells themselves. Mechanical stimuli can affect the endothelial system, and thence the smooth muscle cells *indirectly*; thus an increase in flow rate increases the shear stress on the endothelial cells, causing them to release nitric oxide and evoking **relaxation** of their adjacent muscle cells (Section 13.6). On the other hand, mechanical stimulation of arteries and arterioles can affect their smooth muscle cells *directly*; an increase in pressure stretches the smooth muscle cells and evokes myogenic **contraction** (Section 13.5). Thus two rather similar mechanical stimuli induce *opposite responses* by the muscle of the vascular wall. However, the endothelium-mediated vasodilation occurs most strongly in large arterioles, whereas the direct myogenic contraction is believed to occur particularly in medium-sized arterioles. Kuo *et al.* (1992) argue that these differences in response can be correlated with the particular physiological demands upon these different sites within the vasculature.

At first it was believed that the above **myogenic responses** were **entirely** mediated by endothelium, i.e. not only in large arterioles but also in medium-sized arterioles and muscular arteries. However, by taking great care not to compromise the smooth muscle cells during the removal or impairment of the endothelium, it was shown that the endothelium is not required for normal myogenic responsiveness in medium-sized arterioles, nor in small muscular arteries (Kuo *et al.*, 1992).

Metabolic factors such as decreased concentration of oxygen in the blood plasma can also act both indirectly via the endothelium, and directly on the smooth muscle cells. The responses by the smooth muscle cells to these two control mechanisms may vary in different parts of the vasculature. In small arterioles of less than 20 μm diameter, the metabolic factors act *directly* on the smooth muscle cells, causing vasodilation in response to decreased oxygen. On the other hand, in some arterial vessels metabolic stimuli induce endothelial cells to release vasoactive agents and thus act *indirectly* on the smooth muscle cells.

Observations of this kind on the varying responses to mechanical and metabolic stimuli suggest that the vascular tree is divided into segments, each segment having its own dominant regulating mechanism. The integration of such elaborate control mechanisms seems to be almost incredibly complex, but presumably offers very refined regulation throughout the arterial system.

13.8 Circulatory adjustments during exercise

At the onset of severe exercise there is a mass discharge of the sympathetic nervous system, causing a generalized vasoconstriction of all the innervated blood vessels of the peripheral circulation; this includes all muscular arteries and all arterioles (though not metarterioles, since these are not innervated, Section 13.3.1). This in turn induces an immediate increase in total vascular resistance. Simultaneously, generalized sympathetic stimulation causes venoconstriction that empties the venous reservoirs, thus increasing the venous return to the heart (Section 12.16.3). Sympathetic stimulation also increases the heart rate (Section 22.13) and the force of contraction of the heart (Section 22.16). The combination of increased total vascular resistance and increased cardiac performance causes a great increase in aortic pressure. The systemic circulation is now ready to perform one of its principal functions (Section 12.4.3), i.e. to use its head of pressure to redistribute blood, including that obtained from the venous reservoirs, thus sending more blood to active tissues (skeletal muscle, in this instance) and less to inactive tissues (e.g. gut).

Decreasing the perfusion of **inactive** organs is straightforward, since all that is needed is to maintain the sympathetic vasoconstriction of their arteries. **Increasing** the perfusion of **active** organs (skeletal muscle, in exercise) is more complex: it requires the overruling of the generalized sympathetic vasoconstriction of the arteries and arterioles of the limbs that accompanies the onset of exercise, and the substitution of vasodilation in those vessels.

The series of steps by which vasoconstriction in the exercising limbs is replaced by vasodilation, all the way from the microcirculation to the distributing arteries, has been studied by Segal (1992). **Ascending vasodilation** *begins* at the metarterioles and the smallest arterioles, where it is caused by **metabolic factors**; this is predictable from the fact that these vessels belong to the microcirculation and are therefore in close contact with the metabolically active tissues. Vasodilation then ascends to medium-sized arterioles, to the large arterioles, and finally to the muscular arteries (distributing arteries; Section 12.5.2) that arise from the femoral artery and axillary artery, and supply the individual muscles of the limbs.

The ascent of vasodilation upstream in the medium-sized arterioles up to (and including) the muscular arteries is probably **flow dependent** throughout, i.e. mediated mechanically by increased **shear stress** on the **endothelium** (Section 13.6). The ascent begins with the initial metabolic vasodilation of the smallest arterioles, which increases the shear stress on their endothelial cells. This induces the release from their endothelial cells of a dilator factor such as nitric oxide. The dilator factor *diffuses* into the adjacent smooth muscle cells *including those that are very slightly upstream*, and thus dilates the adjoining medium-sized arterioles and then the large arterioles. Finally the progressively ascending vasodilation increases the shear stress in the distributing (muscular) arteries also, and causes them to dilate as well. It will be noted that the largest arterioles and certainly the distributing (muscular) arteries will be mostly **outside** the surface of the muscles, and are therefore denied access to the local metabolic factors generated in the muscle tissue itself.

Section 13.7 showed that the **peripheral control system** regulating **vascular tone** offers various combinations of mechanisms. These act *directly* on the smooth muscle, or *indirectly* on the smooth muscle via the endothelium, or both directly and indirectly. Segal (1992) believed that, in the contracting gastrocnemius muscle of the cat, the ascending vasodilation from (and including) medium-sized arterioles to the femoral artery, is flow-dependent. It will be based on increased shear stress on the endothelium, caused by the increased flow rate. The endothelial cells then release a vasodilator factor that diffuses a short distance, upstream as well as downstream, to the smooth muscle cells; or there is electrotonic spread of hyperpolarization from the endothelial cells to the smooth muscle cells.

Segal (1992) recognized that the distributing arteries appear to be a critical site for integrating descending sympathetic vasoconstriction with ascending vasodilation. Sympathetic vasoconstriction at this site can dictate the magnitude of muscle flow during exercise. These are muscular arteries, and are likely to be strongly influenced by their sympathetic vasoconstrictor innervation. At this point in the ascending vasodilation, nitric oxide might not prevail over the sympathetic innervation. Therefore it is suggested (Segal, 1992) that the endothelial cells could here act neurally by releasing an agent that acts at α_2-**receptor sites** on the noradrenergic axon terminals (Section 2.37), thus presynaptically blocking the release of noradrenaline from the terminal (Miller, 1992; Kuo *et al.*, 1992). Observations show that, by one mechanism or another, dilation of distributing arteries does take place to a considerable extent (Segal, 1992).

Chapter 14
Capillaries: Lymphatics: Lymphatic Tissues: Immune System: Lymph Nodes: Ducts

Sections III (Lymphatic tissues) and IV (cellular basis of the immune system) of this chapter were co-written by A.S. King and J.B. Dixon.

I   CAPILLARY EXCHANGE

14.1   Mechanisms moving substances across the capillary wall

The endothelial lining and basal lamina of the blood capillary (Section 12.12) act as a selectively permeable membrane, allowing the ready movement across the capillary wall of dissolved gases, water, and small molecule solutes such as sodium, chloride, and potassium ions, but restricting the passage of large molecules such as the plasma proteins. The solution which is formed by the outward transport from the blood capillary is **interstitial fluid** (tissue fluid) (Section 12.2); it contains water, small molecule solutes, gases, and some plasma proteins. Transport can also occur in the opposite direction, **into** the blood capillary, and this inward transport is the principal way of removing interstitial fluid and waste products (the other being drainage by lymphatic capillaries (Section 14.7.1).

Four main mechanisms are involved in the transport of substances across the capillary wall: diffusion, filtration, absorption, and pinocytosis. **Diffusion** (Section 12.3) depends on a concentration gradient of a substance on one side or the other of the capillary wall, the substance being driven from the higher concentration towards the lower concentration. **Filtration** depends on the presence of a hydrostatic pressure gradient across the capillary wall, driving a filtrate from the plasma to the interstitial fluid. Under the influence of the hydrostatic pressure inside the capillary, there is a bulk flow of water and solutes between the blood and the interstitial fluid, across the capillary wall, resembling the passage of a solution through a filter paper. **Absorption** (generally thought of as reabsorption) depends on a high osmotic pressure in the plasma and a low osmotic pressure in the interstitial fluid, thus sucking fluid back into the bloodstream. Absorption also creates bulk flow. **Pinocytosis** depends on the movement or coalescence of intracellular vesicles across the endothelial cell.

The role of **diffusion** across the capillary wall is to meet the needs of cellular metabolism. This includes: the delivery of oxygen, and removal of carbon dioxide and hydrogen ions; delivery of nutrients such as glucose, amino acids, and fatty acids; maintenance of the required concentrations of sodium, chloride, and other ions; and provision or removal of regulatory hormones. Diffusion is by far the most important mechanism of transport of substances across the capillary wall. The role of **filtration** across the capillary wall is mainly to balance the fluid volume of the blood plasma against that of the interstitial fluid; it contributes very little to the exchange of nutrients and waste products. The role of **pinocytosis** is to transport macromolecules across the capillary wall.

There are various other more specialized mechanisms of transport across the plasmalemma. Among these is carrier-mediated transport by **integral proteins** projecting through the plasmalemma. Integral proteins provide ion channels for depolarization and hyperpolarization of **excitable cells**.

14.2 Diffusion across the capillary wall

14.2.1 *The endothelial cell*

Some substances, notably oxygen and carbon dioxide, and many anaesthetic agents, diffuse readily through the endothelial cell. Water also diffuses through by this direct route. However, in general the substances that use this pathway must be of small molecular weight and lipid-soluble in order to pass through the bimolecular phospholipid layer of the plasmalemma. Because of these restrictions, diffusion directly through the endothelial cell accounts for only a relatively small proportion of total diffusion.

14.2.2 *Intercellular clefts*

There is a gap between the adjacent edges of endothelial cells, known as the **intercellular cleft** (Section 12.12.3). The cleft is sealed at scattered spot-like gap junctions, but between and around the gap junctions the cleft is held open by protein–carbohydrate macromolecular complexes similar to those forming the ground substance of the interstitium (Section 12.2). Thus the cleft forms a continuum between the blood plasma and the interstitial fluid, so that at its clefts the capillary wall behaves as though it offers no physical barrier at all to water and its small molecule solutes. Consequently the great majority of the water that is transported across the capillary wall, and all of the water-soluble, lipid-insoluble substances, including glucose, urea, and sodium and chloride ions, diffuse through the cleft. Thus the intercellular clefts account for the great majority of diffusion across the capillary wall (although the rate of diffusion is slower here than by the direct route through the endothelial cell). The clefts are also the main pathway for filtration and reabsorption of water and solutes.

The intercellular clefts are estimated (Guyton, 1986, p. 350) to form only one thousandth of the total surface area of the capillary walls. Nevertheless, the velocity of thermal motion is so great that water molecules diffuse through the capillary wall about 80 times faster than the flow of plasma along the capillary. Thus the water of the plasma is exchanged 80 times with the water in the interstitial fluid while the plasma makes its journey from the beginning to the end of a capillary.

The diffusion of carbon dioxide and oxygen between the cells of the body tissues and the **pulmonary alveoli** requires pressure gradients that are remarkably different, the gradient for carbon dioxide being very small, and that for oxygen very large.

Metabolism of oxygen in the cells of the tissues generates **carbon dioxide**, which diffuses through the interstitial fluid and capillary endothelium into the blood. The P_{CO_2} within the cell is about 46 mmHg (6.1 kPa), whereas the P_{CO_2} in the **interstitial fluid** is about 45 mmHg (6.0 kPa), giving the very small pressure gradient from cell to interstitial fluid of only 1 mmHg (0.1 kPa). The **arterial blood** entering the tissue has a P_{CO_2} of 40 mmHg (5.3 kPa), so there is pressure gradient of 5 mmHg (0.7 kPa) driving the CO_2 from the interstitial fluid into the blood. The P_{CO_2} of the interstitial tissue and venous blood come into equilibrium, so the **venous blood** leaving the tissues has a P_{CO_2} of 45 mmHg (6.0 kPa). On entering the **pulmonary capillaries** the venous blood comes into equilibrium with **alveolar gas**, which has a P_{CO_2} of 40 mmHg (5.3 kPa), so the pressure gradient from pulmonary capillary blood to alveolar air is also 5 mmHg (0.7 kPa). Thus the delivery of carbon dioxide from tissue cell to alveolar gas is achieved by a total pressure gradient of only 6 mmHg (0.8 kPa). Yet equilibrium in the removal of CO_2 is reached when the blood is only about one third of the way through the **pulmonary capillary** (note the similarity to the equally large safety factor in the uptake of oxygen by the pulmonary capillaries, where the uptake of oxygen is completed when the red cells have passed the first third of the pulmonary capillary; Section 6.28).

The pressure gradient in the **diffusion of oxygen** is far greater. **Arterial blood** arriving in the tissues has a P_{O_2} of about 95 mmHg (12.7 kPa). The P_{O_2} in the **interstitial fluid** averages about 40 mmHg (5.3 kPa). Under the influence of this high pressure gradient (55 mmHg; 7.3 kPa) the blood in the capillary rapidly gives up oxygen to the interstitial fluid until its P_{O_2} comes into equilibrium with that of the interstitial fluid; so the venous blood leaving the tissues also has a P_{O_2} of about 40 mmHg (5.3 kPa). The normal **intracellular** P_{O_2} averages about 23 mmHg (3.1 kPa). Therefore the delivery of oxygen from arterial blood to the interior of the cell has a **total pressure gradient** of about $95 - 23$ mmHg, or 72 mmHg ($12.7 - 3.1 = 9.6$ kPa). An intracellular P_{O_2} of about 3 mmHg (0.4 kPa) is normally required to provide fully for the cell metabolism, so the intracellular P_{O_2} of 23 mmHg (3.1 kPa) confers another substantial safety margin.

The great difference between the pressure gradients required for the diffusion of carbon dioxide and that of oxygen arises because carbon dioxide diffuses about 20 times faster than oxygen.

14.2.3 *Fenestrations*

In some tissues such as endocrine organs the inner and outer layers of the plasmalemma fuse into a single thin membrane in circular areas known as fenestrations (Section 12.12.5). Diffusion of macromolecules such as hormones, as well as solutes and water, is presumed to be accelerated through these very thin fenestrations.

14.3 The oxygen–haemoglobin dissociation curve

Oxygen binds to the haemoglobin molecule by a reversible reaction to form oxyhaemoglobin, $Hb + O_2 \leftrightarrow HbO_2$. When the concentration of oxygen is high (high partial pressure), as in the lung, the haemoglobin takes up oxygen. When the concentration of oxygen is low (low partial pressure), as in the tissues, the haemoglobin releases oxygen. If the partial pressure is zero, the haemoglobin gives up all of its oxygen.

For the optimal uptake of oxygen in the lung, a high affinity of haemoglobin for oxygen is advantageous: on the other hand, for the optimal unloading of oxygen in the tissues a low affinity is desirable. In the living animal, the unloading is just as vital as the uptake. There is therefore a conflict of interest between the lung and the tissues.

The amount of oxygen that combines with haemoglobin depends on the partial pressure of oxygen (P_{O_2}) in the blood plasma. The amount of oxygen can be expressed as the **volume of oxygen per 100 ml of blood**. It is more usual, however, to represent the oxygen as **percentage saturation of the arterial haemoglobin**. A plot of percentage saturation against the partial pressure of oxygen gives an oxygen dissociation curve (Fig. 14.1). This turns out to be an S-shaped curve: when the P_{O_2} is high, the slope is almost flat; when the P_{O_2} is low the slope falls steeply. It is the steep lower part that is really the **dissociation** part of the curve, since it represents the **unloading** of oxygen to the tissues. The upper flat part is actually the **association** part of the curve, because it represents the **uptake** of oxygen by the lung.

The oxygen–haemoglobin dissociation curve is sometimes known as the oxygen equilibrium curve, since what the curve actually describes is the level of oxygen binding to haemoglobin when the haemoglobin is in equilibrium with oxygen dissolved in the blood plasma at a given P_{O_2} (Weibel, 1984, p. 147).

When about 97% of the haemoglobin is saturated with oxygen, as in normal arterial blood, the **volume of oxygen per 100 ml of blood** is about 19 ml. In the capillaries in the tissues, the saturation of haemoglobin falls on average to about 75%; at this level of saturation, the volume of oxygen carried by each 100 ml of blood also decreases to about 75% of its original value, and therefore still carries about 14 ml of oxygen. Thus, in average tissues, each 100 ml of blood delivers about 5 ml of oxygen from the lung to the tissues (Guyton, 1986, p. 497).

14.3.1 *Uptake of oxygen by haemoglobin*

At a P_{O_2} of 104 mmHg (13.9 kPa), haemoglobin is about 98% saturated. Since the P_{O_2} of alveolar gas at sea level is about 104 mmHg (Section 6.28.1), it follows that arterial blood leaving the lung in the pulmonary vein is normally almost fully saturated with oxygen. Hyperventilation can raise the P_{O_2} of alveolar gas to about 130 mmHg (17.3 kPa), but this adds a negligible amount of oxygen to each 100 ml of blood.

The uptake mechanism has a large safety margin; the body maintains its alveolar P_{O_2} at a level that is substantially higher than that needed to almost completely saturate the haemoglobin of its arterial blood (Section 11.11.2). Because of the flatness of the association part of the curve, a reduction in the P_{O_2} to 80 mmHg (10.7 kPa) decreases the saturation only very slightly (to about 96%). At an altitude of 10 000 feet (3.3 km), the P_{O_2} of alveolar gas falls slightly below 70 mmHg (9.3 kPa), but even then the arterial oxygen saturation is still about 90% (Fig. 14.1), and this enables a mammal to live at such an altitude. Likewise, if respiratory disease has caused the P_{O_2} of alveolar gas to decrease to slightly below 70 mmHg, an animal will nevertheless have arterial blood that is about 90% saturated.

14.3.2 *Unloading of oxygen*

Arterial blood entering the tissues has a P_{O_2} of about 95 mmHg (12.7 kPa). The P_{O_2} of capillary blood leaving the tissues has fallen on average to

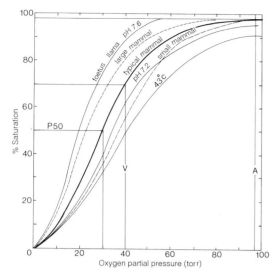

Fig. 14.1   Mammalian oxygen–haemoglobin dissociation curves. The curves plot the percentage saturation of arterial haemoglobin against the gaseous partial pressure of oxygen. The bold line in the middle represents a typical mammal at a normal blood pH of 7.4 and normal body temperature. The other lines represent five variants. In two of these, the curve is shifted to the **left** of that of the typical mammal, i.e. the affinity of haemoglobin for oxygen is increased. This promotes the **uptake of oxygen in the lung**, and occurs in mammals that live in environments where the oxygen supply is relatively deficient through its low partial pressure, e.g. at high altitudes (llama), in underground burrows, and in the fetus. It also occurs (one aspect of the Bohr effect) when the pH of the blood rises (7.6), as in hypocapnia (respiratory alkalosis). The other three curves are shifted to the **right** of that of the typical mammal. This promotes the **unloading of oxygen in the tissues**. A shift to the right occurs during exercise, when the pH of the blood plasma decreases (7.2) due to an increase in CO_2 or lactic acid (the other aspect of the Bohr effect); a shift to the right also occurs during exercise when the temperature of blood in active muscle rises (43°C). Very small mammals have a relatively large resting oxygen consumption. In order to meet the high demand of their tissues for oxygen, the curve shifts to the right (broken line on the right). Large mammals tend to have a relatively low resting oxygen consumption, and their dissociation curve shifts to the left (broken line on the left). Normal values for arterial and venous blood are indicated respectively by A and V. P_{50} is the half saturation pressure, about 30 mmHg (4.0 kPa), when half the oxygen is unloaded. Data for: typical mammal (Tenney, 1977); high altitude and body size (Schmidt-Nielsen, 1990); fetus, temperature, and pH (Comroe, 1975).

about 40 mmHg (5.3 kPa). Figure 14.1 shows that, in a typical mammal (the bold curve), the oxygen saturation at a P_{O_2} of 40 mmHg has decreased on average to about 70%. Thus the capillary blood has unloaded about 26% of its oxygen into the tissues. The steepness of the curve in its middle segment enables the blood to release large volumes of oxygen in response to only relatively small reductions in P_{O_2}.

Although the blood flow to the tissues delivers, on average, about 26% of its oxygen, a far greater proportion is unloaded in skeletal muscle during exercise, and in cardiac muscle.

The various organs differ greatly in the extent to which their capillaries unload oxygen (Tenney, 1977, p. 186). Even when the animal is at rest, the P_{O_2} of the blood in the venous capillaries in the **myocardium** (Section 18.6) decreases to about 23 mmHg (3.1 kPa) (Comroe, 1975, p. 200); this would lower the oxygen saturation to about 30% (bold curve in Fig. 14.1), thus unloading about 68% of its oxygen (Guyton, 1986, p. 296).

In **skeletal musculature** during **heavy exercise** (Guyton, 1986, p. 497), the P_{O_2} of the interstitial tissue, and hence also of the blood in the venous capillaries, falls to about 15 mmHg (2.0 kPa); this would decrease the oxygen saturation to about 15% (bold curve in Fig. 14.1), so that the blood now unloads about 84% of its oxygen. Since 100 ml of arterial blood contain about 19 ml of oxygen, each packet of 100 ml delivers 84% of 19 ml of oxygen, i.e. about 16 ml, to skeletal muscle during heavy exercise; this volume is about three times greater than the 5 ml of oxygen conveyed to average tissues. In addition to this gain in oxygen transport, the cardiac output increases 6- to 7-fold during maximum exercise in human marathon runners. The increase in the volume of transported oxygen, multiplied by the increase in cardiac output, enables the oxygen consumption of skeletal muscle during extreme exercise to increase to a maximum of about 20 times the resting value, which is about the extreme limit for a world class endurance athlete (Guyton, 1986, p. 496).

At a P_{O_2} of about 30 mmHg (4.0 kPa), half the oxygen is unloaded. This value is known as the **half saturation pressure**, or P_{50}.

14.3.3   *Shift to the left*

In Fig. 14.1, on the left side of the dissociation curve for a typical mammal (the bold line), there are two additional curves. These two curves exhibit a shift to the left.

The curve on the extreme left occurs in the blood of mammals living in **environments with a**

relatively low oxygen concentration, i.e. a low partial pressure of oxygen. The haemoglobin of such an animal has a higher affinity for oxygen than the blood of a typical mammal; indeed, blood possessing this curve is nearly fully saturated even when the P_{O_2} is only about 55 mmHg (7.3 kPa). This is advantageous for the *uptake* of oxygen by mammals that live at **high altitude** (for example the llama) or inhabit **burrows**.

The dissociation curve of the mammalian **fetus** has a similar shift to the left (Fig. 14.1, once again the extreme left curve). Fetal blood therefore has a higher affinity for oxygen than maternal blood. This enables the fetus to acquire an adequate supply of oxygen from the maternal blood, across the placenta, even though the blood flow through the placental capillaries is much lower than the flow through the pulmonary capillaries in the postnatal mammal.

The shift to the left in mammals native to **high altitude** is a genetic characteristic, since specimens born and raised at sea level have the same high affinity to oxygen as those born and raised at high altitude (Schmidt-Nielsen, 1990, p. 76). The same shift to the left occurs in that most famous of all athletes (Section 6.1), the bar-headed goose (Fedde, 1990, p. 191). (In contrast, note the surprising shift to the **right** that occurs in people acclimatized to high altitude; see Section 14.3.4.)

The highest P_{O_2} of **fetal arterial blood**, i.e. that leaving the placenta, is only about 30 mmHg (4.0 kPa) (Comroe, 1975, p. 246). To achieve adequate oxygen transport under such impoverished oxygen conditions, the fetus adopts various strategies. (1) Its haemoglobin has a higher affinity for oxygen than does maternal blood. This higher affinity is due partly to a slight difference in fetal haemoglobin, and partly to a difference in organic phosphate within the red cells (Schmidt-Nielsen, 1990, p. 74). Postnatally, fetal haemoglobin is gradually replaced by adult haemoglobin. (2) The fetus has about 20% more erythrocytes per unit volume of blood than an adult (Comroe, 1975, p. 246). (3) The fetus has about 33% more haemoglobin per unit volume of blood than the postnatal mammal; i.e. there are about 20 g of haemoglobin in 100 ml of fetal blood (Comroe, 1975, p. 246), and 15 g in 100 ml of adult blood (Guyton, 1986, p. 497). (4) A rise in the pH of fetal blood (to 7.6 in Fig. 14.1) shifts the dissociation curve to the left, thus increasing its affinity for oxygen. Such a change to an alkaline pH in the fetal blood seems surprising, since the fetal blood in general is loaded with large quantities of CO_2. However, on reaching the placenta (Guyton, 1986, p. 986) much of this CO_2 diffuses into the maternal blood, making the fetal blood more alkaline and the maternal blood more acidic. The shift in the dissociation curve in response to

a change in the pH of the blood is an example of the **Bohr effect**. In this instance, in response to an increase in pH, the Bohr effect shifts the curve to the left, increasing the fetal affinity for oxygen: the Bohr effect works in the opposite direction in the mother, decreasing the affinity to oxygen and thus unloading oxygen from mother to fetus (Guyton, 1986, p. 986).

Figure 14.1 also shows that the blood of **large mammals** (the broken line on the immediate left of the typical mammal) has a shift to the left, i.e. it has a relatively great affinity to oxygen. Large mammals such as a horse have a lower oxygen consumption per unit body mass than very small mammals like a mouse; in principle, the oxygen consumption in mammals decreases consistently as the body mass increases. The greater affinity to oxygen of the blood in large mammals promotes economy in the unloading of oxygen into their tissues. (The oxygen consumption per unit body mass is commonly known as the 'mass-specific oxygen consumption'; see Section 6.26 for use of the term mass-specific.)

It used to be thought that **small mammals** have a higher metabolic rate than large mammals because small mammals have a larger surface area per unit body mass and therefore lose heat faster than larger mammals; to keep warm, they would have to generate metabolic heat at a rate corresponding to their heat loss. However, it turns out that invertebrates, and even some plants, show the same relationship as mammals between body mass and metabolic rate (i.e. smaller mass is associated with higher metabolic rate), and yet temperature regulation is not a problem for these organisms. The explanation of the relationship between body mass and metabolic rate remains uncertain (Schmidt-Nielsen, 1990, p. 197).

What oxygen strategy (Schmidt-Nielsen, 1990, pp. 77, 192) would be predicted for **diving mammals**? Would it be advantageous for the average diving mammal to have a relatively high affinity for oxygen, i.e. a shift to the left in its oxygen dissociation curve? A high affinity would, however, have the drawback of hindering the unloading of oxygen in the tissues during diving, especially in the heart and brain. Moreover the uptake of oxygen in these animals occurs as in terrestrial mammals, i.e. in atmospheric air when the animal surfaces. Consequently there is no advantage in shifting the dissociation curve to either the right or the left in average divers. On the other hand, the largest diving mammals such as the gigantic whales with their immense body mass, gain from their low mass-specific oxygen consumption and the accompanying shift to the left of the oxygen dissociation curve that characterizes large mammals in general (Fig. 14.1). These features enable huge whales to stay submerged for about 2 hours.

14.3.4 *Shift to the right*

On the right side of the dissociation curve for a typical mammal in Fig. 14.1, there are three more curves, all of them typifying a shift to the right, and all of them promoting the unloading of oxygen in the tissues. In other words, a shift to the right means that oxygen becomes less strongly bound to haemoglobin.

The curve on the extreme right of Fig. 14.1 shows the effect of an **increase in blood temperature** to about 43°C. This promotes the unloading of oxygen in active tissues, and especially skeletal muscle during exercise, in response to local heating. You can remind yourself of this mechanism by looking in a mirror on a cold day; your nose goes red (not blue), because the affinity for oxygen is increased by low temperature.

Another of the curves to the right in Fig. 14.1 arises from a **fall in the pH of the blood** to 7.2, caused by an increase in carbon dioxide or lactic acid in the blood plasma. This again favours the unloading of oxygen in active tissues, especially skeletal muscle (Section 22.16.3).

The broken line on the right of Fig. 14.1 illustrates the shift to the right of the dissociation curve in a **small mammal** such as a mouse. Mammals with a small body mass have a relatively high metabolic rate (see also Section 14.3.3). The shift to the right promotes the release of oxygen in their tissues.

> In active skeletal muscle, the **temperature of the blood** rises several degrees, favouring unloading of oxygen (Weibel, 1984, p. 151). In the lungs the temperature of the blood returns to normal, thus restoring the affinity to oxygen.
>
> The shift to the right caused by a decrease in the blood pH is an example of the **Bohr effect**. The Bohr effect can work both ways, since a rise in pH causes a shift to the left (see Section 14.3.3).
>
> Although mammals native to a high altitude habitat have an oxygen dissociation curve with a shift to the left, giving an increased affinity for oxygen (Section 14.3.3), people **acclimatized to high altitude** show a shift to the right. At first sight this appears to be an adverse adaptation, but it has the advantage of aiding the unloading of oxygen in the tissues (Schmidt-Nielsen, 1990, p. 76). The shift to the right develops within a few hours of exposure, due to formation inside the red cells of increased quantities of phosphate compounds, some of which combine with the haemoglobin and thus decrease its affinity for oxygen. Acclimatization includes several other strategies (Guyton, 1986, p. 530): an immediate increase in pulmonary ventilation, which then increases plasma pH by blowing off large volumes of CO_2; a slow increase in haematocrit and blood volume; and increased diffusing

capacity for oxygen in the lungs, due to various factors including recruitment of pulmonary capillaries and increased pulmonary arterial pressure.

14.3.5   *Myoglobin*

Myoglobin is a form of haemoglobin, but does not enter the circulation. It is confined to muscle cells, where it is principally responsible for the dark red colour of red skeletal muscle fibres as opposed to the pallor of white skeletal muscle fibres. **Red skeletal muscle fibres** contract relatively slowly, but generate vigorous and sustained activity: **white skeletal muscle fibres** have a lower content of myoglobin, and offer faster but less durable contraction, mainly from anaerobic glycolysis.

Like blood haemoglobin, myoglobin is almost 100% saturated with oxygen at a P_{O_2} of 100 mmHg (13.3 kPa). But it has a much greater affinity for oxygen than blood haemoglobin. Thus it remains nearly 90% saturated with oxygen even when the P_{O_2} has fallen as low as about 20 mmHg (2.7 kPa). However, between 20 and 0 mmHg it unloads *all* its remaining 80% of oxygen. In skeletal muscle, during severe exercise, the P_{O_2} in the interstitial tissue may fall as low as 15 mmHg (2.0 kPa) (Section 14.3.2). Thus, at low oxygen concentrations of about 20 mmHg (2.7 kPa) downwards, myoglobin may serve as a reserve source of oxygen in contracting skeletal muscle, able to even out fluctuations in the oxygen supply.

For **transport of carbon dioxide** see Section 11.11.1.

14.4   Filtration and reabsorption across the capillary wall

Filtration across the capillary wall takes place mainly through the intercellular clefts (Section 12.12.3).

Filtration depends on a balance between hydrostatic and osmotic forces, according to the **Starling hypothesis** of fluid exchange across capillary walls. The blood plasma in a capillary is under **hydrostatic pressure**, derived from arterial pressure. The interstitial fluid has hydrostatic pressure too, but at a much lower level than that of the plasma. Therefore the effect of hydrostatic pressure is to drive water and solutes out of the plasma and into the interstitial fluid.

The blood plasma also has **osmotic pressure**. This is because the colloidal proteins in the blood plasma do not pass readily through the capillary wall. The osmotic pressure is due only to the plasma proteins, i.e. it is the colloid osmotic pressure and is generally known as the **oncotic pressure**; it is assumed that the smaller molecules in the blood plasma diffuse readily and exert no oncotic pressure in the capillary. The interstitial fluid, too, has oncotic pressure, because some proteins do enter it from the blood plasma. However, the amount of protein in the interstitial fluid is much smaller than that in the plasma; consequently the oncotic pressure of the blood plasma is far higher than that of the interstitial fluid. Therefore the effect of oncotic pressure is to pull water and solutes *back* into the capillary.

The exact values of the hydrostatic and oncotic forces that determine filtration inwards or outwards across the capillary wall are disputed, but the following approximations indicate in principle which way the transport is going. Essentially, all these forces vary only slightly, except one (the hydrostatic pressure in the plasma). Thus the **oncotic pressure in the blood plasma** is about 25 mmHg (3.3 kPa) at both the arterial and the venous end of the capillary. The **hydrostatic pressure and oncotic pressure of the interstitial fluid** are consistently far lower, respectively, than the hydrostatic and oncotic pressures of the blood plasma, the hydrostatic pressure being supposedly about 1–3 mmHg (0.1–0.4 kPa) and the oncotic pressure about 6 mmHg (0.8 kPa) (but these values have recently been challenged, see the advanced text below).

The only substantially variable factor is the **hydrostatic pressure in the capillary**. At the **arterial end of the capillary**, the hydrostatic pressure of the plasma is about 32 mmHg (4.3 kPa); therefore at the **arterial end** of the capillary the hydrostatic pressure of the plasma exceeds the oncotic pressure of the plasma by about 7 mmHg (0.9 kPa) (the **filtration pressure**), so filtration occurs. At the **venous end** of the capillary, the hydrostatic pressure of the plasma has fallen to about 15 mmHg (2.0 kPa) but the oncotic pressure of the plasma remains near 25 mmHg (3.3 kPa); thus the oncotic pressure of the plasma at the venous end

of the capillary exceeds the hydrostatic pressure of the plasma by about 10 mmHg (1.3 kPa) (**the reabsorption pressure**), and reabsorption occurs.

The filtration volume from the arterial end of the capillary is normally almost equalled by the reabsorption volume at the venous end of the capillary. Nevertheless, the forces are not quite balanced, and there is *slightly more filtration than reabsorption*. The small excess of filtration volume (which is known as the **net filtration**) is balanced by the return of fluid to the blood plasma through **lymphatic drainage**. About 90% of the filtrate from the arterial end of the capillaries is returned to the plasma by reabsorption at the venous end of the capillaries. The lymphatics return the remaining 10% of the filtrate (Section 14.7.1).

Osmotic pressure is determined by the number of molecules dissolved in a fluid, rather than by their weight. The plasma proteins include albumin, globulins, and fibrinogen. The molecular weight of **albumin** is much less than that of the other two proteins, and the concentration of albumin in grams per cent is considerably greater. Consequently about three quarters of the total colloid osmotic pressure of plasma arises from the albumin fraction (Guyton, 1986, p. 357).

The concept that **filtration** and **reabsorption** across the capillary are in *near-equilibrium* was suggested at the end of the nineteenth century by E.H. Starling – hence, the **Starling hypothesis**. In principle it still holds good today, but three of the four parameters of the equation on which the balance depends are either not accurately known or disputed (Diana and Fleming, 1979). It is impossible to measure (i) **capillary hydrostatic pressure** and (ii) **interstitial hydrostatic pressure** under absolutely reliable conditions (Guyton, 1986, pp. 353, 354); (iii) the **oncotic pressure of the interstitial fluid** is usually assigned a value of about 6 mmHg (0.8 kPa), but its accuracy is uncertain because of the difficulty in withdrawing samples under normal conditions (Wiederhielm, 1974, p. 135). Estimates of the mean **hydrostatic pressure** in the **venous end of the capillary** vary from 15 mmHg (2.0 kPa) (Wiederhielm, 1974, p. 138) to 10 mmHg (1.3 kPa) (Guyton, 1986, p. 354). Moreover the estimated values for the **interstitial hydrostatic pressure** are particularly controversial.

The classical view is that the (subcutaneous) **interstitial hydrostatic pressure** is slightly positive, being usually between 1 and 3 mmHg (0.1 and 0.4 kPa), but not more than 6.5 mmHg (0.87 kPa), above atmospheric pressure (Catchpole, 1966, p. 626). This value is approximately equal to the interstitial oncotic pressure. Therefore, since these two forces act in opposite directions across the capillary wall, they roughly cancel each other out (Wiederhielm, 1974, p. 136). Recently, however, experiments with porous plastic capsules embedded in the connective tissue have indicated (Guyton, 1986, p. 354) that the interstitial hydrostatic pressure is usually about 6 mmHg (0.8 kPa) *below* atmospheric pressure; part of the evidence for this is the ability to inject vast quantities of fluid into subcutaneous tissues by a pressure gradient of only about 1 mmHg (0.1 kPa). If the hydrostatic interstitial fluid really is *less* than atmospheric, it then **favours** filtration from the capillary instead of opposing it.

The **reabsorption pressure** is normally much lower than the filtration pressure. However, in compensation for this, *venous capillaries* are believed to be *more permeable* than arterial capillaries. They are also *more numerous* than arterial capillaries and hence the *surface area for reabsorption* is larger than that for filtration (Section 12.12) (Guyton, 1986, p. 358).

In the **pulmonary circulation** (Section 17.19) the hydrostatic pressure of the plasma is lower than the oncotic pressure of the plasma along the whole length of the alveolar capillary, and this favours *absorption along the whole length of the capillary* (Scott, 1986, p. 46). The **surface tension** of fluid on the internal surface of the alveolar wall provides an additional force, which strongly favours outward movement of water from the plasma. Normally, however, the **pulmonary surfactant** (Section 6.25) effectively counteracts this outward force. However, if there is insufficient surfactant or the surfactant is inactivated **oedema** develops in the alveoli (Section 17.19.4). Such **pulmonary oedema** can be a serious complication of prematurely-born mammals, particularly human babies and foals.

14.5   Transport across the capillary wall by pinocytosis

The pinocytotic vesicles of the endothelial cells of blood capillaries (Section 12.12.4) play only a small part in the transport of water and its small molecule solutes. However, the transport from plasma to interstitial fluid of the **macromolecules** of the **plasma proteins**, i.e. albumin, globulins, and fibrinogen, appears to be mainly carried out by this pathway across the capillary cells.

Because their mode of transport is largely restricted to micropinocytotic vesicles, the plasma proteins escape from the blood plasma much more slowly than water and its small molecule solutes. Nevertheless, there is a slow but continuous leakage of macromolecules from the plasma into the interstitial fluid. The **globulins**, in particular, **must** pass into the interstitial fluid in order to carry out their immunological function of defending the tissues against infection.

During the course of 1 day, 50% or more of the total amount of protein circulating in the blood is lost from the capillaries and returned to the bloodstream by the lymphatics. Most of the plasma protein that goes through the capillary walls is returned to the blood through the lymphatics.

The plasma proteins are responsible for the oncotic pressure of the blood plasma (about 25 mmHg; 3.3 kPa). Each unit volume of plasma contains about twice the weight of albumin as of globulin. The molecular weight of the albumin molecules is about half that of the globulin molecules. Therefore there are many more albumen molecules than globulin molecules per unit volume of plasma. Since the osmotic pressure is determined by the number of molecules rather than their weight, about 75% of the oncotic pressure of the plasma is derived from the albumin (Guyton, 1986, p. 357).

Morphological investigations, ultrastructural tracer studies, models, and physiological observations, strongly support the role of micropinocytotic vesicles in the capillary exchange of large molecular substances (Diana and Fleming, 1979).

II   LYMPHATIC DRAINAGE

14.6   Microscopic anatomy of lymphatic vessels

14.6.1   *Lymphatic capillaries*

A lymphatic capillary begins as a **blind-ending**, thin-walled tube, often with a bulb-like dilation at its end, and continues into a network of branching and anastomosing tubes. The wall is formed by a thin endothelial cell equipped with pinocytotic vesicles. There is usually no basal lamina to obstruct the uptake of fluid, and pericytes are absent. Adjacent endothelial cells overlap to form intercellular clefts as in a blood capillary (Fig. 12.5, top diagram), but the clefts are not secured by gap junctions and can therefore open more widely than those of blood capillaries. These structural characteristics help lymphatic capillaries to collect interstitial fluid.

The diameter of lymphatic capillaries is more irregular (Fig. 14.2) and larger than that of blood capillaries

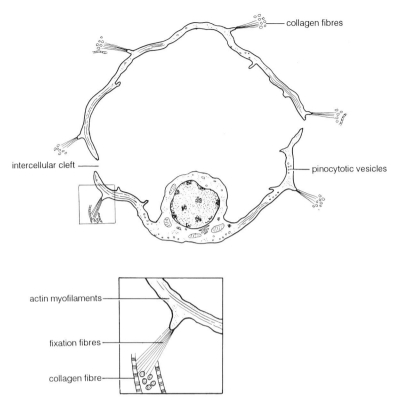

collagen fibres

intercellular cleft

pinocytotic vesicles

actin myofilaments

fixation fibres

collagen fibre

Fig. 14.2   Transverse section through a lymphatic capillary. The wall is formed by thin endothelial cells. Usually basal lamina and pericytes are absent. The ends of adjacent endothelial cells can be interlocked as in blood capillaries (Fig. 12.5, top), creating a narrow intercellular cleft, but there are no gap junctions to secure the cleft. In this lymphatic capillary, the two intercellular clefts have been opened by tension in the surrounding connective tissue, for example in oedema, causing the fixation fibres to pull the endothelial cells apart. The endothelial cells can also be pulled apart by contraction of their actin myofilaments. The widening of the clefts promotes the uptake of interstitial fluid. The diameter of this capillary is about 20 μm.

(Williams *et al.*, 1989, p. 821), ranging from about 10 to 50 μm (Krstic, 1984, p. 236). The endothelial cells that line them have an average thickness of about 3 μm (Rhodin, 1974, p. 372).

When seen in a longitudinal section, the overlapping edge of one endothelial cell over another (as in the blood capillary in Fig. 12.5) projects flexibly into the lumen like a flap, in the direction of flow of the lymph stream; reversal of flow is believed to catch the edge of the flap, which then behaves as a tiny **valve** and prevents regurgitation (Guyton, 1986, p. 361). **Actin myofilaments** run circumferentially in the cytoplasm (Fig. 14.2), and when contracted are believed to cause the endothelial cells to separate from each other and thus open the intercellular cleft, hence augmenting the uptake of interstitial fluid (Krstic, 1984, p. 237). **Fixation fibres** (fibrae fixationes; NH, 1983) (strands of fine fibrils) radiate from the external surface of the endothelial cell and tether it like guy ropes to collagen fibrils in the surrounding connective

tissue (Fig. 14.2); distension of the interstitial tissue causes these guy ropes to pull the endothelial cells away from each other, thus promoting the uptake of lymph (Guyton, 1986, p. 361). Occasional **gap junctions** may obstruct the clefts, but these only occur in a few tissues (Rhodin, 1974, p. 372). **Fenestrations** have been reported in subserous lymphatics.

In the **lacteals** of intestinal villi (so-called because of their milk-white appearance due to the absorption of fat droplets) the intercellular clefts are so wide as to be referred to as 'apertures' (Krstic, 1984, p. 237). The lymphatic capillaries in the lung also are reported to have particularly wide gaps between the endothelial cells (Section 7.8.3).

Lymphatic capillaries are absent from the alveolar walls of the lungs (Section 7.8), the central nervous system, bone marrow, avascular tissues such as the cornea, articular cartilage, and nails (Williams *et al.*, 1989, p. 821), and the intralobular parenchyma of the liver

(Krstic, 1984, p. 236). On the other hand, lymphatic vessels and lymphatic tissue are said to be particularly abundant in tissues that are especially exposed to the external environment (Section 7.8).

In most organs (Schmid-Schönbein and Zweifach, 1994), including the intestinal wall, skeletal muscle, skin, heart, and kidney, the **lymphatic capillaries** are confined *within* the parenchyma proper: the **collecting lymphatics** lie *outside* the parenchyma. This seems to be the best available criterion for distinguishing lymphatic capillaries from collecting lymphatics. The capillaries in the parenchyma form a profuse anastomosing network with few valves (intestinal mucosa and submucosa) or no valves (skeletal muscle), allowing unrestricted flow in all directions. The lymphatic capillary networks in the **intestinal mucosa and submucosa** drain via **small collecting vessels** into **large collecting vessels** at the **mesenteric border**. It is here that **smooth muscle** and true **valves** first appear in intestinal lymphatics, and lymphatic contractions can be regularly observed at this site. In their further passage within the mesentery, the intestinal collecting lymphatics rely entirely on their smooth muscle for propulsion of lymph.

In **skeletal muscle** the majority of **lymphatic capillaries** are closely paired with arterioles. They penetrate along the transverse side branches of the arterioles, but do not reach the blood capillaries. They *lack* smooth muscle. The **collecting lymphatics** lie in the **perimysium**, i.e. outside the muscle parenchyma. In some species these lymphatics have smooth muscle, but in other species all **prenodal collecting lymphatics** of skeletal muscle lack smooth muscle; presumably in these species the skeletal muscle pump gives good propulsion.

The review of Drake and Gabel (1995) indicates that **postnodal collecting lymphatics** typically possess smooth muscle and have valves at intervals of 5–10 mm.

14.6.2 *Lymphatic collecting vessels*

The lymphatic capillaries unite into collecting lymphatic vessels. At first these are simply **endothelial tubes** with a thin covering of fibrous tissue, but **circular smooth muscle cells** presently appear. These vessels converge on larger collecting vessels, that structurally resemble small veins, though with many more **valves**; in the tunica media there are **circular smooth muscle cells** (Fig. 14.4) that help the movement of lymph (Section 14.8). The **thoracic duct** (Section 14.34) resembles a medium-sized vein in its structure, but the smooth muscle in the media is relatively more abundant than in a vein.

The larger collecting lymphatic vessels (Williams *et al.*, 1989, p. 821) possess a tunica intima, tunica media, and tunica adventitia (Fig. 14.4). The circumferential smooth muscle cells in the media are often placed just proximal to a valve, where they have the best opportunity for driving the lymph onward. Elastic fibres form an outer elastic membrane in the media.

The numerous **valves** in lymphatic collecting vessels, as in veins (Section 12.16.2), are formed from the intima, and are semilunar and generally paired. Downstream to the attached edge of each cusp the wall of the vessel is dilated, giving the vessel a beaded appearance when distended, like a vein.

14.7   Functions of lymphatic capillaries

14.7.1 *Drainage of interstitial fluid*

The lymphatic capillaries collect interstitial fluid. As noted in Section 14.4, there is a small overall discrepancy between the outward filtration into the interstitium at the arterial end of the capillary bed, and the inward reabsorption from the interstitium at the venous end, causing more fluid to be pushed out of the blood plasma at the arterial end than returns to the plasma at the venous end. This would result in a progressive accumulation of interstitial fluid, were it not for the collection of interstitial fluid by the lymphatic capillaries. Thus the volume of the lymph that drains from a tissue is the difference between the volume of filtration from the arterial end of the blood capillaries and the volume of reabsorption into the venous end of the blood capillaries; this volume (the net filtration) amounts to about 10% of the filtrate.

Water and its small molecule solutes enter the lymphatic capillaries freely through the **intercellular clefts**. The absence of gap junctions at these clefts, coupled with the lack of a basal lamina and pericytes (Section 14.6.1), causes the interior of the lymphatic capillaries to be virtually in direct continuity with the interstitial fluid: thus lymph can be regarded as simply an extension of the interstitial fluid. Consequently the protein macromolecules which have leaked into the interstitial fluid enter the lymphatic capillaries almost completely unimpeded.

By far the most important function of lymphatics is to prevent the build-up of **protein** in the interstitial fluid. There is a slow but continuous leakage of small amounts of protein from the blood capillaries into the interstitial fluid, probably mainly by pinocytosis (Section 14.5). Only a small proportion of this protein is reabsorbed by the venous ends of the blood capillaries, and therefore protein becomes concentrated in the interstitial fluid before it is collected by the lymphatics. However, an excessive accumulation of protein would increase the oncotic pressure of the interstitial fluid and thus tend to cancel out the oncotic pressure of the plasma in the venous end of the blood capillary: this would diminish the force that causes reabsorption of interstitial fluid into the venous capillaries, and interstitial fluid everywhere would progressively increase in volume – with fatal consequences in a matter of hours.

14.7.2 *Drainage of particles and cells*

Relatively large particles such as injected dyes, bacteria, or cells, are also able to enter the lymphatic capillaries via the intercellular clefts. This pathway is of particular importance to the immunological defences of the body. Lymphocytes and macrophages patrolling the outlying tissues of the body can pick up antigens, enter a lymphatic capillary, and be filtered out in the first lymph node along the course of the lymphatic vessel. There they set up the appropriate cell-mediated or humoral immune responses (Section 14.22).

14.8 Movement of lymph

Lymph is propelled mainly by contractions of the circular **smooth muscle** cells in the walls of collecting lymphatic vessels. This is an *active* (or *intrinsic*) **pumping mechanism**. The contractions are modulated by myogenic **autoregulation**, the smooth muscle cells responding to distension by automatically increasing the force and frequency of their contractions. (Similar autoregulatory contractile responses to mechanical stimuli occur in small arteries and arterioles (Section 13.5).) The numerous valves in collecting lymphatics ensure that lymph is always driven towards the heart.

The intrinsic pumping mechanism is reinforced by two *passive* (or *extrinsic*) **pumping mecha-**

nisms. One of the these is the **muscle pump** in the limbs, which is particularly important in the return of **venous blood** from the limbs (Section 12.16.2); contraction of the muscles in the limb applies pressure to the veins and lymphatics of the limb, and thus forces venous blood and lymph towards the heart, under the guidance of the valves. The second extrinsic mechanism is **breathing**. During inspiration, the rise in intraabdominal pressure and the fall in intrathoracic pressure causes a pressure gradient towards the heart in the lymphatic system, just as it does in the venous system (Section 12.16.3).

Active pumping by the lymphatic smooth muscle is the basis for propulsion of lymph from *most tissues*. *Passive pumping* by the movements of breathing is also important in the *lung* (Section 7.8.1), especially in *pulmonary oedema* (Section 17.26.2).

The mechanisms that pump lymph have been reviewed by McHale (1995). For a long time the propulsion of lymph was believed to be a purely passive process based on the energy imparted to the blood by the heart. But this would require **filtration pressures** in the blood capillaries as high as 30 mmHg (4.0 kPa). Filtration pressure is the difference between the hydrostatic pressure of the plasma in the blood capillaries and the oncotic pressure of the plasma, and this is typically only about 7 mmHg (0.9 kPa) (Section 14.4). Such a filtration pressure does impart a **hydrostatic pressure** to the **interstitial fluid**, and this should drive fluid into the lymphatic capillaries. However, the hydrostatic pressure of the interstitial fluid (which cannot be measured reliably) may be as low as from 1 to 6 mmHg (0.1–0.8 kPa) and could even be about 6 mmHg (0.8 kPa) *below* atmospheric pressure (Section 14.4). The actual pressure in lymphatics is about 0.6 mmHg (0.08 kPa) in ducts near the terminals, but is about 40 mmHg (5.3 kPa) in the larger collecting ducts. Clearly the hydrostatic pressure of the interstitial fluid can contribute little to shifting lymph against such a steep pressure gradient.

It was then thought that the massaging effects of contractions of the limb musculature, and perhaps also of arterial pulsation, could explain the transport of lymph into the great veins at the thoracic inlet against this large uphill gradient. However, actual measurements of lymphatic flow in the limbs of quadruped mammals have failed to demonstrate substantial transport of lymph through the effects of walking.

The most important evidence on lymphatic pumping has come from **isolated segments** of lymphatic vessels. These have demonstrated that lymphatic vessels have an **active (intrinsic) mechanism** that makes these vessels into very effective pumps (Drake and Gabel, 1995). The smooth muscle in the media of collecting lymphatics undergoes peristaltic-type contractions (Schmid-Schönbein and Zweifach, 1994), spontaneous and rhythmical (McHale, 1995). These contractions operate over a wide range of flow rates. The contractions are modulated by myogenic autoregulation; the mechanical stimulus of distension causes an increase in the force and frequency of the spontaneous contractions, thus enabling the pump to overcome increased resistance through gravity or obstruction of nodes by disease.

The smooth muscle has an **adrenergic innervation**. Although the mechanism is not fully understood, stimulation of the splanchnic nerve is known to increase the pumping activity of the ducts and to induce a significant increase in lymph flow; possibly the innervation provides fine tuning (McHale, 1995). The smooth muscle also responds to a variety of humoral agents. Furthermore, as in small blood vessels (Section 13.6), the endothelium of collecting lymphatic vessels appears to release nitric oxide in response to shear stresses caused by the movement of fluid, even though the shear stresses in these vessels are relatively small (Schmid-Schönbein and Zweifach, 1994).

McHale (1995) concluded that 'it is now generally agreed that *intrinsic pumping* of the valved lymphatic vessels is the essential motor for lymph propulsion *in most tissues*' (my italics). One exception to this principle appears to be the **lung** (Drake and Gabel, 1995): active pumping has been shown to be very important in maintaining lymph flow in the *normal* lung, but passive propulsion by the intrathoracic pressure changes during breathing (Section 6.13) appears to be more important if *pulmonary oedema* has already developed.

14.9   Oedema

Oedema is an abnormal accumulation of interstitial fluid. This is caused by an excess of capillary filtration (because of increased capillary pressure or increased capillary permeability), or defective capillary reabsorption (as a result of decreased plasma protein), or a decrease in lymphatic drainage.

In the normal **ground substance** of the interstitium (Section 12.2), nearly all the water is **bound water**: in oedema, the additional water is added to the normally minute vesicles and channels of **free water**.

Localized oedema may be confined to a limited region such as the head, or one limb or even a part of a limb. **Generalized oedema** tends to be conspicuous in the pendent parts of the body, espe-

cially the lower parts of the limbs and the ventral aspect of the abdomen and thorax. **Pulmonary oedema** (oedema of the lung) is considered in Sections 17.25 and 17.26. **Pleural effusion** (oedema of the pleural cavity) is discussed in Section 17.27.

14.9.1   *Increase in capillary pressure*

An excess of filtration is caused by a sustained rise in the hydrostatic pressure of the blood in the capillary. This inevitably distorts the delicate balance between filtration and reabsorption, augmenting the predominance of filtration. Interstitial fluid then accumulates until its hydrostatic pressure increases enough to tip the balance in favour, once again, of reabsorption.

An increase in capillary pressure of the systemic vasculature occurs in **right ventricular failure** (Section 22.17), when the venous return to the right side of the heart is obstructed, as in pulmonary stenosis (Section 15.9). The right ventricle fails and the systemic veins become engorged, thus leading to systemic oedema and abdominal oedema (ascites). Likewise, in **left ventricular heart failure**, as in aortic stenosis (Section 15.10) or mitral insufficiency (Section 15.13), the drainage of the pulmonary veins into the left atrium is obstructed; the pressure in the pulmonary capillaries rises, and ('hydrostatic') pulmonary oedema forms (Section 17.25.3).

> The **central venous pressure** (the pressure in the right atrium) can be raised by a variety of *non-cardiac* intrathoracic disorders, all leading to chronic peripheral oedema. In the horse, for example, these include large cranial mediastinal masses, chronic pleural effusion, and pleural abscesses (Brown, 1989, p. 148).
>
> Large **venous blood clots** are rather common in man (and potentially dangerous, because of embolism; Section 17.9.4), particularly after major abdominal or pelvic surgery (deep vein thrombosis). By obstructing the venous flow towards the heart, they lead to oedema in the region normally drained by the obstructed vein.

14.9.2   *Increased permeability of blood capillaries*

An excess of filtration is also caused by an increase in the permeability of blood capillaries. The commonest reason for an increase in permeability is tissue injury, of mechanical, chemical, thermal, or bacterial origin. It can also result from hypoxia of the endothelium, as in haemorrhagic shock after a major haemorrhage.

The main cause of increased capillary permeability after damage to the tissues appears to be the release of **histamine** and **serotonin** from **mast cells**, in response to the injury. These substances are powerful vasodilators, acting on muscular arteries, arterioles, and metarterioles, and therefore greatly increase the blood flow in the microcirculation; hence the redness of an inflamed area. Histamine also directly increases the permeability of capillary endothelium to water and the small molecule solutes, and also to the protein macromolecules. As a result of all these changes, large quantities of fluid and of small and large molecule solutes escape from the plasma into the interstitial fluid, causing oedema and swelling. In addition, numerous polymorphs adhere to the endothelium and then work their way through the loosened intercellular clefts, particularly in the post-capillary venules. Once through the wall, the polymorphs move relatively easily through the oedematous ground substance, which is less viscous than normal tissue gel (Section 12.2).

In the lung, oedema arising by these processes is known as 'permeability' pulmonary oedema (Section 17.25.4).

> The swelling caused by the increase in the volume of interstitial fluid causes the **fixation fibres** of lymphatic capillaries (Section 14.6.1, Fig. 14.2) to actively separate the edges of the endothelial cells. This increases filtration still further. It also enables inflammatory cells (polymorphonuclear leucocytes) to escape from the blood into the inflamed tissue by **diapedesis**, especially through the wall of postcapillary venules (Section 12.14).

14.9.3 *Decreased plasma protein*

Defective capillary reabsorption occurs if the oncotic pressure of the plasma is lowered. This diminishes the reabsorption of interstitial fluid at the venous end of the capillaries, and hence causes the accumulation of interstitial fluid. The oncotic pressure falls if the protein content of the plasma is decreased. This can arise through: (a) the continual loss of protein in the urine in **chronic kidney disease**; (b) a failure to absorb protein from the gut because of a pathological change in

the intestine (**malabsorption**); (c) **starvation**; or (d) rupture of the thoracic duct (Section 14.34).

A deficiency of plasma protein leading to oedema is known as **hypoproteinaemia**, or more accurately **hypoalbuminaemia** since albumin is the main source of oncotic pressure in the plasma (Section 14.4). In principle (Blood and Studdert, 1988, pp. 324, 470; Brown, 1989, p. 147), hypoalbuminaemia is caused by either deficient synthesis or chronic loss of protein.

A major cause of **deficient synthesis of protein** is **chronic hepatic disease**. The **malabsorption syndrome**, which may be caused by a digestive defect or mucosal abnormality, is another major factor in deficient protein synthesis in both companion and food animals, since it is associated with excessive loss of nutrients in the faeces (Blood and Studdert, 1988, p. 553). The malabsorption syndrome is a major factor in the pathogenesis of parasitic and viral diarrhoeas in food animals, and the undifferentiated chronic diarrhoeas in horses. Moreover, parasites can directly consume the host's protein (Brown, 1989, p. 19).

Chronic loss of protein can arise not only from renal disease but also from chronic **protein-losing enteropathy**, which is associated with excessive loss of plasma proteins into the intestinal lumen in a variety of conditions including congestive heart failure, and gastric or intestinal ulceration (Blood and Studdert, 1988, p. 324).

14.9.4 *Decreased lymphatic drainage*

Local obstruction of lymphatic vessels reduces the drainage of interstitial fluid and leads to **local oedema** in the area drained. The oedema is made worse by the accumulation of protein macromolecules, which increases the oncotic pressure of the oedema fluid. The commonest primary cause of acute local oedema is trauma, leading to increased capillary permeability and initial oedema at the site of the injury, which compresses the outgoing lymphatics. Among other causes of local obstruction is neoplastic invasion of lymph nodes.

In horses, lack of movement when stalled is the commonest cause of swelling and oedema of the limbs (known as 'stocking-up'). It usually disappears after 20 minutes of light exercise. The probable explanation is inactivity of the **muscle pump** (Section 12.16.2), which in the active animal forces the columns of venous blood and lymph vertically through successive segments of the vessels, each segment being guarded by valves. In the immobile animal, absence of the pump decreases lymphatic (and venous) drainage, leading to accumulation of both lymph and venous blood in long vertical columns of fluid with high hydrostatic pressure, and hence to oedema.

Prolonged distension of lymphatic vessels may reach the point when the valves no longer close, i.e. they become incompetent. This allows retrograde flow.

III   LYMPHATIC TISSUES

14.10   Mononuclear phagocyte system

The concept of the mononuclear phagocyte system embraces a diffuse array of 'macrophages'. All of them are large phagocytic cells. (They are distinguished by their size from 'microphages' (Section 7.7.4), which are small phagocytic cells, notably granulocytes.)

For historical reasons, the varieties of cell in the mononuclear phagocyte system were named according to the tissues in which they were found. Thus they include the classical fixed and wandering macrophages (sometimes known as histiocytes) that are found in connective tissues more or less everywhere; they also include the macrophages in specialized sites, such as stellate macrophages (Kupffer cells) in the liver, alveolar macrophages in the lung (Section 7.7.1), microglia in the CNS, splenic macrophages, macrophages lining the lymphatic sinuses of lymph nodes (littoral cells), and dendritic mononuclear phagocytes in lymphonodules, lymph nodes, spleen, thymus, and epidermis.

These cells are characterized by: (1) origin from the bone marrow, via monocytes (Section 12.29); (2) phagocytosis and destruction of both moribund cells and invading particles such as bacteria; and (3) the ability to present antigens to, and thus immunologically activate, T-lymphocytes.

Mononuclear phagocytes ('macrophages') vary in structure according to their state of activity and the tissues they inhabit. Typically, they have an irregular surface with folds and amoeboid protrusions (Figs 6.6, 14.4), abundant rough endoplasmic reticulum, active Golgi complex, many lysosomes, and euchromatic nucleus, all of which indicate active metabolism and continual

synthesis of enzymes. The nucleus is often indented and eccentric in the cell. The splenic macrophage is regarded as a particularly avid phagocyte and destroyer, by means of the cocktail of enzymes in its lysosomes, of living and inert particles that gain entry to the body (Section 14.18.2).

Dendritic mononuclear phagocytes (dendritic cells, for short) differ from the other mononuclear phagocytes in being slender and branched, as their name implies. They are not essentially phagocytic, being capable of only a moderate uptake of particulate material. After such uptake of antigenic particles, however, they have an important function as an antigen-presenting cell, presenting the antigen to resting helper T-lymphocytes (Section 14.30). Dendritic cells occur throughout the lymphatic tissues.

Monocytes are the largest of all leucocytes (up to 20 μm). The large nucleus is kidney shaped, with a characteristic indentation on one side (Fig. 14.4). Monocytes are actively phagocytic.

Monocytes arise in the bone marrow and are released into the general circulation. They pass through the walls of capillaries and venules, penetrate the connective tissue, and establish themselves in various tissues where they become the diverse types of macrophage of the mononuclear phagocyte system.

The mononuclear phagocyte system has replaced the concept of the reticulo-endothelial system. In the *Nomina Histologica* (1994) the classical fixed and wandering macrophages (histiocytes) are now the macrophagocytus stabilis and nomadicus; the monocyte is monocytus. The stellate macrophage in the liver is macrophagocytus stellatus.

Monocytes (monocytus) form between 2 and 8% of the leucocytes. They are actively motile, with strong amoeboid movements. The large nucleus is euchromatic. The abundant cytoplasm contains a well developed Golgi apparatus and many lysosomes. Mitochondria are quite numerous, reflecting high motility. These characteristics are all similar to those of macrophages in general.

Monocytes arise initially from pluripotent haemopoietic stem cells in the bone marrow (Section 12.25), but the subsequent cellular stages in their development are unknown (Section 12.29). After several divisions of stem cells, they are released into the general circulation. Possibly they have to differentiate in order to assume their role as macrophages, but a simpler view is that monocytes are merely macrophages looking for a home;

thus a monocyte is a macrophage in the process of passing (via the blood stream) from the bone marrow where it was formed, to the peripheral tissues where it will function.

Although the cells in the mononuclear phagocyte system are capable of both phagocytosis and the presentation of antigens, they can be divided functionally into two groups (Williams *et al.*, 1989, p. 669). One group is preoccupied with *phagocytosis*, and thus the removal of micro-organisms and dead cells, with the aid of copious lysosomes; this group includes all the cells listed above, except dendritic cells. An example is the **alveolar macrophage** (Section 7.7.1). The other group, i.e. **dendritic cells**, is mainly concerned with the *presentation of antigens* to helper T-lymphocytes. To carry out their function, dendritic cells also have to be capable of taking up particulate matter, but are then largely dedicated to stimulating the immune response of resting helper **T-lymphocytes**; this they do by presenting antigens to the T-lymphocyte by means of the molecules of the **major histocompatibility complex of class II** (MHC II).

There are three types of **dendritic cell**, interdigitating (or paracortical), intraepidermal, and follicular. The **interdigitating** and **intraepidermal dendritic cells** are dedicated primarily to presenting antigens to helper T-lymphocytes and have only subsidiary powers of phagocytosis (Section 14.30.1a). Like mononuclear phagocytes in general, they are *derived* from the bone marrow via monocytes. **Follicular dendritic cells**, on the other hand, are not true antigen-presenting cells because they lack MHC II molecules (Section 14.30.1a).

Interdigitating dendritic cells (Abbas *et al.*, 1994, p. 23) are present in the interstitial tissue of most organs, but are particularly abundant in the thymus-dependent components of lymph nodes and spleen, i.e. in the paracortex of a node and the periarteriolar lymphatic sheath of the spleen. This is the reason for their alternative, and somewhat more meaningful name, '**paracortical' dendritic cell**. Interdigitating (paracortical) cells also occur in the thymus, at the corticomedullary junction (Abbas *et al.*, 1994, p. 169); here they come into contact with maturing thymocytes that have migrated from the cortex and will soon leave the thymus via blood vessels and lymphatics. Their *function* – and it is a function that is central to both humoral and cell-mediated immunity – is to *present antigen to resting helper T-lymphocytes* (Section 14.30.1a). For this purpose they use major histocompatibility molecules of class II (MHC II) (Abbas *et al.*, 1994, p. 123).

Intraepidermal dendritic cells (macrophagocytus intraepidermalis) were previously known as Langerhans cells. They are found in the epidermis, where they bind to *cutaneous antigens* and then migrate via lymphatic vessels to the thymus-dependent paracortex of a regional lymph node. Here their *function* is to *present antigen to resting helper T cells*, expressing the antigen by class II MHC molecules. They may be important in *cell-mediated immunity* to *viral infections of the skin* (Williams *et al.*, 1989, p. 77), e.g. viral fibropapillomata, *ectoparasites* such as ticks, and *epidermal tumours*. It has been suggested (Williams *et al.*, 1989, p. 669) that the interdigitating dendritic cell and intraepidermal dendritic cell may be one and the same cell seen at different points during its migration, and Abbas *et al.* (1994, p. 23) seemed to support this interpretation. These two cells have a similar origin from the bone marrow, and both of them contain the mysterious Birbeck (Langerhans) granule of unknown function.

Follicular dendritic cells occur only in the *germinal centres of lymphonodules* (Abbas *et al.*, 1994, p. 199). The term 'follicular' presumably arose because the lymphonodule had previously been known (*Nomina Anatomica*, 1977) as a 'lymphatic follicle'. These cells are present in all the standard types of lymphonodule, i.e. those in lymph nodes and the spleen, and also in submucosal lymphonodules of the intestine and tracheobronchial tree (Abbas *et al.*, 1994, p. 23). In lymph nodes they are particularly developed in the *light* zone of the germinal centre (Heinen, 1995) The *function* of follicular dendritic cells (Abbas *et al.*, 1994, p. 23) is to *bind antigens* on their surface and '*display*' them there for recognition by *resting B-lymphocytes* (Section 14.28.2).

Cells of the mononuclear phagocyte system have a third *function* in addition to phagocytosis and presentation of antigens, i.e. to **promote tissue repair**. They interact with **fibroblasts**, modulating their growth and hence controlling the deposition of collagen. In this way they make an important contribution to wound healing (Piani *et al.*, 1994).

14.11 Basic microscopic anatomy of lymphatic tissue

Lymphatic (or lymphoid) tissue occurs in various forms, including: 'free' lymphocytes and plasma cells, wandering alone in the tissues; loose accumulations of lymphocytes; lymphonodules (solitary or aggregated); lymph nodes; spleen; tonsils; and thymus.

Except for the free cells and the simplest accumulations, these lymphatic tissues share three basic structural components: (a) a network of **fixed cells** (reticular cells), suspended in (b) **reticular fibres**, with (c) **free cells**, lodged in the network. This meshwork filters out cell debris and micro-organisms, and traps antigens. The same three structural components occur in bone marrow (Section 12.26).

The **fixed cells** are **reticular cells** (reticulocytus). They form a three-dimensional sponge-like network of stellate-shaped cells, interconnected by gap junctions. The functions of the reticular cells are as follows: (1) Phagocytosis of dead cells, infective organisms, and foreign materials such as dust particles When activated to become phagocytic cells, they abandon their reticular fibres, develop pseudopodia for motility, and add to their lysosomes for dealing with ingested material. (2) Trapping antigens on their surface, and thus enabling adjacent B-lymphocytes to encounter antigens. (3) Synthesis of reticular fibres. The **reticular fibres** (fibra reticularis) (Fig. 14.4) are attached to or enclosed by reticular cells. They are generally considered to be small collagen fibres (*Nomina Histologica*, 1994, Annot. 30).

The **free cells** consist mainly of **lymphocytes**, **plasma cells**, and **macrophages**, and are 'free' to wander through the network of fixed cells.

In all of the lymphatic tissues except the thymus, both the fixed cells and the free cells are *derived* exclusively from mesenchyme. In the **thymus** (Section 14.19), only the free cells are of mesenchymal origin: the fixed cells are derived from the endodermal epithelium of the third (and possibly the fourth) pharyngeal pouch. Despite these differences in their developmental source, the fixed cells are, in fact, virtually identical in structure in the thymus and all the other lymphatic tissues, except that in the thymus the fixed cells lack supporting reticular fibres.

14.12 Lymphocytes

Lymphocytes and monocytes are **agranulocytes**, as opposed to granulocytes which are distinguished by their specific granules.

Lymphocytes are loosely classified into **B-lymphocytes** and **T-lymphocytes** according to their origins and their immunological potential, but there are no recognizable *structural* differences between these two groups. The great majority of B- and T-lymphocytes continuously recirculate between the blood, the connective tissues, and lymph. This continuous recirculation maximizes the opportunities for contact with antigens, and also for the contacts with each other that are essential for their immune activation.

Lymphocytes are also classified into **small** and **large lymphocytes**. The **small lymphocyte** forms the majority of lymphocytes in circulating blood. This really is a *small* cell, since (in the domestic mammals) it measures only about 5–10 µm in diameter, and is therefore much the same size as

an erythrocyte (about 4.1–7.5 µm). Each cell contains a densely-staining round nucleus, and a very narrow rim of cytoplasm (Fig. 14.4). The dense staining of the nucleus (caused by very condensed heterochromatin) and the sparseness of the organelles indicate a low metabolic rate. These cells are therefore considered to be in a *'resting' phase, in immunological terms*: 'resting' means *unstimulated by any antigen*. The term 'resting' may seem to suggest total inactivity, but far from doing nothing they are constantly patrolling the fluids and tissues of the body in the search for antigens.

Large lymphocytes are indeed much larger than small lymphocytes, being about three times greater in diameter (up to 25 µm in diameter). They are a mixture of *two populations*, both of which have cytological characteristics that reveal *active synthesis of proteins*, i.e. a pale-staining (euchromatic) nucleus, a large Golgi apparatus, and a basophilic cytoplasm containing many clusters of polyribosomes: These two populations of large lymphocytes (Fig. 14.3A) are either (a) *very immature cells* that are undergoing rapid cell division to form great numbers of small ('resting') lymphocytes – these are '*lymphoblasts*'; or (b) *maturing or mature cells* that have become immunologically 'active' and are undergoing rapid cell division to form B cells and T cells – these are '*immunoblasts*'.

14.12.1 *Terminology*

In the *Nomina Histologica* (1989) the small lymphocyte is lymphocytus parvus and the large lymphocyte is lymphocytus magnus. The term **lymphoblast** has been applied to *both* of the two populations of **large lymphocyte** that are described in the previous paragraph, i.e. to both immature and immunologically mature cells. Krstic (1984, p. 201) totally avoided using it for the *immature* cells; he accepted it as applicable to the *mature* cells, but for these he preferred the term *immunoblast*. Abbas *et al.* (1994, p. 20) applied the term lymphoblast to the *mature* cells only, and did not employ the term immunoblast at all. This appears to be the standard usage in immunology (e.g. see Lackie and Dow, 1989, p. 139). Williams *et al.* (1989, p. 667) confined the term lymphoblast to the *immature* cells, and avoided the term immunoblast altogether (presumably because it is not an official term in the third edition of the *Nomina Histologica*, 1989). In histology, the suffix '-blast' implies active productivity, either of cells or secretions. For

(A)

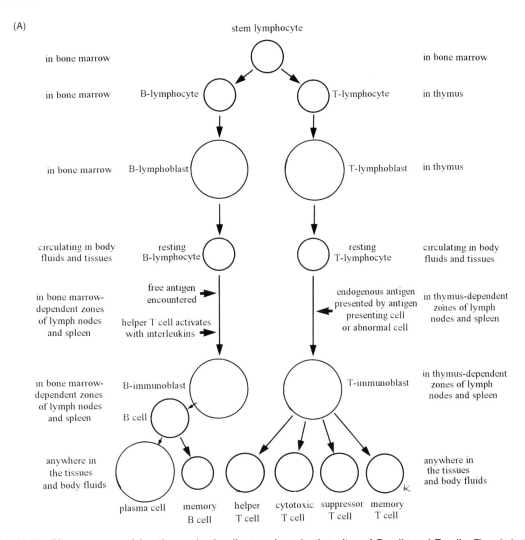

Fig. 14.3A   Diagram summarizing the production lines and production sites of B cells and T cells. The pluripotent lymphopoietic stem cells that produce both the B lineage and the T lineage originate in the bone marrow as stem lymphocytes. The B- and T-lymphoblasts are, histologically, identical large lymphocytes. Functionally, they are immature cells, actively dividing in the bone marrow (B-lymphoblasts) and in the thymus (T-lymphoblasts). They proliferate numerous small lymphocytes, which are functionally 'resting' lymphocytes in the sense that they have not been immunologically activated. After activation by contact with antigen and/or helper T cells, the resting B-lymphocytes become B-immunoblasts and the resting T-lymphocytes become T-immunoblasts. Histologically these are again identical large lymphocytes. Functionally, they are mature cells, rapidly dividing to form B cells (in the bone marrow-dependent lymphatic tissues) and T cells (in the thymus-dependent lymphatic tissues). B cells differentiate into plasma cells and memory B cells. The T cells differentiate into helper, cytotoxic, and memory, and perhaps suppressor T cells.

example, the haemocytoblast proliferates blood cells, whereas the osteoblast secretes osteoid. The term lymphoblast is therefore appropriate for a cell that is proliferating either immature or mature cells. However, to apply it to *both* of these populations of proliferating cells would mean having the same term (lymphoblast)

for two radically different groups of cells. The *Nomina Histologica* adopts lymphoblastus, but unfortunately does so without defining its relationships to immature or mature cells.

To avoid possible confusion in this book, its core material aims (1) to confine **lymphoblast** to the immature line of cells thus following Williams *et al.* (1989, p. 667), and (2) to follow Krstic (1984, p. 201) by applying **immunoblast** to the large cells that proliferate immunologically activated cells. Thus the B-immunoblast generates B cells, which differentiate into plasma cells or memory B cells: the T-immunoblast generates T cells, which differentiate into T helper, T cytotoxic, and T memory cells, and perhaps T suppressor cells. It needs to be re-emphasized, however, that most immunology textbooks seem to do without the term 'immunoblast' altogether; for example Abbas *et al.* (1994, p. 20) use the term *lymphoblast* for the large, immunologically activated, lymphocytes that proliferate B cells and T cells.

In the interests of consistency, a minor convention of **hyphenation** has been adopted. The '-blast' terms are hyphenated throughout this account, i.e. B-lymphoblast and T-lymphoblast, and B-immunoblast and T-immunoblast. Also hyphenated are the '-lymphocyte' term: hence B-lymphocyte and resting B-lymphocyte; and T-lymphocyte and resting T-lymphocyte. In contrast the final cells in the B and T lineages are not hyphenated – thus B cell, plasma cell and B memory cell; and T helper cell, T cytotoxic cell, T suppressor cell, and T memory cell. All of these hyphenated and unhyphenated terms are shown in Fig. 14.3A.

In immunology texts the term *B-lymphocyte* seems generally to be used virtually as a synonym for **B cell**, just as *T-lymphocyte* is treated as a synonym for **T cell**. Yet the reader may wonder whether *lymphocyte* and *cell* might have slightly different connotations. It appears logical to restrict the term *lymphocyte* to relatively immature cells, since the basic stem cell is undeniably a lymphocyte and certainly is not a B cell or T cell. The terms *B cell* and *T cell* (together with B memory cell, and T helper cell, T cytotoxic cell, etc.) could then logically be reserved for cells that are immunologically active (the B cells being engaged in secreting antibodies, and the T cells being occupied in cell-mediated immunity). Although this usage may not be established in the literature, an effort has been made to adopt it consistently in the core material of this book in order to help the inexperienced reader.

Many different terms are used in the immunological literature to indicated the **functional status** of cells in the immune series. For example, **immunological inactivity** is indicated by various adjectives including resting, unstimulated, inactive, uncommitted, naive, and virgin: **immunological activity** is indicated by stimulated, active, activated, committed, immunoreactive, and immunocompetent. Whilst the cognoscenti doubtless have no difficulty with these many descriptive terms, such variations may trouble readers who are new to the subject. In the core material of this book an attempt has been made to consistently use **resting** and **activated**: the resting state is arbitrarily regarded as changing into the activated state when (1) a B-lymphocyte has been converted into a

B-immunoblast by the release of interleukins from a helper T cell, and (2) a T-lymphocyte has been converted into a T-immunoblast by binding to an antigen-presenting cell. In other words, a B-lymphocyte is a 'resting' cell, and a B-immunoblast is an 'activated' cell: likewise, a T-lymphocyte is a 'resting' cell, and a T-immunoblast is an 'activated' cell.

Finally, it may be as well to note that, with one exception, all of the cells of the B-lymphocyte and T-lymphocyte lineages are **indistinguishable histologically**, except for size. In histology they are all lymphocytes, large or small, no matter what their functions may be. The single exception is the **plasma cell**, with its distinctive clock-face nucleus (Section 14.14).

14.12.2 *Developmental origins of lymphocytes*

Like all other types of blood cells, lymphocytes originate *initially* from a (primitive) **totipotent haemopoietic stem cell** (Section 12.25). Late in pregnancy this totipotent stem cell gives rise, in the bone marrow, to two types of **pluripotent stem cell**: (1) a **stem lymphocyte** (Fig. 14.3A) that produces **B-** and **T-lymphocytes**; and (2) a **haemopoietic stem cell** that gives rise to all the other lineages of blood cell (Section 12.25). In the bone marrow, the **B-lymphocyte** (Section 14.12.4) becomes a **B-lymphoblast** (Fig. 14.3A) that proliferates **resting B-lymphocytes**. In the bone marrow-dependent zones of lymph nodes and the spleen, the resting B-lymphocyte differentiates into a **B-immunoblast**, which in turn forms **B cells** (Fig. 14.3A). The **T-lymphocyte** (Section 14.12.5) leaves the bone marrow and enters the thymus, becoming a **T-lymphoblast**. There, it proliferates **resting T-lymphocytes** (thymocytes). These enter thymus-dependent zones of lymph nodes and spleen, and differentiate into **T-immunoblasts**, which then produce the various types of **T cell** (e.g. cytotoxic T cells, helper T cells; Fig. 14.3A).

14.12.3 *Circulation of lymphocytes*

Lymphocytes push their way between the endothelial cells of small blood vessels to enter the connective tissues. After percolating through a tissue they drain into lymphatic capillaries, travel into and through regional lymph nodes, and are duly returned to the blood by the thoracic duct (Section 14.34) and right lymphatic duct (Section 14.36).

Postcapillary venules (Section 12.14) in the inner cortex (i.e. the thymus-dependent zone; Fig. 14.3) of lymph nodes are the main pathway used by **resting T-lymphocytes** to enter lymph nodes from the blood stream (Abbas *et al.*, 1994, pp. 226–229). Because of their exceptionally tall endothelial cells, the postcapillary venules of the inner cortex are known by immunologists as 'high endothelial venules'. Similar venules occur in the lymphonodules associated with mucous membranes, including those of the intestine (Peyer's patches), though not in those of the spleen. The main factor enabling lymphocytes to penetrate these venules is their ability to stick to the endothelium. Lymphocytes going through other parts of the microcirculation normally bounce off the endothelium in a fraction of a second, but when resting T-lymphocytes travel along these particular venules they adhere for several seconds and this evidently gives them just enough time to get their toe in the door between the endothelial cells. The actual attachment is mediated by specific surface proteins.

If resting T-lymphocytes encounter specific antigen in a lymph node they remain there, but otherwise they exit via the efferent lymphatics of the node. Adhesion molecules attract T cells (e.g. cytotoxic T cells, helper T cells) to leave the microcirculation at **sites of inflammation** in the tissues (Abbas *et al.*, 1994, p. 229).

Relatively little is known about the **recirculation and homing of B-lymphocytes** (Abbas *et al.*, 1994, p. 229) However, most of the lymphocytes that home on the aggregated lymphonodules of the intestinal mucosa (Peyer's patches) appear to be B-lymphocytes. Although it is known that large numbers of lymphocytes work their way through the bronchial epithelium to reach the airway, where they can be recovered by bronchial lavage (Section 7.9.3), the mechanisms controlling the homing of lymphocytes to the respiratory mucosa are apparently a major gap in current knowledge; so also is the homing of lymphocytes to the spleen (Abbas *et al.*, 1994, p. 229).

The continual circulation and recirculation of lymphocytes enables them to find and bind to antigens, and this is of critical importance in the immune defences of the body against pathogenic micro-organisms (such as bacteria or parasites) and abnormal host cells (cancerous, or virus invaded).

14.12.4 *B-lymphocytes*

'Resting' B-lymphocytes ('resting' in the immunological sense) are released from the bone marrow. They then wander via the circulation into the connective tissues as free cells (Fig. 14.3A); many enter the general lymphatic tissue, finding their way into solitary and aggregated lymphonodules, and into the lymphonodules of lymph nodes and the spleen.

Since these cells have come directly from the bone marrow, the regions of the lymphatic tissues in which they settle are known as **bone marrow-dependent zones** (Sections 14.17, 14.18.1). Thus the main bone marrow-dependent zone of a lymph node is the **lymphonodule**. Likewise in the spleen the **splenic nodule** is bone marrow-dependent.

In order to make its contribution to the immune defences of the body, the resting B-lymphocyte must now progress through the following four stages (considered in more detail in Section 14.28), generally in a bone marrow-dependent zone in a lymph node or the spleen: (1) The resting B-lymphocyte binds to its antigen, and thus becomes *antigenically stimulated*. (2) The now antigenically stimulated B-lymphocyte is then *activated* by a T helper cell, and so becomes a **B-immunoblast**. (3) The B-immunoblast divides rapidly, forming large numbers of **B cells**. (4) Most of the B cells differentiate into **plasma cells** (Section 14.14), and the remainder differentiate into **memory B cells** (Fig. 14.3A). The plasma cells produce antibodies against the antigen that stimulated the B-lymphocyte in the first place. Memory B cells are very long-lived. Eventually they may rapidly multiply and pump out IgG in response to the same antigen, even after a period of years. Memory B cells form the clinical basis of **active immunization**.

This account of the four stages in the activation of a B-lymphocyte omits one vital trick that the cell has up its sleeve. How can the B-lymphocyte *find* the particular antigen that simulates it in stage 1? The answer is that, during its development from its stem cell, the resting B-lymphocyte forms an enormous number of molecules of antibody which are inserted by their tails (Fc component; Section 14.26) all over the plasmalemma. There the molecules wait with their mouths open, so to speak, ready to bind with the right antigen at any instant during the relentless patrol of the lymphocyte through the body fluids and tissues.

The principal antibody produced by this mechanism is **immunoglobulin G** (IgG), which is the main antibody *circulating* in the blood plasma (Section 14.28). The **lymph nodes** are the principal site of the formation of plasma cells and their IgG. Within the node, the rapid division of the B-immunoblasts that forms the very numerous B cells occurs in **germinal centre** of the (secondary) lymphonodule.

Another series of B-immunoblasts forms B cells that differentiate into plasma cells that produce **immunoglobin A** (IgA). This class of antibody defends all the *mucosal surfaces* of the body (Section 7.13).

It is believed that, after being formed in the bone marrow, the *stem cells* of B-lymphocytes must migrate to a special component of the lymphatic tissues known as the **'bursal' analogue** (Krstic, 1984, p. 45). This tissue, and no other, is somehow able to *induce* the differentiation of the stem cells into B-lymphocytes (Krstic, 1984, p. 58). Once that has happened, the B-lymphocytes can wander into any other component of the lymphatic tissues and proceed with the ultimate differentiation into B-immunoblasts and plasma cells. The B-immunoblast can divide once in about every 6–12 hours, enabling a single cell to produce nearly 5000 daughter cells in 5 days (Abbas *et al.*, 1994, p. 199).

The bursal analogue of mammals may be equivalent to the **cloacal bursa** (bursa of Fabricius) in birds. The cloacal bursa (a diverticulum of the cloaca) is known to be the site in birds where the differentiation of B-lymphocytes from the bone marrow is induced. The 'B' of B-lymphocyte refers strictly to the 'b' of bursa, but the bursal analogue in mammals has not been firmly identified. Some believe (Krstic, 1984, p. 58) that solitary and aggregated lymphonodules in the small intestine (Peyer's patches) can partly undertake this role in mammals, and this is consistent with a *gut* site in both birds and mammals; others conclude (Williams *et al.*, 1989, p. 671) that the bone marrow itself is the site of B-lymphocyte differentiation – in which case, although it may be nice to contemplate birds, there is no need to drag them into this particular problem since the 'B' of B-lymphocyte may perfectly well stand for the 'b' of bone marrow.

The **bone marrow-dependent zone** (Krstic, 1984, pp. 108, 238) of a **lymph node** is the whole of the **outer cortex**, i.e. the lymphonodules plus the diffuse lymphatic tissue between the nodules, and also the **medullary cords** (Fig. 14.3B). The **bone marrow-dependent zone** of the **spleen** (Krstic, 1984, p. 389) is formed by the splenic nodules (especially the mantle but also the germinal centre), and the **marginal zone** of the **white pulp** (Fig. 14.5).

The total number of **antibody molecules** that project from the surface of a resting B-lymphocyte is estimated at about 150 000 (Krstic, 1984, p. 45). The antibody is of the IgM type, and can form complexes with appropriate antigens.

14.12.5   *T-lymphocytes*

The small lymphocytes that are destined to form the T lineage leave the bone marrow as **T-lymphocytes**, enter the general circulation, and migrate to, and colonize, the **thymus**. There, as **T-lymphoblasts** (alias thymocytes), they proliferate **resting T-lymphocytes** (Fig. 14.3A). Resting T-lymphocytes ('resting' in the immunological sense) begin the process of differentiation, acquiring the *potential* to become one or other of the various classes of T cell (i.e. helper, cytotoxic, or memory T cells, or perhaps suppressor T cell) (Section 14.19.5). These processes are especially active during the perinatal phase of the animal's life, so that thymectomy at this stage leads to a progressively fatal inability to mount an effective immune response. The **resting T-lymphocytes** thus formed in the thymus re-enter the circulation, and migrate to the **thymus-dependent zones** of the lymph nodes and spleen (the sites of these zones are summarized in Figs 14.3B and 14.5, in Sections 14.17, 14.18.1, and also in the advanced text immediately below). The cells of the T lineage are probably not activated into fully immunocompetent T cells until they take up residence in these thymus-dependent zones (Section 14.19.5).

The resting T-lymphocytes that have now taken up residence in the thymus-dependent zones of the lymph nodes and spleen, are 'blind' to the antigens that ultimately *activate* them. The antigen has to be 'presented' to them by an *accessory cell*, known as an **antigen-presenting cell (APC)** (Section 14.30). Resting T-lymphocytes with the potential to become helper T cells require a *specialized* antigen-presenting cell, often a macrophage, especially a B cell, and even more particularly a dendritic mononuclear phagocyte (dendritic cell). Cytotoxic T-lymphocytes also require an antigen-presenting cell, but almost any cell in the body can perform this function.

Once the antigen has thus been 'presented' to the resting T-lymphocyte, the T-lymphocyte is *activated*. The resting T-lymphocyte now becomes a **T-immunoblast** (Fig. 14.3A). The T-immunoblast proliferates large numbers of T cells, differentiating into one or other of the three (or four) functional types of T cell, i.e. **helper**, **cytotoxic**, and **memory** (or perhaps a **suppressor**) T cell.

Suppressor T cells have been regarded as a distinct class of T cell, but this is now controversial (Section 14.30.4).

The activation of T-lymphocytes by antigen-presenting cells probably happens mainly in the thymus-dependent zones of the lymphatic tissues. The **thymus-dependent zones** (Krstic, 1984, p. 238) of the lymphatic tissues are: (a) the inner cortex (paracortex) of lymph nodes (Section 14.17; Fig. 14.3B); (b) the periarteriolar lymphatic sheath of the spleen, but excluding the marginal zone (Section 14.18.1; Fig. 14.5); and (c) the internodular regions of the aggregated lymphonodules of the intestine (Peyer's patches). Small numbers of T-lymphocytes are also present in the germinal centres in lymph nodes (Krstic, 1984, p. 169), where they are essential for the activation of B-lymphocytes (which happens in the germinal centre).

14.13 Lymphoblasts and immunoblasts

As noted in Section 14.12.1, large lymphocytes include two very different types of cell – *immature* cells that are rapidly producing small ('resting') lymphocytes, and *mature* cells that are differentiating into immunologically active B cells and T cells. The large lymphocyte that produces the *immature* line of resting lymphocytes is a **lymphoblast**: the large lymphocyte that produces the *mature* line of immunologically active cells is an **immunoblast** (Fig. 14.3A). Although so different functionally, these two types of '-blast' cells are structurally indistinguishable. Each is a large mononuclear cell with the cytological features of a highly productive cell (Section 14.12).

Lymphoblasts are divided into B-lymphoblasts producing B-lymphocytes; and T-lymphoblasts producing T-lymphocytes. B-Lymphoblasts and T-lymphoblasts are structurally identical. Their *production sites* are the bone marrow for B-lymphoblasts, and the thymus for T-lymphoblasts (Fig. 14.3A).

Immunoblasts are divided into **B-immunoblasts**, producing B cells and thence plasma cells and B memory cells (Section 14.28), and **T-immunoblasts**, producing T cells and thence helper, cytotoxic, and memory T cells, and possibly suppressor T cells (Section 14.30). B-immunoblasts and T-immunoblasts are morphologically indistinguishable. Only one cell in these series of cells is histologically distinctive, and that is the plasma cell (Section 14.14).

The *production site* of the B-immunoblasts is in lymphonodules, lymph nodes, and the spleen (strictly, in the bone marrow-dependent zones of these tissues, see Sections 14.17 and 14.18.1). The *production site* of the T-immunoblasts is initially in the thymus, and then in the lymph nodes and

spleen (strictly, in the thymus-dependent zones of these tissues, see Sections 14.17 and 14.18.1).

14.14 Plasma cells

The **plasma cell** is a large cell, about the same size as the monocyte, lymphoblast, and immunoblast (about 20 μm in diameter). A *distinctive histological feature* of this ovoid, basophilic, nongranulated cell is its circular eccentric *nucleus with a 'clock-face' appearance* (Fig. 14.4), caused by radially arranged clumps of dense heterochromatin; sharp-eyed students will see this in the practical laboratory. Another characteristic feature is the huge extent of the rough endoplasmic reticulum, with concentric dilated cisternae (gorged with immunoglobulin).

Plasma cells are *found* in connective tissue everywhere, and in lymph nodes, lymphonodules, and the spleen.

The main *production site* of plasma cells (and the immunoglobulins that they form) is in the germinal centres of the lymphonodules in lymph nodes (Section 14.16). As described in Section 14.12.4, the plasma cell develops through the following cellular sequence: resting B-lymphocyte, B-immunoblast, B cell, and differentiation of B cell into plasma cell (Fig. 14.3A).

Plasma cells are particularly plentiful in sites that are especially vulnerable to penetration by bacteria or foreign proteins and consequently need immediate defence by antibodies, notably the mucous membranes of the body. In these sites they form the **common mucosal immune system** (Section 14.29.2). They are very numerous in the lamina propria of the **tracheobronchial mucosa** (Section 7.9.3) and **intestinal mucosa**. Here, they provide a powerful local defence by synthesizing **immunoglobulin A**. This is released directly into the local tissues. It is transported across the mucous membrane to lie on the *luminal surface*, where it blocks the absorption of microbial toxins and inhibits the adherence of micro-organisms to the epithelium. It thus provides the main immunological defence of the tracheobronchial and intestinal mucosa (Section 7.13). The system is seen in action in mucous membranes, or indeed in any other tissue, where bacteria or foreign proteins have succeeded in gaining access: the resulting inflammation is signalled by the presence of large numbers of plasma cells.

> Plasma cells (plasmacytus) are constant attributes of normal connective tissue, and are formed there by incoming B-immunoblasts (Krstic, 1984, p. 336). However, the lymphonodules of lymph nodes (strictly, *secondary lymphonodules*) are the most important production sites of both plasma cells and IgG (Section 14.28) (Krstic, 1984, p. 237). Plasma cells are also formed in solitary and aggregated lymphonodules, and in the nodules of the **spleen**. In **lymph nodes**, they are present in the germinal centres of the secondary lymphonodules, but only in small numbers, since as soon as they are formed they migrate from the germinal centres into the medullary cords of lymph nodes, where they are numerous (Krstic, 1984, p. 249). In the spleen (Krstic, 1984, p. 389) the germinal centres contain differentiating B-immunoblasts, and therefore include some plasma cells. In all these sites, plasma cells synthesize and release **immunoglobulin G**, which is the principal circulating antibody in the blood plasma (Section 14.28).
>
> Plasma cells defend all the **mucous surfaces** of the body, including not only the intestinal tract and tracheobronchial tree but also the urogenital organs and mammary gland, by the *local* secretion of **IgA** (Section 14.29). Plasma cells and IgA are the basis of the **common mucosal immune system** (Section 14.29.2). Although the plasma cells eventually produce IgA, initially they form IgM; later, isotype switching occurs (Section 14.27.3), thus committing them to IgA.

14.15 Lymphonodule

Individual lymphocytes ('free' lymphocytes), and **diffuse accumulations** of lymphocytes, are scattered along the walls of the alimentary, respiratory, and urogenital tracts, just below the luminal epithelium in the lamina propria of the mucous membrane. Being severely exposed to the external environment, these epithelial surfaces are particularly heavily protected by local lymphatic tissue.

Diffuse accumulations are the simplest expression of lymphatic tissue. The **lymphonodule** is a more organized form of lymphatic tissue. A lymphonodule differs from a diffuse accumulation of lymphocytes by being a compact spherical structure. In its immature form it is a **primary lymphonodule** (lymphonodulus primarius), consisting of small lymphocytes that are uniformly

and densely distributed throughout the characteristic three-dimensional framework of **reticular cells** and **reticular fibres** (Section 14.11). In response to antigenic stimuli, the nodule develops a **germinal centre** (Fig. 14.3B), and is now a **secondary lymphonodule** (lymphonodulus secundarius). The pale germinal centre is surrounded by a dense accumulation of small lymphocytes, the **mantle** (corona) (Fig. 14.3B).

A **solitary lymphonodule** is a single isolated lymphonodule. An **aggregated (multiple) lymphonodule** consists of a cluster of many lymphonodules. Solitary and aggregated lymphonodules are found in the lamina propria of mucous membranes, especially in the alimentary, respiratory, and urogenital systems. Subepithelial aggregated lymphonodules are just visible to the naked eye as white spots on the conjunctiva, on the mucosa of the natural orifices during the clinical examination of a live animal, or on visceral mucosal surfaces at post-mortem or meat inspection. In the small intestine many such nodules (200–400) may be grouped together as a **Peyer's patch**), and are then clearly visible.

The abundant diffuse lymphatic accumulations, and solitary and aggregated nodules, that occur beneath the epithelium of the tracheobronchial tree go by the name of **bronchus-associated lymphoid tissue** (**BALT**) (Section 7.9.2). Similar tissue in the intestine, including Peyer's patches, is known as **gut-associated lymphoid tissue** (**GALT**).

Lymphonodules also occur in the cortex of **lymph nodes** (Section 14.17), in the white pulp of the **spleen** (Section 14.18), and in the **tonsils**.

In all of its sites, i.e. solitary nodules, aggregated nodules, lymph nodes, spleen, and tonsils, the structure of the lymphonodule is essentially the same.

> In the *Nomina Histologica* (1994) a solitary lymphonodule is known as lymphonodulus solitarius. An aggregated (multiple) lymphonodule is lymphonodulus aggregatus. The germinal centre is centrum germinale. The primary and secondary lymphonodules are lymphonodulus primarius and secundarius, respectively.
>
> According to Ham (1974, p. 336) there is no **capsule** around a lymphonodule. However, Krstic (1984, p. 237) reported the presence of a capsule in the form of a thin network of reticular cells, though it is 'almost invisible' because of heavy infiltration with small lymphocytes;

however, it can be seen in semithin sections of splenic nodules (Krstic, 1984, p. 64).

14.16   Germinal centre

This is the central pale zone of a secondary lymphonodule (Fig. 14.3B). It contains relatively large pale cells with abundant cytoplasm. Most of these cells are rapidly dividing **B-immunoblasts** forming **activated B cells** that differentiate into **plasma cells** and memory B cells. There are therefore some plasma cells in the germinal centre of a lymph node as well, although they speedily migrate into the medullary cords. **Helper T cells** are also present, since they are essential for the activation of resting B-lymphocytes. There are also some **macrophages** in the germinal centre.

The rim of the germinal centre is formed by the **mantle**, a darkly staining zone of small lymphocytes.

In a solitary nodule in a subepithelial position, the germinal centre (centrum germinale) tends to become eccentric and to be covered not by a continuous mantle (corona) but by a cap of small lymphocytes that is directed towards the epithelium (Schummer *et al.*, 1981, p. 276).

14.17   Microscopic anatomy of lymph node

A **lymph node** (nodus lymphaticus) (Fig. 14.3B) is typically oval or bean-shaped. The outer surface is formed by a thin connective tissue **capsule** (capsula). This is perforated by **afferent lymphatic**

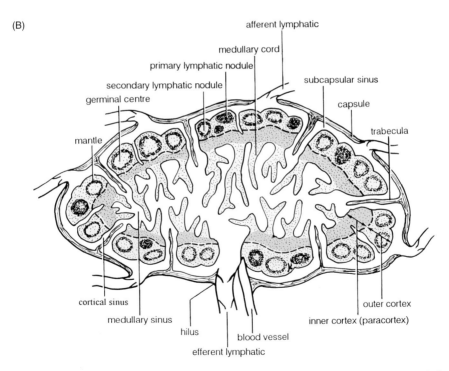

Fig. 14.3B   Schematic longitudinal section through a lymph node. The thin connective tissue capsule is penetrated by afferent lymphatics opening into the subcapsular sinus. The outer cortex contains lymphonodules. Primary nodules are uniformly dark staining. Secondary nodules have been stimulated antigenically, and show a germinal centre surrounded by a dark staining mantle packed with lymphocytes. The inner cortex is directly continuous with the medullary cords. The subcapsular sinus drains through intermediate and medullary sinuses to an efferent lymphatic vessel at the hilus. Dark green, thymus dependent zone. Pale green, bone marrow-dependent zones.

vessels that empty into the **subcapsular sinus**. Thin extensions of the capsule project into the parenchyma as **trabeculae**, which are accompanied by cortical and medullary sinuses.

The structure of the parenchyma is based, as in lymphatic tissue generally (Section 14.11), on a three-dimensional network of interconnected reticular cells supported by reticular fibres, with many free cells of the lymphoid series suspended in the meshes (Fig. 14.4). This parenchymatous meshwork is divided into cortex and medulla.

The **cortex** is differentiated into an **outer cortex** and an **inner cortex** (paracortex). The outer cortex contains **lymphonodules**. The **lymphonodules** have the structure and cell contents that characterize lymphonodules generally, as described in Section 14.15. **Primary nodules** consist of small lymphocytes and are uniformly darkly-stained. **Secondary nodules** have a pale germinal centre, surrounded by the mantle of darkly stained small lymphocytes (Section 14.16). The inner cortex continues without a clear boundary into branching **medullary cords**.

The **medullary cords** are rich in B cells, plasma cells, and macrophages.

The lymphonodules and medullary cords are **bone marrow-dependent**, and are the sites of activation of B-lymphocytes into B-lymphoblasts and their differentiation into B cells and plasma cells. The inner cortex is **thymus-dependent**, and is the site of the activation of T-lymphocytes into T-immunoblasts, and the subsequent differentiation into T helper, T cytotoxic, and T memory cells, and perhaps also suppressor T cells (Section 14.30).

The **subcapsular sinus** connects by **cortical sinuses** to the **medullary sinuses** that ramify between the medullary cords in the depth of the node (Fig. 14.3B). The medullary sinuses finally converge at the **hilus** into an **efferent lymphatic vessel**. Therefore, by means of the sinuses, lymph arriving in the afferent vessels can flow more or less *directly* to the efferent vessel. The lumen of all sinuses is criss-crossed by reticular cells and reticular fibres (Fig. 14.4), which can hold back cells travelling in the lymph. The boundaries of the sinuses are formed by the parenchyma of the node: thus the inner wall of the subcapsular sinus is formed by the outer surface of the cortex, and the cortical and medullary sinuses are delimited

by the parenchyma of the cortex and the medullary cords (Fig. 14.3B). The cells that actually line the sinuses are sometimes known as **littoral cells**, but are probably simply flattened reticular cells. Nevertheless, they belong to the mononuclear phagocyte system, since they remove particulate matter from the lymph as it percolates through the sinuses. In the cortical and medullary sinuses the littoral cells lack a basal lamina, and therefore the walls of these sinuses are quite permeable not only to fluid but also to motile cells such as lymphocytes (Fig. 14.4) and macrophages. Moreover, the parenchyma itself is strung out on its reticular framework (Fig. 14.4). Because of the sponge-like structure of this framework (Section 14.11), some lymph (about 1% of the total entering the node) is able to percolate, though slowly, through the sinus walls and then on through the parenchyma, and so make its way *indirectly* to the hilus. Both the direct and the indirect pathways for lymph are well adapted for filtering out living or inert foreign particles or neoplastic cells from the lymph, thus making an important contribution to immune surveillance.

The afferent and efferent lymphatic vessels have valves ensuring that lymph always moves in a central direction.

If a lymph node drains a site of infection, the whole node increases in size and vascularity. Germinal centres also increase in size and number because of the proliferation of lymphocytes and macrophages. Numerous plasma cells differentiate in the sinuses.

Immunologists (e.g. Abbas *et al.*, 1994, p. 27) have generally retained an older terminology, now discarded by the *Nomina Anatomica Veterinaria* and the revised second edition of the *Nomina Histologica*, both published in 1994. For instance, lymphonodules are commonly known by immunologists as follicles, and the paracortex as the parafollicular area.

The **bone marrow-dependent zone** of the lymph node (Fig. 14.3, and Section 14.12.4) comprises the whole of the **outer cortex** including the lymphonodules (lymphonoduli), and also the **medullary cords** (chordae medullares) (Krstic, 1984, p. 238). The **thymus-dependent zone** of the lymph node (Section 14.12.5) is the inner cortex (paracortex) (Fig. 14.3).

The **pathway of lymph** through the node is reversed in the **pig** (nodus lymphaticus inversus) (Schummer *et al.*, 1981, p. 279). The afferent lymphatic vessels (vas lymphaticum afferens) converge on the hilus, and

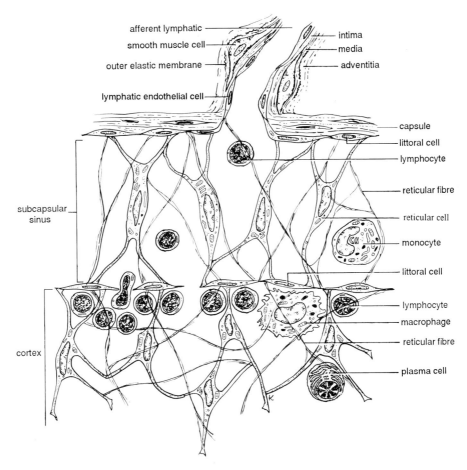

Fig. 14.4 Semischematic view of the microscopic anatomy of the capsule, subcapsular sinus, and periphery of the outer cortex of a lymph node, showing the basic architecture of fixed and free cells. The sinuses and parenchyma are founded on a three-dimensional framework of reticular cells and fine reticular fibres. The reticular cells (fixed cells) are stellate in form. Their processes are attached to each other, to reticular fibres, and to littoral cells lining the sinus. The littoral cells are loosely attached to each other, allowing blood cells and macrophages transit between the sinus and the cortex and vice versa, like the lymphocyte on the left. The cortex is packed with free cells. Only a few are shown, to make the reticular framework visible. The free cells are mostly lymphocytes, with macrophages, plasma cells, and monocytes. The tunica media of the afferent lymphatic vessel has circular smooth muscle cells and an outer elastic membrane.

discharge there into the subcapsular sinus (sinus subcapsularis). The cortex of the node, with lymphonodules, faces the hilus and there meets the incoming lymph. The lymph drains through the centre of the node via cortical sinuses, and then passes into medullary sinuses between medullary cords that abut on the convex periphery of the node. The medullary sinuses open into the subcapsular sinus around the periphery of the node. Multiple efferent lymphatics pierce the capsule and drain the lymph from the subcapsular sinus.

The **blood supply** of a lymph node is derived from a small muscular artery that enters the hilus, passes into trabeculae, and branches into medullary cords. On reaching the cortex, the branches form capillaries that spread into networks around the germinal centres of lymphonodules. The capillaries are drained by specialized **postcapillary venules** (Section 12.14) that run radially through the inner cortex, enter medullary cords, and continue into a vein leaving the hilus. Thus the medullary cords provide a roadway for arterioles on their way to the cortex, and for venules returning towards the hilus; they also carry non-myelinated axons (Krstic, 1984, p. 249).

Haemal lymph nodes (lymphonodus haemalis) (Schummer *et al.*, 1981, p. 280) occur in domestic ruminants and rodents, usually near lymph nodes, and are easily distinguished from lymph nodes by their red-brown colour. They are typically about 1–10 mm long. The parenchyma is founded on a three-dimensional spongy reticular meshwork, typical of lymphatic tissue generally. Lymphonodules with germinal centres are scattered throughout the parenchyma in some species and collected into a cortex in others. There are also medullary cords. Subcapsular, cortical, and medullary sinuses are present.

According to Schummer *et al.* (1981, p. 280), the fundamental difference between a lymph node and a haemal node is that the haemal node has no afferent and efferent lymphatics, and therefore has no flow of lymph through its parenchyma. The subcapsular, cortical, and medullary sinuses are not lymphatic sinuses but **blood sinuses** that are supplied by an artery and drained by a vein. Haemopoietic tissue and numerous red blood cells are present in the parenchyma. The reticular cells phagocytose red cells and store blood pigments. Functionally, haemal nodes would then resemble (a) the spleen in filtering the blood, (b) the bone marrow in performing haemopoiesis, and (c) lymph nodes in producing antibodies.

According to Abu-Hijleh and Scothorne (1996), however, afferent lymphatics and efferent lymphatics are present in the haemal lymph nodes of the rat. They suggested that the numerous erythrocytes in the sinuses might get there via the afferent lymphatics. In their survey of the literature, they found that since 1925 two published papers had denied the existence of afferent lymphatics and four others had confirmed their presence. Evidently the matter requires further attention.

14.18   Spleen

14.18.1   *Microscopic anatomy of the spleen*

The **capsule** of the spleen distributes trabeculae into the parenchyma. Both the capsule and the trabeculae contain elastic fibres and smooth muscle cells (Fig. 14.5). The muscle cells are particularly abundant in carnivores. These elastic and contractile properties make the spleen an important factor in adjustment of the venous return to the heart during stress.

The parenchyma of the spleen is based on the usual three-dimensional framework of **reticular fibres and reticular cells** that typifies lymphatic tissues (Section 14.11). However, unlike other lymphatic tissues the reticular spaces of the parenchyma are occupied by two components, the **white pulp** and the **red pulp** (Fig. 14.5).

The **white pulp** consists essentially of *lymphatic tissue* (the periarteriolar lymphatic sheaths and splenic nodules; Fig. 14.5). The **splenic nodule** has all the structural and functional characteristics of a secondary lymphonodule in a lymph node (Section 14.15) (and is therefore a **bone marrow-dependent zone**). The dark staining **mantle** (corona) of the splenic nodule contains a concentrated mass of **B-lymphocytes**. The **germinal centre** is the pale central zone of the nodule, comprising mainly B-immunoblasts, and B cells differentiating into plasma cells and B memory cells. The splenic nodule is enclosed by a layer of B-lymphocytes and B-immunoblasts called the **marginal zone**, and this layer also extends over the periarteriolar lymphatic sheath (Fig. 14.5). Thus the splenic nodule, together with the marginal zone, are production sites for B-immunoblasts and their progeny of B cells and plasma cells, and hence is a source of **immunoglobulin G**. The splenic nodule and marginal zone are together the **bone marrow-dependent zones of the spleen**.

The **periarteriolar sheath** consists mainly of **T-lymphocytes** and **T-immunoblasts**. The T-immunoblasts proliferate helper T cells, cytotoxic T cells, memory T cells, and perhaps suppressor T cells. The periarteriolar sheath is therefore the **thymus-dependent zone of the spleen**.

The **red pulp** consists essentially of *vascular tissue* (splenic cords and splenic sinuses). Its main component is formed by the **splenic sinuses** and the large volume of venous blood that they contain. The **splenic cords** are not columns of cells as the term implies, but are simply the usual reticular network of lymphatic tissue; blood percolates through this meshwork into the splenic sinuses.

In the horse, dog, and cat the **spleen** is relatively large, well endowed with capsular and trabecular smooth muscle, and poor in white pulp, and the red pulp therefore constitutes an effective blood storage organ. In man the capsule and trabeculae contain relatively few smooth muscle cells and the white pulp is relatively abundant, so blood storage is less significant. The pig and ruminants form an intermediate group (Habel and Biberstein, 1960, p. 133).

The architecture of the white pulp (pulpa alba) of the spleen (lien in the *Nomina Anatomica Veterinaria* (1994), and splen in the *Nomina Histologica* (1994)) is based on the splenic vasculature (Fig. 14.5). At the hilus of the spleen, the splenic artery forms **trabecular arteries** (arteria trabecularis) that run through the trabeculae

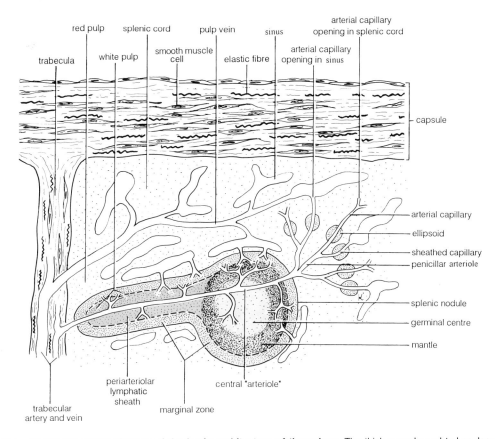

Fig. 14.5 Highly schematic diagram of the basic architecture of the spleen. The thick capsule and trabeculae contain smooth muscle cells and elastic fibres. The trabecular artery forms an arteriole that immediately becomes enclosed within the periarteriolar lymphatic sheath. The sheath ends in a typical lymphonodule, the splenic nodule. Both the sheath and the nodule are surrounded by the marginal zone. The periarteriolar lymphatic sheath, splenic nodule, and marginal zone are the white pulp. The arteriole continues as the central arteriole (central artery) through the edge of the germinal centre. Having supplied capillaries to the nodule, the central arteriole emerges from the nodule and enters the red pulp, branching into about six penicillar arterioles (only three are shown). Each of these divides into two or three sheathed capillaries with a small spindle-shaped cuff of lymphatic tissue (ellipsoid). After the cuff, the vessel continues as a simple arterial capillary. Most arterial capillaries discharge (indirectly) into the splenic cords (open circulation). Others discharge (directly) into the splenic sinuses (closed circulation). The splenic sinuses are irregular channels forming most of the red pulp. They are drained by pulp veins into trabecular veins. The splenic nodule and marginal zone contain resting B-lymphocytes, B-immunoblasts, B cells, and plasma cells. The splenic nodule and marginal zone constitute a bone marrow-dependent zone (pale green). The periarterial lymphatic sheath contains resting T-lymphocytes, T-immunoblasts, and T cells, and constitutes a thymus-dependent zone (dark green).

throughout the organ. The trabecular arteries give rise to arterioles that leave the trabeculae. At the point where an arteriole emerges from a trabecula it becomes a component of the **white pulp**. This is because its tunica adventitia is immediately replaced by a longitudinal cuff of lymphatic tissue, the **periarteriolar lymphatic sheath** (vagina periarterialis lymphatica), which therefore completely encloses the arteriole. This cuff continues along the length of the arteriole until the vessel reaches a **splenic nodule** (lymphonodulus splenicus), which is a

typical spherical lymphonodule. The splenic nodule is reported to be surrounded by a 'capsule' of reticular cells (Krstic, 1984, p. 64). Inside the splenic nodule, the arteriole continues as the '**central artery**': often, however, it is not an artery but an arteriole (see immediately below); nor is it central, for it lies on the *edge* of the germinal centre (Fig. 14.5). The 'central arteriole' supplies capillaries to the nodule. The central arteriole passes right through the nodule and emerges on the other side, where it now enters the red pulp. (In the

Nomina Histologica, 1994, the 'central artery' has become the 'artery of the lymphonodule' (arteria lymphonoduli).)

Although the arterial vessel that branches out from the trabecula is often held to be a muscular artery, Williams *et al.* (1989, p. 829) emphasized that these vessels are 'the finest *arteriolar* branches'.

Having entered the **red pulp**, the central artery abruptly branches into about half a dozen **'penicillar' arterioles** (arteriola penicillares) (Fig. 14.5), so-called because they stick up like the bristles of a brush (Latin: penicillus, a painter's brush); penicillar arterioles are reported to be true end-arterioles – a rare kind of arterial vessel (Section 12.19). Each penicillar artery now divides into two or three **sheathed capillaries** (vagina pericapillaris macrophagiosa) (Fig. 14.5), each being enclosed by a short spindle-shaped cuff of lymphocytes and plasma cells held within a mini-framework of reticular cells and fibres. The sheath of a sheathed capillary is known as an **ellipsoid**, referring to its oval shape. It was previously known as the ellipsoid of Schweigger-Seidel. Ellipsoids are well developed in the carnivores and pig, but not in man (Williams *et al.*, 1989, p. 829). The sheathed capillaries finally continue as simple arterial capillaries (vas capillare terminale).

Most of these **arterial capillaries** end by discharging into the sponge-like reticular meshwork of the **splenic cords** (chorda splenica) (Fig. 14.5); their blood percolates through the splenic cords and eventually drains (essentially indirectly) into the **splenic sinusoids** ('*open circulation*'). The remainder of the arterial capillaries open directly into splenic sinusoids ('*closed circulation*') (Fig. 14.5).

The term **splenic cords** is misleading, since it suggests that the *red pulp* is arranged in orderly elongated columns of cells. On the contrary, the splenic cords, and hence the red pulp, have no obvious overall design, but are a typical, though extensive, continuous three-dimensional sponge-like network of reticular cells and reticular fibres, through which blood percolates. Large numbers of red cells are parked here in the resting animal, thus constituting the reserve of erythrocytes that may be mobilized by sympathetic discharge in the stress of haemorrhage or severe exercise. Among the many other cell types that are strung out on this spongy reticular network, or trapped within its meshes, are the highly phagocytic splenic macrophages, as well as monocytes, lymphocytes, and all the other types of mature blood cells.

The **splenic sinuses** (sinus venularis) are extensive irregular anastomosing channels, forming the bulk of the red pulp and constituting a substantial volume of venous blood. The sinuses are lined by discontinuous endothelial cells devoid of basal lamina, allowing easy exchange of cells and fluids between the blood in the sinuses and blood percolating through the splenic cords. The sinuses empty into **pulp veins** (venae pulpae

rubrae), which drain into **trabecular veins** (vena trabecularis) and thence into **splenic veins** (vena lienalis) at the hilus of the spleen.

There is a special zone of white pulp, called the **marginal zone** (Fig. 14.5). It is a condensation of B-lymphocytes and B cells that encloses both the periarteriolar lymphatic sheath and the mantle of the splenic nodule. The marginal zone seems to represent the major compartment of B cells, i.e. the major bone marrow-dependent zone in the spleen (Krstic, 1984, p. 246).

The distribution of **lymphatic vessels** in the spleen has been controversial. However, such vessels occur not only in the capsule, trabeculae, and white pulp, but also in the red pulp, at least in some species (Williams *et al.*, 1989, p. 832). Blind ending vessels occur in the white pulp, follow the arterial vessels, and exit by efferent lymphatics at the hilus, the flow of lymph therefore running counter to arterial blood. This is a major pathway by which the many lymphocytes formed in the spleen enter the general circulation. Afferent lymphatic vessels draining into the spleen have not been found.

The **bone marrow-dependent** parts (Section 14.12.4) of the spleen (Fig. 14.5) are the whole of the **marginal zone** of the white pulp, and the whole of the splenic nodule, but especially the mantle (Krstic, 1984, p. 389). The lymphocytes of the periarteriolar lymphatic sheath are **thymus-dependent** (Junqueira and Carneiro, 1983, p. 310). Since the spleen lacks the inner (thymus-dependent) cortex of the lymph node, the periarteriolar sheath is the *only* component of the spleen that is thymus-dependent.

14.18.2 *Functions of the spleen*

The spleen is involved in (1) blood storage, (2) removal of worn out erythrocytes, (3) phagocytosis of living particles (bacteria and viruses) and inert particles, (4) immune responses, and (5) production of circulating cells. The spleen is therefore particularly important to the defence of the body. However, it is not indispensable since its functions are taken over by the liver and other lymphatic tissues after splenectomy.

(1) Blood storage

The spleen acts as a contractile reservoir of blood after **haemorrhage** or at the onset of **severe exercise**. In the dog and horse, sympathetic discharge and circulating adrenaline then induce contraction of the **smooth muscle** in the **capsule**, and this decreases the volume of the spleen several-fold. In these athletic species, such contraction not only increases the circulating blood volume, but also ejects numerous resting erythrocytes into the circulating blood, thus greatly enhancing the capacity of the blood for oxygen transport. Conversely, sympathetic inhibition when the body is at rest relaxes the smooth muscle of the capsule and thus allows the spleen to expand, with considerable storage of blood.

The *packed cell volume* or *haematocrit* represents the volume percentage of erythrocytes in whole blood. It is obtained by centrifuging a blood sample, thus separating the cellular elements from the blood plasma and hence indicating the ratio of cell volume to plasma volume. Most of the domestic mammals have a packed cell volume of 38–45% with a mean of 40% (Swenson, 1977, p. 20). In the greyhound and Thoroughbred horse, in contrast to the human athlete, the contraction of the spleen at exercise greatly increases the packed cell volume, i.e. to 60–70% (Snow, 1985), thus producing a substantial increase in the capacity for oxygen transport. A very high haematocrit (about 60%) has been found in the bat (Thomas and Suthers, 1972). The combination of great oxygen transport, large heart size and hence relatively large stroke volume, and a very high heart rate at exercise (Section 22.16), form the cardiovascular basis for the supreme athleticism of the greyhound and Thoroughbred horse (Snow, 1985; Evans, 1994, p. 130). Similar factors represent important adaptations for enabling the bat to achieve the high metabolic rate required by powered flight (Thomas and Suthers, 1972).

(2) *Removal of worn out erythrocytes*

An important component of the mononuclear phagocytic system (Section 14.10) is formed by **splenic macrophages**. These exceptionally voracious phagocytes are distributed throughout the splenic cords of the red pulp and the marginal zone of the white pulp. They avidly remove effete red cells, and with the aid of lysosomes break down haemoglobin into a pigment **bilirubin** that contains no iron, and a protein **ferritin** that does contain iron. The bilirubin circulates in the blood plasma to the liver, where it is taken up by liver cells and excreted in the bile; failure of this process of elimination leads to jaundice. Ferritin circulates in the plasma to the bone marrow, where erythroblasts largely re-use the iron.

(3) *Phagocytosis of living and inert particles*

Of all the phagocytes in the body the **splenic macrophages** are believed to be the most active in the phagocytosis of bacteria, viruses, and inert particles that get into the blood. Their lysosomes contain many powerful enzymes that hydrolyse these bodies, particularly when the enzymes are augmented by the release of **lymphokines** from **helper T cells**.

(4) *Immune responses*

The white pulp of the spleen carries out the same **immune responses** as the cortex and medulla of a lymph node. Thus the resting B-lymphocytes of a splenic nodule respond to antigenic stimuli and to activation by helper T cells by forming B-immunoblasts; in the germinal centre, these proliferate activated B cells which differentiate into plasma cells that release circulating immunoglobulin G.

In order themselves to be activated, the resting T-lymphocytes require an antigen-presenting cell (Section 14.30.1) to present their antigens. This process takes place in the thymus-dependent part of the spleen, i.e. the periarteriolar lymphatic sheath. **Dendritic cells** (Section 14.10) are common antigen-presenting cells in the spleen. Once activated, resting T-lymphocytes differentiate into T-immunoblasts that form the four types of T cell, i.e., helper, cytotoxic, and memory, and perhaps also suppressor T cells, which are responsible for cell-mediated immunity (Section 14.30).

(5) *Production of circulating cells*

In the fetus, the spleen is haemopoietic. The red pulp produces the erythrocyte, granulocyte, monocyte–macrophage, and megakaryocyte–platelet lineages (Sections 12.27–12.30). The white pulp produces B- and T-lymphocyte lineages (Section 12.31). In postnatal life, the red pulp stops making any of these cells. However, the white pulp continues to generate a constant flow of B cells and plasma cells in its bone marrow-dependent zones, and T cells in its thymus-dependent zones; these migrate into the red pulp and enter the sinuses to join the blood stream.

14.19   Thymus

14.19.1 *Developmental anatomy of the thymus*

The **fixed cells** of the thymus, on which the basic framework of the organ is built (Section 14.11), arise from the **endoderm** of the left and right walls of the embryonic **pharynx**. Since its basic framework has arisen bilaterally, the thymus retains signs of being a paired organ in the postnatal animal, especially in the neck and even to some extent in the thorax (see Section 14.19.2).

The **thymocytes** arise as stem lymphocytes from **mesenchyme**. This mesenchyme is at first situated in the yolk sac, then in the liver and spleen, and finally in the bone marrow. Having entered the circulation from the bone marrow and arrived in the thymus (Fig. 14.3A), the stem lymphocytes become T-lymphoblasts, which proliferate T-lymphocytes (now known as thymocytes). Whilst still in the thymus, the T-lymphocytes acquire the *potential* to become helper and cytotoxic T cells, and memory T cells, and possibly suppressor T cells (Section 14.12.2). However, to *complete their differentiation* into these four classes of T cell, they must first migrate to the thymus-dependent zones of the lymphatic tissues (see Section 14.19.5).

In mammals generally (Patten, 1958, p. 425), the thymal **epithelioreticulocytes** (epithelioreticulocyti thymi) that form the basic framework of the thymus are derived from ventral outgrowths of the left and right third and fourth pharyngeal pouches. There seem to be substantial species differences in the contribution made by these two pairs of thymic primordia. In most higher mammals, and certainly in man and pig, the third pair of pouches makes a much more important contribution to the thymus than the fourth. In man, strands of thymic tissue do often arise from the fourth pharyngeal pouch (Williams *et al.*, 1989, p. 833), and a small part of the fourth pouch also contributes to the thymus in the sheep (Noden and de Lahunta, 1985, p. 277).

The earlier literature found no clear evidence that the ectoderm of the third **pharyngeal cleft** also contributes to the developing thymus (Arey, 1958, p. 235). However, most of the embryological evidence (Williams *et al.*, 1989, p. 834) now favours the view that the epithelioreticulocytes are derived from not only the endoderm but also the ectoderm of the third pharyngeal pouch/cleft, with contributions also from the endoderm and ectoderm of the fourth pouch/cleft; the ectoderm seems to be essential for the subsequent lymphopoiesis.

The epithelioreticulocytes probably produce **thymosin** (thymic humoral factor), which initiates the differentiation of T-lymphocytes (see Section 14.19.5).

Like the septum transversum (Section 8.13), the postnatal position of the thymus in the thorax is not attained by a caudal migration of the organ, but by the cranial elongation of the neck of the embryo which leaves behind the heart, septum transversum, and thymus.

14.19.2   *Macroscopic anatomy of the thymus*

The thymus is fully formed in the neonatal animal. It then consists of cervical and thoracic components (Fig. 14.6). The thoracic component is present in all the domestic mammals, and is an essentially midline structure though bilobed in most species. It is situated in the ventral **mediastinum**, cranial to the heart. The cervical component is paired, lying along each side of the trachea, but is absent in some species. From sexual maturity onwards the organ gets smaller and finally disappears.

As would be expected from its paired origin from the embryonic pharynx, the postnatal thymus is essentially a

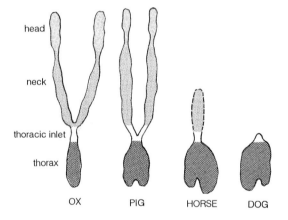

head

neck

thoracic inlet

thorax

OX   PIG   HORSE   DOG

Fig. 14.6 Schematic ventral view diagram of the fully developed thymus of immediately postnatal domestic mammals, showing species variations in macroscopic anatomy. The thymus has three named components. The left and right cervical lobes (light stipple) lie on each side of the cervical trachea. The narrow intermediate lobe (unshaded) lies in the midline and goes through the thoracic inlet. The left and right thoracic lobes (dark stipple) lie in the cranial mediastinum. All species have thoracic lobes, but they blend to varying degrees into a more or less bilobed median structure. In the calf and pig the cervical lobes have a cranial segment (lightest stipple) attached to the pharynx. In the horse the cervical lobes fuse into a single midline structure, but are usually absent (broken line). In the dog only the thoracic lobes are present, the right lobe being larger than the left. In the pig the left and right thoracic lobes are recognizable and symmetrical. In the ox the thoracic lobe is unpaired. In the horse the left thoracic lobe is larger than the right.

paired organ with left and right **cervical lobes** and left and right **thoracic lobes**; the cervical and thoracic lobes are connected by a midline **intermediate lobe** in the narrow space of the thoracic inlet (Fig. 14.6). In the ox and pig the cervical component is larger than the thoracic component, but it is lost in the dog and usually in the horse also (Fig. 14.6). The initially paired thoracic lobes, lying in the cranial mediastinum, tend to be more or less fused, though asymmetrically in the dog and horse. The essentially pharyngeal origin of the thymus also suggests the possible presence of a 'pharyngeal' or 'cranial' component in the postnatal animal. This component (lightest stipple in Fig. 14.6) does occur in the piglet and calf, between the mandibular and parotid salivary glands (Schummer *et al.*, 1981, p. 288).

14.19.3 *Microscopic anatomy of the thymus*

Like that of all the other lymphatic (lymphoid) tissues (Section 14.11), the microscopic anatomy of the parenchyma of the thymus is founded on a network of stellate-shaped **fixed cells**, with **free cells** lodged or moving about in the network.

The surface of the thymus is formed by a connective tissue **capsule**. This gives rise to connective tissue **septa**, which penetrate the cortex and partially divide the organ into irregular **lobules** (Fig. 14.8). A thymic lobule consists of a darkly staining outer cortex and a pale inner medulla; but the medullary parts of adjacent lobules are continuous with each other. The **cortex** stains darkly because it contains dense masses of **thymocytes**, so tightly packed within the network of epithelioreticulocytes that they almost obscure the **interstitial space** enclosed by the network (Fig. 14.7). The origin and future development of thymocytes are reviewed in Section 14.19.5. The **medulla** consists mostly of pale staining epithelioreticulocytes, enclosing an interconnecting network of **interstitial spaces** containing relatively few thymocytes (Fig. 14.7). The interstitial spaces of the cortex and medulla connect with each other (Fig. 14.7), thus allowing movement of cells between the cortex and medulla.

Mononuclear phagocytes (Section 14.10) occur in both the cortex and the medulla (Fig. 14.7). Those in the cortex are strongly phagocytic macrophages, that are busy removing the corpses of rejected T-lymphocytes (Section 14.19.5). Those in the medulla are **interdigitating dendritic cells** (Section 14.10), which are weakly phagocytic

but have the important role of acting as antigen-presenting cells to helper resting T-lymphocytes.

Thymic corpuscles, previously known as Hassal's corpuscles, are scattered throughout the medulla of the thymus (Fig. 14.8). They consist of concentric rings of degenerating epithelioreticulocytes (Fig. 14.7).

In all the other lymphatic tissues, *both* the **fixed cells** *and* the **free cells** are derived exclusively from mesenchyme. In the thymus, only the free cells (thymocytes) are mesenchymal in origin: the fixed cells (thymal epithelioreticulocytes) are *endodermal*, from the epithelium of the third and fourth pharyngeal pouches.

Despite this developmental difference, the **epithelioreticulocytes** (epitheliocyti) have much in common structurally with the **reticular cells** of the other lymphatic organs, such as **lymph nodes** and the **spleen** (compare Fig. 14.7 with Fig. 14.4). The epithelioreticulocytes are stellate in shape. Their slender branched processes are attached to those of their neighbours by cell junctions, thus forming a network (hence 'reticulo-') which enmeshes the free cells (Fig. 14.7). But the epithelioreticulocytes differ structurally from reticular cells in having few, if any, reticular fibres, or any other fibre system, for their support (Junqueira and Carneiro, 1983, p. 301). Also, epithelioreticulocytes appear to have fundamental functions that reticular cells totally lack: thus epithelioreticulocytes evidently play a crucial role in initiating the *differentiation* of T-lymphocytes (Section 14.19.5).

There is evidence for the existence of six functional types of **epithelioreticulocytes** (Williams *et al.*, 1989, p. 834). Those forming the continuous cellular sheet under the capsule and on the septa (type 1 cells) appear to provide a partial **blood–thymus barrier**. Types 1, 2, and 3 are all in the outer cortex, and type 4 is in the inner cortex; some of these contribute to the complete blood–thymus barrier in the cortex. This series of cells shows a graded structure, for example gradations of granular endoplasmic reticulum, correlated with varying functions in the differentiation of the T-lymphocytes (Section 14.19.5) dependent on their position in the cortex. Type 5 cells are in the medulla, and seem relatively undifferentiated. Type 6 cells are those that are associated with thymic corpuscles (corpusculum thymicum).

14.19.4 *Blood–thymus barrier*

The thymic arteries and veins arise from the internal thoracic artery and vein. They enter and leave the parenchyma through the capsule and septa, in the absence of a hilus (Fig. 14.8). Arterioles from the septa run along the corticomedullary

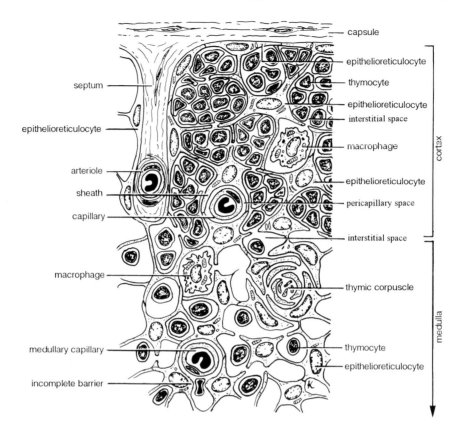

Fig. 14.7   Semischematic view of the microscopic anatomy of the cortex and medulla of the thymus, showing the basic architecture of fixed and free cells. The epithelioreticulocytes (fixed cells) are stellate in form. Their delicate branching processes are attached to each other forming a cellular network. In the cortex, thymocytes are densely packed into the interstitial spaces of the network. In the medulla, thymocytes are much less numerous so that the interstitial spaces are more obvious. Throughout the cortex and medulla the interstitial spaces are interconnected, allowing movement of free cells. The epithelioreticulocytes contribute to a complete pericapillary sheath around cortical capillaries, thus preventing antigenic macromolecules from escaping from the blood plasma. Macrophages remove any antigenic material that does gain access. The medullary capillaries have only an incomplete pericapillary sheath, allowing extensive diffusion of antigens into the medulla. Thymic corpuscles consist of concentric rings of epithelioreticulocytes around a degenerate cell remnant.

junction supplying capillaries to the cortex and medulla (Fig. 14.7).

The inner surface of the capsule, and the surfaces of the septa, are covered with a continuous single layer of **thymic epithelioreticulocytes** (Fig. 14.7). These cells provide a **partial blood–thymus barrier**, which limits access of circulating antigens to the parenchyma. Furthermore, the capillaries in the cortex are surrounded by a closed sheath and pericapillary space, the sheath being formed by epithelioreticulocytes (Fig. 14.7). The capillary endothelium is continuous, and backed by a basal lamina. These sheath-like structures around the

capillaries endow the **cortex** with a **complete blood–thymus barrier**. In the **medulla**, the epithelioreticulocyte sheath around the capillaries is **incomplete** (Fig. 14.7). The complete blood–thymus barrier of the cortex *prevents* antigenic macromolecules from reaching the lymphoblasts in the cortex, but the incomplete epithelioreticulocyte sheath of the capillaries in the medulla allows *extensive diffusion of antigens into the medulla*. Any macromolecules (e.g. experimental tracers) that do escape from the blood plasma and enter the cortex, or diffuse into the cortex from the medulla, are briskly removed by the **cortical**

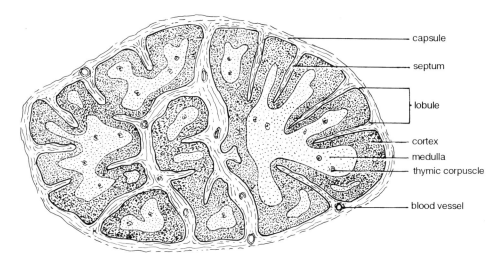

Fig. 14.8 Semischematic view of the microscopic anatomy of a segment of thymus. The capsule forms septa, which create lobules and carry blood vessels. A lobule comprises a dark staining cortex and a pale medulla. The medulla of adjacent lobules blends, forming a continuous branching inner zone. Thymic corpuscles are scattered in the medulla.

macrophages. Thus the thymic cortex and its production line of differentiating resting T-lymphocytes is isolated from antigenic stimuli by a triple barrier, i.e. the continuous sheet of epithelioreticular cells lining the capsule and septa, the periarteriolar and pericapillary sheath, and zealous cortical macrophages. However, once the resting T-lymphocytes have moved into the medulla they are freely exposed to antigens.

The thymus has no afferent lymphatic supply, but **efferent lymphatics** drain the medulla and corticomedullary junction and exit through the capsule.

14.19.5 *T-lymphocyte production cycle*

Stem lymphocytes from the bone marrow enter the cortex of the thymus and become **T-lymphocytes** (Fig. 14.3A). In response to stimulation by the adjacent thymic epithelioreticulocytes, the T-lymphocytes in the cortex are converted into **T-lymphoblasts**. The T-lymphoblasts repeatedly divide mitotically (about every 8 hours), forming **resting T-lymphocytes**. The resulting clones of resting T-lymphocytes ('resting', in the immunological sense) move progressively deeper into the cortex, and onwards into the medulla. Resting T-lymphocytes become much less abundant in the medulla than in the cortex (Fig. 14.7);

this is because most of them leave the thymus through blood vessels and lymphatics in the general region of the **corticomedullary junction**. They then make their way to the **thymus-dependent zones** of the lymph nodes and spleen.

The epithelioreticulocytes also seem to *begin* the induction process which programmes resting T-lymphocytes to differentiate into the various categories of T cells (helper, cytotoxic, memory and, possibly, suppressor T cells). The epithelioreticulocytes probably achieve these effects by releasing a secretion. But at this stage the resting T-lymphocytes are not yet fully immunocompetent (i.e. not fully activated); probably they become fully immunocompetent only when they have left the thymus and become established as T-immunoblasts in their final destinations in the **thymus-dependent zones** of the lymph nodes and spleen (Section 14.12.5).

However, while they are still in the thymus the maturation of resting T-lymphocytes does reach the critical point where they can distinguish between '**self**' and '**non-self**'. Nearly all cells (erythrocytes are a notable exception) expose molecules on their surface that are unique to the individual mammal that owns them. Such a molecular complex is known as a 'major histocompatibility complex of class I' (MHC Class I) (Section 14.19.6). This molecular complex is *invariant* throughout the tissues of a single individual. On the other hand, it varies greatly between all other individuals of the same species, except for genetically identical or very closely related individuals, and especially homozygous ('identical') twins.

A cell that has been infected by a virus, or has become malignant (sometimes they are the same thing) synthesizes peptides that are **virus-specific** or **tumour-specific**. Such a peptide is then transported to the surface of the affected cell where it is *displayed* in *combination* with the class I major histocompatibility molecule (Fig. 14.10B): this is a phenomenon of crucial interest in immunology. The viral or cancerous peptide modifies the molecular characteristics of the MHC, so that the MHC changes from being 'self' to being 'non-self.' This makes it possible for appropriate T cells, by means of their constant immune surveillance, to find, attack, and destroy a cell that bears this alien marker. The T cells that carry out this fatal assault are **cytotoxic T cells** (Section 14.30.3).

A cell from another individual, even from the same species, is a particularly conspicuous target for cytotoxic T cells. In this instance, detection is not achieved because of some subtle structural alteration in the MHC molecule of such a cell through the incorporation of an alien peptide: the *entire* MHC of the grafted cell is different from that of the host cells. Inevitably, this defensive mechanism also destroys surgically transplanted tissues or organs. But we should still be glad of this, since if it were not so, cancer would be catching.

Before it leaves the thymus, *every* new resting T-lymphocyte (thymocyte) is tested to ensure that it can *distinguish between self and non-self*. Thymocytes that fail the test, i.e. those that do 'recognize' (respond to) 'self', are immediately killed. Only those that pass the test are allowed to migrate to the peripheral lymphatic tissues and set up shop in the thymus-dependent zones of the lymph nodes and spleen. As just described, their function in the thymus-dependent zones is to find and destroy faulty or 'non-self' cells, by cell-mediated immune responses (Section 14.30), especially by means of cytotoxic T cells.

It seems likely that only a very small proportion of resting T-lymphocytes (thymocytes) manage to get through this scrutiny (i.e. the test for distin-

guishing 'self' from 'non-self'), which must therefore be even more rigorous than that which decides student entry to a veterinary school. In fact, total success in this screening of potential T cells is vitally important to the health of the animal. T cells that do react to 'self' are a menace, since they thus are programmed to attack the normal tissues of their own body, and this leads to **autoimmune disease**.

Despite **involution** (Section 14.19.7), the thymus continues throughout life to produce resting T-lymphocytes that enter the thymus-dependent zones of the peripheral lymphatic tissues and spleen, form T-immunoblasts there, and thus maintain effective immune responses.

Immunological self-tolerance extends between the antigens of two genetically identical individuals, notably between monozygotic twins. It also occurs between dizygotic twins if they have shared the same placenta (ox, sheep) and consequently exchanged lymphocyte stem cells (Blood and Studdert, 1988, p. 921). Some degree of self-tolerance may even occur within a highly inbred strain of the same species, so that tissue grafts may be accepted by such closely related animals. Grafts between genetically dissimilar members of the same species (isologous grafts) succeed or fail according to the degree of matching of tissue antigens between donor and recipient.

Autoimmune diseases (Blood and Studdert, 1988, p. 83) are rare in large farm animals, only thrombocytopenia, milk allergy, neonatal haemolytic disease in foals, and spermatic granuloma being well known. In dogs and cats, however, they occur quite commonly. Examples include autoimmune haemolytic anaemia and thrombocytopenia, systemic lupus erythematosus, rheumatoid arthritis, glomerulonephritis, lymphocytic thyroiditis, and dermatological diseases of the pemphigus variety.

Williams *et al.* (1989, p. 834) suggested that the **differentiation** and **maturation** of T-lymphocytes within the thymus may be controlled by soluble factors e.g. **thymosin (thymic humoral factor**, a protein containing 108 amino acid residues) released by the thymic epithelioreticulocytes (Krstic, 1984, p. 416). The associated mesenchyme may play an inductive role in the secretion of these factors (Williams *et al.*, 1989, p. 834).

The expression of certain membrane proteins indicates that the differentiation of T cells into helper or cytotoxic T cells has occurred. These proteins act as phenotypic markers distinguishing discrete populations of T cells (Abbas *et al.*, 1994, p. 19). For example most helper T cells express a surface protein known as **CD4**, and most cytotoxic T cells express **CD8** (Section 14.30.3). These CD4 and CD8 molecules are known as

coreceptor molecules (Fig. 14.10). The earliest cells (stem lymphocytes) arriving at the thymus from the bone marrow do not express CD4 or CD8 molecules (Abbas *et al.*, 1994, p. 185). However, the T-lymphoblasts proliferating in the thymic cortex undergo rearrangement of their T cell receptor genes, and experience surface expression of CD4 or CD8 molecules.

The **destruction of erroneous T cells** within the thymus seems to involve one process of positive selection and another process of negative selection (Abbas *et al.*, 1994, pp. 174–186). In **positive selection**, thymocytes that can bind self MHC molecules are selected and permitted to survive. This is advantageous, since thymocytes that *cannot* bind self MHC molecules would be useless because they would be incapable of recognizing the self MHC molecules of antigen-presenting cells (APCs). Therefore positive selection retains useful cells that are able to recognize *foreign* antigen when it is presented on *self* MHC molecules of APCs. However, it also retains potentially harmful T cells that react to *self* antigen presented on *self* MHC molecules of APCs. **Negative selection** eliminates these potentially dangerous cells. Presumably this mechanism of deletion occurs whenever any such thymocyte reacts to a self antigen presented by another thymocyte. Apparently there is also evidence that dendritic cells (the interdigitating variety) within the thymus can present self antigens to, and cause the deletion of, T cells reactive to self antigen. The only cells that then remain are those that react to *foreign* antigen presented on *self* MHC molecules, and it is these that are wanted.

It has been estimated (Williams *et al.*, 1989, p. 838) that between 90% and 99% of thymocytes and their progeny never leave the thymus, i.e. are destroyed because they fail the vital test of distinguishing 'self' from 'non-self'. However, the histological evidence for such mass destruction is rather weak. It has to be assumed that the faulty T-lymphocytes die so rapidly and are so speedily removed by the thymic macrophages that their corpses are seldom seen.

It will be recalled (Section 14.19.4) that although the blood–thymus barrier denies access of blood-borne antigens to the thymic cortex, **blood-borne antigens** do penetrate the thymic **medulla**, and that **dendritic cells** are present in the **medulla**. These facts together indicate that the medulla of the thymus is involved in the antigenic activation of T-lymphocytes. It has therefore been suggested (Williams *et al.*, 1989, p. 835) that perhaps at least part of the thymic medulla may behave as a '*peripheral*' or '*secondary*' component of the lymphatic tissue (as opposed to a *primary* or *central* component, such as the thymic cortex). This would grant the thymic medulla the same functional properties as the **thymus-dependent zones** in the lymph nodes and spleen, where antigenic stimulation renders full immunocompetence to helper, cytotoxic, memory, and perhaps suppressor T cells (Section 14.30). According to this concept, the medulla of the

thymus, or part of it, would be a thymus-dependent zone of the thymus. This concept is further complicated by the observation that occasional germinal centres, complete with mature B-lymphoblasts and plasma cells, are present in the medulla, thus suggesting the presence of a bone marrow-dependent zone as well.

14.19.6 *Major histocompatibility complex*

Cells display molecular complexes on their surfaces. Amongst the most important of these are antigens of the major histocompatibility complexes (MHC), comprising molecules that establish the distinctiveness of the cells of each individual member of a mammalian species. Because of this function, such molecules play a vital role in the immune system. These distinctive molecules are the histocompatibility antigens. They are expressed by the unique genome of the individual animal to which they belong (Williams *et al.*, 1989, p. 835).

The major histocompatibility antigens are a set of plasmalemmal glycoproteins that share the same region of one of the chromosomes (Williams *et al.*, 1989, p. 682), their genes being grouped together as the 'major histocompatibility complex' and expressed in the body as a number of distinctive proteins. Three classes of histocompatibility antigens are recognized: I, II, and III.

The **class I major histocompatibility molecules** display *endogenous* peptide antigens on the surface of macrophages (Section 14.30.1, Fig. 14.10B). They consist of *HLA* genes in man, and the *H2* system in mice; these are subdivided into *A*, *B*, and *C* genes of human *HLA*, and *K*, *D*, and *L* genes of mouse *H2*. *A* and *B* are represented by a number of different alleles; these genes generate a distinctive set of gene products that are expressed at the surfaces of most of the cells of the body. Only one *HLA* sequence is selected from a great possible range during the development of each person, thus bestowing thereafter a unique chemical identity to the cells of that individual.

Class I histocompatibility molecules are the basis of cell-mediated immune reactions by **cytotoxic T cells**. The class I MHC molecules present *endogenous* 'alien' peptide antigens to cytotoxic T cells, i.e. 'alien' peptide antigens that have arisen *inside* the cell, for example from viral or tumour origins (Abbas *et al.*, 1994, p. 129). The cytotoxic T cells recognize and attack cells that present such 'alien' antigens on the cell surface in association with class I MHC molecules (Abbas *et al.*, 1994, p. 129).

The **class II major histocompatibility molecules** display *exogenous* peptide antigens to **helper T cells**, i.e. foreign peptides that have entered the cell from the *outside* (Section 14.30.1, Fig. 14.10A), for example foreign peptides of bacterial or parasitic origin. The class II MHC molecules occur on the surfaces of **antigen-presenting cells** (**APCs**), i.e. interdigitating dendritic cells, macrophages, B cells, etc. (Section 14.28.2). These molecules are anchored into the plasmalemma of the APC. Like the HLA antigens (class I MHC) they are highly variable, and *have a different chemical structure in each individual* within a species. The phagocytic cell (APC) to which they belong engulfs an antigen and partly digests it. The APC then presents digested peptide components, in conjunction with its class II major histocompatibility complex, to a **helper T cell**. Class II antigens are formed by HLDA-DR antigens in man, and H2 Ia antigens in the mouse (Lackie and Dow, 1989, p. 103).

There appears to be a loose genetic linkage between the human *HLA* system and alleles that predispose to a variety of autoimmune diseases, including rheumatoid arthritis and perhaps multiple sclerosis.

The genes for class III MHC components are expressed in various elements of the complement system, as well as some other, non-immune related proteins (Williams *et al.*, 1989, p. 682).

14.19.7 *Involution of the thymus*

The ratio of thymus mass to body mass is greatest around the time of birth, but the organ goes on increasing in mass for a variable number of weeks, months, or years after birth, depending on the species. Probably the absolute mass decreases from sexual maturity onwards, as in man, but the details for the domestic species seem uncertain. Involution in the sense of a natural progressive degeneration probably begins soon after birth, as in man, but is not necessarily accompanied by a reduction in absolute mass.

Involution takes the form of a gradual replacement of thymic tissue by connective tissue and adipose tissue. This replacement is progressive, but nevertheless it is established (at least in man) that the production and differentiation of thymocytes continues throughout life, so that resting T-lymphocytes from the thymus continue to populate the thymus-dependent zones of the peripheral lymphatic tissues.

Involution (in man) begins from the capsule and septa, enters the cortex where it replaces thymocytes, and advances towards the medulla (Williams *et al.*, 1989, p. 836).

Thymectomy (Williams *et al.*, 1989, p. 837) during neonatal and early postnatal life leads to a progressively fatal condition, with hypoplasia of the peripheral lymphatic organs, wasting, and inability to mount an effective immune response. After sexual maturity the main lymphatic tissues are fully established; thymectomy is then less debilitating, but effective responses to novel antigens are eventually reduced.

14.19.8 *Endocrine associations of the thymus*

It had long been suspected that the thymus had some endocrine function, but Schummer *et al.* (1981, p. 285) considered this to be unlikely. However, various endocrine organs do interact with the thymus (Williams *et al.*, 1989, p. 838). Thymectomy in rodents is associated with cellular changes in the adenohypophysis, and levels of circulating luteinizing hormone and follicle stimulating hormone also fall but can be restored by thymic transplantation at birth.

There are many other interactions with endocrine glands (Williams *et al.*, 1989, p. 838). Adrenocorticosteroid hormone inhibits the function of the thymus and causes its involution; the same effect is produced indirectly by adrenocorticotrophic hormone, by stimulating the adrenal cortex to produce glucocorticoid hormones. Male and female sex hormones accelerate thymic involution, whereas castration has the opposite effect (Junqueira and Carneiro, 1983, p. 307). In pregnancy the thymus involutes, but is restored during lactation, possibly through the action of prolactin (Williams *et al.*, 1989, p. 838).

These observations indicate that the immune system and neuroendocrine system are interdependent.

IV CELLULAR BASIS OF THE IMMUNE SYSTEM

14.20 The immune system

Every vertebrate animal has an immune system that saves it from certain death through the activities of hostile bacterial, viral, fungal, and parasitic infectious agents. The system comprises natural immunity and acquired immunity.

Natural immunity is based on defence mechanisms that are *inborn*, i.e. *innate*. These include: (1) physical barriers such as the skin and the mucus carpet of the tracheobronchial tree (Section 7.3); (2) phagocytic cells of the mononuclear phagocyte system (Section 14.10) and also microphages, notably neutrophilic granulocytes (Sections 12.28, 7.7.4); (3) natural killer cells (Section 14.30.5); (4) various blood-borne molecules. All of these resources are in place *before* an attack by pathogenic micro-organisms or foreign macromolecules.

Acquired immunity is based on the secretions of lymphocytes that are induced in direct response to invasion by specific foreign macromolecules. The invading macromolecules are known as **antigens**, and the body's defensive secretions are **antibodies**. The antibodies are designed to eliminate the antigens. For successful defence, the mechanisms of acquired immunity have to be integrated with those of natural immunity.

A first insight into how this system might work arose from the observation that individuals who recovered from certain diseases appeared to be resistant to repeated infection. The idea of vaccination came in the 1770s from a chance remark by a dairymaid to Edward Jenner, a country medical practitioner: 'I can't take smallpox, for I have already had cowpox'. For 20 years Jenner debated whether to take the risk of testing this observation experimentally. Finally, in 1796 he followed the oft-repeated advice of his mentor, John Hunter – 'Why think? Why not try the experiment?' He 'vaccinated' an 8 year old boy, James Phipps, with pus from the hand of a dairymaid, Sarah Nelmes, who had cowpox. Eight weeks later he inoculated the boy with smallpox: no disease appeared. Incidentally this event explains why the word vaccinate comes from vacca, Latin for cow.

> Inoculation against smallpox had been practised in Europe since the beginning of the eighteenth century, and centuries before that in China (Guthrie, 1945, p. 246). In China, powdered crusts from a smallpox case were sniffed or blown into the nose. In Europe, a thread soaked in a smallpox pustule was drawn through a superficial incision or a small scratch. A Quaker physician, Thomas Dimsdale (1712–1800), was so successful with this procedure that the Empress Catherine of Russia invited him to St. Petersburg to inoculate herself and her son. It was a dangerous mission, and arrangements were made to cover his escape if the plan ended in disaster. He inoculated nearly 200 people and all did well, including the Empress who 'has had smallpox in the most desirable manner; which now thank God is over.' He came home with £10 000 in his pocket, a pension of £500, and a Russian baronetcy. However, it was not until Jenner's discovery and the widespread adoption of vaccination that the incidence and mortality of smallpox really began to fall.

14.21 Antigen

Any substance capable of inducing an immune reaction is referred to as an **antigen**. Virtually any macromolecule can induce an immune reaction, provided that it is *foreign* to the recipient. It is, indeed, essential that immune reactions are made *only* in response to antigens that are foreign to the host, and are not made in response to antigens that are a normal constituent of the host itself: otherwise the immune reaction will destroy the host's own cells.

Examples of biochemical materials that are antigenic include macromolecules such as albumins, globulins, bacterial toxins and capsules, viruses, excretory and secretory products of parasitic worms, snake venoms, protozoal cell membranes, and tissue grafts.

The surface of the antigen may combine with a specific antigen-binding receptor site on the surface of a lymphocyte, or with an identical site on the surface of an antibody. The component of the surface of the antigen that does the actual combining is known as the **antigenic determinant** or **epitope**. The molecular configuration of the antigen *fits* the molecular antigen-binding site (Fig. 14.9) as a key fits its lock. In this mechanism, the lymphocyte is responding to the *shape* of the antigen. **Resting B-lymphocytes** appear to recognize antigen mainly by this process.

On the other hand, *all* **resting T-lymphocytes** *must* receive their antibody through the agency of another cell, especially an **antigen-presenting cell** (APC) (Section 14.30). The APC (which is generally a macrophage, dendritic cell, or B cell) engulfs the antigen, breaks it down, and then presents the antigen on its surface as a peptide. Thus the resting T-lymphocyte mainly identifies the antigen by its distinctive *amino acid sequence*, rather than by its shape.

14.22 Immune responses

Immune responses fall into two main classes, humoral and cell-mediated. Humoral antibody responses require resting B-lymphocytes, and thence B-immunoblasts, to produce B cells (Fig. 14.3A). The B cells then form plasma cells that produce antibodies. Antibodies circulate in the body fluids and bind specifically to the antigen that stimulated their production, thus leading to the elimination of the antigen. Cell-mediated immune responses require resting T-lymphocytes to form T-immunoblasts, and thence T cells of sev-

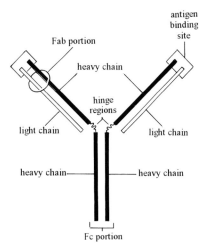

antigen binding site

Fab portion

heavy chain

hinge regions

light chain   light chain

heavy chain ——— ——— heavy chain

Fc portion

Fig. 14.9   Highly schematic diagram of a Y-shaped antibody molecule. It has two identical antigen-binding sites, one at the tip of each arm of the Y. The tail of the molecule (i.e. the handle of the Y) can attach the antibody to a cell. Two hinge regions enable each arm to swing from or towards the axis of the Y, when binding to an antigen. The antibody molecule has two identical halves, consisting of four polypeptide chains, two light and two heavy. The left and right halves of the molecule are held together by sulphydryl linkages. The antibody molecule can be split artificially into three fragments, i.e. two arms and a tail. Each arm is named Fab (**F**ragment **a**ntigen **b**inding, because it includes the antigen binding site); the tail region is known as Fc (because it **c**rystallizes readily).

eral types (Fig. 14.3A). T cells do not employ antibody, but react mainly with foreign antigens on the surface of host cells; the T cell (cytotoxic T cell) then destroys an abnormal host cell, i.e. a host cell that displays a foreign antigen on its cell surface.

> In the **humoral response**, the antigen has arisen *outside* the host cell. For example, the antigen may be a macromolecular toxin released into the blood stream by a bacterium (Section 14.28). The binding of **antibody** to such a circulating antigen can inactivate or destroy the antigen (Williams *et al.*, 1989, p. 672). Alternatively (Alberts *et al.*, 1983, p. 952), the binding of the antigen to antibody can subsequently enhance the ability of phagocytic cells to ingest the antigen. Or it may activate **complement** in the normal blood plasma, which is a series of enzymatic proteins that induce cytolysis and phagocytosis of pathogens (Section 14.28.3).
>
> The **cell mediated response** occurs if the antigen has arisen *within* a host cell. In this case the antigen is beyond the reach of antibodies. For example, the antigen

may have come from a virus that has invaded host cells, or from the 'transformed' cells of a tumour, or from a graft of foreign cells. The antigen will be presented on the surface of a host cell (an **antigen presenting cell**), and the presenting host cell (together with a virus that may have attacked it) will then be destroyed by a **cytotoxic T cell** (Fig. 14.3B; Section 14.30.2). Or the antigen may cause a **delayed type hypersensitivity-related cell** to attract macrophages and stimulate them to destroy the host cell.

14.23   Clonal selection theory

One of the most astounding characteristics of the immune system is that it can respond to the millions of different foreign antigens to which the animal may be exposed in the whole of its lifetime, even including man-made substances that do not occur in nature.

The **clonal selection theory** proposes that, during development, each lymphocyte becomes committed to react with one particular antigen before ever being exposed to it. Each lymphocyte achieves this commitment by developing its own surface receptor proteins that will specifically match this one antigen; if Darwin could have known this, he would certainly have been impressed by such a supreme example of evolutionary power. The binding of the antigen to the receptor *activates* the lymphocyte, causing it to multiply and mature. Thus the lymphocyte system should never be taken by surprise, no matter what the antigen may be, since there is always a lymphocyte there, with its receptor site at the ready. It is because of this that immune responses are antigen-specific. The term 'clonal' (as in 'clonal selection theory') means the *sharing of identical characteristics*: it arises because the lymphocytes must be composed of millions of different families or *clones* of cells. Each clone is descended from a common ancestor. Each ancestral cell is already committed to make one particular, antigen-specific, receptor protein. Therefore every individual cell within a clone is equipped with identical antigen specificity.

> At first it was suggested that the molecular structure of antibodies would be determined by the antigen: folded polypeptide chains at the antigen-binding site would unfold to conform to the molecular structure of the anti-

gen. This was the *instruction hypothesis*. However, protein chemists ruled out the instruction hypothesis, and it was replaced by the *clonal selection theory*.

The specificity of an antigen depends on its molecular structure, and particularly on that of its epitope (Dixon, 1993, p. 6). An antigenic protein molecule may have 18 or more epitopes of which only five or six are exposed on the surface of the molecule. An antibody produced in response to an epitope combines only with that epitope or another of very similar structure. The **specificity** of a protein epitope is determined by its amino acid sequence. The body's ability to recognize antigens is so precise that it can discriminate between two proteins that differ only in a single amino acid or two optical isomers (Alberts *et al.*, 1983, p. 952).

The **antigenicity** of molecules *increases* with the size and number of their epitopes.

14.24   Immunological memory

The immune system has a memory, and this provides an animal with immunity to many viral diseases that lasts long after the initial exposure to the virus. Once an animal is infected with the virus, its immune response appears after a delay of several days, increases rapidly, and then gradually decreases again: this is the **primary immune response**. Reinfection weeks, months, or years later, leads to a quicker, greater, and longer response; this is the **secondary immune response**.

The cellular basis of immunological **memory** arises from **clonal selection**. 'Resting' lymphocytes, belonging to a particular clone, respond to their first exposure to antigen by proliferating and differentiating into two types of cell. (1) **Effector B cells** and **effector T cells**, respond actively to the antigen, the B cells and plasma cells responding by secreting antibody (Section 14.28), and T cells responding by making cell-mediated responses (Section 14.30). (2) **Memory B cells** and **memory T cells** do *not* immediately respond to the antigen by secreting antibody (B cells) or by making cell-mediated responses (T cells). Instead they circulate and recirculate between the blood, the tissues, and lymph; but on a later encounter with the same antigen, even years later, they readily convert to effector B or effector T cells and make a vigorous secondary immune response. Thus the resting, effector, and memory cells all belong to the same clone, and therefore make the same immune responses to the same antigen even if years

have passed since the first exposure. Memory B and memory T cells have a very long life, circulating and recirculating without dividing: in contrast, resting lymphocytes seem to die within weeks or days.

14.25   Avoiding destruction of self

As already noted in Section 14.21, it is essential that immune reactions are *only* made in response to antigens that are *foreign* to the host, and are not made in response to molecules that are a part of the host itself: otherwise the immune reaction will attack the host's own normal cells. It is therefore necessary that the immune system should be able to recognize self, so that it can then accept self and reject non-self. This is known as **immunological tolerance to self**.

At an early stage in development, i.e. *before* they leave the thymus, all newly formed resting T-lymphocytes with receptors that respond to antigenic determinants on *self* molecules are destroyed or suppressed. The elimination of these undesirable T-lymphocytes, i.e. T-lymphocytes that fail to distinguish between self and non-self, is discussed in Section 14.19.5. Failure of this process of elimination leads to **autoimmune disease**.

14.26   Structure of antibodies

Antibodies are proteins. Each antibody molecule is Y-shaped (Fig. 14.9). The tip of each arm of the Y carries an identical site for binding to an antigen (so-called *bivalent* antigen). The two arms are hinged, making the binding to antigens more effective. The tail is used to attach the antibody to a cell. Alternatively, the whole Y-shaped antibody can float free in the body fluids.

The 'bivalent' form of antibodies enables them to form cross-linked antigen molecules into lattices. For a large lattice to form, each antigen must have three or more epitopes. A lattice precipitates out of solution if sufficiently large.

The antibody molecule consists of four polypeptide chains, held together by **disulphide** linkages. Two of the chains are long (heavy chains) and two are short (light chains). Each light chain (L chain) comprises about 220 amino acids, and each heavy chain (H chain) has about twice that number (Alberts *et al.*, 1983, p. 965) – hence its greater length.

The antibody molecule can be split artificially into three parts, i.e. its two arms and its tail. Each arm has its antigen-binding site and is known as an **Fab** fragment (**Fragment antigen binding**). The single tail fragment is called an **Fc** fragment because it readily **c**rystallizes.

There are five variants of heavy chain (α, δ, ε, γ, and μ). They belong, respectively, to the five *classes* of antibodies (IgA, IgD, IgE, IgG, and IgM). These five variants of H chain impart particular characteristics to each of the five classes of antibody. Since the tail of the antibody consists only of H chain (Fig. 14.3A), it is the *tail* of the antigen (Fc) that expresses these characteristics of each class of antibody (Alberts *et al.*, 1983, p. 966). For example the Fc of IgG enables it to bind to the plasmalemma of macrophages and other defensive cells, or to bind to and hence unleash the first component of the complement system (Section 14.28.3).

14.27   Types of immunoglobulins

Five classes of antibodies (or immunoglobulins) are known, immunoglobulin M, G, A, E, and D. They are all secreted by **plasma cells** (Section 14.14). Initially, all antibodies circulate in the body fluids as *circulating antibodies*, and are then known as **soluble antibodies**. Soluble antibodies recognize and bind to antigens (such as bacterial toxins) in the body fluids, thus inactivating or destroying those antigens.

Some circulating antibodies become *secondarily* attached to the plasmalemma of macrophages and a variety of other defensive cells. As stated in Section 14.26, this attachment is made by means of the tail of the antigen (its Fc component). Such an attachment enhances particular defensive functions of these cells, or widens the range of these functions. **Immunoglobulin G (IgG)** is produced in abundance during the secondary immune response, and thus forms the bulk of the circulating antibodies (Section 14.28). It is a Y-shaped molecule (Fig. 14.9), with an antigen binding site on the end of each of its two arms (its two Fab portions). Its tail (Fc component) gives it other functional characteristics, such as binding to macrophages and thus enhancing their performance, and activating the complement system (Section 14.28.3). **Immunoglobulin M (IgM)** is the main antibody secreted into the blood in the early stages of a primary immune response. **Immunoglobulin A (IgA)** is the main antibody in secretions (Section 14.29) – respiratory, intestinal, lacrimal, salivary, and mammary. IgA forms a **common mucosal immune system** (Section 14.29.2) that defends the respiratory system, gastrointestinal tract, and other mucosal systems against infection. **Immunoglobulin E (IgE)** is mainly attached to mast cells, inducing them to release their secretions in the presence of parasites. **Immunoglobulin D (IgD)** is an immunoglobulin on the surface of B cells, where it may contribute to the recognition of antigens.

14.27.1 *Distribution of antibodies*

The distribution of antibodies in the body is restricted to certain cells and fluid compartments (Abbas *et al.*, 1994, p. 34). *The only cells that* **synthesize** *antibodies* are B-lymphocytes and their progeny, especially plasma cells (Section 14.28.1). Consequently antibodies are present within the cytoplasm of B cells (in membrane-bound form), and are also displayed on the surface of B cells. Antibodies secreted by B cells are found in the blood plasma, and smaller amounts find their way into the interstitial fluid; when blood clots, antibodies remain in the residual **serum**, hence the concepts of 'antiserum' and 'serology'. Some other cells (e.g. mast cells; Section 14.27.4) do not synthesize antibody but have specific receptors for binding antibodies to their surface. Antibodies also occur in certain secretory fluids, particularly colostrum (Section 14.28.4).

14.27.2 *Immunoglobulin M*

IgM is the first antibody to be produced by B cells, and indeed *all* B cells begin their career of antibody synthesis by making IgM. However, a B cell that begins by synthesizing IgM can later switch to the production of one other class of antibody, i.e. IgG, IgA, IgE, or IgD, thus focusing on IgG alone or on one of the other antibodies in its potential repertoire. This process is known as isotype switching.

14.27.3 *Isotype switching*

This mechanism (Abbas *et al.*, 1994, p. 85) involves an irreversible rearrangement of the gene products in the heavy chain of the antibody molecule (Section 14.26). The process is not random, but is regulated by helper T cells and their secreted lymphokines. For example, the switch to IgE is stimulated by interleukin-4 (Abbas *et al.*, 1994, p. 86).

14.27.4   *Immunoglobulin E*

IgE is important in the immune defences against parasites. The synthesis of IgE by B cells is regulated by a particular group of helper T cells, which secrete interleukin-4 (IL-4) and interleukin-5 (IL-5). IL-4 induces the required isotype switch from IgM to IgE; IL-5 activates eosinophils.

Mast cells, and their circulating counterparts **basophils**, carry a specific receptor for the Fc component of the IgE molecule. When thus attached to the plasmalemma of a mast cell or basophil, IgE in due course meets, and binds to, its specific antigen. This causes the mast cell to release its granules, containing histamine and an array of other mediators. These substances induce the classic inflammatory response (Section 14.28.3); this damages the host tissues, but presumably also damages the parasite.

The mast cell also releases eosinophil chemotactic factor, which attracts **eosinophils**. Yet more eosinophils are recruited by the interleukin-5 released by helper T cells. Eosinophils are involved in defence against parasites. Their mode of attack on helminths is not clear, but they may secrete **lysosomal enzymes**. Like mast cells they release **vaso-active lipids** (prostaglandins, leukotrienes) from their granules, causing inflammatory changes (J.B. Dixon, 1996, personal communication).

14.27.5   *Immunoglobulin D*

IgD usually remains membrane-bound, and is commonly expressed together with IgM during the early differentiation of a B-lymphocyte (Abbas *et al.*, 1994, p. 85).

14.27.6   *Allergy, anaphylaxis, and hypersensitivity*

Unfortunately the substances released by **mast cells**, **basophils**, and **eosinophils** under the influence of **IgE** (e.g. **histamine**, **serotonin**, **prostaglandins**) can cause not only local inflammation but also severe systemic reactions. The systemic reactions include increased vascular permeability (and hence oedema, swelling of tissues, and decreased blood volume), vasodilation, and bronchial contraction (Abbas *et al.*, 1994, p. 279). These responses can be drastic enough to end in death by cardiovascular collapse and asphyxia. Such conditions are known as **allergy**, **anaphylaxis**, or **hypersensitivity**. In view of these conditions and the threat of autoimmune disease (Section 14.19.5), it seems that the immune defences can only be gained at the cost of some potentially lethal side effects. Evidently the immune system treads a fine line between attacking the invader and damaging the body (Willison, 1996).

14.28   Immunoglobulin G

The formation of IgG goes through several steps. The 'resting' B-lymphocyte must first bind to, and thus be *antigenically stimulated* by, its specific antigen (i.e. the antigen to which it is preprogrammed to respond). It does this by binding directly to antigen which it encounters in the extracellular fluids (blood plasma or interstitial fluid). Next it must be *activated* by a **helper T cell**. Once it has been activated it now becomes a **B-immunoblast** (Section 14.12.4). This proliferates mitotically to form numerous **B cells**. These differentiate into plasma cells and B memory cells. The **plasma cells** mass-produce IgG, forming about three quarters of the total immunoglobulin in the blood serum.

In its soluble antibody form, IgG binds to antigens such as bacterial toxins that are circulating in the body fluids. By binding to them it inactivates or destroys them. Secondarily, its Fc component (tail) binds to specific receptors on the plasmalemma of macrophages and polymorphonuclear leucocytes. Thus armed, macrophages and polymorphs can more effectively find, engulf, and destroy micro-organisms that have become coated with IgG antibodies in response to infection. Furthermore the Fc fragment of IgG binds to the first component of the **complement system** (Section 14.28.3), thus initiating an enzymatic attack that destroys the micro-organism.

14.28.1   *Production of IgG by plasma cells*

The events leading to the production of IgG by B cells and their plasma cells are essentially as follows (Krstic, 1984, p. 45; Grey *et al.*, 1989; von Boehmer and Kisielow, 1991). A protein antigen is carried on a pathogenic organism, or on a toxin produced by such an organism. The organism might be a virus, a bacterium, or even a multicellular parasite. The antigen contacts a group of resting B-lymphocytes. One resting **B-lymphocyte** in this group carries an antigen-receptor molecule on its *surface* that is programmed to respond to this specific antigen, and binds to it, thereby enabling that particular B-lymphocyte to recognize the antigen as foreign. The resting B-lymphocyte interiorizes the molecular complex so formed, breaks down the protein antigen, and then displays a peptide antigen on its surface using a **class II major histocompatibility complex** (class II MHC) (Section 14.19.6).

The resting B-lymphocyte is thus *antigenically stimulated*, but it now needs to be *activated* by a **helper T cell**. This occurs in two steps (Abbas *et al.*, 1994, p. 194). First the antigenically-stimulated resting B-lymphocyte must 'present' the antigen (carried on its plasmalemma by a class II MHC molecule) to (an activated) helper T cell. In so doing, the resting B lymphocyte has assumed the role of an **antigen-presenting cell** (Section 14.30.1). The helper T cell carries on its surface a single molecule – the T cell receptor molecule (TCR) as shown in Figure 14.10 – which has a specificity for the class II MHC of the resting B-lymphocyte, in combination with the antigen that the B-lymphocyte presents. The T cell receptor molecule of the helper T cell binds to the MHC of the antigenically-stimulated B-lymphocyte. The second step in the activation of the B cell then occurs: the helper T cell releases a **lymphokine**, especially interleukin-2, -4, and -5 (Abbas *et al.*, 1994, p. 197). Only when the antigenically-stimulated resting B-lymphocyte is hit by the interleukins is it '*activated*', i.e. converted into a **B-immunoblast**.

This all important process of *activation* of the B-lymphocyte by the helper T cell is considered again in Section 14.30.2. In favourable conditions, the B-immunoblasts can divide every 6 hours, forming great numbers of B cells (Krstic, 1984, p. 45). Most of these B cells differentiate into **plasma cells** (i.e. *effector* B cells; Section 14.24), secreting at first IgM and then IgG. The remainder become **memory B cells**, which respond rapidly to any future contact with the same antigen.

The *main production site* of both plasma cells and IgG (Krstic, 1984, p. 237) is in the bone marrow-dependent zones of the **lymphonodules** of **lymph nodes** (Section 14.14).

The resting B-lymphocyte that has become bound to its antigen and is therefore antigenically stimulated does express IgG on its surface, and can even begin secreting soluble antibody before it interacts with the T helper cell. But the *mass-production of soluble IgG*, at a rate of about 2000 molecules per second, requires the proliferation of differentiated plasma cells that commit nearly all their protein-synthesizing equipment to making antibody and die after only a few days (Alberts *et al.*, 1983, p. 964): this differentiation into plasma cells cannot happen until the antigenically-stimulated resting B-lymphocyte has interacted with the helper T cell.

Although IgG travels throughout the body as **circulating IgG** in the blood, it also makes some contribution to the *local* defence of mucous membranes. This it does by diffusing through the mucosal epithelium. For example, some circulating IgG diffuses through the tracheobronchial epithelium to the luminal surface, but it makes only a minor contribution to the defence of the lung and indeed of other mucosal surfaces. This is probably because it induces a **complement reaction**, and thus causes a local inflammatory reaction that could actually damage the mucosal surface (Section 14.28.3). However, there is

a true, *locally secreted*, form of IgG. This is known as '**secretory**' **IgG**. Secretory IgG is formed relatively abundantly in the lung alveoli, where it contributes to the vital defences of the alveolar wall by enhancing antiviral activities and inhibiting adhesion of bacteria (Section 7.12). Secretory IgG also plays a major role in the defence of the gut of ruminants (Stokes and Bourne, 1989, p. 171).

14.28.2   *Participation of accessory cells in the binding of antigen to B-lymphocytes*

As stated in the preceding section, when a resting B-lymphocyte encounters its specific antigen in the extracellular fluid it can bind to that antigen directly, by means of an antigen-receptor molecule that it expresses on its plasmalemma. Probably this *direct* method of binding is the one that usually operates. However, Abbas *et al.* (1994, p. 23) reported that **follicular dendritic cells** ('trap antigens complexed to antibodies or complement products and display these antigens on their surfaces for recognition by resting B-lymphocytes'. This may seem to suggest that follicular dendritic cells act as true antigen-presenting cells for resting B-lymphocytes, in essentially the same way that interdigitating dendritic cells (and other cells) act as APCs for helper T-lymphocytes (Section 14.30.1a).

However, the 'display' of antigen to a resting B-lymphocyte by a follicular dendritic cell differs in two respects from the 'presentation' of antigen to a helper T-lymphocyte by an antigenically stimulated B-lymphocyte: (1) The 'display' of an antigen to a resting B-lymphocyte is *not* essential for the binding of antigen to that B-lymphocyte, but the 'presentation' of antigen to a helper T-lymphocyte by an antigen-presenting cell *is* essential for the binding of the T cell receptor molecule (TCR) to the MHC of the resting B-lymphocyte. (2) The 'display' of antigen by a follicular dendritic cell to a resting B-lymphocyte is made by a relatively unspecialized antigen-receptor molecule, whereas the 'presentation' of antigen by a resting B-lymphocyte to a helper T cell can only be made by the highly specialized major histocompatibility molecular complex of class II (class II MHC).

In summary, the resting B-lymphocyte probably relies mainly on direct contact with its specific antigen. No doubt the resting B-lymphocyte gratefully accepts the antigen if offered it by an accessory cell, but Abbas *et al.* (1994, p. 203) concluded that there is no evidence that resting B-lymphocytes *need* an accessory cell of any kind in order to recognize an antigen (although Stokes and Bourne (1989, pp. 181–182) described antigen presentation to B cells by the MHC pathway). However, it has been shown that **follicular dendritic cells** are evidently able to store and display antibody-complexed antigens for many years, and they may therefore be important for the periodic restimulation of memory B cells.

14.28.3 Antigen–antibody complex: complement: inflammatory response: opsonization

The combination of IgG with antibody forms an **antigen–antibody complex**, and this has various defensive functions. Firstly it has the beneficial effect (in the intestine and presumably also in the respiratory tract) of stimulating the release of **mucus** from goblet cells and increasing the cleansing activity of that mucus (Stokes and Bourne, 1989, p. 171). Secondly the antigen–antibody complex that forms on the surface of a microorganism interacts with **complement**. This interaction unleashes a biochemical assault on the micro-organism, comprising (Abbas *et al.*, 1994, p. 294): (1) production of a lytic complex causing **lysis** of the micro-organism; (2) release of **opsonins** (see immediately below) that enhance phagocytosis, since mononuclear phagocytes and polymorphonuclear granulocytes (neutrophils, basophils, and eosinophils) express specific receptors for these opsonins and are thus attracted to the site; (3) production of peptides (anaphylatoxins) from fragments of complement, which cause **degranulation of mast cells** with release of histamine and thence increased capillary permeability. Effects (2) and (3) are the **classic inflammatory response**.

The terms **complement** and **opsonin** tend to baffle the beginner. **Complement** is a series of enzymatic proteins found in normal **blood serum**. (Blood serum is the clear straw-coloured fluid that remains after blood has clotted; it therefore lacks blood cells since these are trapped in the clot, and has lost the various proteins involved in clotting, e.g. fibrinogen.) Soon after the discovery of humoral immunity it was observed that fresh serum at body temperature caused agglutination and lysis of bacteria, but if heated to 56°C the serum induced agglutination but not lysis; it was concluded that serum must contain another heat-labile component that assists or '*complements*' the lytic function of antibodies (Abbas *et al.*, 1994, p. 294). It is now known that 'complement' is not a single protein but a complex of at least 15 discrete enzymatic proteins that interact with the antigen–antibody complex to produce lysis when the antigen is an intact cell (Blood and Studdert, 1988, p. 213).

Apparently the most important **opsonins** are (1) antibodies, and (2) the substances derived from complement by its interaction with the antigen–antibody complex, as mentioned above (Lackie and Dow, 1989, p. 172). What does the word 'opsonin' actually mean? Unfortunately there is no way of discerning this from the everyday use of English, since no other word in the language even remotely resembles it. According to the *Shorter Oxford Dictionary* it comes from the Latin 'obsonare', meaning

'to cater' or 'to buy provisions'. A slightly better fit would be 'obsonium', 'food eaten with bread'. This in turn comes from a Greek word, opson (οψον), meaning a *food delicacy*, and here lies the explanation of the term: an opsonin converts a particle into a tasty morsel highly attractive to phagocytes. Gentle reader, I hope you enjoyed this rather delicious etymological digression.

14.28.4 The placenta

In ungulates (Latshaw, 1987, p. 55), the placenta is believed to be effectively **epitheliochorial**, so that six layers of tissue separate the maternal and fetal circulation (uterine endothelium, uterine connective tissue, and uterine epithelium; chorionic epithelium, fetal connective tissue, and fetal endothelium). In carnivores the placenta is **endotheliochorial**, being reduced to four layers, (uterine endothelium, chorionic epithelium, fetal connective tissue, and fetal endothelium). In primates (Noden and de Lahunta, 1985, p. 62) the placenta is **haemochorial** and reduced to only three layers (chorionic epithelium, fetal connective tissue, and fetal endothelium).

The thinness of the primate placenta allows maternal IgG to enter the fetal circulation, but no antibodies are known to cross the placenta of the horse, pig, and ruminants, and only very small amounts cross in carnivores (Latshaw, 1987, p. 72). Therefore in the domestic mammals the neonate must acquire its initial passive immunity via colostrum.

Colostrum (Blood and Studdert, 1988, p. 210) is very rich in antibodies for about a week after birth. The neonate must ingest an adequate amount of colostrum during the first few hours after birth, since only during that period is the intestinal epithelium permeable to the macromolecules of the immunoglobulins. In the horse, pig, and ruminants, IgG predominates; in the dog the main immunoglobulin is IgA.

14.29 Immunoglobulin A: common mucosal immune system

Immunoglobulin A is the only antibody that is readily secreted *through* epithelial cells and *into* the lumen of organs, notably the intestine and tracheobronchial tree.

IgA is formed in response to a specific antigen that has penetrated the epithelial surface of a mucous membrane. The antigen could be a bacterium or a soluble toxin, and the epithelium could belong to any of the mucous membranes and especially those of the alimentary, respiratory, and urinogenital tracts. The area of these intestinal and respiratory mucosal surfaces is immense, allowing correspondingly great exposure to the pathogenic micro-organisms of the external environment. Immune responses are therefore an important factor in the defence of mucous membranes. An outstanding feature of this defence is the massive production of IgA, which accounts for about 60–70% of the daily output of all antibodies.

The formation of IgA is initiated in the same way as the formation of IgG (Section 14.28). An antigen that penetrates the epithelium binds to a resting B-lymphocyte in the submucosa. The B-lymphocyte is then activated by a helper T cell, and now becomes a B-immunoblast (Fig. 14.3A). This proliferates more B-immunoblasts, and these form B cells that differentiate into plasma cells. The plasma cells now undergo an isotype switch (Section 14.27.3) and secrete **IgA** (instead of IgG) into the loose connective tissue beneath the epithelium.

The function of IgA is to provide a local defence of mucous membranes throughout the body, thus constituting the **common mucosal immune system**. Its defensive action consists of preventing toxins and micro-organisms from penetrating mucous membranes. To achieve this objective, IgA is actively transported from the connective tissue *beneath* the epithelium to the *luminal surface* of the mucous membrane. There it both blocks the absorption of toxins, and inhibits the adherence of micro-organisms to the surface of the epithelium.

Although the common mucosal immune system is a major factor in the defence of the mucosal surfaces of the gastrointestinal, respiratory, and urinogenital systems, all of these systems have additional, non-specific 'natural' immune systems (Section 14.20). In the respiratory system these include the mucociliary escalator (Section 7.2), coughing (Section 7.6.2), non-immunological antimicrobial defences such as lysozyme and lactoferrin (Section 7.15), and alveolar and tracheobronchial clearance by phagocytes (Section 7.16). In the gastrointestinal tract these non-specific 'natural' immune systems include the significant bactericidal acidity of the stomach contents, trapping and removal of micro-organisms by the mucous layer covering the intestinal epithelium, incessant and rapid elimination and

renewal of intestinal epithelium, the repeated sweeping out of gut contents by peristalsis, competition from the large numbers of symbiotic normal micro-organisms, and non-immunological antimicrobial defences such as lysozyme secreted into the mucous layer.

14.29.1 *Secretory and circulatory forms of IgA*

Two forms of IgA can be distinguished, one of them 'secretory' and the other 'circulatory'. The **secretory form, SIgA** (Stokes and Bourne, 1989, p. 185), is found in the secretions of mucous membranes. It is a dimer consisting of two monomer IgA molecules. These are linked by two smaller polypeptide chains; one of these is known as the J (for 'joining') component; the other, which is known as the 'secretory' component, is picked up from the surface of the epithelial cells (Alberts *et al.*, 1983, p. 968). The **circulatory form of IgA** is found in the blood plasma (Murray, 1973). It is structurally different from secretory IgA, being a monomer like IgG (Alberts *et al.*, 1983, p. 968). It is less important than the secretory form.

14.29.2 *Common mucosal immune system*

The secretory form of IgA predominates not only in respiratory secretions but also in other external secretions, including gastrointestinal secretions, saliva, tears, colostrum, and milk (Murray, 1973). It is the main immunological component in the strategy of defending the mucous surfaces of the body against foreign material by *exclusion* (Sections 7.1, 14.29.5). It operates within the concept of a **common mucosal immune system**, mediated locally, that is shared by the intestinal, respiratory, and urogenital tracts, and the mammary gland, and controls events at the mucosal surfaces of all these great organ systems (Stokes and Bourne, 1989, p. 176). The mechanisms of this system have been studied mainly in the gastrointestinal tract. Relatively little is known about the other mucosal sites, but it is likely that the principles are basically similar (Abbas *et al.*, 1994, p. 233).

14.29.3 *Formation of IgA*

Antigen in the intestinal lumen or tracheobronchial tree may be soluble (e.g. a bacterial toxin) or particulate (e.g. bacteria or worms, and protozoa in the intestine). Most of the antigens that penetrate the intestinal epithelium enter the lymphatics draining the intestinal mucosa (Abbas *et al.*, 1994, p. 234) and are carried to the lymph nodes of the cranial mesenteric lymphocentre (Section 14.32.5). Here the antigen binds to a molecular receptor site on a B-lymphocyte. By means of interaction with a helper T cell (Section 14.30.2), the B-lymphocyte is then *activated* into a B-immunoblast, which proliferates large numbers of activated B cells. The plasma cells derived from these activated B cells form IgM at first, but then undergo an isotype switch and thereafter secrete IgA (the secretory form). B Cells that have been thus activated in a lymph node of the cranial mesenteric lymph centre may then return to the intestine to populate the lamina propria of the intestinal mucosa.

Some of the macromolecular antigens that penetrate the intestinal epithelium pass directly to the aggregated lymphonodules (Peyer's patches) in the submucosa (Section 14.15). Specialized absorptive cells known as **M cells** are scattered in the intestinal epithelium covering Peyer's patches (Krstic, 1984, p. 247). These cells are actively pinocytotic, and are believed to transport macromolecular antigens across the intestinal epithelium, delivering them close to the numerous resting B-lymphocytes in the submucosal lymphonodules. Although M cells probably play an important role in delivering antigen near to these B-lymphocytes, they do not function as true antigen-presenting cells (APCs) (Abbas *et al.*, 1994, p. 233). Cells similar to M cells are believed to occur in the **bronchial epithelium**, covering bronchial lymphonodules (Section 7.9.2).

14.29.4 *Transport of IgA to the luminal surface*

The transport of IgA from the plasma cell to the surface of the intestinal lumen is not done by passive diffusion, but by an active process involving the so-called **secretory component** (SC). The secretory component is synthesized by mucosal epithelial cells, independently of IgA.

The dimeric IgA molecule secreted by the plasma cells binds to the secretory component (Abbas *et al.*, 1994, p. 234). The secretory component–IgA complex so formed is absorbed into the epithelial cell by pinocytosis, transported across the epithelial cell, and discharged onto the luminal surface by reverse pinocytosis. There, the IgA is released from the complex, into the lumen.

IgA is transported to the lumen of the tracheobronchial tree by a similar mechanism (Stokes and Bourne, 1989, p. 185). It seems likely that the secretory component is synthesized by the serous secretory cells and serous glandular cells of the bronchial mucosa and displayed on the abluminal surface of the bronchial epithelium, where it binds to the IgA (Section 6.2) (Breeze and Wheeldon, 1977, p. 751).

14.29.5 *Role of IgA*

The **antibody-mediated immunity** that results from the expression of IgA (the secretory form) at mucosal surfaces has several aspects, covered collectively (Section 7.1) by the term **immune exclusion** (Stokes and Bourne,

1989, p. 170). Firstly, there is evidence (from the gut) that IgA *reduces the absorption* of soluble antigens such as bacterial toxins across the epithelium. Secondly, IgA seems to *inhibit the binding* of micro-organisms to the epithelium and hence prevents colonization. Furthermore, IgA appears to induce *cell-mediated cytotoxicity* against bacteria. It has also been shown to have antiviral properties (Blood and Studdert, 1988, p. 478).

Unlike IgG, IgA does not activate complement or opsonization (Stokes and Bourne, 1989, p. 170). In general its functions are passive and anti-inflammatory, and avoid the damage to epithelial surfaces that would be caused by the active and inflammatory effects of IgG.

The essentially **local** action of the secretory form of IgA has led to the **local** administration of antigens for **immunization** (Murray, 1973), for example by aerosols in the respiratory system (Blood and Studdert, 1988, p. 478).

14.30 Cell-mediated immunity

T-Lymphocytes eventually differentiate, via T-immunoblasts, into three (or four) functional types of T cell, namely helper T cells, cytotoxic T cells, and memory T cells (and perhaps suppressor T cells). None of these various types of T cell secretes free antibody, but all are involved in cell-mediated immune reactions. The differentiation of T-lymphocytes into one or other of these types (Fig. 14.3A) begins in the thymus (Section 14.19.5). Natural killer cells also contribute to the destruction of various types of target cell.

Helper T cells (and suppressor T cells) are regulatory cells, respectively initiating (and inhibiting) the activities of B- and T-lymphocytes. Helper T cells hold a pre-eminent position in the immune system. This is firstly because B cells *cannot function* until they have been activated by helper T cells (Sections 14.28.1, 14.30.2). By being responsible for the activation of B cells, helper T cells indirectly (but nonetheless effectively) control the production of *all* antibodies, including both IgG and IgA. A failure of helper T cells therefore means that the body loses control of pathogenic organisms that are normally kept in check by its immune defences. The outstanding example of such loss of control is the **human immunodeficiency virus (HIV-1)**, which specifically infects and kills helper T cells, thus leading to **acquired immune deficiency syndrome (AIDS)**. Other viruses, and various other factors including malnutrition, can cause similar though far less lethal immunosuppression. Secondly, helper T cells secrete an array of lymphokines that powerfully enhance the activity of macrophages and the differentiation of cytotoxic T cells, as well as inhibit the replication of viruses (Section 14.31.2).

Cytotoxic T cells (also known as **cytolytic T cells** or **CTLs**) protect the host against viruses and tumours, and are responsible for the rejection of tissue transplants from another individual. Cells that have been invaded by a virus synthesize and display *virus-specific proteins*; likewise cancerous cells synthesize and display *tumour-specific proteins*. Cytotoxic T cells recognize these specific proteins as antigens, and find and destroy the cells that are producing them. Cytotoxic T cells recognize cells of tissue transplants from another individual as foreign and destroy them too. The destruction is achieved by the release from the cytotoxic T cell of (1) a pore-forming protein called *perforin*, and (2) a lymphokine (*lymphotoxin*, Section 14.31.2). Both of these agents cause cytolysis of the target cell (Section 14.30.3). By destroying the cells that house a virus, they deprive the virus of its essential life support; therefore they have a powerful action in *killing viruses*. Like a number of other cells, they also synthesize lymphokines (Section 14.31.2) that *inhibit viral replication*. Furthermore, cytotoxic T cells secrete other lymphokines that strongly *promote macrophage activity*.

Memory T cells have a life span of years, and differentiate into cytotoxic T cells or helper T cells if the same antigen is reintroduced.

In Section 14.12.5, it was noted that **resting T-lymphocytes** are 'blind' to the antigens that stimulate them. This is a fundamental difference between T-lymphocytes and B-lymphocytes. It is possible for a resting B-lymphocyte to bind to, and thus be *antigenically stimulated* by, a specific antigen that it may encounter anywhere in the extracellular fluids (Section 14.28). Such antigens may be *soluble antigens*. In contrast, resting T-lymphocytes are unable to respond to soluble antigens, and are *only able to respond to antigens that are bound to the surfaces of other cells*. Consequently both the resting helper T-lymphocyte and the resting cytotoxic T-lymphocyte must have the antigen 'presented' to it by an *accessory cell*; only then can a resting helper or resting cytotoxic T-lymphocyte recognize and respond to antigen.

This accessory cell is known as an **antigen-presenting cell** (**APC**).

In principle, there are two types of APC, one for resting helper T-lymphocytes and the other for resting cytotoxic T-lymphocytes. (1) The **APCs for resting helper T-lymphocytes** are a group of relatively specialized cells. They are able to take up and digest protein antigens from pathogens such as bacteria and parasites. They then 'present' the antigen to a resting helper T-lymphocyte. (The act of presentation is made by means of a class II major histocompatibility complex, Fig. 14.10A). The resting helper T-lymphocyte is now *activated* into a helper T-immunoblast, and proliferates fully functional helper T cells. The APCs for resting helper T-lymphocytes are the cells of the **mononuclear phagocyte system** (**macrophages** and **dendritic cells**) (Section 14.10). **Resting B-lymphocytes** can also act as APCs to helper T cells. However, the objective of this antigen presentation is entirely different: it is not to activate the helper T cell, but to activate the B-lymphocyte. This interaction between helper T cell and resting B-lymphocyte is essential in order to initiate the mass-production of IgG and IgA by plasma cells (Sections 14.28 and 14.29).

(2) Almost any type of cell (erythrocytes being one exception) can act as an **APC for cytotoxic T-lymphocytes**. This ensures that almost any cell that synthesizes virus-specific or tumour-specific proteins can be recognized and killed by cytotoxic T cells. (This act of presentation is made by a class I major histocompatibility complex (Fig. 14.10B).) The **natural killer cell** (Section 14.30.5) is a lymphocyte-like cell. It attaches itself to certain virus-infected cells, tumour cells, and protozoa, and then releases a cytotoxic protein. Thus, it functions like a cytotoxic T cell, but differs in not needing to be antigenically stimulated.

14.30.1a *Antigen-presenting cells for helper T-lymphocytes*

As just stated, in order to be *activated* the **resting helper T-lymphocyte** requires an antigen to be presented to it on the surface of an antigen-presenting cell (APC). The best-known APC for a resting helper T-lymphocyte is a **macrophage** (Section 14.10), but various other APCs ('specialized' and 'non-professional') for resting helper T-lymphocytes are surveyed at the end of this subsection.

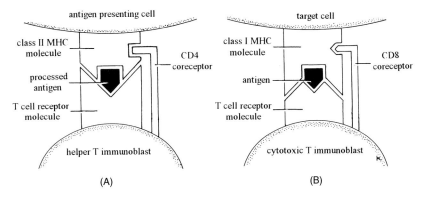

Fig. 14.10 Highly schematic diagram of the molecular components used by antigen-presenting cells (APC) and T cells for displaying and recognizing antigens, and for distinguishing between self and non-self.

A. An antigen-presenting cell, typically a macrophage, has ingested foreign material, broken it down into short fragments, and thus obtained a processed exogenous antigen in the form of a single peptide. It has presented the processed antigen on its cell surface by means of a class II major histocompatibility complex (MHC II) molecule, to a resting T-lymphocyte. The resting T-lymphocyte has used its T cell receptor molecule to recognize, and bind to, the combined antigen and MHC of the antigen presenting cell. The resting T-lymphocyte now becomes a T-immunoblast, and is about to begin repeated mitotic divisions. Since this T-immunoblast carries a CD4 coreceptor molecule, its progeny will be helper T cells.

B. A cell has been infected by a virus, and has formed an abnormal molecule in its cytoplasm. By means of a class I major histocompatibility complex (MHC class I) molecule, the infected cell has presented this endogenous alien molecule as an antigen to a resting T-lymphocyte. The resting T-lymphocyte has used its T cell receptor molecule to recognize, and bind to, the combined antigen and MHC of the infected cell. The resting T-lymphocyte has now been activated into a T-immunoblast, and is about to begin repeated mitotic divisions. Since the T-immunoblast carries a CD8 coreceptor molecule, its progeny will be cytotoxic T cells. The cytotoxic T cells that it produces will search for, and bind to, any cell that displays the alien antigen. The cytotoxic T cells will interpret the combination of alien antigen and MHC class I displayed by such a cell as non-self, and will destroy all such cells.

Based on Boehmer and Kisielow (1991).

The APC endocytoses the protein antigen, breaks it down into short fragments or peptides, and then displays on its surface a single peptide which is now the antigen. Since the antigen that is finally presented to the resting helper T-lymphocyte is always a *broken down fragment* of the original antigen, it follows that the resting helper T-lymphocyte is not essentially interested in antigen *configuration*: instead, the resting helper T-lymphocyte recognizes mainly antigen *composition*, i.e. the sequence of amino acids in the protein chain. This is in contrast to the resting B-lymphocyte, which recognizes antigen mainly by its molecular configuration (Section 14.21).

The peptide antigen of the antigen-presenting cell is now expressed by a molecular complex, the **Class II major histocompatibility complex (class II MHC)**, which presents the antigen on the surface of the APC (Fig. 14.10A). The class **II** MHC displays *exogenous peptide antigens*, i.e. peptides derived from proteins such as bacteria or bacterial toxins that have entered the antigen-presenting cell from the *outside*.

Using its class II MHC, the APC presents the peptide antigen directly to an antigen-specific receptor molecule (a **T cell antigen receptor** or **TCR**) on the surface of a **resting helper T-lymphocyte**. On binding to the antigen by means of its T cell antigen-receptor molecule, the resting helper T-lymphocyte is *activated*. It now becomes

a **helper T-immunoblast** (Fig. 14.0A), and proliferates **helper T cells**.

Two groups of cells are potential APCs for resting helper T-lymphocytes. Firstly there are **specialized antigen-presenting cells**; these have a major capacity for antigen presentation, and possess also a greater or lesser capacity for phagocytosing cellular and microbial debris. It is certain that these cells *do* present antigen to resting helper T-lymphocytes. Secondly, there are many other cells of epithelial or mesenchymal origins, with a wide range of particular functions of their own, which can be *induced* to present antigens. But it is not yet certain to what extent these cells really do present antigen to resting helper T-lymphocytes. Abbas *et al.* (1994, pp. 125, 272) dubbed the specialized cells as '*professional antigen-presenting cells*' and the others as '*non-professional antigen-presenting cells*'.

(1) Specialized ('professional') antigen-presenting cells for helper T-lymphocytes

These include four types of cell. The first two (dendritic cells and macrophages) are members of the mononuclear phagocyte system. (i) **Dendritic cells** (interdigitating and intradermal dendritic cells). These are *true* dendritic cells, and are the most highly specialized APCs (Section 14.10). Although capable of only a moderate uptake of particulate matter, they are extremely efficient at presenting it to helper T-lymphocytes (Abbas *et al.*, 1994, p. 23). **Follicular dendritic cells** are *not* APCs for helper T-lymphocytes; they lack the class II MHC, and simply 'display' antigen to B-lymphocytes (Section 14.28.2). (ii) **Macrophages**. These are the strongly phagocytic cells of the mononuclear phagocyte system. They also present antigens to helper T-lymphocytes, these essentially *exogenous* antigens being derived from pathogens such as bacteria and parasites (Abbas *et al.*, 1994, p. 123). (iii) **B-lymphocytes**. The presentation of antigen by B-lymphocytes to helper T cells is an essential prerequisite to the activation of B cells by helper T cells – the interaction that culminates in the mass-production of IgG and IgA by plasma cells (Section 14.28.1). (iv) **Endothelial cells of venules**. These may be important APCs in cell-mediated immunity (Abbas *et al.*, 1994, p. 125).

All of these four specialized cell types have *two essential characteristics* that enable them to function as APCs for resting helper T-lymphocytes. They must have the ability (a) to endocytose and process exogenous antigens, and (b) to present those antigens by class II MHC molecules (since class II MHC molecules are specifically recognized by helper T-lymphocytes) (Abbas *et al.*, 1994, p. 123).

(2) 'Non-professional' antigen-presenting cells for helper T-lymphocytes

Included in this group is a wide range of epithelial and mesenchymal cells. Important among them are representatives of the mucosal epithelia that are so vulnerable to the external environment, including *intestinal epithelium* (Bland and Whiting, 1993), *bronchial epithelium* (Suda *et al.*, 1995), *uterine epithelium* (Wira and Rossoll, 1995), and *renal epithelium* (Kelley and Singer, 1993). All of these epithelial cells can be induced to follow the same processes as the specialized APCs, i.e. surface binding of exogenous antigen, endocytosis, internal processing, and expression by class II MHC molecules. These antigen-presenting processes are induced by the lymphokine **interferon-γ**, released by helper T cells. However, Abbas *et al.* (1994, p. 125) concluded that the physiological significance of these 'non-professional' APCs remains unclear. For instance, they found no evidence (Abbas *et al.*, 1994, p. 234) that intestinal epithelial cells are capable of presenting antigens to, and stimulating, resting helper T-lymphocytes. On the other hand, presentation of antigen to T cells by bronchial epithelial cells was reported by Suda *et al.* (1995), and to renal tubular epithelial cells by Kelley and Singer (1993).

14.30.1b   Antigen-presenting cells for cytotoxic T-lymphocytes

Resting cytotoxic T-lymphocytes respond only to antigen presented by the **class I major histocompatibility complex** (Fig. 14.10A, Section 14.19.6) (Abbas *et al.*,

1994, p. 120). The class I MHC complex displays *endogenous* peptide antigens, i.e. peptides made from proteins *inside* the cell, and these include virus-specific and tumour-specific peptides. Since almost all cells of the body express class I MHC molecules, any such cell that displays virus-specific or tumour-specific peptides will be detected by a resting cytotoxic T-lymphocyte. This detection will lead to the full maturation of the resting cytotoxic T-lymphocyte into a cytotoxic T-immunoblast, and thence to the proliferation of cytotoxic T cells (Section 14.30.3).

14.30.2   Helper T cells

Helper T cells and cytotoxic T cells express different membrane proteins which act as phenotypic markers (Abbas *et al.*, 1994, p. 19). Most helper T cells express an accessory surface protein known as CD4, and most cytotoxic T cells express a different accessory surface protein known as CD8; consequently helper T cells are often referred to as **CD4 cells**, and cytotoxic cells as **CD8 cells**. ('CD' is short for 'cluster of differentiation'.) The CD4 and CD8 molecules are named *coreceptors*. They act as *adhesion molecules*: CD4 helps to bind the helper T cell to an antigen-presenting cell, and CD8 helps to bind the cytotoxic T cell to a target cell, as shown schematically in Fig. 14.10. The coreceptor molecules may also *transmit signals* between the two cells that they bind (Abbas *et al.*, 1994, pp. 151–153). As stated in Section 14.30.1b, a further fundamental distinction between helper T cells and cytotoxic T cells is that helper T cells respond only to antigen that is presented by MHC class II molecules, whereas cytotoxic T cells respond only to antigen presented by MHC class I molecules.

Helper T cells have a very wide repertoire of cell-mediated immune activities. The *activation of B-lymphocytes* by helper T cells is particularly important, since by inducing the proliferation of plasma cells the helper T cell dominates humoral immunity.

The first step in the full maturation of a resting B-lymphocyte is its antigenic stimulation by an *exogenous agent*, either a toxin or a protein antigen carried on a pathogenic organism (Section 14.28.1). The resting B-lymphocyte binds to the exogenous protein antigen, endocytoses the molecular complex so formed, breaks down the protein antigen, and expresses a peptide antigen on its surface by a class II major histocompatibility complex. An activated helper T cell uses its own T cell antigen-receptor molecule (TCR) to find and bind to the peptide displayed by the class II MHC of the B-lymphocyte. The helper T cell then releases **lymphokines** (interleukin-2, -4, and -5) (Section 14.31.2), and these *activate* the B-lymphocyte to become a B-immunoblast (Section 14.12.4). The B-immunoblast proliferates B cells, and these differentiate into plasma cells secreting antibodies (initially IgM, and then after an isotype switch, IgG or IgA).

Furthermore, helper T cells secrete numerous other **lymphokines** that have a potent influence on antimicrobial defences (Section 14.31.2). Among these lymphokines are powerful activators of mononuclear phagocytes (e.g. interferon-γ) and of polymorphonuclear leucocytes (tumour necrosis factor and lymphotoxin; Section 14.31.2), and lymphokines that enhance the differentiation of cytotoxic T-lymphocytes (interleukin-2).

Thus helper T cells are the one element that influences virtually all other aspects of protective immunity (Dixon, 1993, p. 12).

14.30.3 *Cytotoxic T cells*

Resting cytotoxic T-lymphocytes have undergone partial maturation and selection in the thymus, and are committed to the cytotoxic lineage (these are the 'pre-CTLs' of Abbas *et al.* (1994, p. 272)). They express CD8 coreceptor molecules on their surface and respond to antigen presented by class I MHC molecules. But they are not yet fully differentiated when they leave the thymus, and still lack cytolytic function.

The **full maturation** of a **resting cytotoxic T-lymphocyte**, so that it can perform its cytolytic function, goes through two steps. In the first step the resting cytotoxic T-lymphocyte uses its T cell receptor molecule (TCR) together with its accessory CD8 coreceptor molecule to recognize, and to bind to, the specific antigen presented by the class I MHC molecule of its target cell (Fig. 14.10B). The second step requires the release of a cytokine. Neither the identity nor the cell source of such a cytokine is known (Abbas *et al.*, 1994, p. 272), but interleukin-2 and interferon-γ are likely to be involved, and there seems to be a requirement for helper T cells. Presumably the cell now proliferates, and could then be regarded as a cytotoxic T-immunoblast.

The **differentiation** into a **fully mature cytotoxic T cell** is now completed by the development of (a) membrane-bound cytoplasmic granules containing the protein cytolytic agent (perforin), and (b) a range of lymphokines (particularly interferon-γ, lymphotoxin, and tumour necrosis factor).

The now fully mature cytotoxic T cell is *activated* to perform **cytolysis** by the binding of its TCR–CD complex to the MHC I complex on the target cell (Abbas *et al.*, 1994, p. 273). This triggers the release of the cytolytic granules from the cytotoxic T cell at the point of contact with the target cell, bystander cells being unaffected. The cytolytic cell does not injure itself, but on the contrary is able to kill a sequence of many target cells. Destruction of a cell that harbours a virus not only destroys the virus's life-support system, but also makes the virus accessible to antibodies which can finally eliminate it (von Boehmer and Kisielow, 1991). Cytotoxic T cells will also recognize the class I MHC of cells of foreign tissue transplants as non-self, and destroy them.

14.30.4 *Suppressor T cells*

Suppressor T cells have been regarded as a separate class of T cell, distinct from helper and cytotoxic T cells, and with the function of inhibiting the defensive actions of B cells and other T cells (Williams *et al.*, 1989, p. 674). However, there is now considerable controversy as to whether this suppressor function really is mediated by a discrete class of T cells. It may be more likely that helper and cytotoxic T cells mutually stimulate or inhibit each other by secreting appropriate lymphokines (Abbas *et al.*, 1994, pp. 19, 216).

14.30.5 *Natural killer cells*

The natural killer cell (Williams *et al.*, 1989, p. 674) is a lymphocyte-like cell. It is classified as a 'large granular lymphocyte', but forms only a small percentage of all lymphocyte-like cells. It is not a B or T cell (Abbas *et al.*, 1994, p. 275). These cells function rather like cytotoxic T cells, killing various kinds of target cells, including virus-infected cells, cells from certain tumours especially when haemopoietic, and protozoa. They attach themselves to the target cell, and then release a lethal cytolytic protein from cytoplasmic granules. They can also secrete lymphokines (tumour necrosis factor and interferon-γ).

Natural killer cells differ from T cells in not needing to be antigenically stimulated by an antigen-presenting cell. The molecular structures that natural killer cells recognize on the surfaces of their target cells are not known. Several lymphokines (e.g. interferon-γ) enhance their cytolytic attack on target cells.

Natural killer cells therefore constitute a relatively non-specific means of destroying pathogenic cells. Abbas *et al.* (1994, p. 274) suggested that they are best regarded as phylogenetically primitive cytolytic T cells that have not evolved the specific T cell receptor molecules on their plasmalemma that are essential for antigen recognition.

14.31 Other antimicrobial defences

14.31.1 *Lysozyme*

Lysozyme is a bactericidal enzyme found in serum and tears and on the skin, as well as in respiratory mucus where it is secreted by the underlying epithelium and mucoserous glands. It is also secreted by neutrophil leucocytes and macrophages. It attacks many bacteria, causing bacterial lysis. Lysozyme represents a first line of defence against bacteria, since it is already there and waiting, whereas immunoglobulins and cell-mediated immune responses are formed only after B and T cells have been activated.

Lysozyme and other bactericidal enzymes are nonspecific antibacterial substances. Lysozyme evidently becomes incorporated into respiratory mucus by being secreted beneath, and then diffusing into, the mucous carpet. It appears to be formed (Breeze and Wheeldon, 1977, pp. 716, 751) by the **serous epithelial cells** (Section 6.2) and the cells of the **serous tubules** of the **mucoserous bronchial glands** (Section 6.2) and also by alveolar phagocytes. It attacks many Gram-negative bacteria (Cohen and Gold, 1975, p. 331), causing bacterial lysis.

Lactoferrin is another bactericidal agent found in **tracheobronchial** and various other secretions including milk, tears, and saliva, and in neutrophils. It is an iron-binding protein. It inhibits the growth of bacteria that depend on iron by chelating soluble iron salts (Cohen and Gold, 1975, p. 331).

14.31.2 *Cytokines*

Cytokines are protein hormones, co-ordinating the cells that defend the body against micro-organisms by *natural* and *acquired immunity*. Cytokines that act in natural immunity are produced mainly by cells of the **mononuclear phagocyte system** (Section 14.10), and are therefore known as **monokines**. Those that take part in acquired immunity are produced mainly by activated cells of the **lymphocyte lineage**, and are therefore known as **lymphokines**. Cytokines also include '**chemokines**' that attract **neutrophils**.

Cytokines include interferons, interleukins, tumour necrosis factor, chemokines, lymphotoxin, migration inhibition factor, and colony stimulating factor.

Helper T cells can secrete the following **lymphokines**. *Interleukins-2, -4,* and *-5* activate resting B-lymphocytes into B-immunoblasts (Section 14.28.1). Interleukins-2 and -4 also promote the differentiation of T cells. *Interferon-γ* (Abbas *et al.*, 1994, p. 254) is an activator of macrophages and neutrophils, a stimulator of natural killer cells (Section 14.30.5), an antiviral agent, a possible stimulator of cytotoxic T cell differentiation, and an inducer of class II MHC molecules in 'non-professional' antigen-presenting cells). *Lymphotoxin* is an even more potent activator of neutrophils, and may contribute to the lysis of cells by cytotoxic T cells (Abbas *et al.*, 1994, p. 256).

Cytotoxic T cells also produce **lymphokines**. These include *interferon-γ, lymphotoxin,* and *tumour necrosis factor* (Abbas *et al.*, 1994, p. 273). The tumour necrosis factor powerfully activates neutrophils to kill micro-organisms, and stimulates mononuclear phagocytes to produce their own monokines; it also induces adhesiveness between endothelial cells and neutrophils, monocytes, and lymphocytes, thus contributing importantly to the accumulation of these defensive cells at sites of inflammation (Abbas *et al.*, 1994, p. 246).

Mononuclear phagocytes secrete the following series of potent **monokines** that mediate natural immunity against viral and bacterial infections (Abbas *et al.*, 1994, pp. 243–251). *Type 1 interferon* inhibits the replication of viruses and increases the action of natural killer cells in killing virally infected cells, thus helping substantially to eradicate viral infections. *Tumour necrosis factor* helps the accumulation of defensive cells at sites of inflammation, as just described. *Interleukin-1* has similar biological effects to those of tumour necrosis factor, acting by inducing leucocyte adhesion and causing macrophages to produce monokines that activate neutrophils to kill micro-organisms. *Chemokines* attract neutrophils to sites of acute inflammation.

All of the cytokines mentioned in the three preceding paragraphs *promote* immune responses, and thus are '**pro-inflammatory cytokines**'. Another group has the opposite effect – *inhibition* of immune responses: these are **immunosuppressive cytokines**. Of these, *transforming growth factor-β* (TGF-β) is potentially important because it inhibits many responses of lymphocytes (Abbas *et al.*, 1994, p. 254). For example, it inhibits the maturation of cytotoxic T cells, and counteracts the effects of pro-inflammatory cytokines on polymorphonuclear leucocytes. It is synthesized by helper T cells, some B cells, and mononuclear phagocytes. *Interleukin-10* (Abbas *et al.*, 1994, p. 256) inhibits the pro-inflammatory effects of tumour necrosis factor, interleukin-1, and chemokine. The **immunosuppression** created naturally by these immunosuppressive cytokines is supported **therapeutically**, particularly to prevent **graft rejection**, by various methods (Abbas *et al.*, 1994, p. 347). *Corticosteroids* may lyse T cells, but more probably block the synthesis of pro-inflammatory cytokines by mononuclear phagocytes. *Cyclosporin A*, a fungal peptide metabolite, is the most important immunosuppressive agent in current clinical use (Abbas *et al.*, 1994, p. 348): it blocks the action of IL-2 in inducing the growth and differentiation of T cells.

The above cytokines are only a selection of this large family of proteins that mediate both natural and acquired immunity. A particular cytokine is often produced by several types of cell and may thus be both a lymphokine and a monokine, and one cytokine often acts on many types of cell. The general complexity of cytokines is shown by the fact that the interaction between the T helper cell and the B-lymphocyte (progressing through B-immunoblasts, B cells, plasma cells, and the formation of IgG) requires the integrated action of at least ten agents, i.e. seven types of interleukin, interferon-γ, tumour necrosis factor, and a lymphotoxin (J.B. Dixon, personal communication, 1996).

14.31.3 *Oxidizing agents*

Neutrophils and macrophages release powerful **oxidizing agents** that are lethal, even in very small quantities, to bacteria and fungi (Maly and Schürer-Maly, 1995). These oxidants include superoxide (O_2^-), hydrogen peroxide (H_2O_2), and hydroxyl ions (—OH). The enzyme responsible for generating **superoxide** is known as **NADPH oxidase** (NADPH is nicotinamide adenine dinucleotide phosphate bound with hydrogen). The enzyme is lodged in the membrane of the **phagosome**, which is a cytoplasmic vesicle containing phagocytized material.

Physiological stimuli that activate NADPH oxidase in phagocytes include ingestion of bacteria, immune complexes, lymphokines such as tumour necrosis factor, interferon-γ, and chemotactic peptides (Maly and Schürer-Maly, 1995). The first product of this process is superoxide, but this in turn forms a complex of more potent oxidants including hydrogen peroxide.

Overactivity of NADPH oxidase is involved in a wide variety of **pathophysiological mechanisms** (Maly and Schürer-Maly, 1995), including impairment of T-lymphocytes and cytotoxicity against endothelial cells, and various acute and chronic inflammatory conditions, e.g. bacterial sepsis, rheumatic diseases, and vasculitis.

Superoxide generation, and expression of NADPH oxidase, have now been found in a wide variety of non-phagocytic cell types. These include the granular cells of the **carotid body**, and the cells of neonatal pulmonary **neuroepithelial bodies** (Section 6.12.1), all of which sense oxygen concentration and initiate responses to **hypoxia** (Sections 4.16.4; 19.9.3). It also occurs in B lymphocytes where it has been thoroughly studied at cellular, biochemical, and molecular levels.

14.31.4 *Reactive nitrogen and non-oxidative agents*

Macrophages do not rely solely on oxidants as a direct weapon against micro-organisms, but also employ the reactive **nitric oxide radical** (**NO·**). The production of **NO·** by macrophages is activated by interferon-γ and by endotoxins (Section 13.6). The NO· radical is also highly important in the regulation of vascular tone when released by endothelial cells in response to stress caused by the flow of blood (Section 13.6). Macrophages also utilize a variety of **non-oxidative** agents such as **proteases** and **bactericidal peptides** (Maly and Schürer-Maly, 1995).

14.31.5 *Surfactant*

Surfactant (Section 6.25) has been shown to have a bactericidal effect (Junqueira and Carneiro, 1983, p. 378).

V   LYMPHOCENTRES AND LYMPH NODES

14.32   Lymphocentres

There are many named lymph nodes in the mammalian body, and their presence and site vary with the species. However, the lymph nodes can be grouped into a much smaller number of **lymphocentres**, each occurring in all species and at essentially the same site, and receiving its afferent vessels from the same region in most species. The lymphocentre is therefore a useful simplification.

For clinical and pathological purposes, it is advisable for the veterinarian to be particularly aware of (a) 'key' lymphocentres, i.e. those that receive *all* the drainage from each of the main regions of the body, such as the thorax and abdomen, and (b) individual lymph nodes that are of particular *diagnostic* or *surgical interest*.

The **general characteristics** of named lymph nodes vary with the species. In the ruminants and carnivores, the named nodes are typically represented by a single large elongated node. (For example, the jejunal nodes of the ox are sometimes fused into one continuous node, up to 100 cm in length.) In the pig up to six nodes typically represent one named node, and in the horse up to several dozen from a few millimetres to 1 or 2 cm in diameter are typically assembled together as one named 'lymph node'.

Six major regions of the body are drained by 'key' lymphocentres (Fig. 14.11), namely the head, neck, forelimb, thorax, abdomen, and the hind limb and pelvis together. The lymphocentres that drain the neck and forelimb help to drain the thoracic wall, and thus contribute to the general drainage of the thorax.

14.32.1 *Head*

The key lymphocentre of the head is the **retropharyngeal lymphocentre** (Fig. 14.11). All

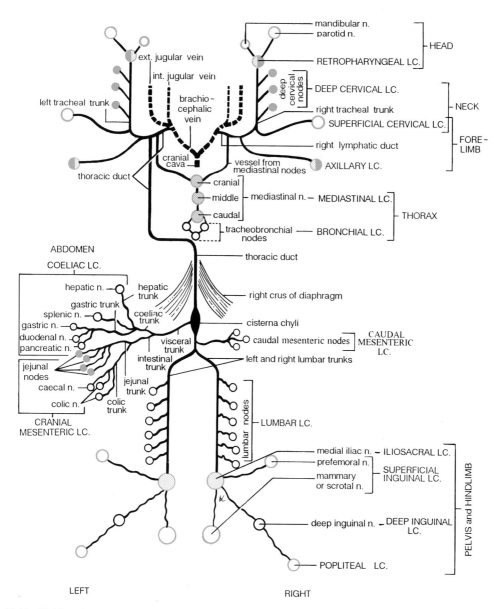

Fig. 14.11 Highly schematic diagram of the lymphocentres that drain the main regions of the body in a hypothetical mammal. Each main region of the body (head, neck, forelimb, thorax, abdomen, hind limb) is drained by one, or often two, 'key' lymphocentres (LC) that ultimately receive all the lymph from that region. These key lymphocentres are: head, retropharyngeal LC; neck, superficial cervical LC and deep cervical LC; forelimb, superficial cervical and axillary LC; thorax, mediastinal LC and bronchial LC; abdomen, coeliac LC and cranial mesenteric LC; pelvic structures and hind limb, iliosacral LC. Four important examples of these key lymphocentres, i.e. retropharyngeal LC, axillary LC, mediastinal LC, and iliosacral LC, are stippled green. Lymph nodes palpable when abnormally enlarged are shown in full green. Nodes half stippled and half green (e.g. retropharyngeal node) are key lymphocentres palpable if enlarged. Lymph nodes shown as green rings are palpable in the normal ox and dog (except that the prefemoral node is present in only a minority of dogs, and the popliteal node is not palpable in the ox). Nodes drawn as black circles are not palpable. The thoracic duct drains the lumbar trunks (pelvis, hindlimb), visceral trunk (gastrointestinal tract), mediastinal nodes (thoracic viscera), and left tracheal trunk (head, neck, forelimb, on the left side). The right lymphatic duct drains the right tracheal duct (head, neck, forelimb, on the right side) and mediastinal nodes (thoracic viscera). All lymph empties into the great veins (broken lines) at the thoracic inlet.

the lymph from the structures of the head eventually drains through it.

14.32.2 Neck

There are two key lymphocentres in the neck, the superficial cervical lymphocentre and the deep cervical lymphocentre.

The skin and superficial muscles drain into the **superficial cervical lymphocentre** cranial to the shoulder joint. A prominent component of this lymphocentre is the **superficial cervical lymph node** (Fig. 14.12), which was previously known as the **prescapular node** – topographically, a much more meaningful name). The deep structures of the neck drain into the **deep cervical lymphocentre**, which extends from the thyroid gland and along the trachea (represented by the **deep cervical lymph nodes** in Fig. 14.11). Both the superficial and the deep cervical lymphocentres on the left and right sides of the neck, including all their nodes, drain respectively into the left and right **tracheal ducts** (Section 14.35.1) (Figs 14.11, 14.12).

The **superficial cervical lymphocentre** (lymphocentrum cervicale superficiale) comprises the relatively prominent superficial cervical (prescapular) node (or nodes, in the horse) which can be palpated cranial to the supraspinatus muscle (Fig. 14.12), and the smaller dorsal, medial, and ventral superficial cervical nodes. These drain the skin and superficial structures of the neck, the thoracic limb, and the thoracic wall. The **deep cervical lymphocentre** (lymphocentrum cervicale profundum) comprises a chain of deep cervical lymph nodes (lymphonodi cervicales profundi) along the left and right side of the trachea (Fig. 14.12), draining the deep cervical structures.

14.32.3 Forelimb

There are two key lymphocentres for the forelimb, the **superficial cervical lymphocentre** and the **axillary lymphocentre**. The skin and muscles of the forelimb drain into these two lymphocentres (Fig. 14.11). The axillary lymphocentre (represented by the **axillary lymph node** in Fig. 14.12) lies in the axillary space, caudal to the shoulder joint. Both of these two key lymphocentres drain into the tracheal duct on the corresponding side (Figs 14.11, 14.12).

Much of the skin and musculature of the forelimb, especially the proximal parts but also many distal structures including even the digital joints, drain into the **superficial cervical lymphocentre** (superficial cervical node) (Figs 14.11, 14.12) (Schummer et al., 1981, pp. 312, 317). Most of the deeper parts of the limb, and some skin, drain into the **axillary lymphocentre** (Schummer et al., 1981, p. 317). The **axillary lymphocentre** (centrum axillare) comprises in all species the various axillary lymph nodes (lymphonodi axillares) in the axilla, and in the horse the cubital nodes (lymphonodi cubitales) lying medio-proximal to the elbow (Schaller et al., 1992, p. 404). The axillary lymphocentre also drains the cranial mammary glands in the bitch (Section 14.33.2).

14.32.4 Thorax

The thoracic viscera (heart, lungs, trachea, oesophagus, and pleura) have two key lymphocentres, the bronchial lymphocentre and the mediastinal lymphocentre. The **bronchial lymphocentre** (represented by the **tracheobronchial lymph nodes** in Fig. 14.11) lies at the bifurcation of the trachea: the **mediastinal lymphocentre** (represented by unpaired **mediastinal lymph nodes** in Fig. 14.11) is in the cranial mediastinum. Both of these lymphocentres drain the heart, lungs, trachea, oesophagus, and pleura, directly. The bronchial lymphocentre itself drains secondarily into the mediastinal centre. The mediastinal lymphocentre is therefore the ultimate filtration point for all the thoracic viscera, a useful generalization for the morbid anatomist and meat inspector. The mediastinal lymphocentre drains into the thoracic duct and right lymphatic duct (Fig. 14.11).

The **mediastinal lymphocentre** (lymphocentrum mediastinale) comprises cranial, middle, and caudal mediastinal nodes (lymphonodi mediastinales – craniales, medii, caudales) (Schaller et al., 1992, p. 406). These nodes are in the cranial, middle, and caudal mediastinum respectively, and are therefore unpaired. The **bronchial lymphocentre** (lymphocentrum bronchale) comprises left, right, middle, and cranial tracheobronchial lymph nodes (Saar and Getty, 1975, pp. 623, 1033, 1349, 1656). The **left tracheobronchial node** (lymphonodus tracheobronchalis sinister) lies on the cranial surface of the left principal bronchus at the bifurcation of the trachea. This is a large node in the ox (about 2.5 cm × 3.5 cm) (Saar and Getty, 1975, p. 1033), but is partly concealed by the arch of the aorta and the left pulmonary artery. The **right tracheobronchial node** (lymphonodus tracheobronchalis dexter) is small and

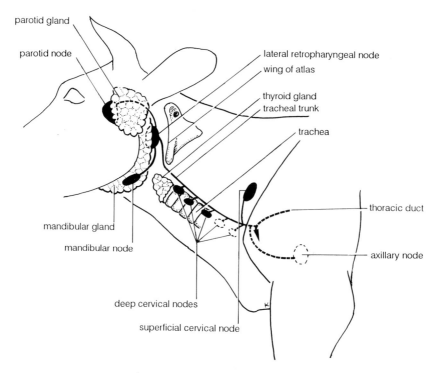

Fig. 14.12 Semidiagrammatic view of the left side of the head, neck, and forelimb of an ox, showing the approximate position of the main lymph nodes and left tracheal duct. The mandibular and parotid nodes can be palpated in the normal animal, and sometimes the lateral retropharyngeal node if the head is extended. All lymph from the head drains through the retropharyngeal lymphocentre. The deep cervical nodes drain the structures related to the trachea; they are not normally palpable. The superficial cervical node is normally palpable along the cranial border of supraspinatus muscle. It drains the neck, thoracic wall, and forelimb. The axillary node lies in the axillary space, caudal to the shoulder. It drains the deep parts of the forelimb. The left tracheal duct empties into the end of the thoracic duct.

inconstant in the ox, on the cranial aspect of the origin of the right principal bronchus from the trachea (de Lahunta and Habel, 1986, p. 200). The **middle tracheobronchial node** lies in the midline, caudal to the tracheal bifurcation. The **cranial tracheobronchial node** occurs in ruminants and the pig, at the right side of the trachea on the ventral aspect of the root of the **tracheal bronchus**. The **pulmonary lymph nodes**, deep in the parenchyma of the lung, are inconstant (Section 7.9.1). The thorax possesses two other lymphocentres, the **dorsal** and **ventral thoracic lymphocentres** (lymphocentrum thoracicum – dorsale, ventrale). These comprise aortic, intercostal (near the heads of the ribs), sternal, and (at the caval foramen in the diaphragm) phrenic nodes, and drain the thoracic walls. Of this group of nodes, the **aortic nodes** (lymphonodi thoracici aortici) are relatively important, since they are often examined in **meat inspection** (Section 14.33).

The lymphatic pathways from the thoracic cavity of the horse, ox, and pig were reviewed by Saar and Getty (1975, pp. 622, 1032, 1349) and those of the dog by Bezuidenhout (1993, p. 717). In all of these species,

lymph from the mediastinum and from the pleura in general flows into all of the four **thoracic lymphocentres**, i.e. the dorsal thoracic, ventral thoracic, mediastinal, and bronchial lymphocentres (see Schaller *et al.*, 1992, p. 406). Some lymph from the caudal regions of the thorax drains into the lumbar lymphocentre (Hare, 1975, p. 132).

14.32.5 *Abdomen*

The abdomen has two key lymphocentres, the **coeliac lymphocentre** and the **cranial mesenteric lymphocentre** (Fig. 14.11), draining the organs supplied by the coeliac and cranial mesenteric arteries, respectively.

14.32.6 *Pelvic structures and hind limb*

These regions have one key lymphocentre, the **iliosacral lymphocentre** (represented by the medial iliac node in Fig. 14.11). All lymph from the pelvic wall, pelvic organs, and the several lesser lymphocentres of the hind limb, drains ultimately through this lymphocentre.

14.33 Lymph nodes of special diagnostic or surgical interest

As stated in Section 14.32, the named lymph nodes in the domestic ruminants and carnivores are typically represented by a single large elongated node. In the pig a group of up to six smaller nodes typically represent one named node, and in the horse up to several dozen small or very small nodes are typically assembled together as one named 'lymph node'. Because of their relatively large size, bovine and canine lymph nodes can be palpated in the normal living animal more readily than equine nodes.

Lymph nodes filter out noxious agents such as bacteria and toxins. The resulting immune response within a node causes it to enlarge and sometimes to become painful on palpation. Detection of an enlarged node by palpation during the **physical examination** of an animal alerts the clinician to possible infection of the tissues or organ drained by that node. At **post-mortem**, the examination of the succession of lymph nodes that drain an infected area enables the pathologist to trace the sequence of events by which an infection has developed and spread, or allows the meat inspector to assess how far infection has involved other tissues; at **meat inspection**, the spread of pathological changes may determine whether the organ alone, or a part or all of the carcase, must be condemned as unfit for human consumption. Neoplastic cells from an organ containing a malignant tumour may be filtered out by the lymph nodes that drain that organ, resulting in the development of secondary tumours (metastases) within these nodes; this possibility may require the **surgeon** to remove not only the primary tumour but also the lymph nodes that drain it. All these procedures are encountered in veterinary practice, and all of them depend on a knowledge of the sites of lymph nodes and of the tissues or organs that they drain.

Many lymph nodes are too small or too deep in the body to be palpated. However, some lymph nodes are **palpable in the normal live animal**. In the head, such nodes include the **mandibular node** in the intermandibular space in the dog, ox, and horse (Fig. 14.12), and the **parotid node** in the ox and dog under the parotid gland (Fig. 14.12), and the **retropharyngeal nodes** in the ox (externally, or through the mouth, though with difficulty). In the neck, the **superficial cervical (prescapular) node** can be palpated in the dog, ox, and horse (Fig. 14.12). In the forelimb the axillary node (Fig. 14.12) is palpable in the dog only. The cubital node is palpable in the normal horse.

In the abdomen of the horse, the **jejunal lymph nodes** can always be palpated per rectum, if the animal is thin. No other nodes are palpable in the thorax and abdomen of the normal animal.

Of the many nodes in the pelvic region and hind limb, only the prefemoral, scrotal, mammary, and popliteal nodes are palpable in normal animals. The very large **prefemoral (subiliac) node** of the ox and horse is easily felt at the cranial aspect of the thigh; this node is absent in the dog. The **mammary nodes** of the cow can be found by lifting the udder from behind and palpating the space between the thighs. Mammary nodes of the mare and bitch can also be palpated. The **scrotal nodes** can be palpated in the dog, stallion, and bull. In the normal animal, the popliteal node is palpable in the dog.

National, and in Europe international, regulations prescribe the compulsory examination by a veterinarian of certain nodes of food animals at **meat inspection**. These regulations may be modified, but Schummer *et al.* (1981, pp. 338–339) report that in principle the following nodes *must* be examined (others are examined in particular circumstances): **Head**: parotid, mandibular, lateral retropharyngeal, and medial retropharyngeal nodes. **Thorax**: cranial, middle, and caudal mediastinal nodes; left, right, middle, and cranial tracheobronchial nodes; aortic nodes. **Abdomen**: gastric nodes (in pig and horse); splenic nodes (in ruminants); hepatic, jejunal, caecal, colic, and caudal mesenteric nodes (in all food species). **Pelvic region**: scrotal and mammary nodes.

The **concept of lymphocentres** offers a useful overview of the lymph nodes of the domestic mammals. However, a veterinarian needing exact knowledge of species variations for pathology, meat inspection, or surgery, cannot avoid referring to more detailed anatomical sources. Fortunately, the study of the topographical anatomy of the lymphatic system in the domestic species has been one of the strong points of veterinary anatomy since the classic investigations at Dresden and Leipzig by Hermann Baum between the two world wars. These researches have formed the basis of two excellent contemporary accounts in English of the systematic anatomy of the lymphatic system, namely that by Saar and Getty in the 1975 edition of *Sisson and Grossman's Anatomy of the Domestic Animals*, and the masterly survey by Schummer *et al.* (1981) in the English translation of Vol. 3 of *Lehrbuch der Anatomie der Haustiere*.

The applied anatomy of the lymph nodes in the domestic mammals has been thoroughly reviewed by de Lahunta and Habel (1986); the following account of applied aspects of nodes in the thoracic region is based on their survey.

14.33.1   *Neck*

The only cervical node that can be palpated in the normal animal is the **superficial cervical node** (prescapular node) (Fig. 14.12). In the **ox**, this is a very large node (about 3 cm × 10 cm), in the groove along the cranial border of the supraspinatus muscle; it can be felt by sliding the fingers away from the supraspinatus muscle and towards the head. In the **dog**, it can be identified by drawing the limb caudally and palpating the cranial border of the supraspinatus muscle, slightly dorsal to the level of the acromion.

14.33.2   *Forelimb*

The **axillary node** can be palpated in the **dog**. If the limb is drawn cranially, the node can be palpated at the level of the shoulder joint over the first intercostal space or second rib (Schummer *et al.*, 1981, p. 342). This node is of interest in mammary carcinoma in the bitch.

14.33.3   *Thorax*

The tracheobronchial and caudal mediastinal nodes of the **bovine 'pluck'** (heart, lungs, and oesophagus) are examined during meat inspection. The node that is most easily examined is the **cranial tracheobronchial node**. This lies at the right side of the trachea on the ventral aspect of the root of the **tracheal bronchus**. The **left tracheobronchial node** is larger, but is concealed by the aorta and left pulmonary trunk, which have to be cut to expose the node.

The **caudal mediastinal nodes** in the **ox** are a group of several nodes, some of which are very large (up to 10 cm long) extending caudally to the diaphragm (Saar and Getty, 1975, p. 1033). Enlargement of this node caused by tuberculosis or lymphosarcoma can compress the

oesophagus and cause choke or bloat; it can also damage the dorsal and ventral vagal trunks and derange gastric motility.

VI   LYMPHATIC DUCTS

14.34   Thoracic duct

The lymphatic vascular system ends by discharging its lymph into one or other of the great veins at the thoracic inlet (Fig. 14.11). In principle the connections occur at the point where the left and right **external jugular veins** join the other great veins; often the connections are into the external jugular vein itself. Thus the **thoracic duct** empties close to the caudal end of the left external jugular vein, and the **right lymphatic duct** ends close to the caudal end of the right external jugular vein.

The thoracic duct (Fig. 14.11) returns lymph from the whole body, except the regions drained by the right lymphatic duct. It begins as a slender dilation, the **cisterna chyli** (Fig. 14.11), lying in the aortic hiatus between the crura of the diaphragm (Fig. 9.5). The thoracic duct continues from the cranial end of the cistern, entering the caudal part of the mediastinum. Caudal to the heart it lies on the right dorsal side of the aorta. At the level of the heart (and therefore at about the fifth thoracic vertebra) it crosses to the left side and dips ventrally. It then passes cranially along the left surface of the thoracic oesophagus (or thoracic trachea) to the thoracic inlet, where it ends by opening into the great veins in the thoracic inlet, as just described. It is thin walled and has many valves.

Usually the **cisterna chyli** lies on the right dorsal aspect of the aorta, between the aorta and the bodies of the lumbar vertebrae (Fig. 9.5). The **thoracic duct** (ductus thoracicus) emerges from the aortic hiatus, and enters the thoracic cavity on the right side of the aorta. The only exception to this node of entry occurs in the ox, in which the duct passes through a gap in the muscle of the right crus of the diaphragm, instead of through the aortic hiatus (Schummer *et al.*, 1981, p. 403). The thoracic duct always arises from the cisterna chyli as a single trunk in the pig and ruminants, but in the horse and dog it is usually double, and in the dog there may be three trunks (Schummer *et al.*, 1981, p. 322). The duct tends to be somewhat plexiform rather than a simple tube. In the dog, horse, and ox, there is often an **ampulla** at its cranial end. In all the domestic species there are about 10–15 **valves** along the course of the duct. The actual **orifice** is closed by a pair of valves, a single valve, or a narrowing of the lumen. Despite the presence of a pair of valves, in the horse at post-mortem there is always a retrograde flow of blood into the duct. **Histologically**, the thoracic duct resembles a medium sized vein, except for being somewhat more muscular (Section 14.6.2).

The **lymph in the thoracic duct** is transparent and slightly yellow in the fasting animal. After a fatty meal it becomes turbid and more yellow, from the presence of minute fatty globules (0.03–0.5 μm in diameter) known as **chylomicrons**. About 80–90% of all **fat** absorbed by the gut is transported to the blood by the thoracic duct in the form of chylomicrons (Guyton, 1986, p. 796). In the small intestine most triglycerides are split into monoglycerides and fatty acids. In the intestinal epithelial cells these are resynthesized into triglycerides which aggregate into globules. The epithelial cells extrude the globules into the interstitial space by exocytosis. From there, the globules enter the lymph in the central lacteal of the intestinal villus, and are now called chylomicrons.

The discontinuous endothelial lining of the hepatic sinusoids (Section 12.13) allows the **liver** to form large quantities of lymph, with a high protein content only slightly less than that of blood plasma. Consequently about half of the total volume of lymph that is formed by the body at rest, and discharged by the thoracic duct into the great veins, comes from the liver (Guyton, 1986, p. 836).

Rupture of the thoracic duct occurs in man, and in the cat and dog. It can be caused by mediastinal surgery, such as incision of the oesophagus, or by trauma such as rupture of the diaphragm through being run over, or by neoplastic invasion. Rupture of the duct causes accumulation of lymph in the mediastinum, followed by bursting of the mediastinal pleura and escape of lymph into either the left or the right pleural cavities, or into both pleural cavities. The loss of protein through the rupture reduces the oncotic pressure of the blood plasma generally, leading to a tendency for oedema (Section 14.9.3).

14.35   Lymphatic trunks draining into thoracic duct

14.35.1   *Left and right tracheal trunks*

The **left tracheal trunk** (truncus trachealis) (Figs 14.11, 14.12) drains the lymph from the left side of the head and neck, the left thoracic wall, and the left forelimb. It descends the neck, starting along the left side of the cervical oesophagus and continuing on the left side of the cervical trachea.

It usually discharges caudally into the end of the thoracic duct, or directly into the left external jugular vein or one of the other great veins at the thoracic inlet.

The **right tracheal trunk** (Fig. 14.11) drains the same territory as the left trunk, but on the *right* side of the head and neck. It runs its whole course in contact with the right side of the trachea. It ends at the thoracic inlet by uniting with the efferent lymphatic vessels from the **superficial cervical lymphocentre** to form the **right lymphatic duct** (Fig. 14.11).

14.35.2   *Left and right efferent vessels from cranial mediastinal lymphocentre*

These pathways (Fig. 14.11) drain lymph from the thoracic viscera into the thoracic duct on the left side, and into the right lymphatic duct on the right side.

14.35.3   *Visceral trunk*

The unpaired visceral trunk (Fig. 14.11) collects lymph from the lymphocentres of the gastrointestinal tract, and empties into the cisterna chyli.

The **visceral trunk** (truncus visceralis) (Schaller *et al.*, 1992, p. 402) receives the coeliac trunk and intestinal trunk (Fig. 14.11). The **coeliac trunk** drains the coeliac lymphocentre by two tributaries, namely the **hepatic trunk** from the hepatic nodes, and the **gastric trunk** from the gastric nodes (Fig. 14.11). The **intestinal trunk** drains the cranial mesenteric lymphocentre, again by two tributaries, one being the **jejunal trunk** from the jejunal nodes, and the other being the **colic trunk** from the colic nodes (Fig. 14.11).

14.35.4   *Lumbar trunks*

The paired lumbar trunks (truncus lumbalis) are formed by the efferent vessels from the left and right **medial iliac lymph nodes** (left and right **iliosacral lymphocentres**), and empty into the cisterna chyli (Fig. 14.11). Since all the lymphocentres of the pelvic region and hind limb drain through the medial iliac lymph nodes (Fig. 14.11), the lumbar trunks drain all the lymph from the caudal parts of the body (pelvic musculature and viscera, external genitalia, the pelvic components of the mammary glands, and the hind limbs). They also drain the **lumbar lymphocentre**, which includes important nodes in the caudo-dorsal region of the abdominal cavity (notably the renal, and gonadal nodes).

14.36   Right lymphatic duct

The **right lymphatic duct** (ductus lymphaticus dexter) is a short vessel formed by the union of the **right tracheal trunk** with the efferent lym-phatic vessel from the **right superficial cervical lymphocentre** (Fig. 14.11). It receives only one tributary, i.e. an efferent vessel (or vessels) from the **mediastinal lymphocentre** (Fig. 14.11). The right lymphatic duct therefore drains the right side of the head and neck, the right forelimb, the right thoracic wall, the parietal and visceral pleura, the lungs, and the heart.

The right lymphatic duct empties into the great veins at the thoracic inlet, near the end of the **right external jugular vein** (Fig. 14.11).

Chapter 15
Development of the Heart and Great Vessels

I DEVELOPMENT OF THE HEART

15.1 Endocardial tubes and simple tubular heart

The heart arises in the mesoderm from the paired endocardial tubes (Fig. 15.1A). At first these two tubes consist of endocardium only, but they soon become enclosed by thickened splanchnic mesoderm (Figs 8.26, 8.27) which adds the **epi-myocardium** (Fig. 8.27). The epi-myocardium differentiates into the thin serous **epicardium** and the thick muscular **myocardium**; the epicardium is also known as the **visceral pericardium** (Fig. 8.28; Section 20.2).

At this early stage, therefore, the primordial heart has a left chamber and a right chamber. However, these paired chambers are quickly lost by the early fusion of the mid-portion of the two endocardial tubes into a midline tubular heart (Figs 8.28, 15.1B). Cranially and caudally the paired primordial tubes persist, forming the paired **ventral aortae** cranially and the paired **vitelline veins** caudally.

> The zone between the developing myocardium and the walls of the endocardial tubes is filled with the **cardiac jelly** (cardioglia) (Fig. 8.28). This is a viscous fluid (Noden and de Lahunta, 1985, p. 232) rich in collagen and glycoproteins, that gives the myocardium enough freedom of movement to act as a pump. It also provides a medium for mesenchymal cells to migrate in order to form connective tissues in the cardiac septa and valves.

15.2 Formation of the sigmoid heart

The simple midline tubular heart now elongates. The ventral aortae and vitelline veins firmly an-chor it cranially and caudally within the pericardial sac. Therefore elongation is only possible by bending the heart into an S-shaped loop, thus forming the **sigmoid** (S-shaped) **heart** (Figs 15.1C, 15.2A). As Fig. 15.2A shows, the main elements of this loop are the primitive bulbus cordis and the primitive ventricle. The loop is therefore known as the **bulboventricular loop**.

At first the bulboventricular loop bulges to the *right* side of the embryo as in Figs 15.1C and 15.2A, but continuous rapid growth then causes it to bulge in the *ventral* direction also, as in Fig. 15.2B. This brings the ventricle into its definitive position, caudoventral to the atrium.

During the formation of the sigmoid heart, the primary subdivisions of the heart become clearly differentiated. The great veins enter the thin-walled **sinus venosus**. The **primitive atrium** develops as a dilated region marked off by external constrictions (Fig. 15.2B). The **primitive ventricle** and **primitive bulbus cordis** together form the bulboventricular loop. The most cranial part of the original cardiac tube continues more or less unchanged into the **truncus arteriosus**, which in turn gives rise to the left and right **ventral aortae**.

Further demands for space cause the two components of the bulboventricular loop, i.e. the primitive ventricle and the primitive bulbus cordis, to become pressed together along the bulboventricular sulcus (Fig. 15.2B); this relationship enables the bulbus to be absorbed into the ventricle.

> Since the S-shaped form of the sigmoid heart bends laterally, vertically, and longitudinally, it is actually a spiralled S, in three dimensions (Arey, 1958, p. 349).
>
> The precise origin of the definitive **right ventricle** is uncertain. Initially the two components of the **bulboventricular loop** (i.e. the primitive bulbus cordis and primitive ventricle) are separated by their walls, along the bulboventricular sulcus. Noden and de

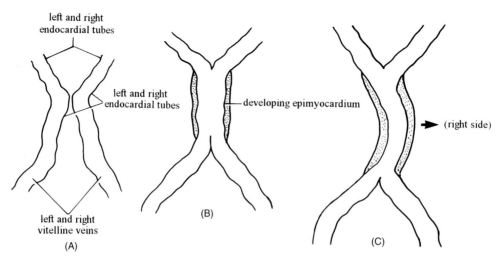

left and right
endocardial tubes

left and right
endocardial tubes

developing epimyocardium

(right side)

left and right
vitelline veins

(A)

(B)

(C)

Fig. 15.1 Schematic dorsal view diagrams showing the formation of the simple tubular heart from the paired endocardial tubes. The endocardial tubes are drawn as though transparent.

A. The left and right endocardial tubes lie parallel with each other, but have almost grown into contact with each other at their cranial ends.

B. The left and right endocardial tubes have fused in their midsection, forming a simple tubular heart in the midline. The wall of the tubular heart is being invested by the developing myocardium. Paired tubes persist at the caudal end as the right and left vitelline veins, and at the cranial end as the right and left ventral aortae.

C. Since the simple tubular heart is anchored at its caudal and cranial ends by the vitelline veins and ventral aortae, elongation begins to force it to bend laterally, to the right side (arrow), foreshadowing the sigmoid heart.

Lahunta (1985, p. 245) suggested that expansion of the primitive ventricle and primitive bulbus forms 'most' of the right ventricle. Arey (1958, p. 351) followed an earlier suggestion (attributed to Keith) that, while the rest of the heart rapidly enlarges, the bulboventricular sulcus either fails to keep pace or actually atrophies, thus leading to the merging of the two chambers. Williams *et al.* (1989, p. 211) concluded that 'it is uncertain whether the definitive right ventricle is solely a derivative of the common ventricle, or of the caudal end of the primitive bulbus, or both'.

The **sinus venosus** receives venous blood from the paired vitelline, common cardinal, and umbilical veins. The venous return progressively increases to the right side of the sinus venosus and diminishes to the left, until finally it all goes to the right side. The right component of the sinus venosus then becomes entirely incorporated into the right atrium, receiving the cranial and caudal caval flows. The left part of the sinus venosus becomes the coronary sinus (Noden and de Lahunta, 1985, p. 238).

The dorsal and ventral **mesocardiums** (Fig. 8.27) are thin and flexible, and the ventral one degenerates anyway (Fig. 8.28), thus allowing the tubular heart to become contorted into its S configuration (Noden and de Lahunta, 1985, p. 235).

15.3 Formation of the four-chambered heart

15.3.1 *Atrioventricular endocardial cushions*

In the sigmoid heart the primitive atrium connects with the primitive ventricle through a common **atrioventricular canal** (Fig. 15.3A). Two buttress-like projections, the cranial and caudal **atrioventricular endocardial cushions**, grow towards each other (Fig. 15.3A) and eventually fuse, thus dividing the original common atrioventricular opening into a **left** and **right atrioventricular canal**.

Endocardial cushion tissue consists of plastic masses of peculiar, loosely organized, modified mesenchyme. It forms the tissue of all the various septa that eventually separate the four chambers of the heart, i.e. not only the atrioventricular cushions but also the interventricular septum, the bulbar septum in the bulbus cordis, and the aorticopulmonary septum in the truncus arteriosus

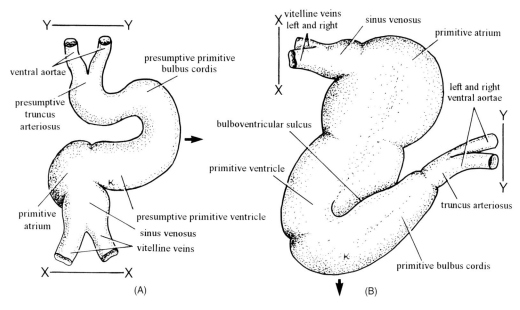

Fig. 15.2   Schematic diagrams showing the bending of the sigmoid heart. A. *Dorsal view* of a stage following soon after that shown in Fig. 15.1C. The developing heart is fixed at its caudal end (X–X) and cranial end (Y–Y). Further elongation has compelled the heart to bend much further *laterally* (to the right, arrow). This brings the (presumptive) primitive ventricle and (presumptive) primitive bulbus cordis to the right side of the heart, in the form of a bulboventricular loop.

B. *Lateral view* of the right side of the sigmoid heart, at a slightly later stage than A. Being still fixed at X–X and Y–Y, the elongating heart has been forced to bend *ventrally* (arrow) as well as to the right. The heart is now clearly S-shaped, in both the horizontal plane and the sagittal plane. The bulboventricular loop becomes very tight. The primitive bulbus cordis is pressed firmly against the right lateral surface of the primitive ventricle, along the bulboventricular sulcus. This close apposition enables the bulbus cordis subsequently to be absorbed into, i.e. become a part of, the ventricle. Slight folds indicate the boundaries of the sinus venosus, primitive atrium, primitive ventricle, primitive bulbus cordis, and truncus arteriosus.

(Patten, 1958, pp. 272, 519, 524). It also produces the aortic and pulmonary semilunar valves, and apparently contributes to the cusps of the atrioventricular valves (Williams *et al.*, 1989, p. 212).

15.3.2   *Interventricular septum*

This septum grows dorsally from the ventral floor of the primitive ventricle (Fig. 15.3A,B), gradually dividing the right ventricle from the left ventricle. Eventually it unites with the atrioventricular endocardial cushions and with the spiral septum (Section 15.3.3). Until this union finally occurs, an **interventricular channel** connects the two ventricles (Fig. 15.3A,B).

Completion of the separation of the left from the right ventricle entails complex contributions from the interventricular septum, the bulbar cushions, and the atrioventricular endocardial cushions (Fig. 15.3A). The fusion of the early interventricular septum with

the atrioventricular endocardial cushions creates a circular **interventricular foramen** at the dorsal edge of the interventricular septum (Fig. 15.4A). This foramen is finally plugged by a contribution from an atrioventricular endocardial cushion (Noden and de Lahunta, 1985, p. 245). The very small area of tissue that finally closes this interventricular gap remains thin and fibrous as the **membranous part** of the definitive interventricular septum (Section 20.10). All the rest of the developing interventricular septum becomes thick myocardium.

15.3.3   *Spiral septum*

The primitive bulbus cordis and the truncus arteriosus become divided into the pulmonary trunk and aorta by the **spiral septum**. This septum becomes structurally continuous with the interventricular septum.

In Fig. 15.3A, the spiral septum looks as if it is developing (from two longitudinal ridges) solely

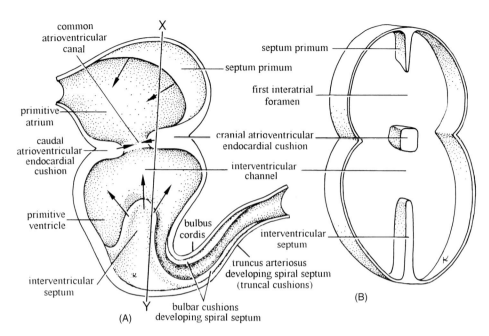

Fig. 15.3 Schematic views of the interior of the developing heart, showing the onset of separation of the left and right chambers. A. The interior of the heart, after removal of its right wall. The cranial and caudal atrioventricular endocardial cushions are advancing towards each other (horizontal arrows), to divide the atrioventricular canal into a right and left channel. The septum primum (first interatrial septum) is descending ventrocaudally (downward arrows) to fuse with the atrioventricular endocardial cushions. The interventricular septum is growing dorsally towards the atrioventricular endocardial cushions (upward arrows). In the bulbus cordis and truncus arteriosus, two spiral ridges (bulbar cushions and truncal cushions) grow towards each other and will fuse to form the spiral septum, thus separating the aorta from the pulmonary trunk. X–Y, the plane of the section in Fig. 15.3B.

B. Transverse section of the developing heart. The section is cut in the plane X–Y in Fig. 15.3A. The septum primum is descending ventrally into the primitive atrium to blend with the atrioventricular endocardial cushions. The interventricular septum is growing dorsally to fuse with the atrioventricular endocardial cushions.

in the *vertical* plane, but in fact the septum rotates along its caudocranial length through about 180°, and is therefore essentially *spiral* as shown in Fig. 15.4A,B. Consequently the pulmonary trunk leaves the right ventricle as a channel in the right half of the truncus arteriosus, but ends up as a channel in the left half: conversely, the aorta leaves the left ventricle as a channel in the left half of the truncus arteriosus, but finishes as a channel in the right half. This spiral arrangement of the septum accounts for the peculiar position of the aorta and pulmonary trunk in relation to the left and right sides of the definitive heart. Thus the pulmonary trunk comes to lie on the *left* side of the definitive heart (Figs 15.6 and 18.1), yet it arises from the *right* ventricle: the aorta lies on the *right* side of the pulmonary trunk, and yet arises from the *left* ventricle.

The **spiral septum** develops in the primitive bulbus cordis and truncus arteriosus of the sigmoid heart (Noden and de Lahunta, 1985, p. 242). It is formed by the growing together of (a) two longitudinal spiral ridges in the bulbus cordis, the **bulbar cushions** (Fig. 15.3A), to form the **bulbar septum**; and (b) two longitudinal spiral ridges in the truncus arteriosus, the **truncal cushions**, to form the **aorticopulmonary septum**. The bulbar septum then becomes continuous (caudocranially) with the aorticopulmonary septum, thus forming the **spiral septum** (Fig. 15.4A,B) dividing the lumen into a pulmonary and an aortic channel.

The mode of formation of the spiral septum is similar in principle to the separation of the right and left atrioventricular channels. Both processes require the fusion of *two* masses of projecting tissue. However, the atrioventricular endocardial cushions are short simple buttresses, whereas the bulbar and truncal cushions are elongated spiral crests.

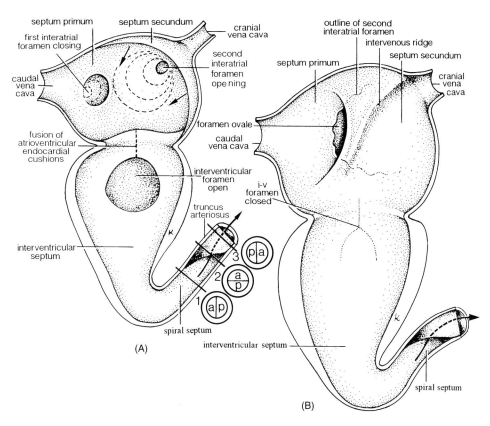

Fig. 15.4 **Schematic views of the interior of the developing right atrium and right ventricle, showing the partitions that separate the right side from the left side of the heart.** The right lateral walls of the right atrium and right ventricle have been removed.

A. The atrioventricular endocardial cushions have fused. The septum primum (first interatrial septum) has almost completely separated the left and right atria, but a small remnant of the first interatrial foramen still allows communication. As the first interatrial foramen closes, the second interatrial foramen opens and progressively widens (rings in broken lines), thus maintaining the communication between the two atria. The septum secundum (second interatrial septum) has begun to descend like a curtain (downward arrows), to the right of the septum primum. The interventricular septum has not yet fused with the atrioventricular endocardial cushions, and therefore an interventricular foramen remains. The truncus arteriosus is divided into the pulmonary trunk and aorta by the spiral septum. The three transverse sections through the bulbus cordis and truncus arteriosus are viewed from their *caudal* aspects, i.e. in the direction of blood flow. They show that the spiral septum has rotated clockwise through 180°. The outflow of the pulmonary trunk (p) from the right ventricle begins on the *right* side of the bulbus cordis (TS 1). The aorta (a) begins on the *left*. Because of the spiral form of the septum, the outflow channel of the pulmonary trunk (arrow) then progresses to the ventral aspect of the truncus (TS 2), and finally emerges on the left aspect of the truncus (TS 3). Thus the pulmonary trunk and aorta change places in the truncus.

B. At this slightly later stage the first interatrial foramen has finally closed. The second interatrial foramen has now attained its full size. It is almost completely covered on its right aspect by the fully developed septum secundum, and has now formed the lumen of the foramen ovale. The septum primum persists as the membranous valvula (flap) of the foramen ovale. The ventricles are now totally separated by closure of the interventricular foramen. An arrow indicates the transfer of the pulmonary trunk from the right side to the left side of the truncus arteriosus. i-v, interventricular.

In its completed form, the spiral septum has rotated through about 180° (Fig. 15.4A, transverse sections 1, 2, and 3). Thus the pulmonary trunk is transferred from its origin from the *right* ventricle, to its exit on the *left* side of the adult heart (Figs 15.6, 20.1): the aorta is trans-ferred from the *left* ventricle to its final position on the *right* aspect of the pulmonary trunk.

The **aortic** and **pulmonary valves** develop as local specializations of the truncal cushions (Patten, 1958, p. 524).

15.3.4 *Interatrial septa*

Two interatrial septa participate in the division of the primitive atrium into the left and right atria. The first interatrial septum, the **septum primum**, descends like a curtain from the craniodorsal part of the primitive atrium, towards the caudal vena cava (Fig. 15.3A,B). It is flexible and membranous, and eventually becomes the **valvula** (flap) of the **foramen ovale** (Fig. 15.5B). The second interatrial septum, the **septum secundum**, descends on the *right* side of the septum primum

(Fig. 15.4A). Its direction of growth is caudoventral, like that of the septum primum. Unlike the septum primum, however, it develops into a thick firm partition; i.e. it becomes the **definitive interatrial septum**.

The caudal edge of the septum secundum, facing the caudal vena cava, has a particularly important function in the fetal circulation: it forms the **crista dividens** (dividing ridge), which splits the oxygenated caudal caval flow into a left stream (via sinistra) and a right stream (via dextra), as in Fig. 15.5B (Section 16.6).

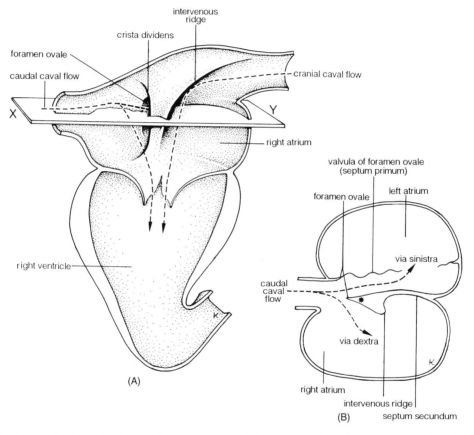

(A)

(B)

Fig. 15.5 Schematic views showing the division of the caudal caval blood flow at the foramen ovale and the ventral deflection of the cranial caval blood flow. A. The interior of the right side of the fetal heart. The oxygenated caudal caval flow strikes the crista dividens, and is split into a left stream which goes through the foramen ovale and enters the left atrium (the via sinistra), and a right stream which enters the right atrium and right ventricle (the via dextra). The deoxygenated cranial caval flow is deflected ventrally into the right ventricle by the concave surface of the intervenous ridge, and thus avoids mixing with the cranial caval flow in the right atrium.

B. A horizontal section through the left and right atria in the plane X–Y in Fig. 15.5A. The caudal caval flow is split by the crista dividens (asterisk). The left stream takes the via sinistra into the left atrium, pushing aside the valvula of the foramen ovale. When the left atrium contracts, the valvula is pressed against the septum secundum, closing the foramen ovale. The right stream takes the via dextra into the right atrium and thence into the right ventricle.

15.3.5 *Interatrial foramina*

In the fetal heart, the interatrial septa allow communication between the left and right atrium by means of three successive interatrial foramina.

The **first interatrial foramen** is formed by the crescentic free edge of the interatrial septum primum, as the septum descends caudoventrally towards the atrioventricular endocardial cushions (Fig. 15.3A). As the septum descends, the first interatrial foramen gets progressively smaller (Fig. 15.4A); it finally closes completely when the septum primum unites with the atrioventricular endocardial cushions.

The **second interatrial foramen** opens as a perforation in the craniodorsal region of the septum primum (Fig. 15.4A,B). It opens just when the first interatrial foramen is about to close, and then enlarges progressively. It becomes the channel of the foramen ovale.

The **foramen ovale** (Fig. 15.4B) is the third and final interatrial foramen. It persists until birth, allowing blood to flow from the right to the left atrium, and then finally closes postnatally (Section 16.20).

15.3.6 *Components of the foramen ovale*

The foramen ovale incorporates the interatrial septum primum and interatrial septum secundum, and the second interatrial foramen (Fig. 15.4B).

The **crista dividens** (dividing ridge) (Figs. 15.5A) is formed by the caudally directed, crescentic free edge of the septum secundum. It is a sharp vertical ridge facing the incoming caudal caval blood (Fig. 15.7). It therefore divides the caudal caval flow into a left stream and a right stream. The left stream takes the left road, the **via sinistra** (Latin: via, road; sinister, left), passing through the foramen ovale into the *left* atrium (Fig. 15.5B). The right stream of caudal caval blood takes the right road, the **via dextra** (Latin: dexter, right), entering the *right* atrium (Fig. 15.5B). The left stream gives the heart and brain a preferential oxygen supply (Section 16.8).

The **valvula** (flap) of the foramen ovale is derived from the septum primum (Fig. 15.5B). In all species it is membranous and flexible. In primates and carnivores it is a simple sheet. In 'ungulates' it is tubular, like a sock with holes where the toes

would be (Figs 15.6, 15.7). This fenestrated sock-like structure in ungulates enables the valvula to form a bung in the foramen ovale and become adherent to the rim of the foramen ovale very soon after birth, thereby quickly eliminating the typical right-to-left shunt in the fetus through the foramen ovale (Section 16.20). In primates and carnivores, fusion of the simple flap to the rim of the foramen ovale postnatally takes much longer than the fusion of the sock-like valvula in ungulates.

In all its forms, the foramen ovale is a one-way valve (Section 16.6) allowing flow from right to left only.

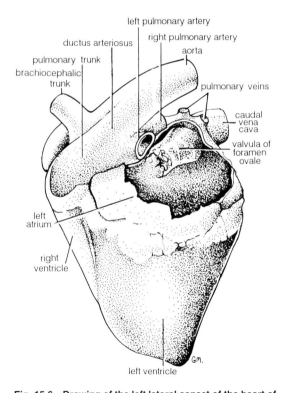

Fig. 15.6 Drawing of the left lateral aspect of the heart of a full term fetal calf, to show the valvula of the foramen ovale and the ductus arteriosus. The wall of the left atrium has been removed to expose the sock-like valvula of the foramen ovale. The peripheral end of the valvula, through which the blood escapes into the left atrium, is perforated by irregular holes. This network of small openings helps the valvula to become anatomically closed soon after birth. The calibre of the ductus arteriosus is similar to that of the aorta.

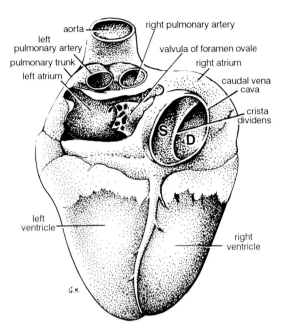

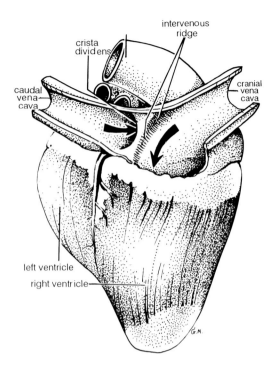

Fig. 15.7 Drawing of the caudal aspect of the heart of a full term fetal calf, to show the crista dividens and the valvula of the foramen ovale. The caudal vena cava has been transected, thus revealing the view presented to a red blood cell as it is about to enter the right atrium. The crescentic edge of the crista dividens offers the erythrocyte a choice between the via dextra (D) into the right atrium, and the via sinistra (S) into the left atrium through the foramen ovale. The wall of the left atrium has been removed to show the sock-like valvula of the foramen ovale, with its perforated end.

Fig. 15.8 Drawing of the right lateral aspect of the heart of a full term fetal calf, to show the crista dividens and intervenous ridge. The lateral walls of the right atrium and cranial and caudal venae cavae have been opened. The intervenous ridge is an arch-like prominence of the interatrial septum. It deflects the cranial caval blood stream into the right ventricle (right arrow), preventing it from colliding in the right atrium with the caudal caval blood stream. Part of the caudal caval blood stream (left arrow) passes to the left of the crista dividens (via sinistra), and therefore goes through the foramen ovale into the left atrium.

15.3.7 *Intervenous ridge*

This is a part of the right surface of the septum secundum (Fig. 15.5A,B). Thus it is a transverse arch, projecting into the cavity of the right atrium from the surface of the definitive interatrial septum (Figs 15.4B, 15.8). The concave aspect of the arch faces *ventrally*, towards the right ventricle. Because of its concavity it deflects the cranial caval blood stream directly into the right ventricle (Fig. 15.5A). It therefore separates the cranial and caudal caval flows (Fig. 15.5A), hence the name 'intervenous' ridge; this is an important function, since it prevents collision, and hence mixing, of the cranial and caudal caval flows in the right atrium (Section 16.8).

The terms crista dividens (dividing ridge), via sinistra, and via dextra are not official terms. They were devised by Barclay, Franklin, and Prichard (1944) in their classic monograph on the fetal circulation, and are retained here because of their functional descriptiveness. Their monograph reported the first cineradiographic observations on fetal blood flow.

The intervenous ridge is the tuberculum intervenosum of the *Nomina Anatomica Veterinaria* (1994).

II DEVELOPMENT OF THE GREAT ARTERIES

15.4 Primordial arteries

In the mammalian embryo, six pairs of aortic arches encircle the pharynx, thus joining the

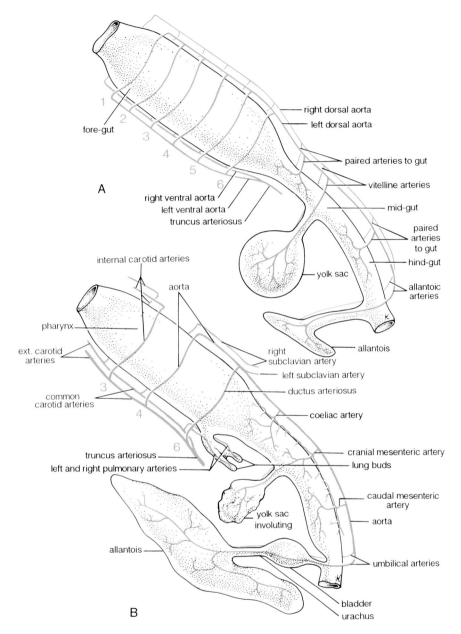

Fig. 15.9 Schematic left lateral views of the developing aortic arches and other principal arteries in the mammal. A. Primordial arteries in a mammalian embryo. Six pairs of aortic arches (1–6) connect the left and right ventral aortae with the left and right dorsal aortae. Paired vitelline and allantoic arteries supply the yolk sac and allantois. Paired arteries supply the gut.

B. Arterial derivatives in a postnatal mammal. The first, second, and fifth pairs of aortic arches disappear. The left and right dorsal aortae fuse caudally to form the single definitive aorta. They drop out between the third and fourth arterial arches; also a short length of the right dorsal aorta is lost caudal to the origin of the right subclavian artery. The remaining arteries are retained and converted as labelled.

paired ventral aortae to the paired dorsal aortae (Figs 15.9A, 15.10A). The paired dorsal aortae give rise to paired vitelline arteries supplying the yolk sac, paired allantoic arteries supplying the allantois, and paired arteries supplying the gut.

15.5   Arteries derived from aortic arches of mammalian embryo

The derivatives of the mammalian aortic arches and other embryonic arteries are shown in Fig. 15.9B and summarized in Fig. 15.10B.

The left and right first, second, and fifth arterial arches make only a fleeting appearance in the early embryo, and contribute nothing.

The left and right **external carotid arteries** arise from extensions of the left and right ventral aortae rostral to arch 3.

The left and right **internal carotid arteries** are derived on each side from aortic arch 3 and from the dorsal aorta cranial to arch 3. The short length of the dorsal aorta between arches 3 and 4 drops out on both sides; this small elimination is functionally important, since it separates the arterial supply to the trunk from the arterial supply to the head in general and the brain in particular.

The left and right **common carotid arteries** develop by elongation of the left and right ventral aortae between arches 3 and 4.

The **aorta** of mammals arises from a sequence of components. The first part is formed by the left ventral aorta (or fused ventral aortae as in Fig.

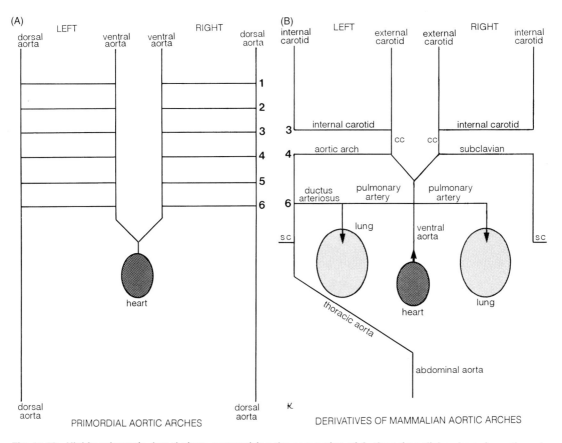

Fig. 15.10 Highly schematic dorsal views summarizing the conversion of A, the primordial embryonic aortic arches into B, definitive arteries in the mammal. 1–6, first to sixth aortic arches. In B, the caudal parts of the left and right ventral aortae have fused to form a midline ventral aorta. The abdominal aorta is formed by the fusion of the left and right dorsal aortae. A short length of the dorsal aorta is lost caudal to the right subclavian artery. cc, common carotid; sc, left and right subclavian arteries.

15.10B), the left fourth aortic arch, and the subsequent part of the left dorsal aorta. A short length of the right dorsal aorta drops out caudal to the root of the right subclavian artery (Fig. 15.10B); caudal to this eliminated segment of the right dorsal aorta, the left and right dorsal aortae fuse into a single midline vessel, and this forms the whole of the remainder of the definitive aorta. If this short segment of the dorsal aorta fails to be eliminated, a vascular ring anomaly occurs (Section 15.15).

The **right subclavian artery** (Fig. 15.9) arises from the right ventral aorta (or fused ventral aortae), right fourth aortic arch, right dorsal aorta between arches 4 and 6, and a short dorsal segmental artery that branches off the right dorsal aorta at about the level of arch 6 (**sc** on the *right* side of Fig. 15.10B). The **left subclavian** arises solely from the corresponding dorsal segmental branch of the left dorsal aorta (**sc** on the *left* side of Fig. 15.10B).

The ventral parts of the left and right sixth aortic arches form the left and right **pulmonary arteries** (Figs 15.9B, 15.10B). The remainder of the right sixth arch contributes nothing in mammals, but the remainder of the left sixth arch forms the **ductus arteriosus** (Fig. 15.10B). In the fetus, the ductus arteriosus allows much of the right ventricular output to bypass the lung and enter the aorta (Section 16.7). In the postnatal mammal the ductus arteriosus becomes the **ligamentum arteriosum**.

The paired allantoic arteries form the paired **umbilical arteries** (Section 16.3). In the fetal circulation these carry venous blood to the *fetal* component of the placenta for metabolic exchange with the *maternal* component of the placenta. In the postnatal mammal the umbilical arteries become the **round ligaments of the bladder**.

When the yolk sac regresses, the paired vitelline arteries resolve themselves into a single **cranial mesenteric artery** (Fig. 15.9B). Similarly, other paired arteries to the gut are converted into the midline **coeliac** and **caudal mesenteric arteries** (Fig. 15.9B).

The six **aortic arches** are components of the six **pharyngeal (branchial) arches** that develop as rings of mesoderm surrounding the embryonic pharynx. Caudal to each pharyngeal arch there is a **pharyngeal cleft** (the homologue of the gill cleft in gill-breathing vertebrates). Each pharyngeal arch contains a pair of **aortic arches**.

In the mammalian embryo all six aortic arches are never present at any one time (Patten, 1958, p. 491). The *first two aortic arches* degenerate before the most caudal aortic arches appear. The *fifth aortic arches* are inconstant, incomplete, and transitory, and disappear in the very early embryo without trace (Arey, 1958, p. 370); all the other components of the fifth pharyngeal (branchial) arch also disappear and contribute nothing to the developing head. Doubts about the genuine existence of a fifth pair of aortic arches are countered by phylogenetic evidence, notably by the persistence of the fifth aortic arches in adults of modern urodele amphibians (Fig. 15.11D; Section 15.6.1).

During the development of the third, fourth, and sixth arterial arches, the most caudal segment of the left and right ventral aortae fuse into a single **ventral aorta** (Fig. 15.10B); this becomes divided into a pulmonary and an aortic channel by the aorticopulmonary septum (Section 15.3.3).

A series of small arteries arise along the length of the dorsal aorta and extend into the dorsal body wall between the somites. These are the **dorsal intersegmental arteries** (Patten, 1958, p. 497). The dorsal intersegmental arteries in the thoracic region lie between the ribs and therefore become the **intercostal arteries**. The dorsal intersegmental artery at the level (usually) of the seventh somite (Noden and de Lahunta, 1985, p. 215) enters the right forelimb bud and becomes the **right subclavian artery**; the corresponding dorsal intersegmental artery on the left side forms the **left subclavian artery** (Figs 15.9B, 15.10B).

The dorsal intersegmental arteries on both sides of the cervical region, cranial to the subclavian arteries, become connected by longitudinal anastomoses to form the **vertebral arteries** (Patten, 1958, p. 499); their intersegmental roots then disappear, leaving the vertebral artery as a branch of the subclavian artery (as on the left side of the pig and carnivores).

15.6 Phylogeny of the heart and aortic arches in vertebrates

15.6.1 *Aortic arches*

A **hypothetical ancestor** of the jawed vertebrates (Gnathostomata, which include all higher vertebrates) is presumed to have possessed six pairs of aortic arches (Romer, 1962, p. 426). Each arch forms an **afferent branchial artery** to a **gill slit**, and continues from the gill slit as an **efferent branchial artery** (Fig. 15.11A). The first aortic arch is never present in a typical form in any living adult vertebrate, although it does occur in the embryo. Consistent with the loss of the first aortic arch, the first gill slit is replaced by the spiracle. Thus in the selachian fish (Fig. 15.11B) and lungfishes (Fig. 15.11C) there are

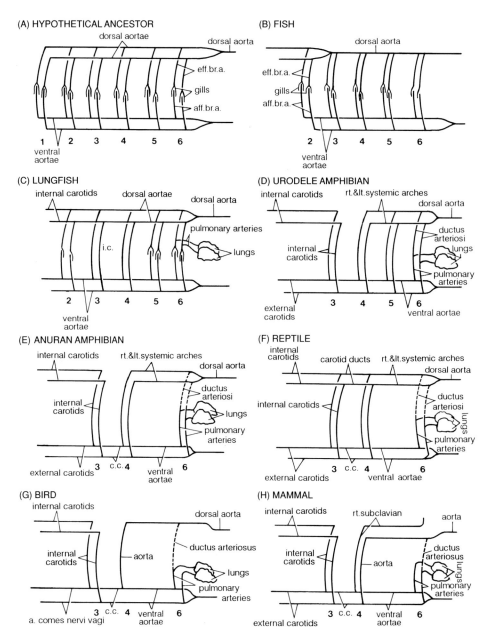

Fig. 15.11 Highly schematic left lateral views of the aortic arches and their derivatives in vertebrates. A, Hypothetical ancestor of the jawed vertebrates; B, selachian fish; C, lungfish; D, urodele amphibian (newt or salamander); E, anuran amphibian (frog or toad); F, reptile (lizard); G, bird; H, mammal. (Redesigned and modified after Goodrich, 1930, pp. 506–528 and Romer, 1962, pp. 424–431.) To enable the homologous pattern of the aortic arches to be recognized more easily in the eight diagrams, the varying degrees of fusion of the left and right ventral aortae are not shown. In selachians (B) the two ventral aortae are actually fused along their whole length into a single midline vessel from which the pairs of aortic arches arise; the left and right dorsal aortae also fuse into a median dorsal aorta. In contrast, in anuran amphibians the fusion of the ventral aortae is limited to a very short length immediately cranial to the heart. In urodele amphibians the ventral aortae are shortened to the point of being almost non-existent, so that the third, fourth, fifth, and sixth arches arise almost directly from the truncus arteriosus. 1–6, First to sixth aortic arches; aff.br.a., afferent branchial artery; c.c., common carotid arteries; eff.br.a., efferent branchial artery; i.c., internal carotid arteries, rt. & lt. systemic arches, right and left systemic arches.

only five aortic arches, 2 to 6 inclusive. In **lungfishes**, gill slits are lost from branchial arches 3 and 4, so aortic arches 3 and 4 run through the gill region without interruption (Fig. 15.11C); this reduction in gill-breathing in lungfishes coincides with the arrival of lung-breathing. However, the pulmonary arteries in lungfishes arise from the sixth aortic arches *distal* to the gill slits (Fig. 15.11C), so that the blood in the sixth arches has already undergone gas exchange in the gills before it reaches the lungs (suggesting a certain lack of confidence in these newfangled respiratory devices).

In **amphibians** the second aortic arch is lost, as well as the first. In tailed amphibians (**urodeles**), i.e. newts and salamanders, the **fifth aortic arch** is present (Fig. 15.11D), but it is absent in the adult of all other land vertebrates (Romer, 1962, p. 429). The **internal** and **external carotid arteries** are present in urodeles (Fig. 15.11D), and in tailless amphibians (**anuran amphibians**), i.e. frogs and toads (Fig. 15.11E). In urodeles the **ventral aortae** are fused and shortened to the point of being almost non-existent, and furthermore the carotid, systemic, and pulmonary arches branch almost directly from the truncus arteriosus (Porter, 1972, p. 64); the common carotid arteries are therefore indistinct in urodeles. The ventral aortae are very short in anuran amphibians also, but slightly more extensive than those of urodeles (Porter, 1972, Fig. 2.40B) so that the common carotid arteries (Fig. 15.11E) are still recognizable (Goodrich, 1930, Fig. 540). The lumen of the short length of the fused ventral aorta in amphibians, and in lungfishes also, is partly divided by the '**spiral valve**' (Section 15.6.2) into two channels (Romer, 1962, pp. 430, 450), one carrying mainly deoxygenated blood to the lungs, and the other carrying mainly oygenated blood to the head and trunk. The flow to the trunk in amphibians is by the **right** and **left systemic arches**, consisting of the right and left fourth aortic arches and right and left dorsal aortae (Fig. 15.11D,E). The dorsal aorta between arches 3 and 4 (which forms the **carotid duct** when present) is lost in anurans and most urodeles (Fig. 15.11D,E). Elimination of this short segment of the dorsal aorta in the higher vertebrates is an important step forward, since it completely separates the arterial supply to the head from that to the trunk (Romer, 1962, p. 428); one benefit of this is that it enables the mammalian embryo to give a preferential oxygen supply to the brain during development (Section 16.8). In amphibians the gills are lost in the adult, and the left and right sixth aortic arches form the **pulmonary artery** and **ductus arteriosus** on each side of the body (Fig. 15.11D,E). In the frog, the pulmonary arteries are, in fact, **pulmo-cutaneous arteries** since they give off special **cutaneous branches** to the skin for gas exchange (Young, 1962, p. 336). The ductus arteriosus on each side remains open in the adult urodele amphibian (Fig. 15.11D), though in a reduced form (Romer, 1962, p. 430). In anuran amphibians (Fig. 15.11E), the ductus arteriosus disappears after

metamorphosis, reminiscent of its closure in the mammal after birth; this is desirable for circulatory efficiency, since a patent ductus arteriosus can produce an arterial-to-venous shunt (Section 15.8).

In some **reptiles** (Fig. 15.11F), but not the crocodiles, the **carotid ducts** persist. All living reptiles retain both the **left** and the **right systemic arches**. Each of these two systemic arches has its own direct opening from a ventricle (Fig. 15.12). The *right* systemic arch opens from the *left* ventricle, and therefore conveys oxygenated arterial blood to the head and trunk (Section 15.6.2); the *left* systemic arch opens mainly from the *right* ventricle, a disadvantageous arrangement since it means that the left systemic arch carries mainly venous blood and is therefore an ineffective artery (Section 15.6.2). **Internal, external**, and **common carotid arteries** (Figs 15.11F, 15.12) are recognizable in reptiles (Goodrich, 1930, Fig. 545). The sixth aortic arches form the left and right **pulmonary arteries** and the left and right **ductus arteriosus** (Fig. 15.11F). The ductus arteriosus on both sides loses its lumen in the adult of most, but not all, extant reptiles. Only one species among all the reptiles, birds, and mammals retains both an open carotid duct and an open ductus arteriosus in the fully developed normal adult, and that is the reptile *Sphenodon* (Goodrich, 1930, p. 525).

Birds have abandoned the system of *paired* (i.e. both left and right) systemic arches, which physiologically is at the best unnecessary and at the worst plainly inefficient. Since birds are descended relatively recently from reptiles it is not surprising that they abandoned the ineffective left systemic arch, and retained the **right fourth aortic arch** as the basis of a **right systemic arch** (Fig. 15.11G), i.e. the systemic arch that in reptiles supplies the trunk with *oxygenated* blood. The **left fourth aortic arch** drops out entirely in birds (Romanoff, 1960, p. 615). The **common carotid** artery is very short on each side. It forms the internal carotid artery and the arteria comes nervi vagi (Baumel, 1993, p. 425), at the thoracic inlet. Consequently the **internal carotid** is as long as the common carotid is short. As in other higher vertebrates, the internal carotid is derived from the third aortic arch and dorsal aorta (Fig. 15.11G). The **arteria comes nervi vagi** is the homologue of the external carotid artery in amphibians, reptiles, and mammals (see Romanoff, 1960, p. 621, and Baumel, 1993, p. 426). The definitive external carotid artery in birds is a new vessel that arises from the internal carotid artery near the mandible; some of its branches anastomose with the arteria comes nervi vagi (Baumel, 1993, pp. 426, 429). The **pulmonary arteries** arise from the right and left sixth aortic arches. The **ductus arteriosus** arises from the *right* sixth arch in order to connect with the **right** dorsal aorta (Fig. 15.11G); it becomes closed in the adult bird.

Like the bird, the **mammal** retains only one systemic arch, but unlike the bird it selects the **left fourth aortic arch** as the foundation of its **left systemic arch**. The **right**

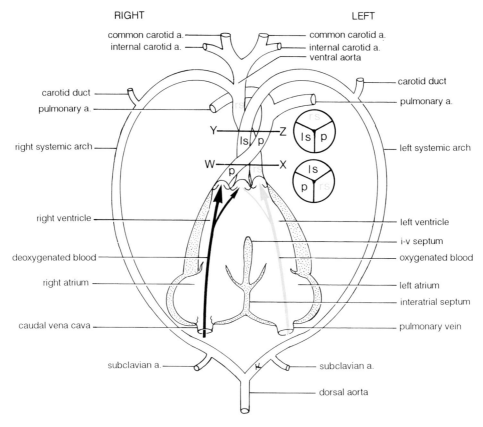

Fig. 15.12 **Ventral view diagram of the heart of all reptiles, except crocodilia, showing the three spiral channels in the truncus arteriosus and their outflows from the left and right ventricles.** W–X, transverse section through the bulbus cordis; Y–Z, transverse section through the truncus arteriosus. Spiral septa divide the outflow from the ventricles into three channels, p to the pulmonary arteries, rs (green) to the right systemic arch, and ls to the left systemic arch. Oxygenated blood from the lungs (green arrow) comes from the lungs and goes through the left atrium and left ventricle into the ventral aorta and right systemic arch to supply the head and trunk. Deoxygenated blood from the body (black arrow) goes through the right atrium and right ventricle mainly into the pulmonary arteries to be oxygenated in the lungs. Deoxygenated blood from the right ventricle also passes directly into the left systemic arch; only a small amount of oxygenated blood from the left ventricle crosses the incomplete interventricular septum and enters the left systemic arch. Therefore the blood in the left systemic arch is mainly deoxygenated, constituting a disadvantageous venous-to-arterial shunt. a., artery; i-v, interventricular. (Adapted from Young, 1962, after Goodrich.)

fourth aortic arch is retained as the basis of the **right subclavian artery** (Fig. 15.11H). The **common** and **external carotid arteries** arise from the ventral aortae, and the **internal carotid arteries** from the third aortic arches and dorsal aortae, as in amphibia and reptiles (Fig. 15.11H). The **pulmonary arteries** arise from the sixth aortic arches. The **ductus arteriosus** is developed from the *left* sixth aortic arch, in order to connect with the **left dorsal aorta** (Fig. 15.11H); it closes after birth (Section 16.21).

15.6.2 *Heart*

Typical **fishes** have a simple S-shaped heart (Romer, 1962, p. 447). It has the same chambers as the **sigmoid**

heart of the mammalian embryo (Fig. 15.2A), i.e. sinus venosus, atrium, ventricle, and bulbus cordis (though the latter is now known as the conus arteriosus). The bulbus cordis continues peripherally into the truncus arteriosus (Goodrich, 1930, Fig. 587) and ventral aorta. Like the heart in the early mammalian embryo (Section 15.1), the sigmoid heart of fish bends to the right and dorsoventrally.

In typical fishes, the gaseous exchanges of respiration take place in **gills**, vascularized by the paired aortic arches. **Lung-breathing** reinforces gill-breathing in lungfish (Fig. 15.11C), and replaces it in amphibians, reptiles, birds, and mammals (Fig. 15.11D, E, F, G and H). For lung breathing to be effective, the oxygenated blood from the lungs must now be separated from the deoxygenated venous blood from the body. This entails partitioning of the heart into left and right chambers.

In **lungfish** and **amphibians** an **interatrial septum** creates a left atrium that receives oxygenated blood from the lungs, and a right atrium that receives typical deoxygenated venous blood. In lungfishes this septum is incomplete. In typical amphibians it is complete, but both of the atria share the same opening into the single ventricle (Romer, 1962, p. 449).

Various structural and functional adaptations have evolved to prevent the oxygenated blood from the left atrium, and the deoxygenated blood from the right atrium, from mixing in the common ventricle of lungfish and amphibians. Extant **lungfish** have developed a partial **interventricular septum**, essentially continuous with the interatrial septum. **Amphibians** have not evolved an interventricular septum at all; however, the classical view is that in amphibians the left and right atrial blood streams are to some extent separated functionally by the spongy structure of the ventricular cavity, although radio-opaque injections evidently fail to confirm this separation (Young, 1962, p. 338). Amphibians have escaped urgent evolutionary pressure to keep the oxygenated pulmonary blood flow separate from the deoxygenated venous blood returning from the body, since (in modern amphibians) much of the gas exchange occurs in the **skin** anyway (Romer, 1962, p. 449). Cutaneous gas exchange means that separation of the right and left atrial blood streams in the amphibian ventricle would not be clearly advantageous. An incomplete interventricular septum does develop in most **reptiles** (Fig. 15.12); however, the gap in the septum is so great that the ventricle is treated by some authorities as a single common chamber (Goodrich, 1930, p. 557), though others (Romer, 1962, p. 449) consider there to be left and right ventricles. In **crocodilians** the septum is almost complete, creating a distinct left ventricle and a distinct right ventricle (Romer, 1962, p. 450). In **birds** and **mammals** the interventricular septum is finally complete, thus at last perfecting the separation of the left from the right ventricle, as first foreshadowed in the lungfish (Goodrich, 1930, p. 555).

The final problem in tetrapods (four footed vertebrates, i.e. amphibians, reptiles, birds, and mammals) is how to divide the blood flow in the **conus arteriosus** (bulbus cordis) and **truncus arteriosus** into a deoxygenated (venous) and an oxygenated (arterial) stream (Romer, 1962, p. 450). The deoxygenated stream must enter the sixth aortic arches and go to the lungs: the oxygenated arterial stream must go to the body and head, principally by the fourth and third aortic arches. In **lungfishes** and **amphibians**, a 'spiral valve' runs the length of the conus arteriosus (bulbus cordis), partly dividing the conus into two channels, a *venous channel* and an *arterial channel*. As in the truncus arteriosus of the mammalian embryo (Section 15.2.3), this spiral septum is formed by the growing together of two

endocardial ridges (Goodrich, 1930, p. 551). As just stated, haemodynamic factors within the heart of lungfish and amphibians are generally believed to direct the deoxygenated blood mainly into the venous channel, and oxygenated blood mainly into the arterial channel (although this has been challenged by the results of radio-opaque injections in amphibians); peripherally, the venous channel then carries its deoxygenated blood mainly to the lungs via the pulmonary (sixth) aortic arches; the arterial channel carries its oxygenated blood mainly to the head via the third aortic arches, and to the trunk via the right and left systemic arches (Fig. 15.11C,D and E). Thus in lungfishes and amphibians the two blood streams may be fairly effectively separated functionally, even though the anatomical partitioning is so imperfect.

In the three highest classes of vertebrates, i.e. **reptiles**, **birds**, and **mammals** (the amniotes), the **truncus arteriosus** develops a **longitudinal spiral septum**, rotating essentially through 180°. The details of its anatomy vary, however, each class evolving its own type of spiral structure (Goodrich, 1930, pp. 558–561).

In **reptiles** the spiral septum possesses an additional ridge, which divides the lumen of the truncus arteriosus into *three* spiral channels (Goodrich, 1930, pp. 560, 576) (see the two transverse sections in Fig. 15.12). Two of these channels (ls and rs) are aortic channels to the trunk, i.e. respectively the **left** and the **right systemic arches** (Fig. 15.11F). Each of these two systemic arches has its own direct opening from a ventricle (Goodrich, 1930, Fig. 587C; Romer, 1962, pp. 449–450). The right systemic arch opens from the left ventricle. The left systemic arch opens mainly from the right ventricle. The third channel in the reptilian truncus arteriosus (p in Fig. 15.12) opens from the right ventricle, and goes to the left and right pulmonary arteries (Fig. 15.11F). In the reptilian heart, the atria are so arranged anatomically that most of their blood is directed into the appropriate ventricle (Romer, 1962, pp. 449–450). Thus deoxygenated (venous) blood that arrives in the right atrium from the body is directed into the right ventricle, and thence mainly into the pulmonary arteries. The oxygenated (arterial) blood that arrives in the left atrium from the lungs is directed into the left ventricle, and thence mainly into the right systemic arch (green arrow in Fig. 15.12). The left systemic arch is less efficient physiologically. It opens largely from the right ventricle, and therefore receives mainly venous blood (black arrow in Fig. 15.12). This amounts to a venous-to-arterial shunt even in crocodiles, where the interventricular septum is almost complete, since venous blood definitely enters the left systemic arch (Romer, 1962, p. 430). The subsequent recirculation to the body of such mainly venous blood is a venous-to-arterial shunt and is therefore physiologically inefficient.

Birds have eradicated this physiological inefficiency by suppressing the left systemic arch completely (Fig. 15.11G). An additional ridge may arise briefly on the spiral septum in the truncus arteriosus as in reptiles (Goodrich, 1930, Fig. 571; Hamilton, 1952, p. 429), but, if so, very early absorption of this ridge soon reduces the channels in the truncus arteriosus to two; the aortic channel continues into the *right* fourth aortic arch; the other (venous) channel leads to the left and right pulmonary arteries.

In **mammals** the **spiral septum** creates two channels in the truncus arteriosus (Section 15.3.3); the aortic channel continues into the *left* fourth aortic arch, forming the definitive aorta, and the other (venous) channel supplies the left and right pulmonary arteries.

As Romer (1962, p. 450) pointed out, the introduction of the lung in advanced fishes (i.e. in the lungfishes) created circulatory problems that the vertebrates found difficult to solve. This difficulty is reflected in the anatomical variability of the solutions. Lungfishes, amphibians, and reptiles have solved it only partly, yet quite effectively. Only birds and mammals have solved it completely.

The progressive evolution in the vertebrate classes of the sigmoid heart, interatrial septum, interventricular septum, spiral aorticopulmonary septum, and aortic arches, over a period of some 400 million years, strikingly resembles the embryonic stages that the mammalian embryo achieves during a mere handful of weeks, and is probably one of the best examples of how ontogeny recapitulates phylogeny.

III CONGENITAL CARDIOVASCULAR DISORDERS

15.7 General characteristics of congenital cardiovascular disorders

Cardiovascular anomalies account for only a small proportion of cardiovascular disorders in domestic mammals, but can be disproportionately stressful to the owners of young companion animals. The commonest anomalies include patent ductus arteriosus, pulmonary stenosis, aortic stenosis, defects in the interventricular septum, and mitral insufficiency.

Such anomalies are characterized by occurring in immature animals. Their clinical effects vary greatly. Multiple defects (e.g. the Fallot tetralogy) can be very debilitating from the outset. Other defects (e.g. aortic stenosis) may initially cause only minimal physiological disturbance, but tend

to progress through a sequence of structural and hence functional changes that culminate in irreversible and fatal damage.

From the very beginning, all of these anomalies generate turbulence in the bloodstream, causing cardiac murmurs with typical sounds and sites (Section 22.7.7). Such a murmur may be recognizable in an otherwise apparently normal young dog brought in for vaccination.

The anatomy and pathophysiology of these cardiovascular defects have been well surveyed by Noden and de Lahunta (1985, pp. 224, 245), Latshaw (1987, p. 223), and Darke (1989).

Congenital cardiovascular disorders, including anomalies of the aortic arches, account for only about 10% of clinical cardiovascular cases in domestic mammals; they are encountered more often in cattle and dogs than in horses and cats, the apparently low occurrence in horses being due to a relatively high early mortality (Noden and de Lahunta, 1985, p. 245). They worry breeders of companion animals faced with the prospect of inherited defects (Darke, 1989).

The commonest defects in the **dog** appear to be **patent ductus arteriosus** and **pulmonary stenosis**; in the **cat** patent ductus arteriosus also occurs, but pulmonary stenosis is rare (Darke, 1989). Defects in the **interventricular septum** are believed to be the commonest cardiac malformation in the domestic species as a whole (Darke, 1989), and in the **sheep** and **horse**, and **cattle** in particular (Noden and de Lahunta, 1985, p. 251; Latshaw, 1987, p. 226); they are also quite common in **cats** (Darke, 1989). **Mitral valve insufficiency** is held to be the commonest cardiac anomaly in the cat (Latshaw, 1987, p. 224). All these anomalies can have serious cardiorespiratory consequences. In the horse and cat, interventricular defects are usually fatal before weaning (Noden and de Lahunta, 1985, p. 251). Defects in the **interatrial septum** occur, but are often virtually harmless functionally.

The clinician may suspect a cardiovascular malformation on the basis of the following signs (Fisher, 1972). The animal will be immature (for example, often under 2 years old in the dog), breathless (especially after exercise), and poorly-developed physically; it may tend to faint and sometimes shows cyanosis of mucous membranes. However, these general signs of heart disease tend to be absent at first. Nearly all of the common cardiovascular anomalies cause clearly audible **cardiac murmurs** with distinctive characteristics, and the source of the murmur can often be identified by the point on the thoracic wall where the intensity is maximal (Darke, 1989): thus in the dog the machinery murmur of a **patent ductus arteriosus** is often concentrated at the base of the heart on the left side; **pulmonary stenosis** has a harsh murmur, and tends to be maximal on the cranial aspect of the left side of the thorax near the sternum; the murmur of **ventricular septal defects** is usually maximal on the right side of the thorax; the softer regurgitant murmur of **mitral dysplasia** tends to be on the left side, well caudal to triceps.

Most of the classical cardiac anomalies have been repaired surgically in dogs. However, cardiac bypass is usually needed, and this requires resources that are generally beyond the means of clients and the facilities of referral services (Darke, 1989).

15.8   Patent ductus arteriosus

In the fetus, the normal ductus arteriosus is a very wide-bore vessel directly connecting the pulmonary trunk to the aorta (Fig. 15.6). The fetal lung offers a high resistance to blood flow. Because of this, the pressure gradient in the fetal ductus arteriosus is from pulmonary trunk to aorta; this enables the ductus to bypass the lungs and divert a large part of the right ventricular output directly to the aorta (Section 16.7).

In the normal postnatal mammal the ductus arteriosus begins to close soon after birth. However, in some species, especially the horse and ox, complete closure is not attained until several days postnatally (Section 16.21). In some individuals, the mechanisms that normally induce postnatal closure of the ductus fail altogether, and it remains permanently open. While the ductus is open the postnatal pressure gradient in the aorta is reversed, i.e. it goes from aorta to pulmonary trunk. This causes a **left-to-right**, or **arterial-to-venous**, **shunt**. The reversal of flow in the ductus arteriosus occurs at the first breath (Section 16.14). It causes turbulence in the ductus arteriosus, which is **continuous** throughout both systole and diastole; this turbulence creates a continuous '**machinery murmur**', so-called because it resembles the rumble of continuously moving machinery.

A left-to-right shunt through the ductus arteriosus does not, in itself, impair the oxygenation of arterial blood or its distribution to the body. However, the lung is now receiving not only all the right ventricular output but also a substantial part of the left ventricular output as well (Section 16.14). The increased flow to the lungs is returned by the pulmonary veins to the left atrium, and this in turn overloads the left ventricle. The left atrium and left ventricle become

dilated and hypertrophied. At this stage in the sequence of changes, cardiorespiratory deterioration in the dog can be arrested by ligation of the offending ductus arteriosus.

In the absence of surgical intervention, the left side of the heart may be unable to keep up with the overloading. If so, blood banks up in the pulmonary veins, and the resulting pulmonary venous congestion leads to a diffusion of fluid from the blood plasma into the lung alveoli (**pulmonary oedema**, Section 17.25). **Respiratory failure** begins (Section 17.29.2). Furthermore, the pulmonary blood vessels are not designed to withstand aortic pressures, and undergo compensatory changes in the thickness of their walls through formation of fibrous tissue with loss of their elasticity. Moreover, the right ventricle has to pump against the high aortic pressure, and therefore responds by dilation and hypertrophy. The result is **pulmonary hypertension**. This may eventually cause the right ventricular pressure to exceed the left ventricular pressure. A **right-to-left shunt** (**venous-to-arterial shunt**) then exists. Arterial blood in the aorta is now diluted by venous blood from the right ventricle, leading to cyanosis of mucous membranes, breathlessness, low exercise tolerance, weakness of the limbs, fainting, and collapse. Thus an insidious sequence of changes has culminated in irreversible damage.

Hypertrophy of the myocardial muscle cells of the left or right ventricle can lead to ischaemia of the myocardium. This is because the enlargement of the muscle cells is not accompanied by the development of additional capillaries to supply the hypertrophied cells (Section 18.3).

A patent ductus arteriosus in the dog can be corrected surgically by ligation, and is the most readily repaired of the cardiac anomalies. However, the wall of the patent ductus tends to become dangerously thin, probably because of the energy released by turbulence, and can easily be fatally ruptured (Darke, 1989).

15.9   Valvular pulmonary stenosis

Pulmonary stenosis is a narrowing of the pulmonary trunk where it opens from the right ventricle. The narrowing is usually caused by fusion of the semilunar cusps of the pulmonary valve (Fig. 15.13B). Because the blood is being forced through an abnormally narrow outlet, its linear

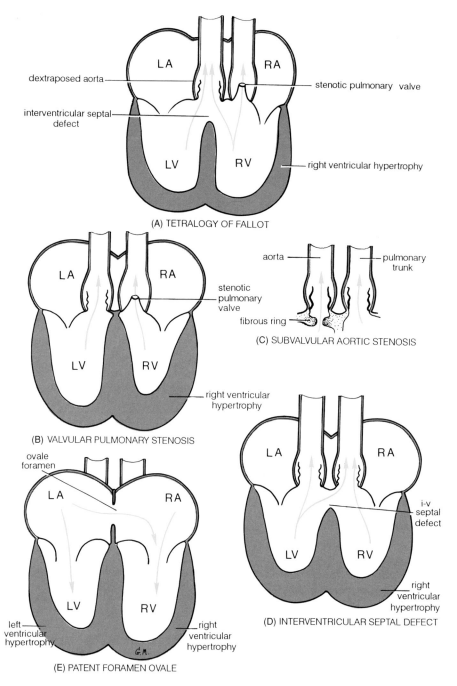

Fig. 15.13 Highly schematic diagrams of common cardiac anomalies. The green arrows indicate blood flow. LA, left atrium; RA, right atrium; LV, left ventricle; RV, right ventricle. i-v, interventricular.

velocity is greatly increased. Consequently the blood stream loses its laminar flow and becomes turbulent, and this causes a loud *systolic murmur* (Section 22.7.7). The increase in the resistance to flow through the valve induces dilation and hypertrophy of the right ventricle, and may end in **right heart failure** (Section 22.17).

There are two main types of pulmonary stenosis. In **valvular stenosis** the three semilunar cusps (valvulae) of the pulmonary trunk become fused together (Fig. 15.13B), and this is the common form of pulmonary stenosis in the dog (Noden and de Lahunta, 1985, p. 249). In **subvalvular pulmonary stenosis** the outflow channel is narrowed by fibrous tissue *proximal* to the valve (as in the subvalvular aortic stenosis shown in Fig. 15.13C).

Right heart failure (Section 22.17) is indicated by weakness, and dyspnoea; there is systemic venous congestion (congestive heart failure) with systemic oedema, and also ascites (accumulation of peritoneal fluid) (Noden and de Lahunta, 1985, p. 249). The turbulence immediately distal to the valve weakens the wall of the sinuses of the pulmonary trunk, causing the trunk to dilate.

The narrowed valve can be dilated by various surgical techniques (Darke, 1989, p. 605), including passing forceps through the valve via an incision in the wall of the right ventricle, or transvenous balloon valvuloplasty. Valvular regurgitation after such surgery of the pulmonary valve is usually not serious.

15.10   Valvular aortic stenosis

Aortic stenosis is usually caused by a fibromuscular constriction of the aorta immediately *proximal* to the aortic valve (Fig. 15.13C), which may reduce the diameter of the channel by about half. The functional consequences of the obstruction resemble those of pulmonary stenosis, in principle. Thus, the increased linear velocity of the blood as it is forced through the narrow entrance to the aorta causes turbulence, with a loud systolic murmur (Section 22.7.7). The ventricle (left, in this instance) becomes dilated and hypertrophies in response to the increased resistance. So long as the hypertrophy succeeds in compensating for the increased resistance, there may be no clinical signs; when this compensation fails, **left heart failure** results, with **pulmonary oedema** and **pleural effusion**, and **respiratory insufficiency** (Section 17.29).

There are two varieties of aortic stenosis, **valvular** and **subvalvular**, as for pulmonary stenosis. Contrary to pulmonary stenosis, however, in the dog the subvalvular form (as described in the preceding paragraph) is the common variety. Aortic stenosis occurs in all of the domestic mammals (Noden and de Lahunta, 1985, p. 250).

Valvular aortic stenosis may lead to *left heart failure* (Section 22.17). Animals with subvalvular aortic stenosis may show minimal signs of circulatory disorder before maturity, but episodes of collapse at exercise may develop in the apparently healthy young adult; sudden death is common, probably from myocardial ischaemia which often provokes ventricular dysrhythmias (Darke, 1989).

Congenital aortic stenosis is often associated with *aortic regurgitation* (Section 22.6, ii).

15.11   Interventricular septal defects

An interventricular septal defect arises from the failure of the final fusion of the interventricular septum with the atrioventricular endocardial cushions and the spiral septum (Section 15.3.2). The defect therefore occurs in the extreme dorsal part of the interventricular septum (Fig. 15.13D). The defects range from a very small hole to a large aperture. At post-mortem, many cattle are reported to have small interventricular septal defects.

If the defect is small, the animal may be clinically normal. Even a small defect, however, does allow the higher left ventricular pressure to create a left-to-right shunt. The animal is therefore likely to have a distinct systolic murmur, because of turbulence in the high velocity stream that the left ventricle forces through the opening. The right ventricle undergoes hypertrophy (Fig. 15.13D) in response to the high pressure flow from the left ventricle, and this may stabilize the problem by preventing the left-to-right shunt.

If the defect is large, a substantial left-to-right shunt may go through the defect and be added to the flow through the lungs. The resulting increase in venous return from the lungs to the left atrium may overload the left side of the heart (as in the left-to-right shunt of a patent ductus arteriosus). This usually leads to **left heart failure** (Section 22.17), with **pulmonary oedema**. There is often pulmonary hypertension as well, because of the high pressure exerted in the lungs by the left ventricle. Eventually right ventricular hypertrophy may reverse the shunt, so that it becomes right-to-left (again, as in patent ductus arteriosus).

> When viewed from within the right ventricle, the defect is found under the cranial edge of the septal cusp (Fig. 20.3) of the right atrioventricular valve; when seen from within the left ventricle, it is lies immediately below the right cusp of the aortic valve (Fig. 20.3) (Latshaw, 1987, p. 227).
>
> Noden and de Lahunta (1985, p. 251) reported interventricular septal defects to be the commonest cardiac malformation in the large domestic mammals, especially cattle. In the horse and cat it is usually fatal before weaning.

15.12   Interatrial septal defects

A simple failure of an otherwise structurally normal foramen ovale to undergo *permanent* (i.e. anatomical) closure after birth is likely to be harmless. The left atrial pressure is considerably higher than the right atrial pressure in the normal adult. During atrial systole the left atrial pressure may reach about 12 mmHg (1.6 kPa) (Fig. 22.1), while the right atrial pressure is less than 5 mmHg (0.7 kPa). Consequently, although the foramen ovale may not be *permanently* obliterated, the pressure gradient from left to right presses its flap (valvula) against the definitive interatrial septum during atrial systole; this closes the foramen ovale during atrial systole, and prevents any left-to-right shunt of oxygenated blood into the right atrium. Usually no clinical abnormality is evident.

If the flap is completely missing and the interatrial communication is wide open, i.e. a **patent foramen ovale** (Fig. 15.13E), giving free communication between the two atria, there is a left-to-right atrial shunt because of the relatively higher systolic pressure in the left atrium. The right atrium and right ventricle are then overloaded by the additional left atrial blood; right atrial and right ventricular hypertrophy result, with the threat of **right heart failure**. The increased venous return from the lungs often overloads the left side of the heart as well.

> Atrial septal defects have been observed in all the domestic mammals, but appear to be very rare in the horse (Noden and de Lahunta, 1985, p. 251).

15.13   Defects in atrioventricular valves

Anomalies in both the left and the right atrioventricular valves have been found in all of the domestic mammals. They are generally known, respectively, as **mitral dysplasia** and **tricuspid dysplasia** (dysplasia is an abnormality in development). The cusps of the valve are too short, and are therefore unable to close the atrioventricular opening during ventricular systole. This failure is known as either **mitral** (left A-V valve or **tricuspid** (right A-V valve) **insufficiency**. Consequently blood regurgitates from ventricle to atrium during ventricular systole, giving a soft regurgitant systolic murmur. As in aortic stenosis (Section 15.10), mitral insufficiency prevents the left ventricle from maintaining an adequate output, and usually leads to **left heart failure** (Section 22.17).

> Mitral and tricuspid dysplasia are also known as mitral and tricuspid **atresia** (atresia means congenital absence or closure of a normal body channel). The resulting insufficiency is also known as mitral or tricuspid **incompetence**. According to Blood and Studdert (1988, pp. 588, 935) in cats mitral dysplasia is rare, whereas tricuspid dysplasia is commonest in cats; according to Latshaw (1987, p. 224) mitral dysplasia is the commonest cardiac anomaly in the cat.
>
> The dysplasia of the valve takes several forms (Latshaw, 1987, p. 224). For example, the cusps themselves may be short and thickened. The chordae tendineae may be absent, so that the cusps are attached directly to the papillary muscles or even to the ventricular wall.
>
> As in aortic stenosis (Section 15.10), the **left heart failure** in mitral insufficiency involves increased pulmonary capillary pressure leading to severe **pulmonary oedema** (Section 17.25.2).

15.14   The Fallot tetralogy

Sometimes several anomalies occur in combination. In the Fallot tetralogy (tetra, four) (Fig. 15.13A) there are four anomalies: (1) valvular pulmonary stenosis; (2) dextraposition of the aorta, so that the mouth of the aorta overrides the interventricular septum thus enabling the aorta to receive blood from *both* ventricles simultaneously; (3) an interventricular septal defect, which makes possible this overriding; and (4) hypertrophy of the right ventricle.

The right ventricle undergoes dilation and hypertrophy in response to (a) the pulmonary stenosis, and (b) the high pressure in the aorta, which has now become the principal outlet of the right ventricle. Since both ventricles have access to the aorta, some deoxygenated blood is always liable to be distributed to the body. As the right ventricular hypertrophy advances, however, so the right ventricular pressure tends to exceed the left ventricular pressure. This gives a frank right-to-left (venous-to-arterial) shunt; increasing volumes of deoxygenated blood now enter the aorta, giving cyanosis of the mucous membranes.

> The Fallot tetralogy occurs in most of the domestic mammals, and particularly in ruminants and dogs (Noden and de Lahunta, 1985, p. 254). Poor exercise tolerance, stunted growth, dyspnoea, and cyanosis are characteristic. It is almost always a lethal defect (Blood and Studdert, 1988, p. 906).
>
> The tetralogy also occurs in man. 'Blue baby' operations have been devised, including the creation of an 'artificial ductus arteriosus'. This can be achieved by anastomosing the left subclavian artery to the pulmonary trunk, thus increasing the volume of oxygenated blood returning from the lungs to the left atrium.

15.15   Vascular ring anomalies

Vascular ring anomalies occur relatively commonly in dogs. They cause no circulatory disorders, but seriously obstruct the oesophagus.

Usually the essential cause is **persistence of the right dorsal aorta** between the point where it normally gives rise to the right subclavian artery and the point of fusion of the left and right dorsal aorta; normally, this short segment of the right dorsal aorta drops out (Section 15.5; Figs 15.9B, 15.10B, 15.11H). The *right* fourth aortic arch and *right* dorsal aorta then form the definitive aorta, as in birds (Fig. 15.11G); the left fourth aortic arch and left dorsal aorta, which should form the definitive mammalian aorta (Figs 15.9B, 15.11H), disappear. The mammalian anomaly is completed by the **ligamentum arteriosum**, which (as it should, in a mammal) arises from the left sixth aortic arch. The developing oesophagus is now trapped in a vascular ring, the ring being formed by the aorta on the right and the ligamentum arteriosum on the left (Fig. 15.14).

Clinical evidence of the ring appears at weaning, when undigested food is consistently vomited immediately after every meal.

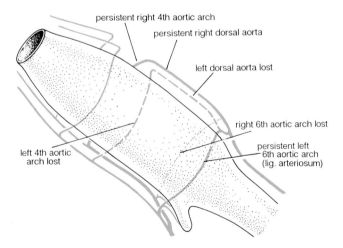

Fig. 15.14   Highly schematic left lateral view of a vascular ring obstruction of the oesophagus. The left fourth aortic arch, which normally forms part of the definitive aorta in mammals, has dropped out, and the right fourth aortic arch has taken its place, forming the aortic arch. The oesophagus is trapped in a ring (heavy green line) formed by the right fourth aortic arch, right dorsal aorta, and ligamentum arteriosum. To identify the other aortic arches shown in the diagram, see Fig. 15.9B. Persistence of the fourth aortic arch and dorsal aorta on both the left and right sides may form another variety of vascular ring. Yet another (hypothetical?) form could arise from persistence of the ligamentum arteriosum on both the left and the right side.

Vascular ring anomalies have been reviewed by Latshaw (1987, p. 200) and Noden and de Lahunta (1985, p. 225). They have been encountered in all domestic mammals, but are commonest in dogs (Noden and de Lahunta, 1985, p. 225). In ruminants they cause dysphagia, regurgitation, and bloat (Blood and Studdert, 1988, p. 63).

In the dog, there is gross dilation of the oesophagus (**megaoesophagus**) cranial to the vascular ring (Noden and de Lahunta, 1985, p. 225). This form of megaoesophagus is restricted to the oesophagus *cranial* to the base of the heart. Barium meal and radiography distinguish it from the megaoesophagus of **oesophageal achalasia** caused by failure of the enteric nervous system, since the latter affects the *whole* of the caudal end of the oesophagus up to and including the cardiac sphincter (Section 3.23.1).

The condition can be relieved in dogs by cutting the ligamentum arteriosum, but the long term prognosis is said to be only fair (Latshaw, 1987, p. 201).

Figure 15.11 shows that developmental errors in the left and right fourth and sixth aortic arches, and in the left and right dorsal aortae, may have the potential to cause several varieties of vascular ring round the oesophagus. (1) All of these vessels could persist, thus forming paired, fully functional, **left** and **right systemic arches** as in amphibians (Fig. 15.11D, E) and reptiles (Figs 15.11F, 15.12). (2) All these vessels could persist, but the systemic arch on the right could lose its function and become a fibrous remnant. Both of these two variants have apparently been reported (Latshaw, 1987, p. 201). (3) The paired sixth aortic arches could persist, dorsal to the points of origin of the left and right pulmonary arteries, forming a ligamentum arteriosum on both the left and right side; this would combine the avian system which retains the right sixth aortic arch as its ductus arteriosus and hence ligamentum arteriosum (Fig. 15.11G), and the mammalian system which retains the left sixth aortic arch as its ductus arteriosum and ligamentum arteriosum (Fig. 15.11H) – but this variant seems to be hypothetical. (4) The aorta could be formed from the **left fourth arch**, and the **right sixth arch** could persist as the ductus arteriosus, thus representing a combination of mammalian (aorta from left fourth arch) and avian (ductus arteriosus from right sixth arch) features; this variety was found in a kitten by McCandlish *et al.* (1984), but was hitherto regarded as no more than another hypothetical possibility.

15.16   Other cardiovascular anomalies

Numerous other varieties of anomaly can occur, through failure of one or other of the many complex processes which occur during development of the heart.

15.16.1   *Transposition of the great arteries*

The **aorticopulmonary septum** (Section 15.3.3) may fail to develop as a **spiral** (Noden and de Lahunta, 1985, p. 254). The effect of this is to connect the aorta to the right ventricle, and the pulmonary artery to the left ventricle. The pulmonary and systemic circulations are then completely isolated from each other, pumping in parallel instead of in series: the right ventricle pumps blood round the body, but the venous blood returns to it via the right atrium, unoxygenated, and then goes round the body again; the left ventricle pumps blood through the lungs, and receives it back again via the left atrium, oxygenated. Such an animal must die immediately after birth.

15.16.2   *Persistent truncus arteriosus*

The **aorticopulmonary septum** (Section 15.3.3) may entirely fail to develop. This retains the common truncus arteriosus, from which both the aorta and the pulmonary arteries arise together. This is usually fatal shortly after birth (Noden and de Lahunta, 1985, p. 254).

15.16.3   *Ectopia cordis*

Occasionally the heart as a whole is displaced to a site essentially on the surface of the body. Usually it lies in the neck region (ectopia cordis cervicalis) (Greek: ek, out of; topos, place). If the paired sternal bars fail to fuse to form the sternum (Section 8.7.6), the heart may lie ventrally outside the thorax (ectopia cordis thoracis) (Noden and de Lahunta, 1985, p. 252). Ectopia cordis is said to be particularly common in the ox (Latshaw, 1987, p. 224).

15.17   Pericardioperitoneal hernia

The possible cause of this hernia by retraction of the liver is outlined in Section 8.15.3.

Because of the subsequent entry of abdominal viscera into the pericardial cavity, this hernia may cause not only digestive disturbances but also cardiac disorders (Blood and Studdert, 1988, pp. 690, 895). Thus compression of the heart (cardiac tamponade) by the invasion of abdominal viscera interferes with heart action and leads to congestive heart failure or sudden death. Surgical correction from an abdominal approach is relatively simple (Darke, 1989).

Chapter 16
Fetal and Neonatal Circulation and Respiration

I FETUS

The transition from fetus to neonate is one of the most dangerous periods in mammalian life.

Hanson *et al.* (1993, Preface, p. x)

16.1 Heart

The fetal cardiac output differs from that of the adult in that the left and right **ventricles** pump in parallel instead of in series. Thus in the **fetus**, the two ventricles pump simultaneously into the same arterial network – this is essentially because the aorta and pulmonary trunk are united by the massive ductus arteriosus (Fig. 16.1). Since they share a common arterial outlet, there is no anatomical limitation to the output of each ventricle. Because the left and right ventricles both pump blood, in parallel, into the shared arterial system, cardiac output in the fetus is considered to be the *sum of the right and left ventricular outputs*; i.e. it is therefore expressed as the **combined ventricular output**.

The term 'cardiac output' is so familiar that physiology textbooks sometimes define it somewhat imprecisely: for example, one leading authority defines it as 'the amount of blood pumped by the heart in a unit period of time'. Logically this amount would include the output of *both* ventricles. However, in the *postnatal animal*, 'cardiac output' should be strictly defined as the output of *one* ventricle only, either the left or the right. The output of the two postnatal ventricles is normally quite similar, since what goes into the right ventricle must in due course come out of the left ventricle. Admittedly the output of the two sides of the heart does vary in the adult in successive ventricular systoles, in response to variations in the venous

return to the atria and the resulting activation of the Frank–Starling mechanism of the heart (Section 21.11). But the only regular difference between the left and right ventricular outputs in the adult is the small excess (typically about 1 or 2%) of the left ventricular output over the right, caused by the bronchial and coronary circulations (Section 18.8).

In the fetus, the **right ventricle** pumps nearly twice as much blood per unit time as the left: thus Fig. 16.1 shows that the right ventricle accounts for about 65% and the **left ventricle** for only about 35% of the combined output of both ventricles together. Hence in the fetus, the right ventricle is doing more work than the left – the opposite to what happens in the postnatal animal.

In all vertebrates the primary determinant of cardiac output is the **total oxygen requirement of the tissues**. The total oxygen requirements of the fetus differ from those of the adult. The adult needs an economic resting oxygen consumption, and a substantial **reserve capacity** to cope with **fight and flight**. The fetus devotes its energetic expenditure almost entirely to **growth**. The energetic cost of this is so great that the fetus uses oxygen at about twice the rate per unit body mass of a resting adult. The combined ventricular output of the fetus is therefore correspondingly high. In fact the combined ventricular output per unit body mass ($ml\,min^{-1}\,kg^{-1}$) of the fetal lamb at the end of pregnancy is about four and a half times greater than the cardiac output (the output of either the left or right ventricle) of the resting adult sheep per unit body mass; for details, see advanced text below.

Because of the huge oxygen demands of tissue growth, the fetal heart operates close to its full capacity all the time. This means that it has no **reserve capacity** (cardiac reserve). This strategy is not too hazardous when living inside a

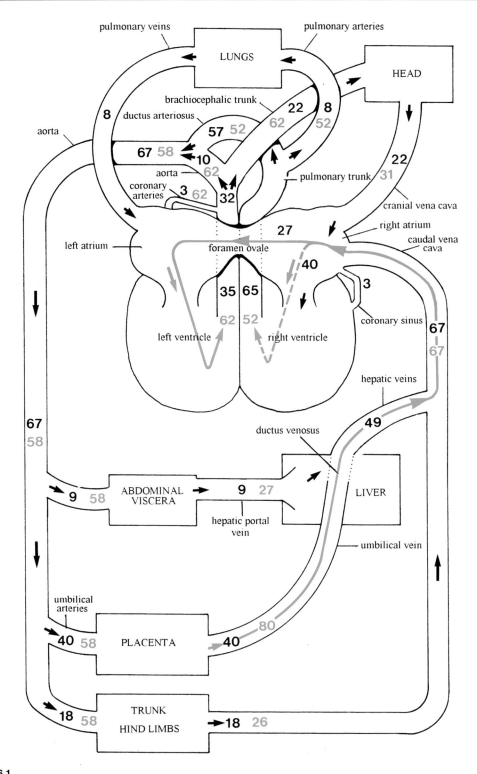

Fig. 16.1

centrally-heated maternal body, with all 'needments' provided. However, the fetus does face some emergencies, particularly **fetal asphyxia** during labour (Section 16.11). In such emergencies, the fetus is unable to increase its cardiac output: it is able to adapt only by vasodilation in the essential organs, especially the brain and heart, and vasoconstriction in the less urgently essential organs such as the abdominal viscera, skeletomuscular system, and skin.

The fetal sheep has been the standard subject for intensive investigation of the anatomy and physiology of the fetal circulation since 1927 (Dawes, 1961; Iwamoto, 1993, p. 199). Initially, whole animal physiological studies were confined to exteriorized fetal lambs, and these led to many important concepts, but the exteriorized fetus undergoes major physiological changes in circulation. Since 1967 (Rudolph and Heymann, 1974) it has become possible to study these aspects of circulation in unanaesthetized fetuses *in utero*. For example, catheters, flow transducers, and pressure transducers can be implanted under anaesthesia at various points in the cardiovascular system of the fetal lamb. The catheters and electrical leads are passed through the uterus and lateral abdominal wall, and attached to the flank of the ewe. After 5 days for recovery, continuous recordings can be made of parameters such as fetal heart rate, arterial pressure, ventricular pressure, and ventricular output in the undisturbed unanaesthetized animal.

Ventricular output in the fetus has been reviewed by Walker (1993, p. 161). In the fetal lamb near term, the combined ventricular output is about $450\,ml\,min^{-1}\,kg^{-1}$ (body mass). Of this, the left ventricle accounts for about 150 ml and the right about 300 ml. These values compare with a resting cardiac output in the adult sheep of about $100\,ml\,min^{-1}\,kg^{-1}$ (i.e. 100 ml for each ventricle) (Walker, 1993, Table 7.1). Figure 16.1 expresses the volume of the left and right ventricular outputs in the fetus as a percent of the total combined output.

In the fetus the two ventricles contract, of course, at the same rate. Since output depends on rate multiplied by stroke volume, it follows that the greater output of the fetal right ventricle than the left ventricle must arise from a greater stroke volume. Estimates indicate a **stroke volume** in the fetal sheep of about $2\,ml\,kg^{-1}$ for the right ventricle, and $1\,ml\,kg^{-1}$ for the left; the **heart rate** of the fetal sheep is about 150 beats per minute. The corresponding values in the adult sheep are: stroke volume of the left and right ventricle $1\,ml\,kg^{-1}$ each, and rate 100 beats per minute. Thus the remarkable pumping performance of the fetal heart is explained by a combination of a high heart rate and a large stroke volume of the right ventricle.

The far greater output of the right ventricle of the fetus than that of the left, should be matched by a greater muscular development of the right ventricle (Harvey, 1628). A survey of the literature on this topic by Kirk *et al.* (1975) revealed conflicting opinions on whether, at birth, the mass of the human right ventricle really is greater than, equal to, or less than the mass of the left ventricle, although the consensus was that the right ventricle does weigh more than the left. Similar observations on near term lambs yielded the opposite conclusion. This is a difficult measurement to make, because of the arbitrary status of the interventricular septum, some authors regarding the septum as a part of the left ventricle and others believing that the ventricles are divided along a natural line of cleavage in the septum. In the neonatal dog, however, the two ventricles can be separated along a clear plane of cleavage in the septum. The weight of the right ventricle of the newborn pup is significantly greater than that of the left (Kirk *et al.*, 1975), thus correlating muscular development with cardiac output.

16.2   Resistance in the fetal circulation

The distribution of blood throughout the body of the normal fetus and newborn mammal is

---

Fig. 16.1   Highly schematic diagram of the fetal circulation, to show the distribution of blood and the saturation of haemoglobin with oxygen in the fetal lamb at full term. The right ventricle pumps 65% and the left ventricle 35% of the combined ventricular outputs. Throughout the diagram, the percentages in black indicate the distribution of the combined left and right ventricular outputs. The values for percentage oxygen saturation are shown in green. The flow of oxygenated blood from the placenta to the heart is indicated by a green line. This flow is laminar, so that the oxygenated blood does not mix with deoxygenated blood in the caudal vena cava. At the right atrium, the caudal caval flow divides into two unequal parts. The larger component of blood (40 'units') goes into the right ventricle. The smaller component (27 'units') goes through the foramen ovale into the left atrium. The smaller component includes most of the oxygenated blood from the placenta (represented by a continuous green line). Consequently the blood entering the aorta has a relatively high O_2 saturation (62%). This blood is distributed by the left ventricle preferentially to the coronary arteries (thus to the myocardium) and to the head (thus to the brain). The larger component of caudal caval blood (represented by a broken green line) contains less of the oxygenated blood from the placenta. Consequently the blood entering the pulmonary trunk has a relatively low oxygen saturation (52%). Oxygen saturation values from Dawes (1961); percentages of cardiac output from Walker (1993, p. 164).

governed by two main resistances. In the fetus, the **placenta** is a **low resistance pathway**: since the umbilical artery is a branch of the aorta (Figs 15.9B, 16.1), the systemic arterial circulation as a whole is a low resistance pathway. On the other hand, the **lungs**, and therefore the pulmonary circulation as a whole, are a **high resistance pathway**. These resistances determine the distribution of blood in the normal fetus: thus the high resistance in the fetal lung causes the diversion of a very large volume of blood to the placenta (Section 16.8.2).

The high vascular resistance of the lungs in the fetus is maintained chiefly by a combination of **mechanical factors** and **vasomotor factors** operated by the **blood gases**. Thus the collapsed state of the fetal lungs, which is maintained until the first breath after birth, compresses the alveolar vasculature. The low P_{O_2} of the blood passing through the alveolar vascular bed maintains arteriolar vasoconstriction (Section 16.8.2), just as it does in poorly ventilated alveoli in the adult lung (Section 17.21.1). The effects of these mechanical and vasomotor factors are reversed in the neonate at the onset of breathing (Section 16.16).

Experimental inflation of the fetal lung induces dilation of the pulmonary vasculature, thus demonstrating the significance of mechanical factors in the regulation of normal fetal pulmonary circulation (Wood, 1993, p. 104). However, the high pulmonary vascular resistance in the fetus can be attributed predominantly to **hypoxic vasoconstriction**; raising the level of fetal blood oxygen *in utero* near term, without inflating the lungs, can increase the pulmonary blood flow to the full level that occurs normally after birth (Walker, 1993, p. 171). The powerful vasoconstriction that sustains the high pulmonary resistance until birth is attributed to the relatively great thickness of the smooth muscle of the small pulmonary arteries (Walker, 1993, p. 170).

16.3   Placenta

The mammalian fetus depends essentially on a **chorioallantoic placenta**. The **chorion** (the outermost of the fetal membranes) is vascularized by the **allantoic arteries** (Fig. 15.9A), which are subsequently named the **umbilical arteries** (Fig. 15.9B).

Oxygenated blood is delivered through the uterine arteries of the mother into the arteries of the *maternal component* of the placenta: deoxygenated venous blood is carried through the fetal umbilical arteries into the arteries of the *fetal component* of the placenta. Minute vascularized processes of the *fetal* chorion (**chorionic villi**) fit intimately into corresponding vascularized depressions in the surface of the *maternal* endometrium, thus allowing exchange of blood gases, electrolytes, and metabolites, and removal of fetal waste products. The placenta therefore functions as the lungs, gut, and kidneys of the fetus. It is also an endocrine organ, producing placental hormones. The fetal placental blood is returned by the **umbilical veins** to the caudal vena cava.

In the basic mammalian chorioallantoic placenta the *fetal* blood is separated from the *maternal* blood by six layers of tissue: (1) the endothelium that lines the allantoic blood vessels, (2) chorioallantoic connective tissue, and (3) chorionic epithelium; and (4) the endometrial epithelium, (5) endometrial connective tissue, and (6) endometrial endothelium. This six-layered structure occurs in all the domestic ungulates, but in carnivores the outer two layers (layers 4 and 5) of the endometrium are eroded.

The barrier of as many as six layers of tissue between the maternal and fetal blood contrasts starkly with the elegant slimness of the blood–gas barrier of the postnatal lung (Section 6.24). Oxygen uptake in the placenta must inevitably be less efficient than oxygen uptake in the lung.

However, various adaptations of the fetal blood do minimize this inefficiency (Section 14.3.3). Notable among these adaptations is the shift to the left of the fetal oxygen dissociation curve; this greatly increases the affinity of fetal haemoglobin for oxygen, even at very low partial pressures of oxygen. Thus the P_{O_2} of fetal blood leaving the placenta is only about 30 mmHg (4.0 kPa), yet its haemoglobin is about 80% saturated with oxygen (Fig. 16.1): in the lung of the adult mammal, a P_{O_2} of 30 mmHg would yield a saturation of only about 50% (Fig. 14.1). Nevertheless, these adaptations can do no more than enable the fetal blood to make the best of a bad job; the functional superiority of the postnatal lung is unmistakable – blood leaving the alveolar wall of the adult lung has a P_{O_2} of about 104 mmHg (13.9 kPa) (Section

6.28.1) and its haemoglobin is about 98% saturated with oxygen (Section 14.3.1).

The structure of the placenta varies in the different groups of eutherian mammals. In the **diffuse placenta** of the horse and pig, the chorionic villi are distributed over the whole surface of the chorion. In the **cotyledonary placenta** of ruminants, the villi are grouped into cup-shaped cotyledons which fit elevated endometrial caruncles, together forming **placentomes**. In the **zonary placenta** of carnivores, the villi form a circular band around the body of the fetus. In the **discoidal placenta** of rodents and primates, the villi are assembled in a single patch.

All six layers of tissue are present in the **epitheliochorial placenta** (placenta epitheliochorialis) of the horse, pig, and ox. It has been reported that the endometrial epithelium is lost in the sheep and goat, giving a **syndesmochorial placenta** (Noden and de Lahunta, 1985, p. 60): but this has been disputed, so that the placenta in these ruminants would then be epitheliochorial (Latshaw, 1987, p. 62). In the **endotheliochorial placenta** (placenta endotheliochorialis) of carnivores the endometrial epithelium and connective tissue are eroded, leaving only four layers. In the **haemochorial placenta** of insectivores, rodents, lagomorphs, and most primates, the maternal blood is in direct contact with the chorion. The ultimate reduction in layers was thought to occur in the **haemoendothelial placenta** of rodents; the maternal blood would then be separated from the fetal blood by only one layer, the fetal endothelium; however, it is now suggested that these placentas are really haemochorial (Latshaw, 1987, p. 55).

A vascular feature of particular importance for placental gas exchange is the **direction of blood flow** in the maternal and fetal vessels (Carter, 1993, p. 119). The optimal relationship for exchange is countercurrent, and this occurs in the mare. In the sheep the relationship is concurrent or crosscurrent. Countercurrent flow occurs in lagomorphs and some rodents.

16.4 Umbilical cord

The umbilical cord (Fig. 16.2) connects the embryo (fetus) to its placenta. The site of connection of the cord to the fetal body is the **umbilicus**.

The umbilical cord is founded on the stalk of the **allantoic sac**, which is a diverticulum of the hind gut (Fig. 15.9). Embedded in the gelatinous connective tissue of the allantoic stalk are the umbilical arteries and umbilical veins. Also embedded there is the thin-walled **urachus**; this is the

part of the allantois that connects the developing urinary bladder with the allantoic cavity (Fig. 15.9B). Early in development, the umbilical cord contains the stalk of the **yolk sac** with its **vitelline vessels**. The ectodermal epithelium and connective tissue of the **amnion** form most of the outer covering of the umbilical cord.

In many species there are two **umbilical veins** in the umbilical cord, which merge at the umbilicus (Fig. 16.2). In all the domestic species there is only one umbilical vein inside the fetus. This ends in the fetal liver at the ductus venosus (Section 16.5; Fig. 16.3). There are two **umbilical arteries** in both the fetal body and the umbilical cord. These arise from the aorta, as the left and right allantoic arteries (Section 15.5; Fig. 15.9). The umbilical arteries have thick muscular walls. The walls of

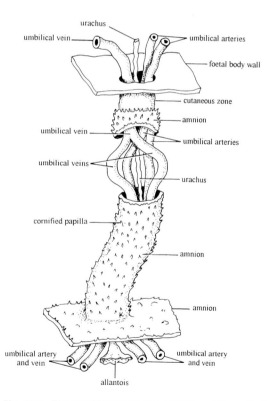

Fig. 16.2 The umbilical cord of a calf fetus at 5 months' gestation, reduced to two thirds natural size. The amniotic covering of the cord has been removed near the body wall, and the gelatinous allantoic connective tissue has been removed. This has enabled the umbilical vessels and urachus to be spread out. Redrawn and modified after Schnorr (1985).

the umbilical vein or veins are equally thick and muscular.

Pulsations are detectable in the umbilical cord in most species, including man. The pulsations arise in the umbilical arteries. They stop if the cord is pulled, presumably because mechanical stimulation of the smooth muscle in the arterial wall induces contraction (Section 16.18). Torsion of the umbilical cord can fatally obstruct umbilical cord blood flow, especially in the foal.

In the ruminants and pig the whole length of the umbilical cord is covered by **amnion**, except for a short **cutaneous zone** at the actual umbilicus (Fig. 16.2). In carnivores the cutaneous zone is hairy (Schnorr, 1985, p. 58). In ruminants the amniotic surface carries **cornified papillae** (Fig. 16.2). In the horse and carnivore the proximal part of the cord (the part nearer to the fetal body) is lined by amniotic epithelium, but the distal part is covered by **allantoic epithelium**, at least initially.

In the calf, lamb, and carnivores, there are two **umbilical veins** in the umbilical cord. At the umbilicus, these merge into the single umbilical vein (Fig. 16.2). In the cord of the other domestic species, the right vein generally regresses leaving only the left vein (Schnorr, 1985, p. 58). In all species the single **umbilical vein** (vena umbilicalis) in the fetal body (Latshaw, 1987, p. 70) is the left vein of the original pair (Section 16.5). The structure of the umbilical veins is quite different from that of ordinary veins, the wall being about as thick and muscular as the umbilical arteries.

The **intraembryonic coelom** (the developing embryonic peritoneal cavity) is continuous during development with **extraembryonic coelom** (Section 8.12.1) in the umbilical cord. This continuity allows a **herniation** of the **intestinal loop** into the umbilical cord during normal development (Fig. 8.30). The intestinal loop carries the stalk of the yolk sac on its apex (Fig. 8.30), and has the **vitelline arteries** in its long axis. The vitelline arteries become the **cranial mesenteric artery** (Section 15.5). Later, the herniated intestinal loop withdraws into the peritoneal cavity of the fetus, and the coelomic cavity in the umbilical cord is obliterated.

In the **foal** at delivery (Rossdale and Mahaffey, 1958) the single vein in the umbilical cord is soft, non-pulsating, and at least **twice** the diameter of either artery. The arteries in the foal feel rather hard and cord-like, and pulsate; often one is thicker than the other, sometimes markedly so. There is a **natural point of rupture** of the umbilical cord, about 1.5 cm **outside** the body wall. According to Whitwell (1975) the point of rupture of the arteries lies up to 6 cm **inside** the foal. The arteries seem to be able to slide in and out of the umbilicus, so that after spontaneous rupture they retract out of view; on the other hand, the veins are not free to move in and out

of the umbilicus, and therefore a lengthy part of their collapsed ruptured ends remains protruding from the umbilicus (Franklin *et al.*, 1946, p. 9). Whitwell (1975) reported that in the allantoic part of the foal's cord there is a persistent vestige of the **extraembryonic coelom**, even up to term, and this contains a remnant of the yolk sac. **Torsion** of the umbilical cord (before birth) appears to be quite common in the foal (Whitwell, 1975). It can obstruct the umbilical vessels, and this she believes to be 'the major cause of foetal death' in foals; respiratory distress is another candidate for this dubious distinction (Section 16.26.1). Torsion of the cord also obstructs the urachus, causing a large distension of the bladder; obstruction of the urachus can also lead to multiple distensions of the urachus which cause it to leak externally through the umbilicus after birth.

The umbilical vessels appear to have no **innervation** (Sexton *et al.*, 1996), except for a small length at the umbilicus (Rudolph and Heymann, 1974, p. 199). The wall of the artery contains not only circular but also longitudinal muscle (Rudolph and Heymann, 1974, p. 199). Histologically, the walls of the umbilical arteries and veins are similar: there are no axons or vasa vasorum, at least in man (Sexton *et al.*, 1996).

A striking feature of the human umbilical cord (Williams *et al.*, 1989, p. 143) is the normal **spiral twisting** of the umbilical vessels. There may be only a few turns, or over 300. A natural assumption is that these twists relate somehow to the great length of the cord and fetal movements, but their cause and functional significance are uncertain. It has been suggested that an additional spiral longitudinal muscle (external in position on the arterial wall) is responsible for the twisting of the umbilical vessels in man, since its removal uncoils the isolated artery (Rudolph and Heymann, 1974, p. 199). In the foal, which also has a long cord, there is very little tendency for the vessels to spiral round each other (Whitwell, 1975).

The **length** of the umbilical cord is absolutely greatest in the horse, measuring 30–95 cm (mean 55 cm) in Thoroughbred foals (Whitwell, 1975), but is also absolutely very long in man, measuring 20–120 cm (Williams *et al.*, 1989, p. 143). Relative to the length of the fetal body (Schnorr, 1985, p. 58), the longest cord is that of the pig, which is equal to body length; horse and dog, half; cat, one third; ox and sheep, one quarter; and goat one sixth of the length of the fetal body.

Umbilical anomalies (Noden and de Lahunta, 1985, p. 308) include **umbilical fistula** (fistula umbilicalis), in which the junction of the stalk of the yolk sac with the intestine persists and remains patent, thus forming an open channel from the intestine which allows faeces to escape from the umbilicus. An **omphalocoele** (omphalocelia) is a hernia of intestines into the umbilical stalk, probably arising from a failure of the intestinal loop to withdraw.

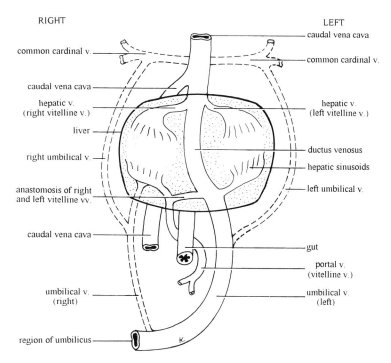

RIGHT

LEFT

caudal vena cava

common cardinal v.

common cardinal v.

caudal vena cava

hepatic v.
(right vitelline v.)

hepatic v.
(left vitelline v.)

liver

ductus venosus

right umbilical v.

hepatic sinusoids

left umbilical v.

anastomosis of right
and left vitelline vv.

caudal vena cava

gut

portal v.
(vitelline v.)

umbilical v.
(right)

umbilical v.
(left)

region of umbilicus

Fig. 16.3   Ventral view diagram of the embryonic liver and developing great veins to show the ductus venosus. The vessels in broken lines disappear or are modified during development. Caudal to the liver, the left and right vitelline veins anastomose to form the portal vein. Within the liver they form the hepatic sinusoids and the hepatic veins draining the sinusoids into the caudal vena cava. The caudal part of the left umbilical vein conveys placental blood to the liver. Nearly half of this oxygenated blood flow is carried by the ductus venosus into the caudal vena cava, bypassing the hepatic sinusoids. The remainder mixes with deoxygenated portal blood in the sinusoids and exits into the caudal vena cava by the hepatic veins. At the heart, most of the oxygenated stream from the ductus venosus goes through the foramen ovale into the left atrium. (Distribution of blood, Walker (1993); embryology, Patten (1958) and Noden and de Lahunta (1985).)

16.5   Ductus venosus

The ductus venosus is a wide venous channel in the liver (Fig. 16.3). It leads directly from the end of the umbilical vein, through the parenchyma of the liver, to empty into the caudal vena cava. Thus it bypasses the hepatic sinusoids and delivers its blood directly into the caudal vena cava.

Oxygenated blood from the placenta returns to the body of the fetus by the **umbilical vein**, which discharges it into the liver (Fig. 16.1). In the liver, nearly half the volume of this oxygenated placental blood enters the ductus venosus, as a laminar flow (Section 6.14); being laminar, it does not mix with the deoxygenated blood from the gastrointestinal tract that enters the liver through the hepatic portal vein (Figs 16.1, 16.3), but con-

tinues as a distinct column of oxygenated blood in the caudal vena cava to the **foramen ovale** (green stream in Fig. 16.1).

The development of the venous system was described by Noden and de Lahunta (1985, p. 258). In the early embryo, the left and right **umbilical veins** pass along the ventral body wall to the **septum transversum**. The liver develops immediately caudal to the septum transversum (Fig. 8.30). The left and right **vitelline veins** enter the septum transversum to drain the yolk sac vasculature into the sinus venosus. The most cranial part of the left vitelline vein disappears, but that of the right vitelline vein forms the hepatic component of the **caudal vena cava**.

Within the liver (Fig. 16.3), the left and right **vitelline veins** (venae vitellinae) form the **hepatic sinusoids**, and drain them into the caudal vena cava; caudal to the liver (Fig. 16.3), anastomoses between the left and right vitelline veins develop around the gut to form the **he-**

patic portal vein and its branches. Also the right vitelline vein anastomoses with the left vitelline vein within the liver (Fig. 16.3). The umbilical veins anastomose with the **hepatic sinusoids** (Fig. 16.3).

The cranial continuations of the left and right umbilical veins to the common cardinal veins drop out, and the caudal segment of the right umbilical vein also degenerates; these eliminations (Fig. 16.3) leave only the **left** umbilical vein (now named **the** umbilical vein) to convey the entire flow from the placenta to the liver.

The **ductus venosus** connects the (left) umbilical vein with the caudal vena cava (Fig. 16.3). In carnivores, ruminants, and primates, the ductus venosus persists until birth; in the horse and pig it disappears during gestation.

In the fetal lamb, the ductus venosus enables about 45% of the blood from the placenta to bypass the hepatic sinusoids (Carter, 1993, p. 126). About 95% of the total flow in the ductus venosus is highly oxygenated placental blood, the remaining 5% being deoxygenated hepatic portal blood (Walker, 1993, p. 166). Laminar flow in the thoracic part of the caudal vena cava projects this stream of highly oxygenated blood from the ductus venosus directly to the **foramen ovale** (the green stream in Fig. 16.1).

The single umbilical vein in the abdomen is retained postnatally as the **round ligament** of the liver (ligamentum teres hepatis), and is suspended in a ventral mesentery named the **falciform ligament** (ligamentum falciforme) (Section 8.13). In some species (including the dog) the falciform ligament becomes a fat depot, and forms an obstacle to midline abdominal incisions between the umbilicus and sternum.

16.6   Foramen ovale

The foramen ovale is a one-way valve (Section 15.3). Its valvula (flap) can be deflected by a stream of blood passing from the right atrium, through the foramen ovale (the via sinistra) and into the left atrium: but a reversal of flow, i.e. from the left atrium towards the right atrium, presses the valvula against the interatrial septum and thus closes the valve (Harvey, 1628, p. 46). The main force that actually causes the flow of blood through the foramen ovale in the fetus is the kinetic energy of the blood stream in the caudal vena cava.

Because of laminar flow, the stream of oxygenated placental blood that has gone through the ductus venosus remains unmixed as it flows along the caudal vena cava. At the entrance of the caudal vena cava into the right atrium, this lamina of oxygenated blood is confronted by the vertical knife-edge of the **crista dividens** (Fig. 15.7). Here, less than half of the caudal caval flow (27 'units' out of the 67 that constitute the caudal caval flow in Fig. 16.1) is deflected to the *left*, through the **foramen ovale** (Sections 15.3.5, 15.3.6), thus taking the *via sinistra* into the left atrium (Fig. 15.5B). However, the all-important point is that this blood contains *most of the lamina of oxygenated blood*. The pathway through the via sinistra that is taken by this oxygenated blood is shown as the continuous green line going through the foramen ovale in Fig. 16.1. The rest of the lamina of oxygenated blood is deflected to the *right* of the crista dividens. It therefore takes the *via dextra* (Fig. 15.5B) into the right atrium and right ventricle (Fig. 16.1, broken green line), where it mixes with deoxygenated blood carried from the **head** by the **cranial vena cava**. Only minimal amounts of *cranial* caval blood go through the foramen ovale into the left atrium.

The oxygenated blood that takes the via sinistra into the left atrium is delivered preferentially by the left ventricle to the **myocardium** (Section 16.8.3) and **brain** (Section 16.8.4).

In his book of 1628 proving the circulation of the blood, William Harvey accurately described how the ductus arteriosus and foramen ovale divert fetal blood from the caudal vena cava to the aorta and away from the lungs until the first breath, after which both channels close so that the blood then goes through the lungs.

Two forces determine the blood flow through the valve of the foramen ovale in the fetus, hydrostatic pressure and kinetic energy (Walker, 1993, p. 168). A very small hydrostatic pressure difference does exist between the two atria in the fetus, the pressure in the right atrium exceeding that in the left (Section 16.8). In the lamb immediately before birth, the pressure in the left atrium is about 6 cm H_2O (0.59 kPa), and that in the caudal vena cava is about 7 cm H_2O (0.69 kPa) (Dawes, 1961, Fig. 8). This gradient favours the opening of the valve, and certainly militates against its closure. However, the kinetic energy of the caudal caval blood stream provides a much greater force, and it is this that maintains flow through the valve (Walker, 1993, p. 168).

In the fetal lamb, discrete streams of well-oxygenated and poorly-oxygenated blood can actually be seen with the naked eye, through the thin wall of the caudal vena cava (Walker, 1993, p. 165).

Figure 16.1 shows that less than half of the **caudal caval flow** goes through the foramen ovale into the left atrium. Thus 67% of the combined cardiac output arrives at the foramen ovale in the caudal vena cava. Of these 67 units, only 27 go through the foramen into the left atrium, and 40 units enter the right atrium and ventricle. However, the oxygenated stream from the placenta and ductus venosus is so preferentially placed in the caudal caval flow that most of it is in the 27 units that pass through the foramen ovale (Walker, 1993, p. 165).

There appear to be no direct measurements of the actual volume of the oxygenated lamina and its division between the via sinistra and via dextra; the evidence that most of it takes the via sinistra is based on values for the oxygen saturation of the blood in the left and right ventricles, following the principles adopted by Dawes (1961) for estimating flow volumes by relative oxygen saturations.

16.7   Ductus arteriosus

The mammalian ductus arteriosus is derived from the left sixth aortic arch (Section 15.5; Fig. 15.9B). In the full term fetus it is a very large artery, connecting the pulmonary trunk to the aortic arch (Fig. 15.6). In fact, examining a transverse section of the ductus and aortic arch together is rather like looking into the end of a double-barrelled shotgun (not a recommended procedure).

Both the pulmonary trunk and the aorta are typical **elastic arteries**, like large arteries in general (Section 12.8). But, despite its huge calibre, the ductus arteriosus is a **muscular artery** (Section 12.9) with powerful smooth muscle in its wall. The capability of the ductus arteriosus to undergo complete constriction is essential, since it must close as soon after birth as possible in order to prevent a left-to-right shunt from aorta to pulmonary trunk (Section 16.21).

The **oxygen saturation** of the blood in the ductus arteriosus is relatively low (52%; Fig. 16.1, values in green). This is because the right ventricle receives a substantial volume of deoxygenated blood from the cranial vena cava, and gains only a minority of the highly oxygenated blood from the placenta (the broken green line in Fig. 16.1).

The ductus arteriosus is perfectly placed to divert the great majority of the right ventricular output away from the lungs and into the aorta, and thence to the placenta, **before** birth. **After** birth, it closes and thus redistributes right ventricular blood away from the aorta and into the lungs. It has one other function: it provides the right ventricle with an '*exercise channel*' (Patten, 1958, p. 530), enabling the fetal ventricle to de-

velop its muscularity in preparation for delivering its entire output to the lungs after birth.

The **calibre** of the ductus arteriosus is similar to that of the aortic arch (Franklin *et al.*, 1946, p. 7). Its huge calibre enables the fetal ductus arteriosus to divert about 88% of the right ventricular output, which is itself very large, directly into the aorta (leaving only about 12% of the right ventricular output for the lungs); the majority of this aortic flow finds its way to the placenta. When this distribution is expressed in terms of the combined ventricular output as in Fig. 16.1, the ductus carries 57% and the lungs receive only 8%.

16.8   Regional distribution of blood in the fetal circulation

The two potential gas exchange organs, the placenta and the lungs, dominate the distribution of blood before and after birth. *Before birth*, the high resistance of the pulmonary circulation diverts blood into the low resistance systemic circulation and placenta, which is the organ of gas exchange in the fetus. The two major shunts that characterize the fetal circulation, namely the foramen ovale and the ductus arteriosus, make this possible by ensuring that most of the right ventricular output bypasses the lungs.

Figure 16.1 summarizes the distribution of the total cardiac output in the fetus (i.e. the combined left and right ventricular outputs). The **right ventricle** accounts for 65%, and the **left ventricle** for 35% of the combined output. Figure 16.1 also shows in green the percentage oxygen saturation of the haemoglobin at various points in the circulation.

The blood pumped from the **left ventricle** has a substantially higher oxygen saturation (62%) than that from the right ventricle (52%). The relatively high value in the left ventricle is due to the preferential flow of oxygenated placental blood (67% saturation) through the *via sinistra* of the foramen ovale and into the left atrium (green arrow through the foramen ovale, in Fig. 16.1). In the left atrium, this oxygenated blood is joined by the small volume (only 8% of combined ventricular output) of deoxygenated blood returning from the lungs by the pulmonary veins. The mixture (now 62% O_2 saturation) leaves the left ventricle and enters the aorta.

The blood in the **right ventricle** comes from three sources, i.e. the caudal vena cava, the cranial vena cava, and the venous drainage of the heart (Fig. 16.1). The volume of the **cranial vena caval flow** is substantial (about 22% of combined ventricular output), and consists of deoxygenated blood (only 31% saturated) from the brain and the head in general. It is important that this deoxygenated cranial caval blood should not collide with the oxygenated caudal caval blood that arrives in the right atrium, since this would disrupt the streamline laminar flow of oxygenated placental blood through the foramen ovale. Collision is prevented by the **intervenous ridge** (Section 15.3.7; Fig. 15.5A), which bounces the cranial caval flow ventrally into the right ventricle. In the right ventricle the deoxygenated cranial caval flow mixes with the minority of the oxygenated lamina (Section 16.6) that takes the via dextra at the foramen ovale (Fig. 15.5B; broken green line in Fig. 16.1). This mixing gives the blood in the right ventricle a lower oxygen saturation (52%) than the blood in the left ventricle.

The large output of the right ventricle (65% of combined cardiac output) must, of course, be preceded by a correspondingly large venous return to the **right atrium**. The relatively small output of the left ventricle (only 35% of combined cardiac output) must be preceded by a correspondingly small venous return to the left atrium. Therefore, before birth, the venous return to the right atrium greatly exceeds the venous return to the left atrium.

There is therefore a right-to-left pressure gradient across the foramen ovale, which is a one-way valve allowing flow only from the right atrium to the left atrium. The right-to-left gradient prevents closure of the foramen ovale, but kinetic energy is the main force that actually creates blood flow through the foramen (Section 16.6). At birth, the gradient across the foramen ovale is reversed, i.e. it becomes left-to-right, and this closes the valve (Section 16.20).

16.8.1   *Placenta*

The fetal **placenta** receives about 40% of the combined cardiac output – by far the largest proportion delivered to any individual organ system in the fetus (Fig. 16.1).

The blood flow in the fetal placenta has been examined by Carter (1993, p. 116). In the sheep, the proportion of fetal cardiac output that goes to the placenta decreases during pregnancy. Thus in the fetal sheep it forms about 50% of the combined ventricular output before the final third of pregnancy, gradually decreasing to about 40% at term; however, there is a progressive absolute increase in flow, due to a fall in the vascular resistance of the placenta and an increase in arterial pressure. But when standardized against body mass, the flow is greater at mid-gestation than at term. The fall in placental resistance is caused (at least in man) by a steady increase in the diameter of the placental vessels. The human placenta at term receives only about 20% of the combined ventricular output.

The **uterine contractions** that occur throughout pregnancy in the ewe have no effect on umbilical blood flow. Similarly, studies in man have revealed no effect of **labour** on the *volume* of flow in the umbilical vein. However, in the second stage of labour (Section 16.12), repeated reductions in uterine blood flow occur frequently, caused by uterine contractions and especially by straining; although the *volume* of umbilical flow may be unchanged, the fetal *oxygen saturation* falls repeatedly during these events, thus subjecting the fetus to varying degrees of hypoxia (Jensen and Berger, 1993, p. 34).

Maternal **exercise** does not cause a major stress to the fetus. Fetal blood gases are unaffected by mild exercise in the ewe, and even prolonged exercise at 70% of maximal maternal oxygen consumption induces no major fetal cardiovascular changes. Umbilical blood flow is maintained in the near-term lamb during acute **maternal hypoxia**, but chronic maternal hypoxia with acidaemia leads to a decline in umbilical flow.

Daily exposure of the ewe and cow to high **ambient temperatures** lowers maternal and fetal placental blood flow, and retards fetal growth. Such fetal stunting produces calves with body mass as much as 20% below normal (Arthur *et al.*, 1982, p. 86).

The placental vasculature is not innervated (Section 16.9).

16.8.2   *Lungs*

Nearly 90% of the **right ventricular output** of the fetus is diverted through the **ductus arteriosus** and into the aorta, and the remaining small volume (only about one tenth) goes to the lungs. The **lungs** therefore receive only a very small proportion (about 8%) of the combined cardiac output (Fig. 16.1).

Even so, this pulmonary volume is far from negligible. It has to be great enough to develop a vascular bed that can accommodate the *entire* output of the right ventricle *almost immediately* after birth: at the same time, the pulmonary vascular bed has to maintain a vascular resistance (Section 16.2) sufficient to limit the pulmonary flow until birth, and thus to divert about 40% of the combined ventricular output to the placenta for oxygenation.

> Although the perfusion of the fetal lung is usually considered to be 'low', the volume of flow in the lamb (about $150\,ml\,min^{-1}\,(100\,g)^{-1}$) (Walker, 1993, p. 170) is not far below that of the fetal brain at term (about $170\,ml\,min^{-1}\,(100\,g)^{-1}$) (Walker, 1993, Fig. 7a), which is regarded as highly perfused (Walker, 1993, p. 170).
>
> If oxygen delivery to the fetus is reduced (by various methods), pulmonary vascular resistance increases and pulmonary blood flow falls to about half of its normal value. This *hypoxaemic vasoconstrictor response* appears to be an important regulatory factor in the fetus, since it has the effect of diverting an increased volume of blood through the ductus arteriosus for oxygenation in the placenta (Iwamoto, 1993, p. 207).

16.8.3 *Myocardium*

The left and right **coronary arteries** are the first branches to arise from the aorta (Section 18.2), arising immediately peripheral to the aortic valve (Fig. 18.1). Therefore they receive typical left ventricular blood (Fig. 16.1). The volume of coronary blood flow in the fetus is relatively small (about 3% of the combined ventricular output), but its quality makes up for its quantity. This blood has come mainly from the placenta, travelling in sequence through the ductus venosus, the via sinistra of the foramen ovale, the left atrium, and the left ventricle (continuous green arrow through the foramen ovale in Fig. 16.1). Together with the blood to the brain, it has the highest oxygen saturation in the fetal arterial system (about 62%; Fig. 16.1).

16.8.4 *Brain*

The brain and the head in general are supplied by the brachiocephalic trunk. This great artery arises from the aortic arch *proximal* to the point where the ductus arteriosus joins the aorta (Fig. 15.6). Therefore the brain, like the heart, receives typical left ventricular blood with high oxygen saturation (about 62%, Fig. 16.1).

16.8.5 *Trunk, abdominal viscera, and limbs*

These regions of the fetus are supplied by the aorta *peripheral* to the point where the aorta is joined by the ductus arteriosus (Fig. 16.1). Therefore this blood is a mixture of a small quantity of well oxygenated left ventricular blood (10% of the combined ventricular output; Fig. 16.1) and a large volume of poorly oxygenated right ventricular blood (57% of the combined ventricular output). This blood therefore has a relatively low oxygen saturation (about 58%; Fig. 16.1).

> Jensen and Berger (1993, p. 25) estimated that the **skeletomuscular system** and **skin** receive about 30% of the combined ventricular output. The small intestine receives about 2.6%, the kidneys about 2.3%, and the adrenal glands about 0.006%.

16.9 Innervation of the fetal cardiovascular system

From about half way through pregnancy, the fetal body has a full equipment of **parasympathetic** and **sympathetic** motor pathways, as well as **chemoreceptor pathways** from the **carotid bodies** and **aortic bodies**, and **baroreceptor pathways** from the **carotid sinus** and **aortic arch**. These act through typical reflex arcs as in the adult animal (Sections 19.12, 19.13), thus contributing to cardiovascular homeostasis. For example, a rise in arterial pressure stimulates baroreceptor endings in the carotid sinus, and induces reflex vagal activity that slows the heart rate. **Vasoactive secretions** also induce vasodilation and vasoconstriction (Sections 13.4), as in postnatal life.

> Activity of the fetal autonomic nervous system has been surveyed by Walker (1993, pp. 1820–185). The **parasympathetic innervation** becomes active first, as would be expected from its role in the conservation of bodily reserves (Section 1.3.2). From about half way through pregnancy, the heart rate of the human fetus declines progressively until term; this is because increasing vagal inhibitory activity gradually dominates a weaker degree of tonic **sympathetic** stimulation. In the lamb the heart rate can be slowed by vagal stimulation before the half-way stage of gestation; sympathetic myocardial innervation begins soon after the half-way stage and continues to develop after birth. In newborn mammals, adrenergic innervation is predictably better

developed in species that are relatively independent at birth.

In addition to parasympathetic and sympathetic neuronal activity, a wide range of **vasoactive substances** (Sections 13.4.2 and 13.6) affect the fetal circulation (Walker, 1993, p. 185). These include the renin–angiotensin system, prostaglandins (produced in the placenta), various endothelial dilators and vasoconstrictors including endothelin, and atrial natriuretic factors.

Arterial baroreceptor pathways in the **carotid sinus nerve** and **aortic nerve** begin to function in the lamb soon after half way through gestation (Walker, 1993, p. 182). From about two thirds of gestation, **arterial chemoreceptors** respond to the falling P_{O_2} of **asphyxia** by inducing reflex bradycardia (Section 19.9.4), increased arterial pressure, and sympathetic vasoconstriction, as in the adult animal.

The **placental vasculature** is not innervated (Carter, 1993, p. 128). Therefore the placental vascular resistance must be controlled by vasoactive secretions. The **ductus venosus** could be subject to neuronal control, but it is not yet known if this shunt participates in the regulation of placental blood flow.

16.10 Respiratory movements in utero

Although the fetus is completely immersed in amniotic fluid, it makes numerous breathing movements all through the last part of pregnancy, thus moving amniotic fluid in and out of the trachea.

In the fetal lamb, rapid irregular respiratory movements (Rudolph and Heymann, 1974, p. 203) occur normally in the last third of gestation. They are present for about 50% of the time. The rate of movement is high (80–100 min^{-1}), but the volume is small displacing only 2–4 ml of tracheal fluid. They cause an increase in fetal oxygen consumption, with a concomitant increase in heart rate, arterial pressure, and placental blood flow (Carter, 1993, p. 122).

The movements are increased in amplitude by hypercapnoea (Carter, 1993, p. 122), and profoundly inhibited by acute fetal hypoxaemia (Bocking, 1993, p. 215).

16.11 Fetal stress and circulatory responses

Asphyxia is the commonest cause of fetal stress. This arises during *normal birth*, from repeated reductions in uterine blood flow caused by uterine contraction, and especially by 'straining' during the phase of expulsion through the pelvic canal. Consequently the fetus is usually born in a state of *'physiological asphyxia'* but this is normally relieved by the first few breaths (Section 16.24). Important additional relief may also be obtained, at least in some species and especially the foal, if the umbilical cord is still intact when the neonate is delivered, since there is then a privileged, though brief, period when the neonate may have *two* sources of oxygen – the placenta as well as the lung.

Because the fetal heart works at virtually full capacity (Section 16.1) it has no reserve for dealing with asphyxia, but protective vasodilation does occur in the most vulnerable organs, notably the brain and myocardium.

During pregnancy, the normal fetus evidently maintains a satisfactory placental blood flow, even during uterine contractions (Section 16.8.1).

In the **second stage of labour** (Section 16.12), voluntary 'straining' coincident with uterine contraction causes repeated reductions in uterine blood flow. The volume of umbilical flow may remain unchanged, but the fetal oxygen saturation falls during such episodes, thus subjecting the fetus to equally frequent hypoxia (Section 16.8.1). During human birth these adverse hypoxic effects on the fetus are more significant if the contractions come very rapidly rather than at well-spaced regular intervals. The term 'physiological asphyxia', describing the state of the fetus at birth, was devised by Dejours (1981, p. 168).

Iwamoto (1993, p. 197) has surveyed the cardiovascular responses of the fetus to acute physiological emergencies, such as **hypoxaemia**, **acidaemia**, and **hypercapnia**, caused for example by obstruction of the uterine artery or umbilical cord (Iwamoto, 1993, p. 201). Umbilical vessels can sometimes become occluded by kinking or torsion of the umbilical cord; in principle, the consequences of this are mismatching of maternal and fetal perfusion, comparable to the mismatching of ventilation and perfusion in the air-breathing lung (Section 6.30.1) (Comroe, 1975, p. 242).

The circulatory responses of the fetus to hypoxia and/or hypercapnia are particularly important for maintaining **fetal homeostasis** (Wood, 1993, p. 108), but the best that the heart can do is maintain its output; this it can achieve, even if the oxygen delivery falls as low as 50%, but more severe levels of hypoxaemia are associated with profound falls in heart rate with reduced stroke volume, leading to death (Iwamoto, 1993, p. 205).

However, a **preferential vasodilation** does occur in the **brain**, **heart**, and **adrenal glands** in asphyxia, although the dilatory mechanism is unknown (Iwamoto, 1993, p. 206). A simultaneous **vasoconstriction** in the **gut**, **kidneys**, **skin**, **muscle**, and **bone** appears to work through sympathetic, adrenergic, and vasopressin mechanisms. There is also **pulmonary vasoconstriction**, though this is not a sympathetic but a local vascular response. All these organs that undergo vasoconstriction can withstand a short-term reduction in oxygen delivery (Wood, 1993, p. 108). Their widespread vasoconstriction increases the total peripheral resistance and hence raises the arterial pressure; this directs the blood secondarily to where it is most urgently needed, i.e. to the heart and brain, and especially to the fetal placenta (Wood, 1993, p. 110). Consequently the blood flow in the all important **umbilical artery** is generally maintained during moderate hypoxia (Iwamoto, 1993, p. 205).

II NEONATE

16.12 Birth

All the domestic mammals generally give birth lying down, on the side (mare and sow) or on the sternum (cow and bitch), but they sometimes do it standing up. The angle of the pelvis in relation to the advancing fetus is likely to be most favourable in the recumbent position.

Species that may carry only one fetus at a time (mare, cow, and ewe) usually deliver it in 'anterior' **presentation**, the forefeet preceding the head. In species that give birth to several fetuses at one labour (sow, bitch, and cat) 'posterior' presentations with the hind feet first are nearly as common as 'anterior' presentations. In all species, delivery of the head through the vulva takes the greatest and longest effort; the rest follows relatively easily.

The **first stage** of labour is essentially a phase of **uterine contractions** with a dilated cervix. In the **second stage** voluntary contractions of the **abdominal muscles**, or '*straining*', are superimposed on uterine contractions. This stage ends in delivery of the fetus. The coordination of the voluntary and involuntary contractions is attained by the uterine contractions, which force the fetal membranes and fetus into the vagina and induce conscious sensations from the vaginal mucosa. These are transmitted by somatic afferent pathways in the **pudendal nerve** (Section 4.14) to the ascending tracts of the spinal cord culminating in the brain. There, the cerebral cortex interprets these sensations as the entry of a foreign body into the vagina, and calls for expulsion. The resulting reflex straining is similar to that induced during defecation. Indeed one lady known to the author concluded that giving birth was like defecating a turnip. In the **third stage of labour** voluntary abdominal contractions tend to stop, but **uterine contractions** continue. Moreover these contractions go like peristaltic waves along the whole length of the uterus in either direction, craniocaudally or caudocranially. These contractions squeeze blood out of the fetal placenta and detach the placenta from the endometrium. The onset of **suckling** augments the uterine contractions of the third stage. Eventually the fetal placenta enters the vagina and is finally forced out by renewed voluntary abdominal contractions. In the mare, the renewed contractions at the end of the third stage are painful, and the mare shows signs of colic immediately after the final expulsion of the membranes.

The manner of **rupture of the umbilical cord** varies with the species. The umbilical cord of the **calf** is so short (Section 16.4) that it often breaks during delivery, but it may remain intact while the hind legs are still in the vagina. The cord of the **pig** is so long that the piglet can suckle while the cord is still intact, and eventually the piglet breaks it by moving about. The **carnivores** usually rupture the cord by biting it. Generally the **foal** has its hind legs up to the hocks still in the vagina, at the end of the mare's expulsive efforts. If not disturbed the mare and foal then rest for about 5–20 minutes, with the cord intact. During this phase, the neonate has two organs of respiration, i.e. the lungs which are rapidly gaining in their capacity for gas exchange, and the placenta which is equally rapidly declining in its capacity. The primary cause of rupture of the cord is the mare getting up. In man the cord is ligated and cut soon after delivery.

Rupture of the umbilical cord in the foal, and indeed in domestic mammals generally, does not require any sort of human intervention in the form of tying or cutting. Contraction of the naturally ruptured umbilical arteries prevents haemorrhage (Section 16.18). Interference with the natural process of foaling by hasty ligation of the cord may be frankly detrimental by depriving the foal of a placental blood transfusion (Section 16.25).

Domestic mammals except the mare eat the 'afterbirth'.

> The **birth of Thoroughbred foals** has been described by Rossdale and Mahaffey (1958). Rupture of the allantochorion, releasing small and eventually large quantities of urine-like fluid, marks the definite onset of parturition. Very soon the shiny, bulging, intact amnion appears at the vulva. Under natural conditions the amnion remains intact until the foal ruptures it by its own movements after delivery. In the UK, stud grooms generally rupture the amnion and peel it from the head as soon as the latter leaves the vulva. This coincides with, or more probably actually induces the first attempts at breathing. Grooms generally interrupt the umbilical cord as soon as they can get at it. They often cut the cord with scissors about 3.5 cm from the foal's abdomen, with or without ligation. Another common practice is to break the cord with a strong pull. Some grooms drag the foal to the mare's head immediately, and this at once ruptures the cord. If there is no interference the mare rests for a while and then ruptures the cord at the natural point by getting up. Separation of the placenta usually starts soon after delivery and is generally complete within the hour.
>
> Welsh pony foals are normally up and running within half an hour of birth. Several hours may elapse in Thoroughbred foals in the UK, though such long delays are apparently less common in Thoroughbred foals born without human assistance in Australia.

16.13 Interruption of placental blood flow during birth

As described in Section 16.11, during normal labour there are repeated reductions in placental blood flow, especially during the expulsive phase; these create severe fetal asphyxia. Soon after delivery the fetal placental circulation begins to decrease, and after some minutes stops altogether through vasoconstriction or rupture of the umbilical arteries. This increases the asphyxia. The normal fetus is therefore born in a state of '**physiological asphyxia**'. In the normal neonate the asphyxia is rapidly relieved by the first breaths after birth (Section 16.24). For as long as the umbilical cord is intact after delivery, placental gas exchange may also be able to contribute to the urgent recovery from asphyxia (Section 16.12), particularly in the foal.

Mechanical stimulation of the intact umbilical arteries, caused for example by pulling or compressing the umbilical cord during birth or at delivery, induces contraction of the arterial walls (Section 16.18); such contraction can be felt if the cord is held in the hand, and disappearance of the normal arterial pulsations (Section 16.4) can be detected. These contractions, as well as the actual compression of the cord while the fetus is being squeezed through the pelvic canal, reduce the oxygen supply to the fetus and allow carbon dioxide to accumulate in the fetal blood. Partial separation of the placenta during birth may also diminish fetal gas exchange.

> When a foal is passing through the pelvic canal its oral mucosa becomes deep purple in colour, indicating severe anoxia. Within seconds of complete delivery the oral mucosa is transformed to a bright pink colour (Rossdale and Mahaffey, 1958). This instant recovery is presumably due to a resumption of placental function, since the umbilical cord would still be intact and the uterus is no longer being compressed by straining.
>
> During normal delivery, arterial O_2 saturation in human infants falls to below 30%. In the foal during normal birth the arterial P_{O_2} falls as low as 15–25 mmHg (2.0–3.3 KPa), the arterial P_{CO_2} rises to 50–70 mmHg (6.7–9.3 KPa), and the pH of arterial blood drops to about 7.1.
>
> In abnormal birth, including compression of the cord or functional failure of the placenta, the pH of fetal arterial blood may even fall below 7.00; at this level of severe acidaemia, cellular damage may occur in the heart, lungs, liver, kidney, and brain (Rossdale, 1972).

16.14 Changes in vascular resistance after birth

In the fetus, the placenta offers a low resistance to blood flow, and the lungs a high resistance (Section 16.2). These resistances determine the distribution of blood throughout the fetal body.

At birth, the taking of the first breath and the loss of the placenta cause these two resistances to be reversed (Fig. 16.4). The **systemic arterial system** now becomes a *high resistance pathway*: the **pulmonary circulation** is converted into a *low resistance pathway*. These changes in resistance bring about an immediate and radical redistribution of blood in the neonate.

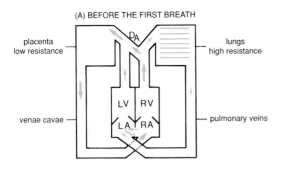

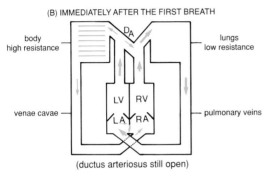

(ductus arteriosus still open)

Fig. 16.4 Diagram summarizing the effects of the vascular resistance of the placenta and lungs on the direction of blood flow before and after the onset of breathing.
A. **Before the first breath.** The placenta is a low resistance pathway. This induces a large flow (large arrow) from the right ventricle (RV) through the ductus arteriosus (DA), and a smaller flow (medium arrow) from the left ventricle (LV); this combined right and left ventricular flow passes through the aorta, placenta and body, venae cavae, and into the right atrium (RA). In the right atrium it promotes a right-to-left shunt which opens the flap (green wavy line) of the foramen ovale. There is a small flow (small arrow) from the right ventricle through the lungs and pulmonary veins, to the left atrium (LA).
B. **Immediately after the first breath and loss of the placenta.** The lungs are now a low resistance pathway. There is a large flow (large arrow) from the right ventricle through the lungs. This is augmented by a substantial flow from the left ventricle through the ductus arteriosus to the lungs (medium arrow). This large combined right and left ventricular flow to the lungs (large arrow) returns in the pulmonary veins to the left atrium. In the left atrium it sets up a left-to-right pressure gradient that closes the flap of the foramen ovale (green wavy line). The majority of left ventricular flow (medium arrow) goes through the body and returns by the venae cavae to the right atrium. Because of the ductus flow, the venous return to the left atrium (large arrow) exceeds that to the right (medium arrow). Therefore, while the ductus is open, the left ventricular output (long arrow) exceeds the right ventricular output (shorter arrow). When the ductus arteriosus closes, the left ventricular flow through the body will finally equal the right ventricular flow through the lungs.

The principal change is the sudden great increase in flow through the **lungs** (Section 16.16). This greatly increases the flow through the pulmonary veins, and hence the venous return to the left atrium (Fig. 16.4B). A *left-to-right* pressure gradient now develops across the **foramen ovale**, closing its flap (Section 16.20).

The loss of the placenta causes the resistance in the systemic arterial system to become greater than the resistance in the pulmonary circulation. This creates a pressure gradient from the aorta to the lungs. Consequently, at the point where the aorta is joined by the **ductus arteriosus**, the aortic flow divides (Fig. 16.4B): most of it continues down the aorta, but about one third of the aortic flow now turns at an acute angle and enters the ductus arteriosus. At the junction of the ductus with the pulmonary trunk (Fig. 15.6), the blood in the ductus makes another acute turn to enter the pulmonary trunk, and then flows to the lungs through the left and right pulmonary arteries. These two acute changes in direction in the blood flow within the neonatal ductus arteriosus create turbulence, and this is audible for a time after birth as a '**machinery murmur**' in most species (Sections 15.8, 22.7.7).

Thus blood continues to flow through the ductus arteriosus for a while after birth. But now this is **left** ventricular blood instead of right, and it flows in the reverse direction to that in the fetus (Fig. 16.4B). Therefore, immediately after the first breath, the ductus arteriosus carries a substantial flow of blood from the left ventricle to the lungs, and this continues until the ductus arteriosus closes, minutes, hours, or days after birth, depending on the species (Section 16.21). The addition of left ventricular blood to the pulmonary circulation augments the already large venous return to the left atrium. Consequently the venous return to the left atrium now substantially exceeds that to the right atrium; this causes a *left-to-right* pressure gradient across the foramen ovale, which functionally closes the foramen (Section 16.20). It also causes the left ventricular output to correspondingly exceed the right – until the ductus arteriosus closes.

In man the left-to-right shunt of left ventricular blood through the ductus arteriosus after birth is substantial, about 35% of the left ventricular output being thus 'stolen' by the lung through the ductus arteriosus (Walker, 1993, p. 175). While the ductus is patent, the left ventricular output exceeds the right by a volume corresponding to the volume of the shunt (left ventricular output, about 250 ml min^{-1} kg^{-1}; right ventricular output, about 175 ml min^{-1} kg^{-1}). In the lamb the ductus arteriosus closes within the first hour of birth, and therefore at that time the left and right ventricular outputs become virtually equal in this species.

16.15   Cardiac output at birth

The rate of **oxygen consumption** per unit body mass of the fetus is about twice that of an adult, up to and including the moment of birth, thus providing for the very high *energetic cost of growth* in the fetus (Section 16.1). This requires a much greater cardiac output (about four and a half times greater in terms of ml min^{-1} kg^{-1}) in the fetus, right up to the time of birth, than in the adult. Remember that cardiac output in the fetus is expressed as the combined output of *both* ventricles, whereas cardiac output in the postnatal mammal is expressed as the output of only *one* ventricle (Section 16.1). One consequence of this huge demand for oxygen is that the fetal heart is constantly working at full capacity, with virtually no reserve output to deal with functional emergencies such as episodes of **asphyxia** during and immediately after birth (Section 16.11).

Throughout the first hours and day or two after birth, the cardiac output (one ventricle) is almost as high as the combined ventricular output in the fetus. This entails a remarkable change in the performance of the left ventricle. Before birth, the output of the left ventricle was only a little more than half that of the right ventricle (35% of the combined ventricular output; Fig. 16.1): immediately after birth, the output of the left ventricle must equal that of the right ventricle. This means that, at birth, the output of the left ventricle instantly has to make an enormous increase of more than two and a half times. Indeed, because a substantial volume of left ventricular blood is diverted through the ductus arteriosus immediately after birth (Section 16.14), the output of the left ventricle *exceeds* that of the right until the ductus closes.

Starting a few days after birth, the cardiac output per kilogram of body mass declines quite rapidly during the next few weeks, finally stabilizing at its adult level. The output of each ventricle is then less than one quarter of the combined ventricular output of the fetus. Thus the heart has now acquired a **cardiac reserve** (Section 22.16) for physiological emergencies.

This progressive and very large reduction in cardiac output per kg of bodymass after birth, from immaturity to maturity, is made possible by the steadily declining energetic demands of *growth*, and by a gradual improvement in *thermoregulation* so that relatively less energy is lost from the surface of the body as heat. (In the normal adult body, about 75–80% of all the energy from food is lost as heat.)

An important clinical consequence of the fetal heart operating at almost its maximal capacity is that the neonate (newborn animal), both human and domestic, is greatly at risk if it has a cardiac disorder. It will be almost impossible to increase its cardiac performance by drug therapy.

Postnatal changes in cardiac output have been reviewed by Walker (1993, p. 180). The high cardiac output **immediately after birth** is required mainly to sustain temporarily the high output that existed before birth, thus providing a platform for the controlled decline after birth.

As noted in Section 16.14, in most species the **ductus arteriosus** is patent for a short time after birth. A substantial volume of left ventricular blood therefore goes through the lungs, and is then added to the venous return to the left atrium. Therefore the *left-to-right* shunt through the ductus arteriosus causes the left ventricular output to substantially exceed the right for a short while after birth. This does not occur in the lamb. In this species the ductus arteriosus closes during the first hour after birth, and consequently the left and right ventricular outputs become equal within the first hour of birth.

The **mass** of the canine *right* ventricle is greater than that of the left at birth (Kirk *et al.*, 1975). However, during the week after birth the *left* ventricle thickens and gains weight much more rapidly than the right, soon assuming its characteristic muscular predominance (Section 16.1).

The fetus has an **oxygen consumption** per unit body mass about twice that of the adult, to provide for the energetic cost of growth. On departing from the cosy intimacy of the uterus, the **neonate** undergoes an increase in oxygen consumption to maintain its body temperature in the rigours of the real world. However, this increase can be accounted for by enhanced extraction of oxygen from arterial blood, and does not require an increased blood flow. The onset of **muscular activity** also increases the oxygen consumption.

During the first week after birth the **cardiac output** of the lamb (left ventricular output) falls to about $300 \, ml \, min^{-1} \, kg^{-1}$ (Walker, 1993, p. 180). This is achieved by a reduction in stroke volume, the rate remaining unchanged. During the next few weeks the cardiac output declines quite rapidly, and then continues to fall more slowly to the postnatal level of about $100 \, ml \, min^{-1} \, kg^{-1}$.

Arterial pressure rises rapidly during the first postnatal week. This is related to the increased resistance of the systemic circulation, following the loss of the low resistance placenta. **Heart rate** falls during this period, because of a decrease in the intrinsic rate of discharge of the sinuatrial node.

Fetal blood is modified to enhance the uptake of oxygen (Section 14.3.3). Postnatal modifications (Comroe, 1975, p. 246) include replacement of high affinity fetal haemoglobin with low affinity adult haemoglobin, thus shifting the oxygen dissociation curve to the right (Fig. 14.1). Also, in man, about 20% of the red blood cells are shed.

Amory *et al.* (1993) remarked on the 'unique fragility' of the newborn human in cardiac diseases. Because the heart of the resting newborn mammal is already pumping virtually at its full capacity, treatment of congenital heart disease with **inotropic drugs** may have little potential benefit. Inotropic drugs (Greek: inion, muscle; tropos, direction; hence muscle-directed – a somewhat unhelpful etymology, see Section 22.8.1) are those that increase the force of muscular contraction, especially cardiac muscle, digitalis glycosides being an example (Blood and Studdert, 1988, p. 489). From their studies on the haemodynamics of normal calves, Amory *et al.* (1993) concluded that inotropic therapy may be ineffective in the newborn calf as well as in neonatal man and sheep.

16.16 Pulmonary circulation

As stated in Section 16.2, the high vascular resistance of the pulmonary circulation in the fetal lung is maintained by the collapsed state of the lung, which mechanically compresses the alveolar vasculature; it is also maintained by the low P_{O_2} of the pulmonary blood, which causes arterial vasoconstriction.

Within minutes of the first breath there is an enormous decrease in pulmonary vascular resistance (to a mere one tenth of its fetal value). This is accompanied by an equally huge increase in pulmonary blood flow (to about ten times its fetal value). The main cause of this profound fall in resistance is the instant flooding of the lung alveoli with oxygen during the first breaths, and the virtually simultaneous increase in the oxygen content of the blood: the increased blood P_{O_2} has a powerful vasodilator effect on the small muscular arteries of the pulmonary vascular beds. The mechanical expansion of the lung with gas also contributes, by relieving the compression of the microvasculature within the collapsed lung; this is achieved by the physical expansion of small vessels and by the unkinking of small pulmonary arteries.

Several other factors contribute to the reduction in pulmonary vascular resistance after the onset of breathing (Walker, 1993, pp. 171, 185). At least some of the mechanical effect of the postnatal rhythmic inflation of the lungs appears to be mediated by dilator **prostaglandins** such as prostocyclin. The **endothelium** plays an important part in vasomotor control in the lung by releasing various vasodilator factors in response to mechanical forces applied to the endothelium by the flowing blood, as it does in the systemic circulation (Section 13.6); potent endothelial vasodilators include the prostaglandin **prostacyclin**, the peptide **bradykinin**, and **endothelium-derived relaxing factor** (EDRF).

The inflation of the *conducting airways* with gas helps the perfusion of the pulmonary vasculature with blood. It has been suggested that, conversely, the perfusion of the pulmonary microvasculature helps the inflation of the *respiratory airways* by *capillary erection*.

16.17 Removal of lung fluid after birth

The fetus is swimming in amniotic fluid, and makes repeated respiratory movements during the last third of pregnancy. It is therefore to be expected that at birth the airways will contain amniotic fluid.

Reabsorption of the fluid in the lung is necessary before the alveolar wall can be fully exposed to the alveolar gases. Removal is very quickly carried out by an increase in pulmonary lymphatic drainage, and presumably by simple drainage into the pharynx.

The volumes of the fetal respiratory movements are in fact small (Section 16.10), and the fluid in the airways may be partly a secretion of the lung itself.

Lauweryns and Baert (1977, p. 641) concluded that although the lung lymphatics dilate and their lymphatic flow greatly increases, the pulmonary blood capillaries should also contribute to the removal of fluid.

16.18   Closure of the umbilical vessels

Closure of the **umbilical arteries** immediately after the umbilical cord is ruptured is of the first importance, since otherwise the neonatal animal would bleed to death.

Forcible rupture of the umbilical cord induces the strongest and most immediate closure. This occurs during natural birth, when the mother rises from recumbency, delivers standing up, or chews the cord, or when the neonate moves away (Section 16.12). Under these conditions the intra-abdominal regions of the umbilical arteries of the neonate are pulled partly out of the abdomen and rupture. Their ends fly back into the abdomen and then immediately become firmly sealed. The remnants of the two umbilical arteries become the left and right **round ligaments of the bladder**.

The actual closure of the ruptured arterial stump is achieved by contraction of the thick layer of smooth muscle of the tunica media. Contraction occurs in direct response to mechanical stimulation. This is a fundamental characteristic of vascular smooth muscle, forming the basis of the myogenic regulation (autoregulation) of vascular tone (Section 13.5). It is also a fundamental protective response of arteries generally (Section 12.21.1).

After rupture of the cord, the ends of the **umbilical veins** immediately close. Since they are about as muscular as the umbilical arteries, the smooth muscle in their walls probably contracts in response to the same stimuli as those that activate the walls of the arteries. Their closed stumps can usually be seen in the torn end of the umbilical cord. After natural rupture the stumps protrude from the umbilicus, then shrivel and drop off.

It might be expected that the **circular muscle** in the tunica media of the umbilical arteries would close the arterial stump, but the circular muscle alone is ineffective (Rudolph and Heymann, 1974, p. 199). Contraction of the **longitudinal smooth muscle** in the wall (and the spiral longitudinal muscle when present as in man, Section 16.4) shortens the stump and causes the intima

to bulge into the lumen, thus helping the circular muscle to produce complete closure.

The contractile response does not depend on a nerve supply. The circular muscle contracts in response to an **increase in P_{O_2}** (as does the muscular wall of the ductus arteriosus; Section 16.21), and is relaxed by a decrease in P_{O_2}. The longitudinal muscle contracts in direct response to the mechanical stimulus of **stretching**. Furthermore the spiral longitudinal muscle of the human umbilical cord is actively constricted by a fall in the ambient **temperature** to about 27°C. The powerful vasoconstrictor **endothelin** (Section 13.6) is released in high concentrations from the endothelium of umbilical vessels and may therefore contribute to constriction of umbilical vessels at birth (Walker, 1993, p. 186).

16.19   Closure of the ductus venosus

The ductus venosus is closed functionally within hours or a few days of birth, depending on the species. Closure seems to occur passively. The decrease in blood flow and blood pressure in the ductus venosus leads to narrowing of its inlet. Permanent obliteration by connective tissue is completed in a few weeks.

In the dog, functional closure occurs on the second or third day after birth, and anatomical closure is complete between the second and sixth days (see Meyer *et al.*, 1995).

A muscular sphincter with autonomic innervation has been described at the junction of the umbilical vein with the ductus venosus (Franklin *et al.*, 1946, p. 9), but the structural evidence for it is controversial (Walker, 1993, p. 167). It has been suggested (see Meyer *et al.*, 1995) that the increased neonatal activity of thromboxane A_2 and decreased activity of prostaglandin E_2 may contribute to the contraction of the ductus venosus, but Walker (1993, p. 167) considered it unlikely that neural or other vasomotor mechanisms play a major role in closure. **Portacaval shunts** arise from a **patent ductus venosus** and other anomalous connections between the portal vein and caudal vena cava, causing portal blood to bypass the liver. This leads to hyperammonaemia, with neurological dysfunction and other clinical signs. Such anomalous shunts occur in the foal and calf, but are commonest in cats and dogs (Noden and de Lahunta, 1985, p. 266).

16.20   Closure of the foramen ovale

The foramen ovale is a one-way valve, allowing only *right-to-left* flow (Section 16.6). In the fetus the foramen ovale is open. This allows most of the *oxygenated lamina* in the caudal vena cava to go from the right side of the heart, through the valve of the foramen ovale, and into the left side of the heart. From there it is distributed preferentially to the myocardium and brain (Section 16.6).

In the **postnatal heart**, such a *right-to-left shunt* would be highly disadvantageous, since it would transfer *deoxygenated* blood from the cranial and caudal venae cavae into the left side of the heart and thence into the systemic arterial circulation. It is therefore desirable that the foramen ovale be closed as soon as possible after birth (Section 15.12).

Functional closure of the foramen ovale immediately after birth is achieved by the changes in the pressure gradients between the right and left atria. These gradients depend on the relative volumes of the venous return to the two atria. In the fetus, the volume of the venous return to the right atrium exceeds that to the left atrium (Fig. 16.4A; Section 16.8). Therefore in the fetus there is a pressure gradient from the right atrium to the left atrium, and this allows the foramen ovale to be open; the kinetic energy of the caudal caval flow then drives the blood stream from right to left through the foramen ovale (Section 16.6).

After birth, the expansion of the pulmonary circulation, including the aortic contribution through the ductus arteriosus, causes the venous return to the left atrium to greatly exceed that to the right atrium (Fig. 16.4B; Section 16.14). Therefore there is now a strong pressure gradient the other way, i.e. from the left atrium to the right atrium, and this functionally closes the foramen ovale by pressing its flap (valvula) against the interatrial septum.

Functional closure of the foramen ovale occurs within the first few breaths after birth. However, in the period immediately after birth, it is always possible for functional closure of the foramen ovale to be reversed by haemodynamic changes, giving a deleterious venous-to-arterial (right-to-left) shunt. The foramen ovale is not securely closed until its valvula is *anatomically fused* to the interatrial septum. This fusion occurs more quickly in 'ungulate' species with a sock-like valvula, than in carnivore and primate species with a sheet-like valvula (Section 15.3.6).

Anatomical closure (Dawes, 1961, p. 152) occurs within a few hours of birth in the foal, and begins towards the end of the first week in the lamb. No signs of permanent closure were seen in Rhesus monkeys 8–12 days old.

In man, anatomical closure does not normally occur before the end of the first year (Walker, 1993, p. 168). *Right-to-left shunts* in the human neonate may persist for several days after birth, and can be induced by normal behaviour such as crying and straining. They can also occur under pathophysiological conditions in which pulmonary vascular resistance is increased or pulmonary blood flow is reduced. About 25% of adults have a small permanent opening, but without shunting or functional handicap.

16.21 Closure of the ductus arteriosus

Despite the fact that it joins an elastic artery (pulmonary trunk) to an elastic artery (aorta), the ductus arteriosus is a massively developed **muscular artery**.

In most species the ductus arteriosus begins to close functionally soon after the onset of breathing, and in some species (especially the lamb) actually completes its closure within a matter of hours. However, in other species the machinery murmur that arises from the turbulence of its reversed blood flow (Section 16.14) can sometimes be heard loudly for hours or days after birth.

Functional closure is achieved by constriction of the powerful smooth muscle in the ductus wall (Section 16.7). The main factor inducing this constriction is the increased P_{O_2} of the blood flowing through the ductus. This relationship between increased P_{O_2} and increased vasoconstriction by the smooth muscle of arterioles and metarterioles is characteristic of the metabolic regulation of vascular tone (Section 13.2.1).

Anatomical closure of the ductus, i.e. permanent obliteration of the lumen, occurs much later, probably months after birth. The surviving remnant becomes the **ligamentum arteriosum**.

Failure of the ductus arteriosus to close may cause serious respiratory and cardiovascular disturbances (Section 15.8).

Functional closure usually takes only a few minutes in guinea pigs and rabbits, an hour in lambs, and up to 15 hours in human babies (Walker, 1993, p. 169). A machinery murmur is difficult to hear in puppies and kittens (Noden and de Lahunta, 1985, p. 224). In the calf and foal it is loud for a period of hours or days after birth; thereafter it becomes fainter and disappears when anatomical obliteration of the lumen has finally taken place (Dawes, 1961, p. 151). **Anatomical closure** is achieved by proliferation of the endothelial lining (Williams *et al.*, 1989, p. 725).

The mechanisms that cause **functional closure** of the ductus arteriosus after birth have been reviewed by Walker (1993, p. 168). Before birth, the ductus arteriosus is kept open by the powerful vasodilator action of circulating *prostaglandins* released by the ductus arteriosus, notably prostaglandin E$_2$. At the onset of breathing, the stimulus for the ductus to constrict is the *increased oxygen tension* of the blood. A balance now ensues, between oxygen-induced vasoconstriction and prostaglandin-induced vasodilation. After normal birth, the circulating prostaglandin E$_2$ undergoes clearance, leaving the oxygen-induced vasoconstriction dominant.

Another factor facilitating functional closure of the ductus is the *fall in pulmonary arterial pressure* after birth. The evidence for this is that the ductus is more constricted at its low pressure end (its pulmonary trunk end) than at its aortic end.

There seems to be no information about the architecture of the smooth muscle in the ductus arteriosus. Presumably it is circular.

Failure of the ductus arteriosus to close may cause serious respiratory and cardiovascular disturbances (Section 15.8).

16.22   Closure of the urachus

The urachus lies in the ventral mesentery of the urinary bladder, and connects the apex of the bladder with the umbilicus (Section 16.4). In the postnatal animal this ventral mesentery becomes the median ligament of the bladder, and attaches the ventral surface of the bladder to the pelvic symphysis and linea alba. Normally the urachus closes and degenerates.

If the urachus fails to close (Noden and de Lahunta, 1985, p. 308) it forms a **patent urachus** or **urachal fistula**. Urine will then be released at the umbilicus, thus giving an entry for infection of the bladder. Persistence of the distal end of the urachus at the umbilicus forms a **urachal umbilical sinus**. If only the proximal end of the urachus remains patent it forms a **bladder diverticulum** which is vulnerable to chronic cystitis.

16.23   Initiation of breathing

From about halfway through gestation, the fetus has a full array of functional autonomic reflex arcs that regulate circulation and respiration; these include arterial baroreceptor and arterial chemoreceptor pathways (Section 16.9). There is no doubt that rising **carbon dioxide** levels and falling **oxygen** levels in the arterial blood at birth are a major factor contributing to the initiation of breathing, just as they contribute to the stimulation of breathing in the adult (Section 11.11). At birth, the neonate is already in a state of moderate asphyxia ('*physiological asphyxia*') (Section 16.13), and this becomes progressively more intense until the first breath is taken.

The newborn mammal is also assailed on all sides by new sensory stimuli. Of these, probably cold is the most powerful stimulus to breathe. A lamb delivered on the frozen turf of a windy moor receives a sharp stimulus to its cutaneous temperature receptors: would you gasp in similar circumstances?

Many afferent stimuli evidently contribute to the onset of breathing (Comroe, 1975, p. 244). Contact with the ground stimulates touch and pain receptors, the body experiences gravity, and the movements of the limbs activate mechanoreceptors in joints and muscles. Sounds assail the ears and light strikes the eyes. However, the application of cold stimuli to the skin (Rudolph and Heymann, 1974, p. 203; Derenne *et al.*, 1978, p. 380), and particularly to the muzzle, seems to be the most important factor in the initiation of breathing; a condom filled with warm amniotic fluid and covering the muzzle of a lamb delays the onset of breathing (Franklin *et al.*, 1946, p. 6). Blowing hard on the chest or tapping the soles of the feet are recommended ways of starting the breathing of a human infant.

16.24   The first breaths

Before the first breath, the airways in the lungs are collapsed and filled with fluid; the respiratory airways (Section 6.1) are therefore subjected to powerful forces of surface tension (Section 6.25). Throughout the later part of gestation, the developing **granular epithelial cells** in the alveolar walls secrete **surfactant** (Section 6.25), which decreases the surface tension in the collapsed fetal alveoli. Even in the presence of surfactant, however, surface tension imposes a formidable energetic cost on the newborn mammal when it takes its first breaths.

The first breaths therefore have to be powerful gasps. The actions of the **inspiratory muscles**, notably the diaphragm (Section 10.8) and particular components of the intercostal muscles (Section 10.9), forcibly expand the thoracic cage, and thus dilate the airways of the lung.

Regulation of the **expiratory phase** of the first gasp is also important. If all the air that has just entered the lung now leaves it, the lungs would revert to their collapsed state with renewed cohesion of the alveolar walls because of surface tension. The second breath would demand an equally huge effort. Repetition of such heavy expenditure of energy quickly exhausts the newborn animal, and this is what happens in the **respiratory distress syndrome of the newborn** (Section 16.26.1).

In the normal neonate, the expiratory phase is so controlled that a reserve volume of gas is built up, from the first gasp onwards. This reserve is the **functional residual capacity** (Fig. 10.5).

The normal neonate is delivered in a state of *physiological asphyxia* (Section 16.13), but this is quickly relieved by the first breaths. For as long as the umbilical cord remains intact after birth, placental gas exchange may also contribute, particularly in the foal (Section 16.11).

The pleural pressure, measured by a balloon in the oesophagus (Section 10.4), falls as low as $80\,cmH_2O$ (7.8 kPa) below atmospheric pressure in the inspiratory phase of the first gasps after birth (Dejours, 1981, p. 170). In resting breathing in a normal adult, the pleural pressure falls to only about $-8\,cmH_2O$ (0.78 kPa) during inspiration.

There is evidence that pulmonary arterial pressure also contributes to the initial inflation of the airways (see Rossdale and Mahaffey, 1958). Air inflation alone of the lungs of stillborn lambs and human babies was unable to produce the normal microanatomy of the aerated lung; liquid perfusion of the pulmonary arteries was also necessary, causing '*capillary erection*' (Section 16.16).

16.25   Placental transfusion

If birth by a domestic mammal is undisturbed, the mother is usually lying on her side or sternum when the neonate is delivered. The body of the neonate is therefore likely to be at a somewhat lower level than that of the uterus, thus allowing blood in the fetal placenta to drain by gravity into the body of the neonate. In other words, the neonate would receive a blood transfusion from the fetal component of its placenta, provided, of course, that the umbilical cord is still intact. In general, the umbilical cord remains intact during a natural delivery, at least while the hind limbs are still in the vagina.

In the Thoroughbred foal it has been the practice, in some countries, to ligate and cut the cord immediately after delivery. However, it is now believed that, by depriving the foal of a valuable component of blood, this action may contribute to the pathogenesis of neonatal disorders (the *respiratory distress syndrome* or the *neonatal maladjustment syndrome*). It is now strongly recommended that, in a normal birth, there should be no human interference with the cord and that rupture of the cord should be left strictly to the natural actions of the mare and foal (see immediately below for further details).

Franklin *et al.* (1946, p. 8) emphasized the apparent physiological benefits of transferring to the neonate as much as possible of the blood in the fetal component of the placenta and umbilical cord.

Rossdale and Mahaffey (1958) reported the following measurements of the volume of blood obtained from the cut stump of the umbilical cord of **Thoroughbred foals**: cord cut within seconds after birth, average about 1 litre; cord cut while still pulsating, $1-5\frac{1}{2}$ minutes after birth, average about 400 ml; cord cut after pulsation ceased, 1–7 minutes after birth, average about 170 ml. They calculated that loss of a litre of cord blood would deprive the foal of about 150 g of haemoglobin and 500 mg of iron.

In the **human neonate** the blood volume at birth is about 300 ml, but another 75 ml (an additional 25%) can be added by leaving the infant attached to the placenta for a few minutes or by 'milking' the blood out of the cord and into the baby (Guyton, 1986, p. 1001).

The loss of these volumes of blood by immediate severance of the cord would seem to be rather disastrous. However, at least in some species including man, the fetus has a higher mass-specific red cell count than the adult, in order to compensate for the low oxygen concentration of fetal blood (Section 14.3.2). Consequently in the 4 weeks after birth the human neonate normally eliminates about 20% of its erythrocytes (Comroe, 1975, p. 246); this causes **physiological jaundice**, since the neonatal liver is unable to conjugate significant quantities of bilirubin for excretion in bile, and bilirubin is therefore deposited in the tissues during the first few days after birth. Also, if the additional 25% of blood volume is transfused from the cord to the human neonate, fluid is lost from the blood plasma into the tissues during the next few hours, restoring the blood volume to the normal value of about 300 ml; some paediatricians believe that, in the human neonate, this extra blood volume may cause mild pulmonary oedema with some degree of respiratory distress (Guyton, 1986, p. 1002). However, in the literature on human paediatrics Rossdale and Mahaffey (1958) found other evidence suggesting that respiratory and neurological syndromes of the human neonate might be linked with the loss of placental transfusion.

Neonatal disorders involving respiratory and neurological signs appeared to be common in **Thoroughbred foals** in European studs, where early severance of the umbilical cord was practised (Rossdale and Mahaffey, 1958). In other equine breeds and in Australian Thoroughbred studs these disorders are almost unknown, but the mares foal with much less or minimal human interference and therefore receive the placental transfusion. It is a striking observation that the human infant and the Thoroughbred foal are the only two species which are routinely interfered with during birth, including early cutting of the cord, and both of these species are subject to rather similar respiratory and neurological syndromes. In view of these findings, Rossdale and Mahaffey (1958) concluded that the rupture of the umbilical cord in horses, particularly Thoroughbreds, should be left entirely to natural processes, thus ensuring transfer of blood from the placenta. In 1972 Rossdale reaffirmed this conclusion.

16.26   Neonatal disorders

Several (non-infective) disorders afflict the neonate. The foal and human infant appear to be particularly vulnerable, but the calf and piglet are also affected. The clinical signs and lesions are respiratory and neurological. In most species the respiratory signs tend to be predominant, and have prompted the terms **respiratory distress syndrome of the newborn (RDS)**, or **hyaline membrane disease**. In Thoroughbred foals the neurological lesions tend to predominate and include severe behavioural abnormalities (e.g. wandering, blindness) thus generating the term **neonatal maladjustment syndrome**.

These two syndromes appear to have much in common (Rossdale and Mahaffey, 1958), and may perhaps be variations on the same theme. Some authors, e.g. Rossdale (1972) and Noden and de Lahunta (1985, p. 287), use respiratory stress syndrome and neonatal maladjustment syndrome as alternative names for the same

condition. However, the pathogeneses of the two conditions may be separable and yet may share features in common. It may then be more useful to follow Sonea (1989, pp. 269 and 271), and distinguish the respiratory distress syndrome as being an essentially respiratory condition, and the neonatal maladjustment syndrome as being an essentially neurological condition with behavioural abnormalities.

16.26.1   *Respiratory distress syndrome of the newborn*

In the USA this condition killed about 30 000 newborn human infants annually, premature infants being particularly susceptible (Hildebrandt, 1974, p. 322). The condition is characterized by abnormally high **surface tension** within the alveoli, collapsed alveoli, filling of alveoli with fluid, and a covering of the walls of the **respiratory airways** with a thickened glassy **hyaline-like membrane** consisting of clotted exudate (Weibel, 1984, p. 264).

The **surface tension** in the lungs of such infants is about four times higher than normal. Within a few hours of birth there is severe dyspnoea, hypoxaemia, and a marked *right-to-left shunt* due to perfusion–ventilation mismatching, with cyanosis. A similar condition occurs in foals (Blood and Studdert, 1988, p. 455), in calves after Caesarean section near to term (Eigenmann *et al.*, 1984), and in piglets as a result of an autosomal recessive genetic trait (Gibson *et al.*, 1976). A characteristic clinical sign of this condition in the human infant, foal, and piglet, is a grunting sound on expiration like a dog barking; this has led to the term '**barker syndrome**'. Many premature animals of domestic species that fail to survive the first few hours after birth are believed to suffer from the respiratory distress syndrome, but are not examined post-mortem to confirm the diagnosis (Noden and de Lahunta, 1985, p. 286). Respiratory disorders are the major cause of death in newborn foals (Sonea, 1989, p. 271).

The underlying abnormality is believed to be a deficiency in the quantity of lung **surfactant** in man (Guyton, 1986, p. 1000), foal (Blood and Studdert, 1988, p. 455), calf (Eigenmann *et al.*, 1984), and piglet (Gibson *et al.*, 1976).

How this deficiency of surfactant occurs is not clear. Since the condition in pigs has an autosomal recessive genetic basis, it could perhaps arise directly from a defect in the formation of surfactant in this species. In mammals generally, surfactant first appears in lung fluids in the later stages of gestation, between 18 and 25 weeks in man and 125 and 130 days in the sheep (Section 5.1), and therefore surfactant probably would be deficient in a sufficiently **premature neonate**.

An alternative explanation is that interruptions of placental blood flow during pregnancy or birth could cause incidents of **asphyxia** of the fetus (Section 16.13), which could induce phases of severe pulmonary vasoconstriction. These could inhibit the secretion of surfactant by the **granular epithelial cells** in the alveolar walls (Section 6.18). The resulting deficiency of surfactant would promote diffusion of fluid from the blood plasma into the lung alveoli (Section 17.19.4). A variant of this theory is that pulmonary vasoconstriction in asphyxia could damage the pulmonary endothelium, causing it to leak **fibrinogen** into the alveolar cavities, where it would clot in combination with the surfactant. This would account for the deficiency of surfactant and the formation of the **hyaline membrane**.

16.26.2 *Neonatal maladjustment syndrome*

This condition occurs in full term Thoroughbred foals during the days immediately following birth (Rossdale, 1972). There is *respiratory distress* with hypoxaemia and hypercapnia, but the main clinical signs are *neurologic*, with hypertonus, blindness, wandering, convulsions, coma, and death, though some foals recover.

Palmer and Rossdale (1976) reported the neuropathology of 18 affected foals. In all the brains the principal lesions extended over the whole of the **cerebral cortex** except the pyriform and hippocampal regions. The neuropathological processes were of two types, ischaemic necrosis and haemorrhage, but both of them could be based on a single pathogenesis, differing only in the severity of the precipitating factor: slight severity would induce relatively protracted perineuronal oedema and ischaemic necrosis; great severity would induce acute vascular permeability, intracranial haemorrhage, and rapid death. The underlying cause of the neuropathological changes appears to be a perinatal circulatory disturbance leading to hypoxia of the brain.

The obvious cause of such perinatal hypoxia of the brain is **asphyxia**, but this could occur in several ways. (1) Perinatal asphyxia could arise from *inadequate blood volume* in the neonate, caused by loss of placental transfusion (Section 16.25). The maladjustment syndrome is particularly prevalent when early interruption of the umbilical cord is practised (Rossdale, 1972), but nevertheless the syndrome does sometimes occur when there has been no human interference; therefore hasty severance of the cord cannot be the only factor (Palmer and Rossdale, 1976). (2) Perinatal asphyxia could be caused by interference with *placental blood flow* during pregnancy; because the fetal heart is normally working close to full capacity, the defences of the fetus against asphyxia *in utero* are limited virtually to preferential vasodilation of the brain (Section 16.11). Severe asphyxia can also occur during *birth* (Section 16.13). However, foals with maladjustment syndrome have usually experienced a simple uncomplicated birth. (3) The perinatal asphyxia could be secondary to *deficient uptake of oxygen* by the lungs after birth. The foals do show respiratory distress, and this could arise from *insufficient surfactant*. The respiratory distress could also arise from defective perfusion of the pulmonary microvasculature (*failure of capillary erection*, Section 16.24), caused by reduced blood volume because of the loss of placental transfusion (Noden and de Lahunta, 1985, p. 287). The pathogenesis of the maladjustment syndrome remains uncertain (Palmer and Rossdale, 1976).

Chapter 17
Circulation in the Lungs

There are two circulatory systems in the lung, pulmonary and bronchial. The **pulmonary circulation** is a large volume system, with a low pressure input from the pulmonary trunk, carrying venous blood to the lungs: the **bronchial circulation** is a low volume system, with a high pressure input from the aorta, conveying arterial blood to the lungs.

The function of the pulmonary circulation is to carry mixed venous blood to the lung for gas exchange, and then to return it to the left side of the heart as arterialized blood.

The role of the bronchial arteries is to carry arterialized blood from the systemic arterial system to the tissues of the bronchial tree in order to supply their metabolic needs. The resulting deoxygenated bronchial blood should ideally be returned to the right side of the heart as venous blood, but by an apparent quirk of evolution it is returned to the wrong side of the heart, i.e. to the left side, thus creating a small but recognizable right-to-left (venous-to-arterial) shunt.

Although the bronchial arteries are rather insignificant in the normal animal, they are exceptionally responsive to pathological changes and contribute to the defence of the lung if the pulmonary arteries are occluded or if oedema arises in the lungs or pleural cavities.

The early Greek and Roman anatomists seem to have overlooked the bronchial arteries, but Leonardo da Vinci (circa AD 1513) gave a drawing, annotated in his usual mirror writing, which showed them on the bronchial tree apparently of an ox (Daly and Hebb, 1966, p. 42). His drawing included a cavitation lesion, probably tuberculous, surrounded by distorted branches of the bronchial artery (Baier, 1986), thus anticipating our present awareness of the extraordinary sensitivity of the bronchial circulation to pathological changes in the lung.

Because of its involvement with the pulmonary circulation in health and disease, the bronchial circulation has attracted a good deal of attention. Unfortunately its anatomy is very variable between species and within the same species, and indeed much more so than that of most of the other distinctive circulatory beds such as the coronary, cerebral, splanchnic, renal, and pulmonary circulations; this variability has caused difficulties in experimental design and interpretation of results (Aviado, 1965, p. 186).

I BRONCHIAL CIRCULATION

17.1 Anatomical source of the bronchial arteries

The left and right **bronchial arteries** arise from **bronchoesophageal arteries**. The latter are formed from several alternative sources within the thorax, depending on the species. The main sources in man and the domestic mammals are the thoracic aorta itself between segments T4 and T7, or the right **dorsal intercostal arteries** in the same segments (Fig. 17.1). As their name implies, the bronchoesophageal arteries supply **bronchial arteries** to the bronchi and **oesophageal branches** to the thoracic oesophagus.

The flow in the bronchial arteries (rami bronchales) clearly comes *predominantly* from the aorta or its dorsal intercostal arteries, but is evidently supplemented by other sources. According to Baier (1986), there are usually extensive anastomoses, apparently in the region of the hilus of the lung, with an assortment of extrapulmonary circulatory systems in man. These include the coronary, oesophageal, thyroid, thymic, subclavian, vertebral, and pericardiophrenic arteries. Some of these are predictable, e.g. oesophageal anastomoses. One of the commonest appears to be that with the internal thoracic artery (Daly and Hebb, 1966, p. 46). Such *subsidiary* anastomoses are seldom mentioned in domestic mammals, but anastomoses with the internal thoracic and pericardial arteries are known to occur in the dog (Aviado, 1965, p. 191).

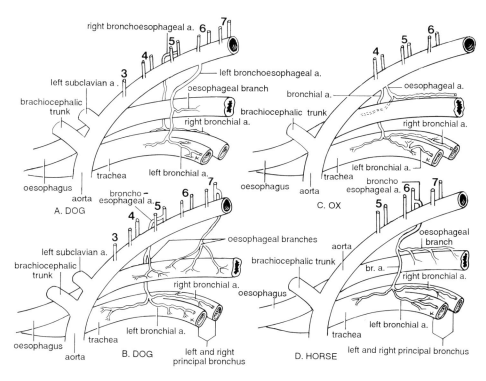

Fig. 17.1 **Diagrams showing species variations in the origins of the bronchoesophageal arteries.** The diagrams are left lateral views, not to scale. Also shown are the first (i.e. most cranial) of the dorsal aortic intercostal arteries in each species. A. Dog: based on Ghoshal (1975, p. 1631) and Schummer *et al.* (1981, Figs 94, 95). B. Dog: based on Evans (1993, Fig. 11-50). C. Ox: based on Ghoshal (1975, p. 981) and Schummer *et al.* (1981, Fig. 155). D. Horse: based mainly on O'Callaghan *et al.* (1987b), and also on Ghoshal (1975, p. 595) and Schummer *et al.* (1981, Fig. 103).

In man (Williams *et al.*, 1989, p. 1285) smaller bronchial arteries arise from the thoracic aorta; one of these may pass to the lung in the **pulmonary ligament**, and is of surgical significance in pulmonary lobectomy. O'Callaghan *et al.* (1987a) noted very large (3–6 mm diameter) bronchial arteries in the pulmonary ligament of the horse; their anatomical source was not established, but was probably aortic.

A comprehensive account of the bronchial arteries in the domestic mammals was given by Ghoshal (1975).

17.1.1 *Horse*

Ghoshal (1975, p. 595) described the bronchoesophageal artery (a. bronchoesophagea) in this species as an unpaired trunk, arising from the thoracic aorta immediately caudal to the first pair of aortic dorsal intercostal arteries, i.e. the fifth dorsal intercostal arteries. Each of the first two pairs of aortic intercostal arteries in this species usually springs from a common stem (Ghoshal, 1975, p. 598), and when this happens the bronchoesophageal artery may share the first or second

of these common stems. In some specimens there is no bronchoesophageal artery as such, because the (unpaired) **bronchial** and **oesophageal** arteries arise separately; Daly and Hebb (1966, p. 48) also mentioned this variant, adding that these two arteries arise from the common stem shared by the sixth dorsal intercostal arteries.

In studies of the bronchoesophageal artery in the live horse, Fowler *et al.* (1963) reported the artery to be formed from the *dorsal* wall of the aorta, although (unspecified) variations were encountered. However, Schummer *et al.* (1981, Fig. 103) clearly showed it springing from the *ventral* wall.

In 19 out of 21 horses affected with exercise-induced pulmonary haemorrhage O'Callaghan *et al.* (1987b) found that the bronchoesophageal artery arose about 0.5–2 cm along the caudal wall of the right sixth intercostal artery, as in Fig. 17.1D.

Once formed (Ghoshal, 1975, p. 595), the bronchoesophageal artery proceeds ventrally across the right side of the aorta (Fig. 17.1D). At the oesophagus, it divides into the oesophageal branch and bronchial branch. The **oesophageal branch** (ramus esophageus) runs along the dorsal wall of the oesophagus in the caudal mediastinum, supplying the oesophagus, mediastinal lymph nodes, and mediastinal pleura, and anastomoses caudally with the oesophageal branch of the left gastric artery. The **bronchial branch** crosses the left surface of the oesophagus, to the tracheal bifurcation. There it divides into the **right** and **left bronchial arteries**, which accompany the dorsal surfaces of the right and left principal bronchi and their branches. When the bronchial artery and oesophageal artery arise independently from the common trunk of the sixth dorsal intercostal arteries, the bronchial artery divides at the tracheal bifurcation to supply both lungs (Daly and Hebb, 1966, p. 48).

McLaughlin *et al.* (1961) reported the presence of a very large additional bronchial artery that accompanied the pulmonary artery rather than the principal bronchus, and supplied blood directly to the alveolar capillaries (Section 17.2).

17.1.2   *Ruminants*

In the **ox** (Fig. 17.1C), the bronchial and oesophageal arteries often arise as separate unpaired trunks (Zietzschmann, 1943, p. 703; Ghoshal, 1975, p. 981). Ghoshal stated their origin to be 'from the wall of the thoracic aorta'. Schummer *et al.* (1981, Fig. 155) showed the two arteries arising very close together from the ventral wall of the aorta, as in Fig. 17.1C. The bronchial artery goes across the right surface of the oesophagus to reach the bifurcation of the trachea, where it forms tracheal branches and divides into the **left** and **right** **bronchial arteries** accompanying the bronchial tree (Fig. 17.1C). The **oesophageal artery** divides into a cranial branch on the right side of the oesophagus, and a larger caudal branch; the latter runs along the dorsal surface of the oesophagus to the oesophageal hiatus supplying the oesophagus, the caudal mediastinal lymph nodes, the mediastinal pleura, and the pericardium.

In the **sheep** (Ghoshal, 1975, p. 1012) the bronchoesophageal artery is usually an unpaired common trunk, arising from the ventral wall (Charan *et al.*, 1984) of the thoracic aorta at the level of the fifth intercostal space. In Charan's casts it was 0.5–1.5 cm long and 1.0–2.5 mm in diameter. On reaching the dorsal surface of the oesophagus, it divides into the **bronchial artery** and the **oesophageal artery**. In some specimens these arise from the aorta as two independent unpaired trunks. The bronchial artery crosses the left surface of the oesophagus to reach the tracheal bifurcation. Here, it divides into four branches, forming a **lateral** and **medial bronchial artery** which descend the whole length of the dorsal aspect of each principal bronchus (Zietzschmann, 1943, p. 703; Schummer *et al.*, 1981, Fig. 100). Otherwise the courses and general distribution of the bronchial and oesophageal branches are the same as in the ox. Charan *et al.* (1984) confirmed this account from observations on 18 sheep, except that they found the origin of the

bronchoesophageal artery from the ventral wall of the aorta to be at the level of the sixth intercostal space. Also they identified not only two, but sometimes three, bronchial arteries descending each principal bronchus; these anastomosed freely, distributed branches to each bronchial branch, and could be traced as far as the terminal bronchioles.

17.1.3   *Pig*

The bronchoesophageal system is somewhat reduced in the pig (Zeitzschmann, 1943, p. 709), in that the *oesophageal component* is reduced to only two fine twigs, which are restricted to the region of the oesophagus at the base of the heart (Schummer *et al.*, 1981, p. 123). The unpaired **bronchial artery** arises from the aorta in the usual way (Ghoshal, 1975, p. 1326). The initial course of the **bronchial artery** is also unusual, in that it crosses the left aspect of the trachea and joins the *ventral* aspect of the bifurcation (Zeitzschmann, 1943, p. 709); only rarely does it approach the bifurcation by the dorsal aspect as in other species. At the bifurcation it forms a **medial** and a **lateral bronchial artery** on each principal bronchus as in the sheep, though these are apparently on the ventral rather than the dorsal surface of the bronchus.

17.1.4   *Dog*

There is much intraspecific variation in this species. Ghoshal (1975, p. 1631) and Schummer *et al.* (1981, p. 123) agreed that the bronchoesophageal artery is paired; they derived the left artery from the aorta at about the level of the sixth dorsal intercostal arteries, and the right artery from the fifth (or sixth) right dorsal intercostal artery (Fig. 17.1A). In some specimens both arteries spring independently, either from the aorta or from dorsal intercostal arteries. Schummer *et al.* (1981, Fig. 94) showed the left bronchoesophageal artery crossing and supplying the left surface of the oesophagus with **oesophageal arteries**, and then distributing **bronchial arteries** to the left principal bronchus and its branches, and sending also a few twigs to the trachea (Fig. 17.1A); the right bronchoesophageal artery traverses the right surface of the oesophagus, which it supplies with **oesophageal arteries**, and then forms **bronchial arteries** ramifying on the right principal bronchus and its branches and supplying also the caudal end of the trachea (Fig. 17.1A).

Evans (1993, p. 646) described only a single (i.e. unpaired) bronchoesophageal artery, arising usually from the right fifth dorsal intercostal artery (Fig. 17.1B). After crossing the right surface of the aorta and the right surface of the oesophagus, it joined the dorsal aspect of the tracheal bifurcation. Here it formed **left** and **right** **bronchial arteries** ramifying on the left and right principal bronchi, with branches to the trachea. Evans (1993,

p. 646) also showed an unpaired **oesophageal artery** arising from the right seventh dorsal intercostal artery and supplying the oesophagus (Fig. 17.1B). Among further variations reported in the literature, Evans (1993, p. 646) included a branch from the right fifth or sixth dorsal intercostal that supplied the right lung (this would correspond to the right bronchoesophageal artery shown in Fig. 17.1A); the left lung was supplied by a single branch from the *left* sixth dorsal intercostal artery. Daly and Hebb (1966, p. 47) also mentioned this variant; if confirmed, it would be a rare instance of a *left* intercostal artery contributing to the bronchoesophageal system.

17.2 Course of bronchial arteries on the bronchial tree

Taking a winding course, the left bronchial artery forms two arteries that lie on and follow the left principal bronchus. The two arteries anastomose repeatedly by short transverse, ladder-like connections. The two arteries give off two corresponding branches that supply each branch of the bronchial tree. The right bronchial artery follows the right principal bronchus and its branches in the same way.

In mammals generally, the left and right bronchial arteries eventually lose their identity in the region of the **respiratory bronchioles**.

The bronchial arteries and their branches tend to look large, because they have unusually thick muscular walls (Fig. 6.3B).

It is widely agreed (Krahl, 1964, p. 271; Daly and Hebb, 1966, p. 57; Baier, 1986; Williams *et al.*, 1989, p. 1285) that, in mammals generally, the bronchial arteries can be followed to the smaller bronchioles, but as soon as alveoli appear along the walls of the respiratory bronchioles the bronchial arteries are no longer distinctly recognizable.

Normal bronchial arteries (Harris and Heath, 1962, pp. 254, 277) have very thick muscular walls, so that they appear almost occluded in histological sections. The muscle is basically circular, but in man may include an eccentric column of longitudinal muscle adjacent to the intima. The circular muscle of the arterioles is thicker than that of typical systemic arterioles, and much thinner than that of pulmonary arterioles.

In most mammals, the main course is typically on the *dorsal* aspect of the bronchi (Fig. 6.3B), with smaller vessels on the *ventral* surface, causing some authorities (e.g. Daly and Hebb, 1966, p. 46, and Aviado, 1965, p. 191) to refer to **dorsal** and **ventral bronchial arteries**. The pig seems to be exceptional in having its main bronchial

arterial vessels on the *ventral* surface (Section 17.1.3). In the other species the smaller ventral vessels evidently arise from subsidiary anastomoses of the bronchial circulation, especially from the internal thoracic and pericardiophrenic arteries (Aviado, 1965, p. 191).

There are typically two, and sometimes three, main trunks on the dorsal surface of the principal bronchus (Daly and Hebb, 1966, p. 57; Baier, 1986); these are presumably the well-attested **medial** and **lateral bronchial arteries** of the sheep (Section 17.1.2). The many transverse anastomoses between the two trunks form an irregular arterial network on the bronchial surface.

Clearly the bronchial arteries are about as far from being *end-arteries* as any arterial system can be. This is the exact opposite of the pulmonary arteries (Section 17.14), which are true end-arteries (Liebow *et al.*, 1950).

McLaughlin *et al.* (1961) noted an unusually large number of bronchial arteries in the pulmonary parenchyma of the **horse**. This was accounted for primarily by the presence of an **additional bronchial artery** that closely accompanied the pulmonary artery rather than the principal bronchus. Incidentally, this extra artery could be followed to the parenchyma, where it provided blood directly to the alveolar capillaries. The additional artery had a very large diameter, in its distal regions attaining one-fourth to one-fifth the diameter of the satellite pulmonary artery. Its great size ruled out the possibility that it belonged to the system of vasa vasorum of the pulmonary arteries.

The presence in the horse of a significant distribution of bronchial arteries to the capillary bed of the exchange tissue may be a factor in the destruction of the alveolar walls that occurs in **alveolar emphysema** in this species (Section 7.19.3).

17.3 Distribution of bronchial arteries within the lung tissues

As they follow the bronchial tree, the bronchial arteries supply innumerable small branches to all the tissues within the **airway walls** of the **conducting airways** (bronchi and bronchioles). They also extend to the **respiratory airways**, but in mammals generally they only go as far as the respiratory bronchioles (Section 17.7).

The main tissues supplied in the airway wall are the bronchial mucosa, bronchial smooth muscle, bronchial cartilage, and bronchial mucous and serous glands. The outer and inner blood-vascular plexuses in the bronchial walls (Section 17.6), which are of special functional importance in providing the bronchus with hydraulic 'give' (Section 6.13), get their blood from the bronchial arteries.

The connective tissues of the **interlobular septa** (Section 5.8) are another component supplied by the bronchial arteries.

Along their course the bronchial arteries give a series of **vasa vasorum** to the accompanying pulmonary arteries and a few to the pulmonary veins. The intrapulmonary nerves and ganglia of the **vagal bronchial rami** (Section 3.11.4) accompany the bronchial arteries. They receive arterial twigs that pierce the epineurium and run between the axon bundles.

The few **pulmonary lymph nodes** on the principal bronchus (Section 7.9.1) obtain their blood supply from the bronchial arteries. So also do the very abundant **lymphatic nodules** of the bronchus-associated lymphoid tissue (**BALT**), which play such a vital part in the defence of the bronchial mucosa by locally secreted immunoglobulin A (Sections 7.9.2, 7.13).

In the horse, additional branches of the bronchial arteries are believed to supply the alveolar capillary bed (Section 17.2).

17.4 Distribution of the bronchial arteries to the pleura

The **parietal pleura** is supplied by regional systemic arteries, particularly the intercostal arteries (Section 9.9).

The **pulmonary (visceral) pleura** is supplied by either the bronchial or the pulmonary arteries. In most species the pulmonary pleura gets its arterial supply from the bronchial arteries (Section 9.9).

In the region of the hilus of the lung, **hilar pleural arteries** arise directly from branches of the bronchial arteries in the region of the tracheal bifurcation, i.e. before the bronchial arteries disappear below the surface of the lung.

In the depth of the lung, the bronchial arteries form branches that accompany the **interlobular septa**. In most species the interlobular septa continue to the surface of the lung, giving the familiar marbled appearance of the lungs of the pig and ox (Section 5.8). The interlobular septa carry **interlobular pleural branches** of the bronchial arteries to the surface of the lung, where they ramify in the vascular stratum of the **pulmonary (visceral) pleura**.

In most species the visceral pleura is very vascular, and is anyway more vascular than the parietal pleura (Section 9.7). The great vascularity of the visceral pleura enables it to absorb **pleural effusion** from the pleural cavity (Section 17.27.2).

The species that receive their arterial supply to the visceral pleura from the bronchial arteries include the ox, sheep, pig, horse, and man, these being species with a thick, highly vascularized pleura. In the dog, cat, and Rhesus monkey, there are no true interlobular septa (Section 5.8). Therefore in these species, branches of the bronchial artery do not reach the surface of the lung. The blood supply of the pulmonary (visceral) pleura, which is thin and poorly vascularized, is taken over by the **pulmonary artery** (Aviado, 1965, p. 191), except for some hilar branches of the **bronchial artery**. In the guinea pig, rat, and mouse, the blood supply to the pulmonary pleura is also from the pulmonary arteries. See Section 9.7 for further details of species variations.

It was reported in the earlier literature (see Daly and Hebb, 1966, p. 53) that, in the horse, the pleural branches of the bronchial artery that supply the pulmonary pleura are large, thick-walled, and contain a great amount of smooth muscle. O'Callaghan *et al.* (1987a) have now shown that, in horses affected by exercise-induced pulmonary haemorrhage (EIPH), the pleural branches of the bronchial artery become extremely prominent and thickened (Section 17.28.2) with a diameter of up to 6 mm. EIPH in the horse is so common that the earlier observations on supposedly normal lungs may have been made on affected lungs.

17.5 Venous drainage of the bronchial circulation: azygos veins

Venous blood from the tissues of the first one or two generations of bronchi drains into the **azygos venous system** by true **bronchial veins** (Fig. 17.2); these bronchi are extrapulmonary, at the **hilus** of the lung. The azygos venous system empties into the **right atrium**. Slightly less than one third of the bronchial blood flow takes this route.

The tissues of the remaining generations of bronchi, bronchioles, and respiratory bronchioles have no true bronchial veins. Instead, they drain via the bronchial vascular plexuses (Section 17.6) into bronchopulmonary veins (Section 17.6.3) that are tributaries of the **pulmonary veins** (Figs 6.3, 17.2), and thence into the **left atrium**. Rather more than two thirds of the bronchial venous blood drains by this pathway. This constitutes a

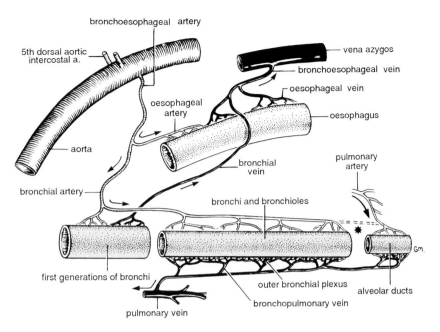

Fig. 17.2 Highly schematic diagram showing the structures supplied and drained by the bronchial arteries and bronchial veins in a hypothetical mammal. In most mammals the bronchial arteries lose their identity at the respiratory bronchioles, but continue there (asterisk) to supply capillary beds which they share with the pulmonary arteries. The venous drainage of the first one or two generations of bronchi, which are essentially extrapulmonary, is by bronchial veins into the azygos vein and thence into the right atrium. The venous drainage of the rest of the bronchial tree is by bronchopulmonary veins into tributaries of the pulmonary veins and so into the left atrium.

small **venous-to-arterial shunt** (Section 17.10). The small coronary veins (Section 18.8) add to this shunt, which is typically about 1 or 2% of cardiac output.

The venous drainage of the pulmonary pleura is into the pulmonary veins, regardless of whether the arterial supply is from the bronchial or pulmonary arteries.

The **right azygos vein** (vena azygos dextra) (Fig. 17.5) occurs in the carnivores, ruminants, horse, and sometimes in the pig. It receives the **bronchoesophageal vein** (v. broncho-esophagea) (paired in carnivores and unpaired in the horse), which is formed by **bronchial** and **oesophageal veins** (vv. bronchales, oesophageales). The right azygos vein drains into the cranial vena cava, close to the right atrium (Schummer *et al.*, 1981, p. 185). The **left azygos vein** (v. azygos sinistra) occurs in the pig and ruminants, and receives separate **bronchial** and **oesophageal veins** (Simoens, 1992, pp. 338, 340). It drains into the **coronary sinus** (Schummer *et al.*, 1981, p. 186). The **dorsal intercostal veins** drain into the azygos veins (Section 8.16.2). **Intervertebral veins** drain the **external** and **inter-**

nal **vertebral venous plexuses** into the azygos veins (Simoens, 1992, pp. 338, 340).

In the dog (and probably also man)(Daly and Hebb, 1966, p. 59), there is an extensive **venous plexus** at the root of the lung, draining into the right azygos vein. This plexus receives not only the more dorsal and larger bronchial veins but also oesophageal, mediastinal, and pericardial veins, together with veins from the mediastinal lymph nodes and the vasa vasorum of the pulmonary artery. The smaller more ventral bronchial veins evidently drain mainly into the internal thoracic vein. The more dorsal and larger bronchial veins sometimes bypass the venous plexus and drain directly into the right azygos vein.

This already elaborate plexus of systemic veins at the root of the lung is further complicated, at least in man, by anastomosing with the pulmonary veins. This means that venous blood from a large variety of systemic structures (including the principal bronchi) may find its way into the left atrium (Daly and Hebb, 1966, p. 60).

There seems to be a conspiracy of silence about the venous drainage of the **visceral pleura**, even in the most advanced anatomical reference works. This is all the more surprising for the reason that the mechanisms of **pleural effusion** depend on the venous drainage of the pleura (Section 17.27.2). Daly and Hebb (1966, p. 388) alone gave a reasonably full account. They explicitly stated that in species with a thick visceral pleura (i.e. man, horse, ox, goat, and pig) the drainage is into the **pulmonary veins** via veins that run in the **interlobular septa**. The visceral pleura in the region of the hilus probably drains into the azygos system as well as into the pulmonary veins (see Williams *et al.*, 1989, p. 1285). The drainage in species with a thin visceral pleura (i.e. the dog, cat, and Rhesus monkey) seems not to be directly stated anywhere; however, again it is virtually certain to be into the pulmonary veins, since the arterial supply in these species is via the pulmonary arteries (whereas it is via the bronchial arteries in species with a thick visceral pleura).

Daly and his co-workers estimated experimentally in the anaesthetized dog what fraction of the bronchial arterial flow went to the left atrium (via the bronchial vascular plexuses and their drainage into the tributaries of the pulmonary veins), and what fraction went (via the azygos vein) to the right atrium (Daly and Hebb, 1966, p. 70). In their experimental preparation, only the bronchial artery was perfused, with no flow through the pulmonary artery. The mean ratio of the volume of bronchial blood returned to the left atrium to the volume returned to the right atrium was about 3.4:1 (range 1.4:1 to 7:1). In other words, under these experimental conditions about 30% of the bronchial output went to the extrapulmonary part of the bronchial tree, and 70% was distributed to the smaller bronchi. Investigations in the late 1980s have shown that the proportion of the bronchial arterial blood that goes to the airways is more than double that supplying the other intrapulmonary structures and the visceral pleura (Butler, 1991).

17.6   The bronchial blood-vascular plexuses

As described in Section 17.2, the bronchial arteries follow a winding course along the outer walls (Fig. 6.3B) of the whole length of all bronchi, giving off many branches as they go. These arterial branches form the **outer** and **inner bronchial blood-vascular plexuses** (Fig. 6.3B). The outer and inner bronchial blood-vascular plexuses are major components of the **peribronchial sheath** (Section 6.13).

17.6.1   *Outer bronchial blood-vascular plexus*

This plexus forms an outer thick sleeve of fine blood vessels enclosing the whole length of every bronchus (Fig. 6.3B).

The plexus consists of freely anastomosing arterial and venous capillaries, and venules, in the outer part of the wall of each bronchus. Since the blood-vascular components of this plexus all belong to the microcirculation (Section 12.7), this is really a *microvascular* plexus. Its vessels are suspended in the three-dimensional framework of fine collagen and elastic fibres of the **fibrous continuum** (Section 6.9). A plexus of **lymphatic vessels** is also interspersed within the blood capillary meshwork of the blood-vascular plexus (Fig. 6.3B).

The outer surface of the outer bronchial blood-vascular plexus blends with the alveoli of the surrounding exchange tissue (Fig. 6.3B). All over this surface, the capillaries of the outer bronchial blood-vascular plexus anastomose directly with the capillaries of the alveolar walls, thus forming extensive anastomotic continuity at the capillary level between the bronchial and pulmonary circulations (Section 17.8).

The outer bronchial blood-vascular plexus and the fibrous continuum that holds it form a large part of the **peribronchial sheath** (Section 6.13; Fig. 6.3B, green). (The arterial and arteriolar branches of the pulmonary artery in the lung parenchyma are also enclosed in vascular sleeves, constituting the **periarterial sheath** – also green in Fig. 6.3B (Section 6.13) – but this periarterial sheath is composed solely of *lymphatic* vessels.)

17.6.2   *Inner bronchial blood-vascular plexus*

At its deep surface, i.e. its surface nearer to the bronchial lumen, the outer bronchial blood-vascular plexus anastomoses with the **inner bronchial blood-vascular plexus**. The inner plexus lies in the tunica mucosa between the cartilage plates of the bronchus and the bronchial epithelium (Fig. 6.3B). Like the outer plexus, it consists of blood capillaries and venules (i.e. it is another **microvascular plexus**). Again like the outer plexus, it also includes a network of numerous fine lymphatic channels.

The blood-vascular and lymphatic plexuses in the peribronchial and periarterial sheaths confer *hydraulic 'give'* to the walls of the bronchi, arteries, and arterioles, thus enabling the diameters of the bronchi, arteries, and arterioles to be regulated independently of inspiration and expiration (Section 6.13). The bronchial vascular plexuses, and particularly the inner one, play an important part in the removal of **pulmonary oedema** (Section 17.26.4).

The architecture of the outer and inner blood-vascular plexuses of the bronchial wall has been clarified by scanning electron microscopy. In the studies of Charan *et al.* (1984) on the lung of the sheep, the outer bronchial plexus is seen to be formed by branches of the **bronchial arteries**. In the periphery of the plexus the capillaries of the bronchial arteries become continuous with the capillaries in the adjoining alveolar walls; this is shown unmistakably by the scanning micrographs of Guntheroth *et al.* (1982). In the scans of Charan *et al.* (1984), individual capillaries in the outermost parts of the outer plexus can be followed to their anastomoses with the adjacent alveolar capillaries.

The inner bronchial vascular plexus was envisaged by Krahl (1964, p. 251) as lying between the cartilage plates and the bronchial smooth muscle. However, with the scanning electron microscope Charan *et al.* (1984) were able to see small arterioles that crossed the muscle layer and thus extended the inner plexus as far as the epithelium. This means that the inner plexus is really a *mucosal* plexus, (as stated by Williams *et al.*, 1989, p. 1285).

Krahl (1964, p. 271) and Daly and Hebb (1966, p. 60) interpreted the outer and inner bronchial blood-vascular plexuses as being essentially 'venous': on the other hand, Williams *et al.* (1989, p. 1285) referred to them as 'capillary plexuses'. Charan *et al.* (1984) regarded the vessels of the inner plexus as being basically 'capillaries', though their diameters ranged from 5 to 50 µm, so that larger vessels are almost certainly postcapillary venules (Section 12.14). But all of these vessels are unquestionably 'microvascular', and belong to the **microcirculation** of the blood-vascular system (Section 12.7).

Daly and Hebb (1966, p. 60) themselves seem to have been the first to use distinctive names for the two bronchial blood-vascular plexuses; perhaps unhappily, they gave the term 'superficial' to the inner plexus, and 'deep' to the outer plexus.

The bronchial vascular plexuses are appropriately situated and constructed to contribute to the removal of pulmonary oedema from the bronchial walls and bronchial lumen, and from the cuffs of oedema that may form around the bronchi (Section 17.26.4): their microvascular and lymphatic constituents reabsorb excess fluid.

17.6.3 *Bronchopulmonary veins*

At each point where a bronchus divides or gives off a branch, the outer and inner bronchial

blood-vascular plexuses converge to form a **bronchopulmonary vein** (Fig. 6.3B). Each bronchopulmonary vein is a tributary of the pulmonary vein; i.e. it conveys *bronchial* blood into the *pulmonary* vein (Fig. 17.2), hence the name 'bronchopulmonary'.

The term **bronchopulmonary vein** was given in 1858 by Le Fort, one of the pioneers of pulmonary morphology (Daly and Hebb, 1966, p. 60), to the venous channels that drain the outer and inner bronchial plexuses into tributaries of the pulmonary veins. Daly and Hebb re-introduced this term.

17.7 Blood supply of the terminal airways

It is widely agreed that the capillary beds of the **respiratory bronchioles** are *shared* by the bronchial arteries and the pulmonary arteries in mammals generally. Thus the terminal meshwork of capillaries on the respiratory bronchioles anastomoses with alveolar capillaries to form a *common capillary network* (at the level of the asterisk in Fig. 17.2). In mammals generally, peripheral to the respiratory bronchioles the alveolar capillaries are supplied by the pulmonary artery only.

Many of the earlier investigators were convinced that part of the capillary networks of the **exchange tissue** is supplied by the bronchial arteries (Daly and Hebb, 1966, p. 57). Materials injected into the bronchial arteries do easily make their way into alveolar capillaries, but injections into the pulmonary artery equally easily reach the bronchial blood-vascular plexuses. Such observations are readily explained by microvascular anastomoses between the outer blood-vascular plexus and the surrounding alveolar capillaries (Section 17.6.1), and by the shared capillaries of the respiratory bronchioles.

However, McLaughlin *et al.* (1961) found that in the horse the bronchial artery really does provide a significant blood supply directly to the alveolar capillary bed (Section 17.2). After re-evaluating the evidence for man, they also suggested that the human and equine lung are structurally similar in this as well as other respects. These observations by McLaughlin *et al.* (1961) on the equine bronchial circulation are potentially important to an understanding of the pathogenesis of alveolar emphysema associated with chronic obstructive pulmonary disease in horses (Section 7.19), and therefore merit careful confirmation.

17.8   Normal anastomoses between the bronchial and pulmonary circulations

The two systems are certainly connected: a dye injected into the bronchial artery is returned simultaneously to both the right atrium and the left atrium. As already stated, it reaches the *right* atrium by draining through the **bronchial veins** from the first one or two orders of bronchi, and thence through the **azygos venous system** (Section 17.5).

It reaches the *left* atrium via three routes: (1) the **bronchial blood-vascular plexuses** and their drainage (by the bronchopulmonary veins) into tributaries of the pulmonary veins (Section 17.6.3); (2) the **capillary anastomoses** between the outer bronchial blood vascular plexuses and the adjoining alveolar capillaries (Section 17.6.1); and (3) the **shared terminal capillary networks** common to both the bronchial and the pulmonary arteries (Section 17.7).

Of these three routes to the left atrium, the second is probably the most important functionally. Its significance is that it provides a bypass enabling the bronchial arteries to take over perfusion of the alveolar walls if branches of the pulmonary arteries become pathologically obstructed, e.g. by a pulmonary embolus (Section 17.9.4).

Anastomoses between the bronchial and pulmonary circulations have potential physiological and pathological significance, and have therefore generated a vast amount of literature during the last two centuries of anatomical research (Krahl, 1964, p. 271).

The first and third of the three anastomotic pathways to the left atrium outlined above are generally accepted (Daly and Hebb, 1966, p. 61). The second (capillary anastomoses at the surface of the outer bronchial blood-vascular plexus) has received relatively little attention because it is only through scanning electron microscopy during the last two or three decades that its exploration has been possible.

There is a fourth anastomotic possibility, namely *precapillary anastomoses*, i.e. anastomoses between the bronchial and pulmonary arteries (bronchi-pulmonary arterial anastomoses). Pathophysiologically this is a particularly attractive concept, since it would be the best way for the bronchial arteries to take over perfusion of exchange tissue after obstruction of pulmonary arterial branches. The presence of such **bronchopulmonary arte-** rial anastomoses in *pathological lungs* is not disputed (Section 17.9), but their existence in *normal healthy lungs* has been particularly hotly debated. Daly and Hebb (1966, p. 61) were 'never' able to demonstrate them in laboratory animals 'to their complete satisfaction', and cited (in their Table IV) six investigations of seven species including man in which such anastomoses could not be found. Charan *et al.* (1984) saw 'only a few' such anastomoses in the sheep with the scanning microscope. On the other hand, Krahl's view (1964, p. 273) was that 'there can be no doubt of their existence', having been observed 'in several different species of animals'.

In 1942, von Hayek (1960, p. 282) proposed a particularly elaborate version of bronchopulmonary arterial anastomosis in the normal human lung. This he named Sperrarterien (German: Sperr, barrier), because the anastomosis supposedly has powerful muscular walls which could enable it to be selectively perfused by either the pulmonary artery or the bronchial artery. He claimed that the anastomotic channel gave off branches to alveolar capillaries and branches to the bronchial venous plexus; these branches could be perfused from either end of the anastomotic channel, i.e. by either the pulmonary artery at one end or the bronchial artery at the other. His book of 1960 contains a distressingly baffling account and diagrams of this mechanism. Krahl (1964, p. 273) believed in it, but Daly and Hebb (1966, p. 66) were unimpressed.

McLaughlin *et al.* (1961) found no bronchial artery–pulmonary artery (or arteriolar) anastomoses (bronchopulmonary arterial anastomoses) in the dog, cat, and Rhesus monkey, 'a small number' in the ox, sheep, and pig, and one in the horse; however, they argued for the existence of functional anastomoses between the bronchial and pulmonary artery under muscular control (e.g. von Hayek's Sperrarterien), thus providing 'demand shunts'.

Aviado (1965, p. 189) pointed out that W.S. Miller, one of the main authorities in this field, interpreted any anatomical connections of bronchial to pulmonary arteries as no more than **vasa vasorum**. This was supported by several workers who injected particulate masses into the bronchial arteries and found that particles with diameters of 14–30 μm could not pass directly into the pulmonary artery.

The anatomical basis for bronchial artery–pulmonary artery anastomoses (bronchopulmonary arterial anastomoses) in normal lungs remains unsure.

17.9   Proliferation of the bronchial circulation in pathological tissues

The lung has extraordinary powers of withstanding ischaemia, as caused for example by obstruction to a branch of the pulmonary artery. How does it manage this?

In response to such an obstruction, the bronchial circulation has the capacity (a) to enlarge, and (b) to generate new vessels (**angiogenesis**; Section 12.20). The bronchial arteries dilate and enlarge their overall size, and thus increase their flow rate. At the same time, they proliferate new vasculature mainly in the form of **bronchopulmonary arterial anastomoses**. The increased bronchial blood flow by-passes the obstructed pulmonary artery by going through the anastomoses, and then perfuses the pulmonary artery beyond the obstruction.

The increase in flow rate happens within minutes of a sudden pulmonary obstruction, and new blood vessels are evident after only a few days. Within weeks or months the bronchial circulation takes over from the pulmonary circulation where this has failed because of the obstruction.

So responsive are the bronchial arteries to pathological stimuli that it is almost impossible to eliminate these vessels from the bronchial wall; for example, ligation of a bronchial artery is rapidly followed by the sprouting of collaterals (Harris and Heath, 1962, p. 252).

The remarkable angiogenic capacity of the bronchial circulation, and especially its ability to proliferate bronchopulmonary arterial anastomoses under pathological conditions, may have a bearing on the disagreement among anatomists about the occurrence of bronchopulmonary arterial anastomoses in 'normal' lungs (Section 17.8). Some leading investigators of circulatory anatomy in the lung (see Daly and Hebb, 1966, p. 66) have indeed expressed doubts about the existence of bronchopulmonary arterial anastomoses (bronchial artery–pulmonary anastomoses) in the *normal* lung.

Commenting as pulmonary pathologists on bronchopulmonary anastomoses in general, Harris and Heath (1962, p. 257) affirmed that 'the great majority of them are acquired in association with diseases of the heart or lung but very rarely they are congenital'. Von Hayek's 'Sperrarterien' were regarded by Harris and Heath (1962, p. 256) 'as abnormal sclerosed bronchial arteries'. This suggests the possibility that the bronchopulmonary arterial anastomoses found by other investigators in supposedly normal tissues were really responses to pathological changes. Harris and Heath (1962, p. 277) conceded, however, that it is difficult to distinguish normal from abnormal bronchial arteries, since the normal arteries are very thick-walled and appear almost occluded.

17.9.1 *Angiogenic factors*

Angiogenic factors that mediate angiogenesis by bronchial arteries in particular have not been identified with certainty (Butler, 1991). However, adaptive and defensive angiogenesis elsewhere in the systemic vasculature is well known, including in the repair of damaged tissues, and appears to be mediated by angiogenic factors released from macrophages, activated T-lymphocytes, and local cells such as mast cells and platelets (Section 12.20). **Endothelial growth factor** and the local release of **heparin** have been proposed as essentials for the development of new capillary buds from existing endothelium (see O'Callaghan *et al.*, 1987c).

17.9.2 *Stimuli for pathological bronchopulmonary arterial anastomoses*

The two main stimuli for the angiogenesis of **bronchopulmonary anastomoses** appear to be obstruction of the blood flow through the pulmonary artery or its branches, and the formation of new tissue in the lungs (Harris and Heath, 1962, p. 257). An example of the first of these two stimuli is the severe pulmonary oligaemia (deficient blood volume in the lung) that occurs in conditions of generalized pulmonary occlusion such as **pulmonary stenosis** (Section 15.9), **tricuspid dysplasia** (Section 15.13), and the **Fallot tetralogy** (Section 15.14): these disorders are usually characterized (in man) by extensive bronchopulmonary arterial anastomoses.

The formation of **inflammatory** or **neoplastic tissue** is thought to be an even greater stimulus for the production of bronchopulmonary arterial anastomoses, as in **bronchiectasis**, **lung abscess**, and **bronchial carcinoma** (Harris and Heath, 1962, p. 258); the operative stimulus in these conditions may be the increased oxygen demand of lymphoid or neoplastic tissue.

17.9.3 *Mode of formation of pathological bronchopulmonary arterial anastomoses*

Several possible processes may form these anastomoses (Harris and Heath, 1962, p. 259). (a) In the granulation tissue of pneumonia, organizing capillaries may come from both the bronchial and the pulmonary arteries; the capillaries join and become anastomotic channels. (b) If a large branch of a pulmonary artery becomes occluded, its vasa vasorum (derived from a bronchial artery) proliferate, dilate, penetrate the intima, and so recanalize the lumen. (c) In view of the uncertainty about the existence of normal bronchopulmonary anastomoses, the possibility remains that some of these anastomoses in pathological tissue may simply be enlargements of pre-existing normal anastomoses.

17.9.4   *Pulmonary embolism and infarction*

The rapid enlargement and angiogenesis of the bronchial circulation in response to ischaemia explains why **pulmonary infarction** rarely follows pulmonary arterial occlusion, an observation that has been made repeatedly since the middle of the last century; clinically, pulmonary infarction occurs in less than 10% of cases of pulmonary embolism in man (Jindal *et al.*, 1984). (An infarct is an area of necrosis caused by occlusion of the blood supply.)

Within 5 minutes of obstructing the branch of the pulmonary artery to a lobe of the lung in the dog, there is a marked increase in the flow rate through its bronchial arteries (Jindal *et al.*, 1984). This is not simply a passive response to the fall in pulmonary pressure, but appears to be an active vasodilation of bronchial arteries apparently caused by the release of local vasodilator substances (Jindal *et al.*, 1984). Three months after ligation of such a branch of the pulmonary artery, the bronchial arteries have grown to ten times their normal size (Harris and Heath, 1962, p. 258); there also seems to be extensive **angiogenesis** in the form of many bronchopulmonary arterial anastomoses.

Pulmonary embolism is the sudden blocking of the pulmonary artery or its branches by an embolus swept in by the blood flow. The **embolus** (plug) is usually a **thrombus** (a blood clot formed inside an intact blood vessel) but can be a piece of tissue, a globule of fat, an air bubble, a cluster of tumour cells, or one of many other objects transportable by the blood stream.

In man, massive **pulmonary embolism** by a single large blood clot is a familiar and dangerous clinical emergency. Typically the clot forms in the veins of the legs or pelvic cavity during a period of immobility after surgery. A large part of the clot, or all of it, becomes detached, particularly when the patient first walks after prolonged bed rest. The clot is carried to the right side of the heart and thence to the pulmonary trunk. If very large it may lodge at the bifurcation of the pulmonary trunk into the left and right pulmonary arteries. Blocking of the pulmonary trunk or both of the main pulmonary arteries simultaneously is quickly fatal. Blocking of the left or right pulmonary arteries is not immediately fatal, since the other lung can accommodate all of the right ventricular output; the bronchial arterial system on the blocked side rapidly increases its blood flow by immediate vasodilation and angiogenic production of bronchopulmonary arterial anastomoses, thus maintaining the viability of the airway tissues. Usually the bronchial perfusion prevents the formation of a pulmonary infarct, as already stated, although small infarcts are sometimes seen (Harris and Heath, 1962, p. 320). However, if the bronchial flow is decreased (as in an experimental preparation) infarcts occur rather consistently (see Jindal *et al.*, 1984). **Diffuse pulmonary embolism** is caused by showers of small emboli, for example fat globules from traumatized fatty tissue.

Blockage of one or several large branches of the pulmonary arterial system, or of many small branches, causes a steep rise in pulmonary resistance with a corresponding increase in pulmonary arterial pressure, i.e. primary pulmonary hypertension (Section 17.22). The clot tends to get bigger, and extend into yet more pulmonary branches. Death may follow from acute right ventricular failure (right heart failure, Section 22.17) (Harris and Heath, 1962, p. 318; Guyton, 1986, p. 293).

17.9.5   *Alveolar emphysema*

Destruction of the alveolar walls, giving alveolar emphysema (Section 7.19) occurs in all the domestic mammals, and is particularly important in the horse and man. Various factors have been considered as contributors to its development in the horse. One possible factor is ischaemia of the alveolar wall arising from obstruction of either the bronchial arterial supply or the alveolar capillaries, leading to extensive destruction of alveolar epithelial cells (Section 7.19.3).

It has been observed in man (Butler, 1991) that, despite their extensive ramifications, the bronchial arteries can be completely blocked with few noticeable ischaemic changes. The mildness of this response to obstruction is believed to be explained by the ability of the pulmonary arteries to take over perfusion of the bronchial circulation, presumably by the many capillary networks that the two systems share. Indeed, local blockage of the bronchial circulation is sometimes performed in man to treat **haemoptysis** (coughing or spitting of blood from the respiratory tract), without creating any obvious problems.

Harris and Heath (1962, p. 277) observed that the bronchial vasculature is 'often normal' in alveolar emphysema in man. On the other hand, they cited other reports that in emphysema in man many bronchial arteries were narrowed or even obliterated by hypertrophy of the media and fibrosis of the intima. However, as already mentioned at the beginning of this section, Harris and Heath (1962, p. 277) found that normal bronchial arteries are so thick-walled and apparently occluded that it is difficult to decide whether or not they are pathological. Also chronic inflammation of small bronchi may lead to occlusion of the bronchial arteries. On the whole, the evidence seems not to support the proposition that ischaemia of the bronchial arteries is a major factor in the development of alveolar emphysema (Section 7.19.3).

17.10   Distribution, volume, and pressure in the bronchial circulation

The venous drainage of the first one or two generations of branches of the bronchial tree empties via the azygos venous system into the right atrium. The rest of the bronchial tree as far as the respiratory bronchioles, together with alveolar capillaries shared with the pulmonary arteries, drains into tributaries of the pulmonary veins (Section 17.5), and therefore empties into the left atrium; these latter regions are much more extensive than the first two generations of bronchi, and therefore it is to be expected that most of the bronchial blood (more than two thirds) will go to the left atrium (Section 17.5).

The **flow rate** through the *normal* bronchial arteries is small. The main trunks of the bronchial artery or arteries, at their origins from the aorta or intercostal arteries, are only small vessels. On the other hand, the **volume** of the vascular bed supplied by the bronchial arteries is disproportionately large, since it resembles a river delta with multiple channels.

The **pressure** in the main trunks of the bronchial arteries is aortic. But in the long meandering multiple channels of the bronchial vasculature the **resistance** to flow must be great. Consequently the pressure in the outlying regions of the bronchial microvasculature is bound to be low. Since the bronchial and pulmonary microvasculatures anastomose so very extensively, the pressures in their peripheral territories must be equally low.

If there are *pathological conditions* in the lung, all this may change profoundly. The great capacity of the bronchial vasculature for dilation, enlargement, and proliferation (Section 17.9) must allow substantial increases in its peripheral pressure and flow rate, thus enabling bronchial arterial blood to take over the perfusion of large areas of capillaries previously perfused by the pulmonary circulation. The combination of the driving force of aortic pressure and angiogenicity endows the bronchial vasculature with ideal flexibility for its role as a reserve circulation.

It is a curious feature of the normal bronchial circulation that about two thirds of its blood flow starts from the left ventricle and returns to the left atrium. A simplified way of thinking of this is to regard the left side of the heart as constantly circulating a small volume of blood which need never pass through the right side of the heart. Because of the bronchial circulation, the output of the left ventricle is consistently greater than that of the right ventricle; the small coronary veins (Section 18.9) also add to this minor imbalance.

The excess of the left output over the right is small but measurable, amounting to about 1 or 2% of cardiac output. These are approximate values for **normal** lungs. In pathological lungs with enlarged bronchial arteries and copious proliferation of bronchopulmonary arterial anastomoses (Section 17.9) the values will be much higher.

It would be nice to know accurately how great the **difference between the right and left ventricular outputs** really is. Daly and Hebb (1966, p. 79) reviewed many different experimental techniques used in attempts to answer this question. Preferably the difference should be measured on intact animals, and these (dogs) gave estimates ranging from 1.2% to 8.3% of cardiac output. In sheep, Baier (1986) found a range of 0.3 to 3.3%, mean 1.2%. The wide range of the estimates shows that the problem is far from solved. Daly and Hebb (1996) pointed out that the tendency is for authorities to accept the lowest estimates of bronchial flow (in the normal lung), for example less than 1% (Butler, 1991) or about 1–2% (Smith and Hamlin, 1977, p. 142; Guyton, 1986, p. 287).

Measurements obtained by perfusing both the bronchial vascular system and the pulmonary vascular system, separately and simultaneously, at varying flow rates and pressures (Daly and Hebb, 1966, p. 74), give some idea of the *extremes* of flow that can pass through the bronchial pathway. They showed that from 2.8 to 12.5% of the flow into the left atrium could come through the bronchial pathway, depending on the perfusion volumes and pressures. As would be expected, the bronchial flow increased when the pulmonary flow decreased, and vice versa. These observations appear to be a useful guide to what the bronchial circulation could do in pathological situations where the pulmonary circulation is diminished. If the normal bronchial vasculature can permit such a large flow, the pathological bronchial vasculature with its enlargements and proliferative anastomoses should be capable of a very generous flow.

It is not known how much blood normally passes through the capillary beds common to the bronchial and pulmonary circulations, nor is there any direct evidence to show which way it generally goes. The direction of flow depends on the relative pressures in the aorta and pulmonary artery; in theory, vasomotor control of the pulmonary vasculature could adjust the direction, but the autonomic regulation of the pulmonary circulation seems to be of rather little functional significance (Section 17.21.4).

The return of bronchial blood, which is venous blood, to the *left* side of the heart, constitutes a *venous-to-arterial shunt*. Since the volume of bronchial flow is small in the normal animal, the shunt probably is normally insignificant, though in the pathological lung this might not be so. In many mammals (Daly and Hebb, 1966, p. 87) the oxygen saturation of left atrial blood is only about 95% at most, so there is an admixture of venous blood from somewhere. If the bronchial venous return to the left atrium forms only 1% of the left ventricular output, it cannot account for the whole of this venous admixture, and the main explanation is more likely to be perfusion–ventilation mismatching (Section 6.30). Nevertheless, Daly and Hebb (1966, p. 88) considered that 'an appreciable fraction of the venous blood which enters the left atrium will be due to bronchopulmonary blood even if the lowest estimates of its volume are assumed'.

It is a useful maxim in biology that almost every structure conveys some functional advantage, but no functional advantage has been suggested for draining most of the bronchial circulation into the wrong side of the heart; actually this is functionally disadvantageous, since it discharges venous blood into the oxygenated blood of the left atrium, and therefore creates a venous-to-arterial shunt. Venous-to-arterial shunts are something that vertebrates have painstakingly eliminated during their evolution; an example is the suppression by birds and mammals of one or other of the paired **systemic arches** of **reptiles** (Section 15.6.1). However, some structures are inherited from ancestors that had good use for them, but are useless to their contemporary owners. When such structures are clearly on the way out functionally, they are usually obviously vestigial, for example the second and fourth metacarpal bones of the horse. But the bronchial circulation of mammals is far from vestigial. The discharge of most of it into the **left** side of the heart is therefore a riddle. In situations of this kind, it usually turns out that there *is* an adaptational advantage (i.e. a useful function) but we do not know enough to recognize it.

17.11 Autonomic regulation of the bronchial vasculature

Sympathetic and vagal fibres surround and enter the walls of the bronchial arteries. The sympathetic fibres are said to be vasoconstrictor, and the vagal fibres vasodilator, but little is known of their functional significance.

Vagal and sympathetic fibres reach the bronchial tree through the **pulmonary plexus** at the root of the lung (Sections 2.11, 3.11.4).

The innervation of the bronchial arteries was found to be denser than that of the pulmonary arteries (Daly and Hebb, 1966, p. 55), the innervation of the latter being of apparently minor functional importance (Guyton, 1986, p. 289). Crosby *et al.* (1962, p. 531) reported that stimulation of the vagus induced vasodilation of the bronchial vessels and that stimulation of the sympathetic fibres resulted in vasoconstriction. Infusion with acetylcholine increases bronchial blood flow, a response blocked by atropine; adrenaline decreases blood flow. The venous drainage of the bronchial circulation seems to be more reactive to these substances, and may be the site of autonomic regulation (Baier, 1986).

II PULMONARY CIRCULATION

The pulmonary circulation was correctly recognized in 1553 by Servetus, 63 years before Harvey resolved the whole circulation of the blood. The current doctrine at the time of Servetus was that the blood passed from the left ventricle to the right ventricle through pores in the interventricular septum, as proclaimed by Galen (AD 130–200). In the early seventeenth century two famous professors at Leyden were so convinced of this that they pierced the septum with fine stilettes before demonstrating the heart to medical students. Servetus established that the blood from the right ventricle traversed the lungs, where it received 'the divine spirit', and then went to the left ventricle. Since it was not politically acceptable at that time to deny orthodoxy, Servetus was charged with heresy and duly burnt at the stake (Tenney, 1991). A little learning is a dangerous thing – apparently a *lot* can even be lethal.

17.12 Design requirements of the pulmonary vasculature

The pulmonary circulation is unique among the organ circulations: the entire cardiac output is pumped through it, and its components (the lungs) therefore receive a blood supply vastly in excess of their metabolic requirements. No other single organ circulation receives such a high blood flow per unit mass of tissue. The total flow in the systemic circulation is similar, but is divided between many different organs.

Unlike the systemic circulation, the pulmonary circulation has no need of a high *head of pressure* for driving blood into distant regions of the body. Nor need it have powerful **arterial musculature** for selectively shutting down the flow against high pressure, so as to divert blood away from inactive or non-vital organs. However, it does require enough muscular control to enable perfusion to match ventilation.

The **design requirements** of the pulmonary vasculature therefore demand the following: (1) low resistance, to economize on the energetic cost of pumping very large volumes of blood; (2) large capacitance, for accommodating high rates of blood flow especially during exercise; and (3) sufficient smooth muscle in the arterial and arteriolar walls to control regional flow within the lung.

The vessels of the pulmonary circulation should therefore be short and wide for low resistance, thin-walled for capacitance, but equipped with minimal smooth muscle for control (Section 17.16).

17.13   The pulmonary trunk

The **pulmonary trunk** carries venous blood to the lungs. It arises from the **right** ventricle, but because of the **spiral septum** in the embryo (Section 15.3.3) it lies on the *left* side of the cranial aspect of the heart (Fig. 20.1).

It is a very short vessel, lying on the left side of the aorta (Figs 17.3, 20.1). Ventral to the tracheal bifurcation, it divides into the left and right pulmonary arteries (Fig. 17.4). Just before it divides, it is joined to the aorta by the **ligamentum arteriosum** (Fig. 20.1), the remnant of the embryonic ductus arteriosus (Fig. 15.6).

The part of the right ventricle that forms the pulmonary trunk (truncus pulmonalis) is known strictly as the conus arteriosus. The opening from the **conus arteriosus** into the pulmonary trunk is the **ostium of the pulmonary trunk**. The first part of the pulmonary trunk is slightly dilated by the three **sinuses of the pulmonary trunk** (sinus trunci pulmonalis), which are related to the three cusps (valvulae) of the **pulmonary valve** (Fig. 20.5).

The pulmonary trunk is an elastic artery (Section 12.8). Its wall is less than one third as thick as that of the aorta (Smith and Hamlin, 1977, p. 142).

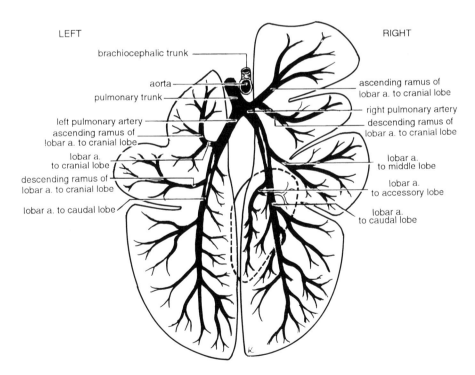

Fig. 17.3   Dorsal view diagram of the pulmonary arteries in a ruminant. Each lobe of the left and right lung is supplied by a lobar branch of the left or right pulmonary artery. The left cranial lobe and the right cranial lobe are divided, and therefore have an ascending and a descending ramus of their lobar artery. The ascending and descending rami to the left cranial lobe may arise separately from the left pulmonary artery as in the diagram. Based on Simoens (1992, p. 243).

17.14   Left and right pulmonary arteries

The **left pulmonary artery** enters the **hilus** of the left lung (Fig. 5.3; Section 5.5). The **right pulmonary artery** enters the **hilus** of the right lung. Having penetrated into the lung, the left and right pulmonary arteries form **lobar arteries** that accompany the lobar bronchus to each lobe of each lung (Fig. 17.4).

The left and right pulmonary arteries accompany the conducting airways of the bronchial tree as far as the respiratory bronchioles. Just as the airways form a tree, so also do the arteries. The two trees are almost perfectly 'congruent', which means that if one be superimposed on the other, the two of them coincide almost completely. In other words, every branch that comes off the bronchial tree takes with it a satellite branch of a pulmonary artery.

At the periphery of the bronchial tree, every bronchiole is still accompanied by its own small arterial branch. At the point where a terminal bronchiole approaches its respiratory bronchiole or alveolar duct, its accompanying arterial branch breaks down into **pulmonary arterioles**.

The arterioles continue into the **pulmonary capillaries** in the alveolar walls (Section 6.7.4). This is the richest capillary network in the body. The segments of this meshwork are so short that the gaps between the capillaries are smaller than the capillaries themselves (Fig. 6.6B). When the surface of an alveolar wall is viewed in a living lung, the flow through the **alveolar capillary network** resembles a thin flat sheet of moving blood.

In summary, each lobar branch of the pulmonary artery strictly follows its lobar bronchus, but yields it no branches until the first alveoli appear in the walls of the respiratory bronchioles. Thus the pulmonary arteries are true **end-arteries** (Section 12.19). On the other hand, the **bronchial arteries** supply typically two trunks to each lobar bronchus, and these anastomose with each other by transverse ladder-like anastomoses and supply branches to the bronchial tissues along the whole length of the bronchus (Section 17.3); thus the bronchial arteries are the very opposite to end-arteries.

Throughout their course in company with the branches of the bronchial tree, each pulmonary lobar artery and pulmonary arteriole is enclosed in a **periarterial sheath** (Fig. 6.3B). This is an outer flexible sleeve of connective tissue, in which is suspended a lymphatic plexus (Section 6.13). The connective tissue of the sheath belongs to the **fibrous continuum** of the lung (Section 6.9). When the thoracic cage and lungs expand during inspiration, the fibres of the continuum stretch the walls of the arteries and arterioles longitudinally and radially, thus tending to expand their capacity. However, by filling or emptying, the lymphatic plexus in the sheath imparts *hydraulic 'give'* to the vascular wall. This makes it possible for the smooth muscle in the arterial and arteriolar wall to regulate the internal diameter, and hence the resistance of the vessel, independently of the traction of the fibrous continuum during each breath.

The **right pulmonary artery** (a. pulmonalis dextra) has to pass ventral to the trachea in order to reach the right lung (Fig. 17.4).

In all the domestic species the left lung has two lobes, a cranial lobe and a caudal lobe (Section 5.6; 1 and 2 in the left lungs, in Fig. 5.4). Therefore the **left pulmonary artery** (a. pulmonalis sinistra) (Simoens, 1992, p. 242) forms a **lobar branch to the left cranial lobe** (ramus lobi cranialis) and a **lobar branch to the left caudal lobe** (ramus lobi caudalis). Since the cranial lobe is divided into two parts (except in the horse) the lobar branch of the pulmonary artery to the left cranial lobe forms an **ascending ramus** (r. ascendens) and a **descending ramus** (r. descendens); these two rami may arise separately from the left pulmonary artery, as in Fig. 17.3. The ascending and descending rami are absent in the horse (Simoens, 1992, p. 242).

Except in the horse, the right lung has four lobes (cranial, middle, caudal, and accessory lobes) and these receive four lobar bronchi (1, 2, 3, and 4, right, in Fig. 5.4). Therefore the **right pulmonary artery** (Simoens, 1992, p. 242) has four **lobar branches**, (1) to the right cranial lobe (r. lobi cranialis), (2) to the right middle lobe (r. lobi medii), (3) to the right caudal lobe (r. lobi caudalis), and (4) to the accessory lobe (r. lobi accessorii) (Fig. 17.4). In the right lung of the horse the middle lobe is usually not distinct, so there is only a cranial lobe, a caudal lobe, and an accessory lobe, each with its lobar branch of the pulmonary artery.

In species with a **tracheal bronchus** (ruminants and pig) (Section 5.6.1), before entering the lung the right pulmonary artery gives off the **branch to the right cranial lobe**. This branch runs cranially outside the lung and

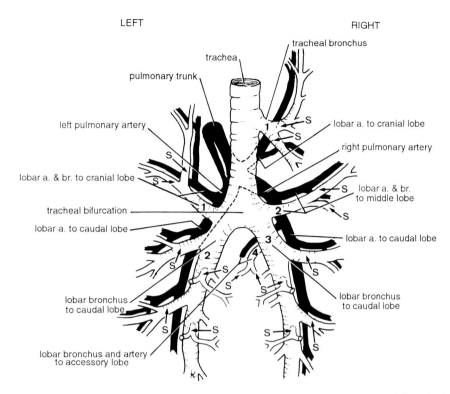

Fig. 17.4 Dorsal view diagram of the tracheal bifurcation and division of the pulmonary trunk into the left and right pulmonary arteries of the pig, to show the general relationships of the lobar arteries to the lobar bronchi. The tracheal bifurcation and its bronchi lie dorsal to the pulmonary vessels. Arteries running cranially tend to be medial to their related bronchi; arteries running laterally or obliquely tend to be cranial to their bronchi; arteries running caudally tend to be lateral to their bronchi. The lobar artery to the right cranial lobe passes cranially along the trachea, outside the lung, before joining the tracheal bronchus and entering the lung. The tracheal bifurcation forms the right and left principal bronchi. The lobar bronchi are numbered 1 to 4 in the right lung, and 1 and 2 in the left lung, as in Fig. 5.4, pig. S indicates the sixteen segmental bronchi (10 in the right lung and 6 in the left) described by Hare (1975, p. 1295) in this species. a., artery; br, bronchus. Anatomical material kindly supplied by Dr W.C.D. Hare.

along the trachea to join the **tracheal bronchus** (Fig. 17.4) (Schummer *et al.*, 1981, p. 71). In ruminants, the right cranial lobe is divided, and therefore the lobar branch of the right pulmonary artery to the right cranial lobe forms an **ascending** and a **descending ramus** (Fig. 17.3).

In principle (Hare, 1975, p. 141), **lobar arteries** running cranially are medial to their related lobar bronchus, lobar arteries running laterally or obliquely are cranial to their related lobar bronchus, and lobar arteries running caudally are lateral to their related lobar bronchus (Fig. 17.4).

In histological sections, the **small muscular arteries** of the pulmonary artery lie in contact with the small bronchi to which they are related, so that their **periarterial** and **peribronchial sheaths** fuse where they touch as in Fig. 6.3B (see Daly and Hebb, 1966, Fig. 1.18 and p. 26). The position of the small veins that are tributaries of

the pulmonary veins varies with the species (Section 17.15).

In the dog, cat, guinea pig, rat, and mouse the **pulmonary (visceral) pleura** (Section 9.9) is supplied solely by the pulmonary arteries (Daly and Hebb, 1966, p. 54).

17.15 Pulmonary veins and their tributaries

The pulmonary arteries are based on a left pulmonary artery and a right pulmonary artery, but corresponding left and right pulmonary veins are lacking. Instead, each **lobe** of the lung tends to have its own **pulmonary vein**, which leaves the hilus of the lung and enters independently through the roof of the left atrium. Therefore the number of pulmonary veins usually corresponds to the number of lung lobes.

Hence the basic pattern in the domestic mammals is six pulmonary veins: two from the left lung, i.e. one from the cranial and one from the caudal lobe (Fig. 20.1); and four from the right lung, i.e. one from each of the cranial, middle, caudal, and accessory lobes (Fig. 17.5). However, variations occur within and between species.

Veins lying within the parenchyma of the lung drain the oxygenated blood that leaves the capillaries of the alveolar walls. These veins are **tributaries of the pulmonary veins** (Fig. 6.3B). All such tributaries are suspended in a sheath of loose connective tissue, but this sheath lacks the rich lymphatic plexus that characterizes the **periarterial**

sheath (Section 6.13). Consequently, with each respiratory cycle, the pulmonary veins and their tributaries expand and fill during inspiration, and then contract and empty during expiration. The overall effect of this cyclic expansion and contraction is that breathing promotes the return of oxygenated blood to the left atrium.

Small **bronchopulmonary veins** lie on the outer surface of the peribronchial sheath of each bronchus (Fig. 6.3B). These veins drain blood (deoxygenated) from the outer and inner bronchial blood-vascular plexuses (Section 17.6.3).

The *basic pattern* of six **pulmonary veins** (venae pulmonales) to the six lobes of the lung is relatively clear in the dog (Schummer *et al.*, 1981, p. 184), as in Fig. 17.5. In the other domestic species the pattern tends to be

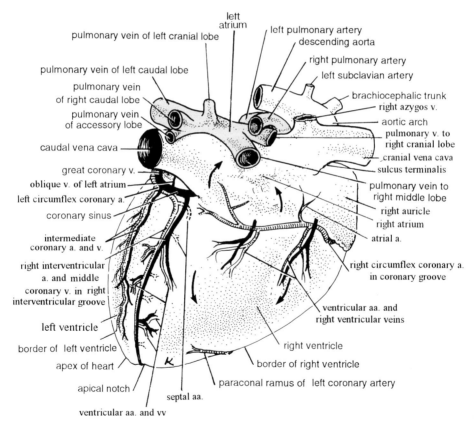

Fig. 17.5 Right lateral view of the heart of a dog, to show the pulmonary veins and coronary vessels. There is one pulmonary vein to each of the four lobes of the right lung and the two lobes of the left lung. The four curved arrows indicate the presence of venae cordis minimae (small coronary veins) draining directly into the lumens of the right atrium and right ventricle; similar small coronary veins empty into the left atrium and left ventricle. Adapted from anatomical data of Simoens (1992, p. 339B) and Nickel *et al.* (1973, p. 44).

somewhat blurred by two lung lobes (or even more than two) sharing one pulmonary vein. The ox has only one large and two or three small veins (Schummer *et al.*, 1981, p. 184). In the horse there are five to nine (Ghoshal, 1975, p. 561). In man there are four, two on each side (Williams *et al.*, 1989, p. 708). These variations arise for developmental reasons (Schummer *et al.*, 1981, p. 26). The pulmonary veins arise as vessels which drain the various branches of the lung buds and converge into a single common trunk that enters the left atrium dorsally (Patten, 1958, p. 512). As the heart grows this trunk vessel is gradually absorbed into the atrial wall. Consequently several of its original branches eventually open directly into the definitive atrium.

In the domestic carnivores and horse (McLaughlin *et al.*, 1961), and in man (Williams *et al.*, 1989, p. 1284), the pulmonary veins and their tributaries are not congruent with the bronchial tree within the substance of the lung (Weibel, 1984, p. 287). Thus in these species, the veins travel independently through the lung parenchyma as in Fig. 6.3B. In man, for example, they lie about midway between the bronchus–artery combinations; only as they reach the hilus of the lung do the veins ultimately accompany the arteries and bronchi (Williams *et al.*, 1989, p. 1284). On the other hand, in the ox, sheep, and pig, even the small veins tend to stay close to the small bronchi and arteries throughout the lung (McLaughlin *et al.*, 1961).

The pulmonary veins are said to be devoid of valves (Schummer *et al.*, 1981, p. 184).

17.16   Structural design of the pulmonary vasculature: resistance to flow

Because of the relatively small size of the lungs and the relatively short distances over which the blood must be transported, the **larger branches** of the **pulmonary arteries** are very much *shorter* than those of typical systemic arteries. They are also *wider* than the corresponding systemic arteries. The **small pulmonary arteries** and **arterioles**, too, are relatively *shorter*, and have *thinner walls* and a *wider lumen* than their systemic counterparts.

The walls of the pulmonary arterial vessels are thin because their **tunica media** contains relatively little smooth muscle. The comparatively wide calibres and thin walls with little musculature, cause the **pulmonary arteries** and pulmonary arterioles to look, histologically, rather like systemic veins of similar calibre. But despite the thinness of their walls, they have enough **smooth muscle** to regulate the flow within them (Section 17.21), such

regulation being made possible by the hydraulic 'give' imparted by the **periarterial sheath** (Section 17.14). The **pulmonary capillaries**, too, are shorter and wider than systemic capillaries.

The **pulmonary veins** are short, but their walls are similar to those of systemic veins.

The overall effect of these structural characteristics is that the **resistance** to flow in the pulmonary circulation is much lower than in the systemic circulation, thus meeting the first design requirement of the pulmonary vasculature (Section 17.12). In the systemic circulation most of the resistance comes from the arterioles, with their generous equipment of musculature (Section 12.10). In the pulmonary vasculature the resistance is more evenly distributed, the arteries, capillaries, and veins all contributing. Since the resistance is low, the **pulmonary arterial pressure** is also low.

The larger branches of the pulmonary arteries are **elastic arteries** (Section 12.8), the tunica media containing more elastic tissue than smooth muscle cells, though not much of either (Daly and Hebb, 1966, p. 23). These are **conducting arteries** (Section 12.5.2), arising directly from the heart and simply conveying blood to the lung and its lobes. As the arteries get smaller, the media is still thin but contains relatively more muscle cells and relatively less elastic elements. Thus these vessels are now **distributing arteries** (Section 12.5.2); by means of the muscle in the media, they have the ability to regulate the distribution (Section 17.21) of blood so as to achieve optimal gas exchange.

Daly and Hebb (1966, pp. 23–26) reviewed species variations in the structure of the muscular arteries and arterioles of the pulmonary circulation. In man, **muscular** pulmonary arteries (Section 12.9) range between 1 mm and 100 μm in diameter. In the dog, ox, pig, and horse the muscular media extends much further down the arterial tree, and is still distinct in arterioles of only 20–30 μm diameter. Among these various species, the ox and pig have the most muscular arteriolar walls (Smith and Hamlin, 1977, p. 148). Species differences in the muscularity of the pulmonary arterial vasculature 'correlate well' with vasomotor activity (Smith and Hamlin, 1977, p. 143). In the rabbit and guinea pig there are sphincter-like thickenings of the muscular media, suggesting the possibility of completely shutting off the pulmonary blood supply to local regions of the lung; such thickenings are absent in the domestic carnivores, rat, mouse, and monkey.

It has been reported (see Comroe, 1975, p. 142) that (in man) the walls of quite large pulmonary arterioles, up to 50 μm in diameter, are so thin that they participate in gaseous exchanges, and contain bright red oxygenated blood where mixed venous blood would be expected.

17.17   Capacitance of the pulmonary circulation: the venous reservoir

Veins in general are **capacitance vessels** (Section 12.5.2). Vascular capacitance reflects the quantity of blood that can be stored in a component of the circulatory system per unit rise in pressure. The capacitance characteristics of veins arise from their ability to change their shape in response to small increases in transmural pressure (Section 12.16.3); this means that veins have a high compliance (Section 6.31). The structure of the walls of the pulmonary veins, and hence their capacitance, are similar to those of systemic veins.

In the pulmonary circulation, however, capacitance is not provided by the veins alone: the exceptional thinness, and hence extreme flexibility, of all the pulmonary blood vessels gives the *whole* of the pulmonary vasculature an important capacitance function. This function is provided by both the arterial and the venous vasculature about equally, in contrast to the systemic circulation where capacitance is provided mainly by the veins.

The high compliance of the pulmonary vasculature meets the second of the design requirements outlined in Section 17.12, namely large capacitance to accommodate rates of blood flow that are at all times very high and often suddenly greatly increased as at exercise (Section 17.21.2).

The veins of the body form a *venous reservoir*, storing about two thirds of the total blood volume (Section 12.16.3). The lungs hold about 10% of the total blood volume.

In general, adrenergic venoconstriction rapidly mobilizes blood from the venous reservoirs in response to a fall in arterial pressure, as after haemorrhage, under the control of baroreceptor reflexes (Section 13.3.5), and at the onset of exercise (Section 22.16). The venous reservoirs include the lungs (Section 12.16.3).

In haemodynamic terms, the **capacitance** of a vascular component is the total volume of blood that it contains per unit rise in pressure (Guyton, 1986, p. 214).

The lung of man contains about 450 ml of blood, of which only about 15% is in the capillaries (Guyton, 1986, p. 288). Scott (1986, p. 73) noted that the sympathetic innervation of the lung has little influence on resistance, but does have 'important effects' on the capacitance of the pulmonary circulation.

17.18   Pressures in the pulmonary circulation

Since the resistance in the pulmonary circulation is low, the pressure is also low. Actual figures are apt to strain the mind of the overloaded veterinary student, but blood pressure and oncotic pressure control so many functions in the lungs, normal and pathological, that the following data are worth inspection.

17.18.1   *Pressures at rest*

In the resting mammal the pressure in the pulmonary trunk is generally only about one sixth of that in the aorta. For example, in a medium-sized adult mammal such as a dog or man at rest, the **pulmonary systolic pressure** is only about 20 mmHg (2.7 kPa) (dog) and 25 mmHg (3.3 kPa) (man), the **pulmonary diastolic pressure** is about 8 mmHg (1.1 kPa) (man) and 10 mmHg (1.3 kPa) (dog), and the systolic and diastolic values in the aorta are about 120 and 80 mmHg (16.0 and 10.7 kPa). In man the **mean pulmonary arterial pressure** (for definition, see advanced text below) is about 15 mmHg (2.0 kPa) and the **mean systemic arterial pressure** is about 100 mmHg (13.3 kPa); the pressure in the **pulmonary capillaries** is about 7 mmHg (0.9 kPa), whilst the pressure in **systemic capillaries** ranges from about 32 mmHg (4.3 kPa) at the arterial end, down to about 15 mmHg (2.0 kPa) at the venous end (Section 14.4).

The low resistance, and hence the low pressure, in the pulmonary circulation allows the right ventricle to do much less work than the left ventricle, so that the action of the *postnatal* right ventricle is energetically economic: thus the structural adaptations of the pulmonary vasculature fully meet the first of the design requirements of the pulmonary circulation, i.e. energetic economy (Section 17.12). Remember, however, that the *fetal heart* lacks this privilege, since the fetal right ventricle does much more work than the left (Section 16.1).

The values for **pulmonary systolic pressure** in the dog are low compared with those of other mammals. Smith and Hamlin (1977, Table 12.1) gave the following values (mmHg): dog, 21 (2.8 kPa); man, 22 (2.9 kPa); cat, 26–36 (3.5–4.8 kPa); cow, 33–46 (4.4–6.1 kPa); pig, 40 (5.3 kPa); horse, 25–51 (3.3–6.8 kPa). **Pulmonary diastolic pressures** (mmHg): man, 9 (1.2 kPa); dog, 10 (1.3 kPa); cat, 15–17 (2.0–2.3 kPa); pig, 9–20 (1.2–2.7 kPa); cow, 19–21 (2.5–2.8 kPa); horse, 14–28 (1.9–3.7 kPa).

The **mean arterial pressure** is not the average of systolic and diastolic pressures, but is the average pressure throughout the whole of the pulse cycle. Since the pressure is usually slightly nearer to the diastolic than to the systolic pressure during most of the pulse cycle, the mean pressure is somewhat lower than the mean of systolic and diastolic pressures. It reflects the average pressure that is driving blood through the circulation, and is therefore an important indicator of blood flow through the tissues (Guyton, 1986, p. 244).

The **pulse pressure** is the difference between systolic and diastolic pressure. The normal pulse pressure in the pulmonary arteries is about $25 - 8 = 17$ mmHg $(3.3 - 1.1 = 2.2$ kPa) in a medium-sized mammal (e.g. man), and $120 - 80 = 40$ mmHg $(16.0 - 10.7 = 5.3$ kPa) in the systemic arteries.

The **left atrial pressure** can be estimated in the intact live animal by passing a catheter through the right heart and into the pulmonary artery. The catheter is then pushed on until its tip wedges tightly in a small artery in the lung, stopping its flow. The blood beyond the tip of the catheter is continuous with capillary blood, which is continuous with left atrial blood. The pressure measured at the tip of the catheter is called the **pulmonary wedge pressure**, and (in man) is normally about 5 mmHg (0.7 kPa) (Guyton, 1986, p. 288). It is believed to be about 3 mmHg (0.4 kPa) greater (in man) than the **mean left atrial pressure** (which is therefore about 2 mmHg (0.3 kPa), and a few millimetres of mercury less than the mean pulmonary capillary pressure (thus establishing the necessary pressure gradient from pulmonary capillaries to left atrium).

The **mean pulmonary capillary pressure** is assumed to be intermediate between the mean pulmonary arterial pressure and the mean left atrial pressure, a value between 5 and 10 mmHg (0.7 and 1.3 kPa) appearing reasonable (Smith and Hamlin, 1977, p. 146). The mean pulmonary capillary pressure in man is estimated to be about 7 mmHg (0.9 kPa) (Guyton, 1986, p. 291).

Pulmonary wedge pressures have been measured in horses at rest and at exercise (Manohar *et al.*, 1993). The values obtained at rest (about 17 mmHg (2.3 kPa)) were about three times higher than in man. However, the mean pulmonary arterial pressure in the horse at rest is evidently about 28 mmHg (3.7 kPa) (Smith and Hamlin,

1977, Table 12.1), i.e. about twice the value of 15 mmHg (2.0 kPa) in man (Guyton, 1986, p. 288).

Pulmonary wedge pressures have been severely criticized for their possible inaccuracy (see Daly and Hebb, 1966, p. 132).

17.18.2 *Pulmonary pressures during exercise*

Exercise requires an increase in cardiac output, and an increase in cardiac output requires an increase in pulmonary arterial pressure. Cardiac output in, for example, a man at rest is about 5 litres min^{-1}, and this is driven by a normal mean pulmonary arterial pressure of less than 15 mmHg (2.0 kPa). During moderately heavy exercise the cardiac output could increase about fivefold to about 25 litres min^{-1}. This would require a pulmonary arterial pressure of about 35 mmHg (4.7 kPa); the pulmonary capillary pressure would then be around the critical level where it would exceed the pulmonary oncotic pressure, so that the onset of pulmonary oedema might be expected (Section 17.25.1).

In **horses**, the pulmonary pressures are extremely high during strenuous exercise. Racehorses have been selectively bred for supreme muscular development, matched by an immense cardiac output exceeding that of the elite human athlete by 100% in terms of ml min^{-1} kg^{-1} (body mass) (Section 17.28.4). In galloping Thoroughbreds the mean pulmonary arterial pressure may exceed 100 mmHg (13.3 kPa), with mean pulmonary capillary pressures of over 70 mmHg (9.3 kPa). These huge pressures in racehorses seem not to cause pulmonary oedema, but unfortunately they do become embroiled in the very serious problem of **exercise-induced pulmonary haemorrhage** (**EIPH**) (Section 17.28.1).

Very severe exercise (Section 6.26.5), for example racing cycling by a trained athlete (in steady state, as opposed to a short sprint), entails about a 13-fold increase in oxygen consumption (McArdle *et al.*, 1981, p. 489). An athletic dog running on a treadmill also experiences a 13-fold increase in oxygen consumption; this would require a sixfold increase in cardiac output (Weibel, 1984, p. 388). To achieve such a high cardiac output, pulmonary arterial pressure would have to rise far above 35 mmHg (4.7 kPa) (see Scott, 1986, Fig. 6.1). The maximum cardiac output in a human athlete is about 30–35 litres min^{-1}, i.e. about five to seven times the resting value (Guyton, 1986, p. 272).

Direct measurements on **horses** on a treadmill by Manohar and his colleagues (Manohar *et al.*, 1993) have shown the mean pulmonary pressure to be about 30 mmHg (4.0 kPa) at rest and over 90 mmHg (12.0 kPa) when galloping, indicating that the mean pulmonary capillary pressure during strenuous exercise in the horse is near 79 mmHg (10.5 kPa). Other workers have recorded even higher values in galloping Thoroughbreds, the mean pulmonary arterial pressure being as high as 120 mmHg (16.0 kPa) and the mean left atrial pressure being 70 mmHg (9.3 kPa) (West and Mathieu-Costello, 1994). These extremely high values are nothing short of astounding, and must be vastly greater than the oncotic pressure of the blood plasma. West and Mathieu-Costello (1994) remarked that 'when traditional mammalian physiologists are informed that the mean left atrial pressure in a galloping racehorse can be as high as 70 Torr, the usual reaction is complete disbelief'.

17.19   Filtration and reabsorption across the pulmonary capillary wall

The dynamics of filtration and reabsorption across the capillary wall in the systemic circulation are considered in Section 14.4. The general principles are the same in the pulmonary circulation. Filtration and reabsorption depend primarily on the balance between the hydrostatic and oncotic forces acting on the blood plasma.

In the **systemic circulation**, the hydrostatic pressure of the plasma exceeds the oncotic pressure of the plasma at the *arterial end* of the capillary (thus creating the filtration pressure), and therefore filtration occurs there: at the *venous end* of the capillary, the oncotic pressure of the plasma exceeds the hydrostatic pressure of the plasma (thus creating the **reabsorption pressure**), and therefore reabsorption occurs there. The interstitial fluid exerts its own hydrostatic and oncotic pressures, but according to long held views these two opposing forces virtually cancel each other out.

In the **pulmonary circulation**, the hydrostatic pressure is so much lower than in the systemic circulation that the oncotic pressure is generally believed to exceed the hydrostatic pressure along the whole length of the capillary. Thus the capillary pressure in the pulmonary circulation of man is only about 7 mmHg (0.9 kPa) (Section 17.18) (compared with about 32–15 mmHg (4.3–2.0 kPa)

at the beginning and end respectively of a capillary in the systemic circulation; Section 14.4). The oncotic pressure is, of course, similar in both circulations, i.e. about 28 mmHg (3.7 kPa) in man and 20 mmHg (2.7 kPa) in the dog. The hydrostatic pressure in the interstitial fluid in the alveolar wall is supposed to be atmospheric. Since, all the way along the capillary, the hydrostatic pressure difference forcing fluid out is so much less than the oncotic pressure pulling fluid in, fluid should be reabsorbed *along the whole length* of the pulmonary capillary, instead of being filtered at the arterial end and reabsorbed at the venous end as in the systemic circulation.

An increase in the hydrostatic pressure can lead to excessive filtration, resulting in a potentially fatal accumulation of fluid in the pulmonary alveoli (**pulmonary oedema**; Section 17.25.1). The above classic version of these forces assumes that an increase in the pulmonary capillary pressure from 7 mmHg (0.9 kPa) to about 30 mmHg (4.0 kPa) would be required to cause the filtration force to exceed the reabsorption force of oncotic pressure (about 28 mmHg (3.7 kPa)), and if this happens pulmonary oedema should begin. However, this would require a large rise in the pulmonary capillary pressure, and it is therefore generally held that there is a correspondingly *large safety margin* of about 23 mmHg (3.1 kPa) before significant pulmonary oedema arises (Guyton, 1986, p. 292; Scott, 1986, p. 70).

> In the above classic version of the forces acting on the blood plasma of pulmonary capillaries, the large excess of oncotic over hydrostatic forces suggests that there should be no filtration at all across the pulmonary capillary wall. In fact, there is normally a small but steady filtration of fluid into the interstitium of the alveolar wall (Guyton, 1986, p. 372). The explanation for this appears to lie in a closer appraisal of the hydrostatic, oncotic, and surface forces in the alveolar interstitial fluid, as follows.

17.19.1   *Hydrostatic pressure in alveolar interstitial fluid*

Hitherto, the hydrostatic pressure of the alveolar interstitial fluid has usually been regarded as 'close to atmospheric pressure' (Scott, 1986, p. 70), or has been assumed to be 'atmospheric' (West, 1975, p. 47). Guyton (1986, p. 371) called attention to measurements indicating that the hydrostatic pressure of the alveolar interstitial fluid is *strongly negative*, i.e. about -8 mmHg (-1.1 kPa) (compared with -5 mmHg (-0.7 kPa) in subcutaneous tissues). Guyton (1986, pp. 292, 372) appeared to attribute this negative pressure to (a) the strong and continual osmotic tendency of the plasma to dehydrate the interstitial spaces of the alveolar walls, and (b) to the sucking of fluid into the pulmonary lymphatics. Clearly a strongly negative hydrostatic interstitial pressure would indeed be a powerful force in favour of filtration. However, he conceded (Guyton, 1986, p. 356) that some physiologists believe that, throughout the body, the connective tissue fibres are strong enough to maintain *positive* compression of the fluids in the interstitial spaces all the time.

17.19.2   Oncotic pressure in alveolar interstitial fluid

Guyton (1986, p. 371) also noted that the alveolar capillaries are relatively leaky to protein molecules (Section 6.19), thus giving the alveolar interstitial fluid an unusually high oncotic pressure, i.e. about 14 mmHg (1.9 kPa) (compared with about 6 mmHg (0.8 kPa) in other tissues). This, too, would strongly favour filtration.

17.19.3   Revised balance of filtration and reabsorption forces

On the basis of these values, Guyton (1986, p. 371) then derived the following balance of forces across the pulmonary capillary in man. Outward forces: capillary hydrostatic pressure, 7 mmHg (0.9 kPa); oncotic pressure of interstitial fluid, 14 mmHg (1.9 kPa); negative hydrostatic pressure of interstitial fluid, 8 mmHg (1.1 kPa); total, 29 mmHg (3.9 kPa). Inward forces: capillary oncotic pressure, 28 mmHg (3.7 kPa). Net force in favour of filtration, 1 mmHg (0.1 kPa).

This revised balance of forces across the pulmonary capillary explains the steady filtration of fluid into the alveolar interstitium, as shown by the continuous drainage of lymph away from the exchange tissue in the **peribronchovascular lymphatic pathway** (Section 7.8.1); in the normal mature unanaesthetized sheep this flow amounts to about 10 ml h^{-1} (Smith and Hamlin, 1977, p. 146).

Unfortunately, whilst the revised balance sheet solves the problem of the steady flow of fluid through the alveolar interstitium, it creates another difficulty: the *safety margin* against the formation of pulmonary oedema, which was thought to be a comforting 23 mmHg (3.1 kPa), now disappears altogether. However, this problem can almost certainly be resolved by a re-evaluation of the mechanisms that drain fluid from the alveolar interstitium (Section 17.26.2).

17.19.4   Other forces contributing to filtration and reabsorption

Several other factors complicate the balance of forces across the pulmonary capillary (Hildebrandt, 1974, p. 312). (1) Increased airway resistance. This occurs in chronic obstructive pulmonary disease and causes an increase in the forces applied by the inspiratory muscles, so that during inspiration the pleural pressure falls below normal values. The fall in pressure is transmitted to the alveoli by parenchymal stress, and becomes an additional factor favouring filtration and oedema. (2) Diminished compliance of the lung. This arises, for example, from deposition of fibrous tissue. It has the same effect as increased airway resistance, favouring filtration and oedema. (3) Blocked pulmonary lymphatics. This could be caused by scar tissue or a neoplasm, favouring accumulation of fluid and oedema. (4) Leakage of protein through damaged capillary endothelium. This can result from many causes, including infections and noxious gases (Section 17.25.3). It increases the oncotic pressure of the alveolar interstitial fluid, and decreases the oncotic pressure of the pulmonary capillary, thus favouring filtration and oedema. (5) Diminished surfactant. This is the underlying defect in the respiratory distress syndrome of the newborn. Increased surface tension at the alveolar wall favours filtration and leads to pulmonary oedema (Weibel, 1984, p. 334). (6) Gravity and posture. The pulmonary capillary pressure is higher in pendent parts of the lung, favouring filtration and oedema in those regions (Butler, 1991).

17.19.5   A third fluid compartment in pulmonary tissue

Weibel (1984, p. 331) pointed out that, although Starling's law must hold in principle for the pulmonary capillary, conditions in the lung are not as simple as in the systemic connective tissues. Instead of being a two-compartment system (plasma and interstitial fluid), the lung is a *three-compartment system*: two cellular barriers (endothelium and epithelium) separate *three* extracellular fluid spaces (blood plasma, interstitial fluid, and fluid lining the luminal surface of the alveolar wall). A complete analysis therefore requires three hydrostatic and three oncotic pressures.

Moreover the hydrostatic pressures of the fluid lining the alveolar wall vary, being either outward into the lumen or inward into the alveolar interstitium, depending on the curvature of the wall. Figures 6.6A and B show that the alveolar wall covering each capillary is convex, bulging into the lumen, but *between* the capillaries the alveolar wall is concave, forming 'intercapillary pits' (Weibel, 1984, p. 332). Each pit contains a pool of lining fluid (referred to as hypophase; Section 6.21). In these pits, the hydrostatic pressure gradient is appreciable; this gradient is greatly influenced by surface tension, and therefore surfactant has an important protective function here by reducing the suction exerted by the surface forces over the pits (Weibel, 1984, p. 333).

For an integrated analysis of alveolar micromechanics, taking into account the actions of surface tension on the fibrous continuum, see Weibel (1984, p. 325).

17.20   Capillary transit time

The total **capillary blood volume** in the pulmonary circulation is quite small at rest, being approximately equal to the ventricular stroke volume. Therefore the **capillary transit time** in the animal at rest is about equal to the duration of ventricular systole. So in a mammal with a resting heart rate of about 70 beats per minute, the erythrocyte goes through the pulmonary capillary in less than a second (about 0.8 s). In the normal lung, oxygen is fully taken up and carbon dioxide fully released by the time that the erythrocyte has traversed the first third of the capillary.

17.21   Regulation of the pulmonary microcirculation

The thin walls of pulmonary arteries and arterioles possess very little smooth muscle (Section 17.16). Nevertheless, pulmonary arterial pressure is so low that even small amounts of smooth muscle can decrease the vascular diameter. This allows vasoconstriction to shunt blood from poorly ventilated alveoli to well ventilated alveoli, thus correcting a mismatch of ventilation and perfusion. Conversely, inhibition of vasoconstrictor tone permits the opening during exercise of many capillaries that are closed when the body is at rest (capillary recruitment; Section 6.29).

17.21.1   *Autoregulation of perfusion–ventilation matching*

As in the systemic microcirculation, local metabolic factors dominate the flow through the pulmonary capillaries by autoregulation. Thus **alveolar hypoxia** (and to a lesser extent **alveolar hypercapnia**, i.e. increased CO_2) is a powerful

vasoconstrictor stimulus; by constricting pulmonary arteries and arterioles, it shunts blood from the capillaries of poorly ventilated alveoli to the capillaries of well ventilated alveoli, thus matching perfusion with ventilation (Section 6.29). Hence oxygen regulates its own uptake by the pulmonary capillaries, by locally adjusting perfusion to match ventilation. Note that this *vasoconstrictor* response to *hypoxia* in the pulmonary microcirculation is the *reverse* of the *vasodilator* response to *local hypoxia* in the systemic microcirculation (Section 13.2.1). The mechanism of this vasoconstrictor response in the pulmonary arterial vasculature is not fully understood.

It is generally accepted (Smith and Hamlin, 1977, p. 147; Scott, 1986, p. 73) that the vasomotor control of the pulmonary microcirculation in response to hypoxia (as in the systemic microcirculation) is achieved by the regulation of small arteries and arterioles, but Hanson *et al.* (1989) believed it to be an exclusively capillary phenomenon.

Until very recently it has not been known how the hypoxia acts on the pulmonary arterial wall (Scott, 1986, p. 73). It may work through the release of **vasoactive substances**, **kinins** and **histamine** being possible agents. The release of **serotonin** from the cells of the **neuro-epithelial bodies** has also been suspected (Section 4.16.4). Alternatively (Section 6.30.3) it may work through the recently discovered O_2-sensitive K^+ channels in the smooth muscle cells of the pulmonary arterial wall (Lopez-Barneo, 1994) (Section 19.9.3); these cause contraction in response to hypoxia. Whatever the mechanism, it operates in isolated lungs from which all the nerves have been removed (Comroe, 1975, p. 156). It is unlikely that the autonomic nervous system participates significantly in the control of the pulmonary circulation (Section 17.21.4).

17.21.2   *Autoregulation of perfusion during exercise: capillary recruitment*

During **severe exercise** the oxygen consumption of the body may increase 20-fold. This demands an appropriate increase in right ventricular output (cardiac output); in a trained athlete, the cardiac output can go up by five to seven times above the resting value, to about 30–35 litres min^{-1}. The resulting increase in the perfusion of the alveolar vasculature is obtained by **capillary recruitment** (Section 6.29): alveolar capillaries that were closed become opened (Fig. 6.10B), and capillaries that were already open become dilated.

Despite this huge increase in blood flow through the lung, changes in pulmonary **arterial pressure** are minimal as exercise progresses. A moderate increase in pulmonary flow is actually accompanied by a fall in **resistance** due to the opening of capillaries that were previously closed, so that the pressure rises very little. At still higher flow rates the resistance falls even further, due to distension of the open capillaries, so here again there is only a small rise in pressure. For example, in man a normal resting cardiac output of about 5 litres min^{-1} requires a normal mean pulmonary arterial pressure of less than 15 mmHg (2.0 kPa). A mere 30% increase in mean pulmonary pressure (to about 20 mmHg (2.7 kPa)) is accompanied by a 300% increase in flow rate (to about 16 litres min^{-1}). A flow rate of about 25 litres min^{-1} (an increase of about fivefold above the resting output) requires a pulmonary arterial pressure of about 35 mmHg (4.7 kPa): this is approaching the critical level where pulmonary capillary pressure exceeds oncotic pressure.

This relationship in exercise between increasing pulmonary flow rate and the recruitment and dilation of pulmonary capillaries is a form of autoregulation. It has the extremely useful effect of allowing a huge rise in cardiac output whilst automatically restraining the rise in pulmonary arterial pressure. In so doing, it fends off the potential disaster of pulmonary oedema: the oncotic pressure of the blood (in man) is about 28 mmHg (3.7 kPa) (Section 17.19), so when the pulmonary capillary pressure exceeds this value, pulmonary oedema may begin to form (Section 17.25.1).

17.21.3 *Pulmonary hypertension of high altitude*

In mammals kept at high altitude there is **alveolar hypoxia**. The resulting automatic vasoconstrictor response of the pulmonary arteries and arterioles to the hypoxia, which is normally so advantageous in correcting ventilation–perfusion mismatching, now acts against the homeostasis of the animal. The resistance of the whole pulmonary circulation rises, and **pulmonary hypertension** results (Section 17.22). When this happens, the right ventricle at first hypertrophies and then dilates, with sys-

temic venous congestion, subcutaneous oedema, and accumulation of peritoneal fluid (ascites); in short, right heart failure (Section 22.17). Return to normal altitude reverses the hypertension.

Mammals with relatively muscular pulmonary arterial vasculature, notably the ox and pig (Section 17.16), are the most vulnerable to the pulmonary hypertension of altitude (Smith and Hamlin, 1977, p. 148). The condition in cattle is known as **brisket disease** because of pendent oedematous swelling of the brisket.

In man, remaining for too long at high altitude causes **chronic mountain sickness** (Guyton, 1986, p. 532). The pulmonary hypertension is exacerbated by a very high red cell count, which increases the viscosity of the blood several-fold and thus decreases the blood flow and delivery of oxygen to the tissues. Right heart failure can lead to death, but after returning to low altitude recovery is usual.

17.21.4 *Autonomic nervous system*

The pulmonary arteries and veins are innervated by the sympathetic (Section 2.10.3) and parasympathetic nervous systems (Section 3.11.4). Stimulation of the sympathetic pathways causes a slight **vasoconstriction**, and therefore a slight increase in resistance; stimulation of the vagus causes a slight decrease in resistance. The vasoconstrictor response of pulmonary arterial vessels to sympathetic stimulation is very much weaker than the powerful vasoconstrictor action of sympathetic stimulation on systemic arterial vasculature (Section 13.3). It is said, however, that sympathetic stimulation does have quite a significant effect on the **capacitance** of the pulmonary veins, presumably decreasing it by venoconstriction.

It is doubtful whether the autonomic nervous system has any major function in the normal control of the pulmonary circulation.

After over a century of research, opinion in the late 1960s was still sharply divided between those believing that the pulmonary vasculature has a motor autonomic innervation, and others holding that the vessels have no innervation or that nerve fibres are too few for effective control (see Hebb, 1969). Histologists were, in general, persuaded that there is an innervation, but the case was weakened by artefacts and technical inconsistencies (see Daly and Hebb, 1966, p. 97). Histochemistry and electron microscopy then established that, although there are species variations, in mammals generally both the pulmonary arteries and the pulmonary veins are unquestionably innervated with cholinergic and adrenergic fibres (Hebb, 1969). The adrenergic supply tends to be more abundant than the cholinergic, particularly in the veins.

Vasomotor responses of the pulmonary circulation to the injection of **catecholamines** in perfused isolated lungs are consistent with the presence of an adrenergic system within the lung (Smith and Hamlin, 1977, p. 147).

17.22 Primary pulmonary hypertension

Pulmonary hypertension is a generalized rise in pressure throughout the pulmonary arterial vasculature. It may be secondary to left heart failure (Section 22.17), arising for example from aortic stenosis. Or pulmonary hypertension can be primary, and is then essentially due to restriction of the pulmonary vascular bed. Such restriction can arise from vasoconstriction (high altitude, Section 17.21.3), obstruction of pulmonary vessels (pulmonary embolism, Sections 12.22, 17.24), or destruction of pulmonary vessels (alveolar emphysema, Section 7.19).

The mechanism of primary pulmonary hypertension is multifactorial, one mechanism often recruiting another (Smith and Hamlin, 1977, p. 148). For instance, an additional obstructive factor at high altitude (mountain sickness) is the great increase in red blood cells, which increases the viscosity of the blood severalfold (Guyton, 1986, p. 532). Another obstructive factor can be heartworm disease in dogs and many other species, by means of mature worms up to 15 cm long, fragments of parasites, or blood clots, in the pulmonary vascular pathways (Smith and Hamlin, 1977, p. 148).

17.23 Effects of gravity on perfusion of the pulmonary vasculature

The computed tomography scans in Figs 24.8 and 24.9 show that the outlet of the right ventricle into the pulmonary trunk in a dog lying on its sternum is slightly dorsal to the centre of the thoracic cavity. Therefore about half the volume of the lung, both left and right, is dorsal to the opening of the ventricle into the pulmonary trunk. Similarly, in the standing horse in Fig. 24.7, of the four radiographic fields 1 and 2, and half of 4, are dorsal to the outlet into the pulmonary trunk.

In the quadruped and the human biped, standing and at rest, all of these extensive regions of the lung that are *dorsal* (cranial, in man) to the opening of the right ventricle into the pulmonary trunk are uphill from the heart, and therefore have to be perfused against the force of gravity. In a circulatory system in which the driving pressure is as low as it is in the pulmonary system, this matters. Since the pulmonary systolic arterial pressure in mammals generally is only about 20–40 mmHg (2.7–5.3 kPa) (Section 17.18), the blood will have difficulty in reaching the most dorsal level of the lung in a large standing quadruped, or in reaching the most cranial level of the lung in a standing man.

For example, if the most dorsal part of the lung of a large standing quadruped at rest were 30 cm dorsal to the outlet from the right ventricle, a pulmonary arterial pressure of 30×0.74 mmHg, i.e. 22 mmHg (2.9 kPa), would be required to reach it against the force of gravity; if the systolic pulmonary pressure were only 20 mmHg (2.7 kPa), no blood at all would reach this part of such a lung. (To convert centimetres of water to millimetres of mercury, multiply by 0.74.) On the other hand, the ventral parts of the lung are downhill from the heart. If the most ventral level of the lung were 30 cm ventral to the right ventricular outlet, it would be very well perfused by blood, at a pressure of 42 mmHg (5.6 kPa) (20 mmHg (2.7 kPa) due to right ventricular systolic pressure and 22 mmHg (2.9 kPa) caused by gravity).

Thus in a standing horse or ox with a large dorsoventral measurement of the thoracic cavity, the force of gravity is great enough to cause considerable inequalities in perfusion of the alveolar capillaries, the dorsal parts of the lung being much less well perfused than the ventral. In the normal animal, however, such inequalities in perfusion are not very significant functionally, since alveolar ventilation is also less in the dorsal than in the ventral parts of the lung, so that ventilation and perfusion may still be nearly matched.

In large quadrupeds such as the horse and ox, the forces of gravity induce serious **mismatching** of ventilation and perfusion during **lateral recumbency**, with a major venous-to-arterial shunt (Section 6.30).

In a man standing at rest, the perfusion of the base of the lungs is about 10 times greater than that of the apex (Scott, 1986, p. 72). Furthermore (Guyton, 1986, p. 491) the ventilation/perfusion ratio at the apex is about three times greater than the ideal value, giving some alveolar dead space. At the base of the lung it is 0.6 times less than the ideal value, and therefore here the blood is not fully oxygenated, giving a venous-to-arterial shunt. Therefore gravity slightly decreases the effectiveness of gas exchange at the apex and base of the lung. At exercise, however, the increased pulmonary arterial pressure perfuses the apex satisfactorily, and the overall effectiveness of gas exchange becomes nearly optimal.

Positive pressure breathing adds to the difficulty in effectively perfusing the lung. By raising the pressure of the gas in the alveoli, a positive pressure pump compresses the capillaries in the alveolar walls. The right ventricle then has to increase its systolic pressure in order to overcome this (transmural) pressure and perfuse the alveolar capillaries. Positive pressure pumps have safety valves that prevent the pressure from rising or falling beyond certain limits. Sustained forced expiration, as in prolonged **abdominal straining**, also obstructs perfusion by raising the transmural pressure in the capillaries.

17.24 Filter action of the pulmonary circulation

As a result of trauma, natural processes, or even therapeutic measures, small particles (notably small blood clots, fat cells, and air bubbles) may enter the venous side of the systemic circulation. Such **emboli** fail to traverse the pulmonary capillaries, and are thus intercepted before they can enter the systemic circulation and block vessels in potentially more dangerous sites such as the cerebral and coronary circulations.

The resting mammal has far more pulmonary capillaries than are needed for effective gaseous exchanges, so some of these can safely be sacrificed to protect other vascular beds. In fact lung tissue is able to survive moderate embolism without undergoing significant cell damage (**infarcts**). The abundant normal anastomoses between pulmonary capillaries, and between bronchial capillaries and pulmonary capillaries (Section 17.8), and the extraordinary angiogenic powers of the bronchial arterial system in pathological lung tissues (Section 17.9), substantially protect the lung against the effects of plugging of pulmonary arteries and arterioles (Section 17.9.4).

Furthermore, there is evidence that the pulmonary circulation may possess additional special mechanisms for removing or recanalizing small plugs (Section 17.9.3). These mechanisms have not been fully elucidated, but may include the presence of special lytic enzymes (Section 12.22) and an abundance of macrophages. The discovery of **pulmonary intravascular macrophages** (Section 7.7.3) introduces another possible mechanism.

It is likely that many small emboli do occur and are continuously filtered out by the pulmonary microcirculation during the normal existence of an individual, without clinical signs. **Mast cells** (Section 12.23.3) are particularly numerous around the alveolar capillaries. By releasing **heparin** they may prevent any further growth of blood clots that have been filtered out. There is, of course, a limit to this capacity to deal with obstructions, and massive pulmonary embolism can cause severe pulmonary hypertension with fatal right heart failure (Section 17.9.4).

III PULMONARY OEDEMA: PLEURAL EFFUSION: PULMONARY HAEMORRHAGE

17.25 Formation of pulmonary oedema

Pulmonary oedema is an accumulation of fluid in the *walls* of alveoli, of bronchi, and of pulmonary blood vessels, and in the *lumens* of alveoli, bronchioles, and bronchi.

By increasing the thickness of the alveolar wall, and then breaking through into the alveolar lumen and flooding the terminal bronchioles, pulmonary oedema becomes a major factor causing **respiratory insufficiency** (Section 17.29).

The stages in the formation of pulmonary oedema have been reviewed by Weibel (1984, p. 333) and Butler (1991). The first sites to show it are the interstitial spaces of the **peribronchial** and **periarterial sheaths**, and the longitudinal **cuffs** of fluid around these sheaths (Baier, 1986; Butler, 1991). This is known as **interstitial oedema** (Weibel, 1984, p. 334). Although it is a secondary event, pulmonary oedema nevertheless appears early in the interstitium of the **alveolar walls** (Comroe, 1975, p. 161).

The resulting pressure in the alveolar interstitium evidently causes gaping of the **tight junctions** that normally attach the alveolar epithelial cells to each other (Section 6.17), thus allowing leakage into the alveolar lumen (Butler, 1991). Moreover, the ultrathin **alveolar epithelial cell** (Section 6.17) has such small tensile strength that the slightest positive pressure in the interstitium causes cell rupture. Therefore, except in the mildest cases of pulmonary oedema, the oedema fluid always finds its way into the alveolar lumen (Guyton, 1986, p. 393). Having once entered the alveolar lumen it backs up into the terminal bronchioles.

17.25.1 *Dynamics of pulmonary oedema*

The dynamics of normal filtration and reabsorption of fluid across the capillary wall in the pulmonary circulation depend on the balance between the hydrostatic and oncotic pressures acting on the blood plasma within the capillaries, as outlined in Section 17.19.

In a normal *resting* mammal, the oncotic pressure (about 28 mmHg (3.7 kPa) in man) is usually believed to substantially exceed the hydrostatic pressure (about 7 mmHg (0.9 kPa)) (Section 17.19) throughout the whole length of the pulmonary capillaries. The classic interpretation of the effects of these forces on the blood plasma in the pulmonary capillaries is that fluid is constantly being *reabsorbed along the whole length of the capillary*.

It is also assumed that the hydrostatic pressure in the pulmonary capillaries, i.e. the capillary pressure, would have to be raised above the oncotic pressure of the plasma before filtration would exceed reabsorption and oedema would form. This would require an increase of pulmonary capillary pressure from a normal resting level of about 7 mmHg (0.9 kPa) to about 30 mmHg (4.0 kPa). It is therefore assumed that there is a large **hydrostatic safety factor** of about 23 mmHg (3.1 kPa) before the danger of pulmonary oedema arises.

It is believed that, even during **exercise**, the oncotic pressure may still exceed the hydrostatic pressure in the pulmonary capillaries. This is because recruitment and dilation of capillaries enables the pulmonary vasculature to accommodate very large increases in flow volume at the cost of only small increases in pressure (Section 17.21.2). For example, in man an increase of **mean pulmonary arterial pressure** from a resting value of about 15 mmHg (2.0 kPa) to an exercise value of about 20 mmHg (2.7 kPa) increases the right ventricular output (and hence the pulmonary flow rate) by about 400%. Since the pulmonary capillary pressure would still be appreciably lower than the mean pulmonary arterial pressure, it is assumed that the pulmonary circulation has a generous **safety margin** before oedema would begin to form, sufficient to permit at least moderate exercise.

Nevertheless, under pathological conditions it is possible for the balance of forces across the wall of the pulmonary capillary to be seriously disturbed. Elevation of pulmonary capillary pressure is particularly dangerous, and can give rise to **'hydrostatic' pulmonary oedema**. Furthermore, the proper operation of the filtration and reabsorption forces across the capillary wall depends on the integrity of the capillary endothelium; an abnormal increase in endothelial permeability can lead to **'permeability' pulmonary oedema**.

17.25.2 *Hydrostatic pulmonary oedema*

Under some pathological conditions, the hydrostatic pressure in the pulmonary capillaries (i.e. the pulmonary capillary pressure) may increase so much that it really does exceed the oncotic pressure. The volume of fluid that is filtered out of the pulmonary capillaries would then exceed that reabsorbed into them. Fluid would therefore accumulate in both the conducting and the **respiratory airways**, forming pulmonary oedema. This can be called 'hydrostatic' pulmonary oedema.

What abnormal conditions cause such a rise in the hydrostatic pressure (filtration pressure) in the pulmonary capillaries? In principle, these are conditions that overload the left atrium, causing (a) **pulmonary venous congestion**, (b) **increased hydrostatic pressure** in the pulmonary veins, and thence (c) in the **pulmonary capillaries** also, and finally (d) **left heart failure** (Section 22.17). Examples of such conditions are **patent ductus arteriosus** (Section 15.8), **aortic stenosis** (Section 15.10), large **interventricular septal defects** (Section 15.11), and **mitral insufficiency** (Section 15.13).

There is circumstantial evidence (Baier, 1986) that the **bronchial circulation** plays a significant role in the formation of hydrostatic oedema. It is believed that oedema in the walls of bronchi and blood vessels (peribronchial and perivascular cuffing) may arise *locally* from the capillaries and venules of the **peribronchial** and **perivascular sheaths**, rather than by the backing up of fluid released into the alveolar lumen from the alveolar capillaries.

The anatomical basis for this is as follows: (1) the outermost capillaries of the **outer bronchial blood-vascular plexus** anastomose directly with the pulmonary capillaries of the surrounding exchange tissue (Section 17.6.1); (2) the bronchial and pulmonary circulations share capillary beds at the level of respiratory bronchioles (Section 17.7); (3) especially significant is the fact that the inner and outer peribronchial blood-vascular plexuses drain into the pulmonary veins (via **bronchopulmonary veins**), and therefore overloading of the left atrium will increase the hydrostatic pressure in the bronchial blood-vascular plexuses.

17.25.3   *Permeability pulmonary oedema*

Under certain other abnormal conditions, the permeability of the endothelium of the pulmonary capillaries may increase. This causes the filtration process to outrun the reabsorption process, so that pulmonary oedema again accumulates. Hence this has been called 'permeability' pulmonary oedema.

An abnormal increase in the **permeability** of the capillary endothelium arises from local damage to the **endothelium** of the pulmonary or bronchial capillaries. Examples are bacterial and viral infections causing pneumonia and bronchitis, inhalation of irritant gases, aspiration of foreign material, and ingestion of poisons. The damaging effects on the airways of infection and noxious gases are discussed in Sections 7.17, 7.18, and 7.19.

Respired **allergens** such as pollen and fungal spores are another cause of permeability oedema arising from capillary damage. The allergens provoke the release of **histamine** from mast cells, and the histamine increases the permeability of the profuse capillary networks in the **bronchial blood-vascular plexuses**. The result is flooding of the bronchial lumen with oedema, and the formation of cuffs of oedema around the bronchi.

The histamine also causes **bronchoconstriction** (Section 7.20) in **chronic obstructive pulmonary disease** in many species.

Observations suggest that bronchial oedema arising from increased capillary permeability, caused by the release of **histamine** in response to respiratory antigens, is likely to arise from the capillaries and venules of the **bronchial vascular plexuses** rather than from the pulmonary capillaries (see Baier, 1986; Butler, 1991).

17.25.4   *Functional effects of pulmonary oedema*

What are the functional consequences of pulmonary oedema? Oedema in the lumen of the **conducting airways** increases the resistance to air flow, and thus causes **airway obstruction**.

Oedema within the **alveolar lumen** forms a barrier of fluid between the alveolar air and the alveolar wall. Oedema within the **alveolar wall** increases the diffusion distance between the gas in the alveolar lumen and the blood in the alveolar capillaries. These obstructions **impede gas exchange**. There will then be a mismatch of perfusion and ventilation (Section 6.30.1); some venous blood will be inadequately exposed to alveolar gas, giving a **venous-to-arterial shunt**. Severe and widespread pulmonary oedema can produce a critical level of venous-to-arterial shunting, leading to **fatal hypoxia**: the victim drowns in its own oedema.

17.26   Mechanisms protecting the airways against pulmonary oedema

The following multiple mechanisms interact to keep the airways properly damp, whilst at the same time countering the constant threat of pulmonary oedema. The first two of these mechanisms (hydrostatic safety factor, and lymphatic drainage from alveoli) are probably the main mechanisms responsible for avoiding the formation of pulmonary oedema. The third (ejection by coughing) is an important emergency mechanism if pulmonary oedema has actually occurred.

Accounts of the mechanisms that control pulmonary oedema tend to emphasize the significance of the hydrostatic safety factor (Section 17.25.1). Admittedly, the general responsiveness of lymphatic drainage to impending breakdown of the hydrostatic safety factor is acknowledged, for example by Guyton (1986, p. 292) when calling attention to 'the extremely rapid run-off of fluid from the pulmonary interstitial spaces through the lymphatics' during a chronic elevation of pulmonary capillary pressure. However, the absence of lymphatic capillaries from the alveolar walls is an understandable obstacle to accepting lymphatic drainage as a highly significant factor in the control of pulmonary oedema.

Fortunately this obstacle can be largely overcome by recognition of the existence and distribution of **alveolar interstitial channels** (Sections 6.20, 17.26.2). At present there tends to be no more than a vague awareness of these mysterious pathways in the alveolar wall. For example, consider Baier (1986): 'According to a generally accepted view, the *connective tissue spaces* surrounding bronchial and pulmonary vessels *are continuous with the pulmonary interstitium*, and therefore interstitial oedema *extends into these spaces*' (my italics). The integrated morphological and physiological survey by Weibel (1984, pp. 331–334) has given a rather better idea of the structure and function of alveolar interstitial channels and their relationships to the fibrous continuum of the lung (Section 6.20). On the control of pulmonary oedema Weibel (1984, p. 334) concluded: 'The design features of the tissue, namely the restriction of spaces and the establishment of *drainage channels*, are *just as important* as a proper balance between the various forces that affect fluid movements.' (The italics are mine).

In addition to the hydrostatic factor, lymphatic drainage, and coughing, four other mechanisms protect the airways against pulmonary oedema (Sections 17.26.4–17.26.7). These are reabsorption of fluid by the bronchial vascular plexuses, reabsorption by the lymphatics of the pulmonary pleura, transfer of fluid by the granular epithelial cell from the alveolar lumen to the interstitium of the alveolar wall, and surfactant. The first three of these are believed to make a substantial contribution.

17.26.1   *Hydrostatic safety factor*

As stated in Section 17.25.1, the basic capillary dynamics of the normal resting mammal ensure that the *oncotic pressure* (about 28 mmHg (3.7 kPa) in man) exceeds the *hydrostatic pressure* (about 7 mmHg (0.9 kPa) in man) throughout the whole length of the pulmonary capillary (Section 17.19). It is therefore generally assumed that pulmonary oedema will not form until the hydrostatic pressure clearly **exceeds** the oncotic pressure, and that there is therefore a substantial **safety factor** (of about 23 mmHg (3.1 kPa) in man).

Experimental and clinical observations appear to support this hypothesis. Experimentally in the dog, no oedema develops in response to a progressive rise in left atrial pressure until the pulmonary capillary pressure exceeds the oncotic pressure of the blood plasma by about 3 mmHg (0.4 kPa). In man, pulmonary oedema usually does not develop until the pulmonary capillary pressure reaches 30 mmHg (4.0 kPa).

The effects of moderate exercise are also consistent with these findings. Thus, as already stated in Section 17.25.1, in man an increase of mean pulmonary arterial pressure from a resting value of about 15 mmHg (2.0 kPa) to an exercise value of about 30 mmHg (4.0 kPa) increases the right ventricular output (and hence the pulmonary flow rate) by about 400%, to 22 l min^{-1}. This allows strenuous exercise without formation of pulmonary oedema.

Cardiac pressures in **exercising racehorses**, however, strain one's faith in the dominance of the hydrostatic safety factor. In the galloping Thoroughbred, the **mean pulmonary arterial pressure** has been found to exceed 100 mmHg (13.3 kPa), with **mean pulmonary capillary pressures** of well over 70 mmHg (9.3 kPa) (Section 17.18.2). The oncotic pressure of equine plasma is believed to be similar to that of other mammals (C.M. Brown, personal communication, 1994), i.e. presumably about 28 mmHg (3.7 kPa). If so, the pulmonary capillary pressure in the exercising racehorse must then so grossly exceed the oncotic pressure of the blood plasma that the animal should swiftly drown in pulmonary oedema. Yet there is no evidence of pulmonary oedema.

Clearly, other protective mechanisms must be at work in the Thoroughbred, and amongst these the prime candidate is surely drainage through the alveolar interstitial channels and thence the pulmonary lymphatics.

In **man** lethal pulmonary oedema can occur within 20–30 minutes if the pulmonary capillary pressure rises 25–30 mmHg (2.7–4.0 kPa) above the safety factor level of about 28 mmHg (3.7 kPa). Thus in acute left heart failure, in which the pulmonary capillary pressure may rise as high as 50 mmHg (6.7 kPa), death from acute pulmonary oedema often follows in less than half an hour (Guyton, 1986, p. 373).

17.26.2   *Drainage by alveolar interstitial channels and pulmonary lymphatics*

Intuitively, lymphatic drainage seems an improbable protection against pulmonary oedema. After all, there are no lymphatic capillaries in the alveolar wall: the nearest available pulmonary lymphatics are in the walls of respiratory bronchioles. However, there are irregular anastomosing **alveolar interstitial channels** in the alveolar wall, between the longitudinal fibres of the fibrous continuum (Section 6.20), and these are well placed to act as drainage channels from the alveolar walls. Just as the *fibres* of the fibrous continuum are continuous through the alveolar walls and onto the bronchial tree, so also are the alveolar interstitial channels continuous through the alveolar walls and onto the bronchial tree. Eventually, therefore, the alveolar interstitial channels meet the blind ends of the **lymphatic capillaries** in the walls of **respiratory bronchioles** (Section 7.8). Here, the fluid from the alveolar interstitial channels bathes the ends of the lymphatic capillaries. Since there are gaps between the endothelial cells that line the lymphatic capillaries, the fluid in the alveolar interstitial channels then becomes continuous with the fluid in the lymphatic capillaries.

The lymphatic capillaries of the respiratory bronchioles continue into the peribronchial and perivascular lymphatic plexuses of the **peribronchial lymphatic pathway** (Section 7.8.1).

The onward movement of fluid through the alveolar interstitial channels and peribronchial lymphatic pathway is achieved by the integration of three mechanisms: (a) the contraction of smooth muscle in the walls of the lymphatics (b) the intermittent compression of the lymphatic vessels caused by the movements of breathing, and (c) the unidirectional flow controlled by the valves in the peribronchial lymphatic vessels.

The **alveolar interstitial channels** on which this drainage pathway depends were elucidated by Weibel (1984, pp. 331–334), as already stated above.

There is an additional minor element of autoregulation in the drainage of interstitial fluid by the alveolar interstitial channels. Drainage of the fluid simultaneously removes the protein that has escaped across the leaky endothelial cells of the pulmonary capillaries (Section 6.19). Removal of this protein decreases the oncotic pressure of the interstitial fluid, and therefore automatically increases the reabsorption of fluid into the pulmonary capillaries (Guyton, 1986, p. 372).

Experimental observations on **dogs** (Guyton, 1986, p. 292) show that, if the pulmonary capillary pressure is *sustained* for 2 weeks at levels about 15 mmHg (2.0 kPa) above that usually inducing oedema, the pulmonary

lymphatics enlarge and increase their flow 20-fold above normal. Similarly, clinical observations in **man** indicate that *chronic* pulmonary capillary pressures as high as 45 mmHg (6.0 kPa) sometimes do not induce pulmonary oedema.

Such observations indicate that, in dog and man, the lymphatic drainage of the alveoli is highly adaptable to the load placed upon it.

The existence in the **racehorse** of huge pulmonary capillary pressures without pulmonary oedema suggests that in these animals drainage by the interstitial channels into the pulmonary lymphatics is very much more effective than had hitherto been suspected.

17.26.3 *Coughing*

The defensive reflex of coughing is an important reserve mechanism for clearing the airways of excess respiratory secretions and fluids (Section 7.6.2).

17.26.4 *Reabsorption by the outer and inner bronchial blood-vascular plexuses*

The bronchial blood-vascular plexuses belong essentially to the bronchial circulation (Section 17.6). The outer plexus encloses the whole length of each bronchus in a sleeve of freely anastomosing arterial, venous, and lymphatic capillaries; the inner plexus has a similar composition but lies in the tunica mucosa, under the bronchial epithelium. The two plexuses anastomose in the bronchial wall at the level of the bronchial cartilages.

The profuse arteriovenous microvasculature of these two plexuses is in close contact with any oedema within the peribronchial and perivascular sheaths, which is where pulmonary oedema begins (Section 17.25.1). The cuffs of oedema that in due course enclose the bronchi are, of course, in contact with the outer surface of the outer plexus. Fluid that actually floods the bronchial lumen is close to the inner plexus. Fluid is also carried mouthward by the mucociliary escalator, and can be reabsorbed into the inner bronchial blood-vascular plexus throughout its journey up the bronchial tree.

Both the outer and the inner bronchial blood-vascular plexuses are well-placed to reabsorb bronchial oedema into their venous capillaries and venules, and into their intermeshed lymphatic vessels.

The bronchial circulation was, indeed, found by Butler (1991) to be involved in reabsorption of pulmonary oedema by means of the bronchial blood-vascular plexuses. Clinically, much of the fluid washed into the larger airways during bronchial lavage is not recovered, and yet morphological and functional observations immediately after lavage usually disclose no evidence of residual fluid. In 1873, Colin instilled 25 litres of water into the trachea of a horse but found no evidence of lung injury 6 hours later.

17.26.5 Lymphatics of the pulmonary pleura

These form an anastomosing lymphatic network over the whole surface of the lung. It is generally believed that little, if any, fluid is removed from the lung by the lymphatics of the pulmonary pleura. However, Drake and Gabel (1995) have shown that lung fluid may be cleared via the pleural cavity, even if the lungs themselves are not oedematous; if there is pulmonary oedema a lot of lung fluid is cleared through the pulmonary (visceral) pleura (Section 7.8.2).

17.26.6 Transport of water by the granular epithelial cell

The granular epithelial cell actively pumps sodium from the alveolar fluid into the alveolar interstitium, and water follows by osmosis (Section 6.18).

17.26.7 Surfactant

Increased surface tension at the alveolar lumen because of diminished surfactant favours filtration from the alveolar capillaries and promotes pulmonary oedema (Section 17.19.4). The presence of surfactant in proper quantities is therefore a protective factor against oedema.

17.26.8 Micropinocytosis by the alveolar epithelial cell

Micropinocytotic vesicles in the alveolar epithelial cell may transport alveolar oedema from the alveolar lumen to the interstitium of the alveolar wall (Weibel, 1984, p. 252) (Section 6.17).

17.27 Formation of pleural effusion

Pleural effusion is the pathological accumulation of fluid in the pleural cavity.

Pleural fluid diffuses in and out of the pleural cavity, through the pulmonary (visceral) and parietal pleura. Normally the pleural cavity is occupied by only a thin film of pleural fluid (Section 9.6), but if the production or removal of this fluid is disturbed its quantity may increase until the lung is collapsed. The dynamics of the filtration and reabsorption of pleural fluid depend on the balance between the *hydrostatic* and *oncotic* forces acting on the blood plasma in the capillaries of the pulmonary and parietal pleura. The principles are similar to those that control the formation and reabsorption of pulmonary oedema (Section 17.19): if the hydrostatic pressure in the pleural microvasculature exceeds the oncotic pressure, pleural effusion will result.

17.27.1 Hydrostatic pressure relationships in the pleural microcirculation

In most of the domestic mammals and man the arterial supply to the pulmonary (visceral) pleura comes from the bronchial arteries, via branches that run in the interlobular septa (Section 17.4). In the other domestic species (dog and cat) the supply comes from the pulmonary arteries.

These species variations might suggest that the pressure in the arterioles of the **pulmonary pleura** would be high in most of the domestic species, and low in the cat and dog, since the bronchial arteries belong to the high pressure systemic arterial system whereas the pulmonary arteries are a low pressure system (Section 17.18). However, the wandering channels of the bronchial arteries and their abundant anastomoses with the pulmonary microvasculature ensure that the pressures in the bronchial and pulmonary microvasculatures are equally low (Section 17.10). Consequently, in all these species, the hydrostatic pressure that drives the filtration of pleural fluid from the blood vessels of the pulmonary pleura is *pulmonary pressure*, and is correspondingly low.

The arterial supply to the **parietal pleura** is provided by intercostal arteries and other regional systemic arteries (Section 9.9). The hydrostatic pressure in these parietal pleural vessels is *systemic*, and is therefore substantially higher than the pressures in the microvasculature of the pulmonary pleura.

The venous drainage of the pulmonary pleura is into the pulmonary veins in all species (Section 17.5). The venous drainage of the parietal pleura is by intercostal and other satellite systemic veins (Section 9.9).

Because of its *vascular stratum* (Section 17.4), the pulmonary pleura is much more vascular than the parietal pleura and is therefore better equipped than the parietal pleura for filtration and reabsorption of pleural fluid.

17.27.2 Reabsorption of pleural fluid by the pleural microcirculation

Pleural fluid is reabsorbed by rich capillary networks in the vascular stratum of the **pulmonary (visceral) pleura**. As stated in Section 17.27.1, the hydrostatic pressure in these blood capillaries of the pulmonary pleura is essentially pulmonary arterial pressure, and in the resting animal is therefore only about 7 mmHg (0.9 kPa). The oncotic pressure in these capillaries is about 28 mmHg (3.7 kPa), i.e. much higher than the hydrostatic pressure. Consequently there is normally a pressure of about 21 mmHg (2.8 kPa) in favour of reabsorption throughout the whole length of the capillaries in the pulmonary pleura. This absorptive force contributes to the subatmospheric pressure in the pleural cavity (Section 10.4), and to the liquid coupling of the lung to the thoracic wall (Section 10.5).

In the blood capillaries of the **parietal pleura**, the hydrostatic pressure is governed by systemic arterial pressure. The pressure is therefore relatively high, i.e. about 32 mmHg (4.3 kPa) at the arterial end of the capillary (Section 14.4), so that filtration occurs at the arterial end of the capillary and reabsorption at the venous end only.

Because of their low hydrostatic pressure, the blood capillaries of the pulmonary (visceral) pleura are an important route for the reabsorption of pleural fluid (Section 9.7), though perhaps not as important as the lymphatics of the pulmonary pleura (Section 17.27.4).

17.27.3 Conditions leading to pleural effusion

The basic rationale of pleural effusion is the same as that of 'hydrostatic' pulmonary oedema – the hydrostatic pressure in the capillaries of the pulmonary (visceral) pleura would have to exceed the oncotic pressure (Section 17.25.2). The basic cause of this increase in hydrostatic pressure is, once again, overloading of the left atrium, resulting in pulmonary venous congestion, increased hydrostatic pressure in the pulmonary veins, and hence increased hydrostatic pressure in the veins

of the pulmonary pleura. This is **left heart failure** (Section 22.17), activated for example by aortic stenosis, major interventricular defects, or mitral insufficiency. *Since such conditions also lead to pulmonary oedema, pleural effusion is usually associated clinically with pulmonary oedema.*

There has been a long-standing controversy (Butler, 1991) as to whether pleural effusions (in man) arise from left or right heart failure. It has now been shown that left heart failure (Section 22.17) is usually the culprit. Nevertheless, the high systemic venous pressure of right heart failure raises the hydrostatic pressure in the capillaries of the parietal pleura, and may therefore directly induce the formation of fluid from the parietal pleura. It may also form fluid indirectly, by impairing the drainage of the parietal pleural lymphatics (Section 9.10) into the great veins at the thoracic inlet via the thoracic duct and right lymphatic duct (Section 14.36).

17.27.4 Lymphatic drainage of pleural effusion

The submesothelial connective tissue of both the pulmonary (visceral) and the parietal pleura contains lymphatic vessels (Section 9.7), but the lymphatics of the pulmonary pleura are particularly well-developed. They form a network of profusely anastomosing channels all over the surface of the lung, draining not only the pulmonary pleura but also the alveoli immediately beneath the pleura. These abundant lymphatic networks in the pulmonary pleura are probably the main pathway for the removal of pleural effusions (Section 9.7).

Each expiration raises the intrapleural pressure, forcing a small volume of fluid into the pleural lymphatics and moving the lymph towards the related lymph nodes.

The lymphatics of the pulmonary pleura drain mainly into the **tracheobronchial lymph nodes**; those of the parietal pleura discharge into the various regional lymph nodes, notably the **intercostal** and **sternal nodes** (Section 9.10).

The impression given by reviews up to the 1970s, e.g. Agostoni and Mead (1964, p. 402) and Wang (1975), was that the rich *blood capillary networks* in the pulmonary (visceral) pleura formed the principal pathway for the normal drainage of plural fluid, but the emphasis has recently shifted towards the *lymphatics* of the pulmonary pleura. Thus Drake and Gabel (1995) concluded that it is the **lymphatics of the pulmonary pleura** that keep the volume of pleural liquid at a minimum in the normal lung, and remove excess fluid if pleural effusion forms (Section 9.7).

Although the lymphatics of the parietal pleura are less abundant than those of the pulmonary pleura, it is claimed that they possess stomata. These are gaps between the mesothelial cells on the surface of the parietal pleura, which open directly into the lymphatic vessels beneath the mesothelium. It is uncertain whether the stomata are permanent structures. They may contribute to the removal of pleural effusions, but are mainly responsible for the extraction of particles from the pleural cavity (Section 9.7).

17.28 Exercise-induced pulmonary haemorrhage

17.28.1 *Exercise-induced pulmonary haemorrhage in the horse (EIPH)*

EIPH is characterized by haemorrhage from the lung in horses after racing. It is recognized by tracheobronchial endoscopy, but a few cases bleed overtly from the nose (epistaxis). The condition may affect the large majority of the population of Thoroughbred and Standardbred racing horses, preventing them from realizing their full racing potential. It is one of the most serious veterinary problems facing the horse-racing industry today, and is also of exceptional physiological interest.

The bleeding occurs from numerous small foci along the dorsal border of both lungs, but particularly at the dorsocaudal region of the caudal lobe of each lung.

EIPS occurs in horses that undergo relatively short bursts of very severe exercise, thus experiencing the maximum changes in systemic and pulmonary blood pressures, ventilatory load, and physical stress (O'Callaghan *et al.*, 1987b). It is very common in racehorses, a reported incidence being 96 out of 117 Thoroughbred racehorses that had been retired from racing (see O'Callaghan *et al.*, 1987a). Fifty per cent or more of the Thoroughbred and Standardbred racing populations are believed to be subclinically affected. Tracheal washings (Whitwell and Greet, 1984) even suggest that essentially *all* Thoroughbreds in training bleed into their lungs. It is reported that the condition does not occur in

horses engaged in lower grade activities such as endurance rides (see O'Callaghan *et al.*, 1987b).

Massive fatal haemorrhage may occur during or immediately after racing, but is uncommon; obvious bleeding from the nose does not happen in most cases, and distress is unusual (O'Callaghan, 1989, p. 109). The main significance of the condition is that it *reduces potential athletic performance*, and that its progressive nature makes the impairment worse with time (O'Callaghan *et al.*, 1987c).

17.28.2 *Anatomical source of the haemorrhage in the horse*

From which vessels does the haemorrhage come? One strongly supported view is that it comes from branches of the **bronchial arteries**, but it has also been proposed that the **pulmonary capillaries** are a more likely source, and the physiological and histopathological arguments for this are very convincing, if not decisive.

Is the haemorrhage from the bronchial arteries?

According to this hypothesis (O'Callaghan *et al.*, 1987c), the primary pathological features are bilaterally symmetrical multiple foci of bronchiolitis (small airway disease) in the caudal lobe of the left and right lung. The lesions are concentrated at the dorsocaudal angle of the lung, but progressively extend cranially along the whole length of the dorsal border to the level of the hilus in the severest cases (O'Callaghan *et al.*, 1987a). The affected areas are usually, though not always, stained brown by alveolar macrophages enclosing large amounts of haemosiderin, and include zones of fibrosis and destruction of lung parenchyma; these changes are interpreted as the results of previous haemorrhage and inflammation. However, some of the areas of small airway disease show no evidence of haemorrhage, indicating that haemorrhage may be **secondary** to the bronchiolitis.

In the affected regions there is intense proliferation of the bronchial arterial vasculature, including extensive anastomoses of the bronchial arteries with the pulmonary arterial vasculature (bronchopulmonary arterial anastomoses). The walls of the pleural branches of the bronchial arteries supplying the pulmonary (visceral) pleura become greatly thickened by proliferation of their smooth muscle. The bronchial arterial circulation now dominates the pulmonary arterial circulation. But there is also proliferation of the bronchial arteries in the small airway lesions that show no signs of haemorrhage, thus indicating that proliferation of the bronchial arteries begins **before** haemorrhage occurs. Angiogenesis, in the form of arterial proliferation and the development of bronchopulmonary arterial anastomoses, is a well-attested response of the bronchial arteries to pathological stimuli (Section 17.9).

Thoracic scintigraphy (Section 24.17) shows mismatching of ventilation and perfusion, the affected areas being markedly underperfused by the pulmonary arteries and moderately underventilated.

O'Callaghan *et al.* (1987c) proposed the following pathogenesis of EIPH. The process starts with multiple focal lesions of bronchiolitis (small airway disease). The most likely cause of this is a low grade respiratory virus. Airway obstruction develops in the affected area (presumably through 'permeability pulmonary oedema'; Section 17.25.3). The proliferation of the bronchial arteries is a response to the bronchiolitis. If the horse is now treated appropriately and not exercised, the inflammatory response wanes and little if any permanent damage to the lung results. But if the horse is repeatedly and intensively exercised, airway obstruction could lead to localized hypoxia in the exchange tissue served by the affected bronchioles. This would stimulate further angiogenesis. At this point, minor local haemorrhages might begin. They probably occur at 'the advancing margin of new vascular growth beneath the epithelium of inflamed alveolar ducts and alveolar septae' (O'Callaghan *et al.*, 1987c). The haemorrhage attracts macrophages, and these contribute further damage by releasing lysozymes and other cytotoxic factors. A vicious cycle is now established, in which repeated exercise creating hypoxia in more extensive areas of the lung may lead to further multiple foci of bleeding.

Some aspects of this pathogenesis seem uncertain. Why are the lesions so strictly limited to the *dorsal* region of the caudal lobe? This suggests a gravitational factor, but how would it work? Where exactly does the bleeding come from? O'Callaghan *et al.* (1987b) were unable to demonstrate ruptured bronchial arteries or arterioles. Why should bleeding from the bronchial arteries happen anyway? The bronchial arteries generally have unusually thick muscular walls (Section 17.2), even more so when responding to pathological stimuli (Section 17.9).

Is the haemorrhage from the pulmonary arteries?

Manohar *et al.* (1993) and West *et al.* (1993) proposed that the pulmonary vasculature is more likely to be the source of the haemorrhage than the bronchial vasculature, basing their argument on physiological evidence and ultrastructural observations.

Measurements by Manohar *et al.* (1993) on horses during strenuous exercise on a treadmill showed that the right ventricular systolic pressure rises to the remarkable value of nearly 100 mmHg (13.3 kPa). Also mean pulmonary arterial pressures as high as 120 mmHg (16.0 kPa)

have been recorded by Jones *et al.* (1992) in galloping Thoroughbreds, with mean left atrial pressures of 70 mmHg (9.3 kPa). The usual reaction of classical mammalian physiologists to these values is 'complete disbelief' (West and Mathieu-Costello, 1994). The right ventricular systolic pressure at rest in normal healthy ponies is about 40 mmHg (5.3 kPa) (Manohar *et al.*, 1993). Pulmonary wedge pressure in horses during strenuous exercise was measured by Manohar *et al.* (1993) at about 65 mmHg (8.7 kPa). From these pulmonary pressures they estimated the **mean pulmonary capillary pressure** in horses during strenuous exercise to be near 79 mmHg (10.5 kPa).

In severe exercise the **transmural pressure** in the **pulmonary capillaries** (i.e. the pressure across the capillary wall) will be even greater than the pulmonary capillary pressure (i.e. the pressure inside the capillary). This is due to the fall in *pleural pressure* (Section 10.4) that occurs during inspiration. (The linkage between pleural pressure and alveolar pressure during breathing can be expressed as transpulmonary, or transmural, pressure; Section 10.4.4). During the hyperpnoea of severe exercise, pleural pressure in galloping Thoroughbreds falls as low as −20 mmHg (−2.7 kPa) (Section 10.4.1). Furthermore, the pressure at the arterial end of the pulmonary capillaries will be higher than the mean pressure. For all these reasons, West and Mathieu-Costello (1994) believe that some pulmonary capillaries in the galloping Thoroughbred will be subjected to transmural pressures well above 100 mmHg (13.3 kPa).

Pulmonary capillaries subjected to **transmural pressures** exceeding 79 mmHg (10.5 kPa) must surely be in danger of rupture. Experimental observations have shown extensive disruption of pulmonary capillary endothelium at transmural capillary pressures of 40 mmHg (5.3 kPa) in the rabbit lung and at 70 mmHg (9.3 kPa) in the dog lung, this phenomenon being known as 'stress failure of the pulmonary capillaries'; ultrastructural studies have shown similar stress failure of pulmonary capillaries in racehorses after galloping, with disrupted endothelial and alveolar epithelial cells, erythrocytes in the alveolar interstitium, proteinaceous fluid and erythrocytes in the alveolar lumen, and oedema in the alveolar interstitium (West *et al.*, 1993).

But why are the pulmonary haemorrhages concentrated in the **dorsal** part of the lung? The transmural pulmonary capillary pressure in the standing animal would be very much higher in the **ventral** parts of the lung, because of *gravitational factors* (Section 17.23). Manohar *et al.* (1993) acknowledged this difficulty. They could only suggest that alveoli in the dorsal part of the lung may have (unrecognized) structural peculiarities making their capillaries relatively vulnerable; or that lower pleural pressures in the dorsal part of the thorax create greater transmural capillary pressures there, particularly during the hyperpnoea of severe exercise.

Possible stress failure of pulmonary capillaries in the pathogenesis of exercise induced pulmonary haemorrhage in horses (EIPH)

Although not all questions yet have answers, stress failure of pulmonary capillaries is being increasingly recognized as the probable mechanism of EIPH. The ruptured pulmonary capillaries and the erythrocytes in the alveolar interstitium are compelling, if not decisive, evidence for the pulmonary capillary as the source of haemorrhage.

17.28.3   *Exercise-induced pulmonary haemorrhage in other species*

Exercise-induced pulmonary haemorrhage has been reported in racing **camels** and racing **greyhounds**. Fortunately it does not occur in the racing human animal.

Camel racing is a traditional sport in the Gulf area (Akbar *et al.*, 1994). Some camels show streaks of blood around the nostrils after racing, or have unexpectedly poor racing performance. Tracheobronchial endoscopy of 20 such camels disclosed blood in the lower respiratory tract in six animals. The tracheal washings of all six of them contained erythrocytes and macrophages containing haemosiderin. The incidence in this small sample of camels appeared to be similar to that in Standardbred horses, but lower than in racing Thoroughbreds. The occurrence of EIPH in greyhounds was reported by King *et al.* (1990).

17.28.4   *Selective breeding and exercise-induced pulmonary haemorrhage*

It appears likely that selective breeding of supremely athletic racing horses with ever more powerful muscles of locomotion, and possibly also similar racing camels and greyhounds, has generated too great a cardiac output. The essence of the problem then lies in the difficulty of filling the left side of the heart.

A huge cardiac output requires an equally huge left ventricular input. The difficulty of achieving this is compounded by the very fast heart rate with a very short diastolic interval, and the massive hypertrophy of the left ventricular myocardium which causes the left ventricle to lose compliance. Powerful left atrial contraction is now needed to fill the stiff left ventricle in the short time available between beats. Unfortunately the high pressure thus developed during left atrial systole must in-

evitably back up into the pulmonary capillary beds, where it causes mean pulmonary capillary pressures of over 70 mmHg (9.3 kPa) (Section 17.18.2). Such pressures evidently prove too great for the ultrathin microvasculature of the blood–gas barrier: stress failure of the capillary endothelium is the result.

West *et al.* (1993) have pointed out that Thoroughbred horses have been selectively bred for supreme athletic performance for four centuries, largely on the basis of four stallions. The modern animal has a maximal oxygen consumption of up to $180 \, \text{ml} \, \text{min}^{-1} \, \text{kg}^{-1}$, which is over twice the $80 \, \text{ml} \, \text{min}^{-1} \, \text{kg}^{-1}$ of the elite human athlete; the cardiac output can exceed $750 \, \text{ml} \, \text{min}^{-1} \, \text{kg}^{-1}$, again nearly exceeding by a factor of two the $400 \, \text{ml} \, \text{min}^{-1} \, \text{kg}^{-1}$ of the human athlete; the maximum heart rate is about $240 \, \text{min}^{-1}$, compared with a maximum of about $185 \, \text{min}^{-1}$ in man. To achieve this phenomenal cardiac performance, the Thoroughbred racehorse must employ an enormously high pressure to fill the left side of its heart, and this accounts for left atrial pressures as great as 70 mmHg (9.3 kPa). Since there has to be a pressure gradient from the pulmonary capillaries to the left atrium, the pressure in the pulmonary capillaries must be even higher, the transmural pressures perhaps surpassing even 100 mmHg (13.3 kPa). These massive pressures evidently exceed the stress tolerance of pulmonary capillaries.

The racing greyhound, and presumably the racing camel, have also been artificially selected for high cardiac performance, and may have outrun the strength of their pulmonary capillaries. The elite human athlete has not been selectively bred, but arises through Darwinist natural selection; consequently the checks and balances of survival of the fittest ensure the elimination of individuals with dangerously high left atrial and pulmonary pressures.

It is possible to get carried away with enthusiasm for 'improvement' of a domestic species. The immense modern turkey, selected for early and rapid growth of the pectoral muscles, has an unfortunate habit of dropping dead when handled, probably because of an insufficient capacity for gas exchange. The modern domestic fowl also appears to have been 'overengineered' to a point closely approaching pulmonary inadequacy, thus predisposing to the now worldwide problem of broiler ascites (Vidyadaran *et al.*, 1987, 1990). A 'sudden death syndrome' has also appeared in the modern pig (Section 20.4).

17.29   Respiratory insufficiency

Normal tissues require a continual renewal of their oxygen supply. This is because the body has virtually no stored oxygen to draw on during complete anoxia or asphyxia. Respiratory insufficiency is a condition in which **respiration** (the exchange of oxygen and carbon dioxide between the atmosphere and the cells of the body) fails to fully support the tissues of the body. Three main varieties of abnormality cause **respiratory insufficiency**: (i) conditions that lead to inadequate ventilation of alveoli; (ii) conditions that decrease gaseous diffusion across the blood–gas barrier; and (iii) conditions that impair the transport of oxygen from the lungs to the tissues.

Several terms are commonly used to indicate a diminished supply of oxygen. **Anoxia** strictly means a total lack of oxygen. **Hypoxia** signifies a decrease in oxygen to below normal levels – in inspired gas, or alveolar gas, or blood, or tissues. **Hypoxaemia** refers to a decrease in the oxygen saturation of haemoglobin, or a decrease in the partial pressure of oxygen (P_{O_2}), or both, of systemic arterial blood. **Anaemia** is a condition in which the oxygen saturation and partial pressure of systemic arterial blood may be normal, but the volume of oxygen per unit volume of blood is below normal; therefore anaemia is really a type of hypoxaemia.

A man of average body mass has only about 1.55 litres of oxygen in his whole body – enough to last him for not much more than about 6 minutes, if it could be appropriately distributed (Comroe, 1975, p. 200). Many abnormal conditions causing respiratory insufficiency are encountered throughout this book, but the following is a summary of the main examples.

17.29.1 *Abnormal conditions leading to inadequate ventilation of alveoli*

Lesions in the medulla oblongata or cervicothoracic spinal cord caused by trauma, tumours, or infections may **disrupt the inspiratory drive pathway** and severely impair breathing (Section 11.3). The medullary respiratory centre tends to be depressed by general anaesthetics (Guyton, 1986, p. 518).

Failure of the mucociliary escalator of the bronchial tree can cause severe airway obstruction by accumulation of mucus; this leads to marked impairment of alveolar ventilation, with serious ventilation–perfusion mismatching and a pronounced venous-to-arterial shunt (Section 7.17).

Decreased pulmonary compliance has similar effects, lessening alveolar ventilation and causing ventilation–perfusion mismatching (Section 6.31). Pulmonary compliance is decreased in alveolar emphysema by the loss of elastic fibres from the disrupted alveolar walls and the laying down of fibrous scar tissue (Section 7.19). Pulmonary compliance is also decreased by hard tumours or abscesses in the lung.

Bronchoconstriction (bronchial spasm) may produce a severe increase in airway resistance and hence diminish the flow of air through the conducting airways and into the respiratory airways (alveoli) (Section 7.20).

Collapse of a lung by pneumothorax (Section 10.3) or pleural oedema (Section 17.27) hinders the normal dilation of the airways during inspiration.

17.29.2 *Abnormal conditions decreasing gaseous diffusion across the blood–gas barrier*

The structural factors controlling the volume of oxygen that diffuses across the blood–gas barrier are the surface area of the barrier, the thickness of the barrier, and the volume of blood in the pulmonary capillaries. These factors determine the anatomical and physiological diffusing capacities of the lung (Sections 6.26.5; 6.27). Therefore any abnormal conditions that reduce the area of the barrier or increase its thickness, or diminish the volume of pulmonary capillary blood, will decrease the diffusing capacity of the lung.

The **surface area** of the barrier and the **volume of blood** circulating in its pulmonary capillaries, are directly reduced by the destruction of alveolar walls in **alveolar emphysema** (Section 7.19). Lung cancer and the lesions of pulmonary tuberculosis can have the same destructive effects on the alveolar walls. Filling of alveoli by pulmonary oedema indirectly reduces the surface area by preventing air from contacting the barrier.

The **thickness of the blood–gas barrier** is increased by the laying down of fibrous scar tissue in **alveolar emphysema**. It is also directly increased in the initial stage of **pulmonary oedema** (Section 17.25), when the oedema invades the alveolar wall; it is indirectly increased when the oedema breaks through the alveolar wall and lines the alveolar lumen. A common cause of pulmonary oedema is left heart failure (Section 22.17). **Pneumonia** from bacterial infection of the alveoli is a major cause of increased barrier thickness. Bacterial toxins damage the endothelium of the pulmonary capillaries, greatly increasing permeability to oedema and inflammatory cells; the barrier is thus directly thickened, and breakthrough into the alveolar lumen indirectly thickens the barrier still further. The infection spreads from alveolus to alveolus, and may eventually lead to 'consolidation' of large areas of the lung by fluid and cellular debris (Guyton, 1986, p. 520).

17.29.3 *Abnormal conditions decreasing oxygen transport by the blood from lungs to tissues*

Anaemia decreases the transport of oxygen to the tissues. It is characterized by an abnormally low number or volume of erythrocytes, or a less than normal quantity of haemoglobin in the blood. Its causes include haemorrhage, depression of erythropoiesis, autoimmune destruction of erythrocytes, injury to erythrocytes by drugs, nutritional deficiency, and blood sucking parasites.

Carbon monoxide has an affinity for haemoglobin over 200 times greater than that of oxygen, and combines at the same site on the haemoglobin molecule as does oxygen. Therefore at a partial pressure of only 0.4 mmHg (0.05 kPa) in the alveoli, it competes on even terms with oxygen when oxygen is at a partial pressure of about 100 mmHg (13.3 kPa) (Guyton, 1986, p. 500). At a partial pressure of about 7 mmHg (0.93 kPa) (about 0.1% in air), carbon monoxide can form a lethal combination with haemoglobin.

Decreased blood flow arising from impaired cardiac output or from defects in peripheral vasomotor control can lower the transport of oxygen to the tissues.

Poisoning of cellular enzymes can prevent the unloading of oxygen into the tissues. For example, cyanide poisoning completely blocks the action of cytochrome oxidase, and thus prevents cells from using oxygen even when it is abundantly available (Guyton, 1986, p. 522).

Chapter 18
Coronary Circulation

The cardiac muscle cell has a very high oxidative metabolic rate. In contrast to the skeletal muscle cell, it has little anaerobic metabolic capacity and therefore cannot incur an oxygen debt that can be paid back during the short rest between each systole. Consequently the myocardium demands a very rich blood supply by the coronary circulation: indeed the coronary blood vessels and their contents form about half the mass of the living myocardium. The coronary circulation in the resting animal (dog or man) accounts for about 4–5% of the total cardiac output, and yet the heart forms only about 0.6% of the total body mass of a mammal.

18.1 Basic design of the coronary arteries and their branches

The arrangement of the coronary arteries is essentially bilaterally symmetrical.

The design is based on the **left coronary artery** supplying the left side of the heart, and the **right coronary artery** supplying the right side. Each of these two coronary arteries has an **interventricular artery** and a **circumflex artery**. All of these vessels are visible on the surface of the heart.

The ventricular region of the left side of the heart has a distinct dorsoventral groove, the **left interventricular groove**. This descends from the base of the heart to the conical apex of the heart (Fig. 20.1), separating the right ventricle cranially from the left ventricle caudally. This groove carries the **left interventricular artery**. The right side of the heart (Fig. 17.5) has a similar dorsoventral groove, the **right interventricular groove**, separating the right ventricle cranially from the left ventricle caudally and housing the **right interventricular artery**.

The left and right circumflex arteries lie in the circular **coronary groove** that separates the atria dorsally from the ventricles ventrally, and thus encircle the heart.

The left and right coronary arteries and their interventricular and circumflex branches supply the myocardium by three groups of smaller branches, i.e. **ventricular**, **septal**, and **atrial arteries**. These form a dense microcirculation between the cardiac muscle cells (Section 18.3).

18.1.1 Ventricular arteries

The **left** and **right interventricular arteries** supply both of the ventricles with **ventricular arteries** (Figs 17.5, 20.1). The **left** and **right circumflex arteries** also supply **ventricular arteries**, directed towards the apex of the heart (Figs 17.5, 20.1).

18.1.2 Septal arteries

The massive musculature of the interventricular septum is supplied by many **septal arteries**. The **interventricular septum** (Section 20.10) extends across the heart, between the left and right interventricular grooves (Fig. 18.2). Since the two interventricular grooves house the two interventricular arteries, the **left** and **right interventricular arteries** form the septal arteries, directed essentially at right angles to the surface of the heart. Examples of septal arteries are shown (*in broken lines*) in Figs 17.5 and 20.1.

18.1.3 Atrial arteries

Because the **left** and **right circumflex arteries** are continuously adjacent to the atria, they supply atrial arteries to the left and right atria, directed essentially dorsally (Figs 17.5, 20.1).

18.1.4 *Species variations*

The bilaterally symmetrical design of the coronary arteries (as described above) occurs in the horse and pig. In the other domestic species the symmetry of the pattern is disturbed by variations in the **right interventricular artery**. In the dog for example, which is often the main anatomical model, and also in ruminants, the **right interventricular artery** is formed from the *left* coronary artery (Fig. 17.5), instead of from the right coronary artery as in the bilaterally symmetrical plan.

Among the domestic mammals the main **interspecific variation** in the arteries of the heart occurs in the **right interventricular artery** (as just stated). There are consequent variations in the arterial supply to the interventricular septum and the ventricular myocardium (Section 18.1.5).

In all the domestic species except apparently the horse, the **intermediate artery** (ramus intermedius of the left coronary artery), and the **intermediate vein** (ramus intermedius of the great coronary vein) descend on the caudal border of the left ventricle (Simoens, 1992, pp. 242, 338).

18.1.5 *Left ventricle and interventricular septum: arterial supply*

The myocardium of the left ventricle and interventricular septum together provide the main pump of the postnatal heart, driving blood over the large distances and high resistances that characterize the systemic circulation (Section 12.4.3). The arterial supply of these two great masses of myocardium is therefore of particular functional importance.

In mammals in general (including man), regardless of interspecific variations, the *main supply* of blood to the myocardium of the left ventricle and interventricular septum is always from the **left** coronary artery. Indeed in some species (e.g. dog and ruminants) the left coronary artery is the *sole* supplier.

18.1.6 *Extent of distribution of left and right coronary arteries*

In the **horse** and **pig** (Fig. 18.2A) the **left coronary artery** supplies (1) most, *but not all*, of the interventricular septum, (2) *most*, but not all, of the left ventricular myocardium, and (3) only a *small part* of the right ven-

tricular myocardium. The **right coronary artery**, which in these species gives rise to the *right interventricular artery*, supplies (1) part of the interventricular septum, (2) regions of the left ventricular myocardium adjoining the right interventricular groove, and (3) most of the right ventricular myocardium. Thus in the horse and pig, both of the coronary arteries contribute more or less substantially to the supply of the septal and ventricular myocardium. This is known as a **bilateral type of coronary supply** (Schummer *et al.*, 1981, p. 39). The right coronary artery is relatively better developed in these species, being a similar-sized vessel if not slightly bigger than the left coronary artery.

In the **dog** and **ruminants** (Fig. 18.2B) the **left coronary artery** supplies (1) the *whole* of the massive interventricular septum; (2) *all* of the left ventricular myocardium; and (3) by means of its *left* and *right* interventricular arteries, those *regions* of the *right* ventricular myocardium that adjoin the left and right interventricular grooves. The ventricular distribution of the **right coronary artery** is restricted to the *remainder* of the right ventricular myocardium. Thus in the dog and ruminants the left coronary artery, through forming not only the left interventricular artery but also the right, has a very much greater myocardial distribution than the right. This is known as a *left coronary type of supply* (Schummer *et al.*, 1981, p. 39). In these species, the left coronary artery is anatomically an appreciably larger vessel than the right, and carries about 80% of the total coronary arterial flow (Smith and Hamlin, 1977, p. 140).

As Fig. 18.2 shows, in **both** types of supply, the **total area** of myocardium supplied by the left coronary artery is larger than that supplied by the right coronary artery; this is because the walls of the left ventricle and interventricular septum are so much thicker than those of the right ventricle. In other words, the *volume* of myocardium supplied by the **left** coronary is *always* greater than that supplied by the right coronary artery.

In the **cat** 50% of specimens have the left coronary type of supply, 30% have the bilateral type of supply, and about 12% have two right interventricular arteries one from the left and the other from the right coronary artery (Schummer *et al.*, 1981, p. 48).

In **man** (Williams *et al.*, 1989, pp. 728, 731) and **other primates** (Smith and Hamlin, 1977, p. 140) the right coronary artery is relatively well developed. The commonest pattern in man is the bilateral type, similar to that of the horse and pig. The right coronary artery in man then forms the (homologue of the) right interventricular artery. In human cardiology this is termed 'right dominance'. Quite often, however, the left coronary artery forms this vessel, as in the dog and ruminants, giving 'left dominance'. In 'balanced dominance' both the left and right coronary arteries contribute homologues of the right interventricular artery. These

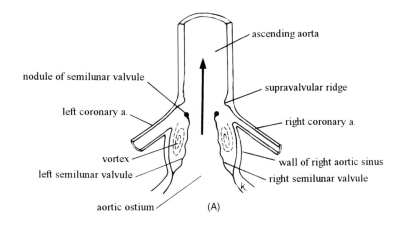

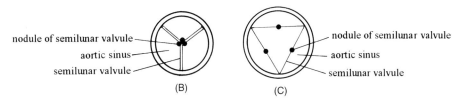

Fig. 18.1 Diagrams of the aortic valve.

A. **Longitudinal section of the aortic valve of the dog during the ejection phase of ventricular systole to show the origin of the coronary arteries.** Immediately peripheral to the aortic ostium (the opening of the aorta from the left ventricle) the aorta expands into the aortic bulb. The aortic bulb is formed by three bulges, the left, right, and septal aortic sinuses, bounded respectively by the left, right, and septal semilunar valvules (cusps) of the aortic valve.

The left coronary artery arises from the left aortic sinus, and the right coronary artery from the right aortic sinus. The left artery is substantially larger than the right in the dog and ruminants, but the right is similar in size or larger in the pig and horse. The angle of origin of the coronary arteries from the aorta (somewhat exaggerated in the diagram) is against the direction of systolic blood flow (arrow).

The aortic wall is thickened just peripheral to the openings of the coronary arteries, forming the supravalvular ridge. The semilunar valvules of the aortic valve extend almost to the openings of the coronary arteries. However, during ventricular systole vortices form in the three aortic sinuses; these hold the valvules away from the aortic wall and leave the entrance to the coronary arteries uncovered.

B. **Semidiagrammatic view of the aortic (or pulmonary) valve when closed during ventricular diastole, as seen from inside the vessel immediately peripheral to the aortic valve.** The three valvules are tightly apposed in a triradiate form, their three nodules sealing the centre of the aperture.

C. **Semidiagrammatic view of the aortic (or pulmonary) valve when open during the ejection phase of ventricular systole, as seen from inside the vessel immediately peripheral to the aortic valve.** The elasticity of the wall allows the aorta to expand during ejection. The resulting enlargement of its diameter has increased the circumference of the aorta at the free borders of the semilunar valvules. The increased circumference draws taut the free borders of the valvules, making the lumen of the valve triangular in shape.

three patterns resemble the three variants that occur in the cat. Williams *et al.* (1989, p. 731) emphasized, however, that the concept of 'dominance' is misleading, because in the human heart the **left** coronary artery almost always supplies **a greater volume of tissue than the right** – as was pointed out above for the domestic species.

18.1.7 *Nomenclature*

The left interventricular artery is strictly known as the **paraconal** interventricular artery (ramus interventricularis paraconalis), and the right as the **subsinuosal** interventricular artery (ramus interventricularis subsinuosus).

The fourth edition of the NAV (1994), as expressed by Schaller *et al.* (1992, p. 242) applies the term '**circumflex ramus**' to the 'continuation of A. coronaria sinistra into the left and caudal parts of the sulcus coronarius', but not to the similar continuation of the A. coronaria dextra into the **right** part of the sulcus coronarius; this means that the term circumflex ramus of the right coronary artery has officially lapsed. However, the monograph by Schummer *et al.* (1981, p. 39), which has long been an authority on the circulatory anatomy of the domestic mammals, retains 'right circumflex ramus'. Since it expresses one of the basic components of the arteries of the heart, the term is again retained here, though modified to right circumflex 'artery'.

The NAV (1994) applies the term 'artery' to the left and right coronary arteries only. All the components and branches of these two trunks are referred to as 'rami', i.e.

interventricular, circumflex, septal, and intermediate rami.

The NAV (1994) and NA (1989) do not name the individual aortic sinuses, and this creates difficulties when describing the origins of the left and right coronary arteries from the aorta. Following Gabella (1996), the three sinuses have been named here according to their semilunar valvules, i.e. left, right, and septal aortic sinuses (Figs 18.1A, 20.2).

18.2 Anatomical origin of the coronary arteries from the aorta

The two coronary arteries, left and right, are the first branches of the aorta. They arise from the

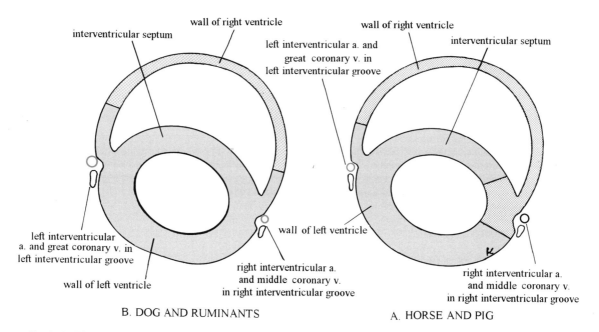

Fig. 18.2 Diagrammatic dorsal views of horizontal sections through the ventricles of A the horse and pig, and B the dog and ruminants, to summarize the distribution of the left and right coronary arteries. The sections are cut just ventral to the coronary groove. The green area is supplied by branches of the left coronary artery (green rings) and the grey area by branches of the right coronary artery (black ring).

In A (the horse and pig) the left coronary artery supplies most of the interventricular septum and left ventricular myocardium. However, in these species the right coronary artery has a relatively large myocardial distribution, because it forms the right interventricular artery. Thus the right coronary artery shares the supply of the interventricular septum, and also supplies a region of the right aspect of the left ventricle, i.e. the region adjoining the right interventricular groove. This is known as a bilateral type of coronary supply. Nevertheless the left coronary still supplies a somewhat greater volume of myocardium than the right coronary artery.

In B (the dog and ruminants) the left coronary artery supplies the whole of the interventricular septum and left ventricle. Because the left coronary artery in these species forms the right interventricular artery, it also supplies the region of the right ventricle adjoining the right interventricular groove. Thus in the dog and ruminants the left coronary artery supplies a much greater volume of myocardium than the right coronary artery. This is known as a left coronary type of supply (Schummer *et al.*, 1981, p. 39).

aortic bulb. This is the root of the aorta, and is the site of the **aortic valve** (Section 20.10). The wall of the aorta is slightly expanded at the aortic bulb by three bulges known as the three **aortic sinuses** (Figs 18.1A, 20.2). The left coronary artery opens from the left aortic sinus (Fig. 20.5), and the right coronary artery from the right aortic sinus (Fig. 18.1A).

Since the aortic bulb is sited in the very centre of the base of the heart, the left and right coronary arteries have at first to pass laterally (Fig. 20.2) beneath the left and right **auricles** respectively (Figs 17.5, 20.1) to reach the left and right parts of the coronary groove.

The **left coronary artery** then divides into the **left circumflex artery** and the **left interventricular artery** (Fig. 20.1). The **right coronary artery** goes round the right side of the heart as the **right circumflex artery** (Fig. 17.5) and (in some species, Section 18.1) ends as the **right interventricular artery**.

The left and right coronary arteries arise, somewhat unusually for large arteries, at a slightly reverse angle in relation to the direction of aortic blood flow during the ejection phase of the cardiac cycle (Fig. 18.1). In the dissection room, the openings of the coronary arteries can be examined on the walls of their two aortic sinuses (sinus aortae): could the semilunar valvules (cusps) of the aortic valve cover the openings of the two coronary arteries while blood is being ejected through the aorta during ventricular systole, thus obstructing the entry of blood into the coronary arteries? This idea was proposed by Thebesius in the early eighteenth century (Williams *et al.*, 1989, p. 727). In the canine heart (personal observations) the valvules can almost be pulled over the arterial openings, and in man (Williams *et al.*, 1989, p. 727) the related valvule (valvula semilunaris dextra) does extend over the right coronary opening in about 10%, and over the left coronary opening in about 15% of specimens.

However, for two reasons the possibility that the valvules could cover the openings of the coronary arteries has no significant functional effect on the entry of blood into the coronary arteries. Firstly, the walls of the aortic sinuses are strongly fibrous at the very beginning of the aorta, i.e. at the **aortic ostium** (ostium aortae), and therefore almost undilatable there. But the walls become progressively more elastic as the aortic bulb (bulbus aortae) transforms into the ascending aorta (aorta ascendens); this increasing elasticity allows the aorta to expand in response to the increase in pressure during the ejection phase of ventricular systole (Fig. 18.1C). At the level of the free edges of the semilunar valvules, the radius of the aortic bulb therefore increases by about

16% during the ejection phase (Williams *et al.*, 1989, p. 712; this enlarges the circumference of this part of the aorta during ejection, thus drawing the three valvules taut and making the valvular lumen triangular (Fig. 18.1C). Therefore, in the living heart during the ejection phase of ventricular systole, the semilunar valvules cannot flatten themselves over the openings into the coronary arteries. Secondly, during the ejection phase of ventricular systole, blood enters the aortic sinuses and forms vortices that help to hold the valvules away from the aortic wall (Williams *et al.*, 1989, p. 712), as in Fig. 18.1A.

18.3   Microcirculation of the heart

The circumflex and interventricular arteries are visible on the surface of the heart, lying deep to the epicardium and more or less embedded in fat depending on nutrition and species. The ventricular, septal, and atrial branches arise approximately at right angles from the circumflex and interventricular arteries, and then immediately penetrate the myocardium.

Within the myocardium, the arteries branch extensively, forming an exceptionally dense **microcirculation** of arterioles and capillaries. The most vascular part of the myocardium is its innermost layer, adjacent to the endocardium. Here, there is a particularly extensive plexus of arterioles and capillaries (subendocardial plexus).

In the myocardium generally, there is at least one capillary for each cardiac muscle cell (Fig. 18.3), and many cells are in contact with two or three capillaries. The capillaries run parallel with the cells. At rest only about half of the capillaries are open. Additional capillaries are *recruited* if the metabolic rate increases, as during exercise.

The ventricular myocardium accounts for about 3–5% of the cardiac output at rest, although the heart forms only about 0.6% of the total body mass (Section 20.4). The flow goes up about 10-fold during severe exercise.

The **total blood flow through the ventricular myocardium** in the pony accounts for about 3% of the cardiac output at rest and about 4% during maximum exertion (Evans, 1994, p. 140). In the dog (Smith and Hamlin, 1977, p. 140) the resting value is 4–5%, with a 10-fold increase in flow volume during severe exertion.

The **arterial vasculature** of the human heart can be resolved into three systems (Guyton, 1986, p. 296). (1)

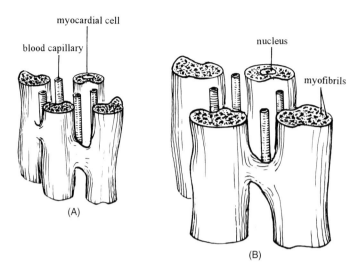

Fig. 18.3 Diagram showing the spatial and numerical relationships between cardiac muscle cells and their blood capillaries. The capillaries lie in the endomysial connective tissue, between and essentially parallel to the cardiac muscle cells. Cardiac muscle cells (and hence also the cardiac muscle fibres that they form) are essentially cylindrical, but since they give rise to branches that anastomose with other cardiac muscle cells (Fig. 21.1), their overall appearance is of irregular anastomosing cylinders. The irregular speckles on the transected surfaces of the cells are myofibrils, visible in histological sections.

A. **Normal adult myocardium.** The ratio of capillaries to cardiac muscle cells is 1 : 1.

B. **Hypertrophied myocardium.** The ratio of capillaries to cardiac muscle cells remains 1 : 1, but the volume of the cardiac muscle cells is greatly increased when hypertrophied; therefore each capillary must now deliver oxygen to more tissue over greater distances. This creates a serious complication in cardiac diseases such as aortic regurgitation in which the myocardium becomes extremely hypertrophied. In trained endurance athletes the myocardium is again hypertrophied, but to a much lesser extent so that the capillaries are fully able to supply their **cardiac muscle** cells. (After Wearn, 1940.)

The **subepicardial** or **extramural system** consists of the circumflex and interventricular arteries. These are large 'distributing arteries' (Section 12.5), subepicardial in position, that distribute the blood to the various components of the heart. (2) The **intramuscular** or **intramural system** is formed by the branches of the subepicardial arteries. These branches supply arterioles and capillaries that form a middle vascular zone of the myocardium. These components of the microcirculation are contained within the **endomysium** (Section 21.3). (3) The **subendocardial system** is a plexus of arterioles and arterial capillaries immediately beneath the endocardium, and is more extensive than the intramuscular system. The existence of these three systems seems not to have been described in domestic mammals. However, it is likely that similar broad distinctions exist. For instance, experimental observations reported by Schaper *et al.* (1988) have shown that a 'subendocardial plexus' is the source of proliferation of collaterals in the dog and pig as well as in man, after chronic coronary occlusion.

In the pig and to some extent in the carnivores and sheep, but not in the ox and horse, the **subepicardial vessels** (deep to the epicardium) are in some places bridged by thin strips of myocardial tissue (Schummer *et al.*, 1981, p. 38).

The richness of the **capillary networks** surrounding cardiac muscle cells is said to be unsurpassed by any other tissue in the body (Hoff, 1949, p. 682). Rival claims, however, are made for the synaptic zones of association areas in the central nervous system, for the alveolar walls in the lung (Section 6.7.4), and for the carotid body (Section 19.7.2). Probably the density of the capillaries in the lung alveoli is in fact unexcelled, but the capillaries in the alveolar wall are essentially in only two dimensions, whereas those of the heart, brain tissue, and carotid body are in three dimensions.

The **capillary density** is about 3300 capillaries per square millimetre in the normal human myocardium, but there are only 400 capillaries in the same area of skeletal muscle (Feigl, 1974, p. 248). Both cardiac and skeletal muscle cells have about one capillary per cell, but the cross-sectional diameter of the cardiac cell is only about 17–20 µm, whereas that of the skeletal muscle cell is about 50 µm, and this accounts for the difference in capillary densities. The greater surface area of capillaries per unit area of myocardial tissue and a relatively greater capillary permeability, are estimated to render myocardial capillaries almost 15 times more effective than skeletal muscle capillaries in exchanging small molecules.

The **ratio of blood capillaries to each cardiac muscle cell** in man (van Citters, 1966, p. 691) is highest at birth (about 6:1); it decreases rapidly during early postnatal development and then more slowly, reaching 1:1 by about 10 years. The number of cardiac muscle cells is still increasing in the neonate, but in many species including man mitoses are scarce after about 2 weeks following parturition (Bishop and van Vleet, 1979). Thereafter, further myocardial enlargement is achieved almost solely by hypertrophy of the cardiac muscle cells (Section 21.1.2).

It is generally assumed that, in man, the 1:1 ratio remains unchanged from adolescence to advanced old age. It is also believed that the ratio is held at 1:1 in **cardiac hypertrophy** (Fig. 18.3B), induced either by **athletic training** or by **disease** involving ventricular hypertension (Section 20.4). Since the volume of the individual cardiac muscle cells then increases, each capillary is now required to supply more tissue over longer distances; this is not a problem in the athletic heart, but by critically impairing the rate of oxygen delivery (Jokl and Jokl, 1977) it becomes a serious adverse factor in cardiac diseases involving massive myocardial hypertrophy, for example **aortic stenosis** (Section 15.10) or **aortic regurgitation**.

Morphometric studies by Mall *et al.* (1987), Mattfeldt *et al.* (1985), and Mattfeldt and Mall (1987) in the rat have reinforced these general findings on the ratio of capillaries to cardiac muscle cells. They also confirmed an earlier idea that an increase in the proportion of capillaries to cardiac muscle cells can be induced by **mild exercise**, the increase being caused by the growth of new capillaries. Furthermore they found an increase during **normal growth** of the immature animal. These authors conclude that changes in the ratio of capillaries to muscle cells are not quite such a rare event as was hitherto supposed.

It might be wondered whether the hypertrophy of cardiac muscle cells that occurs in **endurance athletes**, human and other mammals, might lead to deficient oxygenation during extreme exertion because of the fixed 1:1 ratio of capillaries to cardiac muscle cells.

The proposition that heart strain could result from maximal violent exercise was entertainingly reviewed by Jokl and Jokl (1976). Probably inspired by the unfortunate demise of the marathon runner who dropped dead in the market square of Athens in 490 BC after delivering the news of the Athenian victory over the Persians, the concept of '**athlete's heart**' was widely accepted by the medical profession even until the 1930s. Various medical authorities in the last two decades of the nineteenth century expounded 'the dangers to the heart of organized games in schools', the occurrence of 'heart strain from exercise', and 'the vulnerability of the heart of young boys'. A letter to a London newspaper in 1901 by four eminent doctors condemned all runs over 1 mile by high school boys. Girls were never mentioned. It was said that a horse should 'sweat', a man should 'perspire', but a lady should do no more than 'glow'. More than fifty papers were published in biomedical journals between 1910 and 1912, mostly containing warnings that exercise can cause heart disease. The turning point came in 1935 when one medical author analysed the medical records of 16 000 school boys and another reviewed the entire literature on the heart and sport in England. No clinical or post-mortem evidence was uncovered to show that exercise can cause heart disease. It is now known that the hearts of young athletes, particularly girls, have a remarkable ability to adapt to strenuous exercise.

Some fatal heart attacks do, of course, occur in young people during or after strenuous exercise. In about half of them evidence of pre-existing pathological change has been obtained. Routine medical examination of athletes is imperative. Jokl and Jokl (1977) concluded that 'the **normal** heart is invulnerable to exercise'.

Although **myocardial hypertrophy** occurs in endurance athletes (Section 20.4), the degree of hypertrophy is much less than in, for example, aortic regurgitation where the mass of the left ventricle increases four- or fivefold (Guyton, 1986, p. 319). Such a pathological heart may weigh more than 1000 g, whereas the athlete's heart never exceeds 500 g (Jokl and Jokl, 1977). Evidently the athletic hypertrophy, unlike the pathological hypertrophy, never oversteps the limitations in oxygen delivery imposed by the 1:1 ratio of capillaries to cardiac muscle cells.

Those who habitually lie down until the urge to take exercise has passed off might like to know that they probably have a small heart. Doubtless health freaks would labelled this as a 'couch potato's heart'.

18.4 Flow in the coronary arteries during systole and diastole

The viability of the myocardium depends mainly on the optimal perfusion of the **subendocardial arterial plexus**, since this is the most vascular zone of the myocardium (Section 18.3).

The left and right coronary arteries arise from the root of the aorta, and therefore the pressure within them is close to aortic pressure. This provides good perfusion of the myocardium of the **atria** and **right ventricle** during ventricular systole. In the left ventricle, however, pressure relationships affect perfusion.

The **myocardium** of the **left ventricle** squeezes the blood in its lumen in order to achieve ejection pressure. In so doing, it simultaneously squeezes its own vasculature (Feigl, 1974, p. 250). This almost completely closes the subendocardial arterial plexus, causing its blood flow to fall almost to zero. Consequently the arterial flow in the myocardium of the left ventricle falls to a low level during ventricular systole. On the other hand, during ventricular diastole the left ventricular myocardium relaxes. This releases the compression of its vasculature, and thus allows blood to flow rapidly through the left ventricular myocardium during the whole of ventricular **diastole**. This differs from all other arterial beds throughout the body. The reverse angle of the left coronary artery at its origin from the aorta may favour its filling during ventricular diastole.

During ventricular systole, a **pressure gradient** develops within the tissue of the **ventricular myocardium** (Guyton, 1986, p. 296). The muscle next to the endocardium squeezes the blood in the intraventricular cavity of the heart. The muscle in the middle layer of the myocardium also applies pressure to the blood in the cavity, but can only do so by simultaneously squeezing the muscle adjacent to the endocardium. The muscle in the outermost layer of the myocardium applies further pressure to the blood in the cavity, and at the same time squeezes the muscle in the middle and subendocardial layers. The pressure in the outermost (subepicardial) layer of the myocardium is not much greater than atmospheric; however, the pressure in the subendocardial layer of myocardium is only slightly less than the pressure in the intraventricular cavity (Guyton, 1986, p. 296), or is even slightly greater than the pressure in the cavity (Feigl, 1974, p. 250). Therefore, the arterioles and capillaries in the **subendocardial arterial plexus** of the **left ventricle** are almost closed or are actually shut during ventricular systole.

In the dog (and supposedly also in man; Guyton, 1986, p. 295), the volume of blood flowing through the left coronary artery and thence through the **myocardium of the left ventricle** falls to zero during the **isovolumetric phase** of ventricular systole (van Citters, 1966, p. 693). During the **onset of ejection** a significant volume of flow resumes in the left ventricular myocardium. However, in the resting animal the **mean volume of flow** in the left ventricular myocardium throughout ventricular systole is usually less than 25% of that during ventricular diastole (van Citters, 1966, p. 694).

The review by van Citters (1966, p. 694) showed that, since the **right ventricular pressure** is much lower than the left, the intramural pressure is never great enough to close down the myocardial vasculature in the right ventricle, and that the relationship of flow to systole and diastole in the **right coronary artery** is the same as in any other artery. But according to Guyton (1976, p. 296), the flow in the capillaries of the right ventricle does undergo

phasic changes in relation to the cardiac cycle that are similar to those in the left ventricle, though less marked.

Although it is well known that flow in the left coronary artery does decrease markedly during ventricular systole, the mechanism is not quite as clear as the above account suggests (Hoffman, 1995). The pressure differences in the subendocardial and subepicardial vessels should indeed obstruct subendocardial flow and permit subepicardial flow. However, this hypothesis foundered when it was discovered that little if any forward systolic flow occurs in *small distal epicardial arteries*. Other theories have been advanced (e.g. a vascular elastance theory), but it is evident that myocardial flow is considerably more complicated than was once believed.

18.5 Metabolic regulation of coronary blood flow

About 50% of the myocardial capillaries are open under normal resting conditions. Whenever the energetic cost of contraction increases, the rate of coronary blood flow simultaneously goes up. The increase in flow is accomplished by the dilation of capillaries that are already open, and by the opening of closed capillaries, i.e. **capillary recruitment**. Conversely the rate of coronary flow immediately decreases when myocardial activity decreases. How are these instant local adjustments achieved?

The mechanism is essentially the same as in tissues generally throughout the body, and skeletal muscle in particular. The smooth muscle in the arteries and arterioles of the resting heart is maintained in a state of **basal tone** (Section 13.1): an inhibition of this tone induces vasodilation, and an increase in tone causes vasoconstriction. In the myocardium and tissues generally, local **metabolic regulation** (Section 13.2.1) is mainly responsible for this adjustment of basal tone of arterial vasculature. Neural and hormonal factors play only a minor role.

The coronary circulation is particularly sensitive to **myocardial oxygen tension**, and therefore the regulation of coronary blood flow is dominated by the demand for oxygen. The oxygen concentration in the myocardium falls if the oxygen consumption of the myocardium rises: therefore an increase in myocardial oxygen consumption induces an immediate coronary vasodilation, and vice versa. Alternatively, a decrease in the oxygen supply to cardiac muscle cells, arising for example from a fall in arterial pressure, also induces an immediate coronary vasodilation. This automatic adjustment of coronary blood flow (and hence cardiac muscle oxygen supply) in order to immediately match the oxygen demands of the myocardium, is a basic principle of cardiac physiology and an example of **autoregulation**. It operates entirely effectively, regardless of whether the cardiac muscle innervation is eliminated or intact.

As in the arterial vasculature of tissues generally (Section 13.2.1), the response of the smooth muscle of the cardiac muscle vasculature to changing levels of oxygen may be either direct or indirect. In a **direct response** a local deficiency of oxygen would act directly on the smooth muscle in the walls of the cardiac muscle arterial vasculature, thus weakening its contraction and passively inducing vasodilation. In the **indirect response** the falling oxygen tension in the cardiac muscle vessels would induce the release of a **vasodilator substance** (a mediator); this substance would inhibit the smooth muscle of the cardiac muscle arterial vasculature, thus causing cardiac muscle vasodilation. It is not known whether the direct or the indirect mechanism prevails in the heart.

The myocardium of the **resting** heart removes 65–70% of the oxygen from its arterial blood (Guyton, 1986, p. 296), giving a P_{O_2} of coronary venous blood of only about 20 mmHg (2.7 kPa). This is the highest normal oxygen utilization coefficient in all body tissues (Smith and Hamlyn, 1977, p. 140), yielding the lowest venous P_{O_2} in the resting body (Feigl, 1974, p. 252). (In typical tissues, the capillary blood unloads only about 26% of its oxygen, though the blood in skeletal muscle in heavy exercise yields about 84% of its oxygen (Section 14.3.2). Even in the **resting** heart, not much oxygen remains after the blood has gone through the myocardium, and therefore any substantial increase in oxygen demand caused by an increase in cardiac muscle activity can only be met by a corresponding increase in coronary blood flow (Guyton, 1986, p. 296). During severe exercise, the coronary blood flow increases more than 10-fold in the dog (Smith and Hamlin, 1977, p. 140), and 3–4-fold in man (Guyton, 1986, p. 295).

In the **indirect response** to a local fall in the cardiac muscle oxygen level, it is very likely that more than one, and possibly several, mediators are involved in the subsequent adjustment of blood flow (Gewirtz, 1991). Possible mediators include carbon dioxide, hydrogen ions, potassium ions, bradykinin, and perhaps prostaglandins

(Guyton, 1986, p. 297), but the coronary circulation is not particularly sensitive to carbon dioxide levels and lactic acid (Feigl, 1974, p. 252). Two substances appear to have the greatest potential for vasodilation of the coronary arterial vasculature; these are adenosine and nitric oxide (Section 13.2.1).

If the cardiac muscle oxygen supply falls, much of the ATP in the cardiac muscle cells is degraded to **adenosine** and released into the cardiac muscle interstitial fluid. There the adenosine inhibits the tone of the smooth muscle in the adjacent coronary arterial vasculature thus causing vasodilation, and is then immediately destroyed (Guyton, 1986, p. 296). The formation of cardiac muscle adenosine increases in response to either a decrease in the oxygen supply or an increase in cardiac oxygen consumption (Belardinelli and Shryock, 1992).

Nitric oxide (or endothelium-derived relaxing factor; Section 13.6) is synthesized from L-arginine in vascular endothelial cells by the enzyme nitric oxide synthase. Nitric oxide inhibits the tone of the adjacent vascular smooth muscle and is a powerful vasodilator. Dikranian et al. (1994) found nitric oxide synthase in nearly all the endothelial cells of the coronary artery in the rat, co-localized with several vasoactive peptides, thus indicating that nitric oxide has an important role in the regulation of coronary blood flow. Although the release of nitric oxide from endothelial cells is generally activated by the shearing stress of blood passing over the endothelium (Section 13.6), and there is evidence for this in the coronary circulation (see Dikranian et al., 1994), metabolic factors are also effective stimuli for release (Section 13.6).

Both the direct and the indirect mechanism of metabolic regulation have **objections** (Guyton, 1986, p. 297). Only minute quantities of oxygen are needed by the smooth muscle of the coronary arterial vasculature to sustain full contraction, and this raises doubts about the direct mechanism. The indirect mechanism is questioned by the observation that neutralization of metabolic mediators, including adenosine, does not prevent coronary vasodilation in response to increased cardiac muscle activity; also the vasodilator response seems able to outlast the reserves of adenosine.

18.6   Neural regulation of coronary blood flow

The coronary arterial vasculature possesses a quite elaborate autonomic vasomotor nerve supply. This innervation is capable of modifying coronary blood flow, but any such changes are largely overruled by the process of metabolic regulation outlined in Section 18.5.

Vasoconstriction is mediated by sympathetic adrenergic fibres acting on α-adrenoreceptors

(Section 13.3.2). **Vasodilation** is effected by two varieties of vasomotor fibre: (1) sympathetic adrenergic fibres acting on β_2-adrenoreceptors (Section 13.3.2), and (2) parasympathetic cholinergic fibres (Section 3.11.3).

It will be recalled that there are two varieties of β-adrenoreceptors (Section 2.33.1). **Beta$_1$-adrenoreceptors** excite cardiac muscle cells, increasing the rate and force of cardiac contraction; **β_2-adrenoreceptors** inhibit vascular smooth muscle. Stimulation of the sympathetic nerves to the heart excites both β_1- and β_2-adrenoreceptors. The result is an increase in coronary blood flow. This appears to indicate that the sympathetic nerve supply to the coronary arterial vasculature is essentially vasodilator, which would be different in principle from the usual effect of sympathetic stimulation of blood vessels. However, when the β_1-adrenoreceptors in the myocardium are stimulated, the activity of the myocardium is stimulated; this creates a fall in myocardial oxygen concentration, which in turn activates the **metabolic regulation** of the coronary vasculature (Section 18.5) and induces strong coronary vasodilation. If the β_1-adrenoreceptors are first blocked by appropriate drugs, sympathetic stimulation results consistently in vasoconstriction as in circulatory systems generally (Scott, 1986, p. 75).

In the **subepicardial arteries** α-adrenoreceptors predominate, but in the **myocardial arterial vasculature** β_2-adrenoreceptors are in the majority. The broad effect of sympathetic stimulation of vasomotor pathways to the coronary arterial system could therefore be either vasoconstriction (alpha mediated) or vasodilation (beta$_2$ mediated), but the outcome is usually only **weak vasoconstriction** (Guyton, 1986, p. 298); this response can in turn be reversed by alpha blocking agents (Feigl, 1974, p. 257). As pointed out in Section 13.3.2, it is functionally advantageous that the coronary (and cerebral) circulations should be exempted from the massive sympathetic vasoconstrictor discharge that characterizes the sudden onset of **severe exercise** as in fight and flight.

The **parasympathetic vasomotor fibres** have a vasodilator action when stimulated, provided that the heart is electrically paced to prevent bradycardia (Feigl, 1974, p. 257). Their functional significance remains obscure. They may be important in **cardiac infarction** by inducing reflex vasodilation (Scott, 1986, p. 76).

18.7 Hormonal regulation of coronary blood flow

Noradrenaline causes coronary vasoconstriction, and **adrenaline** induces vasodilation.

The smooth muscle of the coronary arterial vasculature has both α- and β_2-adrenoreceptors. **Noradrenaline** acts on the α-adrenoreceptors to produce vasoconstriction. In principle, **adrenaline** can act on the α-adrenoreceptors to give vasoconstriction, or on the β_2-adrenoreceptors to induce vasodilation. However, in the heart the beta response predominates at all concentrations of adrenaline, so that adrenaline always evokes coronary vasodilation (Scott, 1986, p. 67).

18.8 Venous drainage of the heart

Most of the venous blood of the coronary circulation drains through atrial and ventricular veins into the **great coronary vein** and **coronary sinus**. The great coronary vein and coronary sinus lie in the coronary groove (Fig. 20.1; Section 20.6), the coronary sinus being simply a direct continuation of the great coronary vein (Fig. 17.5). The coronary sinus ends by opening into the right atrium, ventral to the opening of the caudal vena cava (Fig. 21.10).

The **small coronary veins** are numerous very small veins that open directly into all four chambers of the heart. Those that empty into the left atrium and left ventricle constitute a **right-to-left shunt** (venous-to-arterial shunt, or venous admixture) (Section 6.30.1), diluting oxygenated blood with venous blood; this has been directly observed endoscopically in the left ventricle of the rat, jets of dark venous blood being visible as they spurt into the bright red oxygenated blood. The bronchial circulation adds to this venous-to-arterial shunt (Section 17.5). Together, the small coronary veins and bronchial veins cause the left ventricular output to exceed the right by about 1 or 2%.

The atrial and ventricular tributaries of the **great coronary vein** (vena cordis magna) and **coronary sinus** (sinus coronarius) drain all of the heart, *except* the cranial two thirds of the right ventricle and relatively insignificant areas of atrial and ventricular myocardium that drain via the small coronary veins (venae cordis minimae). Since the coronary sinus drains such a large part of the heart, it is not surprising that it carries about 75% of the total coronary flow (Guyton, 1986, p. 295). As already stated (Section 18.5), the myocardium of the *resting* heart removes most of the oxygen from its arterial blood (Guyton, 1986, p. 296). Consequently the P_{O_2} of coronary venous blood is only about 20 mmHg (2.7 kPa), this being the lowest venous P_{O_2} in the resting body (Feigl, 1974, p. 252).

The cranial two thirds of the right ventricle are drained by the **right ventricular veins** (Fig. 17.5). These were known as right distal ventricular veins by Schummer *et al*. (1981, e.g. Fig. 39). The NAV (1994) now refers to them as the venae cordis dextrae. They sometimes unite into a single trunk lying in the right coronary groove (Schummer *et al*., 1981, p. 40), which is then a satellite of the right circumflex coronary artery.

The **great coronary vein** (vena cordis magna) begins by ascending the left (paraconal) interventricular sulcus as a satellite of the left interventricular coronary artery, and continues round the left coronary groove as the satellite of the left circumflex coronary artery (Fig. 20.1). The great coronary vein becomes the coronary sinus at the entry of the oblique vein of the left atrium in the horse and dog, and at the entry of the left vena azygos in the pig and ruminants (Schummer *et al*., 1981, p. 40).

The **coronary sinus** has three named tributaries. (1) The **intermediate coronary vein** (ramus intermedius) ascends the caudal aspect of the left ventricle accompanying the intermediate coronary artery (Figs 17.5, 20.1). (2) The **oblique vein of the left atrium** (vena obliqua atrii sinistri) (Fig. 17.5) is the small remnant of the embryonic left common cardinal vein. Finally, as the coronary sinus connects with the right atrium, it receives (3) the large **middle coronary vein** (vena cordis media), which ascends the right (subsinuosal) interventricular groove as a satellite of the right interventricular coronary artery (Fig. 17.5). The **valve of the coronary sinus** (valvula sinus coronarii) is a semilunar fold at the orifice of the coronary sinus, but it may be indistinct or absent, especially in the horse (Simoens 1992, p. 238).

The **small coronary veins** (venae cordis minimae) were first described by that sharp-eyed eighteenth century anatomist, Thebesius, mentioned in Section 18.2, and have been known ever since as the **Thebesian veins**. Venous drainage via the small coronary veins into the left ventricle is slight, because of the unfavourable pressure gradients, but is relatively great into the right ventricle (Feigl, 1974, p. 249). According to Williams *et al*. (1989, p. 703) these veins are most numerous on the interventricular septum in man, but Schummer *et al*. (1981, p. 40) reported the greatest numbers on the atrial walls and fewer on the ventricular walls. Since some of the small coronary veins open directly into the ventricles it has been suggested that, in coronary arterial obstruction, they might carry a retrograde flow of blood from the ventricular lumen to the myocardium.

Extensive anastomoses have been found at all levels of the venous circulation of the heart, amounting to a veritable venous plexus (Williams *et al*., 1989, p. 793). These anastomoses connect adjacent veins, and form connections between the tributaries of the coronary sinus and the tributaries of the right ventricular veins. The coronary veins also connect with **extracardiac vessels**, especially the vasa vasorum of the great vessels arising from the heart.

The nomenclature of the veins of the heart presents difficulties in ordinary usage, such as teaching. We have 'coronary' arteries and a 'coronary' sinus, and talk freely about the 'coronary' circulation and 'coronary' thrombosis, etc., but we lack 'coronary' veins. Instead, the veins are termed 'venae cordis', i.e. 'veins of the heart'. This is a perfectly logical term, but inconveniently long. The difficulty could be overcome by converting 'of the heart' into an adjective, the nearest translation presumably being 'cardiac'. If so, we would then have 'cardiac veins'. That would give us coronary arteries, coronary sinus, and coronary circulation, but cardiac veins. For simplicity, the account here has adopted 'coronary' throughout, which may be an inferior translation but has the advantage of unifying all elements under the same term – *coronary* arteries, *coronary* veins, *coronary* sinus, *coronary* circulation, and *coronary* disorders.

18.9 Ischaemic heart disease: coronary collateral circulation

Ischaemic heart disease is caused by insufficient coronary blood flow. In Western societies it is the most common cause of death in **man**. About 35% of the population die of it in the USA, and the UK has one of the highest incidences in the world.

In the **domestic mammals**, ischaemic heart disease is not an important problem. However, this is not because typical arterial lesions do not occur in domestic mammals. The whole range of degenerative arterial changes that are found in man are also encountered in domestic mammals, but they seldom have significant clinical effects.

The impairment of coronary blood flow in **man** is characterized by deposits of **lipids** (cholesterol) and aggregations of smooth muscle cells, fibroblasts, and macrophages within the **intima** of the coronary arterial vasculature. These deposits and aggregations form **plaques** that greatly thicken the intima, thus partly or completely obstructing the vascular lumen (Fig. 18.4). Also a plaque tends to break through the luminal surface of the intima (Fig. 18.4) and this initiates the formation of a **thrombus**. (A 'thrombus' forms *inside* an intact blood vessel, whereas a 'blood clot' *seals the wall* of a blood vessel after injury.) The thrombus adds to the occlusion of the vessel, or breaks off to form an **embolus** that plugs a more distal arterial branch. Similar plaques of smooth muscle cells and fibroblasts in the intima (arterio-

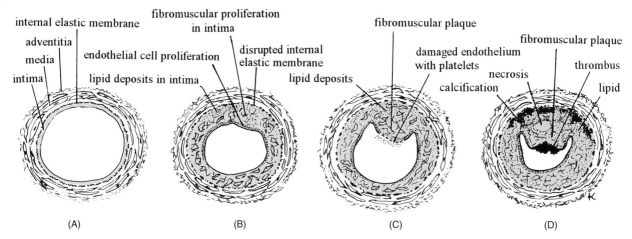

Fig. 18.4   Diagrams showing consecutive stages in the development of an atheromatous plaque in a coronary arteriole in man.

A. **Normal arteriole.** The intima (green) is very thin.

B. **Beginning of plaque formation.** Fragmentation of the internal elastic membrane allows smooth muscle cells from the media to invade the intima. The endothelial cells proliferate. The intima (green) is thickened, reducing the lumen. Lipid (especially cholesterol) begins to be deposited in the intima, at its junction with the media.

C. **Platelets adhere to the plaque.** The endothelium covering the plaque becomes defective, and attracts platelets which attach to the endothelial surface. Deposition of lipids extends throughout the much swollen intima.

D. **Formation of blood clot.** The plaque breaks through the endothelium, fibrin is deposited, blood cells are trapped, and a clot is formed. Areas of necrosis and calcium deposits appear in the plaque. The swollen plaque has largely occluded the lumen.

sclerosis) commonly occur in the coronary arterial vasculature in **dogs**, their frequency increases with age, but is of uncertain clinical importance. Lipid deposits and thrombi are not a significant feature in this species.

In principle, a myocardial zone supplied by an occluded artery experiences **ischaemia** (deficient blood supply). The cardiac muscle cells supplied by that artery can then only contract weakly, or they may die. For survival, the affected zone of myocardium must have an effective collateral circulation.

The presence of a **collateral circulation** (Section 12.18) depends initially on whether or not an artery is an **end-artery**: true end-arteries have no anastomoses whatsoever with any other arteries, and can therefore have no collateral circulation at all. In fact, in **man** the branches of the coronary arterial tree are not true end-arteries but they are **functional end-arteries** (Section 12.19). This means that they *do* have anastomoses at capillary and arteriolar levels (i.e. in the microcirculation). In man this pre-existing collateral circulation immediately dilates in response to the falling oxy-

gen concentration (Section 18.5); but it is unable to sustain the intense metabolic activity of the cardiac muscle cells at normal levels during the first few days after *sudden* occlusion of a coronary arterial vessel. The result may be fatal. However, if coronary occlusion in man is *gradual in onset* rather than abrupt, the collateral circulation may build up by the progressive formation of new arterioles and capillaries, thus protecting the affected area of myocardium and restoring or even maintaining its blood flow at normal levels.

Among the domestic mammals, the **dog** has a much better (pre-existing) coronary collateral circulation than man. In the dog it rapidly provides a highly effective blood flow if there is experimental coronary occlusion. The **pig** has virtually no anatomically demonstrable pre-existing collateral coronary circulation.

To summarize, the build-up of a collateral circulation in the heart occurs in two stages. The first is the immediate dilation of any pre-existing collateral circulation, though in man this is often not fully effective. The second is the progressive proliferation, during the subsequent weeks or months, of new capillaries and arterioles into a new collateral circulation, i.e. **angiogenesis** (Section 12.20).

18.9.1 *Pathological changes in the coronary arterial wall*

Arteriosclerosis is characterized (Kelly, 1989) by the proliferation in the **intima** of arteries and arterioles of **plaques** composed of fibrous tissue and of smooth muscle cells; the muscle cells invade from the media, following fragmentation of the internal elastic membrane. The fibrosis may be accompanied by degeneration with cystic clefts, and calcium may be precipitated, making the arterial wall very hard (hence the term 'sclerosis', meaning hardening). Affected arteries lose much of their distensibility. Also the plaques may have defective endothelium, causing thrombi to form. These changes are dangerously common in **man** (Guyton, 1986, p. 826).

Arteriosclerotic lesions (Kelly, 1989) are common in both the subepicardial and the myocardial (intramural) arterial vasculature of the **dog**. They lead to progressive stenosis, particularly in the intramural arteries of the left ventricle in the ageing dog, and result in focal ischaemic atrophy of cardiac muscle cells in the subendocardial zone. **Atheroma** (deposition of lipids in the plaques) is *not* a typical feature in this species, and **thrombosis** is rare. Arteriosclerotic lesions are of uncertain functional significance in the dog. Nevertheless, 'it is difficult not to suspect that severe and extensive coronary arteriosclerosis may compromise cardiac muscle function and cardiac reserve' (Kelly, 1989).

Perhaps the normal presence in the coronary vasculature of the dog of an exceptionally effective **pre-existing collateral circulation** (see below) may explain why these commonly occurring lesions have few if any clinically recognizable effects in this species. Kelly *et al.* (1992) noted reports, based on experimental fluid mechanics in tubes and observations on human patients and experimental animals, showing that a reduction in luminal diameter of at least 75% is required to compromise coronary blood flow significantly. Since the resistance to fluid flow is inversely proportional to the fourth power of the radius of a tube (Section 6.14), a reduction of the lumen by 75% would create a formidable impedance. However, an active pre-existing collateral circulation may be able to conceal the effects of even such severe obstruction.

The term **atherosclerosis** is given to the deposition of serum lipids (especially cholesterol) within the intima of the arterial or arteriolar wall and includes the tissue responses to these lipid deposits (Kelly, 1989, p. 80). In **man** (Fig. 18.4) these responses entail the initial fragmentation of the internal elastic membrane (Jokl, 1977), and the subsequent invasion of the intima by smooth muscle cells from the media; there is also proliferation of

endothelial cells (Guyton, 1986, p. 826), together with infiltration by macrophages, necrosis, fibrosis, and calcification (Kelly, 1989). The deposition of lipids tends to build up from the junction of the intima with the media (Jokl, 1977). The whole aggregation, i.e. lipids plus cells, greatly thickens the intima and constitutes an **atheromatous plaque** or **atheroma**. (The word atheroma is, surprisingly, derived from the Greek word for groats, i.e. crushed grain or the porridge made therefrom.) The plaque substantially diminishes the lumen of the vessel (Fig. 18.4) and may even close it completely. The endothelial cells covering the plaque become damaged (Fig. 18.4), allowing the plaque to break through to the lumen; platelets then bind to the exposed surface of the plaque, fibrin is deposited, blood cells become trapped, and a thrombus forms (Guyton, 1986, p. 299).

In **man** these atheromatous changes are extremely common in the coronary arterial vasculature, and are of great pathological and clinical importance. They do occur in the elderly **dog** though only rarely, in association with the hypothyroidism of thyroid atrophy (thyroxine being involved in the normal utilization of cholesterol); they are not clinically and pathologically important in this species (Kelly, 1989). They can be made to occur in the pig experimentally by a combination of a high cholesterol diet and endothelial damage (White *et al.*, 1988). Atherosclerosis may also be a factor in aortic rupture in turkeys, which is a serious cause of mortality in that species.

18.9.2 *Formative process of atherosclerosis*

Although arteriosclerosis and atherosclerosis are so very prevalent in man, the mechanisms by which they arise remain uncertain (Guyton, 1986, p. 826). Attention has turned away from the effects of excessive quantities of cholesterol in the blood and focused on events taking place in the **endothelium** and **intima**.

In both man (Schwartz, 1989) and the dog (Kelly, 1989), the lesions in the vascular walls are associated particularly with bifurcations, openings of side branches, and sites of curvature, all of these being places where blood flow is turbulent. The **endothelial cells** of blood vessels recognize the mechanical signals of **shear stress**, and respond by releasing a veritable array of biogenic agents (Section 13.6). These include vasodilator nitric oxide (which also has cytotoxic functions, e.g. against bacteria and tumour cells), peptide vasoconstrictors, and a prostacyclin (PGI_2) which may be involved in clotting mechanisms.

Platelets release various substances (Section 12.21.2), including prostaglandins, phospholipids that activate clotting, fibrin-stabilizing factor, and the mitogen platelet-derived growth factor (PDGF) that activates proliferation of smooth muscle. The adhesive glycoprotein receptors (glycoprotein Ib-IX and IIb–IIIa) on the platelet surface, and their binding to the von Willebrand factor (vWF) of platelets and of endothelial cells to cause **adhesion** and **aggregation** of platelets at the damaged vascular wall, are discussed in Section 12.21.2).

Although the turbulence in the blood flow at arterial divisions, branches, and curvatures is associated with the onset of endothelial damage, the adhesion and aggregation of platelets tends to occur immediately *downstream* from these sites. Here the shear stress in the blood stream is lower, thus making it easier for platelets to become attached to the vascular wall. Therefore it is at these points that atheromatous plaques are prone to form (Ross and McIntire, 1995).

Together, the endothelial cells and platelets produce a cocktail of agents involved in the development of atheromatous plaques (for review, see Schwartz *et al.*, 1989), the process being enhanced by an excess of cholesterol circulating in the blood (Guyton, 1986, p. 827).

18.9.3   *Development of collateral circulation in coronary arteries*

If a branch of a coronary artery of man is suddenly occluded in man (Guyton, 1986, p. 299), the pre-existing **collateral circulation**, such as it is, dilates within a few seconds, but the resulting flow is only about half that required to sustain the viability of the cardiac muscle cells. In the first hours the cardiac muscle cells may therefore outrun their oxygen supply. Some cells are then only able to contract weakly, others stop functioning altogether, and yet others may die (forming an **infarct**). Such ischaemic areas of the myocardium may induce **fibrillation** of the heart (Section 21.23.2), and this is a common cause of death after coronary occlusion. There is no further dilation of the collateral circulation for 8–24 hours. An increase in the collateral blood flow then resumes, doubling after 2 or 3 days and achieving a normal coronary flow in the previously ischaemic zone in about a month.

If the occlusion in man occurs slowly over a period of years, as may happen in **atherosclerosis**, the collateral circulation may develop simultaneously and prevent an acute coronary incident. With increasing age, however, the atherosclerosis may eventually overtake the collateral supply, or may even involve the collateral vasculature itself. If so, the cardiac output progressively declines, and may finally fall below survival levels.

It is generally agreed that **pre-existing collateral anastomoses** occur at all levels of the coronary arterial tree in man, i.e. subepicardial, myocardial, and subendocardial, but these anastomoses are restricted to vessels with a calibre of *only 200 μm or less* (Williams *et al.*, 1989, p. 731), i.e. arterioles, metarterioles, and capillaries. In man, an important part of this collateral circulation lies in the **subendocardial system** of arterial vasculature (Schaper *et al.*, 1988), where there is already a dense arterial plexus in the normal coronary circula-

tion (Section 18.3). There are also **extracardiac anastomoses** with pericardial arteries and with vasa vasorum of the great arteries leaving the heart, but the effectiveness of these after coronary occlusion has occurred is unpredictable (Williams *et al.*, 1989, p. 731).

In the search for experimental models applicable to the human coronary circulation, the effects of **acute** coronary occlusion have been investigated in several mammalian species, as reported in the comprehensive review by Schaper *et al.* (1988). The species differences are diverse and substantial. **Guinea pigs** have such a well-developed pre-existing collateral circulation that they experience no infarcts at all after acute occlusion. The pre-existing collateral circulation of the **canine heart** is also relatively well-developed and comes into action much faster than that of the human heart; its collaterals are mainly subepicardial, as opposed to the mainly subendocardial collaterals in man. The **pig** and some strains of **rabbit** are just the opposite, having virtually no demonstrable pre-existing collateral circulation and readily producing infarcts. **Rats** have some pre-existing collaterals but they are functionally ineffective.

The effects of **chronic** coronary occlusion on the growth of a collateral circulation by angiogenesis has been investigated experimentally only in the dog and pig. In the dog the collateral circulation develops so perfectly that it seems functionally equivalent to the large arteries that it replaces, and this makes this species a doubtful model for the clinical condition in man. The pig heart is judged to be a much better clinical model for man, but experimentally is subject to technical difficulties (Schaper *et al.*, 1988).

Regular **exercise** is often regarded as an important factor in preventing ischaemic heart disease in man, and exercise is also regarded as useful in rehabilitation after recovery from myocardial infarction. However, Schaper *et al.* (1988) were unable to find conclusive evidence in support of these propositions from reported clinical data, although they conceded that anecdotal and inferential evidence does support them. They also found the experimental data on exercise in the dog and pig to be contradictory.

Experimental studies during the last three decades have made important new advances in understanding **how collateral circulations develop**. It seems to be generally accepted (e.g. Guyton, 1986, p. 299) that the acute response to sudden coronary occlusion is **dilation** of the **pre-existing** arteriolar and capillary anastomoses, occurring within a few seconds but conveying less than half the required volume of blood flow; presumably this immediate dilation is induced by the usual metabolic regulation (Section 18.5). On the other hand, the restoration of full flow volume within about a month after acute occlusion, or the maintenance of flow during months or years of chronic occlusion, is achieved by **angiogenesis** (Section 12.20), i.e. by the growth of new arterioles and capillaries.

The key to this vascular growth (Schaper *et al.*, 1988) is believed to be the release of **polypeptide growth factors** and their interaction with **molecular receptors** on endothelial and smooth muscle cells. Some fibroblast growth factors (e.g. $\alpha + \beta$ FGF) induce a mitogenic response in both endothelial and smooth muscle cells. One of the best known vascular growth factors comes from **bovine neural tissue**; this growth factor induces proliferation of endothelial cells, particularly after it has been **potentiated** by **heparin**. It has been noted that sprouting capillaries are often accompanied by mast cells, the local source of heparin. It has now been shown that $\alpha + \beta$ FGF is stored near the cell membrane of endothelial and smooth muscle cells, but is unavailable to receptors under normal physiological conditions.

Vascular endothelial and smooth muscle cells express receptors for these heparin-binding growth factors. Heparin-binding growth factors have been found in the cardiac tissue of the pig, dog, and ox. It is believed that repetitive or progressive ischaemia causes reversible or irreversible damage to the cell membrane, which thus releases the growth factor. The growth factor, potentiated by binding to heparin, then occupies the receptors on the endothelial and smooth muscle cells of the microcirculation in the ischaemic area, and angiogenesis ensues.

Progress in these investigations may open the possibility of treating clinical coronary patients with growth factors injected via a catheter into the coronary arteries (Schaper *et al.*, 1988).

Chapter 19
Arterial Baroreceptors and Chemoreceptors

19.1 Control of arterial pressure: basic principles

In the normal mammal arterial pressure remains within a narrow range, even during a wide variety of postures and physiological conditions. Substantial modifications in arterial pressure are induced only by *maximal* changes in muscular activity. In ordinary **exercise** the mean arterial pressure rises only slightly, even when the energy expenditure is greatly increased.

Control of arterial pressure is essential to the maintenance of a constant internal environment, i.e. to **homeostasis** (Section 12.1). Cellular survival depends on a constant internal environment. This in turn requires control of the composition of the **interstitial fluid**, which is a filtrate of blood plasma (Section 12.2). Arterial pressure controls the composition of the interstitial fluid, by ensuring the adequate circulation of the blood. Blood plasma is then continually transported to and from the tissues, thus maintaining the fuel supply of the cells and removing waste products.

Maintenance of arterial pressure is also essential in order to guarantee the necessary blood supply to essential organs such as the brain and heart.

Arterial pressure is modified by reflexes that are initiated by **baroreceptors** that respond to pressure changes within the arterial system.

19.2 Sites of arterial baroreceptor and chemoreceptor zones

Baroreceptor and chemoreceptor zones occur primitively on the roots of all of the six pairs of **arterial arches** that arise from the embryonic left and right ventral aortae. However, only the third, fourth, and sixth pairs of arterial arches persist postnatally in mammals (Section 15.5). Therefore in the **mature mammal** the baro- and chemo-receptor zones are located on the roots of the **left** and **right internal carotid arteries** (the left and right third arterial arches respectively), the roots of the **arch of the aorta** and the **right subclavian artery** (the left and right fourth arches), and the roots of the left and right **pulmonary arteries** (the left and right sixth arches). (See Fig. 15.10 for the sites where these arteries spring from the embryonic left and right ventral aortae.)

Each of these receptor sites has two structurally specialized zones, both zones being richly supplied by autonomic afferent nerve endings: (1) a highly elastic **baroreceptor zone**, innervated by many **mechanoreceptor endings** and responding to variations in arterial pressure; (2) a **chemoreceptor zone** supplied by abundant **chemoreceptor endings** and responding to variations in the concentrations of carbon dioxide and hydrogen ions in the blood, and particularly the concentration of oxygen.

Of these various baro- and chemoreceptors, the most important are those on the internal carotid arteries and the arch of the aorta. On the internal carotid artery, the baroreceptor zone is known as the **carotid sinus**, and the chemoreceptor zone is the **carotid body**. On the arch of the aorta, the baroreceptor zone is not designated by a special name, but the component parts of the chemoreceptor zone are referred to collectively as the **aortic bodies**.

The attractive concept that **special sensory zones** are sited on each pair of the primordial vertebrate **arterial arches** was developed by comparative anatomists and physiologists. Young (1962, p. 161) and Le Gros Clark (1965, p. 224) reported that pressure receptors in the **branchial arteries** of **elasmobranch fish** give rise to nerve impulses in the vagus at each systole, which are increased by raising the arterial pressure and reflexly slow the heart and respiration; it was suggested by Young that 'these reflexes are presumably the ancestors of the carotid sinus (sinus caroticus) and similar reflexes of land vertebrates'. Adams (1958, p. 221) cited reports by Lutz and Wyman (1932a,b) of cardiac and respiratory reflexes elicited from the branchial arteries of elasmobranch fish.

In a review of the topic, Comroe (1964, p. 561) stated that the concept of **pressure receptor zones** in the vertebrate **arterial arches** (branchial arches) originated from Koch (1931). Comroe noted that the additional presence of **chemoreceptor zones** in *each* of the persisting arterial arches was suggested by his colleague C.F. Schmidt in 1938, the proposition being that the effects of anoxia and increased carbon dioxide on the carotid body (glomus caroticus) and aortic bodies (corpora paraaortica) might represent survival in air-breathing adult mammals of a reflex gill system in fishes, where direct contact occurs between the environment and blood flowing through the gill arches. Krogh (1941, p. 43) reported that the gill movements of fishes are far more sensitive to decreased oxygen tension than to increased carbon dioxide tension in the water.

Such inheritance by mammals of branchial arch chemoreceptors of fishes requires the presence of chemoreceptor tissue in the arterial arches of the mammalian embryo, but unfortunately Boyd (1937) failed to discover any such tissue. Furthermore, Adams (1958, pp. 212–214) was unable to find conclusive evidence in the literature for the presence in the aortic arches of **amphibians** of reflexogenic zones homologous to the carotid sinus and carotid body of mammals, although various workers have suggested that the well-known **carotid labyrinth** might be the functional homologue of the mammalian carotid sinus and/or carotid body. Adams (1958, pp. 184–200) found rather better evidence for the appropriate homologies in the major groups of **reptiles**, but again it was inconclusive. After similar uncertainties, it has now been shown that **birds** do have a carotid sinus and carotid body associated with the third pair of aortic arches, and baro- and chemoreceptor zones associated with the fourth and sixth aortic arches (Abdel-Magied and King, 1978; Abdel-Magied *et al.*, 1982; Taha and King, 1986).

In summary, it has to be conceded that the concept that baro- and chemoreceptor zones on the roots of the aortic arches can be traced throughout the vertebrate classes has not yet been firmly established. However, it is a useful working hypothesis, since it enables the location, structure, and function of these receptor zones to be predicted.

19.3 Anatomy of the mammalian carotid sinus

The **carotid sinus** is located on the origin of the **internal carotid artery**, i.e. at the point where the internal carotid artery arises from the peripheral end of the common carotid artery. At this site, the sinus forms a more or less distinct dilation (Fig. 19.1). It receives a bundle of **baroreceptor nerve fibres** (autonomic afferent fibres) by means of the **carotid sinus nerve** of the glossopharyngeal nerve (Fig. 4.3; Section 4.17.1; Figs 19.1, 19.2).

The wall of the carotid sinus shows two structural modifications. (1) The tunica media is converted into **elastic tissue**, even though the internal and common carotid arteries are muscular arteries in which the tunica media consists of layers of smooth muscle cells (Section 12.9.1). Compared with the adjoining arterial walls, the wall of the sinus feels soft and extremely thin. The greater elasticity of its wall enables the sinus to expand in response to any increase in arterial pressure. (2) The tunica adventitia is much thickened, in order to accommodate a very rich network of **afferent baroreceptor axonal endings** from the carotid sinus nerve (Section 4.17.1).

The **baroreceptor responses** of these endings to changes in arterial pressure are considered in Section 19.4.

19.3.1 Ultrastructure of baroreceptor endings

Electron microscopic observations (Section 4.17.1) reveal presumptive **baroreceptor nerve endings** in the wall of the carotid sinus (Knoche *et al.*, 1980). Their ultrastructural characteristics include profiles with a very large diameter, great numbers of mitochondria, a surface largely devoid of Schwann cell covering, and dense bodies and myelin bodies consistent with a rapid turnover of axoplasm. Presumptive aminergic or peptidergic **efferent nerve endings**, typified by large or small dense-cored vesicles, have also been found in the wall of the carotid sinus, often sharing a Schwann cell with the presumptive baroreceptor ending (Knoche and Kienecker, 1977): these could modulate the activity of the baroreceptor (Section 4.17.1).

19.3.2 Species variations in anatomy of carotid sinus

The carotid sinus (sinus caroticus) is often, but not always, visible as an arterial dilation in the mammalian cadaver. Ask-Upmark (1935, p. 95) found it to be particularly conspicuous in some species, for example in the hedgehog (*Erinaceus europeus*), and recognizable in the dog (Fig. 19.1) and cat (Fig. 19.2); in the horse it is

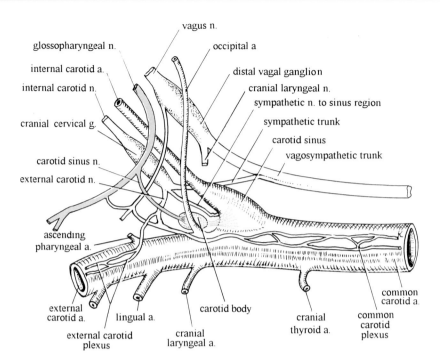

Fig. 19.1 Lateral view of the left carotid sinus region of the dog. The carotid sinus in this species is typical of mammals generally. It is a recognizable dilation on the root of the internal carotid artery. Peripheral to the sinus, the internal carotid continues rostrally as a normal muscular artery. The occipital artery may arise from the external carotid artery as shown, or more often from a common trunk with the ascending pharyngeal artery. The carotid body is about 2 mm long, and lodged in the bifurcation of the common carotid artery into the internal and external carotid arteries. Its arterial supply tends to be multiple from the nearest arteries, principally the occipital and ascending pharyngeal arteries but also from the external carotid. The carotid sinus nerve is a branch of the glossopharyngeal nerve (green). Its fibres ensheath the carotid body and then fan out to supply the carotid sinus. Sympathetic fibres from the cranial cervical ganglion can be followed to the region of the sinus. Sympathetic plexuses accompany the external and common carotid arteries. Redrawn and modified after Adams (1958) and Simoens (1992).

usually not discernible (A.S. King, personal observation). In the *living animal*, however, including the horse, the sinus becomes a distinct distension at every heart beat, as would be expected from its elasticity. Presumably the sinus is more likely to show in the dead animal if fixation is by arterial perfusion. In man (see Adams, 1958, p. 63), the sinus is visible in 80–94% of cadavers: when visible, it is entirely restricted to the internal carotid artery in about 65% of specimens; in 30% it includes the end of the common carotid; in 5% the external carotid is also involved.

Eckberg and Fritsch (1993) agreed with Heymans *et al.* (1933, p. 20) that the **baroreceptor endings** of the sinus wall are restricted mainly to the tunica adventitia, as claimed originally by de Castro (1926, 1928). Adams (1958, p. 43) noted that others found fibres in the tunica media also, and this location is affirmed by Scher (1974, p. 150). However, Adams (1958, p. 43) believed fibres in the media to be efferent rather than afferent. The innervation by baroreceptor endings is not restricted to the

origin of the internal carotid, but may extend also to the origin of the **occipital artery** (a. occipitalis) (Heymans *et al.*, 1933, p. 20; Ask-Upmark, 1935, p. 39). This particularly applies to mammals such as the cat, goat, and hedgehog, in which the occipital artery shares a common origin with the internal carotid artery (Ask-Upmark, 1935, p. 96).

In some species, including the **sheep** and **ox** (Baldwin and Bell, 1963) and the **cat** (Davis and Story, 1943), the lumen of the proximal two thirds of the **internal carotid artery** is obliterated in the weeks or months after birth. There is evidence (Adams, 1958, p. 111) that a similar obliteration occurs in the **pig**. In textbooks of veterinary anatomy (e.g. Schummer *et al.*, 1981, and Dyce *et al.*, 1987) this regression of the internal carotid artery in the pig is not mentioned, and the artery is considered to be fully developed. Nanda (1975, p. 1315), mentioned a report of replacement of the internal carotid by the ascending pharyngeal artery in this species, but nevertheless concluded that the internal carotid artery has a

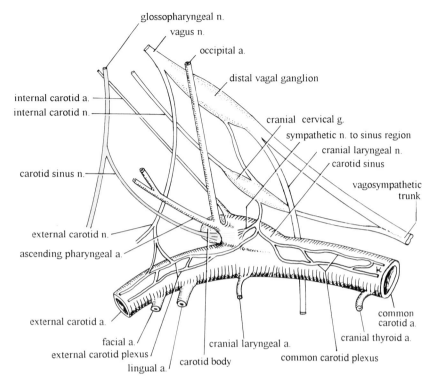

Fig. 19.2 Lateral view of the left carotid sinus region of the cat. In the cat the lumen of the internal carotid artery becomes obliterated in the weeks or months after birth, converting the artery into a slender strand. However, the root of the artery remains patent forming a short nipple-like enlargement, and this is the carotid sinus. The occipital and ascending pharyngeal arteries usually arise from a very short common trunk that springs from the angle between the carotid sinus and the external carotid artery. The carotid body is about 1.3 mm long rostrocaudally and 1.5 mm dorsoventrally. It receives its blood supply from the occipital-ascending pharyngeal trunk, or from the occipital artery. The carotid sinus nerve is a branch of the glossopharyngeal nerve (green). Its fibres spread out over the carotid body and continue onto the carotid sinus. The cranial cervical ganglion supplies the carotid body with sympathetic fibres, some of which can be followed to the vicinity of the carotid sinus. Redrawn and modified after Adams (1958) and Simoens (1992).

typical distribution in the pig. Simoens (1992, p. 270), in his authoritative survey of veterinary anatomical nomenclature for the arterial system, explicitly stated that the extracranial segment of the internal carotid artery of the pig regresses as in the ruminants and the cat. On the basis of a thorough review of the literature, Adams (1958, p. 111) concluded that 'it is certain' that the vessel in the pig that is usually called the internal carotid artery 'is not the true internal carotid'. Adams (1958, p. 113) argued that: (1) the so-called internal carotid artery in the pig is really the **ascending pharyngeal artery** (a. pharyngea ascendens); (2) the sinus region must involve the common trunk which gives rise to the occipital and ascending pharyngeal arteries, and possibly the internal carotid as well; and (3) there is experimental evidence that this ill-defined carotid sinus region in the pig is indeed innervated by the usual carotid sinus branch of

the glossopharyngeal nerve, and responds to variations in arterial pressure in the typical manner.

Adams (1958, p. 119) concluded that in the **adult ox** the **occipital artery** arises from the peripheral end of the common carotid by a short bulbous trunk. This dilated region (Fig. 19.3) is the carotid sinus (Simoens, 1992, Fig. D of p. 271). The dilated region (the sinus) gives rise to the **ascending pharyngeal artery**. Shortly after the point of origin of the ascending pharyngeal artery, the dilated region in the **new-born calf** gives off the slender but still patent **internal carotid artery**. De Castro believed that in the adult ox the sinus with its receptor endings is transferred to the origin of the **occipital artery** (see Ask-Upmark, 1935, p. 96). However, as Adams (1958, p. 43) pointed out, others have shown that the 'sinus' of the ox is more strictly located on the unobliterated origin of the common **occipital-internal carotid trunk** (Fig. 19.3).

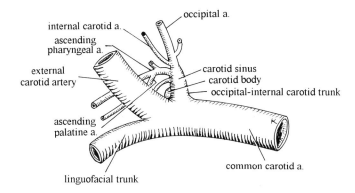

Fig. 19.3   Lateral view of the left carotid sinus of the ox. In the ox the internal carotid and occipital arteries arise by a common trunk. The lumen of the internal carotid artery becomes obliterated by about 18 months of age, converting the artery into a fibrous cord. However, the root of the common trunk of the internal carotid and occipital arteries tends to form a spindle-shaped dilation, the carotid sinus. The carotid body is multilobular and up to 6 mm long. It is apparently vascularized by the first branches from the common trunk of the internal carotid and occipital arteries. It is assumed that the carotid sinus nerve of the glossopharyngeal nerve supplies the carotid sinus, but detailed information on the innervation of the sinus in this species seems not to be available. Redrawn and modified after Adams (1958), and Simoens (1992).

Hovelacque *et al.* (1930) reported that, as in the ox, the carotid sinus and its receptor endings in the **cat** are transferred to the common occipital-internal carotid trunk (Fig. 19.2).

The **cranial cervical ganglion** of the sympathetic system forms the **internal carotid nerve** and the **external carotid nerve** (Figs 19.1, 19.2). The main function of these sympathetic nerves is to supply vasomotor, piloerector, and sudomotor fibres for distribution throughout the head, using the arteries as a roadway (Section 2.24.1). Nevertheless, some of these fibres enter the wall of the carotid sinus, and it has been suggested that sympathetic fibres, or circulating adrenergic hormones, might modulate baroreceptor sensitivity (Section 19.4.7).

19.3.3   *Other carotid baroreceptors*

Histological evidence for six baroreceptor zones in the common carotid artery of the cat was found by Boss and Green (1954).

19.4   Physiology of the carotid sinus

If the pressure increases inside the internal carotid artery, or for that matter inside any artery, the diameter of that artery also increases. However, the special elastic conversion of the tunic media in the wall of the carotid sinus amplifies the increase in the diameter of the sinus.

The increase in the diameter of the sinus stretches the baroreceptor endings in its wall. Since the receptor endings ramify in the adventitia, where the wall has its greatest circumference, the stretching of the nerve endings is maximized. The mechanical distortion of the nerve endings of the baroreceptor axons causes the discharge of action potentials. Thus the baroreceptors are mechanoreceptors that transduce pressure changes into nerve impulses.

In the normal living mammal, the rate of discharge of the baroreceptor axon is directly proportional to the degree of stretching of its receptor endings. Thus in Fig. 19.4A, a single baroreceptor axon is discharging during the pulse waves caused by normal ventricular systole and diastole. The rate of discharge progressively increases as the pressure rises during systole, and progressively decreases as the pressure falls during diastole.

19.5   Projections of baroreceptor axons to cardiovascular centre

By means of their central projections (Section 19.12), the baroreceptor axons continuously inform the cardiovascular 'centre' in the brainstem about any rise or fall in arterial pressure.

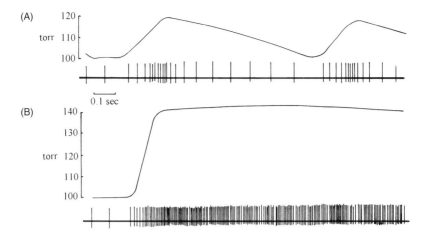

Fig. 19.4   Activity of a single baroreceptor axon from the carotid sinus. In A and B, the upper trace shows the pressure in the carotid sinus and the lower record shows the activity of the single axon, each vertical line being the spike of an action potential.

A. Blood is circulating through the carotid sinus in the normal manner. Each rise in arterial pressure is due to ventricular systole. A burst of impulses accompanies each systolic rise. The frequency of discharge of the impulses is directly related to the pressure.

B. The carotid sinus has been isolated and is being perfused at controlled pressure. The pressure is increased from 100 mmHg (13.3 kPa) and then held at a static pressure of 140 mmHg (18.7 kPa). At this sustained pressure the frequency of discharge is more or less constant. However, there is a slight slowing of the rate of discharge. This indicates adaptation of the axon, but the degree of adaptation is small. This is a slowly-adapting fibre.

As just stated, a rise in arterial pressure excites the baroreceptors. This excitation acts on the cardiovascular 'centre', and reflexly causes a *fall* in arterial pressure (Section 19.12). Conversely, a fall in arterial pressure induces the cardiovascular 'centre' to bring about an *increase* in arterial pressure (by sympathetic excitation; Section 19.12). Thus the arterial baroreceptor reflexes are **negative feedback mechanisms** for regulating arterial pressure.

19.5.1   *What does the baroreceptor ending actually measure?*

By enclosing the carotid sinus of the living animal in a rigid cast it can be shown that the baroreceptors do not respond *directly* to pressure. Although the pressure inside the artery may increase, the cast prevents the sinus from distending and there is then no change in the activity of the baroreceptor axons (Scott, 1986, p. 91). Thus baroreceptors are mechanoreceptors that actually measure *length*, not pressure.

19.5.2   *Reflex responses to pressure on the neck*

In almost all conscious humans (Hoff, 1949, p. 667), it is possible to elicit a 'carotid sinus reflex' mechanically by pressing strongly on the neck over the carotid sinus region. This excites the baroreceptors, and can cause a fall of as much as 20 mmHg (2.7 kPa) in arterial pressure in a normal person or even stop the heart if there are pathological changes in the wall of the sinus (Section 19.5.9).

19.5.3   *Relationships between axonal discharge rate and pressure within the sinus*

The properties of the baroreceptor axons of the normal carotid sinus can best be demonstrated experimentally in an isolated carotid sinus, in which the major arterial branches have been tied off but the pressure can be changed by a hydraulic system.

If the pressure in an isolated sinus is increased in progressive steps, the relationship of the pressure in the sinus to the **discharge rate** of a baroreceptor axon is **linear** over the range of normal arterial pressure (Scott, 1986, p. 92). This is known as the **static response** of the baroreceptor axons. Thus, within the range of normal arterial pressures, either a rise or a fall in pressure will predictably change the total baroreceptor discharge. Below a certain **threshold pressure**, however, a baroreceptor axon falls silent (Scher, 1974, p. 151). This threshold varies, but in some baroreceptor axons may be as low as 30 mmHg (4.0 kPa). When rising pressure reaches the threshold, the baroreceptor axon strikes in at a rate of about 20 impulses per second, and from there onward increases its rate of discharge roughly in proportion to further increases in pressure, so long as the pressure remains within the normal range. At pressures above the normal range, further increases in pressure induce much smaller increments in the rate of discharge (Scott, 1986, p. 92), and finally the discharge rate reaches a maximum at a pressure of about 220 mmHg (29.3 kPa) or higher (Scher, 1974, p. 151).

19.5.4 *Adaptation*

During static discharge, carotid baroreceptor axons experience some degree of **adaptation**. Thus in Fig. 19.4B, an isolated carotid sinus is being perfused by its artificial hydraulic system at a pressure that rises steeply from 100 mmHg (13.3 kPa) and is then held at a static level of 140 mmHg (18.7 kPa). The rate of discharge of the baroreceptor axon increases sharply as the pressure rises, and is then maintained steadily while the pressure is held statically at 140 mmHg (18.7 kPa). During the static phase the discharge rate does decrease slightly, this decrease being known as adaptation. Carotid sinus baroreceptors belong to the class of **slowly adapting mechanoreceptors**, as do the bronchial stretch receptors that mediate the inflation reflex (Section 11.4; Fig. 11.2C).

19.5.5 *Effect of rate of pressure change on axonal discharge rate*

Carotid sinus baroreceptors respond not only to the static level of the pressure within the sinus, but also to the **rate of pressure change** (Scher, 1974, p. 152). The beating of the heart normally imposes pulsatile pressure changes on the baroreceptors of the carotid sinus. Such phasic changes in pressure can be mimicked by a hydraulic system attached to an isolated sinus. The baroreceptor axon discharges progressively faster as the rate of pressure change increases. Like adaptation, sensitivity to the rate of change of the stimulus is a characteristic of **mechanoreceptors** in general.

19.5.6 *Resetting of baroreceptors*

Carotid sinus baroreceptors **reset** themselves to the prevalent level of arterial pressure (Eckberg and Fritsch, 1993). For example (Guyton, 1986, p. 249), if the pressure in the live animal rises from about 100 mmHg (13.3 kPa) to a mean of about 200 mmHg (26.7 kPa) and is then sustained at that abnormally high level, the discharge rate of a baroreceptor axon immediately increases greatly. But during the next 1 or 2 days the discharge rate slowly returns to normal, and remains there even if the mean arterial pressure is still 200 mmHg (26.7 kPa). Conversely, if the arterial pressure falls well

below the normal level and is sustained there, the discharge rate at first decreases greatly but then gradually regains its normal rate. Thus the baroreceptors of the carotid sinus provide the cardiovascular centre in the brainstem with information that enables the centre to adjust arterial pressure in response to *short term* fluctuations in pressure; but because of resetting, the sinus baroreceptors are ineffective for the *long term* regulation of arterial pressure.

19.5.7 *Modulation of baroreceptor sensitivity*

Several mechanisms have been proposed for the **modulation** of baroreceptor sensitivity. (1) **Sympathetic vasomotor fibres** in the walls of the carotid sinus and carotid arteries, or circulating **catecholamines** (Section 19.3.1) might change the sensitivity of the receptors (see Chapleau *et al.*, 1991), or alter the diameter of the vessels, but these actions are controversial (Scher, 1974, p. 152). (2) The presumptive **peptidergic efferent axons** that are so closely associated with the presumptive baroreceptor endings (Sections 4.17.1 and 19.3.1) could modulate the stimulus threshold of a baroreceptor ending (Knoche and Addicks, 1976). This would be an example of postjunctional neuromodulation (Section 2.37). (3) **Ionic mechanisms**, such as variations in the extracellular concentration of ions (Na^+, Ca^{2+}, K^+), may also modulate the sensitivity of baroreceptors to deformation (see Chapleau *et al.*, 1991). (4) **Prostacyclin** (PGI_2), released from **endothelial cells** in response to shearing stress and other stimuli (Section 13.6), exerts an excitatory effect on baroreceptors and thus contributes to increased baroreceptor activity during increases in pressure (Chapleau *et al.*, 1991). Dysfunction of endothelial cells appears to be a major factor in the cause of **chronic hypertension** (Section 13.6). This is believed to result from impaired production of prostacyclin, which in turn is followed by decreased baroreceptor sensitivity.

19.5.8 *Types of baroreceptor fibre*

There are two types of baroreceptor axon (Scott, 1986, p. 92), small diameter, slowly-conducting, higher threshold, **unmyelinated C-fibres**, and larger diameter, lower threshold, faster-conducting **myelinated A-fibres**. The receptor endings belonging to these two types of fibre differ in their sensitivity and threshold. At low pressures more of the low threshold A-fibres fire, but at high pressures more of the higher threshold C-fibres become active. The A-fibres that respond especially to lower pressures are more sensitive to a change in pressure than the C-fibres. Therefore at lower pressures, when the activity of A-fibres predominates, a given change in pressure induces a greater overall alteration in the baroreceptor discharge rate than at higher pressures when greater numbers of the less sensitive C-fibres are active.

19.5.9 *Pathophysiology of the carotid sinus*

Since the first published anatomical account of the carotid sinus in 1811, it has been known that the sinus in man is a predilection site of **arteriosclerosis** (Adams, 1958, p. 64). Pathological thickening of the tunica intima of the sinus wall sometimes occurs even in teenagers, and atheroma and calcification occur frequently when the carotid arteries are unaffected elsewhere.

Baroreceptor sensitivity is impaired in **arteriosclerosis** and **chronic hypertension** (Chapleau *et al.*, 1991). The decrease in baroreceptor sensitivity in **arteriosclerosis** is usually attributed to reduced distensibility of the sinus due to hardening of its wall, and possibly also to frank degeneration of the baroreceptor endings. There is now further evidence that the impairment of baroreceptor sensitivity is augmented by endothelial dysfunction, which leads to decreased formation of **prostacyclin**; since prostacyclin normally has an excitatory effect on baroreceptors (Section 19.5.7) reduction of prostacyclin diminishes baroreceptor sensitivity. It is believed that dysfunction of the endothelium is also a major factor in **chronic hypertension**. This again is because the decreased production of prostacyclin reduces baroreceptor activity.

If calcified arteriosclerotic plaques have developed, the carotid sinus reflex in response to pressure on the neck (Section 19.5.2) can be so strong that the person may lose consciousness, or the heart may even stop altogether (Guyton, 1986, p. 249). Usually vagal escape allows the heart to restart, but some individuals die of cardiac arrest. The condition is known as the **carotid sinus syndrome**. In such individuals, a tight collar may be enough to cause fainting (**carotid sinus syncope**).

19.6   Anatomy and physiology of aortic baroreceptors

Baroreceptor nerve endings are present in the walls of several of the great arteries near the heart (Fig. 19.5). The most important of these receptors lie in the wall of the **arch of the aorta**, and there are others in the origin of the **right subclavian artery**. These two sites are consistent, respectively, with the evolution of baro- and chemoreceptor sites on the roots of the left fourth and right fourth primitive aortic arches (Section 19.2).

All of these are **elastic arteries** (Section 12.8). They therefore have highly elastic walls, and can follow the pulsatile changes in arterial pressure; they have no need of any special elastic modification of their walls, such as the elastic transformation in the tunica media of the carotid sinus (Section 19.3).

The afferent axons belonging to these receptor endings form a bundle of axons known as the **aortic nerve** (depressor nerve) (Section 4.17.1). In most mammals this bundle of axons is buried in the vagus nerve (Figs 3.3, 19.7A, 19.8); its fibres emerge from the left vagus at the heart in order to supply the arch of the aorta (Fig. 19.5), and from the right vagus to supply the root of the right subclavian artery. In a few species these fibres form a fully-independent aortic nerve (Section 19.10.4; Fig. 19.7B).

The baroreceptor fibres of the aortic nerve are mechanoreceptors with the same **physiological properties** as the baroreceptor fibres of the carotid sinus nerve. Thus their baroreceptor endings transduce changes in arterial pressure into axonal action potentials, discharging in a linear relationship to changes in pressure.

19.6.1   *Site of baroreceptor endings*

The baroreceptor endings of the **aorta** and **right subclavian artery** form branching networks mainly in the **tunica adventitia**.

Baroreceptor endings have been found in the walls of **other arteries** between the carotid sinus and aorta, including the origins of the left subclavian artery and the cranial thyroid artery, and the common carotid artery itself (Scott, 1986, p. 90; and see Scher, 1974, p. 148).

19.6.2   *Physiological characteristics of aortic baroreceptors*

Aortic baroreceptors differ slightly from carotid baroreceptors (Scott, 1986, p. 93). They tend to have a higher threshold, and a lower sensitivity to rate of change of pressure. This may reflect the occurrence of much higher **pulse pressures** (the difference between systolic and diastolic pressure) in the thin-walled carotid sinus, as compared with those in the thick-walled elastic arteries such as the aorta. Or these characteristics of the aortic baroreceptors may be due to a higher proportion of C-fibres (with relatively higher threshold and lower sensitivity) than A-fibres.

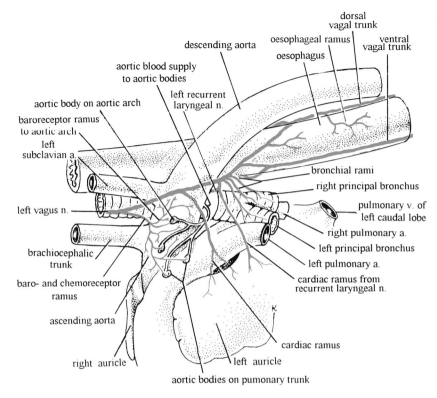

Fig. 19.5 **Semidiagrammatic left craniolateral view of the aortic arch and pulmonary trunk of the immature dog, to show aortic bodies.** In the puppy there are about 20 aortic bodies. Most of them are on the caudoventral aspect of the aortic arch and pulmonary trunk, and cannot be seen in this view. Those shown here are enlarged about twofold, to show their arterial supply from the aortic arch and innervation from the vagus nerve (green).

19.6.3 *Pulmonary baroreceptors*

There is also physiological evidence for baroreceptor activity in the **pulmonary arteries** (Coleridge and Kidd, 1960; Bevan, 1967), where they were categorized as 'low pressure' baroreceptors. This site is consistent with the evolution of receptor sites on the left and right *sixth* aortic arches. However, ultrastructural evidence for baroreceptor endings in the pulmonary arteries appears to be lacking. The receptors of the pulmonary arteries function in essentially the same way as the receptors in the systemic arteries (Guyton, 1986, p. 250): they inhibit the vasomotor centre and thus reflexly decrease arterial pressure.

19.7 Macroscopic anatomy of the carotid body

The mammalian **carotid body** is a small nodule a few millimetres long, embedded in the angle formed by the terminal division of the common carotid artery into the external carotid, internal carotid, and occipital arteries (Figs 19.1–19.3). In the live animal, the carotid body is pink in colour, reflecting its exceptionally rich vascularity (Section 19.7.2).

The **arterial supply** of the carotid body comes directly from one or other of the adjacent terminal branches of the common carotid artery (Fig. 19.8).

The **nerve supply** of the carotid body consists of (autonomic afferent) **chemoreceptor fibres** conveyed by the **carotid sinus nerve** from the glossopharyngeal cranial nerve (Figs 19.1–19.3) (Section 4.17.2).

The macroscopic anatomy of the mammalian carotid body (glomus caroticum) has been summarized by Comroe (1964, p. 558), and extensively surveyed throughout the mammalian orders by Adams (1958, pp.

46–123). Although the carotid body is always present on both sides of the body, it may be overlooked because it is sometimes broken up into separate microscopic lobules scattered among the terminal branches of the common carotid artery (Adams, 1958, p. 46), or it may lie half a centimetre or so cranial to the end of the common carotid artery.

19.7.1 *Dimensions*

The size of the carotid body varies more or less in proportion to the size of the species (Adams, 1958, pp. 84–121): for example mouse, $0.3\,mm \times 0.2\,mm \times 0.15\,mm$; cat, $1.3\,mm \times 1.5\,mm \times 1.2\,mm$; dog, $2\,mm \times 1.5\,mm$; pig, $3.5\,mm \times 1.5\,mm \times 1.0\,mm$; ox, up to $6\,mm \times 3\,mm$; horse, up to $9\,mm \times 4\,mm \times 2\,mm$, though it is not uncommonly divided into two or three separate masses in this species.

19.7.2 *Blood supply*

In many (if not most) mammals the **arterial supply** to the carotid body comes from the occipital or ascending pharyngeal arteries, although in **man** the supply is usually from the bifurcation of the common carotid or from the external carotid (Adams, 1958, pp. 54–55). In the **cat** the arterial supply arises from the occipital artery, or from a common occipito-ascending pharyngeal trunk; in the **dog** it comes from the occipital artery or ascending pharyngeal artery; in the rabbit, it arises from branches of the external carotid, internal carotid, or the bifurcation of the common carotid artery (Comroe, 1964, p. 559). Intraspecific variations in the blood supply are the rule rather than the exception, and collateral circulations occur between the vessels that have access to the carotid body, so that vascular 'isolation' of the carotid body is difficult to achieve experimentally.

The **venous drainage** collects into a plexus covering the surface of the carotid body, and then drains from the cranial pole of the carotid body (the opposite end to the entry of the arteries) by several smaller veins into one or other of the larger venous trunks in the vicinity, such as the pharyngeal, laryngeal, or lingual veins, and the internal jugular vein in the dog.

After sympathetic denervation of the carotid body of the dog, the rate of blood flow through the carotid body, with normal arterial pressure, is about $40\,mm^3\,min^{-1}$. This appears to be an insignificant flow, but when standardized against tissue mass is really a huge value ($2000\,ml\,min^{-1}\,(100\,g)^{-1}$ (Comroe, 1964, p. 599)), which competes with the alveolar wall (Section 6.7.4), myocardium (Section 18.3), and synaptic zones of association areas of the central nervous system, for the title of the most vascular tissue in the body. The flow rate for the kidney, which is the greatest among the larger organs supplied by the systemic circulation, is only $400\,ml\,min^{-1}\,(100\,g)^{-1}$ (Scher, 1974, p. 160).

See also Section 19.9 for evidence that the 'venous' blood draining from the carotid body has a P_{O_2} nearly equal to that of arterial blood.

19.7.3 *Innervation*

The **nerves** associated with the carotid body consist of an intricate meshwork of branches from the glossopharyngeal nerve, vagus nerve, cranial cervical sympathetic ganglion, and sometimes the hypoglossal nerve. For almost 200 years after the original discovery of the carotid body in the first half of the eighteenth century (Adams, 1958, p. 56), researches seemed to show that the **sympathetic fibres** in this plexus are the principal factor controlling the function of the carotid body; supposedly the sympathetic fibres innervated glandular cells in the carotid body that secrete a vasomotor substance, perhaps parasympathomimetic with a hypotensive action. Interest in the **glossopharyngeal component** of the carotid sinus nerve network had been negligible. In the 1920s, however, it emerged that afferent impulses are generated by the carotid sinus and carotid body; de Castro (1926, 1928) showed that the glossopharyngeal nerve carries the *afferent* fibres from the carotid body, and that it is therefore the glossopharyngeal nerve that is of paramount functional importance in the innervation of the carotid body. Although many other nerve fibres seem to spread out on the carotid body, most of them merely traverse it on their way to other regions, notably the sympathetic pathways that pass to the great arteries of the head and neck.

Baroreceptor fibres from the carotid sinus join the chemoreceptor fibres from the carotid body, thus forming the **carotid sinus nerve** (ramus sinus carotici) of the glossopharyngeal nerve. The cell station of these afferent autonomic axons is in the distal glossopharyngeal ganglion (Section 4.17.1). In the horse, the carotid sinus nerve runs across the wall of the guttural pouch (diverticulum tubae auditivae), which thus forms a transparent background to the nerve.

19.7.4 *Development*

The carotid body arises from the mesenchyme of the third pharyngeal (branchial) arch. In the horse, a nodule of cartilage, ossified with age, is closely attached to the artery supplying the carotid body (see Adams, 1958, p. 107). Unlike the calcified areas that occur in the walls of arteries as a result of pathological changes (Sections 18.9.1; 19.5.9), this structure is a constant feature of the normal horse, and can be seen in the embryo where it is presumably a part of the cartilage of the third pharyngeal arch.

19.8 Microscopic anatomy of the carotid body

The tissue of the carotid body consists of granular cells, numerous axonal endings supported by sustentacular cells, and an exceptionally rich microcirculation of fenestrated blood capillaries and sinusoids (Fig. 19.6). The axonal endings belong to autonomic afferent axons with an arterial chemoreceptor function. These chemoreceptor fibres form one of the two great functional components of the **carotid sinus nerve** of the glossopharyngeal nerve, the other component being the baroreceptor axons (Section 19.3). The chemoreceptor axons are excited particularly by a fall in the oxygen content of the blood (Section 19.9).

The actual chemoreceptor function is believed to be carried out by the granular cells. They trans-mit their excitation to their adjacent axonal endings by means of synaptic contacts (Fig. 19.6).

The microscopic anatomy of the carotid body and its ultrastructural innervation was reviewed by Verna (1973) and Williams *et al.* (1989, p. 1473). The surface of the organ is enclosed in a connective tissue capsule. The two types of cell in the carotid body, granular cell (endocrinocytus granularis) and sustentacular cell (epithelioidocytus sustenans), are also known respectively as **type I** and **type II** cells. The **granular cells** (Fig. 19.6) are characterized by membrane-bound, dense-cored, granular vesicles, about 100 nm in diameter. The **sustentacular cells** partly enclose the granular cells, and quite often trap **axonal endings** against the granular cells (Fig. 19.6). A rich network of fenestrated **blood capillaries** or **sinusoids** ramifies among the cells and the axonal endings, thus accounting for the exceptionally great vascularity of the carotid body (Section 19.7.2).

It is generally accepted (Williams *et al.*, 1989, p. 1473) that the **granular cells** form paired **reciprocal synapses** with the **axonal endings** (Fig. 19.6), as shown by Morgan

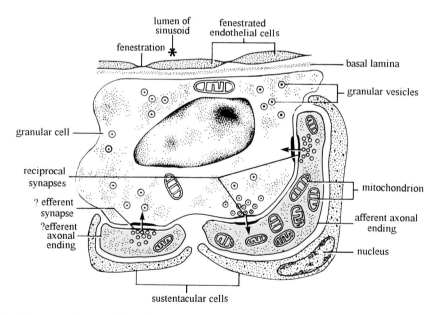

Fig. 19.6 Semidiagrammatic view of the ultrastructure of the cells and axonal endings of the carotid body. Two types of cell are present. Axonal endings are green. The granular cell is probably the chemoreceptor. In response to hypoxia, its dense-cored granular vesicles release catecholamines at synapses with afferent axonal endings (arrow pointing *into* the axonal ending on the *right* side of the diagram). The afferent axonal endings also have reciprocal synapses of uncertain function (arrow pointing *out of* the granular cell on the right). If they exist at all, efferent axonal endings are present only in very small numbers (*left* side of the diagram). The relatively slender sustentacular cells closely support the axonal endings. The sustentacular cell has no synapses or specialized organelles. A rich blood supply is provided by abundant capillaries and sinusoids. Fenestrated endothelial cells minimize the diffusion pathway of blood-borne stimuli from blood to granular cell. The proportions of the cells are not drawn to scale, the granular cells being many times larger than the sustentacular cells and axonal endings.

et al. (1975). Of these paired synapses, one has an accumulation of vesicles in the granular cell and a post-synaptic thickening on the axonal ending, suggesting transmission from cell to axon followed by *afferent* axonal projection to the central nervous system: the other synapse has an accumulation of vesicles in the axonal ending and a postsynaptic thickening on the granular cell, suggesting transmission from axon to cell. Reciprocal synapses have also been found between granular cells (McDonald and Mitchell, 1975). Degeneration experiments (McDonald and Mitchell, 1975) and autoradiographic labelling (Fidone *et al.*, 1977; Smith and Mills, 1981) have demonstrated that the vast majority (over 95%) of the axonal endings in the carotid body are in fact *afferent* (Williams *et al.*, 1989, p. 1473), with their cell stations in the distal glossopharyngeal ganglion (Section 4.17.2); discordant observations suggesting that many of the axonal endings are efferent were obtained from denervation experiments by Biscoe *et al.* (1970), but these could be accounted for by transganglionic degeneration (Abdel-Magied and King, 1982).

A sparse population of **parasympathetic** and **sympathetic ganglion cells** has been found near the surface of the carotid body, but any such *efferent* neurons are presumed to be vasomotor to the arterioles in the microcirculation of the carotid body (Williams *et al.*, 1989, p. 1473). A small number of *efferent* axonal endings may make presynaptic contacts with afferent axons, and would then presumably be inhibitory to the afferent axons.

The **sustentacular cells** are glial in nature and lack specialized organelles (Gonzales *et al.*, 1992). Sustentacular cells have no synaptic contacts with either axonal endings or granular cells, and contain no secretory granules.

19.9 Physiology of the carotid body

The overall function of the carotid body is to initiate reflexes that maintain the homeostasis of oxygen, carbon dioxide, and hydrogen ions within the internal environment of the body, and to adjust the supply of oxygen to the tissues to meet the demands of exercise and high altitude.

The granular cells of the carotid body are excited by a fall in the P_{O_2} of the blood, and also by a rise in the P_{CO_2} or the concentration of hydrogen ions in the blood. This excitation is transmitted, by means of synaptic contacts (Fig. 19.6), to the adjacent axonal endings. The reflex pathway (Section 19.13) then projects into the **medullary respiratory centre** in the brainstem (Figs 11.1, 19.8), and thence to the muscles of respiration via the

inspiratory drive pathway (Section 11.3). Thus these responses lead to a reflex increase in breathing (and hence in alveolar ventilation).

The excitation of arterial chemoreceptor endings by a **fall in P_{O_2}** is the *only* mechanism that activates an increase in breathing in response to a *reduction in the oxygen content* of the blood. Nevertheless, the effect of decreased arterial P_{O_2} on breathing is almost insignificant, *when the lungs are normal*. This is because an increase in ventilation in response to falling arterial P_{O_2} normally removes CO_2 from the blood, and thus diminishes by far the most powerful stimulus to breathing (Section 11.11.1), i.e. the direct stimulus of CO_2 on the **central chemoreceptor area** of the brain stem. (See Section 19.9.2 for pathological conditions in which the increase in ventilation does *not* diminish arterial CO_2, so that a fall in P_{O_2} *does* induce a strong increase in ventilation.)

The excitation of the carotid body chemoreceptor endings in response to an increase in blood CO_2 or a decrease in blood pH is relatively unimportant, because of the much more powerful effects of these changes directly on the central chemoreceptor area.

The carotid body (and aortic bodies, Section 19.10) are so highly vascularized that the 'venous' blood draining from them has a P_{O_2} nearly equal to that of arterial blood. Moreover, whilst circulating through the carotid body the blood traverses capillaries and sinusoids lined by **fenestrated endothelium**, thus minimizing the diffusion pathway for blood-borne stimuli. Therefore these arterial chemoreceptors are essentially assessing *arterial P_{O_2}*.

19.9.1 *Regulation of breathing by arterial chemoreceptors*

The chemoreceptor axons of the carotid body (and aortic bodies) are tonically active, with a low discharge frequency in a typical axon of about $2s^{-1}$ at a normal arterial blood P_{O_2} of about 100 mmHg (13.3 kPa), P_{CO_2} of 40 mmHg (5.3 kPa), and pH of 7.4 (Gonzales *et al.*, 1992). The discharge rate increases when the arterial P_{O_2} falls, or when the P_{CO_2} increases or pH decreases. The discharge rate is particularly responsive to changes in P_{O_2} between 60 and 30 mmHg (4.0 kPa), where the oxygen saturation of arterial haemoglobin decreases rapidly (Fig. 14.1). However, the respiratory response to a falling arterial P_{O_2} is actually rather weak. A fall to about

60 mmHg (8.0 kPa) has a negligible effect on alveolar ventilation. If the fall continues to about 40 mmHg (5.3 kPa), alveolar ventilation increases by a factor of only about 1.5, although a P_{O_2} of 40 down to 20 mmHg (5.3 to 2.7 kPa) is incompatible with life for more than a few minutes. In contrast, doubling the arterial P_{CO_2} from a normal value of 40 mmHg to about 80 mmHg (5.3 to 10.7 kPa) increases alveolar ventilation by a factor of about 10.

19.9.2 Pathological conditions in which oxygen strongly regulates breathing

Gas exchange across the alveolar wall is diminished in **alveolar emphysema**, through loss of alveolar capillaries and deposition of fibrous tissue in the remaining alveolar wall (Section 7.19). Gas exchange is also decreased if fluid accumulates in the alveolar lumen as in **pulmonary oedema** (Section 17.25). Since CO_2 exchange is now diminished as well as O_2 exchange, the increase in ventilation caused by the excitatory action on the carotid body chemoreceptors of falling arterial P_{O_2} does not cause a simultaneous reduction of arterial P_{CO_2} and hydrogen ion concentration. On the contrary, the P_{CO_2} and hydrogen ion concentration tend to increase. Therefore the excitatory effect of oxygen lack on breathing is no longer masked by the inhibitory effect of falling arterial CO_2 and hydrogen ion concentration. Under these pathological circumstances the excitation of arterial chemoreceptors can cause a five- to sevenfold excitation of alveolar ventilation (Guyton, 1986, p. 510).

19.9.3 The transducer mechanism

Despite intensive investigations in recent decades, the carotid body has still not fully yielded the secret of how it transduces chemical changes into neuronal activity. The small size and complicated structure of the carotid body have caused even the *location* of the chemosensitive element, let alone the *transducer mechanism* itself, to be hotly disputed.

Three possible elements in the carotid body have been postulated by various research groups as the actual chemoreceptor: (1) the afferent axonal ending, (2) the granular cell, or (3) the sustentacular cell (see Williams *et al.*, 1989, p. 1473). (**1**) The **afferent axonal ending** may be directly excited by a fall in arterial P_{O_2}, the rate of axonal discharge being somehow modulated by the reciprocal synapse on the granular cell. (**2**) The **granular cell** may be directly excited by a fall in arterial P_{O_2}, and may then release a transmitter substance from its granular vesicles in order to drive the axonal ending. (**3**) The **sustentacular cell** may respond to a fall in arterial P_{O_2}, and initiate the discharge of any axonal ending with which it is in contact.

In the last decade, however, a general consensus has developed that the **granular cell** is, in fact, the key element in chemotransduction (Lopez-Barneo *et al.*, 1993). It is, of course, well-known that these cells have cytosolic granules containing catecholamines (and therefore belong to the **APUD** system; Section 2.40), secrete dopamine and other putative transmitters in response to membrane depolarization and hypoxia, and make synapses with the afferent endings of the carotid sinus nerve. These characteristics had persuaded many workers, since de Castro's report of 1928, that the granular cell is likely to be the primary sensory element. Yet the granular cell appeared to be non-excitable, since regenerative electrical activity could not be detected after impaling the cell with a glass microelectrode. However, the patch–clamp technique, which gives low-resistance electrical accessibility to the cell's interior without severely damaging the cell membrane, has proved that granular cells are indeed electrically excitable: they do have large voltage-dependent Na^+, Ca^{2+}, and K^+ currents, and can generate action potentials repetitively: the granular cell has **O_2-sensitive K^+ channels**, their activity being selectively and reversibly inhibited by low P_{O_2}. Thus direct evidence for the chemoreceptive function of the granular cell is at last available (Lopez-Barneo, 1994). In contrast, K^+ currents in the **sustentacular cell** are unaffected by hypoxia. Incidentally, O_2-sensitive K^+ channels have also been found in the **smooth muscle cells** of the pulmonary arteries, thus contributing to the pulmonary vasoconstriction in hypoxic alveoli (Sections 6.30.3, 17.21.1), and in the cells of the **neuroepithelial bodies** of the lung (Section 6.12.1) (Lopez-Barneo, 1994).

The detection of O_2 by the K^+ channels is the first step in a sequence of events triggered by variations in ambient O_2 (Lopez-Barneo, 1994). As in other secretory cells, excitation–secretion coupling appears to depend on Ca^{2+} influx through voltage-gated channels of the plasma membrane; variations in cytosolic Ca^{2+} in turn determine the rate of transmitter release, and hence the level of the resulting excitation of the afferent axons in the chemoreceptor component of the carotid sinus nerve.

Gonzales *et al.* (1992) suggested the following **model for transduction** by the granular cell of the carotid body. Low P_{O_2} inhibits the K^+ channels. This produces the initial depolarization required to activate the voltage-dependent Ca^{2+} channels, and entry of Ca^{2+} then follows. Simultaneous activation of Na^+ channels provides a fast recruitment of Ca^{2+} channels, thus potentiating the entry of Ca^{2+} and the release of neurotransmitters. Ca^{2+}-dependent K^+ channels contribute to cell repolarization. It has been shown that the granular cell releases dopamine in proportion to the intensity of hypoxic or acidic stimulation, and that the release response is paralleled by the electrical activity in the carotid sinus nerve: in other words, the release of neurotransmitter drives the afferent axonal endings. Presumably the release of dopamine by the granular cell occurs at the cell-to-axon component of the **reciprocal synapse** (Fig. 19.6). The role of the axon-to-cell component of the reciprocal synapses still remains unresolved. A recent addition to the model is the suggestion that a haem-linked NADPH oxidase could be the actual oxygen sensor (Acker and Xue, 1995), the production of hydrogen peroxide by the enzyme being diminished during low P_{O_2} stimulation. (See Section 14.31.3 for the production by NADPH of superoxide and thence H_2O_2.)

In competition with this model, it has been proposed that the P_{O_2}-dependent release of neurotransmitter depends on the release of calcium from *intracellular* calcium stores such as the **mitochondria** of the granular cell (Biscoe and Duchen, 1990; Lahiri, 1994). For instance, an apparently low affinity of cytochrome aa_3 for oxygen might lead to loss of calcium from the mitochondria of the granular cell, and hence induce a rise in intracellular calcium during hypoxia. However, Acker and Xue (1995) concluded from the experimental data that hypoxia promotes a rise of intracellular calcium in the granular cells principally through voltage-gated calcium entry, and not by mitochondrial release.

19.9.4 *Regulation of arterial pressure*

The chemoreceptors in the carotid body and aortic bodies respond to a **fall in the oxygen concentration** in arterial blood, or to a rise in the concentration of carbon dioxide or hydrogen ions above normal, by causing a **reflex increase in arterial pressure**. This increase enables the cardiovascular system to transport more oxygen and remove excess carbon dioxide and hydrogen ions from the tissues of the body (Guyton, 1986, p. 250).

The arterial chemoreceptors in the carotid body and aortic bodies also respond to a **fall in arterial pressure**. If the arterial pressure falls below a critical level, the blood flow within the carotid (and aortic) bodies decreases, and this lowers the availability of oxygen to the granular cells; at the same time, the concentration of carbon dioxide and hydrogen ions in the bodies increases because they are now less well washed out by the slow flow of blood. These changes in the blood result in an increased discharge rate in the chemoreceptor axons of the bodies. Some of these axons project to the **medullary cardiovascular 'centre'** in the brainstem (Fig. 19.8). The chemoreceptor signals excite the cardiovascular centre and thus induce a **reflex rise in arterial pressure**. However, this reflex is not a powerful factor in the regulation of arterial pressure, since it only comes strongly into play when the arterial pressure falls below 80 mmHg (10.7 kPa) (Guyton, 1986, p. 250).

The reflex rise in arterial pressure following chemoreceptor stimulation (Comroe, 1975, p. 46; Scott, 1986, p. 98) is achieved by sympathetic excitation leading to a generalized **vasoconstriction**. There is also **tachycardia**. However, the *direct* effect of stimulating the arterial

chemoreceptors is actually **bradycardia**, not tachycardia. The tachycardia is an *indirect* response that overrides the primary bradycardia; the tachycardia results from a respiratory reflex, activated by the increased inflation of the lung that occurs during the increase in ventilation induced by stimulation of the arterial chemoreceptors. The *direct* bradycardia is accompanied by a *direct* negative inotropic effect on the left ventricle, though this, too, is masked by an *indirect* increase in left ventricular performance resulting from the increased inflation of the lung.

19.10 Anatomy of aortic bodies and other ancillary arterial chemoreceptors

During hypoxia the **carotid bodies** provide most of the chemoreceptor input that stimulates breathing. Significant contributions also come from lesser arterial chemoreceptors, the most important of these being the **aortic bodies**.

The **aortic bodies** are small clusters of chemoreceptor tissue, not easily seen without the microscope. Most of them lie on the surfaces of the aortic arch and pulmonary trunk (Fig. 19.5), and there are a few on the root of the right subclavian artery. These sites are consistent with the principle that baroreceptor and chemoreceptor zones lie on the roots of the embryonic arterial arches, since the aorta and right subclavian arteries are derived from the fourth pair of arches and the pulmonary arteries from the sixth pair (Section 19.2).

The **microscopic anatomy** of the aortic bodies is similar to that of the carotid body (Section 19.8). It is therefore characterized by granular cells, sustentacular cells, afferent axonal endings, and very abundant capillaries and sinusoids.

The **arterial supply** comes from the nearest component of the *systemic* circulation, typically from the aorta itself (Fig. 19.5).

The **nerve supply** of the aortic bodies consists essentially of chemoreceptor afferent axons, as does the nerve supply of the carotid body. The fibres from the aortic bodies travel through the vagus nerve (Fig. 19.7A), except in the few species that have a separate **aortic nerve** (Fig. 19.7B). The cell station is in the distal vagal ganglion.

The main functions of the ancillary arterial chemoreceptors are the same as those of the

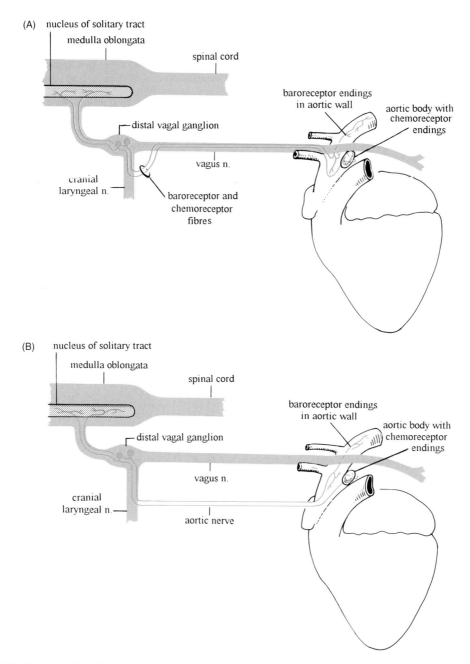

Fig. 19.7 Diagrams showing the course of the aortic nerve fibres.

A. **Semi-independent aortic nerve.** In some mammals the aortic nerve fibres are contained entirely in the vagus, as in Fig. 19.8. In most mammals, however, the aortic nerve fibres (green) ascend the neck within the vagus nerve, but make a loop to join the cranial laryngeal nerve and then return to the vagus as in this diagram. The aortic nerve is then semi-independent.

B. **Fully-independent aortic nerve.** In the rabbit the baroreceptor axons from the aortic arch (green) ascend the neck as a separate aortic nerve, joining the recurrent laryngeal nerve and then continuing centrally within the vagus nerve. This peculiarity in the rabbit enabled the function of the aortic nerve to be discovered more than half a century before that of the far more conspicuous carotid sinus nerve. Because electrical stimulation of the central stump of the cut aortic nerve causes a slowing of the heart and a fall in arterial pressure, the nerve was at first named the 'depressor nerve'. A similar independent form of aortic nerve occurs in the cat on the left side, and has been found in a few other species. The relative proportions of the structures in these diagrams are not to scale.

carotid body. In general, they contribute to the homeostasis of oxygen, carbon dioxide, and hydrogen ions; in particular, they promote an increase in the ventilation of the lung in response to a fall in the oxygen supply to the tissues.

19.10.1 *Terminology for aortic bodies*

Comroe (1964, p. 572) called attention to the many names that have been given to the **aortic bodies** (corpora paraaortica). He advocated the use of 'aortic bodies', for the simple reason that the term 'carotid body' has come into general use and the 'aortic bodies' have the same structure and function. He pointed out that 'bodies' is preferable to '**paraganglia**', because the carotid and aortic bodies have an essentially *receptor* function, whereas the paraganglia are primarily a source of endocrine secretions and therefore have an essentially *effector* function. At the same time, he pointed out that '**glomus**' is not a satisfactory term, since a glomus is essentially a *vascular* structure, whilst it is the *sensory* and not the vascular elements that distinguish the chemoreceptor organs. Mitchell (1953, p. 34) explicitly warned against confusing the paraganglia of the chromaffin system with the carotid body and (what he called) the 'aortic arch bodies' of the autonomic afferent system. However, Mitchell (1953) applied the term 'aortic bodies' to the paraganglia on the aorta: the use of 'aortic arch bodies' and 'aortic bodies' for two totally different structures is surely not advisable. Williams *et al.* (1989, p. 1472) used the term para-aortic bodies for the components of the *chromaffin system* that lie on the *abdominal* aorta, and therefore allocated these structures to the paraganglia (thus departing from the *Nomina Anatomica*, see below): the chemoreceptor bodies on the arch of the aorta were relegated by Williams *et al.* (1989) to 'other small bodies', and not given a specific name.

The nomenclaturists could have clarified this confusion. For the chemoreceptor structures, the *Nomina Anatomica Veterinaria* (1994) adopted glomus caroticum and corpora paraaortica: the *Nomina Histologica* (1994) adopted glomus caroticum, and glomus aorticum and glomus pulmonale. Schaller *et al.* (1992, p. 244) followed the NAV and adopted glomus caroticum and corpora paraaortica; they referred to the *chemoreceptor* characteristics of the glomus caroticum, but defined the corpora paraaortica as *paraganglia*. Thus the NAV and NH have two different names for the same structure (corpora paraaortica and glomus aorticum), and the NH has a third term (glomus pulmonale) which no longer has a physiological basis (see Section 19.10.3). The *Nomina Anatomica* (1989, p. 54) listed corpora para-aortica (hyphenated), placing the term under arcus aortae (and thus divorcing it from the paraganglia, in contrast to Williams *et al.*, 1989).

19.10.2 *Species variations in aortic bodies*

The aortic bodies are not much more than clumps of cells. Consequently their **number** and **location** are difficult to establish, and have been carefully studied in very few species. Comroe (1964, p. 572) assembled the relevant literature, mainly on man, dog, and cat. The dog and cat have well developed aortic bodies, but the mouse and rat have very poorly developed or no aortic bodies (Comroe, 1964, p. 578).

In the **puppy** Nonidez (1937) found about 20 aortic bodies on the arch of the aorta and pulmonary trunk, about 15 of these being scattered over the ventrocaudal aspect of these great trunks; about half a dozen others lay on the dorsocranial aspect as in Fig. 19.5. One or two more were seen on the root of the right subclavian artery. There seems to be great variation within the same species.

The chemoreceptor functions of the **aortic bodies** are of physiological interest, the term 'aortic bodies' being in general use by physiologists (e.g. Smith and Hamlin, 1977, p. 115; Tenney, 1977, p. 196). But the aortic (paraaortic) bodies get rather short shrift in the principal reference works on veterinary anatomy, being omitted, described superficially, or mentioned briefly among paraganglia. A notable exception is the account by Stromberg (1993, p. 791), who incidentally is not averse to the term 'aortic bodies'.

19.10.3 *Blood supply of aortic bodies*

This topic has attracted considerable debate. The close association of aortic bodies with the pulmonary trunk raises the attractive possibility that the blood gases in the mixed venous blood entering the pulmonary circulation might be monitored by chemoreceptors. This led to the concept of a '**glomus pulmonale**' in the adult mammal, a term introduced by Krahl in 1962 and implying a new group of *pulmonary* arterial chemoreceptors (see Comroe, 1964, p. 577).

The developing sixth aortic arch does indeed supply a **pulmonary arterial branch** to aortic bodies on the pulmonary trunk, but in only the *fetus* or *neonate*, as in the human fetus and neonatal kitten (Comroe, 1964, p. 574). However, in the late human fetus the pulmonary arterial supply to these structures is supplemented by branches from the *systemic circulation*, usually from the **left coronary artery**. After birth, the pulmonary arterial branch regresses completely in these species. In young kittens there is a transitional stage between the pulmonary and **systemic arterial** supplies, during which the blood supply is switched from the pulmonary artery to the aorta, this being achieved by intimal proliferation that occludes the pulmonary opening. Comroe (1964, p. 574) pointed out that the occasional presence in the adult cat of a pulmonary vessel represents the persistence of a fetal state, as does a patent ductus arteriosus; thus the disappearance of the pulmonary arterial supply to the aortic bodies should be included among the cardiovascular structural changes that normally occur around the time of birth. Comroe (1964, p. 577; 1975, p. 36) confirmed that experimental perfusion of the adult pulmonary circulation has produced no convincing physiological evidence for the presence of chemoreceptors. The notion of a 'glomus pulmonale' is therefore now generally accepted by physiologists as invalid, and the term has fallen into disuse in the physiological literature although it is retained by the *Nomina Histologica* (1994).

In the adult **dog** the **arterial supply** to the aortic bodies is by a small branch of the **ascending aorta**; in the adult **cat** and **man** it comes from the **coronary artery**, usually the left (Comroe, 1964, pp. 572, 574).

The **venous drainage** of the aortic bodies is always by small veins emptying into the cranial vena cava, either directly or via the left costocervical vein (Comroe, 1964, p. 574).

19.10.4 *Nerve supply of aortic bodies: aortic nerve*

In a few mammalian species the **aortic nerve** or **depressor nerve** (n. depressor) runs from the aortic region as an independent nerve, joining the root of the cranial laryngeal nerve and then continuing centrally in the vagus nerve (Fig. 19.7B). King (1957) named this variant a **fully-independent aortic nerve**. It occurs in the **rabbit**, on both sides of the neck, a disposition that led to its lucky discovery in 1866 by E. Cyon, then a postgraduate student (King, 1956a). Reprimanded for idleness and threatened with dismissal by Professor K.F. Ludwig, his supervisor and Director of the Leipzig Institute of Physiology, Cyon put stimulating electrodes under all the nerves he could find in a rabbit's neck. One of them induced a profound fall in arterial pressure when its central stump was stimulated: this was the **aortic nerve**, or 'depressor nerve' as Cyon and Ludwig named it. This discovery of an afferent control mechanism for regulating arterial pressure was one of the outstanding physiological events of the century. It preceded by over half a century the discovery of the similar function of the **carotid sinus nerve** by Hering and his postgraduate student E. Koch (contemporaries of these events affirmed that Koch made the discovery and Hering got the credit), although the carotid sinus nerve is anatomically so much more conspicuous than the aortic nerve throughout the mammalian orders. The discovery of the depressor nerve and its functions transformed Cyon's status from impending disgrace to one of instant fame. In 1870, he was awarded the Gold Medal of the Paris Academy, and 2 years later at the age of only 29 was appointed to the Chair of Anatomy and Physiology in the Medical School at St. Petersburg. A fully independent aortic nerve also occurs on the left side of the **cat**, and a similar

form has been found in the **badger** (*Meles meles*) (Amoroso *et al.*, 1951). Grau (1943, p. 964) found evidence in the literature for its occurrence in the **pig** also.

It is stated (e.g. Mitchell, 1953, p. 251; Comroe, 1964, p. 574) that, in species lacking an independent aortic nerve, the afferent fibres from the aortic bodies are usually incorporated within the **recurrent laryngeal nerve**. This seems to have originated from an anatomical study published at the beginning of the nineteenth century, and appears to lack physiological confirmation. Anatomical observations on a large number of domestic and wild species within the orders Carnivora, Perissodactyla, Artiodactyla, Rodentia, Insectivora and Primates by several authors between 1880 and 1924 (see Heymans *et al.*, 1933, p. 11; Grau, 1943, p. 965, and King, 1957) suggested that the afferent fibres from the aorta typically ascend the neck in the main trunk of the vagus nerve as far as the root of the **cranial laryngeal nerve**. Here they briefly detach themselves from the vagus, join the cranial laryngeal nerve, and then immediately return to the vagus nerve (Fig. 19.7B). King (1957) referred to this as a **semi-independent aortic nerve**. Physiological support for this pathway appears to be absent in most species. However, in the horse electrical stimulation showed the entire contingent of afferent baroreceptor fibres of the aortic nerve to be dispersed throughout the main trunk of the vagus nerve in the cranial part of the neck as in Fig. 19.8 (King, 1957). On the left side, but not on the right, a substantial proportion of these fibres make a detour through the fan-like root of the cranial laryngeal nerve much as in Fig. 19.7A, thus foreshadowing the tendency for independence of the nerve on the left side in other species.

19.10.5 *Anatomy of other ancillary arterial chemoreceptors*

Comroe (1964, pp. 576–579) surveyed the evidence for the existence of other arterial chemoreceptors. The most convincing seem to be small **abdominal bodies**, identical histologically with the carotid body, lying on the right vagus nerve and the gastric artery in the abdomen of the mouse and rat, generally between the diaphragm and the coeliac plexus. Sinclair (1987) cited experimental evidence that the afferent pathway enters the vagus nerves immediately caudal to their emergence from the diaphragm. Abdominal bodies have not been found in species such as the dog and cat which have well-developed aortic bodies.

Some of the major branches of the external carotid arteries of the rat, cat, and rabbit, appear to be accompanied by chemoreceptor bodies, innervated by the glossopharyngeal nerve (though not by the carotid sinus nerve itself) (Sinclair, 1987). These could reasonably be known as **cervical bodies**. After denervation of the carotid bodies, and of all possible chemoreceptor bodies in the thorax and abdomen, there is still a residual ventilatory response to hypoxia in the rat attributable to 'cervical bodies'.

A **coccygeal body** consisting of 'epithelioid cells' and sinusoidal capillaries is related to the coccyx in man and coccygeal vertebrae in many mammals (Williams *et al.*, 1989, p. 1475). Histologically it has no clear affiliation to either the chromaffin system or the carotid body. Details of innervation, ultrastructure, and function are awaited.

A **tympanic body** (**jugular glomus**) occurs in the adventitia of the internal jugular vein near the tympanic membrane. Histologically it resembles the carotid body and may have a similar function (Williams *et al.*, 1989, p. 1475).

Physiological evidence for a chemoreceptor function has been obtained for these ancillary structures (Section 19.11).

19.11 Physiology of aortic bodies and other ancillary arterial chemoreceptors

The aortic bodies and the other ancillary arterial chemoreceptors function like the carotid body, by stimulating breathing in response to a fall in the P_{O_2}, and increase in the concentration of CO_2 and hydrogen ions, in arterial blood.

The evidence for the **respiratory function** of the ancillary arterial chemoreceptors is based on denervation experiments in small laboratory mammals. Progressive denervation of the carotid bodies, 'cervical bodies', aortic bodies, and abdominal bodies has shown that all of them contribute to the regulation of breathing, but the carotid bodies dominate; the ancillary arterial chemoreceptor tissues (Sinclair, 1987) seem to provide a safety margin, thus constituting an *inherent redundancy* similar to the apparent over-provision of diffusion shown by the anatomical diffusing capacity of the lung for oxygen (Section 6.27).

After apparently total denervation, there is still a residual stimulation of breathing in severe hypoxia in the goat, calf, dog, cat, rabbit, and rat. This may arise from as yet unrecognized arterial chemoreceptor tissues; or it may be of central origin, and would then be contrary to the classical central depression of hypoxia.

The **cardiovascular responses** to stimulation of the chemoreceptors of the aortic bodies differ somewhat from those of the carotid body. Stimulation of the carotid body is followed by a rise in arterial pressure with tachycardia. But the tachycardia is a respiratory reflex, arising *indirectly* from the increased inflation of the lung and masking a direct bradycardia (Section 19.9.4). Simulation of the aortic bodies causes a *direct* reflex tachycardia and a positive inotropic effect on the myocardium

(Scott, 1986, p. 98). Furthermore stimulation of the aortic bodies in the dog produces pulmonary vasoconstriction, whereas stimulation of the carotid body does not (Comroe, 1975, p. 47).

19.12 Central neuronal pathways of arterial baroreceptor reflexes

The baroreceptor reflex arc (Fig. 19.8) comprises (i) an *afferent component*, arising from the carotid sinus and aortic arch and projecting to the brainstem, (ii) a *central component* in the brainstem, integrating the afferent input with the efferent output, and (iii) an *efferent component*, consisting of the autonomic efferent output to the heart and blood vessels.

The *afferent component* consists of **primary afferent neurons** (Section 1.4). The axons of the neurons form the carotid sinus nerve and the aortic nerve. The **carotid sinus nerve** (Section 19.7.3) is a branch of the glossopharyngeal cranial nerve (Figs 19.1, 19.2). The baroreceptor endings are in the wall of the carotid sinus or aortic arch, and are excited by a rise in arterial pressure (Section 19.4). The baroreceptor neurons of the carotid sinus nerve have their cell stations in the distal glossopharyngeal ganglion (Section 4.17.1), and project their axons centrally into the beginning of the *central component*, i.e. into the nucleus of the solitary tract (Fig. 19.8). The baroreceptor fibres of the **aortic nerve** ascend the neck either in the vagus (Fig. 19.8), or as an independent nerve (Fig. 19.7B). They have their cell stations in the distal vagal ganglion (Section 4.17.1), and project their axons centrally into the nucleus of the solitary tract (Fig. 19.8).

The **nucleus of the solitary tract** is the autonomic afferent nucleus of the brainstem (Sections 1.5, 11.7). It receives the many incoming autonomic afferent projections from the body. Some of its neurons make synapses with the incoming baroreceptor axons. These neurons of the nucleus of the solitary tract now form the second neuron in the baroreceptor reflex arc. They project their axons into the 'cardiovascular centre' of the brainstem (Fig. 19.8).

In the '**cardiovascular centre**', the baroreceptor reflex pathway divides into two; one of these becomes an essentially parasympathetic, and the

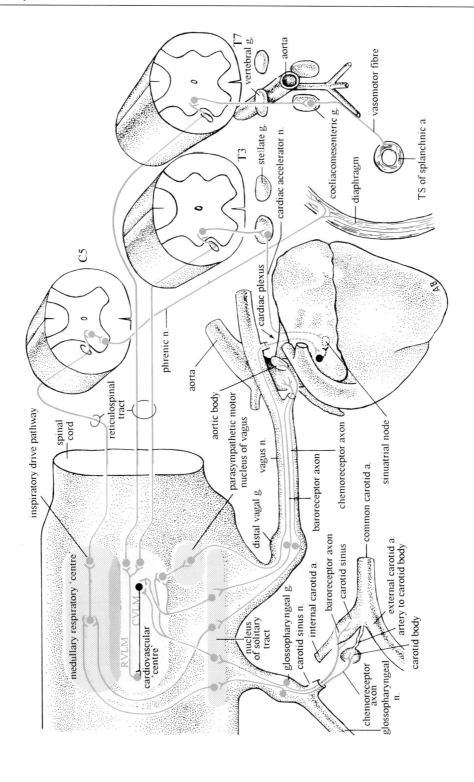

other an essentially sympathetic pathway. The *parasympathetic pathway* consists of neurons that project into the **parasympathetic nucleus of the vagus** (Fig. 19.8), where they make synapses with **preganglionic cardiac vagal neurons**. These preganglionic neurons form the **parasympathetic** part of the *efferent component of the baroreceptor reflex*. Their axons descend through the **vagus nerve** and into the **cardiac plexus**, to the region of the **sinuatrial node** (Fig. 19.8). Near the node, the preganglionic cardiac vagal axons synapse with the short **postganglionic cardiac vagal neurons** that project mainly upon the **nodal cells** of the sinuatrial node (and also on the myocardium). Of this chain of neurons from the baroreceptor endings to the sinuatrial node (schematically, five in number in Fig. 19.8), the first four are *excitatory* in function. Therefore excitation of the baroreceptor endings in the carotid sinus or aortic arch culminates in excitation of the postganglionic cardiac vagal neuron that projects onto the nodal cell in the sinuatrial node. The postganglionic cardiac vagal neuron *inhibits* the nodal cell in the sinuatrial node, thus slowing the heart (Section 22.8.2).

The *sympathetic pathway* in the 'cardiovascular centre' begins with an *inhibitory* neuron (black in Fig. 19.8). This neuron projects onto an excitatory neuron in the 'cardiovascular centre'. The excitatory neuron in turn projects onto the **sympathetic** part of the *efferent component* of the baroreceptor reflex. This consists of two columns of sympathetic axons that descend through the spinal cord in the reticulospinal tract (Fig. 19.8) as two functionally distinct groups, one *cardiac* and the other *vasomotor*.

The *cardiac* sympathetic fibres make synapses with preganglionic neurons in the **lateral horn** of the first five segments of the thoracic spinal cord. These preganglionic neurons then synapse with sympathetic postganglionic neurons in the **stellate ganglion** or in the sympathetic vertebral ganglia of the fourth and fifth thoracic segments (Fig. 19.8). The axons of the postganglionic neurons have their effector endings close to the nodal cells of the sinuatrial node and atrioventricular node, and also close to the cardiac muscle cells of the atrial and ventricular myocardium (Section 22.8.1). Their function is to increase the rate and force of cardiac contraction. They are sometimes known as **cardiac accelerator fibres** (Section 2.10.1).

The *vasomotor* sympathetic fibres make synapses with preganglionic neurons in the **lateral horn** of the spinal cord of thoracic segments 6–10; the axons of these preganglionic neurons make synapses in the **coeliacomesenteric ganglion** with postganglionic neurons. The axons of the postganglionic neurons are vasomotor fibres,

Fig. 19.8 Schematic wiring diagram of the arterial baroreceptor and chemoreceptor reflexes. Excitatory neurons are green: only two neurons are inhibitory, and these are black. Two baroreceptor reflex arcs are shown, one from the carotid sinus and the other from the aortic arch. The afferent baroreceptor neuron innervating the carotid sinus projects through the carotid sinus nerve to its cell station in the distal glossopharyngeal ganglion, and from there to the nucleus of the solitary tract, where the first synapse in the reflex arc occurs. The afferent baroreceptor neuron innervating the aortic arch projects through the vagus nerve to its cell station in the distal vagal ganglion, and from there to the first synapse in the arc in the nucleus of the solitary tract. In both of the baroreceptor arcs, the second neuron (in the nucleus of the solitary tract) projects into the caudal region of the 'cardiovascular centre' (a region known as the caudal ventrolateral medulla, CVLM). Here the pathway of the arc divides. The parasympathetic pathway projects onto preganglionic neurons in the parasympathetic nucleus of the vagus. These neurons send their axons through the vagus and cardiac plexus to synapse with inhibitory postganglionic vagal fibres innervating the sinuatrial node, and thus slow the heart. The sympathetic pathway synapses with an inhibitory neuron (black). This projects into the rostral part of the 'cardiovascular centre' (a region known as the rostral ventrolateral medulla, RVLM). Here it inhibits the excitatory neuron at the top of the sympathetic cardiac accelerator and vasomotor pathways, that culminate in postganglionic neurons in the stellate and coeliacomesenteric ganglia. Inhibition of these sympathetic pathways slows the heart and causes splanchnic vasodilation. Note that the axons innervating the sinuatrial node are drawn as broken lines to show that they are on the right atrium, and not the left atrium as the diagram seems to suggest.

Two chemoreceptor reflex arcs are shown, one from the carotid body and the other from an aortic body. The neuronal pathways are essentially the same as for the baroreceptors, as far as the projections into the nucleus of the solitary tract. From the nucleus of the solitary tract, neurons project into the medullary respiratory 'centre' (again, in the rostral ventrolateral medulla, RVLM). Then a short neuron projects to the top of the inspiratory drive pathway, followed by a sequence of neurons to the ventral horn in cervical segments C5, 6, and 7 and hence to the phrenic nerve, or to the thoracic ventral horn and intercostal nerves. The reticulospinal pathway to the ventral horn may be contralateral as in Fig. 11.1.

supplying the vasculature of the gastrointestinal tract (the so-called splanchnic vascular bed). Their function is to cause vasoconstriction throughout the splanchnic vascular bed (Section 13.3.2), by means of appropriate adjustments of resting sympathetic tone (Section 13.3.3).

In these two chains of neurons that end in sympathetic projections to the heart and blood vessels (schematically, seven in each chain in Fig. 19.8), all of them are *excitatory* except the third (the black one, in Fig. 19.8) which is *inhibitory*. This means that excitation of the first two by baroreceptor stimulation in the carotid sinus or aortic arch, stimulates the third, *inhibitory*, neuron in the 'cardiovascular centre'. This inhibitory neuron now inhibits the activity of the rest of the neurons in both chains, and thus slows the heart and dilates the vasculature of the gastrointestinal tract.

Thus both the parasympathetic and the sympathetic elements in the *efferent component* of the baroreceptor reflex have the function of restoring an *elevated* arterial pressure to normal levels. The baroreceptor reflex is therefore an example of negative feedback.

On the other hand, if arterial pressure *falls* (for example, as a result of haemorrhage), the rate of discharge of the baroreceptor fibres in the carotid sinus and aortic arch decreases. The vagal pathway from the parasympathetic vagal nucleus to the sinuatrial node then becomes less active, thus reducing vagal inhibition of the heart. Consequently the heart rate goes up. At the same time, the inhibitory neuron in the sympathetic efferent pathway to the heart and gastrointestinal vasculature becomes less active. This lifts the brake off the tonic activity of the sympathetic vasomotor pathways. Consequently the peripheral arterial resistance increases. Simultaneously the splanchnic and cutaneous veins of the venous reservoirs (Section 12.16.3) are constricted, thus increasing the venous return to the heart (Section 13.3.5). The combination of increased heart rate, increased peripheral resistance, and increased venous return, *restores* the falling arterial pressure to its normal level.

By correcting either a rise or a fall in arterial pressure, the baroreceptor reflex carries out its basic function of contributing to homeostasis (Section 19.1).

The concept of a '**centre**' within the central nervous system signifies a fairly well circumscribed region with a particular function (Section 1.5). Respiratory, cardiac, vasomotor and other functional 'centres' in the brain have often been postulated to express the results of physiological experiments based, for example, on focal stimulation or ablation. Williams *et al.* (1989, p. 996) regarded the functional relationships attributed to particular reticular nuclei as speculative. Brodal (1981, p. 753) remarked that the concept of 'centres' is 'becoming less and less attractive and less acceptable as our insight into the organization of the nervous system increases'. Such doubts seem particularly applicable to 'centres' in the reticular formation, in view of the overwhelming complications of its multisynaptic connections. However, the term is retained here for descriptive convenience.

Aspects of the central component of the baroreceptor pathway were reviewed by Sved and Gordon (1994). The baroreceptor axons project into a discrete part of the **nucleus of the solitary tract**. From there, there is an excitatory projection into the **reticular formation** of the **caudal ventrolateral medulla**, but this may well be polysynaptic rather than monosynaptic, although it is shown as monosynaptic in Fig. 19.8. Inhibitory neurons project from the caudal ventrolateral medulla to the **rostral ventrolateral medulla**, which is a reticular formation just caudal to the motor nucleus of the facial nerve. This inhibitory pathway is probably monosynaptic, as shown in Fig. 19.8. The most likely **neurotransmitter** in this inhibitory link is the inhibitory amino acid, GABA; the neurotransmitter of the excitatory synapses appears to be another amino acid, glutamate.

The **nucleus of the solitary tract** also receives an afferent input from higher centres, by means of descending projections (Tenney, 1993). These arise especially from the defence area of the **hypothalamus**. When stimulated by conditions of *fight and flight*, the hypothalamic projections inhibit the input from the peripheral baroreceptors (e.g. from the carotid sinus). This inhibition permits a rise in heart rate and arterial pressure, as at the onset of exercise.

The **reticular formation** of the rostral ventrolateral medulla has emerged as a region of the brainstem that is critically involved in the central neural control of both circulation and respiration (Kuwaki *et al.*, 1995); this region may even contain the answer to the riddle (Section 11.2) – where is the rhythm of breathing generated? The rostral ventrolateral medulla is the top of the excitatory **sympathetic pathway** that descends through the spinal cord in a reticulospinal tract (Fig. 19.8) to activate the sympathetic preganglionic neurons in the thoracic lateral horn that regulate cardiac and vasomotor tone. Also the rostral ventrolateral medulla lies immediately dorsal to, and in direct contact with, the **central chemoreceptor area**, which is the ventral surface of this particular region of the medulla oblongata

(Section 11.10); vasomotor neurons in the rostral ventrolateral medulla project dendritic connections within the central chemoreceptor area (Kuwaki *et al.*, 1995).

The **parasympathetic vagal pathway** is uncertain in several aspects. The site of its divergence from the baroreceptor reflex pathway is unsure. In Fig. 19.8 the divergence is represented as an indirect polysynaptic relay from the nucleus of the solitary tract to the reticular formation of the caudal ventrolateral medulla, and from there to the preganglionic cell body in the **parasympathetic nucleus of the vagus** (nucleus parasympathicus nervi vagi). It may, however, be a direct relay from the nucleus of the solitary tract to the preganglionic neuronal cell body (Sved and Gordon, 1994). A further source of dispute is the actual **site of the preganglionic cardiac cell bodies**. The earlier literature was reviewed by Brodal (1981, p. 702). The classical neuroanatomical view is that the neurons of the autonomic efferent component of the vagus, including of course its cardiac efferent fibres, have their cell station in the **parasympathetic nucleus of the vagus** (also known as the **dorsal motor nucleus of the vagus**); the **nucleus ambiguus** is regarded as a special visceral efferent nucleus, innervating the striated 'branchial' musculature of the pharynx and larynx. In the last four decades, however, some experiments based on degeneration, labelling, and stimulation have indicated that vagal cardiac neurons may originate in the **nucleus ambiguus**; on the other hand, other similar experiments have confirmed their location in the parasympathetic vagal nucleus. In a survey of this dispute, Williams *et al.* (1989, p. 1114) acknowledged the claims on behalf of the nucleus ambiguus, but nevertheless stated that the dorsal motor nucleus of the vagus distributes motor fibres to the heart. Sven and Gordon (1994) concluded that the vagal preganglionic neurons are situated 'primarily' in the nucleus ambiguus, but conceded that the parasympathetic component of the baroreceptor reflex has been less extensively studied than the sympathetic component.

19.13   Central neuronal pathways of arterial chemoreceptor reflexes

Like the baroreceptor reflex arc, the chemoreceptor reflex arc (Fig. 19.8) comprises (i) an *afferent component*, arising from the carotid body and aortic bodies and projecting to the brainstem, (ii) a *central component* in the brainstem, integrating the afferent input with the efferent output, and (iii) an *efferent component*, consisting of the efferent output to the inspiratory muscles.

The *afferent component* is formed by the carotid sinus nerve and the aortic nerve (Fig. 19.8). The chemoreceptor neurons of the carotid body project their axons through the carotid sinus nerve to the distal glossopharyngeal ganglion, and from there to the beginning of the *central component* of the reflex arc, i.e. to the **nucleus of the solitary tract**; the chemoreceptor neurons of the aortic bodies project their axons through the aortic nerve to the distal vagal ganglion, and from there to the nucleus of the solitary tract (Fig. 19.8). In the nucleus of the solitary tract the axons of the chemoreceptor neurons make synapses with neurons that project into the **medullary respiratory 'centre'** (Section 11.2). Here they excite the *efferent component* of the chemoreceptor reflex by stimulating the neurons at the top of the **inspiratory drive pathway** (Sections 11.2, 11.3), and thus activate the diaphragm and inspiratory intercostal muscles through the **phrenic nerve** (Fig. 19.8) and **intercostal nerves**.

By inducing an increase in breathing in response to a fall in the oxygen concentration in the blood, or to a rise in the concentration of CO_2 or hydrogen ions, the arterial chemoreceptors contribute to homeostasis.

Yamada *et al.* (1988) concluded from the literature that the dorsolateral marginal zone of the nucleus of the solitary tract is the central terminal site of the chemoreceptor fibres of the carotid sinus nerve. The bilateral or contralateral disposition, and monosynaptic connections, of the inspiratory neurons in the reticulospinal tracts are considered in Section 11.3.

Chapter 20
Anatomy of the Heart

20.1 The work of the heart

The heart has a short diastolic rest after each systole, but otherwise cannot stop even on Sundays.

The work performed by the human heart at rest in 1 hour is roughly equivalent to raising 100 kg to the ceiling of a room, 4.2 m high. During severe exercise the work output of the heart may increase 6–8-fold. This formidable energetic task obviously requires an equally remarkable blood supply. At rest, the coronary circulation takes between 3 and 5% of the total cardiac output (Section 18.3), and yet this is a very small organ forming only about 0.6% of the total body mass of a mammal (Section 20.4).

Calculations by Muir (1971, p. 3) estimated the work of the resting human heart to be 4.12 kilojoules per hour. During very severe exercise, work per hour may increase to 35 kJ. Four hours of heavy work would therefore require 140 kJ. The remaining 20 hours of the day at rest would entail about 82 kJ. The total work of the heart during a 24 hour day could then be about 222 kJ, or 6216 kJ for a month. The lettering on a packet of castor sugar informs us that 100 g yields about 1700 kJ; therefore work of 6216 kJ is equivalent to the energy in about 366 g of sugar. A trip to the supermarket in 1998 would buy you 1 kg of sugar for about 89 pence, so the cost of 366 g would be about 33 pence or $0.5. So the human heart is an impressive machine: it costs about 33 pence a month to run, repairs itself as it goes along, and is expected to work continuously for three score years and ten.

By far the largest part of the energy that the heart converts into work is used to transport the blood from the veins at low pressure to the arteries at high pressure: this is *potential energy* expressed as *pressure*. Expenditure of energy is also needed to accelerate the blood into the arteries: this is *kinetic energy*, expressed as *blood flow*. The kinetic energy of the left ventricle normally accounts for only about 1% of its total work. However, if the aortic valve is stenosed (Section 15.10) the blood may have to be forced through at such high velocity that 50% of the total work output is required to create the kinetic energy of blood flow (Guyton, 1986, p. 157).

20.2 Pericardium

In the embryo, the pleura and the pericardium arise side by side, from (a) the splanchnic mesoderm that suspends the endocardial tubes (Fig. 8.27), and (b) the pleuropericardial folds (Figs 8.27, 8.28) that project from the somatic mesoderm of the lateral body wall (Sections 8.12.1, 8.12.2).

Having shared common embryonic origins, so the pleura and pericardium have similar anatomical relationships to the organs that they envelop in the fully developed body. Thus the anatomical relationship of the pericardium to the heart is essentially the same as the relationship of the pleura to the lung. The pericardium is a **serous sac** deeply invaginated by the heart, just as the serous pleural sac is invaginated by the lung (Section 9.1). The term 'serous' is appropriate for both of these membranes, because the sac is closed and its lining is a simple squamous epithelium.

The inner wall of the pericardial sac coats the surface of the heart and is conveniently known as the **visceral pericardium**. At the neck of the pericardial sac, the visceral pericardium continues into the outer wall of the sac, the **parietal pericardium**, by means of a mesentery-like connection (Fig. 9.1). The visceral pleura blends with the surface of the lung and is named the pulmonary pleura: similarly, the visceral pericardium blends with the surface of the heart. This blending is so intimate that the visceral pericardium is regarded as an integral part of the wall of the heart, and consequently is often known as the **epicardium**.

The external surface of the parietal pericardium is reinforced by a strong layer of fibroelastic tissue, the **fibrous pericardium**. The outer surface of the fibrous pericardium is in turn attached by connective tissue to the **pericardiac pleura** of the **mediastinum** (Fig. 9.1).

The **pericardial cavity** is normally occupied by a thin film of (serous) **pericardial fluid**, just as the pleural cavity is occupied by a thin film of (serous) pleural fluid (Section 9.6). The pericardial fluid and pleural fluid have important lubricatory functions, enabling the visceral and parietal layers of their membranes to slide over each other during every cardiac and respiratory cycle. The pericardial and pleural fluids share the same pressure changes during the respiratory cycle (Section 10.4). At rest the pressure is below atmospheric, falling lower during inspiration and rising above atmospheric during forced expiration. The fall in pressure during inspiration is transmitted to the heart, promoting an increase in venous return.

The **cardiac notch** (Fig. 5.5) is the gap in the ventral border of the left and right lungs that allows the pericardium to make contact with the thoracic wall (Section 5.6.2). In some species, fluid can be withdrawn from the pericardial cavity through the cardiac notch by pericardiocentesis (Section 25.2) or pericardiotomy (Section 25.4). The cardiac notch also provides a useful 'acoustic window' for echocardiography (Section 24.15).

The formal *nomenclature* for the **pericardium**, as adopted by the NAV of 1994, approaches the term from a different standpoint from that of the terminology used above. The pericardium is considered to comprise two main components, the fibrous pericardium (pericardium fibrosum) and the serous pericardium (pericardium serosum) (see Schaller *et al.*, 1992, p. 234). The **serous pericardium** is said to be divided into a **parietal lamina** (lamina parietalis) and a **visceral lamina** (lamina visceralis), which correspond respectively to the parietal pericardium and visceral pericardium, as above. These terms for the pericardium are shown in Fig. 8.29.

Dorsally the pericardium continues over the great vessels, enclosing the aorta, the pulmonary trunk as far as the bifurcation into the left and right pulmonary arteries, and the caudal vena cava, but not the pulmonary veins (Getty, 1975, p. 165). By means of dorsal extensions of the fibrous pericardium beyond the aorta and onto the dorsal region of the **endothoracic fascia** (Section 9.8), the pericardium suspends the heart from the vertebral column (Schummer *et al.*, 1981, p. 16). A tunnel-shaped part of the pericardial cavity, the **sinus transversus pericardii**, extends between the fused aorta and pulmonary trunk on the one hand, and the adjacent walls of the atria on the other (Simoens, 1992, p. 234).

Ventrally the fibrous pericardium escapes from the ventral mediastinum between the left and right sheets of mediastinal pleurae, and attaches to the endothoracic fascia of the sternum as the paired **sternopericardiac ligaments** of ruminants, and the midline **sternopericardiac ligament** of the horse; in the carnivores and pig, the **phrenicopericardiac ligament** (Section 9.4) likewise escapes from the caudal mediastinum, and attaches to the diaphragm (Simoens, 1992, p. 234). These ligaments anchor the heart in position, ventrally and caudally. For the relationships of these ligaments to the mediastinum, see Section 9.4.

There are differences of opinion about whether or not the pericardial sac is distensible. The main histological element of the **fibrous pericardium** is dense collagenous connective tissue (Williams *et al.*, 1989, p. 696). However, this is apparently arranged in several strata, the fibres of which run in various directions (Schummer *et al.*, 1981, p. 16), intermingled with a considerable quantity of elastic fibres (Krstik, 1984, p. 322). Such structure might allow some stretching. However, the fibrous pericardium has been described as 'non-distensible' (Muir, 1971), although Williams *et al.* (1989, p. 695) regarded this idea as 'entirely speculative'. Nevertheless the strong collagenous structure of the fibrous pericardium must inevitably limit the immediate distension of the normal pericardial sac. On the other hand, there can be no doubt whatever that the sac distends if the heart undergoes *gradual* hypertrophy through athletic training or pathology (Section 20.4).

Inflammation of the pericardium (**pericarditis**) may lead to an accumulation of fluid in the pericardial cavity (cavum pericardii); suppurative pericarditis is relatively common in cattle following traumatic reticulitis (Section 25.4). **Pericardial effusion** may also arise from haemorrhage into the pericardial sac, originating from trauma or bleeding from neoplasms. **Cardiac tamponade** (compression of the heart) caused by pericardial effusions may cause the pressure in the pericardial cavity to become critically high, exceeding the diastolic pressure in the right atrium and/or preventing the ventricles from accepting a full load of blood. Chronic cardiac tamponade may lead to right heart failure, and acute tamponade may lower cardiac output to the point of collapse or death (Darke *et al.*, 1996, p. 123). **Pericardiocentesis** (Section 25.2) is required for both diagnosis and treatment of pericardial effusions.

Pericardioperitoneal hernia (Section 8.14.3) can arise from a congenital defect in the ventral part of the diaphragm, allowing abdominal viscera to enter the pericardial cavity and to disturb cardiac or digestive functions. The condition is relatively common in the cat (Darke *et al.*, 1996, p. 123).

20.3 Functional organization of the heart

20.3.1 *Primer pumps and power pumps*

The heart consists of four separate pumps, i.e. two **primer pumps** and two **power pumps**. The left and right **atria** are the primer pumps. By their contraction they top up the filling of the ventricles thus increasing the effectiveness of the ventricles. The left and right **ventricles** are the power pumps. By their contraction they provide the major source of power for driving blood through the systemic and pulmonary vascular systems. Physiologically and clinically the right atrium and right ventricle together are often referred to as the *right heart*, and the left atrium and left ventricle as the *left heart*, as in right heart failure and left heart failure (Section 22.17).

20.3.2 *Atria*

The left and right atria act mainly as reservoirs for the filling of the ventricles. The (postnatal) **right atrium** receives deoxygenated blood from the veins of the systemic circulation, via the cranial and caudal venae cavae and the coronary and bronchial inflow. The blood goes through the right atrioventricular ostium, guarded by the three cusps of the right atrioventricular (tricuspid) valve, and thus into the right ventricle. The (postnatal) **left atrium** receives oxygenated blood from the lungs via the pulmonary veins. It also receives a small volume of deoxygenated blood from the small coronary veins and bronchial veins, constituting a venous-to-arterial shunt (Section 18.8). Left atrial blood passes through the left atrioventricular ostium, guarded by the two cusps of the left atrioventricular (mitral or bicuspid) valve, and so into the left ventricle.

20.3.3 *Ventricles*

Contraction of the **right ventricle** closes the right atrioventricular valve and then, as the pressure continues to rise, opens the pulmonary valve. Blood now flows via the conus arteriosus, through the ostium of the pulmonary trunk, past the three sinuses of the pulmonary trunk, and into the pulmonary arteries. Since the pulmonary circulation in the postnatal animal is a low resistance pathway (Section 17.12), the right ventricle operates at low pressures.

Contraction of the **left ventricle** closes the left atrioventricular valve, and shortly afterwards opens the aortic valve. Blood now flows through the aortic ostium, past the three aortic sinuses but also into the coronary arteries, and onwards into all the rest of the vast systemic arterial tree. The postnatal systemic circulation is a high resistance pathway, and therefore the left ventricle operates at much higher pressures than the right ventricle.

20.3.4 *Transition of the heart at birth*

At the beginning of Chapter 16 some remarkable functional differences between prenatal and postnatal hearts were mentioned. In the *prenatal* heart, the two ventricles pump *in parallel* (Section 16.1). They share a common arterial outlet into the same arterial network: it is a *shared* arterial network, because the massive ductus arteriosus directly unites the systemic arterial bed with the pulmonary arterial bed (Fig. 16.1). The sharing of the arterial network makes it possible for the prenatal left and right ventricles to pump vastly different volumes of blood per unit time. In fact the **right ventricle** pumps nearly twice as much blood per unit time as the left. Therefore before birth, the right ventricle is doing much more work than the left (Section 16.1).

Shortly after birth (within the first hour in the lamb), the output of the left ventricle equals that of the right (Section 16.15). Indeed in the *immediately* postnatal animal the left ventricular output briefly though substantially exceeds the right – until the ductus arteriosus closes (Section 16.21). As soon as the ductus arteriosus closes, the two ventricles are pumping *in series*. From now on, in the normal heart the mean output per unit time of each ventricle is essentially the same, since with two pumps in series what goes into the right side must come out of the left. There is, however, a small excess of left ventricular output over right (about 1 or 2%), caused by the bronchial and coronary circulations (Section 18.8).

After the first breath several other cardiovascular parameters change. (1) The inflation of the lung instantly converts the pulmonary circulation into a low resistance pathway, whereas the loss of the placenta converts the systemic circulation into a high resistance pathway (Section 16.14). Consequently the work load of the two ventricles is now reversed – the left ventricle is suddenly doing much more work than the right. (2) In response to this change in energetic demand, the myocardium of the left ventricle becomes much thicker than that of the right (Section 16.15). (3) The energetic cost of embryonic tissue growth, which caused the heart to work at full capacity throughout gestation and renders the neonate vulnerable to physiological stress (Section 16.1), now begins to decline relatively; this allows the neonatal cardiac output (the output of the left ventricle) per kilogram of body mass to *decrease* rapidly to less than one quarter of the combined left and right ventricular output of the fetus (Section 16.15). Such reduction in the postnatal cardiac output enables the heart to build up reserves for dealing with physiological emergencies.

The total volume of blood makes a complete circuit through the whole circulatory system, systemic and pulmonary, about once a minute at rest and (in man) up to six times a minute at exercise.

20.4   Size of the heart

The heart is disconcertingly small, considering its responsibilities. In **mammals in general** it typically forms only about 0.6% of the total body mass. Despite this small value, the myocardium accounts for at least 3% of cardiac output (Section 18.3), a mass-specific value that is about sixfold greater than the mass-specific value of the size of the heart itself.

In the **greyhound** and **Thoroughbred horse** the mass of the heart relative to total body mass is about twice as great as that of mammals in general (i.e. it is about 1% of the total body mass). This value increases still further in response to the energetic demands of **athletic training**, reaching at least 1.1% in greyhounds and Thoroughbreds. The relatively large mass of the heart in these two athletic breeds produces a relatively *large stroke volume*.

Much greater enlargement of the heart (to about two and a half times its normal mass) can occur in **disease conditions** that overload the left ventricle, such as aortic stenosis (Section 15.10).

These increases in heart mass can be achieved *only* by **hypertrophy** of pre-existing muscle cells. The *total number of cardiac muscle cells* increases progressively up to the time of birth, but in the first 1 or 2 weeks after birth mitosis slows down and then virtually stops. After that, there is virtually no addition of new muscle cells in the normal heart. Thus the postnatal myocardium has no power whatever of regeneration (Section 21.1.3).

Schmidt-Nielsen (1990, p. 102) reported data for a range of mammals, great and small, showing that the average mass of the mammalian heart is about 0.59% of the body mass. Schummer *et al.* (1981, pp. 43–63) assembled the following measurements for the domestic mammals: dog, 0.73% in 14 breeds; cat, 0.5%; pig, 0.30% in five breeds; ox, 0.52% in 15 cattle; horse, 0.78% in 104 animals, with the lowest value of 0.6% in heavy draft horses, 0.62–0.99% in the lighter breeds, and the highest value of 1.04% in Thoroughbreds. Steward *et al.* (1975) found a range of 0.73–0.82% in normal dogs. Evans (1994, p. 130) reported a mean value of 0.94% for untrained and 1.1% for trained Thoroughbreds. Snow (1985) noted a value of 1.2% in greyhounds. Clearly the more energetic domestic species such as the **dog** and **horse** have much larger hearts (relative to body size) than the other domestic species.

The very small size of the heart in the **pig** may be a factor in the '*sudden death syndrome*' in this species (Dyce *et al.*, 1987, p. 743). Selective breeding for early maturation in pigs seems to have caused body mass to have outrun cardiac performance, especially in fat breeds.

The large cardiac **stroke volume** that comes from the huge heart of the racing breeds (greyhound and Thoroughbred), combined with an exceptionally **high haematocrit** (Section 14.18.1) and **fast heart rate** (Section 22.16.3), provides the cardiovascular basis for their elite athleticism (Snow, 1985).

In **bats**, the heart is again very large. Estimates in three species are 0.78% of body mass (Carpenter, 1985), 0.85% (Lechner, 1985), and 0.9% (Thomas and Suthers, 1972). The large stroke volume that this provides is consistent with the very high haematocrit (Section 14.18.2), the extreme energetic demands of flight, and the exceptionally great aerobic capacity of bats (Section 6.26.5).

In **man**, the average mass of the heart is said to be about 300 g in males and about 250 g in females, forming about 0.45% of the body mass in males and 0.40% in females (see Williams *et al.*, 1989, p. 700). In elite human **endurance athletes** such as marathon runners the heart mass increases by about 40% (or even 50%, Guyton, 1986, p. 273), but never exceeds 500 g (Jokl and Jokl, 1977); a value of 500 g would represent about 0.75% of body mass, an increase of 66%. The chambers of the heart also enlarge by about 40% (Guyton, 1986, p. 1016), increasing the **stroke volume** of endurance athletes by as much as 40% at rest and nearly 50% at its maximum, and yielding a maximum **cardiac output** about 40% greater than that of the untrained person. It is reported (Fox, 1984, Fig. 9.7) that, in **non-endurance athletes** such as shot putters and wrestlers, there is hypertrophy of the ventricular myocardium but no enlargement of the heart chambers. Surprisingly, no difference is found in the heart mass of **horses** in racing training for 2 months compared with 19 months, indicating that the hypertrophy in response to training is not gradual but occurs abruptly at the onset of training (Evans, 1994, p. 130).

The above measurements suggest that in athletic species in training the cardiac muscle cells experience a massive **hypertrophy**. The coronary microcirculation copes successfully with hypertrophy resulting from athletic training (Section 18.3). Much greater hypertrophy of the muscle cells may occur in cardiac disease. In **aortic stenosis** or **aortic insufficiency**, the mass of the human left ventricle may increase four- or fivefold, increasing the mass of the heart to 800 g (Guyton, 1986, p. 324) or even 1000 g (Jokl and Jokl, 1977) (Section 18.3).

Since the ratio of blood capillaries to cardiac muscle cells remains constant throughout life at about 1:1, it is theoretically possible that hypertrophy might cause the muscle cells to outrun the capacity of their blood capillaries to supply them with oxygen. This apparently never happens in the heart of athletes (Section 18.3). However, it does become a serious adverse factor in the massive hypertrophy of aortic stenosis or aortic regurgitation.

20.5   Position of the heart

The heart lies in the mediastinum (Section 9.4; Fig. 9.1). In principle, the heart of the domestic mammals is situated between the third and sixth ribs. This area of the lateral thoracic wall is largely covered by the triceps muscle (Section 23.3; Fig. 23.1). The dorsal boundary of the heart lies approximately on a horizontal plane drawn through the centre of the first rib (Figs 23.5, 24.7, 25.2). The caudal boundary is the dome of the diaphragm (Figs 23.4, 24.5), and the ventral boundary is the sternum (Figs 24.5, 24.8). Because the right lung is larger than the left (Section 5.5), most of the heart lies to the left of the midline, and therefore the left surface of the heart is nearer to the thoracic wall than the right (Figs 24.8, 25.1). The long axis of the heart is virtually vertical in the horse (Fig. 23.3), almost vertical in the ruminants (Fig. 23.4), and progressively more oblique in the pig, dog (Fig. 23.5), and cat.

These anatomical relationships affect the clinical examination of the heart by percussion (Section 23.9), auscultation (Section 23.10), and palpation (Section 23.11).

Species variations in the position of the heart are summarized by Schummer *et al.* (1981, p. 19). The heart sometimes lies between ribs 4 and 7 in the dog, and commonly does so in the cat. In the ox the caudal limit is often the fifth rib, and in the sheep and goat the limits are typically the second to the fifth rib. In the horse the cranial limit may extend to the second rib.

The proportion of the heart that lies to the left of the midline is estimated to be 71% in the ox, 60% in the horse, and 57% in the dog.

The cranial angle between the sternum and the long axis of the heart is about 40° in the dog and 25–30° in the cat.

20.6   External features of the heart

The heart (Figs 17.5, 20.1) has the shape of a cone, slightly flattened on each side. The **base** of the heart is a low dome formed by the left and right atria, and is the most dorsal part of the heart. The *great veins*, systemic and pulmonary, *enter* the base of the heart, and the *great arteries*, aortic and pulmonary, *emerge* from it. The heart is held in position by these great vessels, but otherwise lies entirely free within the **pericardium** (Section 20.2). The base of the heart (i.e. the atria) is separated from the ventricles by the **coronary groove** containing the main coronary vessels.

Each atrium has a blind diverticulum, the auricle. On the cranial aspect of the left side of the heart, the two auricles curve round the origin of the pulmonary trunk though without entirely covering it (Fig. 20.1). However, they do completely enclose the origin of the aorta. The right auricle forms the most cranial part of the heart. The edges of both auricles are more or less deeply notched, depending on the species.

The left and right ventricles fuse together to form a cone. The line along which the ventricles blend is visible as a **left interventricular groove** on the left side of the heart and a **right interventricular groove** on the right; these two grooves carry left and right interventricular branches of the coronary arteries and veins (Section 18.1.1). The left and right interventricular

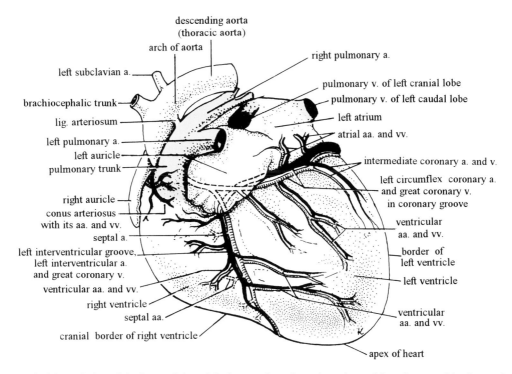

Fig. 20.1   Left lateral view of the heart of the adult dog, to show the atria and ventricles, the great blood vessels, and the coronary vasculature. Although this is the left side of the heart, the right ventricle is visible because it forms the cranial surface of the heart and then continues into the pulmonary trunk on the left side of the heart. The right auricle curls round the cranial surface of the heart, so that it too is visible in this left view. The aorta emerges from the base of the heart on the right side of the pulmonary trunk. The apex of the heart is formed by the left ventricle. The left interventricular groove separates the right and left ventricles. It contains the left interventricular artery and the beginning of the great coronary vein. The left part of the coronary groove separates the left atrium from the left ventricle. It contains the left circumflex coronary artery and the continuation of the great coronary vein. In green are the pulmonary trunk and pulmonary arteries, and the pulmonary veins draining the left lung into the left atrium. Septal arteries arising from the left interventricular artery, supplying the interventricular septum, are shown in broken lines.

grooves correspond with the position of the interventricular septum (Fig. 18.2). The **apex** of the heart is the tip of the cone, and is a part of the left ventricle.

The **left surface** of the heart is formed mainly by the left atrium and left ventricle, but the right ventricle and right auricle extend round the cranial surface of the heart and therefore also contribute substantially to the left surface (Fig. 20.1). The **right surface** is formed mainly by the right atrium and right ventricle, but the left ventricle extends round the caudal surface of the heart and therefore also contributes to the right surface (Fig. 17.5). The position of the *right* ventricle and its pulmonary trunk on the *left* side of the definitive heart, is caused by the growth of the spiral

septum in the embryo (Section 15.3.3). The **cranial border** of the right ventricle is convex. The **caudal border** of the left ventricle is slightly convex in the domestic carnivores (Fig. 24.5), almost straight and vertical in the horse, and slightly concave in ruminants. In the ox the concavity of the caudal border follows the contour of the dome of the diaphragm; in this species the close proximity of the caudal border to the diaphragm brings the pericardium near to the reticulum, thus predisposing to penetration of the pericardium by foreign bodies from the reticulum (Section 25.4).

The pericardium and heart, with the left and right phrenic nerves and vagus nerves as they cross the heart, occupy the **middle mediastinum** (Section 9.4). The **coro-**

nary groove (sulcus coronarius) encircles the heart, except at the conus arteriosus and pulmonary trunk (Fig. 20.1).

The left interventricular groove is known in the NAV (1994) as the **sulcus interventricularis paraconalis**, because it descends from the sulcus coronarius along the *conus* arteriosus; the right interventricular groove is known as the **sulcus interventricularis subsinuosus**, because it descends from the sulcus coronarius ventral to the *sinus* venarum cavarum and *sinus* coronarius. The NAV gives even more difficult names to the left and right surfaces of the heart, again on topographical grounds. Thus the left surface of the heart is named the **auricular surface** (facies auricularis), because both the *left and right auricle* (auriculi atrii) are represented on the left side of the heart; the right surface of the heart is named the **atrial surface** (facies atrialis), apparently because this is the 'heart surface on the side of the atrial mass' (Schaller *et al.*, 1992).

The **apical cardiac notch** (incisura apicis cordis) is an indentation on the cranial aspect of the ventricles, at the ventral end of the left (and right, Fig. 17.5) interventricular groove.

In all of the domestic species except the horse (Simeons, 1992, p. 242), a longitudinal groove descends on the caudal border of the left ventricle; this carries the intermediate branch (ramus intermedius) of the left coronary artery and vein (Figs 17.5, 20.1).

The usage of the term the base of the heart (**basis cordis**) varies. Schummer *et al.* (1982, p. 16) defined it as 'an imaginary plane running through the coronary groove'. Williams *et al.* (1989, p. 701) noted a number of different anatomical and clinical usages in human medicine, and pointed out that the plane of the coronary sulcus should be termed the base of the *ventricles*, as opposed to the base of the heart. The NAV, as presented by Schaller *et al.* (1992, p. 234), defines the base of the heart as the dorsocranially or dorsally directed surface of the heart, delimited by the sulcus coronarius, and this definition is adopted here.

20.7   Right atrium

In all the domestic species the right atrium has four main openings. (1) The cranial **vena cava** drains the systemic veins from the cranial part of the body, entering the atrium at its cranial end (Fig. 17.5). (2) The **caudal vena cava** returns venous blood from the caudal part of the body, into the caudal part of the atrium. (3) The **coronary sinus** returns venous blood from the heart itself, opening immediately ventral to the opening of the caudal vena cava (Fig. 17.5). (4) The **right atrioventricular ostium**, guarded by the right

atrioventricular valve, transfers venous blood from the right atrium to the right ventricle (Fig. 20.2). **Small coronary veins** (Section 18.8) open directly through the atrial wall through numerous small foramina.

The **right auricle** is a blind diverticulum, opening from the cranial end of the right atrium (Fig. 17.5) and winding round the cranial aspect of the heart. The ventral border of the auricle is notched. The **internal wall** of the atrium is smooth, but that of the auricle is interlaced with muscular ridges, the **pectinate muscles**.

Vestiges of the fetal circulation include the fossa ovalis and intervenous ridge. The **fossa ovalis** is the remnant of the **foramen ovale**, visible as an oval depression on the interatrial septum at the opening of the caudal vena cava. Sometimes the valvule of the foramen ovale fails to fuse completely to the rim of the foramen, leaving a small and clinically harmless opening in the interatrial septum; total absence of the valvule creates a large interatrial defect, leading to a left-to-right shunt and right heart failure (Section 15.12). The **intervenous ridge** remains essentially as it is in the fetal heart (Section 15.3.7), i.e. a transverse arch projecting ventrally from the dorsal wall of the atrium, between the cranial and caudal venae cavae (Fig. 15.8); it continues to direct blood from the cranial vena cava into the atrioventricular ostium, as in the fetal heart.

The intervenous ridge is the **tuberculum intervenosum** of the NAV (1994). Another embryonic remnant is the **crista terminalis** (Fig. 17.5). This is a muscular ridge on the internal surface of the right atrium (atrium dextrum); it indicates a boundary, though poorly defined, between the dome-like *dorsal roof* of the atrium that receives the ostia of the cranial and caudal venae cavae, and the *ventral part* of the atrium (the 'atrium proper' of Simoens (1992, p. 238), or 'true atrium' of Schummer *et al.* (1981, p. 25)) that opens into the right atrioventricular ostium. On the outside of the atrium, the crista terminalis is repeated by an indistinct groove, the **sulcus terminalis** (Fig. 17.5). The crista terminalis and sulcus terminalis mark the junction of the embryonic sinus venosus with the primitive atrium. Since the dome-like roof of the atrium has been derived from the sinus venosus, this region of the definitive right atrium is named the **sinus venarum cavarum** in the NAV (1994). Most of the **pectinate muscles** (musculi pectinati) radiate from the crista terminalis (Simoens, 1992, p. 238). The fossa ovalis has a more or less prominent margin, the **limbus fossae ovalis**.

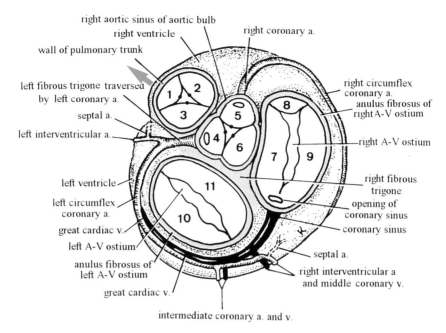

Fig. 20.2 Semidiagrammatic dorsal view of the base of the canine heart after removal of the atria, to show the main coronary blood vessels, the aortic, pulmonary, left atrioventricular, and right atrioventricular valves, and parts of the fibrous skeleton of the heart. The aortic bulb has been transected. It shows three bulges. These are the three aortic sinuses, guarded by the three valvules of the aortic valve. The valvules of the aortic valve are: 4, left; 5, right; 6, septal. The left coronary artery arises from the left aortic sinus, and the right coronary artery arises from the right aortic sinus. The left and right coronary arteries pass laterally to enter the coronary groove on the left and right sides of the heart respectively. The valvules of the pulmonary trunk are: 1, intermediate; 2, right; 3, left. The cusps of the right atrioventricular valve are: 7, septal; 8, angular; 9, parietal. The cusps of the left atrioventricular valve are: 10, parietal; 11, septal (Simoens, 1992, p. 237). Elements of the fibrous skeleton of the heart (simplified) are shown in green. These include the right and left fibrous trigones, and the anulus fibrosus of the left and right atrioventricular ostia. The entire walls of the aortic and pulmonary ostia are not in themselves a part of the fibrous skeleton, although shown here in green, but the wall of each of these ostia does contain a coronet-like anulus fibrosus, which is a part of the fibrous skeleton (see Fig. 20.7). The green arrow indicates the cranial aspect (see Barone, 1996, Fig. 28).

The orifice of the caudal vena cava (ostium venae cavae caudalis) has a valve-like fold (**valvula venae cavae caudalis**), which often disappears in adults and is absent in the foal; the orifice of the coronary sinus also has a semilunar fold (**valvula sinus coronarii**), and this too may be indistinct or absent, especially in the horse (Simoens, 1992, p. 238).

The **right azygos vein** (v. azygos dextra), which occurs in the carnivores, ruminants, horse, and sometimes the pig, enters the cranial vena cava near the right atrium, or opens directly into the roof of the right atrium (Dyce *et al.*, 1987, p. 217). The left azygos vein (v. azygos sinistra), which is present in the ruminants and pig, drains into the coronary sinus.

Evans (1993, p. 590) summarized the territory drained by the great systemic veins as follows. Cranial vena cava: head, neck, forelimbs, ventral thoracic wall, and the adjacent part of the abdominal wall. Caudal vena cava: abdominal viscera, part of the abdominal wall, and the hind limbs. Right azygos vein: part of the lumbar region, and the caudal three-quarters of the thoracic wall, and to these must be added the venous drainage of the bronchial circulation and oesophagus (Section 17.5).

20.8 Right ventricle: right atrioventricular and pulmonary valves

The right atrium connects to the right ventricle through the right atrioventricular opening. The opening is guarded by the **right atrioventricular valve**. The valve consists of three thin, almost transparent, flap-like **cusps** (leaflets) – hence the alternative name of **tricuspid valve**. Each cusp is attached to the fibrous ring that forms the rim of the atrioventricular ostium (Fig. 20.2). The free edge of each cusp is restrained by **chordae tendineae**. The chordae tendineae arise from **papillary muscles** that project from the internal surface of the ventricular wall (Fig. 20.3).

The right atrioventricular valve closes during ventricular systole. The rise in pressure during ventricular systole opens the pulmonary valve, allowing blood to flow into the pulmonary trunk and thence into the lungs. The **pulmonary valve** consists of three **semilunar valvules** forming three pockets (1, 2, and 3 in Fig. 20.2). The abrupt fall in ventricular pressure at the end of ventricular systole causes a sudden pressure gradient from pulmonary trunk to right ventricle. This fills the pockets and so closes the pulmonary valve by tight apposition of the three valvules, as shown for the aortic valve in Fig. 18.1. The working of the valves is discussed further in Section 22.6. Since the pulmonary circulation is a low pressure system (Section 17.12), the wall of the right ventricle need only be about half as thick as that of the left ventricle (Fig. 20.3).

A rounded bundle of tissue crosses the lumen of the ventricle from the interventricular septum to the lateral wall. This is the **right septomarginal trabecula** (Fig. 20.3). Several other similar but smaller bundles, branching and anastomosing, are usually present. In general, these bundles tend to pass from the interventricular septum to the base of the papillary muscles. They were previously called **moderator bands**, under the mistaken impression that they prevent over-distension. It is now known that they distribute conducting fibres to the papillary muscles, thus indicating the possibility of some degree of active control of the atrioventricular valve.

The thick muscular **interventricular septum** (Section 20.10) separates the right and left ventricles (Fig. 20.3).

Evans (1993, p. 596) and Darke *et al.* (1996, Fig. 9.2) maintained that the right atrioventricular valve of the dog and cat is not tricuspid as in the other domestic species and man, but has only two cusps. Ghoshal (1975, p. 1597) described the carnivore right atrioventricular valve as consisting 'basically of two cusps, parietal and septal, with three or four intervening secondary cusps'. Schummer *et al.* (1981, Figs 27, 30) show and label three cusps in all the domestic species, including the dog and cat. Dyce *et al.* (1987, p. 218) make no mention of species

variations in the tricuspid form. The NAV, as interpreted by Simoens (1992, p. 238), accepts three cusps as a uniform feature. In his authoritative survey of angiology, Barone (1996, pp. 35, 95) makes it clear that only in the rabbit among the veterinary species does the right atrioventricular valve definitely have only two cusps. The difference of opinion about the tricuspid or bicuspid form of the right atrioventricular valve in carnivores simply reflects the rather ill-defined boundaries of the small angular cusp in these species.

The root of the pulmonary trunk is slightly increased in diameter in the region of the pulmonary valve. This dilation is caused by three bulges in the wall of the trunk, corresponding to the three semilunar valvules; these are known as the **sinuses of the pulmonary trunk** (sinus trunci pulmonales). These sinuses resemble the three sinuses (sinus aortae) of the aortic bulb (bulbus aortae) (Fig. 18.1), but are less distinct. According to Dyce *et al.* (1987, p. 500) *fenestrations* often appear in the middle region of the valvulae of the pulmonary valve in the horse, but seem to have little if any functional significance.

The lumen of the right ventricle is crescentic in transverse section (Fig. 18.2). The ventricular cavity is arbitrarily divided into two functional components, an inflow channel and an outflow channel (Schummer *et al.*, 1981, p. 27). The *inflow channel* (Fig. 20.3) extends from the right atrioventricular opening (ostium atrioventriculare dextrum) into the ventricle; Williams *et al.* (1989, p. 703) considered it to end ventrally at the **septomarginal trabecula** (trabecula septomarginalis) (Fig. 20.3). The surface of the inflow channel is rendered irregular by the **trabeculae carneae**, which are subendocardial myocardial ridges on the ventricular wall that protrude into the lumen, and by the presence of the papillary muscles (Fig. 20.3). The *outflow channel* lacks a well-defined starting point, but Schummer *et al.* (1981, p. 31) regarded the channel as consisting 'mainly of the conus arteriosus' (Fig. 20.1) and this is consistent with Williams *et al.* (1989, p. 703) who considered the channel to begin at the septomarginal trabecula. The conus arteriosus has no papillary muscles and no trabeculae carneae, and therefore has smooth walls. The smoothness of the walls of the outflow channel is presumed to promote the velocity of ejection. It has been suggested (see Dyce *et al.*, 1987, p. 218) that the irregular surface of the inflow channel may reduce turbulence, but it should have the opposite effect. Williams *et al.* (1989, p. 703) believed that its lack of smoothness may 'assist' in slowing the entry of blood during early systole (as indeed is very likely), but no functional advantage of this was suggested. Similar considerations apply to the inflow and outflow channels of the left ventricle (Section 20.10).

The right ventricle has three **papillary muscles** (Schummer *et al.*, 1981, p. 30). Usually two arise from the interventricular septum. Of these, one lies on the septum immediately ventral to the pulmonary trunk (Fig. 20.3)

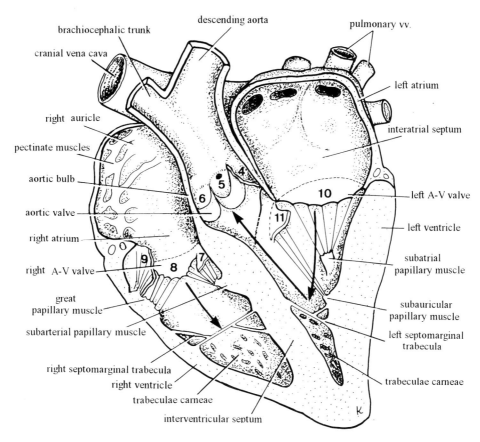

Fig. 20.3 Semidiagrammatic sagittal section through a horse's heart: left lateral view of the right half. The section has passed through the left atrium and left ventricle, the aorta and the aortic valve, the interventricular septum, and the right atrium and right ventricle: the section has missed the pulmonary trunk and pulmonary valve. 10 and 11 are the two cusps of the left atrioventricular valve (10, attached to the outer wall, hence parietal cusp; 11, attached to the interventricular septum, hence septal cusp). The septal cusp (11) separates the left atrioventricular ostium from the aortic ostium; it therefore also separates the rough-walled inflow channel of the left ventricle (ventrally directed arrow) from the smooth-walled outflow channel (dorsally directed arrow). Most of the septal cusp (11) was removed when the heart was cut. The two papillary muscles of the left ventricle (one lying ventral to the left atrium, hence named subatrial; the other ventral to the left auricle, hence subauricular) are on the outer wall of the ventricle. Their chordae tendineae attach to the free edges of the two left atrioventricular cusps. The septomarginal trabecula is a bundle of muscle and conducting tissue, running across the lumen of the left ventricle from septum to outer wall. It is regarded as the end of the inflow channel and the beginning of the outflow channel. Ventral to the septomarginal trabecula the wall shows a sponge-like meshwork of muscular ridges, the trabeculae carneae. The aortic valve is guarded by three semilunar valvules (4, left, largely removed when the heart was cut; 5, right; 6, septal). Just dorsal to 5 is the opening into the right coronary artery. The internal wall of the right auricle carries a well-developed meshwork of pectinate muscles. 7, 8, and 9 are the cusps of the right atrioventricular valve (7, septal, attached to the interventricular septum and largely removed; 9, parietal, attached to the outer wall and also largely removed; and 8, angular, the smallest, situated in the angle between the other two). Three papillary muscles distribute chordae tendineae to the three cusps of the right atrioventricular valve. Two are on the interventricular septum (one near the pulmonary trunk, hence subarterial; a small cluster also on the septum but removed in this section; and a large one, hence 'great', on the outer wall). The left and right inflow channels are shown by ventrally directed arrows. The (arbitrary) ventral limit of each inflow channel is the septomarginal trabecula of conducting tissue passing from interventricular septum to outer wall. The numbering of the cusps and semilunar valvules of the atrioventricular and aortic valves is the same as in Fig. 20.2.

and is therefore named the **subarterial papillary muscle** (musculus papillaris subarteriosus); the other is a cluster of smaller muscles, known therefore as the **small papillary muscles** (musculi papillares parvi), situated more caudally on the septum. The third papillary muscle arises from the outer (parietal) wall of the ventricle; being considerably larger than the others, it is called the **great papillary muscle** (musculus papillaris magnus) (Fig. 20.3). Sometimes all three papillary muscles are on the interventricular septum, especially in carnivores.

The papillary muscles form the tendinous cords (**chordae tendineae**). These fan out to attach to the **cusps** (leaflets) of the atrioventricular valve (Fig. 20.3). Some of them join the *free edge* of a cusp, and at least in the dog these are mainly the smaller cords (Evans, 1993, p. 593). Because of the attachments of the chordae, the free edge is irregular and notched (Fig. 20.4). Most of the chordae, including the larger ones, attach to the *ventricular* surface of the cusp which is relatively rough. The smoother *inflow* surface (atrial surface) of the cusp is then available to make perfect contact with another cusp during full valve closure (Williams *et al.*, 1989, p. 706). It is the atrial surface that makes contact, the reason being that the cusps float down into the ventricular cavity during ventricular diastole, i.e. before the valve closes (Section 22.6.1). Incidentally, as Salmons (1995, p. 1485) pointed out, 'cuspis' is a misnomer by the NA (1989) since it means 'point', particularly of a spear; the leaflets are not cuspid, i.e. pointed in form.

The basic component of a **cusp** is a thin underlying collagenous membrane, both surfaces of which are covered by endocardium (Schummer *et al.*, 1981, p. 30). The fibres of this membrane are continuous with those of the fibrous ring (anulus fibrosus) that surrounds the right atrioventricular ostium (Fig. 20.2). The fibres of the membrane are in turn linked to the fibres of the tendinous cords, which again are covered by endocardium. A **nerve network** derived from the subendocardial plexus has been reported in the atrioventricular valves, especially near the attachments of the chordae tendineae, the right atrioventricular valve being better innervated than the left (Evans, 1993, p. 596). Some **blood vessels** have been observed in the cusps of the atrioventricular valves, but the vascularity is low and the tissue is considered to be sustained mainly by the blood passing over the valves (Evans, 1993, p. 596).

The **septal cusp** (cuspis septalis) is attached to the anulus fibrosus at the interventricular septum (7 in Fig. 20.2). The **parietal cusp** (cuspis parietalis) originates from the outer (parietal) wall of the ventricle (9 in Fig. 20.2). The **angular cusp** (cuspis angularis), which is the smallest, lies in the angle between the other two cusps (8 in Fig. 20.2). The three main cusps can form secondary cusps.

As Fig. 20.4 shows, the relationships between cusps, chordae tendineae, and papillary muscles are such that each papillary muscle modulates the movements of *two* cusps.

The three **semilunar valvules** (valvulae semilunares) of the **valve of the pulmonary trunk** (valva trunci pulmonalis) are referred to as leaflets in some works on pathology (e.g. Darke *et al.*, 1996, p. 80). They are named topographically. Thus in Fig. 20.2, valvule 2 is the right valvule, 3 is the left valvule, and 1 is the intermediate valvule between the other two. Each valvule (Schummer *et al.*, 1981, p. 31) has a slightly thickened free border, with a small **nodule** (nodulus valvulae semilunaris) on the mid-point (Fig. 18.1). On either side of the nodule there is a crescentic transparent zone, the **lunula valvulae semilunaris**.

The structure of the valvule is similar in principle to that of an atrioventricular cusp, consisting of a layer of collagen fibres sandwiched between two layers of endothelium. At the lunula the fibrous layer is tenuous (Salmons, 1995, p. 1488).

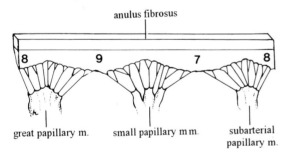

anulus fibrosus

8   9   7   8

great papillary m.   small papillary m.m.   subarterial papillary m.

Fig. 20.4 Diagram of the cusps, chordae tendineae, and papillary muscles of the right atrioventricular valve. The three cusps have been dissected out in a continuous strip, still attached to the anulus fibrosus of the atrioventricular ostium. The angular cusp (8) has been transected, and the strip of three cusps has then been straightened out. The fibres of the anulus fibrosus are continuous with the fibrous membrane on which the cusps are founded. The fibres of the membrane are in turn linked to the fibres of the chordae tendineae. Each cusp is secured by chordae tendineae from two papillary muscles, or each papillary muscle secures two cusps. 7, Septal cusp; 9, parietal cusp. The numbering of the cusps is the same as in Fig. 20.2.

20.9   Left atrium

The left atrium receives the arterial blood that drains from the lungs via the **pulmonary veins**. The basic pattern in the domestic mammals is six pulmonary veins altogether, two from the left lung and four from the right, although there are species variations (Section 17.15). As in the right atrium, **small coronary veins** also empty into the left atrium through small foramina (Section 18.8).

The **left auricle** is a blind diverticulum, slightly overlapping the pulmonary trunk (Fig. 20.1). Its ventral border is notched like that of the right auricle. The internal surface of the auricle has **pectinate muscles** like the right auricle. The rest of the atrium has a smooth internal wall.

The site of fusion of the valvula (flap) of the fetal foramen ovale (Section 15.3.6) may be visible on the interatrial septum.

20.10 Left ventricle: left atrioventricular and aortic valves

The left atrium connects to the left ventricle via the left atrioventricular ostium. The ostium is guarded by the **left atrioventricular valve**. The valve consists of two **cusps**, and therefore has the alternative name of **bicuspid valve** (or mitral valve, after a bishop's mitre). As in the right atrium, each cusp is attached to the fibrous rim of the atrioventricular opening (Fig. 20.2), and the free edge of the cusp connects to **papillary muscles** by **chordae tendineae** (Fig. 20.3).

Like the pulmonary valve, the **aortic valve** consists of three **semilunar valvules** (4, 5, and 6 in Figs 20.2 and 20.3). The increase in ventricular pressure at the onset of ventricular systole closes the left atrioventricular valve and opens the aortic valve. At the end of ventricular systole the steep pressure gradient from aorta to left ventricle closes the aortic valve by apposing the three semilunar valvules in a triradiate form (Fig. 18.1). The root of the aorta at the site of the aortic valve is expanded into the **aortic bulb** (Fig. 20.3) by three bulges, the **aortic sinuses**. The sinuses correspond to the position of the three semilunar valvules (Fig. 18.1), and can be named according to the valvules. Thus the left aortic sinus is related to the left semilunar valvule of the aortic valve (Figs 20.2, 20.5), and the right aortic sinus is related to the right semilunar valvule (Fig. 18.1). The left coronary artery opens from the left aortic sinus, and the right coronary artery from the right aortic sinus (Section 18.2).

Because the systemic circulation is a high pressure system, the wall of the left ventricle is about two or even three times as thick as the right ventricle (Figs 18.2, 20.3). Likewise the cusps of the left atrioventricular valve and the semilunar valvules of the aortic valve are much stronger and thicker than those of the right side of the heart.

As in the right ventricle, one large **trabecula septomarginalis** and several smaller ones traverse the ventricular lumen from the interventricular septum to the base of the papillary muscles on the lateral wall (Fig. 20.3). They supply conducting fibres to the papillary muscles and thus help to coordinate the functions of the left atrioventricular valve (Section 22.6).

The thick muscular **interventricular septum** (Fig. 20.3) is formed by the combined walls of the two ventricles. Its surface facing into the lumen of the left ventricle is concave, thus completing the circular profile of the ventricle as seen in a horizontal section, whereas the surface facing into the lumen of the right ventricle is convex (Fig. 18.2).

In the fixed cadaver, the cavity of the left ventricle looks much smaller than that of the right ventricle, but this is thought to be an artefact caused by post-mortem contraction of its much stronger musculature (Getty, 1975, p. 165).

As in the right ventricle (Section 20.8), the *outflow channel* of the left ventricle is smooth. The walls of the *inflow channel* (Fig. 20.3), however, are very irregular because of the presence of very strong **trabeculae carneae** as well as prominent papillary muscles.

The general structure and relationships between the cusps, chordae tendineae, and papillary muscles of the left atrioventricular valve are the same in principle as for the right atrioventricular valve. Both of the cusps blend with the anulus fibrosus of the atrioventricular ostium (Fig. 20.2). The **septal cusp** (11, in Figs 20.2 and 20.3) is attached in the region of the interventricular septum, and the **parietal cusp** (10, in Figs 20.2 and 20.3) to the lateral wall. Accessory cusps are usually present (Getty, 1975, p. 167). As in the right ventricle, there is the same number of cusps as papillary muscles, but each papillary muscle shares two cusps (Fig. 20.4). Both of the two papillary muscles are a part of the outer wall of the left ventricle (Fig. 20.3): the **subatrial papillary muscle** (musculus papillaris subatrialis) is so called because it lies towards the right side of the ventricle and is therefore ventral to the left atrium; the **subauricular papillary muscle** (musculus papillaris subauricularis) is further cranial and to the left, and is therefore ventral to the left auricle.

The structure of the aortic valve is the same in principle as that of the pulmonary valve, except for being stronger. Salmons (1995, p. 1488) emphasized that the concept of a single circular aortic annulus to support the aortic (and pulmonary) semilunar valvules is incorrect, since (in man, at least) there is no continuous circular collagenous skeleton supporting the entire attachment of all three semilunar valvules: each semicircular valvule is attached to a semicircular fibrous thickening in the wall of the aortic bulb. This difficult and doubtless contentious matter is discussed in Section 20.12.

The **interventricular septum** has two components. The **muscular part** (pars muscularis), which is by far the larger part, is thick myocardium formed by the combined walls of the two ventricles. The **membranous part** (pars membranacea) is a small inconspicuous area in the extreme dorsal part of the septum, just ventral to the aortic valve on the left side and the septal cusp of the right atrioventricular valve on the right (Evans, 1993, p. 596). It is collagenous, but thin (Williams *et al.*, 1989, p. 709) and can be seen by transmitted light (Evans, 1993, p. 596). It marks the site of the final closure of the embryonic interventricular foramen by endocardial cushion tissue (Section 15.3.2). This is the site of congenital interventricular defects, which are reported to be one of the commonest cardiac malformations in domestic mammals, especially in cattle (Section 15.11). The high incidence in cattle may be inconsistent with the claim by Schummer *et al.* (1981, p. 21) that the pars membranacea does not occur in the ox.

Neither the NAV (1994) nor the NA (1989) distinguishes the three aortic sinuses by individual terms. This is inconvenient for describing the origins of the left and right coronary arteries. In the 38th edition of *Gray's Anatomy*, Gabella (1996, p. 1505) has named the three sinuses according to their semilunar valvules, and this principle has been adopted here (i.e. left, right, and septal aortic sinuses).

20.11   Species characteristics of hearts

The ability to identify the species from which a heart has been obtained may be needed in the post-mortem room or abattoir. Usually this is readily done by looking at the **lungs**, which are generally attached to the heart with the liver, thus forming the '*pluck*'. For forensic purposes, serological tests would be conclusive.

It can be difficult to identify the species by the external characteristics of the heart alone, but the following distinguishing features may be useful as a check list.

Size can be unhelpful, since the animal may have been immature. **Fatty tissue** lying beneath the epicardium in the coronary and longitudinal grooves is a good guide. For example, the horse and Channel Island breeds of cattle have yellow fat, whereas other breeds of cattle and also sheep have hard white fat. In cattle the fat is very extensive both in and beyond the grooves. In the horse the fat is soft to the point of being almost oily. The texture of fat varies with temperature, however, being softer when warm and harder when cold.

Shape gives some guidance. The hearts of ruminant species and deep-chested breeds of dog tend to be the most elongated and pointed, whereas the hearts of the barrel-chested dog, and the pig and cat, tend to be relatively rounded. **Notches** are particularly distinct on the borders of both of the auricles in the ox, but are indistinct on the border of the left auricle of the horse. The two fully formed **ossa cordis** in the ox are distinctive, though other species also have islands of hard tissue in the cardiac fibrous skeleton (Section 20.12). The origin of the **left subclavian artery** from the arch of the aorta (Fig. 20.1) distinguishes the carnivore and pig, whereas the origin from the brachiocephalic trunk characterizes the ruminants and horse.

Distinguishing details of the heart of the domestic species were surveyed by Schummer *et al.* (1981, pp. 41, 68–70). The coronary and azygos vasculature provide quite precise criteria.

The right interventricular artery (ramus interventriculus subsinuosus) is formed by the *left* **coronary artery** in the dog (Fig. 17.5) and ruminants, and by the *right* coronary artery in the pig and horse (Section 18.1.4). In all species except the horse, a longitudinal groove descends the caudal border of the left ventricle carrying the ramus intermedius of the left coronary artery and vein (Figs 17.5, 20.1).

The ruminant species have both a right and a left **vena azygos**, the right draining into the cranial vena cava and the left into the coronary sinus. The carnivores and horses have only a right azygos vein, draining into the cranial venal cava or the roof of the right atrium. The pig usually has only a left azygos vein, draining into the coronary sinus.

The differing **shapes of the heart** were summarized by Barone (1996, Chapter 1, part VIII). The equine heart is clearly conical, flattened on either side, with a bluntly pointed apex and a relatively large base. The ruminant heart is a narrower cone with a relatively more extensive base, compared with the horse. The heart of the pig is less clearly conical than the preceding hearts, the apex being blunt and rounded. The carnivore heart is almost globular.

20.12   Cardiac fibrous skeleton

The atria are separated from the ventricles by a distinct *fibrous plate* (Fig. 20.5), known as the **cardiac fibrous skeleton**. The plate is perforated by five essential holes, one for each of the four **valves** of the heart and one more for the **atrioventricular bundle** (Section 21.19.3). Each of the four valves is firmly attached to the rim of its hole in the plate.

In the zone surrounding the aortic valve the fibrous tissue of the plate is reinforced by *cartilage* or *bone*. In the ox two separate bones (the **ossa cordis**) develop at this site. The sheep has one os cordis deep in the interatrial septum, and sometimes a second bone.

The main function of the fibrous plate is to separate the myocardial cells of the atria from those of the ventricles. The purpose of this is to ensure *electrophysiological discontinuity* between these two great groups of cardiac muscle cells, except by means of the interventricular bundle. Without the plate, the atrial muscle cells would directly excite the ventricular muscle cells. This would have the functional disadvantage that the *base of each ventricle would contract before the apex*, which would be as inefficient as squeezing a tube of toothpaste from the top instead of the bottom.

At an *elementary* level, the cardiac fibrous skeleton is often visualized in simple two-dimensional terms, i.e. as a more or less flat plate of fibrous tissue perforated by the four cardiac valves, the plate lying in the same plane as the coronary sulcus. This flat plate is said to consist of (Figs 20.2, 20.5): (1) two roughly triangular fibrous areas, the **left** and **right fibrous trigones** (trigona fibrosa), the left one lying between the aortic ostium and the left atrioventricular ostium, and the right one lying midway between the aortic ostium and the left and the right atrioventricular ostia; and (2) four fibrous rings, the **anuli fibrosi**, each forming respectively a uniform fibrous ring around the aortic ostium, the ostium of the pulmonary trunk, the left atrioventricular ostium, and the right atrioventricular ostium. These four simple fibrous rings are visualized as providing the attachments for the flap-like valvules of each of the four valves.

Actually the fibrous skeleton, at least in man, is much more complex than this suggests (see Williams *et al.*, 1989, p. 715; Salmons, 1995, p. 1492). The time-honoured

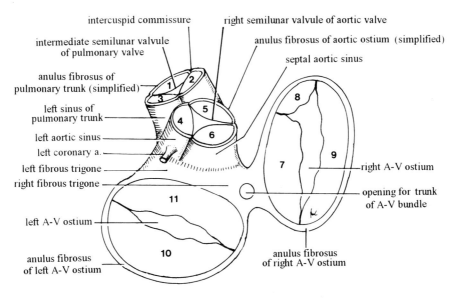

Fig. 20.5   Simplified dorsal view of the fibrous plate that separates the atria from the ventricles. The orientation is similar to that in Fig. 20.2. The aortic and pulmonary ostia, and the left and right atrioventricular ostia, are shown here to be surrounded by simple rings of fibrous tissue, and each such ring is labelled as the anulus fibrosus of its respective ostium (based on Simoens, 1992, p. 237). The anuli fibrosi of the aortic, pulmonary, and left atrioventricular ostia are connected by two flat areas of fibrous tissue, the left and right fibrous trigones. The four anuli fibrosi and the two fibrous trigones are shown as though they all lie roughly in the same plane, as in Fig. 20.2. Actually the anuli and trigones are probably not in the same plane, and the aortic and pulmonary anuli are not simple rings but resemble three-pointed coronets (Fig. 20.6).

terms 'trigone' and 'anulus' are misleading: the trigones are not simple two-dimensional triangular areas, and the anuli fibrosi are not simple two-dimensional rings. Moreover, the four valves depart considerably from a single plane. Hence the two trigones and the four fibrous rings constitute a *three-dimensional framework* for supporting the valves. However, the trigones and rings are fully interconnected structurally (Fig. 20.5) and are thus totally integrated in their function: together, they provide a framework which is deformable, and yet stable enough to hold the valves together, during the powerful forces imposed on them throughout the cardiac cycle.

The architecture of the fibrous skeleton seems to have been quite fully elucidated in man (see Williams *et al.*, 1989, p. 715, and Salmons, 1995, p. 1493). Similarities to man can be recognized readily in the account given by Evans (1993, p. 592) for the dog, but the similarities are less clear in the descriptions given by Schummer *et al.* (1981, p. 20) for this species and some other domestic mammals, which emphasize the *independence* rather than the *integration* of the component parts. In the apparent absence of clear, detailed, descriptions of the fibrous skeleton in the domestic mammals, the following account draws upon that for **man** by Williams *et al.* (1989, p. 715).

The **aortic ostium** is at the centre of the four valvular ostia (Fig. 20.2), and it is its fibrous skeleton that provides the complicated anchorage for the other three ostia (Fig. 20.7). The key to this anchorage is the **anulus fibrosus of the aortic ostium** (aortic anulus fibrosus).

However, this structure is far from being the *simple fibrous ring* around the aortic ostium that Fig. 20.5 suggests. As Salmons (1995, p. 1488) puts it for man, 'Although the aortic valve, like the pulmonary valve, is often described as possessing an annulus in continuity with the fibrous skeleton, *there is no complete collagenous ring supporting the attachments of the leaflets.*' Instead, the **aortic anulus fibrosus** consists of *semicircular fibroelastic thickenings* linked together in the wall of the aortic bulb. Each of these semicircular thickenings attaches the semicircular border of a **semilunar valvule** to the aortic wall. Since there are three semilunar valvules in the aortic valve (4, 5, and 6 in Fig. 20.5), there are three such semicircular thickenings in the walls of the three aortic sinuses (4, 5, and 6 in Fig. 20.6). To fit its valvule, each thickening has to be essentially semicircular, with a 'high point' at each end forming its two **zeniths**, and a 'low point' in the middle forming its **nadir** (Fig. 20.6). The zeniths of adjacent semicircles fuse at the three **intercuspid commissures** of the valve (an intercuspid commissure occurs where the rims of two adjacent valvules meet, as in Fig. 20.5). Therefore, when assembled into the wall of the aortic ostium, the three semicircular thickenings resemble a three-pointed coronet (Fig. 20.6). The three-pointed coronet in the wall of the aortic ostium constitutes (for lack of a better term) the '*anulus fibrosus*' of the aortic ostium; likewise the similar three-pointed coronet in the pulmonary valve constitutes the '*anulus fibrosus*' of the ostium of the pulmonary trunk. (These definitions are consistent with

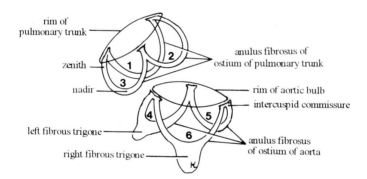

Fig. 20.6 Schematic left dorsal view of the anuli fibrosi of the ostia of the aorta and pulmonary trunk. These two ostia are not in the same plane, but are almost at right angles to each other. The walls of both of these ostia contain three semicircular fibroelastic thickenings. Each of these thickenings provides an attachment for the semicircular border of a semilunar valvule. Each semicircular thickening has a high point (zenith) at each end and a low point (nadir) in its middle. The zeniths are joined together at intercuspid commissures, thus forming a three-pointed coronet. This coronet is the anulus fibrosus. The anulus fibrosus of the aortic ostium is more massive than the anulus fibrosus of the ostium of the pulmonary trunk. The low point (nadir) of the semicircular thickening that belongs to the septal valvule (6) of the aortic valve is extensively widened to form the right fibrous trigone. The nadir of the thickening belonging to the left valvule (4) of the aortic valve is also somewhat widened to form the smaller left fibrous trigone. In the absence of details of the anuli fibrosi of the domestic mammals, the diagram is based on reconstructions of the anuli fibrosi of the human heart (Williams *et al.*, 1989, p. 716). 1, 2 and 3 indicate the semilunar valvules of the valve of the pulmonary trunk (1 intermediate, 2 right, and 3 left). 4, 5, and 6 indicate the semilunar valvules of the aortic valve (4 left, 5 right, and 6 septal).

those of Evans (1993, p. 592), but are more complex than those given by Schummer *et al.* (1981, p. 20) and Simoens (1992, p. 236), which emphasize a *ring-like* rather than the *coronet* form of the anulus fibrosus.)

The semicircular thickening belonging to the *septal valvule* of the aortic valve (valvule 6 in Fig. 20.5) is the focal point that locks together the other components of the fibrous skeleton. Its 'nadir' is massively enlarged (Fig. 20.6), measuring about 2 cm $\times$ 1 cm $\times$ 0.5 cm in man. Because of the flat triangular appearance of this enlarged nadir when sectioned in a slice across the heart in the plane of the coronary sulcus, earlier anatomists named it the **right fibrous trigone** (triangle), but it is now often known as the **central fibrous body** (Williams *et al.*, 1989, p. 716). The nadir of the semicircular thickening of the *left valvule* of the aortic valve (valvule 4 in Fig. 20.5) also consists of a more or less triangular enlargement, the **left fibrous trigone** (Fig. 20.6). Both the right fibrous trigone and the left fibrous trigone contain islands of cartilage in the dog (Evans, 1993, p. 592), and similar islands of cartilage (cartilago cordis) are also present in the trigones of the horse, ox, and pig, with varying ossification (Schummer *et al.*, 1981, pp. 69, 70). This ossification is expressed as two fully-formed **ossa cordis** in the ox (Schummer *et al.*, 1981, p. 21), and one or sometimes two ossa cordis in the sheep (Frink and Merrick, 1974).

As shown in Fig. 20.7, the **right fibrous trigone** (central fibrous body) is in direct contact with (and is attached to) the **anulus fibrosus** of both the **left** and the **right atrioventricular ostium**. Thus the right fibrous trigone secures the left and right atrioventricular ostia to the aortic ostium. The **left fibrous trigone** is also in direct contact with (and attached to) the anulus fibrosus of the left atrioventricular ostium (Fig. 20.7), and thus helps to secure the left atrioventricular ostium to the aortic ostium. The ostium of the pulmonary valve is somewhat distant from the other valvular ostia; also it is not in the same plane as any of them, and indeed is almost at right angles to the aortic ostium (Figs 20.5, 20.7). Nevertheless, it is integrated into the rest of the fibrous skeleton by a collagenous band, the **ligament of the conus arteriosus** (Williams *et al.*, 1989, p. 715; Evans, 1993, p. 593) (or infundibular tendon; Williams *et al.*, 1989, p. 716) that tethers it to the semicircular thickening of the right valvule (valvule 5) of the aortic ostium (Fig. 20.7); this cord is a powerful bond that prevents the aorta and pulmonary trunks from being torn apart during ventricular systole, yet at the same time allows them to twist one upon the other as the blood is forced through. The conus arteriosus is the part of the right ventricle that gives rise to the pulmonary trunk (Fig. 20.1; Section 20.3.3); in the NA (1989), though not in the NAV (1994),

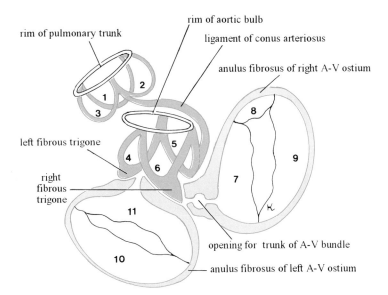

Fig. 20.7   Schematic left dorsal view of the fibrous skeleton of the human heart. The right fibrous trigone fuses to the anuli fibrosi of the left and right atrioventricular ostia. The left fibrous trigone fuses to the anulus fibrosus of the left atrioventricular ostium. Thus the two fibrous trigones unite the aortic ostium, the left atrioventricular ostium, and the right atrioventricular ostium into a strong but flexible fibrous skeleton. The ostium of the pulmonary trunk is distant from the other three ostia and in a different plane, but is secured to the aortic ostium by a fibrous band, the ligament of the conus arteriosus. This prevents the aorta and pulmonary trunks from being torn apart during ventricular systole, but allows them to move independently as the blood is forced through. In the absence of details of the architecture of the fibrous skeleton of the heart of domestic mammals, the diagram is based on the fibrous skeleton of the human heart (Williams *et al.*, 1989, p. 716).

infundibulum is given as an official alternative to conus arteriosus.

Why should the four valvular ostia need such complicated interconnections? The aortic root (aortic bulb) is repeatedly subjected to a formidable surge of pressure at each ventricular systole, and the root of the pulmonary trunk receives a simultaneous, though much smaller, surge; furthermore, the roots of the aorta and pulmonary trunk curve away from each other, more or less at right angles. Anyone who has laid a coiled garden hose at his feet and then turned the tap fully on knows how forcefully the curvature of the pipe changes; the end of a fireman's hose requires two men to hold it off the ground and direct its flow horizontally. In its central position, the aortic ostium relies on its multiple moorings to the other three ostia to avoid being torn from its anchorage. At the same time, the elasticity of these moorings allows deformation of the four ostia, with bulging and twisting as the pressures within them abruptly and repeatedly fluctuate.

The *functions* of the fibrous skeleton of the heart can now be summarized. (1) It ensures electrophysiological discontinuity between the atrial and ventricular myocardium, except via the interventricular bundle; (2) it provides attachments for the ventricular and atrial myocardium; and (3) it holds together, strongly yet flexibly, the aortic, pulmonary, left atrioventricular, and right atrioventricular ostia.

In **lower vertebrates** the musculature of the atria is freely continuous with the ventricular myocardium around the atrioventricular canal (Le Gros Clark, 1965, p. 160).

20.13 Lymphatics of the heart

Lymphatic drainage of the wall of the heart begins in lymphatic capillaries in the endomysium, and empties into the bronchial and mediastinal lymphocentres (Section 14.32.4).

In all the domestic mammals (Schummer *et al.*, 1981, p. 41), there are subendocardial, myocardial, and subepicardial **lymphatic plexuses** in the atrial and ventricular walls. Most of these plexuses follow blood vessels running towards the coronary groove. The main collecting point is where the paraconal interventricular sulcus enters the coronary groove (Section 20.6). From there, the larger ducts drain mainly into the bronchial lymphocentre and its tracheobronchial nodes, and/or into the cranial mediastinal nodes. Minor species variations have been reported.

The **coronary arterial and venous vasculature** are considered in Chapter 18.

Chapter 21
Contractile Mechanism of the Heart

Section 21.16 of this chapter (Excitation-contraction coupling) was written by S.C. O'Neill.

I   THE CONTRACTILE CELL

21.1   Cardiac muscle cell: cardiac muscle fibre

21.1.1   *General structure*

The cellular unit of cardiac muscle is the **cardiac muscle cell**. It is a very large cell, essentially cylindrical in shape, but usually has one or more branches. The cells and their branches join other cells at **intercalated discs** (Fig. 21.1), thus forming a network of branching cylindrical cells (Fig. 18.3).

The **cytoplasm** of cardiac (and skeletal) muscle cells is often known as **sarcoplasm**. The contractile elements are the **myofibrils**, and these form the main component of the cytoplasm. The myofibrils are separated by the usual cytoplasmic organelles, although the mitochondria are exceptionally numerous (Fig. 21.2) as is predictable from the extreme energy expenditure of these cells. One or two nuclei are present in each cell (Fig. 21.1).

The cardiac (and skeletal) muscle cell is a typical excitable cell (Section 21.15). An essential design requirement is the rapid transmission of an action potential throughout all of its cytoplasm. For this function it has evolved tubular invaginations of its plasmalemma known as **T-tubules** (Section 21.12), which convey the action potential throughout the interior of the cell (Section 21.14).

On the arrival of the action potential, calcium ions have to be delivered instantly to the myofibrils in order to activate the immediate interaction between the thick and thin filaments. Therefore a second essential design requirement is a mechanism for the instant delivery of calcium

ions to the myofibrils, and the subsequent rapid removal of these ions. For this function, the cardiac (and skeletal) muscle cell has adapted the smooth endoplasmic reticulum into the **sarcoplasmic reticulum** (Section 21.13).

A sequence of cardiac muscle cells joined together end to end by intercalated discs constitutes a **cardiac muscle fibre** (Fig. 21.1).

The cardiac muscle cell is the myocytus cardiacus of the *Nomina Histologica* (1994).

All myocardial cells are large cells, with a diameter of 10–20 μm in man (Krstic, 1984, p. 65) and 10 μm in the horse and ox (Schummer *et al.*, 1981, p. 37), **ventricular cells** being larger than atrial cells. **Atrial cells** have few or no T-tubules, but otherwise their cytoplasm is essentially similar to that of ventricular cells (Salmons, 1995, p. 764); the insufficiency of T-tubules for delivering the action potential in atrial cells is compensated functionally by the sarcoplasmic reticulum (Section 21.13). Atrial cardiac muscle cells, and especially those of the right atrium (Guyton, 1986, p. 427), do have one distinctive feature around the poles of their nuclei, namely dense membrane-bound granules containing the precursor of **atrial natriuretic factor** (Section 22.9.3).

Because of its multicellular structure and anastomosing branches, the **cardiac muscle fibre** (myofibra) is a difficult structural concept. In contrast, the **skeletal muscle fibre** is a single elongated multinucleated **skeletal muscle cell** (myocytus skeletalis) with clear-cut boundaries. The skeletal muscle fibre is therefore the convenient cellular unit of skeletal muscle (Williams *et al.*, 1989, p. 546). The NH (1994, p. 41) pointed out that myofibra (cardiac muscle fibre) is not a synonym for myocytus cardiacus (cardiac muscle cell), although it is occasionally used as such (e.g. Scott, 1986, p. 2).

Adjacent myofibrils (Section 21.5) are separated by numerous **mitochondria** (Fig. 21.2). The mitochondria are accompanied by sarcoplasmic reticulum (Fig. 21.8), and also by granular material including large **glycogen** deposits and **lipofuscin**, together with **lipid droplets** and occasional **lysosomes** (Krstic, 1984, p. 65). The presence of so many mitochondria, with closely spaced cristae,

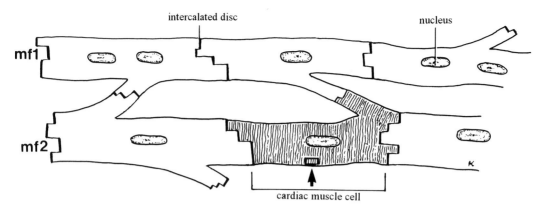

Fig. 21.1   Diagrammatic longitudinal section of cardiac muscle cells, to show their basic form. The cells have irregular branches which are joined to the branches of other cells by intercalated discs, thus forming an anastomosing network of cells. A cord of cells attached to each other by intercalated discs constitutes a cardiac muscle fibre, two fibres (MF1 and 2) being shown here. Because of its multicellular structure and its ramifying and anastomosing branches, the cardiac muscle fibre is a difficult concept. The intercalated discs are shaped like steps. The transverse part of each step that runs at right angles to the long axis of the cell (the 'tread' of the step) has desmosomes that bind the two consecutive cells together; the part of the step that runs parallel with the long axis of the cell (the 'riser' of the step) has gap junctions that provide electrical coupling between the two cells. In histological sections the risers are not visible but the treads are distinct, as indicated in the diagram by their relatively greater thickness. Unlike the multinucleated skeletal muscle cell, the cardiac muscle cell has only one or two nuclei. The dark transverse striations represent A bands and the light striations I bands of sarcomeres, as seen in a histological section stained with haematoxylin and eosin. The small oblong area indicated by the arrow is enlarged in Fig. 21.1.

together with abundant glycogen and strong positive re-actions to **oxidative enzymes**, reflects the extremely high energetic demands of cardiac muscle (Williams *et al.*, 1989, p. 557). Mitochondria and granular deposits are particularly abundant around the poles of the nucleus of the cardiac muscle cell. The mitochondria contain the tricarboxylic acid cycle enzymes and the iron-containing cytochrome pigments of electron transfer chains. Together, these aerobically metabolize lactate, free fatty acids, and glucose, and produce the ATP which the myofilaments utilize to provide energy for their operation.

Opinions among card-bearing histologists are about evenly divided as to whether or not the myofibril is a constituent of the cytoplasm of the cardiac muscle cell. If not, what is it – simply a myofibril? Since myosin and actin are constituents of the cytoplasm of many cells besides muscle cells (Sections 21.6, 21.7), they would seem to be legitimate components of the cardiac muscle cytoplasm.

21.1.2   *Hypertrophy of cardiac muscle cells*

The cardiac muscle cells of endurance athletes respond to the demands of exercise by massive hypertrophy. This greatly increases the overall mass of the heart (by as much as about 40% in human marathon runners). Disease conditions

that overload the heart, such as aortic stenosis or aortic regurgitation, can increase the heart to about two and a half times its normal mass (Section 20.4).

In all such circumstances, the enlargement of the heart is solely due to hypertrophy of cardiac muscle cells. There is no increase in the number of cells.

In both the left and the right ventricle (Salmons, 1995, p. 771), the hypertrophy of cardiac muscle cells is achieved by parallel accretion of myofilaments, amounting even to the addition of new sarcomeres both in series and in parallel.

21.1.3   *Absence of regeneration of cardiac muscle cells*

The satellite cells of skeletal muscle can produce regeneration of skeletal muscle cells, but cardiac muscle totally lacks any capacity for regeneration. The myocardium can do no better than replace areas of dead cells with scar tissue.

Cardiac muscle cells proliferate in the fetus, but within 1 or 2 weeks following birth mitosis slows down and then stops altogether (Bishop and van Vleet, 1979). Cardiac muscle is therefore incapable of regeneration. The cells in the neonatal heart must last for a lifetime.

21.2   Intercalated disc

Intercalated discs join a sequence of cardiac muscle cells to one another, thus forming a cardiac muscle fibre (Fig. 21.1). These junctions always occur at the Z line. The disc has a step-like form. The *transverse part* of the step (the 'tread', at right angles to the long axis of the cell) is covered with short blunt projections that interlock with corresponding shallow hollows on the following cell (Fig. 21.8). At these interdigitations the apposing plasmalemmas are strongly reinforced by **desmosomes**. These membrane specializations stick the cells together, thus enabling them to transmit the force of contraction. Also the **actin filaments** of the sarcomere are firmly anchored in the desmosomes.

In the *vertical part* of the step (the 'riser', in the long axis of the cell), the plasmalemma has **gap junctions** (nexi) that provide electrical coupling between the two adjoining cells.

The **gap junctions** (macula communicans) allow relatively free diffusion of ions from one cell to the other, thus lowering the electrical resistance to about one four hundredth of the resistance through all other parts of the plasmalemma. Therefore action potentials and contraction spread readily throughout the myocardium (Guyton, 1986, p. 151). Thus cardiac muscle behaves electrically as a **syncitium**: however, structurally it is *not* a syncitium, since a syncitium is a multinuclear mass of cells that are not separated by cell membranes.

The myocardium is divided by the **fibrous skeleton** of the heart into two electrophysiological components, one atrial and the other ventricular, connected by the **atrioventricular bundle** (Section 21.19.3).

The adherence across the intercalated disc is dependent on Ca^{2+}, since washing with calcium-free solutions causes the cells to come apart (Muir, 1971, p. 8).

21.3   Endomysium

This is an irregular fine connective tissue that fills the interstitial spaces between cardiac muscle cells. It contains vast number of **blood capillaries** (Fig. 18.3), making cardiac muscle one of the most vascular tissues in the body (Section 18.3).

Many **lymphatic capillaries** are present throughout all components of the heart wall.

Nerve fibres are also present.

Lymphatic capillaries ramify in the cardiac endomysium, unlike the endomysium of skeletal muscle (Salmons, 1995, p. 770). The distribution and performance of these lymphatics was reviewed by Feigl (1974, p. 249). The myocardium has a rich lymphatic plexus of capillaries and larger vessels with valves. This myocardial plexus connects with subepicardial and subendocardial plexuses. Even the mitral and tricuspid valves are supplied with lymphatics. In the dog, cardiac lymphatic flow is about $3\,ml\,h^{-1}$. The total protein in cardiac lymph is about 75% of that in plasma. Potassium, sodium, and chloride concentrations are essentially the same as in plasma.

The larger tracts of cardiac muscle cells are parcelled into fasciculi by **perimysium**, as in skeletal muscle. This tissue is most conspicuous around the fibrous skeleton of the heart (Salmons, 1995, p. 764).

21.4   Sarcomere

The sarcomere is the smallest contractile unit, and hence the powerhouse, of cardiac (and skeletal) muscle. An understanding of how its sliding filaments produce the force of contraction provides the key to the automatic adjustment of stroke volume in response to the degree of filling of the normal atrium or ventricle (the Frank–Starling mechanism of the heart, Section 21.11), and an insight into the pathophysiology of cardiac dilation (Section 21.11.2).

The sarcomere consists of protein filaments, the **myofilaments**. These are of two types, **thick myofilaments** and **thin myofilaments**. The thick filaments are formed by **myosin molecules**, and the thin filaments by **actin molecules**. These filaments lie parallel to each other in the long axis of the cell (Figs 21.2, 21.3). The sarcomere is limited at each end by the **Z line** (Fig. 21.3). The **thin filaments** are anchored to the Z line at one end, and interdigitate with the thick filaments at their other end. The **thick filament** has regularly-spaced projections on either side (Fig. 21.3); each of these projections carries an enlarged (double) head (Fig. 21.5), which forms a cross-bridge with the adjacent actin filament during contraction.

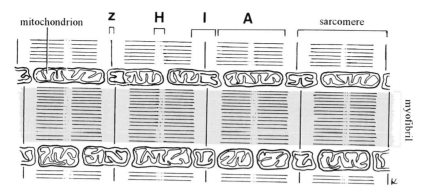

Fig. 21.2 Diagrammatic longitudinal section through part of a cardiac muscle cell, to show a myofibril, sarcomeres, and the alternating light and dark bands of sarcomeres. The field shown is the small area indicated by the arrow in Fig. 21.1. Here it is seen as in an electron micrograph at low magnification. The A bands represent the dark transverse striations in Fig. 21.1, and the I bands represent the light striations in Fig. 21.1. Each sarcomere extends between two dark Z lines. The Z line bisects each light I band. The H band bisects the dark A band. The sarcomere consists of thick and thin myofilaments arranged in the long axis of the cell. Only the thick myofilaments are shown here, represented by the dark parallel lines in the A band of each sarcomere; the thin myofilaments would be indistinct at this magnification. The myofilaments are organized into myofibrils. A myofibril is a longitudinal chain of sarcomeres, joined end-to-end at the Z lines. Four sarcomeres of a myofibril are shown in green. A myofibril extends throughout the whole length of its muscle cell, being attached to the intercalated disc at each end of the cell. Myofibrils are separated from each other by lines of mitochondria. The myofilaments and Z lines of adjacent myofibrils tend to be slightly out of register.

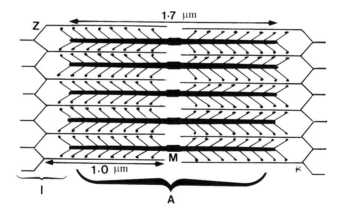

Fig. 21.3 Diagram showing the relationships between thick and thin myofilaments in a sarcomere of a cardiac muscle cell. The I band contains only thin (actin) filaments. The A band consists mainly of thick (myosin) filaments, plus overlapping parts of thin filaments. The H band contains only thick filaments here, but may also contain thin filaments as in stages E, F, and G of Fig. 21.9. The M line is caused by an enlargement of the middle segment of the thick filament. The thin filament is attached to the Z line at one end and unattached at its other end. It is about 1 μm in length. The thick filament is unattached at both ends. It is about 1.7 μm in length. The thick and thin filaments remain essentially unaltered in length during contraction and relaxation. The thick filament contains the rod-like tails of myosin molecules. The heads of these molecules project radially, and form cross-bridges with the actin molecules of the interdigitating thin filaments. The cross-bridges cause the thin filaments to slide towards the centre of the sarcomere during contraction, thus pulling the two Z lines towards the centre of their sarcomere. The relative positions of the thin and thick filaments in this diagram are similar to those in stage C of Fig. 21.9 (the 'rest' position). Thus they offer the maximum number of cross-bridges, and would therefore produce maximum tension if activated.

21.4.1 *Bands and lines of the sarcomere*

Longitudinal sections of cardiac muscle stained by haematoxylin show alternating light and dark bands (Fig. 21.2). The pale **I band** (stria I) contains only those parts of the thin filaments that are not overlapping the thick filaments (Fig. 21.3); it is bisected by the dark **Z line** (linea Z). The Z line is caused by the intermeshing of thin filaments on either side of the Z line, the precise structure of the Z line being uncertain (Krstic, 1984, p. 448). The dark **A band** (stria A) consists mainly of thick filaments together with the overlapping parts of the thin filaments. The pale **H band** (stria H) is sometimes visible across the centre of the A band; it contains only thick filaments. An alternative name for the H band is zona lucida. The I and H bands change their length during contraction, getting shorter as the thin filaments slide over the thick, and disappearing altogether in strong contraction (stage F in Fig. 21.9); the A band stays the same length, except if contraction becomes so excessive that the thick filament becomes crumpled (Stage G in Fig. 21.9). The dark **M line** (linea M) transects the H band; it is formed by the central thickened segment of the myosin filament (Fig. 21.3).

The I band is also known as the **isotropic disc** (discus isotropicus) because it does not alter polarized light. The A band is birefringent in polarized light, and is therefore also known as the **anisotropic disc** (discus anisotropicus).

The essentially hexagonal arrangement of the filaments in transverse sections is shown in Fig. 21.4. At the M line the myosin filaments are connected to each other by transversely orientated, intermediate-sized, desmin microfilaments (Krstic, 1984, p. 268); actin filaments are evidently able to pass between these interconnecting

filaments when they overlap the M line in advanced contraction (stage E in Fig. 21.9).

21.5 Myofibril

The cardiac muscle cell (like the skeletal muscle cell) is organized into **myofibrils**. A myofibril consists of a chain of sarcomeres joined to each other, end-to-end, at their Z lines (Fig. 21.2). The myofibril extends throughout the whole length of the cardiac and skeletal muscle cell, and is attached to the intercalated disc at both ends of the cell.

Adjacent myofibrils are separated by lines of mitochondria (Fig. 21.2), together with the network of fine tubules belonging to the sarcoplasmic reticulum. The T tubule system also passes between myofibrils, though transversely (Fig. 21.8). The mitochondria and their accompanying tissues occupy a fairly large space, so that the myofibrils seen with the light microscope in transverse sections of cardiac muscle stand out quite distinctly (Fig. 18.3). The mitochondria between the myofibrils are very numerous, indicative of the extreme energy expenditure of cardiac muscle which demands large amounts of ATP formed by mitochondria.

The filaments of adjacent myofibrils tend to be slightly out of register with each other (Fig. 21.2).

21.6 Molecular structure of the thick myofilament

The thick filament consists of rod-like molecules of myosin, bound together in a cylindrical bundle (Fig. 21.5). The **myosin molecule** consists of two peptide chains twisted together to form a **double helix** (Fig. 21.6) (the actin molecule is also a double helix; Section 21.7). At one end of the myosin molecule the double helix bends out of the thick filaments as an **arm**, on the end of which are *two* globular **heads** each formed by the folding of its own helical chain (Fig. 21.6). The head is the region where the actin-binding site is located. The remainder of the myosin molecule is known as the **tail**, and this is embedded in the cylindrical bundle that forms the body of the thick filament.

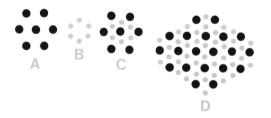

Fig. 21.4 Diagrams showing the content and relationships of the thick and thin myofilaments in the bands and lines of a sarcomere.

A. **Transverse section through the H line.** Only thick filaments are present. They are arranged in a hexagon around a central thick filament. The M line resembles this pattern, except that each of its myosin filaments is connected to its six neighbouring myosin filaments by a short fibril.

B. **Transverse section through the I band.** Only thin filaments are present. They are arranged in a hexagon.

C, D. Transverse sections through the A band. Both thick and thin filaments are present, in hexagonal patterns.

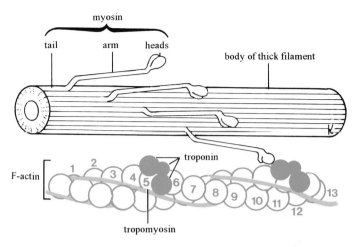

Fig. 21.5   Schematic diagram of a thick and a thin myofilament, showing the molecular structure of the thin (actin) myofilament. The two filaments shown in this diagram are orientated as in the *right* half of the sarcomere in Fig. 21.3; thus the midpoint of the thick (myosin) filament would be to the left. Myosin is a rod-like molecule. The myosin molecules are bound together in a bundle, thus forming the body of the thick filament. One end of each myosin molecule (the end nearer to the Z line) projects radially out of the bundle as the arm, and this carries two globular heads. The remainder of the myosin molecule is known as the tail; the tail is elongated, and embedded in the body of the thick filament. The principal component of the thin filament is formed by two intertwined spiral strands of F-actin (**F**ilamentous actin). Each of these spirals consists of polymerized polypeptide molecules of G-actin (**G**lobular actin) (green circles). There are about 13 G-actin subunits (1–13) in each revolution of F-actin. It is these subunits that carry the sites for binding with the myosin heads, thus producing muscle contraction. In each of the two grooves between these two intertwined spirals of F-actin lies a narrow spiral strand of tropomyosin molecules (pale green strand). The tropomyosin strand blocks the binding sites on the globular actin subunits, thus preventing the formation of myosin–actin bridges. At regular intervals along the tropomyosin strand, there occurs a complex of three troponin subunits (solid green discs). One of these troponin subunits (troponin-T) is bound to the tropomyosin strand. The other two troponin subunits are troponin-C (having an affinity to calcium), and troponin-I. When Ca^{2+} ions bind to the troponin-C, the tropomyosin molecule is displaced, thus exposing the binding sites and allowing myosin–actin bridges to form.

At the M line, tails of myosin molecules abut on each other, end-to-end, and then run towards opposite ends of the sarcomere. The arms of all myosin molecules are therefore directed *away* from the M line and *towards* the Z line. Consequently in the midregion of the thick filament, there are no arms and heads.

The attachment of the tail to the arm is flexible, and the attachment of the arm to the head is also flexible. These flexible points act as hinges (arrows in Fig. 21.6), allowing the arms and their heads to be moved so as to attach to or disengage from the active sites of an actin molecule.

The structure and function of the thick filament (myofilamentum crassum) and myosin molecule have been surveyed by Guyton (1986, p. 123) and Salmons (1995, p. 742). It is estimated that about 274 myosin molecules form the thick filament, each molecule being about 1.6–1.8 µm long. The molecule comprises six

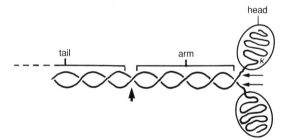

Fig. 21.6   Schematic diagram of a myosin molecule. The myosin molecule consists of two peptide molecules in a double helix. The tail of the myosin molecule is a rod-like structure embedded in the cylindrical body of the thick filament; the end of the tail is directed towards the M line. The arm of the myosin molecule, which is directed towards the Z line, projects out of the thick filament. The arm is hinged at the large arrow. At the free end of the arm, there are two flexible globular heads each formed mainly by the folding of its own helical chain. Each head is hinged at the small arrow. The head is the part of the molecule where the hydrolysis of ATP occurs, and the myosin–actin bridge is formed.

polypeptide chains, two of them heavy chains and four of them light chains. A subfragment of heavy meromysin (HMM-S1) forms the two heads. HMM-S1 contains all the enzymatic and actin-binding elements of the intact myosin molecule that are required for producing force and movement. It seems likely that the two heads can act independently, even binding to different thin (actin) filaments (Salmons, 1995, p. 743).

Myosin can be extracted from almost every cell type in the vertebrate body (Alberts *et al.*, 1983, p. 553), including not only muscle cells but myoepithelial cells, ordinary epithelial cells, and nerve cells.

21.7 Molecular structure of the thin myofilament

The thin filament is formed by three proteins, F-actin (**F**ilamentous actin), tropomyosin, and troponin (Fig. 21.5). The main component is **F-actin**. The F-actin molecule consists of two strands wound round each other in a double helix, like the myosin molecule. Each strand consists of a sequence of globular polypeptide molecules (dark green circles in Fig. 21.5), and it is these subunits that carry the sites for binding with the myosin heads. **Tropomyosin** takes the form of two slender protein strands (pale green in Fig. 21.5) that wind spirally round the two grooves formed by the apposition of the two F-actin strands. Partly superimposed on the tropomyosin strand at regular intervals is another protein, **troponin**, consisting of a complex of three globular subunits (solid dark green in Fig. 21.5). Tropomyosin and troponin regulate the binding sites of the myosin-actin cross-bridges (Section 21.8).

The total length of the spiral **F-actin** strand is about 1.0 μm (Salmons, 1995, p. 744) Its polymerized globular subunits (or monomers) are known as **G-actin** (**G**lobular actin). F-actin completes one revolution in about 70 nm. There are about 13 G-actin molecules (the numbered dark green circles in Fig. 21.5) in one complete revolution of F-actin. According to Guyton (1986, p. 124) one molecule of ADP is attached to each G-actin molecule, thus giving each G-actin subunit a binding site for a myosin–actin cross-bridge (Junqueira and Carneiro, 1983, p. 229). The binding sites on the two F-actin strands are staggered, giving a binding site on the thin filament (myofilamentum tenue) at estimated intervals of 2.7 nm.

Tropomyosin and troponin play a major role in the control of contraction (Section 21.8), and are therefore known as *regulatory* proteins. For every seven G-actin subunits there is one molecule each of tropomyosin and troponin (Salmons, 1995, p. 745).

The **tropomyosin** strand (pale green in Fig. 21.5) consists of tropomyosin polymers. It is a rod-like molecule, about 41 nm long, overlapping slightly with the next successive molecule. Each of the two tropomyosin strands is evidently loosely attached to the groove between the two F-actin strands; this attachment occurs in such a way that, at rest, the tropomyosin strand *physically covers the binding sites on the G-actin subunits, thus preventing myosin–actin interaction* (Guyton, 1986, p. 124).

The **troponin** complex consists of three subunits (solid green in Fig. 21.5), arranged along the actin filament at regular intervals of about 40 nm (Krstic, 1984, p. 430). Each of the three subunits is named according to its function (Salmons, 1995, p. 745). Troponin-**T** binds to tropomyosin (in Fig. 21.5 this is the solid green subunit that is in contact with the tropomyosin strand). Troponin-**C** has an affinity for calcium. Troponin-**I** has a strong affinity for actin, and inhibits the myosin–actin binding (Junqueira and Carneiro, 1983, p. 229).

Actin is present in a large variety of cells (Krstic, 1984, p. 5).

21.8 Interaction between myosin and actin

The interaction between myosin and actin forms the **cross-bridges** between the thick and thin filaments.

Hydrolysis of adenosine triphosphate (ATP) to adenosine diphosphate (ADP) and inorganic phosphate supplies the energy that produces contraction; the enzyme required for this process, an ATPase, is an inherent component of the cross-bridge.

In relaxed muscle, the active sites on the actin are inhibited by tropomyosin, presumably by obstructing access to, or even physically covering, the active sites. Troponin provides a calcium-sensitive switch that removes the inhibitory action of tropomyosin, and thus induces the interaction between myosin and actin. There is a sudden increase in the concentration of free Ca^{2+} in the cytoplasm of the muscle cell (Section 21.16). The calcium ions bind to the troponin. The troponin then undergoes a conformational change that apparently causes the tropomyosin to roll deeper into the two grooves between the two actin strands (Section 21.7). This exposes the binding sites on the actin strands: actin–myosin cross-bridges then form, and contraction occurs. Thus the calcium ions *inhibit* the inhibitory effect of tropomyosin – *disinhibition*, in neurological terms.

> The energy changes that take place during the interaction between myosin and actin at the cross-bridges have been summarized by Salmons (1995, p. 741). After the cleavage of ATP, both the ADP and the inorganic phosphate remain bound to the cross-bridge, with the result that although binding occurs it is weak and reversible. Next, the inorganic phosphate is released, and muscle is *activated* by the calcium ions, thus dislodging tropomyosin and exposing binding sites on the F-actin: the *power stroke* results. To achieve relaxation, a fresh molecule of ATP is made available at the binding site, and this causes the cross-bridge to detach and reset to its original condition. If the fresh ATP fails to arrive – as in death – the contracted state continues, giving rigor mortis. If the muscle remains activated, the formation of bridges can be repeated at the rate of about $1–3\,s^{-1}$.

21.9 Walk-along theory of contraction

Repeated cycles of attachment and detachment of cross-bridges occur at a succession of binding sites along the thin filament. In active muscle, many cross-bridges can operate asynchronously, thus causing a continuous pull on the thin filaments.

Figure 21.7 shows how the *walk-along* mechanism of contraction might work.

Three myosin molecules are shown. The one furthest to the right is in a relaxed state, with its arm and head in position 1 so that its head is detached from any cross-bridge. The myosin molecule in the middle is busy contracting. Its hinges between tail and arm and between arm and head, have brought its myosin head in contact with the thin filament, forming a cross-bridge at position 2. Further hinging between the arm and the head has then moved this cross-bridge to position 3, thus pulling the thin filament to the left. The myosin molecule on the left has been restored to the resting state, with its head detached from a cross-bridge (in position 1). Each myosin molecule operates independently. Its head can bend repeatedly, attaching and detaching cross-bridges, thus 'walking along' the thin filament. In so doing it drags the thin filament ever closer to the midpoint of the thick filament – i.e. it causes contraction.

Obviously, the greater the number of cross-bridges the greater the force of contraction. However, the availability of binding sites varies as the relative positions of the thick and thin filaments change. Some positions of the thick and thin filaments provide an optimum number of

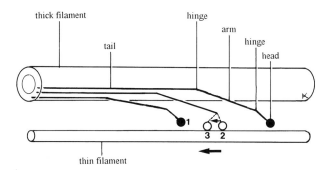

Fig. 21.7 Diagram illustrating the walk-along theory of contraction. The orientation of the thin and the thick filament in this diagram is the same as in Fig. 21.5, i.e. the midpoint of the thick filament is to the left. Three myosin molecules are shown. The one on the right is resting, since its head is not in contact with the thin filament (position 1). The myosin molecule in the middle has flexed the hinge between its tail and its arm, and this has brought its head in contact with the thin filament and made a cross-bridge at position 2; the hinge between its head and arm then flexes, and this is the power stroke moving the cross-bridge to the left to position 3 (small arrow). The myosin molecule on the left has completed its power stroke, detached its head from a cross-bridge, and straightened the hinge between its tail and its arm, thus restoring its head to position 1 at rest. Therefore, while the thick filament has remained stationary, the thin filament has been moved towards the midpoint of the thick filament (large arrow): a small degree of contraction of the sarcomere has occurred. Cross-bridges form and detach in continuous cycles, independently of each other, at many points along the two filaments. The greater the number of cross-bridges, the greater the force of contraction.

cross-bridges, but in others the number is diminished (Section 21.10).

21.10   Length–tension relationships

The force of contraction of cardiac muscle is related to the extent to which the sarcomeres are stretched. Maximum force is generated when the thin filaments fully overlap all those parts of the thick filament which possess the radiating heads

of the myosin molecules (positions C and D of Fig. 21.9); *at these two sarcomere lengths the maximum possible number of cross-bridges is available.* Any further shortening from position D does not make any more myosin heads available. On the contrary, shortening to positions E and F causes the thin filaments to overlap the M line and hence to interfere with the formation of cross-bridges in the other half of the sarcomere, and this results in a fall in tension. At position F the thick filament hits the Z line. Continued shortening of the

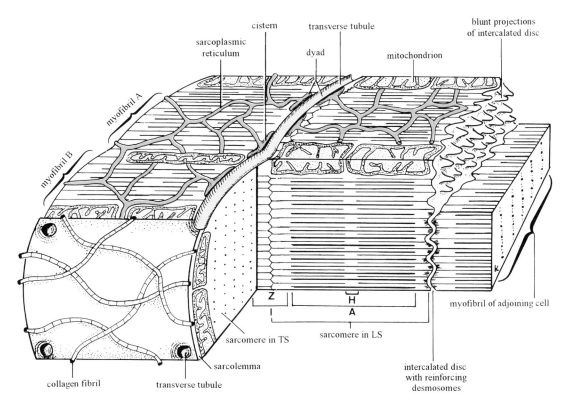

Fig. 21.8   Three-dimensional diagram of part of a cardiac muscle cell, showing myofibrils, sarcomeres and their myofilaments, and transverse tubules and sarcoplasmic reticulum. On the right, an intercalated disc marks the boundary between two cardiac muscle cells. The short blunt projections of the intercalated disc interlock with corresponding hollows on the adjoining cell. Desmosomes attach the projections to the hollows. The cell to the left of the intercalated disc shows two parallel myofibrils, myofibrils A and B, which are largely separated by mitochondria. To the right of centre, one of the sarcomeres of myofibril B has been cut in longitudinal section. Its myofilaments are in the 'rest' position, as in Fig. 21.3. To the left of centre, the next consecutive sarcomere of myofibril A has been cut transversely through the I band, so that only its thin filaments are seen in its cut surface as in Fig. 21.4B. A transverse tubule (light green) arises as a funnel-shaped invagination of the sarcolemma. It penetrates the sarcoplasm at right angles to the cell surface, at the level of a Z line. The T-tubule has a larger diameter than the tubules of the sarcoplasmic reticulum. The fine tubules of the sarcoplasmic reticulum (dark green) more or less enclose the myofibrils. Terminal cisterns of sarcoplasmic reticulum are closely applied to transverse tubules, forming dyads. At the periphery of the cell, a tubule of the sarcoplasmic reticulum is seen passing beneath the sarcolemma. The sarcolemma, which is a typical plasmalemma, is covered by a fine network of collagen fibrils.

sarcomere from position F progressively crumples the thick filament; this adds more resistance to shortening and also reduces the number of available cross-bridges still further. Consequently tension falls profoundly, reaching zero in position G where the thick filament is substantially crumpled and the thin filaments are interfering with each other along their entire lengths.

Normal cardiac sarcomeres operate only over the ascending part of the curve in Fig. 21.9, on a range extending from a point about half way between positions G and F, to a final limit at position C. This means that when contraction of

the ventricles (ventricular systole) is completed, the ventricular sarcomeres have shortened to about half way between G and F. Ventricular diastole follows, with progressive stretching of the ventricle due to venous return. If the venous return be only moderate, as at rest, this may stretch the ventricular sarcomeres to a position somewhere between F and E. Since not all of the cross-bridges are then available, the force produced during the subsequent ventricular systole would be well below the maximum, and of course the volume of blood to be pumped would be relatively small. On the other hand, if the venous

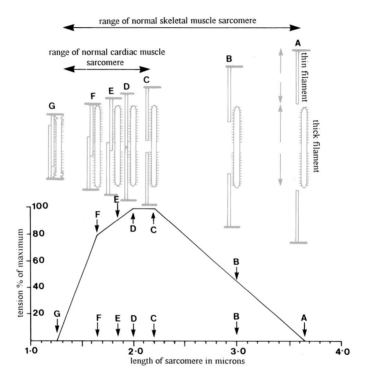

Fig. 21.9 Diagram of thick and thin filaments, illustrating the relationship between length and tension in a sarcomere. Seven possible stages (A–G) of the isometric response to stimulation of a skeletal muscle sarcomere are shown. The tension curve has an ascending limb (G–C), and a descending limb (C–A). Sarcomeres of *normal* **cardiac muscle** operate *only* over the ascending limb, from a maximum length of about 2.2 μm to a minimum of about 1.5 μm, i.e. essentially within stages C, D, and E, and slightly below F. Based on Muir (1971). **A.** Since the thick and thin filaments do not overlap at all, no myosin–actin bridges can occur, so tension is zero. **B.** Nearly half of the possible myosin–actin bridges are in action, and therefore tension is nearly 50%. **C.** The maximum number of bridges is available, so tension is maximal – in both skeletal and cardiac sarcomeres. **D.** The maximum number of bridges is still available, and therefore there is no change in tension between C and D. **E.** The thin filaments overlap, and extend beyond the midpoint of the thick filament. Beyond the midpoint, the thin filaments overlap the M line and hence interfere with the formation of cross-bridges in the other half of the sarcomere. Tension therefore decreases. **F.** The thick filament impinges at both of its ends on the Z lines. This would add to the resistance to shortening. Continued shortening crumples the ends of the thick filaments, thus amplifying the resistance to further shortening and decreasing yet again the number of available cross-bridges.

return were suddenly to be greatly increased, the ventricular sarcomeres may be stretched to positions D or C: now the maximum number of cross-bridges is available, and would therefore enable ventricular systole to develop much greater force and pump a much larger volume of blood.

These relationships between sarcomere length and the tension produced during contraction were established by Gordon *et al.* (1966) on skeletal muscle, the measurements being made under conditions in which the muscle is unable to shorten (isometric contraction). Isolated myocardial muscle strips display similar relationships between length and tension, and these relationships are assumed to extend to the whole ventricle (Thornburg and Morton, 1993, p. 147).

In the *normal* heart the sarcomeres operate only within the range of about 1.5–2.2 μm, yielding 32% tension at full contraction. This range is less than that of the skeletal sarcomere, which works from 3.6 to 1.5 μm with 58% tension at full contraction (Muir, 1971, p. 7).

21.11 Control of stroke volume: the Frank–Starling mechanism

The *stroke volume* is the volume of blood ejected by a ventricle in one systole. The relationships between the length of the sarcomere and the tension it produces during contraction suggest a mechanism by which the heart could automatically increase or decrease its stroke volume in response to an increase or a decrease in the volume of blood that it receives. This mechanism was elaborated by Frank and Starling at the beginning of the twentieth century. It proposed simply that the normal heart automatically pumps out whatever volume of blood is put into it. Thus the heart modulates its stroke volume according to the rate of venous return.

The *venous return* (the volume of blood arriving in the right atrium per minute) varies from moment to moment, for example through *changes in posture* (getting up or lying down) and *movements of the limbs* (the muscle pump; Section 12.16.2), and *breathing* (cyclic fluctuations in intrathoracic and intraabdominal–abdominal pressure; Section 10.4.1). The varying venous return to the right atrium is passed on to the right ventricle, and the right ventricle adjusts its stroke volume accordingly; and so on, to the left atrium and left ventricle.

At rest, the volume of venous blood thus entering the right ventricle is small enough for its sarcomeres to operate around the lower end of the slope between F and E in Fig. 21.9. A transient increase in venous return, caused for example by a change of posture, may stretch the sarcomeres of the right ventricle nearer to position E than to position F. The resulting increase in force produced by the stretched sarcomeres then enables the right ventricle automatically to pump out this increased volume of blood. Corresponding adjustments then follow in the *left side* of the heart: thus the mechanism automatically maintains an essentially equal output from the right and left sides of the heart. The whole essence of the Frank–Starling mechanism is therefore that it *provides autoregulation of stroke volume in response to variations in venous return*. Thus the heart operates on entirely different principles from a typical reciprocating mechanical pump: the mechanical pump has a fixed stroke volume, but the heart continually adjusts its stroke volume in order to cope with the variations in its input.

The same length–tension mechanism enables the heart to adjust its output to *changes in the peripheral resistance* of the systemic arterial circulation. If the peripheral resistance rises suddenly, the force developed by the next systole of the left ventricle may be insufficient to eject its previous stroke volume into the aorta. If so, a corresponding volume of blood is retained in the left ventricle. To this is added the volume supplied by the next atrial systole. The left ventricle is now relatively stretched, and its sarcomeres automatically respond with correspondingly greater force.

The Frank–Starling mechanism is therefore able to increase the cardiac output automatically, and without increasing the heart rate. This meets the animal's circulatory requirements at rest. **At exercise**, however, the energetic demands of the muscles require the cardiac output to be increased about four- or fivefold. This can only be achieved by greatly increasing the heart rate, and this requires activation of the autonomic nervous system (Section 22.16).

Stretching of the sarcomeres beyond position C, towards B and A in Fig. 21.9, results in a progressive reduction of available cross-bridges and hence a progressive fall in tension. This is known as the *descending limb* of the length–tension curve. Pathological *dilation* of a heart chamber would be expected to take it to the descending limb. Dilation of the left atrium and left ventricle occurs with a **patent ductus arteriosus** (Section 15.8), and dilation of the right ventricle occurs with **pulmonary stenosis** (Section 15.9), two common cardiovascular defects in the dog (Section 15.7). A failure to correct the increasing dilation should make the ventricular contractions in these conditions progressively weaker because of the loss of actin–myosin bridges inherent in the descending limb.

21.11.1   *The Starling law of the heart*

Using the length–tension relationships derived by Frank in 1895 from the isolated frog heart, and combining these with his own observations on the canine heart–lung preparation, Starling derived the concept in 1915 that 'the mechanical energy set free on passage from the resting to the contracted state depends on the length of the muscle fibres'. From this concept it was postulated that a progressive increase in venous return would induce a progressive increase in stroke volume with each successive cardiac cycle. The stroke volume would level off at a new outflow rate. Theoretically, the cardiac output could thus be increased without an increase in heart rate (Rushmer, 1966, p. 647).

For many years this attractively simple concept was regarded as the dominant mechanism controlling cardiovascular adjustment, not only in *health* when at rest and at exercise, but also in *disease*, It became known as 'the Starling law of the heart'. This still holds as a valuable principle for the normal heart at rest. However, it is now clear that regulation of the heart is dominated during **exercise** by the autonomic nervous system and autonomic hormones (Section 22.16). For that reason it is better to rename the Starling law as the **Frank–Starling mechanism** (Rushmer, 1966, p. 648).

21.11.2   *The pathologically dilated heart*

The functional significance of the loss of actin–myosin cross-bridges in the pathologically dilated heart is difficult to assess. According to Elzinga (1992), Starling suggested that when a heart was so distended that it arrived at the descending limb it had in fact failed: it was a normal heart that was overfilled and could no longer cope with its venous return. This interpretation of the pathogenesis of cardiac failure attracted clinical attention in human medicine between 1940 and 1960. However, Elzinga (1992) pointed out that experimental demonstrations of the descending limb in the supposedly normal heart by stretching the myocardium beyond the range of 2.4–2.6 µm are difficult to interpret. For instance, such stretching may cause irreversible structural damage to the cardiac muscle cells. Also, in a heart–lung preparation, removal of the pericardium may allow the heart to dilate, thus inducing atrioventricular incompetence. Elzinga (1992) concluded that the descending limb (presumably meaning the loss of cross-bridges in the descending limb) may play only 'a minor role' in most pathological myocardial conditions.

If a loss of cross-bridges (as in the descending limb of the length–tension curve) does contribute to the failure of the heart, it would perhaps be most likely to do so in cardiac disorders that entail severe dilation of heart chambers. **Dilated cardiac myopathy**, which occurs in almost all domestic species and especially the dog, is characterized by ventricular and atrial dilation with depressed systolic function (Darke *et al.*, 1996, p. 98). It is not difficult to visualize that some of the myocardium could enter the descending limb. However, there must presumably have been some primary disorder, such as necrosis of cardiac muscle cells (e.g. following parvovirus infection in the dog), ingestion of toxic substances (e.g. monensin in horses), deficiencies of essential substances (e.g. selenium in cattle and pigs), or myocardial ischaemia. Therefore it would obviously be too simplistic to attribute the failure of the dilated heart primarily to the sliding apart of the thick and thin filaments to between stages C and B in the descending limb, and consequent loss of cross-bridges according to the Starling law of the heart. Even so, Muir (1971, p. 7) may be justified in at least concluding from the Frank–Starling mechanism that 'if a diseased heart is dilated it is weakened and made liable to further distension'.

21.12   Transverse tubule

The plasmalemma (sarcolemma) of the cardiac muscle cell is invaginated into the cytoplasm of the cell to form a system of **transverse (T) tubules**. T-tubules are therefore extensions of the extracellular space. Starting as funnel-shaped openings, T-tubules enter the cytoplasm of the cardiac muscle cell at the level of the Z line, at right angles to the surface (Fig. 21.8). They penetrate deeply between and around the sarcomeres. This enables them to perform their function – to conduct the action potential into the very depths of the cell (Section 21.14).

They are closely applied to dilated cisterns of the sarcoplasmic reticulum, thus forming paired tubules (dyads) (Fig. 21.8). The close apposition of the membranes of the T-tubule and sarcoplasmic reticulum at the dyad enables the release and removal of calcium ions during the action potential.

The T-tubules (tubulus transversus) of **cardiac muscle cells** have a much wider lumen than those of skeletal muscle cells, the diameter being five times greater and the volume 25 times greater (Guyton, 1986, p. 152). The basal lamina of the sarcolemma extends inside the T-tubule as a thin intratubular coating (Kristic, 1984, p. 65); the abundant mucopolysaccharides of the basal lamina are negatively charged and bind a large store of calcium ions. Hence good reserves of calcium ions are always available for diffusion into the cardiac muscle cell when the action potential occurs on the T-tubule.

The **skeletal muscle cell** has *two* T-tubules to each sarcomere, there being one T-tubule at the junction of the A band with the I band at each end of the sarcomere: each T-tubule is therefore in close contact with the point of interaction between the actin and myosin filaments, i.e. optimally placed for fast contraction. The cardiac muscle cell has its T-tubule at the Z line, at the junction between adjacent sarcomeres, so that one tubule is shared by two sarcomeres. Being at the Z line, the tubule is further away from the interaction between the myofilaments, and this may be consistent with the relatively slower contraction of the cardiac sarcomere while the calcium ions diffuse from the Z line to the middle of the sarcomere. Instead of dyads, skeletal muscle cells have **triads**, consisting of a T-tubule with a terminal cistern of sarcoplasmic reticulum on each side.

The cardiac muscle cells of **non-mammalian vertebrates** lack T-tubules (Salmons, 1995, p. 767).

Atrial cardiac muscle cells (Section 21.1) have few, or even no T-tubules (Salmons, 1995, p. 764). This means that atrial cardiac muscle cells partly, or even entirely, lack the standard equipment for transmitting the action potential to the depths of the cell, but the sarcoplasmic reticulum takes over this function; the close apposition of plasmalemma to cisterns of the sarcoplasmic reticulum (where clusters of calcium channels lie at the interface between plasmalemma and sarcoplasmic reticulum) presumably makes an important contribution to this function. Atrial muscle cells are smaller in cross-section than ventricular muscle cells (Section 21.1), and this in itself helps the distribution of the action potential to all parts of the cell.

21.13 Sarcoplasmic reticulum

The sarcoplasmic reticulum is an internal network of fine tubules, more or less enclosing individual myofibrils (Fig. 21.8). Its main function is to store, release, and retrieve calcium ions engaged in activating the sliding mechanism of the thick and thin filaments during myocardial contraction (Section 21.16).

The sarcoplasmic reticulum is, in fact, a variant of smooth endoplasmic reticulum (Krstic, 1984, p. 365). It is not as regular in its form, and is less well-developed, in cardiac than in skeletal sarcomeres (Junqueira and Carneiro, 1983, p. 241).

Small dilated cisterns of sarcoplasmic reticulum make contact with both the sarcolemma (Feigl, 1974, p. 42) and the T-tubules (Salmons, 1995, p. 767). The contact with the sarcolemma brings 'trigger calcium' from the interstitial fluid into contact with the sarcoplasmic reticulum; this takes place via clusters of **calcium channels** in the sarcolemma (Section 21.16.2), these sarcolemmal channels being assembled opposite **clusters** of similar **calcium channels** in the membranous wall of the sarcoplasmic reticulum. The contact between the sarcoplasmic reticulum and the T-tubules is concerned with exciting the release of calcium from the sarcoplasmic reticulum in order to activate contraction. At the dyads, **clusters of calcium channels** on the T-tubule are associated with clusters on the sarcoplasmic reticulum. The sites of these channels are spanned by structures known as **junctional processes** (Salmons, 1995, p. 767). The sarcoplasmic reticulum that bears these junctional processes has been named the **junctional sarcoplasmic reticulum** to distinguish it from the **free sarcoplasmic reticulum** that forms the ordinary network of smooth-surfaced tubules.

21.14 The cardiac impulse: general principles

The cardiac impulse originates from the sinuatrial node (Section 21.19.1). The impulse depolarizes the plasmalemma of a cardiac muscle cell. The plasmalemma (i.e. sarcolemma) not only covers the *surface* of the cell, but it also penetrates into the very *depths* of the cell by means of its T-tubules. In the interior of the cell, the T-tubules are in close contact with the sarcoplasmic reticulum. The sarcoplasmic reticulum embraces groups of myofilaments.

The plasmalemma is depolarized both on the surface of the cell and in the interior of the cell by means of the T-tubules. This depolarization stimulates the release of calcium from the sarcoplasmic reticulum into the cytoplasm of the muscle cell. When the concentration of calcium in the cytoplasm rises to the required level, the ATPase of the myosin–actin junctions is activated, and a contraction is induced. During the subsequent diastole, the calcium is pumped out of the cytoplasm of the muscle cell by the sarcoplasmic reticulum, and the cell relaxes.

Calcium also enters the cytoplasm directly from the interstitial fluid. It enters during the action potential, and then leaves the cell via the Na/Ca exchange and Ca ATPase in the sarcolemma. Nevertheless the sarcoplasmic reticulum is the most important source and sink of calcium (Section 21.16.1).

21.15   The cardiac muscle cell: a typical excitable cell

All three types of muscle cell (smooth, skeletal, and cardiac) share the basic functional characteristics of an **excitable cell** as exemplified by the nerve cell. Thus they exhibit a membrane potential, action potential, absolute refractory period, relative refractory period, recovery, and conduction velocity.

The **membrane potential** (resting potential) of cardiac muscle cells is about 85–95 mV negative with respect to the outside of the cell. The inrush of Na^{2+} ions – *depolarization* – that causes the **action potential** occurs initially through fast-acting sodium ion channels, as in skeletal muscle; this instantly alters the potential within the cell by about 110 mV, to about +20 mV. After the initial spike the membrane remains on a plateau of depolarization for up to another 0.3 s, and this is an **absolute refractory period** during which the cell cannot receive or initiate another potential.

The **absolute refractory period** of the cardiac muscle cell of man lasts about 50 times longer than that of the skeletal muscle cell, and in the heart of large mammals it extends for over 400 ms (Muir, 1971, p. 15). Thus it prevents the sustained contraction (tetanus) that is useful in skeletal muscle but would be potentially lethal in the heart. The relatively very long duration of the absolute refractory period in the cardiac muscle cell is due (Guyton, 1986, p. 151) firstly to the presence of slowly-acting calcium–sodium channels, which open relatively slowly but stay open to admit both sodium and calcium ions throughout the plateau of depolarization; the skeletal muscle cell lacks these slowly-acting channels. Secondly it is due to a fivefold decrease in the permeability of potassium ion channels throughout the plateau, thus opposing *repolarization*; skeletal muscle cells lack this feature. At the end of the absolute refractory period there is a brief **relative refractory period**, in which the

muscle cell can be excited but only with difficulty. In the **recovery phase** at the end of the plateau, the slow sodium–calcium channels close, the potassium channels open, potassium ions are rapidly lost from the cell, and the membrane abruptly *repolarizes*.

The **conduction velocity** of cardiac muscle cells is only about $0.5\,\mathrm{m\,s^{-1}}$, in contrast to the $120\,\mathrm{m/s^{-1}}$ of a large myelinated axon.

21.16   Excitation–contraction coupling

It is an essential design requirement of a contractile cell that when it contracts it should do so uniformly and not piecemeal. The usual method evolved by the body for exciting an excitable cell is to apply an appropriate stimulus (electrical, mechanical, or chemical) to the outer surface of that cell, i.e. to its **plasmalemma**. The electrical stimulus of the cardiac impulse could indeed excite an action potential on the plasmalemma of the cardiac muscle cell, but this is such a very large cell that there would be virtually no flow of current in the depth of its cytoplasm. This difficulty has been overcome by the evolution of the **T-tubule** (Section 21.12), which carries the plasmalemma, and hence the action potential, deep into the interior of the cell.

The arrival of the action potential throughout the interior of the cardiac (or skeletal) muscle cell excites the release of **calcium ions** into the cytoplasm. The calcium ions diffuse rapidly into the **myofibrils**, where they activate the sliding mechanism of the **actin** and **myosin filaments** (Section 21.8) and hence cause *contraction* of the myocardium. At the end of the plateau of the action potential, the flow of calcium ions into the muscle cell is abruptly arrested.

The *force of contraction* is modulated by varying the amount of calcium released into the cardiac muscle cell: an increase in calcium makes more actin–myosin cross-bridges available by displacing tropomyosin. The adrenergic innervation of the cardiac muscle cell increases the force of contraction by means of this mechanism.

Relaxation is achieved by returning the calcium ions to the interior of the sarcoplasmic reticulum, and by transporting calcium out of the cell via the T-tubules.

21.16.1 *Sources of calcium ions*

Two sources of calcium ions are available to the cytoplasm of the cardiac muscle cell.

(a) *Sarcoplasmic reticulum*

Since the small terminal expansions (dyads) of the sarcoplasmic reticulum (Section 21.12) are intimately applied to the T-tubules (Fig. 21.8), the action potential on the T-tubules readily excites the sarcoplasmic reticulum. This causes the sarcoplasmic reticulum to release calcium ions into the cytoplasm of the cardiac muscle cell (as it does in the skeletal muscle cell).

(b) *T-tubule and interstitial fluid*

Large quantities of calcium ions are stored within the T-tubules, by binding with abundant mucopolysaccharides (Guyton, 1986, p. 152). This calcium is released by the action potential of the T-tubule. Since the interstitial fluid percolates into the T-tubule, the concentration of calcium ions in the interstitial fluid necessarily influences strongly the strength of contraction of cardiac muscle. This not a factor in the skeletal muscle cell, which depends almost entirely on calcium ions supplied by the sarcoplasmic reticulum (Guyton, 1986, p. 153); the sarcoplasmic reticulum of the skeletal muscle cell has very voluminous terminal cisterns which give it a much greater volume than that of the cardiac muscle cell (Williams *et al.*, 1989, p. 551).

These several sources of calcium make varying contributions to the activation of the contractile proteins of the ventricles, depending on the species. The rat relies much more on the release of calcium from the sarcoplasmic reticulum than does the rabbit (Bers, 1989).

21.16.2 *Mechanism of release of calcium ions from sarcoplasmic reticulum*

In the region of the **dyads**, both the sarcoplasmic reticulum and the T-tubule carry calcium channels, and these are associated together in clusters. The calcium release channels on the cell membrane of the sarcoplasmic reticulum are gated, on their cytoplasmic face, by calcium ions. The activation of these channels produces a **calcium-induced release of calcium** from the sarcoplasmic reticulum.

The trigger for this calcium-induced calcium release is calcium that comes from the interstitial fluid. Such 'trigger calcium' has first to pass through the plasmalemma of the T-tubule, using **voltage-gated calcium channels**. These voltage-gated channels are opened by depolarization during the plateau of the action potential. Since the calcium channels of the plasmalemma are arranged in clusters opposite to clusters of calcium channels on the cell membrane of the sarcoplasmic reticulum, the 'trigger calcium' is ideally placed to activate the release of

calcium from the sarcoplasmic reticulum. Evidence for the calcium-induced release of calcium has been obtained from single cardiac muscle cells, after these cells have had their cell membrane effectively removed (Fabiato, 1985); brief increases in the concentration of calcium around these cells lead them to release their calcium, without any intervention of electrical stimulation. However, the concept of 'calcium-induced calcium release' implies positive feedback. The mechanism should therefore be an all-or-none process, but it is not: in fact, the force of contraction of the cardiac muscle cell can be modulated by the amount of calcium released from the sarcoplasmic reticulum (Section 21.16.3).

21.16.3 *Modulation of the force of contraction*

For effective function, each beat of the heart should activate *all* of its muscle cells, *once* only. Unlike skeletal muscle, cardiac muscle cannot increase its force by recruiting more fibres. However, the mechanism of calcium-induced calcium release does allow the force of contraction to be modulated. During basal activity of the heart (Salmons, 1995, p. 767), the amount of Ca^{2+} bound to troponin-C during each systole induces less than half-maximal activation of the contractile mechanism. A reserve of force can therefore be mobilized by increasing the Ca^{2+} bound to troponin-C. Changing the amplitude of the calcium inflow into the cell during the action potential alters the amount of calcium released from the sarcoplasmic reticulum, and (after a delay) the calcium content of the sarcoplasmic reticulum.

This, in fact, is the basis of the mechanism by which the **adrenergic stimulation** of cardiac muscle achieves its positive inotropic effect. After the **β_1-adrenoreceptor** and its associated GTP-binding proteins have been activated, cAMP is produced by adenylate cyclase leading apparently to the activation of cAMP-dependent protein kinase A. The kinase phosphorylates calcium channels (L-type) in the surface membrane of the sarcoplasmic reticulum, and also phospholamban (which is a protein in the sarcoplasmic reticulum that inhibits the calcium pump of the sarcoplasmic reticulum). This phosphorylation leads to (a) a greater influx of calcium from the sarcoplasmic reticulum into the sarcoplasm during the action potential, and (b) a faster return of calcium into the sarcoplasmic reticulum when the action potential ends (Section 21.16.4). By increasing (i) the trigger and the calcium available to the sarcoplasmic reticulum (via the action on the L-type calcium channel), and (ii) the calcium content of the sarcoplasmic reticulum (via the action on phospholamban and the calcium pump of the sarcoplasmic reticulum), the *force* of contraction is increased. Thus these Ca^{2+} movements provide an automatic mechanism for matching an increase in heart rate with a progressive increase in contractile force (Salmons, 1995, p. 767). Billman (1992) stated that **α-adrenergic**

fibres act synergistically with **β_1-adrenergic pathways**, stimulating cardiac cellular excitability by inducing a rise in cytosolic calcium levels and thus increasing contractile force.

Since β_1 stimulation also increases the *heart rate*, the increased rate of pumping of calcium into the sarcoplasmic reticulum between beats may be important in creating a diastolic period of optimum duration, and hence in maintaining an appropriate time for ventricular filling, i.e. the increased rate of pumping of calcium into the sarcoplasmic reticulum gives a faster relaxation of the muscle thus helping to maintain the interval between contractions. An increase in heart rate alone cannot sustain an increase in cardiac output, since the filling time is correspondingly decreased; if the filling time is decreased each beat ejects less blood in proportion to the increase in rate, and cardiac output remains unchanged.

21.16.4   *Relaxation*

Calcium ions are returned to the interior of the sarcoplasmic reticulum by an active **calcium pump**. Calcium ions are moved against a large concentration gradient (perhaps as high as millimolar inside the sarcoplasmic reticulum). The necessary energy is obtained from the hydrolysis of ATP by the sarcoplasmic reticulum, the active agent being the ATPase known as calcium ATPase. This is present in high concentration as an integral membrane protein of the sarcoplasmic reticulum, and is dedicated to calcium pumping. The action of this pump is modulated by **phospholamban**; the inhibitory action of this protein on the pump is removed by phosphorylation, as in the mechanism for β_1-adrenergic stimulation (Section 21.16.3).

Calcium ions are also transported out of the cell via the T-tubules, against a large concentration gradient, by two sarcolemmal systems: a calcium ATPase harnesses the energy from hydrolysis of ATP, and a Na/Ca exchanger uses the energy derived from the entry of three sodium ions into the cell down their concentration gradient.

Under stable conditions the amount of calcium transported out of the cell will equal that which entered during the action potential that triggered release. The amount returned to the sarcoplasmic reticulum will equal that which was released initially from the sarcoplasmic reticulum.

21.16.5   *Role of the intercalated disc*

The cardiac muscle cells are joined end-to-end by **intercalated discs** (Section 21.2), consisting of desmosomes alternating with gap junctions.

The **gap junctions** (macula communicans) are sites of low electrical resistance enabling successive muscle cells to be electrically coupled. Thus excitation and contraction spread rapidly along tracts of interconnected cells. The myocardium therefore behaves electrically as a syncitium, although it is not a syncitium structurally.

II   THE CONDUCTING SYSTEM OF THE HEART

21.17   Origin of the heart beat

All parts of the heart possess an inherent capacity for rhythmic contraction, independent of nerve supply. William Harvey demonstrated this in 1628 by cutting a heart of a frog into small pieces and observing that each fragment continued to beat. He also made another shrewd observation from the same experiment: atrial components beat much faster than ventricular. Evidently the rate of the heart beat as a whole is decided by the part with the fastest frequency.

During the next two centuries there was a debate about how the beat actually starts. Is it neurogenic or myogenic? The discovery of nerve cells (vagal) in the wall of the heart swung the argument in favour of a nervous origin. However, by the end of the nineteenth century conclusive evidence for a **myogenic origin** came from various researches, and especially from the observation that the heart starts beating in the embryo *before* any nervous tissue has reached it. It was then accepted that the nerves only *modify* the beat.

How does the cardiac muscle cell achieve **spontaneous excitation**? An electrical potential across the cell membrane (plasmalemma) is present in essentially all animal and plant cells. The inside of the cell is negative with respect to the outside, and this is the **membrane potential**. The source of this potential is the unequal distribution of ions inside and outside the cell, and particularly of K^+ ions outside. The essential cause of the unequal distribution is the relatively very great permeability of the plasmalemma to K^+ ions, and its relatively low permeability to Na^+ and all other ions. The K^+ ions pass through until their tendency to diffuse is balanced by the negative charge created by the organic cations that are left behind. The cell is now *polarized*. In a resting nerve cell and resting skeletal muscle cell the negative charge inside the cell is stabilized by the sodium–potassium pump, which trades Na^+ ions for K^+ ions at the plasmalemma. Only when a nerve impulse arrives, will ion channels open and freely admit Na^+ ions to the interior of the cell. This *depolarizes* the cell, briefly making the inside positive with respect to the outside, and an **action potential** (in a nerve cell) or **contraction** (in a skeletal muscle cell) results.

In a **resting cardiac muscle cell**, the stabilizing processes at the cell membrane are relatively imperfect, allowing a slow inward leakage of Na^+ ions. This causes the membrane potential to rise progressively to the threshold voltage. When this point has been reached, the sodium channels open and depolarization occurs, causing the cardiac muscle cell to contract. Smooth muscle cells tend to have a similar 'leakiness' of the plasmalemma, again giving rise to spontaneous contractions.

Recovery after an action potential in a cardiac muscle cell is similar to that in other excitable cells. While the inside of the cell is *positively* charged during the action potential, K^+ ions take advantage of the permeability of the potassium ion channels, and stream out of the cell in very large numbers, thus restoring the negativity inside the cell. Sodium and potassium ions are then exchanged across the plasmalemma by the sodium–potassium pump, and the original 'resting' ionic relationships are restored.

21.18 Rhythmic mechanism of the sinuatrial node

As already mentioned, Harvey noticed that atrial cells beat faster than ventricular cells. The fastest rhythmicity evidently arises in a small focus of cardiac cells in the wall of the right atrium, near the entry of the cranial vena cava. This is the **sinuatrial node** (S-A node), or '**pacemaker**' of the heart. The normal heart rhythm originating in the sinuatrial node is known as the **sinus rhythm**. The inherent rate of the sinus rhythm varies with changes in vagal or sympathetic tone (Section 22.13).

What characteristics endow the S-A node with its exceptionally fast rhythmicity? The (resting) membrane potential of excitable cells is around 60–95 mV negative, depending on the tissue. The membrane potential of the cells of the S-A node (*nodal myocytes*) appears to be one of the least negative among excitable cells, i.e. as little as -50 mV, which is about 40 mV less negative than that of the ventricular muscle cell. Moreover the plasmalemma (cell membrane) of the sinuatrial cell is exceptional in that it allows a *continual slow inward leak of sodium ions*. This causes the membrane potential of the cells of the S-A node to become progressively less negative during diastole, until it very soon reaches the threshold voltage (about -40 mV) where the sodium channels open and the action potential occurs.

All other cardiac muscle cells undergo similar ionic changes, but the gap between their resting potential and action potential is much greater, and their leakage rate of sodium is much slower. Inevitably, therefore, they take longer to reach an action potential, i.e. their frequency of contraction is slower.

Dudel (1978, p. 22) gave the following approximate numbers of **ions** on either side of a section of plasmalemma $1\,\mu m \times 1\,nm$ in area of a nerve cell or skeletal muscle cell during the resting potential. Outside the cell: K^+, 2000; Na^+, 108000; Cl^-, 110000. Inside the cell: K^+, 100000; Na^+, 10000; Cl^-, 2200; protein anions, 107800. The protein anions are too big to go through the plasmalemma.

Approximate **resting potentials** of normal excitable cells (Guyton, 1986, pp. 127, 141, 151) are as follows: cardiac muscle cell, -90 mV; skeletal muscle cell, -90 mV; large myelinated nerve fibre, -90 mV; smooth muscle cell, -60 mV.

21.19 Anatomy of the cardiac conducting system

The components of the cardiac conducting system are (i) the sinuatrial node, (ii) the atrioventricular node, (iii) the atrioventricular bundle comprising the trunk and the right and left crura, and (iv) the subendocardial plexus of cardiac conducting fibres (Purkinje fibres). All of these components consist of modified cardiac muscle cells. They are all capable of generating action potentials and hence contraction, but some (nodal myocytes; Section 21.20.1) are dedicated to the *generation* of impulses, whereas others (conducting myocytes, alias Purkinje cells; Section 21.20.3) are dedicated to the *conduction* of impulses. The basic anatomy of these conducting pathways is illustrated in Fig. 21.10.

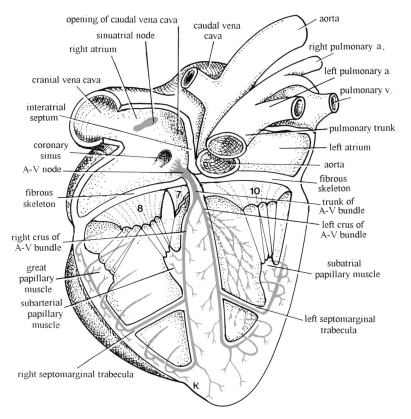

Fig. 21.10 Highly schematic diagram summarizing the anatomy of the conducting system of the heart. The left cranial aspect of the heart is shown. The heart has been somewhat rotated about its long axis, moving its cranial surface slightly to the left. This makes it possible to see down the cranial vena cava and into the right atrium, as far as the opening of the coronary sinus and caudal vena cava. The cranial walls of the right atrium and right ventricle have been excised, together with the root of the pulmonary trunk and the root of the aorta. The position of the **sinuatrial node** in the lateral wall of the right atrium, near the opening of the cranial vena cava, is now exposed. The club-shaped **atrioventricular node** is embedded in the interatrial septum, where the septum joins the floor of the right atrium, close to the opening of the coronary sinus. The **trunk** of the atrioventricular bundle penetrates the fibrous plate (schematic only) that separates the atria from the ventricles, and then continues into the interventricular septum. After a short course in the dorsal part of the septum, it divides into the left crus and right crus of the atrioventricular bundle. The two crura and their main branches are subendocardial in position. The **right crus** is a narrow discrete bundle of fascicles. It passes ventrally down the interventricular septum, supplying the papillary muscles on the interventricular septum, the interventricular septum itself, and the right ventricular myocardium in the region of the apex of the heart. It sends a major branch into the right septomarginal trabecula. This branch supplies the great papillary muscle of the right ventricle, and it also forms recurved subendocardial branches that supply the rest of the right ventricular wall. The **left crus** immediately forms a flattened subendocardial sheet of interlacing branches. These spread over the internal surface of the ventricle. A substantial branch soon goes into the left septomarginal trabecula to supply the papillary muscles of the left ventricle. Fine filaments and recurving branches reach all other parts of the left ventricle and its associated interventricular septum. 7, Septal cusp, and 8, angular cusp, of right atrioventricular valve; 10, parietal cusp of left atrioventricular valve.

21.19.1 *Sinuatrial node*

The sinuatrial node is a small mass of rather ordinary looking cells, **nodal myocytes**, embedded in the lateral wall of the right atrium, at the junction of the atrial wall with the cranial vena cava (Fig. 21.10). The S-A node is the *pace-maker* of the heart, reaching action potentials more quickly than all other parts of the conducting system (Section 21.17). Its action potentials spread directly into the surrounding atrial myocardium, reaching all of the right and left atrial myocardia and finally the atrioventricular node as well.

The sinuatrial node (nodus sinuatrialis) was first seen by a leading anatomist, Sir Arthur Keith, and a young student, Martin Flack, in a mole's heart on a farm in Kent in 1906 (Muir, 1971, p. 13). It was subsequently found in more than 15 other mammalian species, including man and domestic mammals.

The S-A node is embedded within the sulcus terminalis of the right atrium (Fig. 17.5). In man at least, it is *subepicardial* (Salmons, 1995, p. 1496), rather than subendocardial like the rest of the conducting system. In large domestic mammals it tends to be paler than the surrounding atrial musculature, and visible to the naked eye (Schummer *et al.*, 1981, p. 35): in man this is because it is covered by a plaque of subepicardial fat. In the smaller mammalian species it can only be identified microscopically.

Veterinary sources seem reluctant to estimate the dimensions of the S-A node. In man, however, it is stated to be about 10–20 mm long (Salmons, 1995, p. 769), or 15 mm × 3 mm × 1 mm (Guyton, 1986, p. 165).

In the sheep (Frink and Merrick, 1974) the S-A node is always supplied by the right coronary artery. Schummer *et al.* (1981, p. 35) hinted at a circular disposition of the node around its blood supply, and Salmons (1995, p. 1496) explicitly described the presence of a *central artery* in man.

There has been a long-running dispute about the possible presence of specialized bundles of atrial myocardial cells that conduct the impulse from the S-A to the A-V node. Guyton (1986, p. 167) affirmed that the impulse does spread directly throughout the entire atrial muscle mass, but reported the presence of three specialized bundles of atrial muscle fibres resembling ventricular conducting fibres. These conduct at about three times the speed of ordinary atrial muscle fibres. However, Salmons (1995, p. 1500) concluded that modern workers have dismissed the presence of *structurally specialized* conducting pathways between the S-A and A-V nodes; instead, it is believed to be the packing and geometrical arrangement of fibres along well-organized atrial muscle bundles, such as the crista terminalis and fossa ovalis, that are responsible for these *preferential pathways* of relatively rapid conduction.

21.19.2 *Atrioventricular node*

The atrioventricular node is a club-shaped mass of cells, these again being nodal myocytes, identical to the nodal myocytes of the S-A node. The A-V node is embedded in the interatrial septum, where the septum joins the floor of the right atrium and is therefore close to the opening of the coronary sinus (Fig. 21.10). Although the A-V node is itself an *atrial* structure, it forms the root of an extensive tree of conducting tissue that pervades the whole of the left and right ventricles and their papillary muscles.

Since the A-V node is fully equipped with nodal myocytes, it has an inherent capacity to generate rhythmic contractions of the heart. Normally, however, the sinuatrial node is the dominant pacemaker, but the A-V node is the pacemaker with the second highest inherent rate.

Immediately ventral to the atrioventricular node (nodus atrioventricularis) is the septal cusp of the right atrioventricular valve (Fig. 21.10). In the ox, the node lies against the large os cordis.

The difficulty in finding the dimensions of the A-V node in the literature is the opposite to the difficulty mentioned above with the S-A node. Sources on human anatomy are reluctant, but Schummer *et al.* (1981, p. 35) gave some figures: dog, 3–4 mm × 1–2 mm; horse 6–10 mm × 5–7 mm, and ox 8–13 mm × 6–8 mm.

If A-V nodal myocytes become the dominant pacemaker, as in a third degree atrioventricular heart block (Section 21.23.2), the human heart beats at about 40–60 times a minute (Guyton, 1986, p. 169), and that of domestic species at about 40–50 per minute (Hamlin and Smith, 1977, p. 77).

21.19.3 *Atrioventricular bundle*

It will be remembered that, for the heart to work properly in the living animal, the atria have to be isolated electrophysiologically from the ventricles, and that this vital function is carried out by the fibrous skeleton of the heart (Section 20.12). Since the A-V node is stuck on the wrong side of the line, the first part of the A-V bundle, the **trunk**, must begin by piercing the fibrous skeleton of the heart (Fig. 20.7), and this it does where the floor of the right atrium joins the interatrial septum (Fig. 21.10). The A-V bundle then emerges in the dorsal extremity of the interventricular septum, and immediately divides into right and left crura.

The **right crus** is relatively simple in its form, since it runs ventrally in the interventricular septum as a *discrete trunk*, subendocardially, to the apex of the heart and beyond (Fig. 21.10). On the way it gives its first major clusters of branches to the two **papillary muscles** that arise from the interventricular septum. It also supplies branches to the interventricular septum itself. Its second major branch goes to the **right septomarginal trabecula** (and to any subsidiary septomarginal trabeculae associated with it), crosses the lumen of the right ventricle, and supplies the very large **papillary muscle** on the lateral wall of the right ventricle as well the outer wall of the ventricle itself.

The **left crus** breaks down almost immediately into a *flattened subendocardial leash* of ramifying branches (Fig. 21.10). Major branches cross the ventricular lumen in the **left septomarginal trabecula** and its lesser septomarginal trabeculae, supplying first of all the two **papillary muscles** on the outer wall of the left ventricle and then curving back to reach all parts of the ventricle.

> The trunk of the A-V bundle enters the interventricular septum at the attachment of the septal cusp of the right atrioventricular valve. This is also the site of the *membranous part* of the interventricular septum (Section 20.10) (Schummer *et al.*, 1981, p. 36).

21.19.4 *Subendocardial plexus*

This component is the final extension of the left and right crura to all parts of the two ventricles. It consists of a *network* of subendocardial conducting myofibres (Purkinje fibres), which proceed imperceptibly into the cardiac muscle cells.

> The individual fibre bundles of the subendocardial plexus are loosely enclosed in a connective tissue sheath. Fluid injected into the space beneath the sheath extends all over the plexus, making it possible to visualize the entire plexus, especially in ungulates (Schummer *et al.*, 1981, p. 37).

21.20 Histology of the cardiac conducting system

As already stated at the beginning of Section 21.19, all the cells of the conducting system are modified cardiac muscle cells, capable of generating and conducting impulses. However, in the intact heart they resolve themselves into three functional groups: (i) nodal myocytes, that *generate impulses*; (ii) transitional cells, that *form a link* with nodal myocytes, and in so doing contribute to the all-important delay between atrial and ventricular systole; and (iii) conducting myocytes (Purkinje cells and their fibres), that *conduct impulses* all over the ventricles. These functional

variations are reflected in structural differences between these cells.

21.20.1 *Nodal myocyte*

The nodal cell is the main component of both the S-A and the A-V node. It is a rather ordinary looking cell, small, more or less oval, and lacking most of the striking features that immediately characterize a myocardial muscle cell. The only anatomical feature suggesting its myocardial lineage is an occasional disorganized fragment of a myofibril.

> The nodal myocyte (myocytus nodalis) has a similar structure in both the S-A and the A-V node (Salmons, 1995, p. 769).
>
> The cell is about 10 μm wide and up to 25 μm long (Krstic, 1984, p. 293). It has no T-tubules or intercalated discs, attachments to neighbouring cells being by numerous zonulae adherentes. The nucleus is pale, and globular or elongated. The clear cytoplasm contains several large mitochondria, but little endoplasmic reticulum. Salmons (1995, p. 769) noted that glycogen is scarce, but Krstic (1984, p. 293) reported considerable amounts. The large euchromatic nucleus, and perhaps a substantial quantity of glycogen, hint at the underlying activity of the cell.
>
> In cardiac muscle, two types of ion channels admit sodium, namely **fast sodium channels** and **slow calcium–sodium channels** (Guyton, 1986, p. 166). The slow calcium–sodium channels are an important source of the calcium ions essential for the contraction of cardiac muscle. However, the lesser negativity of resting nodal myocytes (Section 21.18) largely closes the fast sodium channels. Since only slow calcium–sodium channels are then available, the action potential in the S-A nodal myocytes *develops more gradually* than in standard ventricular myocardial cells.

21.20.2 *Transitional cells*

Together with nodal myocytes, transitional cells form the sinuatrial and atrioventricular nodes. In the S-A node, the two types of cell mingle, but in the A-V node, the transitional cell is strategically placed between the atrial myocardial cell and the nodal cell.

The essential feature of the transitional cell is its very slender form, only half the width of the nodal cell. Being so slim it has a very slow conduction velocity, and this is a substantial factor in providing the critical delay needed at the A-V node (Section 21.21).

> The **transitional cell** is so-named by Salmons (1995, p. 769) and seems to be the 'junctional fibre' of Guyton (1986, p. 167), but is not recognized by the *Nomina Histologica* of 1994. It is only about 7 μm wide and not much more than 10 μm long (Krstic, 1984, p. 426). It has no T-tubules or intercalated discs, its end-to-end attachments being mostly by zonulae adherentes. However, unlike the nodal cell, the transitional cell is unmistakably a cardiac muscle cell since it contains many myofibrils, although these are not rigorously longitudinal but also spiral and transverse.
>
> In the S-A node the transitional cells simply link nodal cells with other cells. In the A-V node, however, transitional cells are in the majority and surround the nodal cells, the latter being concentrated in the centre of the node (Salmons, 1995, p. 769). The transitional cell therefore seems to be the link between the atrial myocardial cell and the nodal cell. Gap junctions are notably scarce between the transitional cells and nodal cells, and connexin (a major protein of gap junctions) is absent. The narrow calibre of transitional cells and the lack of gap junctions all contribute to the delay in transmission of the impulse from transitional cell to nodal cell, and hence across the A-V node as a whole (Section 21.21). According to Krstic (1984, p. 426), transitional cells also connect conducting myocytes with myocardial cells.

21.20.3 *Conducting myocytes*

These are the cells traditionally known as **Purkinje cells**. Their most significant anatomical feature is their very large diameter – several times greater than that of an ordinary myocardial cell. This provides them with a conduction velocity that is several times faster than that of the ordinary cardiac muscle cell, enabling them to activate the almost immediate contraction of the entire myocardium of both ventricles.

Conducting myofibres, also known as **Purkinje fibres**, are simply longitudinal chains of single conducting myocytes, joined end-to-end by fully developed intercalated discs with extensive gap junctions. Conducting fibres are the main component of the **atrioventricular bundle**. Groups of fibres within the A-V bundle, and even single fibres, are separated from the surrounding myocardium by their connective tissue sheaths. They are essentially *subendocardial* in their course across the ventricular wall.

The terminal branches of the conducting (Purkinje) myofibres finally penetrate into the myocardium of the ventricles. Here they lose their distinctive structure and blend into the cardiac muscle cells.

> The diameter of the conducting myocyte (myocytus conducens cardiacus) is exceptionally large in 'ungulates' (Schummer *et al.*, 1981, p. 37), reaching 80–100 μm in the horse and ox. In man, it is about 30 μm (Salmons, 1995, p. 769) to 50 μm (Krstic, 1984, p. 350). For comparison, the diameter of the ordinary cardiac muscle cell is about 10–20 μm in man (Krstic, 1984, p. 65) and 10 μm in the horse and ox (Schummer *et al.*, 1981, p. 37).
>
> The conducting myocyte is also conspicuous microscopically because of its relatively pale central area of cytoplasm caused by the concentration of myofibrils around the periphery of the cell. There are no T-tubules, but intercalated discs are fully developed and incorporate extensive gap junctions at both the ends and the sides (Salmons, 1995, p. 769).
>
> The terminal branches of the conducting myofibres (myofibra conducens cardiaca) penetrate about one third of the ventricular myocardium (Guyton, 1986, p. 168) before finally blending with the ventricular muscle cells (Salmons, 1995, p. 769).

21.20.4 *Autonomic innervation of the conducting system*

Many postganglionic sympathetic nerve fibres (Section 2.10.1), and postganglionic parasympathetic (vagal) cell bodies and their nerve fibres (Section 3.11.3) are associated with the sinuatrial and atrioventricular nodes (Sections 22.8.1 and 22.8.2).

21.21 Factors controlling transmission of the cardiac impulse

These factors can now be summarized. The initial fast rate of discharge by the **pacemaker**, i.e. the nodal cells of the sinuatrial node, is due to the relatively low negativity of these cells when at rest (-50 mV compared with -90 mV of ventricular myocardial cells) and the steady inward leak of sodium ions (Section 21.18).

The delay at the **atrioventricular node** arises especially from the very small calibre, and hence the very low conduction velocity, of the transitional cells (Section 21.20.2).

> Further factors in the delay at the A-V node are, (a) the scarcity of gap junctions between the transitional and

nodal cells (Section 21.20.2); (b) the lesser negativity of both the transitional cells and the nodal cells when resting, which slows the rate of development of their action potential (Section 20.20.1) (Guyton, 1986, p. 168).

The rapid transmission from the beginning to the end of the **atrioventricular bundle** is caused by, (a) the huge calibre, and hence the very fast conduction velocity, of the conducting myocyte (Section 21.20.3), and (b) the presence of many gap junctions between the conducting myocytes (Section 21.20.3).

The relatively slow transmission across the **atrial myocardium**, and across the **ventricular myocardium** from the end of the conducting (Purkinje) fibres, arises from the intermediate calibre, and hence the intermediate conduction velocity, of the ordinary cardiac muscle cell.

The following **conduction velocities** (Guyton, 1986, pp. 167–169) quantify these variations: (i) ordinary atrial and ventricular cardiac muscle cell, 0.3–0.5 m s^{-1}; (ii) preferential pathways across the atrial myocardium, 1.0 m s^{-1}; (iii) transitional cells, 0.02 m s^{-1}; (iv) nodal cells, 0.1 m s^{-1}; (v) conducting (Purkinje) cells, up to 4.0 m s^{-1}.

21.22 Electrocardiogram

When the heart contracts, a wave of depolarization (the cardiac impulse) passes through the heart. Electrical currents spread from the heart into the surrounding tissues, and small amounts of these currents reach the surface of the body. Such electrical potentials generated by the heart can be recorded as an **electrocardiogram** by electrodes placed on the skin on opposite sides of the heart. Figure 21.11 shows a normal electrocardiogram for a single beat of the heart.

The normal ECG comprises (a) three main wave complexes, designated as the P, QRS, and T waves, and (b) two flat baselines, one between the P and the QRS waves, and the other between the QRS and T waves.

The following general points make it easier to interpret the waves and baselines of the ECG. (i) Current only flows to the surface of the body (thus forming the three wave complexes) when cardiac muscle is partly polarized and partly depolarized. (2) No changes of potential are recorded (thus giving a flat baseline in the electrocardiogram)

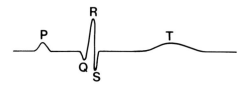

Fig. 21.11 Normal electrocardiogram. The P wave is caused by repolarization of the atria. Between the P wave and the QRS complex the baseline is flat (isoelectric period). During this 'silent' period the atria are continuously contracting, and this produces a plateau of sustained depolarization with no recordable changes in potential. The QRS complex is generated by depolarization of the ventricles. Between the QRS complex and the T wave there is a second isoelectric period, during which the ventricles contract in a plateau of sustained depolarization without recordable changes in potential. The T wave arises from the repolarization of the ventricles to their resting state. The atria repolarize during the QRS complex, and this may show as an atrial T wave but is usually concealed by the much larger QRS deflection. Potentials generated by depolarization and repolarization of the conducting system are in general too small to be recorded on an ECG.

when cardiac muscle is either completely polarized or completely depolarized. (3) The number of cells in the tissues of the conducting system itself is so low that the potentials they generate are too small to be recorded, and therefore the discharges of the sinuatrial node, the atrioventricular node, and the conducting (Purkinje) myofibres of the atrioventricular bundle, are not seen.

The initial upright, low, rounded deflection is the **P wave** (Fig. 21.11). This is caused by the depolarization of the atrial myocardium. Contraction of the atria begins immediately after the onset of the P wave and ends at the QRS complex, the timing of these events being visible in Fig. 22.1. Atrial depolarization spreads from the S-A node like the concentric ripples after a stone is thrown into the centre of a pond, traversing first the right atrium and then the left.

The second deflection is the **QRS complex**. This results from the depolarization of the ventricular myocardium. The contraction of the ventricular myocardium begins almost immediately after the onset of the QRS complex, at about the R component (for timing, see Fig. 22.1).

The third deflection, the **T wave**, is produced by the repolarization of the ventricular myocardium to the resting state. Repolarization takes a relatively long time, so that some fibres are still contracted a few milliseconds after the end of the T wave.

21.22.1 *Isoelectric period*

The initial phase of depolarization (contraction) of cardiac muscle cells is followed by a prolonged **plateau**, i.e. an absolute refractory period (Section 21.15). During the plateau all cells are in nearly the same depolarized state, so that the membrane potential changes little. Between the end of the P wave and the beginning of the QRS complex there is a plateau while the atrial muscle is continuously depolarized; therefore during this period the normal ECG shows a flat baseline, or **isoelectric** ('silent') **period** (Scher, 1974, p. 80).

Likewise, between the S wave and the T wave the ventricular muscle is continuously depolarized, thus giving a second isoelectric period.

21.22.2 *Depolarization of the conducting system*

The S-A node depolarizes shortly before the onset of the P wave. From the downslope of the P wave to just before the onset of the QRS complex, cells of the **A-V node** and the **trunk** of the **atrioventricular bundle** are depolarizing (Scher, 1974, Fig. 6.10). Likewise, from the QRS complex to some point before the T wave, the **crura** of the atrioventricular bundle are depolarizing. Thus during both of the two isoelectric periods, some part of the conducting system is depolarizing. However, as just stated above, the electrical changes produced by these depolarizations of the conducting system are too small to show on the ECG.

21.22.3 *Repolarization of atrial myocardium and the conducting system*

Repolarization of the **atrial myocardium** occurs during the QRS complex, but the potential is usually concealed by the much larger QRS complex (Guyton, 1986, p. 178). It is sometimes just detectable, and is then known as the **atrial T wave** or **Ta wave** (Scher, 1974, p. 84).

Repolarization of the **conducting system** is also concealed by other cardiac activity. Repolarization of the **S-A node** must occur during the P wave. Repolarization of the **A-V node** and **A-V bundle** presumably occurs while the ventricular myocardium is contracting, i.e. from the QRS complex to some point between S and T.

21.22.4 *Variations in the QRS complex*

The duration, amplitude, and configuration of the QRS complex are variable. The *duration*, which represents the time taken to depolarize both right and left ventricles completely, varies with the size of the heart, which in turn varies with the age of an animal and the thickness of its ventricular walls (Breazile, 1971, p. 243). The *amplitudes* of the QRS deflections in standard limb leads of the horse and domestic ruminants are quite small compared with those of the dog; in the cat the amplitudes are intermediate between the dog and horse (Breazile, 1971, p. 244). The low amplitude in the large species is due to the marked synchronization of ventricular depolarization, which causes waves of depolarization to cancel out and leaves only a slight average depolarization in any particular direction (Breazile, 1971, p. 244). The *configuration* in limb leads of the horse and domestic ruminants is quite variable, with notching and skewing within the same animal as well as in different individuals. These differences are attributed to variations in the topographical anatomy of the heart, and to variations in the position of the heart relative to the limbs to which the electrodes are attached (Breazile, 1971, p. 145).

21.22.5 *Leads*

Several systems of leads can be used to record ECGs, including standard bipolar limb leads and precordial (chest or V) leads (Guyton, 1986, p. 181). Standard recording positions are right lateral recumbency for small animals, and standing with the legs square for large animals (Darke *et al.*, 1996, p. 37).

Standard bipolar limb leads involve three arrays of leads, leads I, II, and III. 'Bipolar' means that each array consists of two specific electrodes. 'Specific' refers to the particular point on the body to which an electrode is attached, in this context either a forelimb or a hind limb. To record *lead I*, the positive terminal of the electrocardiograph is attached to the left forelimb ('arm'), and the negative terminal to the right forelimb; hence lead I records the potential difference between the two forelimbs. To record *lead II*, the positive terminal is attached to the left hind limb, and the negative to the right forelimb. To record *lead III*, the positive terminal is attached to the left hind limb and the negative to the left forelimb. In the horse or ox the left forelimb electrode is often moved to the left thoracic wall over the apex of the heart, and the right forelimb electrode is moved to the mid-cervical jugular furrow (Darke *et al.*, 1996, Fig. 5.2b).

In a **precordial lead** an electrode is placed on one of several points over the heart (V_1, V_2, V_3, etc), and connected to the positive terminal of the electrocardiograph. The negative electrode is connected simultaneously through resistances to the right forelimb (R), left forelimb (L), and left hindlimb (F). Because the precordial electrode is close to the heart, each precordial lead records mainly the electrical potential of the cardiac musculature immediately beneath the electrode. Relatively small abnormalities in the ventricles can then cause marked changes in the ECG.

21.22.6   *Information accessible from the ECG*

The information obtainable from electrocardiography has little to offer towards resolving mechanical problems such as valvular disorders, or elucidating the severity or aetiology of cardiac diseases, but it does provide a specific diagnosis of most cardiac dysrhythmias and conduction abnormalities, and often gives an insight into cardiac enlargements (Darke *et al.*, 1996, p. 37). For instance, in small animals, atrial enlargement (usually left) is indicated by prolongation and increased amplitude of the P wave. Left ventricular enlargement is consistent with prolongation of the QRS complex; increased amplitude of the R wave is typical of left ventricular enlargement. Low voltage QRS complexes are compatible with pericardial or pleural effusion. Abnormalities of the T wave may indicate epicardial or subendocardial injury, e.g. ischaemia, pericarditis.

21.23   Cardiac arrhythmias

This term refers to changes in the rhythm of the heart. Some of these changes occur in the normal animal. Others are frankly abnormal and arise mainly from pathological conditions in the conducting system of the heart.

21.23.1   *Normal arrhythmias*

Familiar examples of **normal arrhythmias** include the slowing of the heart (*bradycardia*) in trained athletes. Such slowing gives the athlete an improved reserve of cardiac output during exercise. On the other hand, the heart goes faster (*tachycardia*) in response to emotional stress. These examples of bradycardia and tachycardia are due to normal adjustments in autonomic influences on the sinuatrial node. Incidentally, the names given to these normal arrhythmias are often preceded by the term 'sinus', examples being *'sinus' bradycardia* and *'sinus' tachycardia*. The designation 'sinus' here signifies the *sinu*atrial node, and not the carotid sinus, although the latter participates in the autonomic control mechanisms of some of these arrhythmias.

Another example of a normal arrhythmia is so-called *sinus arrhythmia*. Most people are aware that their heart rate accelerates during inspiration and decelerates during expiration. The increased rate is due to a decrease in vagal tone and an increase sympathetic tone on the sinuatrial node, and the decreased rate to the reverse effects. Sinus arrhythmia is found not only in man but also in normal domestic mammals.

> Sinus arrhythmia occurs in normal dogs and horses, but is rare in cats (Darke *et al.*, 1996, p. 154). Sinus bradycardia and tachycardia are associated with normal rhythms in domestic mammals, for example in sleep or exercise, but also occur in disorders of impulse formation, e.g. sinus bradycardia in dilated cardiomyopathy, and sinus tachycardia in heart failure (Darke *et al.*, p. 158).
>
> The normal mechanism of *sinus arrhythmia* seems to be far from clear. The basic reason for this is that the mechanical interactions between breathing and circulation have been an exceptionally controversial field for over a century (Mead and Whittenberger, 1964, p. 477). Guyton (1986, p. 198) attributed *sinus arrhythmia* to alternating stimulation and inhibition of baroreceptors, supplemented by a waxing and waning of the Bainbridge reflex. Katz (1992, p. 550) favoured a totally different explanation – stimuli arising from stretch receptors in the lung and thoracic wall. Katz (1992, p. 550) also pointed out that sinus arrhythmia is not only a normal finding in the young person, but is actually a sign of a healthy heart: clock-like regularity of the heart beat indicates that normal control by the autonomic nervous system has been lost, and this is one of the earliest manifestations of heart failure.

21.23.2   *Abnormal arrhythmias*

Abnormal arrhythmias arise from two main causes, namely *disorders of impulse formation* (premature beats, or extrasystoles) and *disorders of conduction* (heart blocks).

One basic principle makes it possible to predict the general behaviour of cardiac arrhythmias. Every cardiac muscle cell is capable of generating impulses at its own inherent rhythm (Section 21.17), but the frequency of impulse generation varies with the cell type (Section 21.20), the frequency normally being highest in the nodal myocytes of the sinuatrial node and declining progressively from the atria to the ventricles; the fastest cell in a line of connected muscle cells is the one that imposes its rhythm on all the others.

Thus if a break occurs somewhere in the conduction pathway, the cells beyond the break will beat at their inherent slower rate; this is known as a **heart block**. Or, if a group of cells develops an abnormally high frequency, it will drive all cells connected with it at that abnormal higher rate; the abnormal cells would be referred to as an **ectopic focus** inducing **premature beats**.

Heart blocks

Heart blocks arise from impairment of the conducting system at some point along its course. Clinically, a heart block is characterized by a disturbance in the relationship between atrial and ventricular contraction.

The block may occur in three possible sites. (1) *Sinuatrial heart block* occurs in the *sinuatrial node* itself. It results in delay in, or total absence of, the atrial beat. In the total absence of the atrial beat, the ventricles continue to beat but only at their own, very slow, rate. (2) *Atrioventricular heart block* occurs in the region of the *atrioventricular node*. Depending on the severity of the lesion, this delays ventricular contraction, or even totally disconnects ventricular from atrial contraction so that the atria and ventricles beat independently. (3) *Bundle branch block, right or left* occurs in either the *right* or *left crus* of the *atrioventricular bundle*. The function of the two crura is to coordinate the impulse so that the right and left ventricles contract synchronously. A lesion in, for example, the right crus causes the right ventricle to contract after the left ventricle.

Heart blocks occur in the domestic mammals in a wide variety of diseases, cardiac and otherwise (Darke *et al.*, 1996, p. 158).

Sinuatrial heart block occurs, for example, in dilated cardiomyopathy.

Three degrees of *atrioventricular heart block* are recognized (Hamlin and Smith, 1977, p. 77). In *first degree heart block* the PR interval is prolonged, so that ventricular contraction is delayed. In *second degree A-V block*, there are more P waves than QRS complexes so that the atria beat two, three, or four times for each ventricular contraction. In *third degree*, or *complete heart block*, the conduction pathway in the atrioventricular node or atrioventricular bundle is so disrupted that the transmission of the impulse from atria to ventricles fails completely. The result is that both the atria and the ventricles beat regularly, but at independent rates; depending on the species, the atria might beat at 100 per minute and the ventricles at 40 per minute (as in man) (Guyton, 1986, p. 199). In man, the atrioventricular node is capable of taking over the role of pacemaker from the sinuatrial node, and sustaining life at 40–50 ventricular beats per minute (Wiggers, 1974, p. 104), though an arti-

ficial pacemaker would be preferred. Causes in domestic mammals include infarction of the A-V node or replacement of it by fibrous tissue (Darke *et al.*, 1996, p. 158).

A bundle branch block is also known as an *intra*ventricular heart block, and also as an *inter*ventricular heart block Bundle branch blocks occur in almost any congenital or acquired disease, including interatrial and interventricular septal defects, pulmonary and aortic stenosis, and cardiomyopathy (Darke *et al.*, 1996, p. 158).

Premature beats

The inherent tendency of cardiac tissue to generate impulses can be accentuated by a minor lesion in the myocardium such as a small local area of ischaemia. A hitherto normal group of myocardial cells can then become a pacemaker, generating a series of *premature beats* which are unduly fast and therefore entirely out of phase with the normal sinuatrial rhythm. Such a zone is known as an *ectopic focus*. It may arise in either the atrial myocardium or in the ventricular myocardium, and may be a single focus or multiple foci.

The premature beats from a single ectopic focus may occur at very high frequency (nearly 300 per minute), and the effect is then known as a *flutter* (atrial or ventricular). If the premature beats arise at such high frequency from multiple foci, the result is known as *fibrillation* (atrial or ventricular).

Ventricular fibrillation totally disrupts the pumping action of the ventricle, and thus stops the circulation of the blood. It is therefore fatal, unless corrected immediately. Sinus rhythm can be restored by *ventricular defibrillation*. This is done by delivering a large current across the entire ventricle, thus simultaneously depolarizing all the cardiac muscle cells of the ventricle and placing them all in the absolute refractory period (Section 21.15); this permits the cells to repolarize simultaneously, and then to respond uniformly to the next impulse released by the sinuatrial node.

Premature beats in the atria are referred to as *supraventricular complexes*, and those in the ventricles as *ventricular complexes* (Hamlin and Smith, 1977, p. 77).

Flutter and *fibrillation* were thought to arise from two possible pathophysiological mechanisms (Katz, 1992, p. 597). Flutter could be explained by a single, rapidly discharging, *ectopic focus*; fibrillation could arise from multiple ectopic foci, rapidly discharging. It is now thought more likely that flutter and fibrillation originate from large circus movements known as *reentrant pathways*.

According to the reentrant theory (Scott, 1986, p. 16) waves of excitation from a rapidly discharging ectopic focus spread along regular circular pathways and arrive back at the starting point just after the refractory period of the ectopic cells is over, so that the impulse is immediately repropagated in the ectopic cells. This is like a kitten whirling round and round to catch its tail. If the pathways are regular pathways, the result will be flutter: if the waves of excitation travel by multiple disorganized circus pathways over the whole of the atrium or the whole of the ventricle, the result will be fibrillation.

Atrial fibrillation occurs in clinically normal horses and giant breeds of dogs, but is also clinically important (Darke *et al.*, 1996, p. 155). It is often associated with atrial enlargement and congestive heart failure. In some cases in cattle and horses it spontaneously reverts to normal sinus rhythm, but otherwise can be managed therapeutically.

Ventricular premature beats, expressed as *ventricular tachycardia*, are encountered in the dog, cat, and horse (Darke *et al.*, 1996, p. 155). They can lead to myocardial ischaemia and culminate in ventricular fibrillation.

Pathogenesis of abnormal impulse production and abnormal conduction

This topic has been reviewed by Billman (1992). In the USA, over 400000 people die of ventricular fibrillation each year. The mechanisms responsible for this the most dangerous derangement of cardiac electrical activity are not fully known. However, it is clear that **alterations in cellular calcium** can contribute significantly to the development of abnormalities in both *impulse generation* and *impulse conduction*, particularly during *myocardial ischaemia*. **Acute myocardial ischaemia** elicits a significant increase in *sympathetic activity* and an even greater reduction in *parasympathetic activity*. Release of catecholamines by sympathetic nerve fibres results in increased influx of calcium from the sarcoplasmic reticulum into the sarcoplasm (Section 21.16.3); the net effect of parasympathetic activation is a reduction in cytosolic calcium. Thus, in myocardial ischaemia, the combination of increased sympathetic and reduced parasympathetic activity would favour the accumulation of cytosolic calcium. Elevations in intracellular calcium can provoke oscillations in the membrane potential of cardiac muscle cells. Thus calcium overload and the resulting calcium-dependent ionic currents can contribute to the development of *ectopic activity* in general and may therefore be a trigger for *ventricular fibrillation* in particular. The calcium ions can also contribute to changes in *impulse conduction*, e.g. heart blocks.

These mechanisms may operate in domestic mammals also, since observations on laboratory mammals have shown elevations of cytosolic calcium in animals particularly susceptible to ventricular fibrillation.

Chapter 22
The Cardiac Cycle

I EVENTS OF THE CARDIAC CYCLE

22.1 General characteristics of the cardiac cycle

The cardiac cycle is the period between the end of one contraction of the heart and the end of the next contraction. The sequence of events in the cardiac cycle is shown in Fig. 22.1.

The left and right atria are two independent *primer pumps*, and the left and right ventricles are two independent *power pumps* (Section 20.3), but the left and right atria contract and relax almost simultaneously, as do the left and right ventricles. Therefore, although the diagram illustrates only the *left atrial cycle* and *left ventricular cycle*, the right atrium and right ventricle are contracting and relaxing at the same time as the left chambers.

During **atrial diastole** blood at first accumulates in the atria, and is then transferred passively into the ventricles. In **atrial systole** blood is actively forced into the ventricles by atrial contraction. The ventricles fill slowly during **ventricular diastole**, and then eject blood into the aorta and pulmonary trunk during **ventricular systole**.

The **atrioventricular valves** close at the onset of ventricular systole, and this coincides with the **first heart sound** as recorded on the phonocardiogram. The **aortic and pulmonary valves** close at the onset of ventricular diastole, and this coincides with the **second heart sound**.

The beginning of atrial systole is marked by the **P wave** of the electrocardiogram (Section 21.22), and the beginning of ventricular systole is synchronized with the **QRS complex**. Since the P wave is caused by the depolarization of the atrial musculature, the P wave begins slightly before atrial systole. Similarly, the QRS complex arises from depolarization of the ventricles, and therefore this complex partly precedes ventricular systole.

22.2 Atrial filling and emptying

At the onset of ventricular systole, the rapid rise in ventricular pressure instantly closes the left and right atrioventricular valves. The atria are now cut off from their ventricles, until ventricular systole ends.

Venous blood pours into the right atrium through the great veins, and oxygenated blood returns from the lungs into the left atrium. Figure 22.1 shows that, during the first half of atrial diastole (while the ventricles are contracting), the pressure in the left atrium falls to a low level, just above zero, and then rises slightly; the pressures in the right atrium are similar. Throughout this period, a large volume of blood accumulates in the atria.

At the end of ventricular systole, the pressure in the ventricles falls precipitously to just below the pressure in the atria. There is now a pressure gradient from atria to ventricles, and therefore the left and right atrioventricular valves open. The blood that has accumulated in the atria moves into the ventricles, and is followed by blood that continues to arrive in the atria throughout ventricular diastole.

At the onset of the P wave, the atria contract. The contraction begins at the junction of the cranial vena cava with the right atrium (the site of the S-A node), and spreads over the right and then the left atrium like a peristaltic wave which 'milks' the blood into the two ventricles. Thus atrial systole briefly raises the atrial pressure, giving the atrial blood a parting thrust into the ventricles.

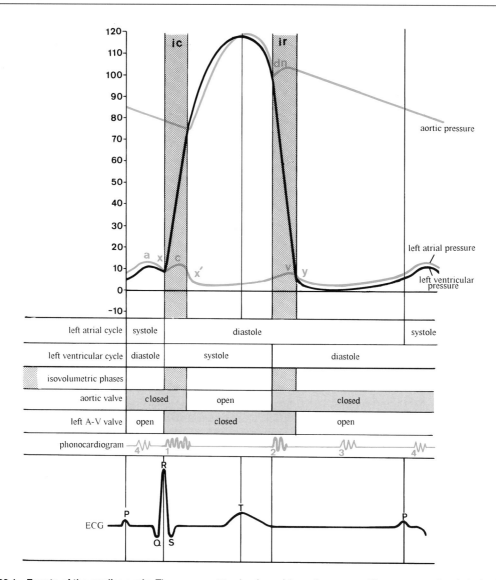

Fig. 22.1 Events of the cardiac cycle. The uppermost tracing (green) is aortic pressure. The wave complex dn is the dicrotic notch, caused by the closure of the aortic valve. At its peak, aortic pressure exceeds ventricular pressure because of conversion of kinetic energy into potential energy. The next tracing (black) is the pressure in the left ventricle. Isometric contraction (ic, stipple) and isometric relaxation (ir, stipple) occur at the beginning and end of left ventricular systole because both the left atrioventricular valve and the aortic valve are closed. Left atrial pressure (green) shows three positive pressure waves, the a wave caused by atrial systole, the c wave by bulging of the left A-V valve, and the v wave by filling of the left atrium. The negative x wave is the dip between the a and c waves, and x′ is a fall in pressure after the c wave. The negative y wave is caused by the opening of the A-V valves. The phonocardiogram tracing (green) records the four heart sounds, 1 being associated with closure of the A-V valves, 2 with closure of the aortic and pulmonary valves, 3 with movement of blood through the open A-V valves during ventricular diastole, and 4 with atrial systole. The electrocardiogram tracing (black) records the P wave caused by depolarization of the atrial myocardium, QRS complex by depolarization of ventricular myocardium, and T wave by repolarization of ventricular myocardium.

The pressure in the right atrium (the central venous pressure) is not governed solely by events in the heart itself, but is strongly influenced by the venous return to the heart from the systemic veins in the normal animal. Various factors can mobilize blood from the **venous reservoirs** including the muscle pump, breathing, and sympathetic venoconstriction (Sections 12.16.2, 12.16.3). Any such rapid inflow of blood from the systemic veins tends to increase the right atrial pressure.

Systole of the right atrium tends to eject blood not only into the right ventricle but also backwards into the venae cavae, where it creates a **jugular pulse** in the normal horse with the head in the erect position, some cattle, and other food animals.

Three positive atrial pressure waves (a, c, and v) and three negative atrial pressure waves (x, x', and y) are recognizable (Fig. 22.1); these are about 3–5 mmHg (0.4–0.7 kPa) in amplitude, and almost identical in both atria (Hamlin and Smith, 1977, p. 84). The *a wave* is caused by atrial systole; the *c wave* coincides with the onset of ventricular systole, and is probably caused mainly by bulging of the closed atrioventricular valve into the atrium; the *v wave* is caused by the final accumulation of blood in the atria, at the end of ventricular systole (Guyton, 1986, p. 154). The negative valley between the a and c waves is known as the x wave. The relatively steep fall in atrial pressure immediately after the c wave (Fig. 22.1) is referred to as the x' wave. It arises from the isovolumetric contraction of the ventricle; this moves the atrioventricular ostium towards the apex of the heart and thus enlarges the atrium, causing the pressure to fall sometimes as low as 5 mmHg (0.7 kPa) below zero (Hamlin and Smith, 1977, p. 83). Immediately after the opening of the A-V valves the atrial pressure falls rapidly, causing the *y wave*.

The right atrium contracts about 0.08 s before the left in the dog, and about 0.16 s in the horse (Hamlin and Smith, 1977, p. 84). The greater asynchrony in the horse is due to the greater distance between the S-A node and the left atrium.

The left and right atria have only a weak capability for emptying themselves into the ventricles. About 70–80% of the blood that enters a ventricle goes in before its atrium contracts; atrial contraction then adds the remainder, thus priming the ventricle for full effectiveness.

At rest, ventricular output is sufficient without atrial priming, but at *exercise* it may not be enough and breathlessness may then result. An increase in venous return at the beginning of minor exercise would distend the atrium, and thus induce the Frank–Starling mechanism, leading automatically to more powerful atrial contraction (Section 21.11).

Atrial contraction does make a major contribution to ventricular filling if the atrioventricular ostium is *obstructed by disease* (for example by mitral stenosis, i.e. narrowing of the left A-V ostium, common in man but rare in domestic mammals; Hamlin and Smith, 1977, p. 99). The pumping action of the atria is then needed to drive blood forcibly into the ventricle against the resistance at the valve. Thus the contractile powers of the atria can be regarded as another example of *inherent redundancy* (Section 19.11). Since narrowing of the atrioventricular ostium will cause more blood to be left behind and this will stretch the atrial wall during the next filling, the increased power of atrial pumping would again be partly dependent on the Frank–Starling mechanism.

Blood and Studdert (1988, p. 507) reported that a small **jugular pulse** is normal in most food animals. De Lahunta and Habel (1986, p. 70) confirmed its presence in some normal cattle; in the normal animal the pulse will usually be eliminated by compressing the cranial end of the vein, since the blood should then drain into the heart. In the normal standing horse with head erect the jugular pulse should be seen on both sides of the neck, near the thoracic inlet (Glazier, 1987). Abnormally prominent pulsations in any species are consistent with incompetence of the tricuspid valve. Continuous distension of the jugular vein indicates right heart failure, pericarditis being a cause in the horse (Glazier, 1987, p. 98) and ox (de Lahunta and Habel, 1986, p. 70). See also Section 23.11.

22.3   Ventricular filling and emptying

The high pressure in the ventricles during ventricular systole keeps the atrioventricular valves closed, and thus permits a large volume of blood to accumulate in the atria. The abrupt fall in ventricular pressure at the end of ventricular systole instantly allows the atrioventricular valves to open. The ventricles then fill rapidly, and are finally topped up by atrial systole.

The onset of ventricular systole immediately reverses the pressure gradient across the atrioventricular valves, abruptly closing them. As ventricular systole builds up, the blood is trapped inside the two ventricles. It cannot escape to the atria because the A-V valves are shut: it cannot enter the aorta or pulmonary trunk because the pressures in these two vessels at first exceed the pressures in the ventricles. The two ventricles now apply increasing pressure to the blood within them, until this pressure slightly exceeds that within the aorta and pulmonary trunk. Throughout this phase, while the pressure in the ventricles is building up, the volume of blood enclosed within the ventricles must remain essentially unchanged since liquid is incompressible; this period of ventricular systole is therefore known as the phase of *isovolumetric contraction* (ic in Fig. 22.1).

Once the pressures in the ventricles exceed those in the aorta and pulmonary trunk, the aortic and pulmonary valves open. A pressure gradient is now established from the ventricles into their arterial outlets, and blood flows into the aorta and pulmonary trunk. This is the *ejection phase* of ventricular systole. The ventricular muscle fibres shorten progressively as the volume of blood in the ventricles decreases. The shortening brings the sarcomeres towards stages E and F of the length–tension plot in Fig. 21.9, and therefore the intraventricular pressure declines progressively as the completion of ventricular systole approaches.

At the end of ventricular systole the ventricles relax suddenly, causing a rapid fall in intraventricular pressure. This creates an immediate pressure gradient from aorta to left ventricle and from pulmonary trunk to right ventricle, and the blood tends to rush back from the aorta and pulmonary trunk into the ventricles. This brief reversal of flow instantly closes the aortic and pulmonary valves (Fig. 18.1). Since the pressure in the ventricles is still high, although falling fast, the atrioventricular valves remain closed as well. Thus once again the blood is trapped within the ventricles. Therefore ventricular diastole begins with a short period when the volume of ventricular blood remains constant; this is therefore known as the phase of *isovolumetric relaxation* of the ventricles (ir in Fig. 22.1). Finally the ventricular pressures fall to their very low diastolic levels, the atrioventricular valves open, and a new cycle of ventricular filling begins.

In the resting heart the ventricles eject only a little more than half of their blood volume. When the heart contracts really strongly, for instance under sympathetic control during severe exercise, the ventricles eject up to 90% of their contents.

The large diameter of the left and right atrioventricular ostia offers a very low resistance to flow, and therefore the opening of the A-V valves is followed by a *phase of rapid filling* of the ventricles. This phase occurs in the first third of ventricular diastole (Guyton, 1986, p. 155)

and takes about 0.1 s (Hamlin and Smith, 1977, p. 84). A further factor apparently contributing to fast ventricular filling in this phase is the elastic recoil of the ventricular wall as it recovers from the muscular contortions of its systole; this is thought to produce ventricular suction (Scher, 1974, p. 109) or 'aspiration' (Hamlin and Smith, 1977, p. 83). During the middle third of ventricular diastole, the rate of ventricular filling slows down to a trickle, derived from the continuing input of blood through the great veins; this slow phase is known as *diastasis*. The last third of ventricular filling is occupied by atrial systole.

During **exercise** the duration of diastasis is diminished. This enables the heart rate to increase without immediately curtailing the time required to fill the ventricles (Section 22.13).

The *isovolumetric phase* of ventricular contraction performs little external work, but potential energy is stored in the ventricle as the pressure increases. The isovolumetric phase is also known as the *isometric phase*, on the grounds that although tension increases there is no shortening of muscle fibres, but in fact the shape of the ventricle changes during systole with shortening from base to apex and an increase in circumference (Guyton, 1986, p. 155). Therefore the isovolumetric contraction of the ventricles is not entirely isometric. Incidentally the distortion of ventricular shape requires external work.

The QRS complex is followed by the onset of vigorous ventricular contraction, after a delay of about 0.02–0.04 s in the dog and 0.08 s in the horse (Hamlin and Smith, 1977, p. 83). Ventricular systole begins with a phase of *rapid ejection*. This occupies approximately only the first third of systole, but accounts for about two thirds of the total volume of blood ejected by the ventricle (Guyton, 1986, p. 155). The peak of pressure during rapid ejection occurs slightly later in the right ventricle than the left, and goes on longer (Hamlin and Smith, 1977, p. 84), thus causing the pulmonary valve to close slightly after the aortic valve. The remaining one third of the ventricular outflow is ejected during the phase of *slow ejection*, throughout the last two thirds of ventricular systole.

The volume of a ventricle when filled at the end of its diastole is known as the *end-diastolic volume*. The fraction of this volume that is ejected during systole is the *ejection fraction*, the actual volume ejected being the *stroke volume*; the remainder in the ventricle after systole is the *end-systolic volume* (Guyton, 1986, p. 155). In **exercise**, an increase in the end-diastolic volume and a decrease in the end-systolic volume augment the stroke volume by about 50% in the human athlete (Guyton, 1986, p. 1016) and Thoroughbred horse (Evans, 1994, p. 136).

22.4   Aortic pressure curve

Contraction of the left ventricle raises the aortic pressure steeply, until the aortic valve opens (Fig.

22.1). The pressure then rises rapidly, because the blood escapes into the aorta. The peak of pressure is followed by a progressive fall associated with the declining length–tension relationships of the sarcomeres as they shorten towards stages E and F of Fig. 21.9.

At the onset of ventricular diastole the aortic blood briefly shoots backwards into the ventricle, but in so doing it instantly closes the aortic valve. Flow then continues along the aorta at a high (though of course declining) pressure, driven by energy stored in the walls of the elastic arteries and large muscular arteries (Section 12.8). This stored energy overcomes the essential intermittency of ventricular pumping, and provides the uninterrupted blood flow required by organs such as the brain that are continuously active metabolically. Thus blood is pumped not only actively by the ventricles, but also passively by the arterial walls.

Pressure changes in the pulmonary trunk and arteries are considered in Section 17.18. The pressure curve in the pulmonary artery resembles that in the aorta, except that the actual pulmonary pressures are only about one sixth as great.

The upward curve of aortic pressure is known as the *anacrotic limb* and the downward curve is the *catacrotic limb* (Hamlin and Smith, 1977, p. 88). The peak of pressure is about 180 mmHg (24.0 kPa) in the dog and about 100 mmHg (13.3 kPa) in the cat (Hamlin and Smith, 1977, p. 88); Blood and Studdert (1988, p. 116) reported 112/77 mmHg (14.9/10.3 kPa) in the horse. At the exact moment during the last part of ventricular systole when ventricular ejection stops and the aortic valve closes, the progressive fall in aortic pressure is suddenly checked, or is actually reversed by a brief rise in aortic pressure; the 'down–up' wave at this point is named the *incisura* or *dicrotic notch* (Fig. 22.1). This is caused by the sudden reverse flow of aortic blood against the closed aortic valve. The anacrotic, catacrotic, and dicrotic waves occur in the pressure curve of the pulmonary trunk as well as that of the aorta, and do so almost synchronously (Hamlin *et al.*, 1974).

Ventricular contraction imparts both kinetic and potential energy to the blood (Hamlin and Smith, 1977, p. 87). The *kinetic energy* is used to overcome the forces of friction between the blood and the endothelial surface of the vascular walls: the *potential energy* is expended as lateral pressure, thus deforming the elastic tissues of the vascular walls, but is then utilized to continue driving the blood passively down the arterial tree.

Common sense would seem to suggest that, throughout ventricular systole, ventricular pressure should ex-

ceed aortic pressure in order to drive blood through the aorta. Figure 22.1, however, shows that the ventricular pressure exceeds aortic pressure only during approximately the first half of the ejection phase (Scher, 1974, p. 108). In the second half, aortic pressure exceeds ventricular. This is because the momentum of the blood represents kinetic energy. As the momentum decreases during the slow phase of ventricular ejection, the kinetic energy is converted into potential energy, i.e. pressure. Consequently the aortic pressure becomes slightly greater than the ventricular pressure.

It would also seem predictable that the pressure in arteries near to the heart should be higher than the pressures in arteries further away from the heart. Actually the systolic pressures in the brachial and femoral arteries can be higher than those in the aorta (Feigl, 1974, p. 119), even by as much as 20–30% (Guyton, 1986, p. 227). This is because primary waves of pressure passing down the arterial tree become superimposed on secondary waves of pressure that are reflected from the walls of smaller arteries and are passing backwards towards the heart along the same vessel; the superimposed waves summate.

The velocity of *blood flow* in an artery is very much less than the *velocity of its pulse wave*. In small arteries the pulse wave may be moving 100-fold faster than the flow wave of the blood itself. Only a very small movement of blood in the aorta is needed to push the peripheral blood onwards and thus cause a pressure wave in distal arteries.

The pressure pulse becomes progressively less pronounced in the small arteries and arterioles, and is almost absent in the capillaries. The main causes of this *damping* of the pressure pulse are vascular elasticity and resistance.

22.5 Myocardial architecture and contractile characteristics

The design requirement of the right and left **atria** is simply to act as two soft flexible bags which fill with blood with minimal resistance, and then empty themselves uniformly and with equally minimal effort. Thus they mainly act passively, first accommodating blood and then transferring it to the ventricles: for this they need only minimal musculature. Essentially, therefore, the myocardial wall of the left and right atria consists of no more than a thin layer of cardiac muscle fibres, so thin as to be in places actually translucent. In certain conditions of stress, however, such as severe exercise or diseased atrioventricular valves with a high resistance to flow, they need a reserve of power. Presumably this requirement is met by the reinforcement of the thin myocardium with some thicker bundles of fibres, such as the **pectinate muscles** (Fig. 20.3).

The design requirement of the **ventricles** is the capability for powerful contraction against substantial resistance. The systemic circulation is a high pressure system, driving long columns of blood through high resistance pathways to metabolically demanding tissues (Section 12.4.3). To meet this requirement the left ventricle must have powerful musculature. On the other hand, the pulmonary circulation is a low pressure system, requiring smaller muscular power in the right ventricle.

It has long been thought that the left and right ventricles have highly distinctive myocardial architectures, and attempts have been made to relate these to their contractile mechanisms.

The lumen of the **right ventricle** is a crescentic cleft between two broad surfaces (Fig. 18.2), one surface being the outer wall of the ventricle and the other being the interventricular septum. The muscle bundles are spiral, but the orientation of the spiral is *mainly circumferential* (Fig. 22.2). Contraction of the muscle of the right ventricle pulls the outer wall of the ventricle towards the interventricular septum, using the apex of the ventricle as a hinge. The action thus *decreases the lumen*, like a pair of bellows (Fig. 22.2). The figure shows that the contraction also decreases the volume by *shortening* the right ventricle; this happens because the interventricular septum, which belongs to the left ventricle but forms one wall of the right ventricle, is shortened by contraction of the left ventricle. The **left ventricle** has a circular lumen enclosed by a thick cylinder of muscle, which includes the interventricular septum. The muscle bundles are mainly longitudinal spirals (Fig. 22.2). As Fig. 22.2 shows, contraction of the muscle of the left ventricle (1) *shortens* the ventricle because of the mainly longitudinal axis of its spiral fibres, and (2) *constricts* the ventricle because of the circumferential element of its spiral fibres. The shortening of the left ventricle and right ventricle is caused by drawing together the atrioventricular ostia and the apices of the ventricles. The shortening, as well as the constriction, or in the case of the right ventricle the bellows action, reduce the volume of the ventricle and thus eject blood.

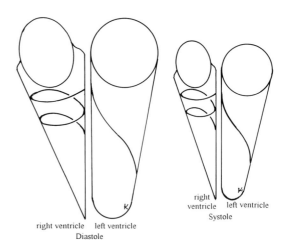

right ventricle   left ventricle
Systole

right ventricle   left ventricle
Diastole

Fig. 22.2 Highly schematic representation of the myocardial emptying of the left and right ventricles. The ventricles are drawn as if viewed from the cranial aspect. The heart on the left is in ventricular diastole, and that on the right is in ventricular systole. In both diagrams, the vertical partition between the ventricles is the interventricular septum. The left ventricular myocardium is a cylinder of muscle bundles. The bundles are spiral, but are orientated mainly in the long axis of the ventricle (sinuous line). They enclose a ventricular lumen that is circular in transverse section (the top of the diagram). The right ventricular myocardium consists of two broad surfaces, seen edge-on in the diagram; the lumen of the right ventricle is crescentic (at the top of the diagram, but drawn as an oval). The two surfaces of the right ventricle, one representing the interventricular septum and the other the outer wall of the right ventricle, are hinged at the apex of the ventricle (the bottom of the diagram). The fibre bundles of the right ventricular myocardium are more less spiral, but their orientation is mainly circumferential (the transverse spiral line). During left ventricular systole, contraction of the spiral muscle of the left ventricle both shortens the ventricle and diminishes its diameter, thus reducing the left ventricular volume. During right ventricular systole, contraction of the essentially circumferential fibres pulls the two ventricular walls together like bellows, thus decreasing the right ventricular lumen. The right ventricle is also shortened, thus still further decreasing the volume of its lumen; the right ventricle is necessarily shortened because the interventricular septum, which is shared by both ventricles, is shortened during left ventricular systole.

The architecture of the myocardium is a difficult topic. Even the thin and relatively **simple atrial myocardium** is uncertain in its arrangement. In man (Salmons, 1995, p. 1494), there is reported to be a thin and incomplete *superficial layer* shared by both atria and forming also the interatrial septum, and a *deep layer* confined to each individual atrium. The deep fibres form loops around the openings of the great veins, and arches over the roofs of the atria. Deep fibres combine to form the thicker myocardial components, notably the **pectinate muscles** in the left and right auricles, and the **intervenous ridge** and **crista terminalis** in the right atrium (Section 20.7).

Similarly, in the domestic species, Schummer *et al.* (1981, p. 22) recognized a *subepicardial layer* (superficial) and a *subendocardial layer* (deep). They designated as *long fibres* those that cover both atria, and *short fibres* those that are confined to one atrium. However, Evans (1993, p. 596) concluded that in the dog the atrial myocardium 'is not divided into distinct layers', except in the interatrial septum where each atrium supplies its own sheet of fibres.

The **ventricular myocardium**, which is inherently far more complex, has been investigated repeatedly. However, the earlier techniques have necessarily been rather crude (Salmons, 1995, p. 1494), beginning with maceration or boiling and ending with dissection or tearing the ventricles apart, so that distinguishing between artefacts and genuine fibre tracts has been difficult. More accurate concepts provided by serial sections have revealed that the origin and insertion of ventricular fibres on the fibrous skeleton have been unduly emphasized. The anatomy of the fibrous skeleton is in itself obscure enough (Section 20.12), but thinking of the myocardium in terms of skeletal muscle, i.e. with its basic attachments to hard tissues, has been actively misleading. 'Thus concepts of ventricular musculature being arranged in tracts which originate at the atrioventricular annulus and insert into the bases of the arterial trunks have little to support them in terms of anatomic fact' (Salmons, 1995, p. 1494). In the same context, Salmons also pointed out that the heart 'is a modified blood vessel', and that therefore the bundles of cardiac muscle fibres are 'attached to their neighbours' rather than to skeletal elements.

Salmons (1995, p. 1494), Evans (1993, p. 596), and Schummer *et al.* (1981, p. 22) agreed that the ventricular myocardium can be divided into *subepicardial* (superficial), *middle*, and *subendocardial* (deep) layers, though Salmons added that this can only be established 'broadly'. From simple inspection after removing the epicardium, Salmons concluded that 'by and large' the *subepicardial fibres* run *circumferentially* around the *right ventricle* and *longitudinally* down the *left ventricle* of the human heart, and then form vortices at the apex of both ventricles so that their fibres are now *subendocardial*; presumably they must be spirals if they have apical vortices, as indicated by Salmons (1995, Figs 10.51, 10.53). The **papillary muscles** are, of course, derived from the subendocardial fibres. The *middle fibres* are circumferential and confined to the left ventricle and interventricular septum, being thickest at the base of the left ventricle. The *interventricular septum* is formed largely by the middle fibres of the left ventricle. The wall of the right ventricle (excluding the septum) consists of subepicardial and subendocardial fibres only. There are major variations from heart to heart.

Both Evans (1993, p. 596) and Schummer *et al.* (1981, p. 22) seem to indicate that in the domestic species all layers of fibres arise from the fibrous skeleton, that the subepicardial layer is spiral and more or less continues into the subendocardial layer at the apical vortex, and that the middle layer is present in both ventricles. The discrepancies between these accounts and those on the myocardial architecture of man may reflect interspecific differences, intraspecific differences, artefacts, or overemphasis on the central role of the fibrous skeleton. However, Schummer *et al.* (1981, p. 22) made this particularly illuminating comment: 'In the musculature of the ventricular wall and septum we differentiate a subepicardial, a middle and a subendocardial layer, but the fibres run between one layer and another in an intricate interlacement. *We are therefore dealing with the same muscle fibres which produce the three layers by merely altering their direction.* We thus have a construction that is in accord with the function of any hollow organ.' Routine inspection of histological sections of the ventricular myocardium does support the notion of erratic fibres rather than clearly organized strata.

Observations of this kind are consistent with Salmons' concept that *structurally the heart is a modified blood vessel* (Salmons, 1995). A spiral organization of the cardiac muscle fibres is consistent with the mainly spiral arrangement of the smooth muscle cells in muscular arteries (Section 12.9.2). Salmons (1995, p. 1495) concluded that much more work must be done to elucidate the true organization of the ventricular fibres.

Unfortunately, these uncertainties about the architecture of the ventricular myocardium make it difficult to see how the mechanism might actually work. However, two anatomical features do appear to give some insight into this question, though the second and more crucial is based on the human heart. Firstly, the lumen of the right ventricle is a crescentic cleft between two broad surfaces (Fig. 18.2), whereas the left ventricle has a circular lumen enclosed by a thick cylinder of muscle fibres (Rushmer, 1966, p. 549). Secondly the cardiac muscle fibres of the ventricular myocardium are *essentially spiral and therefore have both a longitudinal and a circumferential element* (Fig. 22.2), but they run *mainly longitudinally* (i.e. dorsoventrally) down the *left ventricle*, and *mainly circumferentially* (transversely) around the *right ventricle* (Salmons, 1995, p. 1494). These anatomical relationships are consistent with shortening and constriction of the left ventricle as proposed by Hamlin and Smith (1977, p. 81), and the bellows action of the right ventricle postulated by Rushmer (1966, p. 549) and Hamlin and Smith (1977, p. 81).

The shortening of the left ventricle arises from the longitudinal forces of its spiral muscle bundles, which draw the atrioventricular ostium and the apex of the ventricle towards each other, volume being linearly related to length. The constriction of the left ventricle is caused by the circumferential forces of its spiral muscle bundles, a slight reduction in the radius of the lumen being effective since volume is proportional to the square of the radius. Hamlin and Smith (1977, p. 82) adduced cineradiographs of the canine heart showing both constriction and dorsoventral shortening of the left ventricle.

22.6 Valvular mechanisms

The general anatomy of the atrioventricular valves and the aortic and pulmonary valves has been considered with the right ventricle in Section 20.8 and with the left ventricle in Section 20.10. The function of the left and right atrioventricular valves is to prevent blood returning from the ventricles to the left and right atria during ventricular systole. The aortic and pulmonary valves prevent blood from returning from the aorta and pulmonary trunk to the ventricles during ventricular diastole.

All four valves open and close *passively*, in response to pressure gradients. Thus the atrioventricular valves open at the instant when there is a pressure gradient from atria to ventricles, i.e. when the pressure in the atria exceeds that in the ventricles; they close when the pressure in the ventricles exceeds that in the atria. Likewise the aortic and pulmonary valves open when a pressure gradient develops from the ventricles to the aorta or pulmonary artery, and close when the gradient is reversed.

The perfect functioning of the **bicuspid** (left) and **tricuspid** (right) **atrioventricular valves** is governed by the **papillary muscles** and their **chordae tendineae**. Normally, this elaborate musculotendinous apparatus ensures that the **cusps** (leaflets) of the valves, despite their irregular serrated edges, are accurately apposed during ventricular systole, thus ensuring that there is no leakage.

The **aortic valve** is stronger than the **pulmonary valve**, but otherwise the two valves are structurally and functionally similar, with three **semilunar valvules** contained within three **aortic (or pulmonary) sinuses** inside the slightly dilated **aortic bulb** (or root of the **pulmonary trunk**) (Section 20.10; Figs 20.2, 20.3). During ventricular systole, the aortic bulb dilates and the valve opens, but the semilunar valvules are not flattened against the aortic wall (Fig. 18.1A,C). The position of the valvules during ventricular systole, as in Fig. 18.1A, helps their subsequent closure. Thus, when ventricular systole ends, the energy stored in the elastic aortic wall drives blood back towards the ventricle; this brief flow catches the edges of the valvules and fills the pocket-like semilunar valvules with blood, thus shutting the valve (Fig. 18.1B).

22.6.1 *Atrioventricular valves*

The opening and closing of the left and right A-V valves have been reviewed by Salmons (1995, p. 1487). **Opening** of the valves occurs rapidly at the onset of ventricular diastole; the cusps part from each other and project into the ventricular cavity, and blood flows passively from the atria towards the ventricular apex. As this flow diminishes, the cusps begin to float passively together, partly occluding the ostium. Active atrial systole now jets blood towards the ventricular apex, reopening the cusps. As atrial systole ends, the cusps again float rapidly together and the valve **closes**.

Indeed Smetzer *et al.* (1977, p. 97) concluded that 'the A-V valves probably close *solely* (my italics) as a consequence of atrial systole.' They suggested that this (quite surprising) closure immediately after the end of atrial systole, and *before* the onset of ventricular systole, is presumably caused by a transient pressure gradient from ventricle to atrium. But they added the following proviso: if the interval between atrial and ventricular contraction be lengthened, 'the A-V valves close once as a consequence of atrial systole and then drift open again before the onset of ventricular systole.

Closure of the A-V valves is followed by the onset of ventricular systole. The sudden sharp increase in the pressure gradient from ventricles to atria now strongly consolidates the closure of the A-V valves. Tension rises in the papillary muscles, which are among the first myocardial components to receive conducting fibres from the left and right crura of the atrioventricular bundle (Section 21.19.3) via the **septomarginal trabeculae**. As the pressure within the two ventricles rises steeply, the cusps balloon into the atrium. Precisely co-ordinated contraction of the papillary muscle creates exactly the correct tension in the chordae tendineae for promoting perfect apposition of the valvular cusps and maintaining valvular competence. These actions, already elaborate enough, are further complicated by the extreme protean characteristics of the ostia of the A-V valves. The ostia change markedly in position, form, and area during a cardiac cycle. For example, in man, the left valve reduces its orificial area by up to 40% in systole, and at the same time changes its shape from circular to crescentic at the peak of ventricular systole; both valves move ventrally and to the left during systole, and reverse their motion during diastole (Salmons, 1995, p. 1487). The innocent, viewing this apparatus for the first time in the dissection room, would never believe that such a tangle of slender strings, vague muscular projections, and delicate flaps with irregular frilly edges, could ever make a faultless seal. In fact, the echocardiographic experiences of cardiologists show that the atrioventricular valves, and particularly the right atrioventricular valve, are often incompetent in the normal human heart (J. Silas, personal communication, 1997).

The atrioventricular valves are, however, vulnerable to **pathological changes**. Predictably – in view of the hammering it receives from high systemic pressures – the left (bicuspid or mitral) valve is more vulnerable than the right (tricuspid) valve. **Bicuspid (mitral) regurgitation** through a leaking left A-V valve is the most commonly encountered valvular disorder in general veterinary practice (Darke *et al.*, 1996, p. 57). A leaking valve is said to be 'incompetent' or 'insufficient'. *Rupture of chordae tendineae* is one of the principal causes, particularly in horses; other common causes include *dilation of the atrioventricular ostium* associated with volume-overloading of the left ventricle. *Fibrous thickening* of the valve is not uncommon in elderly horses. *Mitral valve dysplasia* based on congenital malformations of the valve (e.g. short, absent, or elongated chordae, or malpositioned or fused papillary muscles) is common in dogs and is also seen in cats. **Tricuspid regurgitation** (Darke *et al.*, 1996, p. 66) can be caused by anomalies and a variety of acquired conditions in dogs, horses, and cattle including gross *hypertrophy of the papillary muscles*.

22.6.2 *Aortic and pulmonary valves*

It can be seen at a glance that the aortic and pulmonary valves, unlike the atrioventricular valves, have a neat design that is obviously going to work. The key feature controlling closure is the triradiate form of the valvular orifice when fully open (Fig. 18.1C). The triradiate form occurs for two reasons. Firstly, the aortic wall is highly elastic in the *peripheral zone* of the aortic (and pulmonary) sinuses; therefore the radius of the artery increases here (the aorta, by about 16% in man) in ventricular systole, and this draws taut the free edges of the semilunar valvules. Secondly, blood always fills the pocket formed by each valvule, and vortices help to keep each pocket open (Salmons, 1995, p. 1489). The nodules of the semilunar valvules seal the triradiate closure.

However, the aortic valve is obliged to endure a more traumatic lifestyle than the left A-V valve. The high pressure at the *end* of ventricular systole closes the aortic valve with a brisk snap, whereas the left A-V valve closes at the *onset* of ventricular systole while pressure is only beginning to rise. Also the blood shoots through the aortic (and pulmonary) valve during ventricular systole

at a much higher velocity than through the atrioventricular valves during atrial systole. Consequently the edges of the semilunar valvules of the aortic and pulmonary valves are subjected to much more mechanical abrasion than are the cusps of the A-V valves (Guyton, 1986, p. 156).

Aortic regurgitation (caused by insufficiency or incompetence of the aortic valve) can arise from various **pathological conditions** (Darke *et al.*, 1996, p. 77). *Fibrous degeneration* of the valve is one of the commonest causes, and is presumably a response to trauma. In horses over 10 years old it can manifest itself commonly as *degenerative linear thickening* or *beading* of the aortic valve, the regurgitation being usually mild but sometimes severe. In all the domestic species aortic regurgitation may be associated with *interventricular septal defects*. These defects arise at the **membranous part** of the interventricular septum (Section 20.10). The membranous part lies just ventral to the aortic valve. Hence a cusp (leaflet) of the aortic valve sometimes prolapses into the interventricular defect. *Congenital aortic stenosis* is often associated with aortic regurgitation.

22.7   Heart sounds

Vibrations are generated by the normal heart, and transmitted as audible sounds to specific sites on the thoracic wall (Section 23.10.1). Sounds are associated with the closure of valves, but not with the opening of valves.

Four normal heart sounds are recognized, all of them being caused by vibration – the vibration of blood, valves, the walls of the heart, and the walls of the aorta and pulmonary trunk.

22.7.1 *First heart sound*

The first sound (S1) is traditionally known as the 'lub' sound. It is usually longer and of lower frequency, than the second sound. It is associated with closure of the A-V valves at the onset of ventricular systole.

Figure 22.1 shows that S1 occurs mainly during the phase of *isometric ventricular contraction*, and this is the key to understanding the vibrations that cause it. Thus at the onset of ventricular systole, the ventricles abruptly force the blood towards the aortic outlet and towards the atrioventricular orifice, at the base of the ventricles. But the atrioventricular and aortic and pulmonary valves are closed, thus trapping the blood within the ventricles. However, there is enough 'give' in the A-V valves, and in the tissues forming the rest of the base of the ventricles, to allow the blood to undergo a brief but rapid acceleration that balloons the closed A-V valves into the atria, this being followed by an instant deceleration: the resulting rebound of blood back into the ventricles sets up vibrations in the walls of the ventricles, in the A-V valves, and in the blood itself, and these vibrations are the main source of the first sound. The subsequent opening of the aortic and pulmonary valves permits renewed acceleration of the blood, and this contributes further vibrations which add to the end of the first heart sound.

The account in Section 22.6.1 (based on Salmons, 1995, p. 1487) of the closing of the atrioventricular valves indicated that after the end of atrial systole the valve closes, and that this happens *before* ventricular systole begins. On the basis of observations on the dog and man by many investigators using various techniques, Luisada *et al.* (1974) confirmed that 'both atrioventricular valves are completely closed at the time of the first rapid vibrations of the first sound'.

Thus the events taking place at the A-V valves at the time of the first heart sound are complicated by the participation of both atrial and ventricular systole. Not surprisingly, therefore, the first sound goes on a long time, and four components can be detected by phonocardiogram (Smetzer *et al.*, 1977, p. 96; Blood and Studdert, 1988, p. 434). The *first component* may arise from vibrations generated by early contractions of the ventricular myocardium; the *second* may come from sudden tension in the left and right A-V valves; the *third* may originate from vibrations caused by the early ejection of blood from the ventricles; the *fourth* may come from rapid ejection by the ventricles. The vibrations of the first and fourth components are of low frequency and low amplitude. The vibrations of the second and third components are of greater frequency and amplitude, and are therefore the most prominent part of the first heart sound. The second and third components tend to occur as distinct entities, thus causing a '*splitting*' or '*doubling*' of the first heart sound, this being audible by auscultation in most normal animals. Because of dilation of the pulmonary trunk through pulmonary hypertension or pulmonary stenosis, the fourth component may be accentuated; it is then known as an 'ejection sound' or 'ejection click', and can sound like a pronounced splitting of S1. Establishing the temporal relationships between S1 and the other sounds enables the timing of murmurs, the identification of 'extra sounds', and the diagnosis of simple arrhythmias.

22.7.2   *Second heart sound*

This is traditionally referred to as the 'dub sound'. It is shorter and has a higher frequency than the first sound.

The second sound (S2) is associated with closure of the aortic and pulmonary valves at the onset of ventricular diastole. The sudden end of ventricular systole, with its precipitous fall in ventricular pressure, allows the blood in the aorta and pulmonary artery to reverse its flow and accelerate towards the ventricles, but the aortic and pulmonary valves bar its way. On impact against the closed aortic and pulmonary valves, the blood abruptly decelerates and then rebounds because of the elasticity of the aortic and pulmonary arterial walls. The vibrations of the walls of these vessels, of the adjacent ventricular walls, and of the blood within them, produce the second heart sound.

Splitting of the second heart sound occurs when the aortic and pulmonary valves close out of phase. This is detectable by auscultation in most normal horses, and in some normal dogs, but (logically) is also characteristic of cardiac disorders in which either the right or the left ventricular cycle is delayed by disease. It occurs during inspiration if the right ventricular cycle is delayed by right bundle branch block, pulmonary stenosis, or pulmonary hypertension, as in the dog; it occurs during expiration in left bundle block or aortic stenosis (Smetzer *et al.*, 1977, p. 98).

In man and some dogs, splitting of S2 is a normal event occurring during inspiration and disappearing during expiration. This because inspiration increases the venous return to the right atrium (Section 13.3.5), and the resulting increase in right ventricular ejection time causes the pulmonary valve to close late; simultaneously, inspiration diminishes venous return to the left atrium (Section 17.15), causing the aortic valve to close early. During expiration, right ventricular ejection time returns to normal, and left ventricular ejection time increases in order to eject the increased volume of blood delivered to the lungs during the previous inspiration.

The frequency of the second heart sound is higher than that of the first heart sound because (1) the mass of blood in the proximal parts of the aorta and pulmonary artery is relatively small compared with the mass of blood in the ventricles, and (2) the aortic and pulmonary valves and their arterial walls have a relatively high elastic modulus compared with the modulus of the ventricular walls. The second heart sound lasts for a shorter time than the first sound because it is likely to be 'damped out' relatively quickly by the elastic vascular wall (Guyton, 1986, p. 317).

22.7.3   Third heart sound

S3 is a very faint ventricular sound associated with the movement of blood from the atria into the ventricle during the first part of ventricular diastole.

> The third sound is of very low frequency, near the limits of the conventional stethoscope (Guyton, 1986, p. 317). The ventricles have a phase of rapid filling which occupies approximately the first third of ventricular diastole (Section 22.3), and it is around the end of this phase that S3 occurs (Smetzer et al., 1977, p. 98; Guyton, 1986, p. 317). The source of the sound is uncertain. It may be caused by vibration in the ventricular walls and blood while the blood pours relatively rapidly into the ventricles, the sound disappearing in the middle of ventricular diastole as the flow from the atria slows down (Guyton, 1986, p. 317).
>
> In cattle (Darke et al., 1996, p. 26), and in many horses (Smetzer et al., 1977, p. 98), S3 is a normal sound. It may be detectable with a phonocardiogram in the normal dog but is rarely audible normally (Smetzer et al., 1977, p. 98), and in small animals usually indicates cardiac disease (Darke et al., 1996, p. 26). In the dog and horse it becomes audible and very intense in congestive heart failure (Smetzer et al., 1977, p. 98).

22.7.4   Fourth heart sound

The fourth heart sound (the 'atrial' heart sound) is associated with atrial systole, and presumably originates from vibrations initiated by the rapid flow of blood into the ventricles.

> S4 is a short sound of very low frequency and intensity (Blood and Studdert, 1988, p. 434). It is a normal sound in cattle (Darke et al., 1996, p. 26), and is commonplace in apparently normal horses (Smetzer, 1977, p. 98). In small animals it generally indicates cardiac disease, usually mitral regurgitation or dilated cardiomyopathy in dogs, and left ventricular hypertrophy in cats (Darke et al., 1996, p. 26).

22.7.5   Diastolic gallop sounds

When the third and fourth heart sounds occur in dogs and cats they form a cadence with S1 and S2 resembling the sound of a galloping horse.

> Atrial and ventricular gallops indicate diastolic dysfunction (Darke et al., 1996, p. 26). They occur mainly in dogs and cats with overload of the left ventricle, e.g. mitral regurgitation or dilated cardiomyopathy in dogs, and left ventricular hypertrophy in cats.

22.7.6   Clicks

A click may be heard between S1 and S2, i.e. associated with ventricular systole.

> A click may occur either early or late in ventricular systole (Smetzer et al., 1977, p. 99). Thus it may be close to S1 and is then an *ejection click*; this is often related to dilation of the aorta or pulmonary artery in the dog. Alternatively a click may be midway between S1 and S2, or close to S2 and therefore late in ventricular systole; this is a *systolic click*. It may indicate mitral incompetence in the dog with prolapse of the valve into the left atrium, but is not uncommon in the normal dog. Glazier (1987) noted that in horses clicks are of unknown cause and are generally regarded as benign. In man they are common, and often associated with mitral prolapse into the left atrium (Glazier, 1987).

22.7.7   Murmurs

Murmurs last longer than heart sounds, and occur during any normally silent interval in the cardiac cycle. They are caused by high velocity turbulent flow or vortices. They may occur during ventricular systole (systolic murmurs), during ventricular diastole (diastolic murmurs), or continuously (continuous murmurs). Some murmurs occur in apparently normal animals, and are then known as 'innocent' or 'benign' murmurs; 'functional' murmurs are those that occur in the absence of structural changes, but the term is also used as a synonym for 'innocent'.

> Murmurs have been reviewed by Smetzer et al. (1977, pp. 99–101). See also Section 23.10.2.

Systolic murmurs
Bicuspid (mitral) insufficiency (regurgitation) (Section 22.6.1) is the commonest cause of systolic murmurs in old animals. *Tricuspid insufficiency (regurgitation)* has similar characteristics. *Congenital pulmonary stenosis* (Section 15.9) is a common cause of loud systolic murmurs in young dogs. *Congenital aortic stenosis* (Section 15.10) gives a similar loud systolic murmur. Systolic murmurs also occur in *congenital* **interventricular septal defect**, because of the high velocity stream forced through the defect by the left ventricle (Section 15.11).

Diastolic murmurs
These murmurs are extremely rare in dogs, but not uncommon in horses. *Aortic insufficiency (regurgitation)* is a common cause of diastolic murmurs in old horses.

Diastolic murmurs from pulmonary insufficiency (regurgitation) are rare in domestic mammals.

Continuous murmurs

In the neonatal ox and horse, the normal reversal of blood flow in the ductus arteriosus at the first breath causes turbulence with a continuous 'machinery' murmur (Section 15.8). In the foal this goes on for about the first 4 days after birth, but a longer period suggests that the normal process of closure of the ductus has failed (Glazier, 1987).

Innocent murmurs

Innocent murmurs, both systolic and diastolic, are not uncommon in apparently normal horses less than 5 years old. Innocent systolic murmurs also occur in apparently normal puppies (Smetzer *et al.*, 1977, pp. 100–101).

22.7.8   Thrill

A thrill is a vibration caused by such violent turbulence that it can be felt by placing the palm of the hand on the thoracic wall.

A *systolic thrill* occurs during ventricular systole in aortic stenosis, pulmonary stenosis, and interventricular septal defect; a *diastolic thrill* is detectable in advanced aortic insufficiency (regurgitation) (Blood and Studdert, 1988, p. 913).

22.7.9   Final thoughts on heart sounds

Streamline flow is silent
Remember that my boys,
But when the flow is turbulent
There's sure to be a noise.
So when your stethoscope picks up
A bruit, murmur, sigh,
Remember that it's turbulence
And you must find out why.

(With grateful thanks to Dr. Alan C. Burton, distinguished cardiac physiologist. At a meeting of the American Physiological Society just after the war, Dr. Burton arranged for this, his doggerel verse, to be sung by a barber-shop quartet of graduate students.)

'The accelerations and decelerations of the cardiovascular structures and of the blood they contain are the cause of all cardiac vibrations, both inaudible and audible.' (Luisada *et al.*, 1974).

22.8   Autonomic regulation of the heart

The sympathetic and parasympathetic motor pathways to the heart regulate the rate and strength of contraction. To obtain the greatest possible control of rate, both sympathetic and parasympathetic motor endings should be especially concentrated in and around the **sinuatrial** and **atrioventricular nodes**, and this is mainly where they are. On the other hand, to regulate the strength of contraction, the sympathetic endings should also be distributed to the **atrial** and particularly to the **ventricular myocardium**, and indeed that is so.

22.8.1   Sympathetic system

The sympathetic motor pathways to the heart consist of a standard preganglionic and postganglionic relay. The preganglionic neurons have their cell station in the first few segments of the thoracic spinal cord (Section 2.9); they release acetylcholine at their endings (Section 2.33.2). The postganglionic neurons have their cell station mainly in the **stellate ganglion** (Section 2.10). Their axons enter the heart via the **cardiac plexus** (Fig. 19.8), releasing noradrenaline at their endings. The cardiac plexus is a profuse network of sympathetic and vagal cardiac nerves (Sections 2.11, 3.11.3).

All cardiac muscle cells experience a slow inward leak of Na^+ ions that causes the membrane potential to rise progressively towards the threshold voltage where an action potential occurs (Section 21.17). The release of noradrenaline from sympathetic motor endings in the vicinity of the sinuatrial node increases the sodium permeability of the nodal cells and therefore accelerates the rise in their membrane potential towards threshold. This induces a modest increase in **heart rate**.

The release of noradrenaline near cardiac muscle cells in the ventricular (and atrial) myocardium increases the amount of Ca^{2+} released into the cytoplasm. The influx of calcium into the cardiac muscle cell displaces tropomyosin, thus making more actin–myosin bridges available (Section 21.8). This increases the **force of contraction** (Section 21.16.3). Infusion of adrenaline and noradrenaline into the blood stream from the **adrenal medulla** similarly increases heart rate and force of contraction.

To summarize, sympathetic stimulation increases (1) the rate of discharge of the sinuatrial node and hence the heart rate, and (2) the force of contraction of the atrial and ventricular myocardium.

Maximum sympathetic stimulation almost triples the *heart rate* and doubles the *force of contraction* (Guyton, 1986, p. 171). Sympathetic stimulation also increases the rate of conduction in the conducting system, and the general excitability of cardiac muscle cells throughout the heart.

Adrenergic fibres are most profusely distributed to the sinuatrial and atrioventricular nodes, and much less densely to the atrial and ventricular myocardium (Salmons, 1995, p. 1500). Adrenergic (and vagal) fibres evidently enter the nodes, but no nerve fibres are seen actually to end on nodal cells (Salmons, 1995, p. 769). Although the sympathetic motor innervation is anatomically bilateral, it is functionally asymmetrical; stimulation of the left stellate ganglion has little effect on heart rate but increases ventricular contractility, whereas stimulation of the right stellate ganglion increases both rate and contractility.

The motor sympathetic pathways to the heart act through β_1-*adrenergic receptors* (Section 2.33). The *resting* cardiac muscle cell has a reserve of force, since the amount of Ca^{2+} bound to troponin-C on the thin (actin) myofilament induces less than half-maximal activation of the contractile mechanism (Section 21.16.3). Greater force during contraction can therefore be attained by increasing the concentration of free Ca^{2+} in the sarcoplasm; more calcium ions then bind to troponin-C, thus displacing more of the tropomyosin and exposing more binding sites on the actin strand (Section 21.8). Adrenergic stimulation releases calcium from the sarcoplasmic reticulum (Section 21.16.3), and thus creates the influx of calcium required for a progressive increase in contractile force.

The force of contraction can, of course, also be increased by stretching the myocardium through increased filling, according to the **Frank–Starling relationship** (Section 21.11). However, increasing the force by sympathetic stimulation is functionally more effective, for two reasons (Scott, 1986, p. 35). First, sympathetic stimulation does not increase the volume of the heart, and therefore the heart will be *smaller* than when it is stretched by filling; the law of Laplace establishes that the tension required to generate a given pressure becomes larger in proportion to the diameter of the heart; therefore the cost in energy and oxygen is less in a small heart than in a stretched heart. Secondly, sympathetic stimulation increases the *velocity* of contraction (and

relaxation); therefore the duration of systole is reduced and more time is available for filling. Maintaining an adequate time for filling is critical when an increase in cardiac output is required (Section 22.13).

The responses to sympathetic stimulation of the heart are gradual, compared with the immediate responses to vagal stimulation (Section 22.8.2) (Smith and Hamlin, 1977, pp. 107, 111). The technical terms for these responses are as follows: positive inotropic effect, for increased force of contraction (negative effect for decrease); positive chronotropic effect, for increased rate of contraction; and positive dromotropic effect, for a shortening of the interval between atrial and ventricular contraction. All of these terms have a classic Greek derivation, and although a well-chosen etymology can be helpful to anyone with a smattering of the classics, 5 minutes with a lexicon will show that the etymology of 'inotropic' (Section 16.15) is almost meaningless and ought to be banned by law.

Stimulation of motor sympathetic pathways to the heart has also been shown to activate α-*adrenoreceptors* (Billman, 1992). The net effect is a rise in the calcium levels of the cardiac muscle cells and an increase in contractile force. Thus α- and β-adrenergic stimulation may act synergistically to elicit an *increased force of contraction*.

Sympathetic tone contributes to the regulation of *rate* in the *resting heart*, but only slightly (Hamlin and Smith, 1977, p. 107); only a small decrease in heart rate follows bilateral removal of the stellate ganglia. However, reflex sympathetic stimulation of the heart is an *important factor when the heart is stressed*: examples are postural changes, haemorrhage, all levels of exercise, emotional stress, and heart disease such as chronic congestive heart failure. Under these conditions, reflex stimulation of the sympathetic cardiac motor pathways increases not only the rate but also the force of contraction, thus yielding an increase in cardiac output.

Sympathetic excitation also acts on the **atrioventricular node**. Here, the increased permeability to sodium ions decreases the conduction time from atrial myocardial cell, through the transitional cell, to the nodal cell, and onward to the atrioventricular bundle (Guyton, 1986, p. 171), and thus shortens the delay in transmission across the A-V node.

22.8.2 *Parasympathetic system*

Cardiac rami from the recurrent laryngeal nerves (Section 3.11.3) distribute vagal preganglionic axons over the left and right atria. These axons make synapses with postganglionic vagal nerve cell bodies in the walls of both atria. The endings of the postganglionic axons are distributed mainly to the sinuatrial and atrioventricular nodes, and some go to the atrial and ventricular myocardium.

Vagal stimulation acts mainly on the **sinuatrial node**. The postganglionic vagal endings release acetylcholine around the nodal cells. This increases the permeability of a nodal cell to potassium ions. The resulting rapid leakage of potassium causes hyperpolarization (increased negativity) of the cell. Hyperpolarization slows down the normal rise in membrane potential caused by the inward leak of sodium ions, so that it now takes longer for the nodal cell to reach the threshold for an action potential. This *slows the heart rate*.

In the **atrioventricular node** vagal stimulation hyperpolarizes the transitional cells (Section 21.20.2), and thus slows transmission of the cardiac impulse into the ventricles.

Strong vagal stimulation can slow the heart to the point where it stops beating, but the rhythm breaks through and the heart starts beating again. This is known as *vagal escape*.

The release of acetylcholine around the **cardiac muscle cells** of the **atrium** decreases intracellular calcium levels and thus depresses their force of contraction (the opposite to the effect of the adrenergic innervation). By weakening atrial contraction, vagal stimulation can *diminish ventricular filling* and thus *indirectly diminish ventricular stroke volume*.

The cardiac efferent vagal fibres from the recurrent laryngeal nerve pass through the **cardiac plexus** (Sections 2.11, 3.11.3), and are then distributed mainly to the sinuatrial and atrioventricular nodes, and much less densely to the atrial and ventricular myocardium (Salmons, 1995, p. 1500). Like the sympathetic pathways, the vagal motor pathways to the heart are more or less bilaterally symmetrical anatomically, but asymmetrical functionally. Thus the right vagus slows the heart mainly via the sinuatrial node, whereas the left vagus acts mainly on the atrioventricular node (Salmons, 1995, p. 769).

In man and most other mammals, **ganglion cells** (i.e. postganglionic vagal nerve cell bodies) are restricted to the atria and interatrial septum (Salmons, 1995, p. 1307). There are many near the nodal borders in the subepicardial tissue, but none actually within the nodes (Salmons, 1995, p. 769). Numerous nerve fibres are present in the nodes but no fibres appear to end on a nodal cell.

Depression of the force of contraction of the **atrial myocardium** by vagal motor pathways (Smith and Hamlin, 1977, p. 110), through a *decrease* in intracellular calcium levels in the cardiac muscle cell (Billman, 1992),

is the opposite action to the release of calcium ions into the cytosol by β_1-adrenergic stimulation. Vagal stimulation apparently has the same direct depressing action on the *ventricular myocardium*, but the effect is insignificant (Scott, 1986, p. 35); presumably this is because the vagal innervation of the ventricular myocardium is sparse (Smith and Hamlin, 1977, p. 111).

The inhibitory action of the vagus on heart rate appears to be continuous (tonic) in the resting heart (Smith and Hamlin, 1977, p. 111), since cutting the vagal cardiac pathway or blocking it with atropine causes a marked increase in heart rate (approximately doubling the rate in the dog and aged horse, and increasing it fourfold in the relatively athletic hare). Thus **vagal tone** (Section 21.18) constitutes a rapid reserve of cardiac acceleration.

The vagal inhibition of the sinuatrial node acts through muscarinic receptors (Katz, 1992, p. 295).

22.8.3 *Integration of sympathetic and parasympathetic systems*

The actions of the sympathetic and parasympathetic pathways to the heart are antagonistic. Simultaneous stimulation of both pathways results in algebraic summation of excitation and inhibition, but the parasympathetic effects begin almost at once and only last a short time, whereas the sympathetic effects take longer to act but last longer. In the normal animal *at rest* both the sympathetic and the parasympathetic pathways are tonically discharging, but the *parasympathetic effects predominate*. When all the nerves to the resting heart are cut, the heart rate is about doubled. On the other hand, during **exercise** and **stress in general**, the sympathetic effects appear to predominate.

The integration of these sympathetic and parasympathetic actions on the heart takes place in the '**cardiovascular centre**' in the brain stem, utilizing *baroreceptor reflex arcs* (Section 19.12). The afferent (sensory) component of these reflex arcs arises from the carotid sinus and aortic arch, and is transmitted to the 'centre' by the **carotid sinus nerve** (Section 19.3) and **aortic nerve** (Section 19.6): the efferent (motor) component is transmitted to the heart by vagal (Section 3.11.3) and sympathetic (Section 2.10.1) pathways.

The reflex slowing of the heart in response to a rise in arterial pressure is mainly a parasympathetic effect; on the other hand, the reflex increase in heart rate after a fall in arterial pressure is a combined parasympathetic and sympathetic effect with some species variations (Smith and Hamlin, 1977, p. 109).

Since the **cardiac nerves** (Section 2.11) are a mixture of sympathetic and vagal fibres, electrical stimulation gives variable results. In normal conditions, when **vagal tone** is high, **sympathetic tone** is low, and vice versa, thus avoiding the cancelling out of their opposing actions (Smith and Hamlin, 1977, p. 111).

22.9 Regulation of blood volume

Blood volume and arterial pressure are related. A slight increase in blood volume causes a substantial increase in cardiac output. In turn, an increase in cardiac output causes an increase in systemic arterial pressure and pulmonary arterial pressure. Therefore the regulation of blood volume is important to the regulation of arterial pressure.

Normally, **blood volume** is rigidly controlled, remaining virtually constant despite marked fluctuations in the daily uptake of fluids, provided always that the uptake is enough to replace unavoidable fluid loss. The basic mechanism for regulating blood volume depends on *renal filtration*. An excessive increase in blood volume increases cardiac output, and hence increases arterial pressure. This in turn increases renal filtration, and thus removes water from the body. A decrease in blood volume below normal has the opposite effect: decreased cardiac output leads to decreased filtration and retention of water. However, these mechanisms take many hours to act.

Three other factors participate in the regulation of blood volume, namely atrial volume receptors, arterial baroreceptors, and the atrial natriuretic factor.

22.9.1 *Atrial volume receptors*

Low pressure stretch receptors in the walls of the left and right atria act as **volume receptors** (Section 4.18.1). By responding to the varying distension of the atrial walls that accompanies an increase or decrease in blood volume, these receptors greatly speed up the adjustment of blood volume. An **increase** in blood volume is largely accommodated in the central veins of the thorax, thus leading to atrial distension. This stimulates the atrial volume receptors, resulting in two reflex renal responses that rapidly return the

blood volume to normal. (1) Projections of the receptors to the cardiovascular centre reflexly *inhibit* sympathetic *vasoconstrictor* pathways to the kidneys (Section 2.14.4). This induces *dilation* of the **afferent arteriole** and hence *increases* the rate of glomerular filtration. At the same time, the dilation of the afferent arteriole increases the hydrostatic pressure in the **peritubular capillaries**, and this impedes the diffusion of water from the tubular filtrate into the blood. Consequently the volume of urine excretion increases, and the blood volume correspondingly *decreases*. Thus the decrease in sympathetic stimulation results in a *decrease* in blood volume. (2) The increase in blood volume stimulates the projections of the atrial volume receptors to the neurohypophysis, causing a reflex *inhibition* of the secretion of **antidiuretic hormone** (**ADH**) by the **neurohypophysis**. By augmenting urine flow, the inhibition of ADH decreases blood volume still further.

Atrial volume receptors may also contribute to the **restoration of blood volume** if there is a rapid **reduction** in volume, for example by acute **haemorrhage**. After an acute haemorrhage the venous return to the heart falls, thus slowing the discharge rate of the atrial volume receptors. This causes three reflex responses that restore the blood volume. (1) The discharge rate of the volume receptors to the cardiovascular centre declines. The falling discharge rate reflexly *excites* the sympathetic motor pathways to the kidney. This excitation has a powerful *constrictor* effect on the **afferent renal arteriole**, thus greatly *reducing* glomerular pressure and glomerular filtration. Simultaneously the pressure in the **peritubular capillaries** falls. The resulting fall in the hydrostatic pressure within these capillaries creates a diffusion gradient from tubule to capillary, and this *increases* the diffusion of water from the tubular filtrate into the blood. Consequently the volume of urine excretion falls, and the blood volume correspondingly *increases*. (2) The reflex excitation of the sympathetic motor pathways to the kidney stimulates the **juxtaglomerular apparatus** (complexus juxtaglomerularis) to release **renin** into the blood (Section 2.14.4). Renin gives rise to **angiotensin**. Angiotensin causes constriction of the **efferent renal arteriole**. Once again this creates a diffusion gradient from tubule to capillary, and favours the return of water to the blood. Also angiotensin (among several other factors) elicits the secretion of **aldosterone** by the **adrenal cortex**. Aldosterone strongly promotes the removal of Na^+ from the filtrate in the renal tubules, and hence also causes the osmotic removal of water from the tubules. The result is that urine output decreases greatly and blood volume increases. (3) The falling discharge rate of the atrial receptors reflexly induces the release of **antidiuretic hormone**, thus reducing urine flow and conserving water.

22.9.2 *Arterial baroreceptors*

The rise in systemic arterial pressure that accompanies an increase in blood volume is detected by the **baroreceptors** of the carotid sinus and aortic arch, and results in a reflex fall in arterial pressure (Sections 19.4, 19.6). Acting through the 'cardiovascular centre', these baroreceptors activate renal and antidiuretic hormone reflexes in the same manner as the atrial receptors, and thus contribute to the regulation of blood volume.

22.9.3 *Natriuretic factor*

The cardiac muscle cells of the atria contain distinctive granules in their cytoplasm. These granules release into the blood stream a hormone known as the **atrial natriuretic factor** (Greek: nitron, soda; oureter, ureter). Release occurs when the atrial walls are stretched by an increase in blood volume. The hormone promotes the loss of sodium, potassium, and water in the urine, thus reducing blood volume.

> The **natriuretic factor** is a peptide hormone, often named **atrial natriuretic peptide**. It was discovered as recently as 1981 and has attracted much interest (Renkin and Tucker, 1996). It is best known for its ability to stimulate the *excretion of salt and water* by the kidneys, and its resulting important role in the regulation of blood volume and arterial pressure. But as a circulating hormone, it also relaxes vascular smooth muscle and is therefore a *vasodilator*; furthermore it *inhibits the renin–angiotensin–aldosterone system* just described above. It therefore provides the **failing myocardium** (Section 22.19.1) with a potent defence mechanism against volume overload, by means of systemic vasodilation, decreased venous return, and reduced blood volume (Winaver *et al.*, 1995). These authors estimated that, on

a molar basis, it is 10000 times more potent than any currently available diuretic agent.

> **Atrial distension** alone is a major stimulus for the secretion of the natriuretic factor by the heart, but there is evidence that the **ventricles** contribute significantly to the circulating levels of the hormone (Ruskoaho and Vuolteenaho, 1993). The natriuretic factor diminishes plasma volume by two mechanisms (Renkin and Tucker, 1996). (i) Protein and fluid move from the plasma into the renal interstitial fluid; (ii) sodium and fluid are excreted by the kidneys. Eventually the fluid released to the interstitium returns to the circulation and is also excreted by the kidneys. The natriuretic and vasodilator effects appear to be mediated by atrial natriuretic peptide receptors on the renal tubule, and by cGMP-dependent processes on vascular smooth muscle cells. By these mechanisms an enlarged blood volume may be restored to a normal volume.

> It has also been found (Oparil and Wyss, 1993) that in the rat brain there are complete systems for the synthesis, processing, and effector expression of natriuretic factor. These occur (predictably) at particularly high levels in regions involved in cardiovascular and blood volume regulation, including the **rostral hypothalamic area** and the **nucleus of the solitary tract**. The natriuretic factor from these sources has been shown to be functionally active in the tonic control of arterial pressure and baroreflex sensitivity.

22.10   Reflex responses to an increase in central venous pressure: Bainbridge reflex

A rise in the *central venous pressure* (the pressure in the right atrium) distends the right atrium and great veins, inducing reflex cardiac acceleration by the **Bainbridge reflex**. The stretch receptors that induce this reflex lie in the walls of the right atrium and great veins, the axons passing through vagal cardiac branches (Section 4.18.2).

> This reflex was first described by Bainbridge in 1915, but its existence has subsequently been controversial and it is, at the best, difficult to demonstrate (Scher, 1974, p. 162). It is presumed to act by inhibiting vagal tone, since it can be abolished by vagal section (Smith and Hamlin, 1977, p. 117). The reflex is thought to relieve an accumulation of blood in the great thoracic veins, the right atrium, the pulmonary circulation, and the left atrium (Guyton, 1986, p. 250). It might also appear to contribute to the increased cardiac performance that occurs at the onset of *exercise* in response to an increase in venous return, but this increase is primarily due to the **Frank–Starling mechanism** (Section 21.11). Furthermore a part

of the increase in heart rate attributed to the Bainbridge reflex can be explained by the *stretching of the sinuatrial node* when the right atrium is distended, since such stretching can increase the heart rate by as much as 15% (Guyton, 1986, p. 250). The actual existence of the Bainbridge reflex has been questioned, since other investigators have been unable to repeat it or have obtained different responses (Scher, 1974, p. 162). Cynics have attributed the Bainbridge reflex to transatlantic one-upmanship (Scher, 1966, p. 674), since it only happens in England. Even if the reflex does exist, its physiological role is not clear (Scott, 1986, p. 96).

II   CARDIAC OUTPUT

22.11   General characteristics of cardiac output

Cardiac output is the volume of blood pumped into the aorta. **Venous return** is the volume of blood that comes back to the right atrium. In principle, the two values are the same, since what goes out of one side of the heart should come in at the other. However, there is a small disparity because most of the bronchial circulation (Section 17.10), and a small part of the coronary circulation (Section 18.8), goes from the left ventricle and back to the left atrium, missing out the right side of the heart. In other words there is a small venous-to-arterial shunt that makes the output of the left ventricle slightly greater than that of the right (about 1 or 2% greater). There are also transient disparities, such as a sudden increase in venous return, caused for example by a change in posture or a deep inspiration, which then has to work its way through the pulmonary circulation into the left heart. Again, a sudden increase in arterial pressure causes a transient decrease in output.

Cardiac output can be regulated by varying the *stroke volume* (the volume of blood ejected at each beat), and/or the *rate* at which the heart beats. Therefore **cardiac output = stroke volume × heart rate**.

The cardiac output is determined by one overriding factor, metabolism: *the cardiac output of a normal animal is virtually proportional to the overall metabolism of its body as a whole*. The same principle of metabolic demand governs the *local* blood flow in the various individual organs. Hence the whole basis of the regulation of cardiac output

is that the tissues of the body control it. By maintaining a pumping capacity that substantially exceeds its venous return, the heart allows the tissues to do the controlling. In response to the demands of its body tissues, the heart can increase its output. This it does by changing either, or both, of the two components of its output – stroke volume and heart rate.

22.12   Stroke volume

Stroke volume is regulated by three main sets of factors, *mechanical*, *neuronal*, and *hormonal*.

The **mechanical factors** involve the concepts of preload and afterload. **Preload** expresses what the ventricle will attempt to shift when it contracts; it therefore represents the degree of filling of the ventricle before ejection begins, i.e. the *end-diastolic volume* of the ventricle. **Afterload** expresses the resistance to ventricular ejection; it therefore represents the aortic pressure. These terms are important in pathophysiology, because in many cardiac disorders the degree of filling of the ventricles (preload) and/or the arterial pressures against which the ventricles must contract (afterload) may have become abnormal.

The essentially mechanical factors that modify stroke volume are those embodied in the **Frank–Starling mechanism** (Section 21.11). It will be recalled that the length of a sarcomere and the tension that it produces when it contracts are related. This length–tension relationship arises from the varying availability of actin–myosin cross-bridges, depending on the overlapping of the thick and thin myofilaments (Fig. 21.9). The practical effect of this relationship is that *the normal heart automatically pumps out whatever volume of blood is put into it* (Section 21.11).

The physical training of *endurance athletes* induces a massive **hypertrophy** of the cardiac muscle cells (Section 20.4). This increases the heart mass (by over 40% in human athletes) and also enlarges the capacity of the chambers of the heart (again by about 40% in human athletes). The result is an increase in stroke volume (of 40–50%).

The **neuronal factors** that modify stroke volume are the effects of the autonomic cardiac innervation on the **force of contraction**, under the control of the '**cardiovascular centre**' in the brain stem (Section 19.12; Fig. 19.8). Excitation of the **sympathetic innervation** induces an influx of Ca^{2+} into the cardiac muscle cells and a consequent displacement of tropomyosin (Section 21.16), and can thus *double the force of contraction*.

Excitation of the **parasympathetic innervation** diminishes the influx of Ca^{2+} into the cardiac muscle cells. This weakens atrial contraction, and thus diminishes ventricular filling and hence ventricular stroke volume.

The increase in ventricular contractile force caused by sympathetic activity increases the ventricular stroke volume by several variables. It enables the ventricle (i) to handle a greater *preload* (greater filling volume), (ii) to empty more completely, and (iii) to do all this against an increased *afterload* (increased aortic pressure). By increasing the speed of contraction, sympathetic stimulation enables the ventricle (iv) to deliver an increased stroke volume, even when the increase in heart rate would otherwise encroach on the time available for ventricular filling.

The **hormonal factors** modifying stroke volume are the effects of circulating catecholamines formed by the adrenal medulla and elsewhere. These hormones have effects on the heart that are similar to those of stimulating the sympathetic cardiac nerves.

The **sympathetic innervation** maintains a slow tonic stimulation of the resting heart. This evokes a **strength of ventricular contraction** that is about 20% greater than the strength when the sympathetic stimulation is entirely blocked (Guyton, 1986, p. 160). Maximal sympathetic stimulation increases the strength of ventricular contraction by about 100%. Maximal **parasympathetic** stimulation reduces the strength of ventricular contraction by about 30%. The sympathetic innervation therefore has a much greater effect than the parasympathetic on contractile strength.

The stroke volume in the resting Thoroughbred horse is about 800–900 ml, or about 2–2.5 ml kg^{-1} body mass, increasing during exercise by about 20–50% (Evans, 1994, p. 136).

22.13 Heart rate

The heart rate of a resting mammal is inherent in its *pacemaker*, the **sinuatrial node** (Section 21.19.1). The rate varies from several hundred beats per minute in very small mammals (from over 300 to 800 in the mouse), down to 30 per minute or less in some horses.

Heart rate can be increased by *decreasing vagal tone*, or by *increasing sympathetic tone*. The increase in rate following a decrease in vagal tone is almost immediate, but lasts only a short time; the increase following sympathetic stimulation is slower in onset, but lasts longer (Section 22.8.3).

The main control of heart rate in the resting animal is mediated by the **baroreceptor reflexes** of the '**cardiovascular centre**' (Section 19.12; Fig. 19.8). A rise in arterial pressure stimulates the carotid sinus nerve and aortic nerve, and this results in a reflex increase in cardiac vagal activity and a decrease in cardiac sympathetic activity. The reverse reflex changes occur if arterial pressure falls.

Maximum sympathetic stimulation as in fight and flight can nearly **triple the heart rate** in man (Section 22.8.1), and in the Thoroughbred horse can increase it fivefold. In general, the faster the heart rate the greater the volume pumped, but as the rate goes up serious limitations to this relationship begin to emerge. The period of diastole between contractions becomes shorter and shorter. Eventually this period is so diminished, despite the increase in the speed of ventricular contraction, that atrial blood does not have enough time to transfer completely to the ventricles. From this point on, further increases in heart rate cause decreases in stroke volume.

Although the sympathetic innervation has a much stronger effect than the parasympathetic innervation on the *strength* of cardiac contraction, the parasympathetic innervation has a substantial effect on *heart rate*. Vagal stimulation can stop the heart altogether, until *vagal escape* occurs (Section 22.8.2).

The approximate mean heart rate per minute of domestic mammals at rest is as follows (Hamlin and Smith, 1977, p. 89): horse, 44; ox, 65; pig, 70; sheep, 75; dog, 115; cat, 120.

In Thoroughbred horses (Evans, 1994, pp. 133–136), from the onset of maximal exercise (after a suitable warm up) a maximum of about 220 beats per minute is reached in little more than about 20 s. Maximal heart rate is not altered by training. After exercise, recovery is usually very rapid in the first minute. Recovery rates are used to assess fitness for endurance rides, poorly performing horses having relatively higher postexercise rates.

22.14   Other factors affecting cardiac output

Some other factors affect the strength of contraction of the heart, and hence the cardiac output. For instance, contraction *weakens* if the supply of *oxygen* to the heart is diminished by deficient respiration, by falling arterial pressure, or by decreased coronary blood flow.

Various *ions* affect cardiac function, especially the cations potassium and calcium, and potentially also sodium. All of these have strong effects on membrane potentials and action potentials, and calcium is critically involved in the contractile process. Therefore the concentrations of these ions may predictably affect cardiac function. *Potassium ions* hyperpolarize excitable cells. Excess potassium in the interstitial fluid therefore weakens the strength of contraction and blocks the conducting system, slowing the heart rate and making the heart flaccid and very dilated. A very large increase in potassium concentration can be fatal. *Excess calcium* has the opposite effects to excess potassium. By exciting the contractile mechanism it throws the heart into spastic contraction. Calcium deficiency causes cardiac flaccidity, like potassium excess.

> *Sodium ions* compete with calcium ions in the contractile process, so that the greater the concentration of sodium ions in the extracellular fluid the less effective calcium becomes in causing contraction (Guyton, 1986, p. 162). However, the concentration of sodium ions in the interstitial fluid probably never becomes high enough to affect the strength of contraction significantly, even in serious pathological conditions. But very low sodium concentration can cause fatal fibrillation.

22.15   Measurement of cardiac output

Cardiac output at rest and during exercise has been measured in horses by various methods. Dye dilution, electromagnetic flow probe, thermodilution, and the direct Fick technique have been employed.

> The Fick measurement is obtained by dividing the oxygen uptake of the lungs in ml per minute, by the difference in oxygen concentration between arterial and mixed venous blood in ml per litre of blood. Values

reported for cardiac output in fit Thoroughbred horses during maximum treadmill exercise are 789 $\pm$ 102 ml/kg/min (355 litres/min) and 534 $\pm$ 54 ml/kg/min (277 litres/min).

22.16   Adjustments of cardiac output during exercise

As was stated in Section 22.11, *the cardiac output of a normal animal is virtually proportional to the overall metabolism of its body as a whole*. Therefore as the work output increases during exercise, so the cardiac output increases in almost linear proportion. In this way, the heart supplies the very large volume of blood and oxygen demanded by the active musculature in intense exercise, as in fight and flight.

The onset of exercise induces an **intense local vasodilation** in the active muscles. This vasodilation (Section 13.2.1) is a response to the local hypoxia that speedily develops in the active muscle, being caused (i) directly by a reduction in the basal tone of the smooth muscle of the arterioles and metarterioles in the active muscle, and (ii) indirectly by the release (from the endothelial cells of small muscular arteries in the active muscle) of vasodilator substances such as *nitric oxide* (Sections 13.6, 13.8). Also a neuronal vasodilator system, operated by *cholinergic sympathetic vasodilator fibres*, initiates the vasodilation in the muscles before the exercise actually begins (Section 13.3.4). The vasodilation in the active musculature creates a low resistance pathway for the flow of large volumes of blood.

The onset of exercise is marked by another important circulatory event. The muscle pump comes into action, producing an immediate increase in **venous return** to the right atrium (Section 12.16.2). Deeper breathing mobilizes blood from the abdominal venous reservoirs (Section 12.16.3).

It was noted during the surveys of the *regulation* of *stroke volume* (Section 22.12) and *heart rate* (Section 22.13) that several quite complex factors are intermingled, some 'mechanical' and others 'neuronal' or 'hormonal'. The **adjustment of cardiac output** enmeshes all these together into highly complex regulatory mechanisms. Nevertheless, the overriding factor determining cardiac output is the **rate of venous return**. In turn, the overriding factor determining the rate of venous return is **sympathetic activity**.

At the onset of exercise the *'cardiovascular centre'* releases a **mass sympathetic discharge** and simultaneously inhibits the parasympathetic pathways to the heart. The sympathetic discharge causes a generalized vasoconstriction of both arterial and venous vasculature, except for the vessels in the active **musculature** since these are strongly dilated by vasodilator factors within the muscles including local hypoxia and adenosine released from the active muscle fibres (Section 13.2.1). The *systemic veins*, and especially the *splanchnic* and *cutaneous* veins, form a major **venous reservoir** (containing over 60% of all the blood in the body; Section 12.16.3). The generalized **venoconstriction** therefore releases a large volume of blood for return to the heart. The generalized **arterial vasoconstriction** temporarily closes down the arterial supply to organs such as the gastrointestinal tract, that are not active during severe exercise. Only the coronary and cerebral arterial systems (in addition to the vessels in the active musculature) escape this general vasoconstriction, the coronary and cerebral vasoconstrictor mechanisms being weak (Section 13.3.2). This exemption is unavoidable – a brain cannot stop working simply because its owner happens to be undergoing severe exercise, and the heart must work overtime under such conditions anyway.

The result of such extensive venous and arterial vasoconstriction is a massive increase in the **venous return** to the heart. The increase in venous return brings into play the Frank–Starling mechanism, thus automatically increasing the stroke volume. As already stated above (Section 22.13), simultaneously the **sympathetic excitation** can nearly *triple the heart rate in man* and can *increase it even fivefold* in the Thoroughbred horse (Section 22.13), and can *double the force of ventricular contraction* (Section 22.12). Combined together, these vascular and cardiac adjustments *vastly increase the cardiac output*. The heart is now fully empowered to redistribute very large volumes of blood to the active skeletal musculature (Section 13.8).

The ability of the heart to increase its output instantly, to meet the demands of exercise, means that it has a substantial **cardiac reserve**. This is defined as the maximum percentage increase in cardiac output that the heart can achieve above its normal resting output (Guyton, 1986, p. 312). Thus, if the heart can increase its output fivefold during exercise (which is a value attainable by a normal young man) it has a cardiac reserve of 400%.

Clearly, however, there has to be a limit to the adaptability of the heart to ever greater demands. There comes a point where the heart can no longer meet the demand for oxygen. The final limitation on the capacity of the body for physical exertion is not the ability of the lung to take up oxygen, but the ability of the heart to transport it to the tissues (Chapman and Mitchell, 1974, p. 91). However, the normal heart is not damaged by the extreme stress of the severest possible exercise: 'the normal heart is invulnerable to exercise' (Section 18.3).

22.16.1   *Adjustments of circulation* before exercise begins

How does the body activate its sympathetic nervous system, and make available an increase in venous return, at the very moment that exercise begins? Actually these adjustments begin slightly *before* the onset of exercise, by four mechanisms.

(a) *Activation of the sympathetic system by the cerebral cortex*

The mental process of merely *contemplating* exercise excites, to a greater or lesser degree depending on the psychological circumstances, a preliminary sympathetic discharge (Guyton, 1986, p. 277), by means of neuronal projections from the cerebral cortex to the *cardiovascular centre* in the brainstem. The result is a preliminary increase in rate and strength of contraction of the heart, and generalized vasoconstriction (which can increase the cardiac output in man by up to 50%, before exercise begins). The conscious recognition of a sudden fight and flight emergency induces an instantaneous and massive preliminary sympathetic discharge, with near maximal preliminary changes in cardiac performance and vasoconstriction.

(b) *Anticipatory vasodilation in the skeletal musculature*

The sympathetic discharge via the cardiovascular centre includes the excitation of *sympathetic cholinergic fibres* supplying the vasculature in skeletal musculature. These induce an anticipatory vasodilation in muscle that is about to become active (Section 13.3.4).

(c) Release of blood from the abdominal venous reservoirs

The body prepares itself for action by creating an initial tenseness that includes contraction of the abdominal musculature. The effect of this is compression of the splanchnic veins and the spleen and liver, all of which are major venous reservoirs. In man this can increase the venous return, and hence cardiac output, by 30–80% within one or two heart beats (Guyton, 1986, p. 277).

(d) Anticipatory stimulation of breathing

Motor pathways from the cerebral cortex drive the *medullary respiratory centre* (Fig. 11.1) to stimulate the muscles of inspiration at, or even slightly before, the onset of exercise (Section 11.14). In addition to providing an anticipatory gas exchange, these respiratory movements increase the venous return to the right atrium (Section 12.16.3).

22.16.2 Redistribution of blood to active musculature

In a normal man, the total blood volume is about 5 litres. In severe exercise about 2 litres of this are immediately made available to the active skeletal musculature (Guyton, 1986, p. 337). This increases the blood flow in that musculature 20–25 fold and its metabolic activity about 50-fold (Guyton, 1986, p. 231). The ascending vasodilation in an exercising limb is induced by a vasodilator factor released by the endothelial cells, notably nitric oxide and/or a factor blocking the release of noradrenaline from sympathetic vasoconstrictor terminals (Section 13.8).

22.16.3 Adjustments of haematocrit and oxygen dissociation curve in exercise

Within the context of this chapter, which is about the heart, the above survey of circulatory adaptations to exercise focuses attention on the adjustment of cardiac output. However, the circulatory system has several other mechanisms for responding to the increased demand for oxygen by the active musculature. For example, in contrast to the human athlete, in the greyhound and Thoroughbred horse the capacity of the blood for oxygen transport is greatly enhanced by contraction of the spleen, which increases the haematocrit to 60–70%. This feature combines with the large size of the heart and relatively large stroke volume, and fast heart rate at exercise, to form the basis for the supreme athleticism of these animals (Section 14.18.2).

The dog is a good model, since it represents a group of predatory carnivores that can generally outrun their prey. Observations by C.R. Taylor on four species of canid running on a treadmill (Weibel, 1984, p. 388) showed that the oxygen consumption increased 13-fold, and cardiac output six-fold (partly through increased stroke volume as well as increased heart rate). Contraction of the spleen raised the haemoglobin content of the blood by over 20%, and thus increased the oxygen content of the blood by 20%. Furthermore the blood in the capillaries picks up CO_2 from the cells causing the pH to drop from about 7.4 to 7.2, and the blood temperature in the working muscle increases by several degrees; these two changes cause a Bohr shift to the right (Section 14.3.4), thus releasing a greater quantity of O_2 from haemoglobin. Through all these factors together, the amount of oxygen delivered to the muscle tissues in these canids could thus be increased by a factor of 2.5.

22.16.4 Cardiac reserve

In the *canid species* mentioned in the preceding paragraph the cardiac output increased to about six times normal, i.e. a cardiac reserve of 500%. The cardiac reserve of a normal human adult is about 400%, and that of a *well-trained human athlete* is about 500% or even 600% (Guyton, 1986, p. 312).

III   THE FAILING HEART

22.17   Definition of the failing heart

It will be recalled that the normal heart pumps out whatever volume of blood enters it (Section 22.12). It will also be recalled that, in the adjustment of cardiac output at the onset of exercise, a principal factor is a massive increase in the **venous return** to the heart (Section 22.16); because the normal heart possesses a very substantial **cardiac reserve** by means of augmenting its stroke volume and rate (Section 22.16), it promptly converts this increase in venous return into a corresponding increase in cardiac output, thus responding to the urgent metabolic demands of exercise.

In **cardiac disease**, however, there may come a point, even in the resting animal, when the volume of the venous return exceeds the volume that the heart is able to pump out. The heart itself has then become the limiting factor in the control of cardiac output. Since the heart is now unable to pump the volume of blood demanded of it, it then becomes a **failing heart**.

In the diseased heart, the output at rest may fall to less than half that of the normal heart. In an acutely damaged heart (as in a severe cardiac infarct in man), this fall in output can occur within a few seconds. In a chronically damaged heart (as in progressive dilated cardiomyopathy in domestic animals) the fall in output may be gradual. Under all these conditions, the heart may have been so damaged that it has no **cardiac reserve** whatsoever. Consequently virtually all capacity for exercise is lost. Exercise or excitement may precipitate collapse into unconsciousness or death.

Clinicians use the terms 'right heart failure' (right ventricular failure) and 'left heart failure' (left ventricular failure). The concept of **right heart failure** is based on an inability of the right ventricle to function effectively, as in *pulmonary stenosis* (Section 15.9) or *pulmonary hypertension* (Sections 17.21.3, 17.22). It is indicated by physical weakness and dyspnoea, together with systemic venous congestion and systemic oedema, and also ascites (accumulation of peritoneal fluid). **Left heart failure**, as in aortic stenosis (Section 15.10) or mitral (bicuspid) insufficiency (Section 15.13), arises from the inability of the left ventricle to sustain a normal output of blood. Being unable to empty adequately, the left ventricle cannot accept an appropriate volume of blood returning from the pulmonary veins via the left atrium. Pulmonary venous congestion results, with substantially increased pulmonary capillary pressure causing major diffusion of fluid into the lung alveoli. Severe *pulmonary oedema* (Section 17.25.2) and *pleural effusion* (Section 17.27.3) will follow, with coughing and dyspnoea. In left ventricular failure, the backing up of blood in the lungs may lead to right ventricular failure also, because the increase in pulmonary resistance induces dilation and hypertrophy of the right ventricle and atrium.

The failing heart can arise from a large variety of cardiac disorders (Noden and de Lahunta, 1985, pp. 45–55; Darke *et al.*, 1996, pp. 98, 123). *Dilated (congestive) cardiomyopathy* of unknown cause occurs in almost all of the domestic mammalian species, and especially the dog. It is characterized by a flabby dilation of the heart chambers, a moderate to severe loss of ventricular myocardial contractility, and exercise intolerance. *Bicuspid regurgitation* caused by failure of the left atrioventricular valve is another very common cause of the failing heart in veterinary practice (Section 22.6.1). *Peri-*

cardial effusion occurs in many species, and may lead to *acute cardiac tamponade* that prevents adequate filling of the right heart and can fatally diminish cardiac output (Section 20.2). In man, though not in the domestic mammals (Section 18.9), ischaemic heart disease is, of course, the major cause of the failing heart.

Congenital cardiac anomalies (Noden and de Lahunta, 1985, pp. 245–55) also can diminish the effectiveness of cardiac pumping. For example *tricuspid insufficiency* (Section 15.13) allows regurgitation of blood from the right ventricle into the right atrium, and *pulmonary stenosis* (Section 15.9) obstructs the output from the right ventricle, both of these conditions leading to a right heart failure. Likewise aortic stenosis (Section 15.10) obstructs the outflow from the left ventricle, thus leading to a left heart failure. See also *patent ductus arteriosus* (Section 15.8), *interventricular defects* (Section 15.11), *interatrial septal defects* (Section 15.12), and the Fallot tetralogy (Section 15.14).

22.18 Compensated heart failure

The body compensates for the fall in cardiac output when the heart is diseased. It does this by two principal mechanisms, stimulation of the myocardium and increased systemic venous pressure.

As in the normal animal, **sympathetic stimulation** increases the heart rate and the force of myocardial contraction, and it also induces a generalized vasoconstriction, including especially venoconstriction (Section 22.16). Even *damaged myocardium* responds to sympathetic stimulation by giving more powerful contraction at a faster rate, and of course any surviving *normal myocardium* responds strongly as in the normal heart. The venoconstriction increases the venous return to the heart and raises the right atrial pressure. The arterial vasoconstriction ensures the distribution of blood to essential regional circulations, notably those of the brain and heart.

The **increase in right atrial pressure** arises partly because the venous return to the heart is dammed back in the great systemic veins. The basic reason for this venous accumulation is that the cardiac output of the diseased heart is diminished, so that it can no longer match the increase in venous return by a corresponding increase in cardiac output. Moreover, the venous engorgement caused by damming back the venous return is greatly augmented by venoconstriction and retention of fluid by the kidneys.

Renal retention of sodium and water arises in all forms of heart failure. There are four mechanisms. (1) *Decreased glomerular filtration*. This occurs indirectly because of the fall in arterial pressure when the heart is failing. But sympathetic constriction of the *afferent* glomerular arterioles directly and strongly reinforces the decrease in glomerular pressure. (2) *Activation of the renin–angiotensin system*. Sympathetic stimulation of the juxtaglomerular apparatus releases renin into the blood, and hence leads to the formation of angiotensin. Angiotensin (one of the most powerful vasoconstrictors known) constricts the *efferent* glomerular arterioles. This reduces the pressure in the *peritubular capillaries* and therefore promotes copious diffusion of water and salt from the renal tubules to the capillaries; on the other hand, waste products (mostly not transferred from the tubules to the capillaries anyway) pass on in the urine. (3) *Aldosterone*. Angiotensin stimulates the secretion of aldosterone by the adrenal cortex. Aldosterone further increases the movement of sodium from the renal tubules, and this in turn leads to transfer of more water to the blood by osmosis. (4) *Antidiuretic hormone (vasopressin)*. Secretion of ADH by the neurohypophysis further increases the transfer of water from the renal tubules to the blood.

Combined together, these cardiac and vascular changes prime the heart with more incoming blood and at a higher filling pressure, than is usual. Thus they help the failing heart to pump an adequate volume of blood. Under these compensatory conditions, the cardiac output may recover to normal levels. This state is known as *compensated heart failure*. But even then, there may be no cardiac reserve. Such an animal could have essentially normal cardiodynamics – but only if it remains at rest.

The high level of sympathetic discharge that characterizes the failing heart is triggered by the falling arterial pressure, activating baroreceptor reflexes (Section 19.5). An acute heart attack in man induces strong sympathetic stimulation within a few seconds. The parasympathetic innervation of the heart is simultaneously inhibited (Guyton, 1986, p. 305).

22.19 Decompensated heart failure

Chronic activation of the compensatory mechanisms may become frankly detrimental. Continual sympathetic stimulation of the heart, together with increased venous return and higher atrial pressures, tend to exhaust the myocardium. General cardiac dilation caused by progressive escalation of the right atrial pressure may cause structural damage to the cardiac muscle cells or may weaken contractility by loss of actin–myosin bridges (Section 21.11.2). The consequence of such events is *decompensated heart failure*, and the eventual outcome is likely to be death.

22.19.1 *Adverse effects of long-term sympathetic stimulation*

There are various detrimental effects (Darke *et al.*, 1996, p. 1).

By increasing the force and rate of contraction, chronic sympathetic stimulation increases the oxygen consumption of the myocardium and predisposes to arrhythmias. Mitral regurgitation is worsened. The generalized systemic arterial vasoconstriction increases the peripheral resistance, and thus adds to the afterload on the heart and further increases the oxygen demands on the heart. Chronic sympathetic stimulation is believed actually to shorten the life span (Darke *et al.*, 1996, p. 1). A natural defence against volume overload appears to be offered by the **natriuretic hormone** (Section 22.9.3).

22.19.2 *Adverse effects of fluid retention: oedema*

Renal retention of fluid can seriously overload the heart (volume overload). The increasing right atrial pressure may augment the capillary pressure enough to cause great loss of fluid into the tissues (Section 14.9.1). Severe oedema in tissues other than the lungs (*peripheral oedema*) then develops in many parts of the body (*congestive heart failure*) (Darke *et al.*, 1996, p. 2). Oedema in the pleural cavity (*pleural effusion*) threatens collapse of the lung (Section 17.27). Oedema in the lungs (*pulmonary oedema*) impairs gas exchange, thus decreasing the oxygen levels in the blood (Section 17.25.5). Progressive oedema reveals decompensation (Guyton, 1986, p. 308).

The main factor in decompensated heart failure is the inability of the heart to pump enough blood to restore the kidneys to normal function (Guyton, 1986, p. 308).

22.19.3 *Principles of treatment of decompensated heart failure*

In man, the compensatory mechanisms may lead to full recovery from a myocardial infarct. Parts of the myocardium may have been destroyed; myocardial cells have no ability to regenerate, but they do have a great capacity for hypertrophy (Section 21.1.2), and this can restore the myocardium to full power.

In the domestic mammals few cardiac disorders can be cured (Darke *et al.*, 1996, p. 3), but avoidance of exercise and excitement makes the most of the compensatory mechanisms. Urgent treatment for progressive decompensated heart failure requires *diuretics* to reduce oedema and prevent chronic retention of sodium and water; this at least allows as much fluid to leave the body as enters it. By lowering the peripheral resistance, *arteriolar vasodilators* reduce ventricular afterload in general and mitral regurgitation in particular, and increase cardiac output. *Venodilators* may reduce venous congestion, particularly pulmonary. *Cardiotonic drugs* such as digitalis and other glycosides have little effect on normal myocardial cells, but in decompensated heart failure they increase contractility by overcoming depression of the calcium mechanism of myocardial contraction (Guyton, 1986, p. 308). However, digoxin has a narrow safety margin (Darke *et al.*, 1996, p. 3), and can easily lead to fibrillation (A.W. Trafford, personal communication, 1996).

Surgical intervention is possible in some cardiac conditions in veterinary practice (Darke *et al.*, 1996, p. 4). Patent ductus arteriosus, pulmonary stenosis (see Section 15.9), and septal defects can be accessible to surgery. Pericardiocentesis can be applied to pericardial effusion and tamponade. Life saving procedures for arrhythmias include pacemakers for heart block.

Part 4
Clinical Aspects of Thoracic Anatomy

A.S. King and C.M. Brown

Chapter 23
Anatomical Principles of the Physical Examination of the Thorax

23.1 Introduction

Clinicians in both veterinary and human medicine routinely carry out a thorough **physical examination of the thorax**, particularly in pulmonary and cardiac auscultation (listening to the lungs and heart). Other diagnostic thoracic procedures include percussion of the lungs and heart, and palpation of the cardiac area. All of these techniques require a working knowledge of the topographical anatomy of the thorax, and especially of the position of the lungs and heart within the thorax.

23.2 General topographical principles

The topographical anatomy of the thorax in the domestic mammals is remarkably constant in its general principles. The one main variant is the **number of ribs**, and this does change the detailed shape of the thorax from species to species. For instance, the thorax of the ox, with only 13 ribs, is relatively short and deep, whereas that of the horse, with 18 ribs, is much longer. The pig, with 14 or 15 ribs, is more or less intermediate in shape. On the other hand, the thorax of the dog, which normally has only 13 ribs, varies greatly with breed, being narrow and deep in greyhounds and wide and shallow in bulldogs. However, despite these variations in shape, the relationships of the lungs and heart to the thoracic skeleton are essentially similar in the domestic mammals, and it is possible to set up a few simple rules which determine the main bony **landmarks** for both **percussion** and **auscultation** of the lungs and heart in all the domestic species.

In man the ventrodorsal (anteroposterior) flattening of the thorax (12 ribs) produces an entirely different thoracic shape, and a tendency for the heart to lie parallel with the sternum rather than vertically or obliquely in the thorax as in the domestic species. Also the thoracic inlet (apertura thoracis cranialis) (Section 8.1) is much more spacious in man, giving a greater margin of safety when disease processes occupy space within the inlet. Many other relationships, however, remain similar to those in the domestic species.

23.3 Anatomical obstacles to percussion and auscultation

There is one anatomical feature which severely restricts the percussion and auscultation of the thorax in all the domestic mammals, and that is the mass of the **triceps brachii muscle** which covers the cranial part of the thoracic wall – a barrier which the human physician is spared. In all the domestic mammals the caudal border of this muscle drops roughly vertically from the caudal angle of the scapula to the olecranon process of the ulna. As a rough guide it may be assumed that the **olecranon process** of the ulna, i.e. the point of the elbow, is fairly close to the **fifth costochondral junction** in all the domestic species when standing. Therefore in all these species *the first five ribs are largely covered by the triceps muscle* (and partly also by the scapula and humerus) (Fig. 23.1). But since the limb is freely movable this relationship is somewhat variable in the live animal, as in Figs 23.2A,B,C.

Although the triceps muscle is an awkward obstacle, it may still be possible to auscultate as far cranially as the third intercostal space in both the large and the small domestic mammals. This can

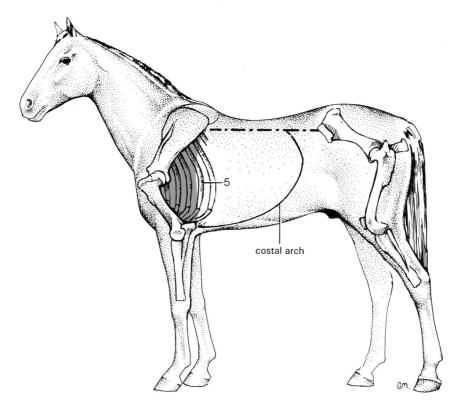

Fig. 23.1 Lateral view of topographical landmarks of the thorax of the horse. In the horse and all the other domestic mammals the triceps muscle covers the area shown in green. The caudal border of this area is formed by an approximately vertical line connecting the caudal angle of the scapula to the olecranon process of the ulna. The olecranon process lies near the fifth costochondral junction. The triceps muscle prevents the percussion and auscultation of the lung cranial to the fifth rib. Since the heart lies from the third to the sixth ribs in all the domestic species, the limb must be drawn forward before the heart can be examined by percussion. Auscultation of the heart also requires the limb to be drawn forward or the bell of the stethoscope to be pushed cranially under the edge of the triceps muscle. The epaxial muscles prevent auscultation of the lungs dorsal to the broken line between the caudal angle of the scapula and the tuber coxae. The costal arch is formed by the costal cartilages of the asternal ribs; together with the last rib, it forms the caudal boundary of the thoracic wall.

be done by drawing the limb cranially (Fig. 23.2C), or by pushing the bell of the stethoscope cranially along the thoracic wall and under the caudal edge of triceps.

In the sheep and pig percussion and auscultation of the thorax are usually unrewarding because of the thick layer of wool in the former and fat in the latter. In fact a thick layer of subcutaneous fat obstructs thoracic auscultation in all species. Obese dogs and horses are difficult to auscultate.

I PHYSICAL EXAMINATION OF THE LUNGS

23.4 External observations

23.4.1 *The pattern of breathing*

In all the domestic species of mammal, as well as man, the inspiratory phase of breathing has a **diaphragmatic component** shown by bulging of

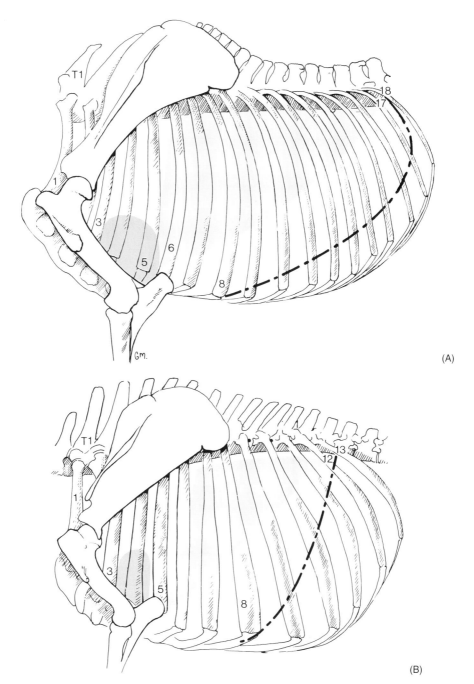

Fig. 23.2 Lateral view diagrams of the left thoracic wall showing the area of cardiac dullness (dark green), the area of percussion and auscultation of the lung (light green), and the costodiaphragmatic line of pleural reflection (broken line): A, horse; B, ox; C, dog. In the standing position the olecranon process is approximately related to the fifth costochondral junction. In C, the limb has been pulled cranially in order to expose the area of cardiac dullness. Although the number of ribs and the shape of the thorax vary, the area of percussion and auscultation of the lungs is bounded by the fifth costochondral junction, the dorsal end of the penultimate intercostal space, and the caudal angle of the scapula. The area is relatively large in the horse and dog, and relatively small in the ox. The area of cardiac dullness lies essentially in the ventral third of the third to the sixth rib (reduced to the fifth rib in the ox). The costodiaphragmatic line of pleural reflection forms the boundary between the pleural and peritoneal cavities. It runs from the eighth costochondral junction to the proximal end of the last rib.

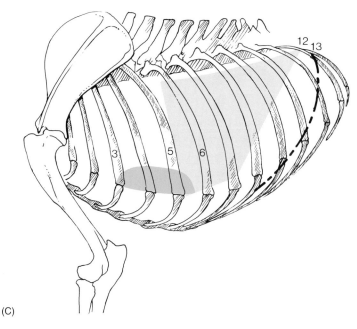

Fig. 23.2 *Continued.*

the abdominal wall, and a **costal component** shown by expansion of the thoracic wall particularly in the caudal half of the thorax (Section 10.8). The main component is diaphragmatic.

Severe pain caused by violent **bruising** of the thoracic wall, a **fractured rib**, or acute **pleuritis** can cause an extremely shallow pattern of breathing. The diaphragmatic component becomes more noticeable, as shown by the increased bulging of the abdominal wall when the abdominal viscera are forced caudally by the straightening of the diaphragm.

On the other hand, the costal component is enhanced if the caudal movement of the diaphragm is resisted by **obesity, peritoneal effusion, pregnancy**, or a large abdominal mass such as a **tumour**. This enhancement is shown by increased excursion of the thoracic wall. The increase is caused by fixation of the tendinous centre, thus allowing the costal component of the diaphragmatic musculature to reverse its action and expand the caudal half of the rib cage. Respiratory distress is often aggravated by obesity.

In the horse, a double expiratory effort is a characteristic sign of **chronic obstructive pulmonary disease** (Section 7.20); hence the term broken wind or heaves. The **costal arch** then tends

to become more prominent, and is known as the **heaves line**.

Respiratory distress (**dyspnoea**) may be revealed by **posture**. Abnormal postures can make the **accessory inspiratory muscles** more efficient (Section 10.10.1). A severely dyspnoeic animal may stand or sit with its mouth open and head extended in order to give the accessory inspiratory muscles of the neck a more powerful action on the rib cage. In the effort to improve the tidal volume the animal may plant its front feet firmly and abduct its elbows, thus activating accessory inspiratory muscles. Dorsal arching of the back spreads the ribs. When sitting, the animal prefers to sit upright (orthopnoea), since gravitation of the abdominal viscera helps the diaphragm to maximize the craniocaudal diameter of the thorax during inspiration (Section 10.6.3). This posture also promotes venous return to the left atrium in right side congestive heart failure as in congenital pulmonary stenosis.

23.4.2 *Examination*

Besides posture and the general pattern of breathing, the shape and size of the thorax should be observed. For instance, in the dog, chronic respiratory disease of long duration may lead to a barrel-shaped thorax.

Systematic **palpation** of the thoracic wall on both sides of the body should reveal signs of **trauma** such as a **broken rib**; a penetrating wound may suggest **pneumothorax**. The presence of severe trauma raises the possibility of **diaphragmatic hernia** (Section 25.13). Tumours of ribs or sternum may be detected; those affecting cartilage may produce only small elevations externally, but grow massively inside the thorax.

For details of the causes, presentation, and clinical evaluation of dyspnoea in the dog, see Reif (1971, p. 78).

23.5 Percussion of the lungs

This technique is based on the principle that a structure filled with air resonates differently, when struck, if compared with a solid structure or a structure filled with fluid.

23.5.1 *Methods for percussion of the lungs*

Percussion depends on the tone and pitch of the sound made by tapping the thoracic wall with the finger, either directly or more usually by striking one of the fingers (generally the middle one) of the other hand. In cattle and horses, percussion is often performed with a rubber-headed hammer (plexor) and a hard flat disc (pleximeter). The pleximeter is placed firmly on the thoracic wall and then struck with the plexor.

The animal should be standing, in order to keep the heart and lungs in their standard relationship. Practice on normal as well as diseased individuals is necessary before abnormalities can be detected.

For anatomical reasons, percussion of the lungs is limited to a restricted area of the thoracic wall (Section 23.7).

23.5.2 *Observations made by percussion of the lungs*

Percussion can reveal abnormalities such as fluid in the pleural cavity (pleural effusion), gas in the pleural cavity (pneumothorax), large areas of consolidation of the lung, and enlargement of the lung (pulmonary emphysema).

Since an **effusion of pleural fluid** maintains a horizontal level, it is possible to detect a definite line where the dullness due to the fluid changes to normal resonance. **Pneumothorax** produces a tympanitic hyper-resonance. Effusion of pleural fluid and pneumothorax cause the lung to collapse progressively as the volume of fluid or gas increases, and if the abnormality is present on only one side the heart is gradually displaced towards the other side. **Consolidated areas of lung**, or pulmonary masses such as **tumours**, are more difficult to detect except when most of a lobe is affected; radiography is more reliable.

In **chronic obstructive lung disease** in horses ('*broken wind*' or '*heaves*') gas may become trapped in distal alveoli (Section 7.19). In severe chronic cases there may also be destruction of alveolar walls, i.e. **alveolar emphysema**. The combination of the trapped gas and emphysema causes an increase in the volume of gas retained within the lung at the end of expiration. The lung therefore remains over-expanded, sometimes to the point of approaching or even reaching the **costodiaphragmatic line of pleural reflection** (Section 23.8), and hence the area of resonance during the expiratory pause is often increased enough to be detected by percussion.

The possible presence of **fenestrations** of the postnatal mediastinum in the horse and carnivores (Section 9.4) suggests that **pneumothorax** and **pleural effusion** may become bilateral in these species. In the dog, pneumothorax is reported to be usually bilateral but pleural effusion may be unilateral (Rutgers, 1989).

23.6 Auscultation of the lungs

23.6.1 *Methods for auscultation of the lungs*

Auscultation, usually with a stethoscope, is the standard method of examining the lungs. Quiet is necessary. It is almost impossible, for example, to auscultate successfully a trembling dog which is standing on a metal table. Breathing should be deep, so that all of the bronchial tree is ventilated; panting and shallow breathing are inadequate. In adult cattle and horses the respiratory rate may be only 12–20 per minute. At these slow rates the velocity of airflow is low, and few if any breathing sounds may be heard, particularly if the animal is fat or has a heavy coat.

The lobes of the lung (or regions of the lungs, in the horse) should be examined systematically on each side. Particular attention should be paid to the most **pendent** regions of the lung, notably the ventral parts of the cranial and middle lobes in the domestic species (Section 5.10.3); secretions tend to pool ventrally, and in dogs with **chronic bronchitis**, for instance, abnormal breath sounds may be restricted to these lobes.

The region of the thoracic wall that is suitable for auscultation of the lungs is the same as the restricted region used for percussion of the lungs.

23.6.2 *Observations made by auscultation of the lungs*

The sounds of breathing are hard to describe, words being no substitute for practice on the live animal. However, as a rough guide in the normal dog, for instance, the **normal sounds** heard over the lungs are described as 'vesicular' and are said to resemble the sound of wind blowing through the trees. These normal sounds are probably caused by the formation of eddies at the branchings of the conducting airways (Section 6.14).

Abnormal lung sounds consist of changes in the normal sounds, or of new sounds not normally heard. A **changed normal sound** may take the form of a decrease in the volume of sound. This can happen when fluid, gas, or tissue is interposed between the lung and the thoracic wall, as in pleural effusion, pneumothorax, or obesity. Sounds will also be decreased when the ventilation of a lobe or a region of the lung has diminished, or when there is no ventilation at all because of consolidation of lung tissue or total obstruction of a major bronchus. On the other hand, normal sounds may be louder when there is increased airflow; for example this may happen in one lung if the other lung has no ventilation, or in an area of normal lung adjacent to a large area of unventilated lung.

Many varieties of **new lung sounds** (i.e. sounds not normally heard) occur in pulmonary diseases, such as gurgles, crackles, whistles, and squeaks. Many explanations of these sounds are possible, including the movement of inflammatory fluids and perhaps even the popping open of small airways. However, the main cause is **turbulent air-flow** (Section 6.14) through bronchi or bronchioles which are narrowed by exudate, by excessive secretion of mucus, by swelling of the bronchial wall from oedema or scar tissue, by spasm of the bronchial muscle, or by any combination or even all of these factors.

> Experienced clinicians may be able to relate certain sounds to particular disease conditions. For example, when the pleurae are roughened by exudate, as in acute **pleuritis**, a characteristic grating or squeaky sound is produced as the roughened surfaces rub against each other, a 'pleural friction rub'; these sounds are usually transitory because the pleural surfaces quickly become separated by liquid exudate.

23.7 Site of percussion and auscultation of the lung

The lung extends over a larger area of the thoracic wall at the peak of inspiration than at the end of expiration; this increase is due to the movement of the lung, during inspiration, into the **costo-diaphragmatic recess** (phrenicocostal sinus) and into the **costomediastinal recess** (Sections 9.6.1, 9.6.2). But it is particularly important clinically to know approximately the normal limits of the area of contact between the lung and the thoracic wall **at the end of expiration**.

Knowledge of these limits is useful because they determine the area in which percussion and auscultation of the lung should be effective in the **normal** animal. In disease, this area may be either increased or decreased, and any such change can be detected by percussion. For example, the area should be **decreased** if abnormal contents occupy the pleural cavity, such as gas (**pneumothorax**) or liquid (**pleural effusion**), since in these conditions the lung is partly collapsed. The area will be **increased** if the lung is enlarged, as in **chronic obstructive lung disease** or severe **alveolar emphysema** in the horse. Anyway, the extent of contact between the lung and the thoracic wall **at the end of expiration** places the ultimate limit on the minimal area which is normally available for percussion and auscultation of the lung: it is this minimal area which provides the basis for percussion and auscultation of the lungs in clinical practice.

In the domestic animals, the area of contact between the thoracic wall and the lung at the end of expiration is roughly triangular, with caudoventral, cranial, and dorsal boundaries. Fortunately these boundaries have much the same topographical relationships to the skeleton in all the domestic species when standing (Figs 23.2A,B,C).

However, because of the variations in the numbers of ribs and in the conformation of the thorax in the different domestic species, the actual size and shape of the area of percussion and auscultation of the lung in the standing animal vary considerably from species to species. The area is very large in the horse (Fig. 23.2A) and surprisingly small in the ox (Fig. 23.2B); in the dog (Fig. 23.2C) and pig it is intermediate in area, relative to the size of the body.

23.7.1   *The caudoventral boundary: the basal border of the lung*

The caudoventral boundary of the area available for auscultation and percussion of the lung is formed by the **basal border** or the **caudal lobe** of the lung (Fig. 5.3; Section 5.5), at the end of a resting expiration. The boundary runs along a line drawn from the **costochondral junction of the fifth rib** to the dorsal end of the **penultimate intercostal space** (Figs 23.2A,B,C). Since the **olecranon process** is close to the fifth costochondral junction, the cranial end of this boundary will usually be near the olecranon process in the standing animal.

> The basal border of the lung is regarded as a straight line in some species (notably the ox; Fig. 23.2B), and curved towards the costal arch in others (especially the horse; Fig. 23.2A). However, for clinical purposes the line can be regarded as virtually straight. The lung is very thin along its caudoventral border and, therefore, even if the caudoventral boundary does curve somewhat beyond this straight line, it is doubtful whether the additional area of lung will be helpful for percussion or auscultation; the thinness of the lung in any such additional area makes it ineffective as a resonance chamber for percussion, and the low velocity of the gas at the lung periphery probably produces little sound.

23.7.2   *The cranial boundary*

The cranial boundary of the area of percussion and auscultation of the lung is the caudal edge of **triceps**. As already stated, in the standing animal this is a line between the caudal angle of the **scapula** and the **fifth costochondral junction** (Figs 23.1, 23.2A,B,C).

23.7.3   *The dorsal boundary*

The dorsal boundary of the area runs roughly parallel to the vertebral column. However, it is considerably restricted by the progressively increasing thickness dorsally of the **epaxial muscles** (longissimus dorsi, etc.). In the horse and ox, the effective dorsal limits for percussion and auscultation lie roughly along a line from the **tuber coxae** to the caudal angle of the **scapula** (Fig. 23.1).

23.8   The costodiaphragmatic line of pleural reflection

This is the line along which the **costal** component of the parietal pleura is reflected from the **lateral thoracic wall** to the **diaphragm**, thus becoming continuous with the **diaphragmatic** component of the parietal pleura (Section 9.6.1). Thus it forms the peripheral limit of the **costodiaphragmatic recess**.

The costodiaphragmatic line of pleural reflection marks the greatest possible expansion of the lung into the costodiaphragmatic recess, but it is said that the normal lung fails to reach the line even when fully expanded (at least in the ox). However, an abnormally dilated lung, as in the horse with **chronic alveolar emphysema** or **chronic obstructive pulmonary disease** (Section 7.19), can reach close to this line, and this abnormal extent can be detected by percussion.

Like other anatomical landmarks in the thorax, the costodiaphragmatic line of pleural reflection has reasonably constant topographical boundaries relative to the skeleton in the domestic species. In all of these animals, it runs approximately from the **eighth costochondral junction** to the proximal end of the **last rib**. In the horse (Fig. 23.2A) and dog (Fig. 23.2C) it follows fairly closely the curve of the **costal arch**, but yet is appreciably craniodorsal to the costal arch (about a hand's breadth in front in a small pony). In the ox (Fig.

23.2B), however, it lies well craniodorsal to the costal arch.

The costodiaphragmatic line is an important line, clinically. It forms the boundary between the pleural and peritoneal cavities, because immediately caudal to it the diaphragm is attached to the thoracic wall. The **peritoneal cavity** can therefore be entered, without damaging the pleura, by penetrating the thoracic wall **caudoventral** to the line (Figs 23.2, 23.3, 23.4). On the other hand, entry to the **pleural cavity**, for example to draw off pleural effusion (**thoracocentesis**; Section 25.1), must be made **craniodorsal** to the line. In the ox, the line is so far cranial to the costal arch that a relatively very large area of the caudal thoracic wall has no contact with the pleural cavity, but the caudal thoracic wall then has correspondingly a much more extensive contact with the peritoneal cavity in this species (Fig. 23.4).

II PHYSICAL EXAMINATION OF THE HEART

23.9 Percussion of the heart

The main objective of percussion of the heart is to establish the size of the heart. The technique is the same as for percussion of the lungs (Section 23.5.1). The size of the heart is correlated with the extent of its contact with the thoracic wall. Where the heart is in direct contact with the thoracic wall, or separated from it by only a thin layer of lung, percussion will reveal an area of dullness which differs from the adjacent areas of resonance where only the lung is in contact with the thoracic wall. This area of comparative dullness is called the **area of cardiac dullness**. An increase in the area of cardiac dullness is consistent with enlargement of the heart or pericardial effusion.

The anatomical factor which mainly determines the area of cardiac dullness is obviously the **position of the heart**. This is virtually the same, relative to the skeleton, in all the domestic species; the heart lies from the **third to the sixth ribs inclusive** in the horse, ox, sheep, pig, and dog, with only minor species variations (Section 20.5).

In the domestic mammals generally, the area of cardiac dullness on the **left** side lies beneath the ventral third of the third, fourth and fifth intercostal spaces (Figs 23.2A, C). The area on the **right** side is usually considerably smaller, being restricted generally to the third and fourth intercostal spaces. The larger size of the left area of cardiac dullness is explained by the substantially greater size of the **right lung** than the left lung in all these species (Section 5.5). The larger size of the right lung forces the heart somewhat to the left side (Fig. 25.1), and therefore brings more of the heart into contact with the left thoracic wall than the right.

Since the triceps brachii muscle covers the region of the thorax that is occupied by the heart, the limb must be drawn cranially when percussion of the heart is attempted. This requirement, coupled with the difficulty in obtaining the cooperation of the animal, restricts the value of cardiac percussion in domestic mammals.

23.9.1 *Methods for percussion of the heart*

The techniques of using fingers, or plexor and pleximeter, for eliciting the sounds of percussion of the heart are the same as those for percussion of the lungs (Section 23.5.1). Some clinicians distinguish an area of absolute cardiac dullness (or superficial dullness), which can be elicited by light percussion. This is considered to correspond to the area of direct contact between the heart and the thoracic wall. An area of relative cardiac dullness (or deep dullness) can be obtained by heavy percussion, and this follows approximately the actual outline of the heart.

23.9.2 *Anatomical basis of the area of cardiac dullness*

Whilst the relationships described above hold good in principle in most species, there is variation in the extent to which the area of contact between heart and left thoracic wall spreads caudally (Schummer *et al.*, 1981, pp. 17–18). In the ox (Figs 5.5, 23.2B) it usually fails to extend beyond the middle of the fourth intercostal space, and therefore in this species the area of contact is entirely covered by the thick body of the triceps muscle; consequently in the ox percussion of the heart is largely impracticable. In the cat, and sometimes even in the dog, the normal heart may reach caudal to the sixth rib, thus extending the area of cardiac dullness to the sixth intercostal space.

The cardiac notch is sometimes regarded as potentially an important anatomical factor determining the size, position, and shape of the area of cardiac dullness. The cardiac notch (Section 5.6.2) is a gap in the cranial part of the ventral border of the lung (CN in Figs 5.3 and 5.4), allowing the heart to make contact with the thoracic wall. It is unlikely to be a major anatomical factor determining the size of the area of cardiac dullness. Firstly, this is because the lung is very thin all round the cardiac notch. Therefore the heart is separated from the thoracic wall by only a very thin sliver of lung over an area which is much larger than the area of the notch itself; most of this larger area evinces cardiac dullness on percussion. Secondly, the cardiac notch must change from moment to moment during breathing, being markedly reduced during inspiration as the lobes of the lung expand into the costomediastinal recess (Section 5.7); despite this, cardiac dullness persists during inspiration. However, the cardiac notch really is significant in echocardiography where it forms an *'acoustic window'* (Section 24.15), and probably also in pericardiocentesis where it may save the lung from damage (Section 25.2).

23.9.3   Observations made by percussion of the heart

Clearly much practice is necessary before changes in the area of cardiac dullness can be recognized, but the skilled clinician can detect certain abnormalities such as enlargement of the heart by this technique. However, experienced clinicians concede that percussion may have a limited value in assessing the outline of the heart; radiography and echocardiography have largely superseded cardiac percussion (Blood and Studdert, 1988, p. 685).

23.10   Auscultation of the heart

The purpose of auscultation of the heart is to detect abnormalities of its action. There are four heart sounds (Section 22.7; Fig. 22.1). The **first sound** (S1) is associated with closure of the A-V valves at the onset of ventricular systole. The **second sound** (S2) is associated with closure of the aortic and pulmonary valves at the onset of ventricular diastole. The **third sound** (S3) is associated with rapid filling of the ventricles in the first part of ventricular diastole, and is very faint. The **fourth sound** (S4) is associated with atrial systole, but is rarely audible in the normal heart (p. 568).

With the aid of a conventional stethoscope the first and second heart sounds can be examined valve by valve, i.e. the pulmonary valve, aortic valve, left atrioventricular valve, and right atrioventricular valve, in sequence.

23.10.1   Anatomical basis of auscultation of the heart

The anatomical landmarks that are used for auscultation of the **valves** obviously depend primarily on the position of the heart within the thorax. As already stated in Section 23.9, the heart has similar bony relations in all the domestic species, i.e. it lies approximately between **ribs 3 and 6**. Since the mass of triceps covers the first five ribs in the domestic mammals (Fig. 23.1), the forelimb must be drawn forward or the chest piece of the stethoscope must be pushed under the caudal edge of triceps.

The valves are situated on the **fibrous skeleton of the heart**, which consists in principle of a fibrous plate separating the atria from the ventricles; the plate is perforated by the four valves (Figs 20.2, 20.5; Section 20.12).

The **dorsoventral levels of the valves** depend on the slope of the heart, and this does vary in the species. In the large animals (horse and ox) the long axis of the heart is approximately **vertical** (Figs 23.3, 23.4), but in the smaller animals (dog and cat) it is **oblique** in relation to the sternum (Fig. 23.5). Because of these varying slopes, the fibrous plate which carries the four valves is essentially parallel with the sternum in the large animals but oblique to the sternum in the cat and dog.

In practice it is found that in the domestic species generally the individual valves are most clearly heard at the following sites: the **pulmonary valve**, at the **left third** intercostal space; the **aortic valve**, at the **left fourth** space; the **left atrioventricular valve**, at the **left fifth** space; and the **right atrioventricular valve** at the **right fourth** space. These sites are summarized in Fig. 23.5, which also approximately indicates the relative dorsoventral levels of each valve in its intercostal space in the dog; the pulmonary valve is relatively far ventral in species with sloping hearts (dog and cat), but is more or less on the same level as the other valves in species with vertical hearts (horse and ox). Despite the value of these preferential sites, auscultation of the heart should be extended over as wide an area as possible, 'inching' the chest piece of the stethoscope around the thorax rather than concentrating on a few special places.

The more precise craniocaudal position of the heart in relation to the ribs varies as follows (Schummer *et al.*, 1981, p. 19): dog, ribs 3–6 (or 4–7); cat, ribs 4–7; pig, ribs 3–6; ox, ribs 3–5 (or 6); sheep and goat, ribs 2–5; horse, ribs 3–6.

Sounds arising from valve function or disease are not necessarily heard most clearly at the point on the thoracic wall that is most directly opposite the actual source of the sound; this may be partly due to the unpredictability of the conduction of sound by tissues of varying texture and density. Besides this factor, however, the place where a valve sound is loudest is usually

where (a) the vessel, or chamber of the heart, in which that valve lies is nearest to the surface of the body, (b) the valve is as far away as possible from the other valves, and (c) the blood flow is 'downstream' from the valve, so that the blood conducts the sound from the valve to the surface (Gardner *et al.*, 1960, p. 440).

The best sites for hearing sounds associated with valvular lesions in the dog have been reported in principle by Ettinger (1971, p. 89) and in detail by Gompf (1988, pp. 34–35). The aortic valve is heard at the fourth left intercostal space, slightly below a line drawn through the point of the shoulder, this region being referred to as the

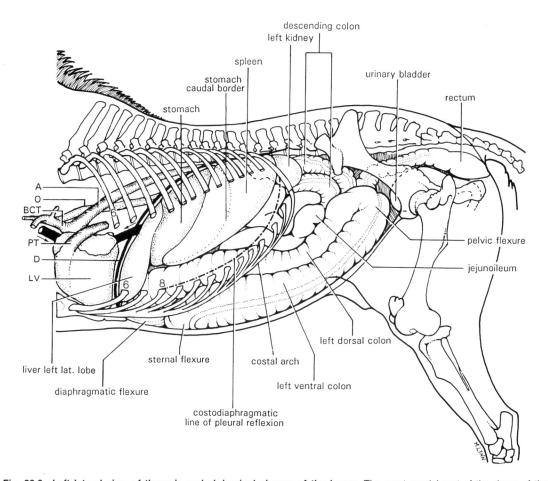

Fig. 23.3 Left lateral view of thoracic and abdominal viscera of the horse. The most cranial part of the dome of the diaphragm, shown in median section, reaches the level of about rib 6. The caudal border of the heart is close to the diaphragm, and therefore also reaches the level of about rib 6. The costodiaphragmatic line (of pleural reflection) runs from the eighth costochondral junction to the proximal end of the last rib. Entry to the pleural cavity is made cranial to this line, whereas entry to the peritoneal cavity is made caudal to it. The cranial and caudal venae cavae (black) are indicated, respectively, by a caudally and cranially directed arrow corresponding to the direction of blood flow. The caudal vena cava passes through the caval foramen in the tendinous centre of the diaphragm. The oesophageal hiatus and aortic hiatus of the diaphragm are progressively dorsal to the caval foramen. A, aorta; BCT, brachiocephalic trunk; D, diaphragm cupola; LV, left ventricle; O, oesophagus; PT, pulmonary trunk.

'aortic area'. The pulmonary valve is also best heard on the left side at the second to fourth intercostal spaces, but its sounds can be heard on both sides and also more cranially and ventrally than the aortic sounds. Sounds from the left atrioventricular valve are loudest at the left fifth intercostal space, dorsal to the middle of its lower third, the 'mitral area'. The right atrioventricular valve is most audible at the right fourth intercostal space, at the level of the costochondral junction, the 'tricuspid area'; this relatively ventral site may be associated with a tendency for the plate-like fibrous skeleton of the heart to be rotated ventrally on the right, thus placing the right atrioventricular valve at a more ventral level than the left valve (Fig. 25.1).

23.10.2 *Observations made by auscultation of the heart*

Words are not much use for describing heart sounds, and there is no substitute for practice at listening to normal and abnormal hearts. However, as a rough guide to the **normal sounds**, it can be said that the **first heart sound** (S1) is normally a long low-frequency sound, while the **second** (S2) is normally a shorter sound of higher frequency, giving the classical **lub–dub** followed by a pause. The sounds are louder in thin animals and muffled

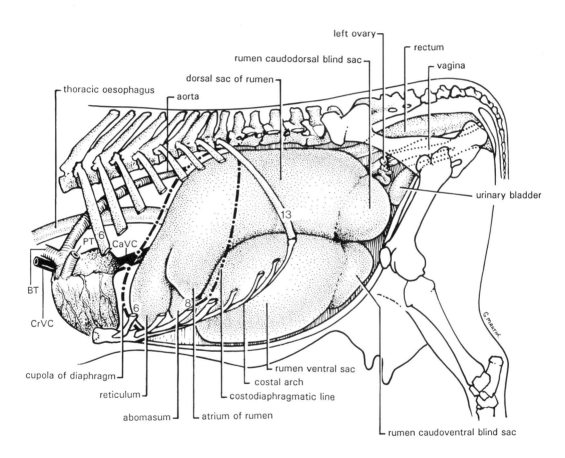

Fig. 23.4 Left lateral view of thoracic and abdominal viscera of the ox. The most cranial part of the dome of the diaphragm, shown in median section, reaches the level of about rib 6. The caudal border of the heart is close to the diaphragm, and therefore also reaches the level of about rib 6. The reticulum is in contact with the caudal surface of the diaphragm. The distance between the reticulum and the parietal pericardium is therefore only 1–2 cm. The costodiaphragmatic line (of pleural reflection) runs from the eighth costochondral junction to the proximal end of the last rib. Entry to the pleural cavity is made cranial to this line, whereas entry to the peritoneal cavity is made cranial to it. BT, brachiocephalic trunk; CaVC, caudal vena cava; CrVC, cranial vena cava; PT, pulmonary trunk.

in fat animals. Various devices are available for amplifying sound, so that all four heart sounds can be recorded (as in Fig. 24.14). It has been recommended that both sides of the thorax should be auscultated using the bell chest piece to accentuate low frequency sounds, and the diaphragm chest piece to accentuate high frequencies.

Abnormal sounds include changes in the volume of sound. Thus greater **loudness** of the first and second sounds tends to occur in certain diseases such as **anaemia**; on the other hand, **muffling** tends to happen in other abnormal conditions, such as **fluid effusion** in the pleural or pericardial cavity and **emphysema** of the lung.

Murmurs are sounds caused by vibration due to turbulent blood flow (Section 22.7.7). **Systolic murmurs** begin after the first heart sound, and end before or with the second heart sound; since the first sound marks the onset of ventricular systole, a systolic murmur signals turbulence occurring

during ventricular systole. **Diastolic murmurs** begin after the second heart sound, and end before or with the first heart sound; they reveal turbulence during ventricular diastole. There are also **continuous murmurs** which go on throughout systole and diastole, thus indicating turbulence throughout the whole cardiac cycle. In addition the first or second heart sound may be **split**, causing two similar sounds in rapid succession.

The length of the intervals between sounds is important diagnostically.

In the normal dog only the first and second heart sounds can be auscultated with a conventional stethoscope (Ettinger, 1971, p. 89); S3 and S4 generally indicate heart disease in small animals (Darke *et al.*, 1996, p. 26). In some normal horses only the first two sounds are audible, but in most normal horses three heart sounds can be heard, S1 and S2 plus either S3 or S4; in some normal horses all four sounds may be heard (Glazier, 1987). In cattle, S3 and S4 are normal (Darke *et al.*, 1996, p. 26).

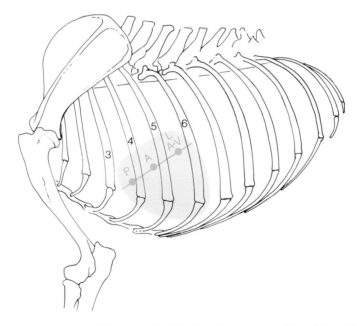

Fig. 23.5   Lateral view diagram of the left thoracic wall of the dog showing the relationships of the heart and its valves to the ribs. In all the domestic species, the heart (green area) lies between ribs 3 and 6. The valves lie in the fibrous skeleton of the heart, which is represented here as an oblique green line, carrying the pulmonary valve (P), the aortic valve (A), and the atrioventricular valves (A-V). In all the species the pulmonary valve is related to the third intercostal space, the aortic valve to the fourth intercostal space, and the left atrioventricular valve (LA-V) to the left fifth intercostal space. The right atrioventricular valve is related to the right fourth intercostal space. In the dog and cat the long axis of the heart typically slopes obliquely, and this causes the pulmonary valve to be nearer to the sternum than the left atrioventricular valve, as in the diagram; in the horse and ox the long axis of the heart is more nearly vertical, and this places the pulmonary valve on much the same dorsoventral level as the atrioventricular valves.

Highly sensitive microphones can be used to pick up sound, allowing the four heart sounds to be displayed on a chart recorder, i.e. **phonocardiography** (Fig. 24.14). Sound can also be picked up by a device on the end of a catheter, i.e. a **phonocatheter**; one of these was in use in the oesophagus in Fig. 24.8.

23.11 Palpation of the heart

In man, dog, cat, foal, calf, and lamb the **normal heart beat** can be felt through the left thoracic wall by palpation. In normal adults of the large domestic mammals it is less readily detectable, but can be felt in many horses and cattle by placing the flat of the hand on the left thoracic wall just above the olecranon process. When evident, the impact of the beat is called the **apex beat** (or point of maximal pulsation). In species with no hair or only a short fine coat (e.g. man, short-haired dog) the apex beat can be seen as well as felt.

The apex beat occurs towards the end of ventricular systole. At this stage of the cardiac cycle the heart rotates, thus bringing the apex of the heart into sudden forcible contact with the thoracic wall; this contact causes the apex beat.

The **site of the apex beat** in the dog typically falls somewhere within a zone between the fourth and sixth intercostal spaces on the **left** side, and especially over the fifth space, just dorsal to the sternal border. Assessment of the apex beat may enable diagnosis of cardiac enlargement.

In the dog and cat, the apex beat can be detected not only on the left but also on the right side, over the fourth and fifth intercostal spaces (Schummer *et al.*, 1981, p. 45). It is particularly obvious in thin narrow-chested athletic breeds of dog (Evans and Christensen, 1979, p. 637). In the cat, the beat is best palpated on the left side between ribs 4 and 6, and at the fifth rib on the right side (Schummer *et al.*, 1981, p. 45). In the horse, it is best felt over the left fifth intercostal space, and can also be detected at the third and fourth (Schummer *et al.*, 1981, p. 64). In the ox, it is most obvious at the left fourth intercostal space, and may be recognizable at the right fourth space (Schummer *et al.*, 1981, p. 57). In man, it usually lies in the fourth or fifth intercostal spaces about 6 or 7 cm to the left of the midline.

In pathological conditions, notably **enlargement of the heart**, both the **force** of the apex beat and the **area of it** may increase. The **position** of the apex beat may change. This can happen if the heart is enlarged or displaced by abnormal structures within the thorax (Ettinger, 1971, p. 88). However, it should be emphasized that, in man particularly, the site of the apex beat normally varies considerably from one person to another.

Palpation can also reveal a **thrill** or **vibration** (Section 22.7.8), which can be felt in the horse by placing the palm of the hand on the thoracic wall. This would suggest severe turbulence and an advanced cardiac murmur; a murmur accompanied by a thrill is usually pathological (Glazier, 1987).

In the **horse** the **external jugular vein** should be examined and palpated with the head in the normal standing position (Glazier, 1987). A **jugular pulse** is normally visible near the thoracic inlet (Section 22.2). Abnormally prominent pulsations extending further up the neck may be associated with **mitral insufficiency** and **right ventricular dilation**. Distension (cording) of the vein without abnormal pulsations may occur in **right ventricular heart failure** or constrictive pericarditis. Distension without pulsation may arise from thrombosis of the vein, or from obstructed flow in the cranial vena cava caused by a cranial mediastinal neoplasm or abscess.

In the **dog** (Ettinger, 1971, p. 87), distension of the **external jugular**, **cephalic**, and **saphenous veins** suggests a generalized increase in venous pressure. This could occur in **right ventricular heart failure** or **pericardial effusion**. Pulsations of the external jugular veins indicate heart failure or cardiac arrhythmia.

Chapter 24
Anatomical Principles of Diagnostic Imaging of the Thorax

24.1 Imaging techniques and their role in anatomy

Imaging is the production of visual images of structures deep within the intact body. The most widely used imaging technique in veterinary medicine is that based on X-rays. Several other imaging techniques are widely used in human medicine, and some of them are being adopted in veterinary medicine. These include **computerized tomography (CT)**, **ultrasonography**, **scintigraphy**, **thermography**, and **magnetic resonance imaging (MRI)**. Many veterinary schools have capabilities for CT, ultrasonography, and scintigraphy, and access to MRI equipment.

All these techniques have the great advantage of being non-invasive, causing little or no injury to the body (provided rigorous precautions are taken against accidental over-exposure to ionizing radiation), and are therefore of great diagnostic value to the clinician. However, clinicians emphasize that imaging techniques are not a substitute for the thorough physical examination of the animal by observation, palpation, and auscultation. But imaging techniques can greatly enhance these skills, by confirming the existence of suspected abnormalities and by revealing details of structural and functional changes caused by disease.

The greatly increasing use of, and continual improvements in, imaging technologies have caused a revaluation of anatomy in clinical studies. Topographical anatomy had declined in importance in the biomedical curriculum. However, it is difficult or impossible to obtain full diagnostic value from imaging without a good grasp of the three dimensional topographical relationships of the relevant structures.

24.2 General principles of radiographic technique

Film can be exposed to the ionizing radiation of the X-ray beam in order to make records of internal structures of the body. Rays that penetrate the body cause decomposition of the silver halide crystals in the film emulsion, forming minute particles of silver. The deposition of silver particles causes black specks in the emulsion, the number of which depends on the intensity of the X-irradiation reaching the film. Tissues penetrated by X-rays are described as radiolucent. Gases are very **radiolucent** and fatty tissue moderately radiolucent. On radiographs, radiolucent structures appear black or a shade of dark grey.

Rays that are absorbed by particular tissues do not change the silver bromide crystals. When the film is fixed these crystals are removed, leaving the film white. Such tissues are **radiopaque**. Bone and calcium deposits are moderately radiopaque. Blood, cartilage, connective tissue, muscle, and water are less radiopaque than bone. Compounds that contain elements such as barium and iodine, which have high atomic weights, are highly radiopaque. On radiographs, radiopaque structures appear white or a shade of pale grey.

A **plain radiograph (straight radiograph)** is one taken without the administration of a contrast medium or the use of any other special effects; it enables pre-existing opacities or translucencies to be identified. **Contrast media** are substances introduced into a structure to increase the contrast with adjacent tissues. **Radiopaque contrast media** include organic iodine compounds and barium sulphate. **Radiolucent contrast media** are gases such as air, oxygen, and carbon dioxide. Barium sulphate is used for gastrointestinal radiography, including the oesophagus. Iodinated contrast media are used in cardiovascular radiography to reveal the chambers of the heart and the great blood vessels.

Film density, or the density of a radiograph, is indicated by the degree of blackness of the film when viewed. The blacker the film the denser it is. **Tissue density** refers to the radiopacity of a particular tissue, relatively radiopaque tissues such as bone having high tissue density. Note that, on radiographs, **dense film** is *black* but **dense tissue** is *white*.

The **contrast** of a radiograph comprises the **differences in film density** of the structures that it shows. Differences in film density should reveal the varying tissue densities of these structures. By controlling contrast, a skilled radiographer can produce thoracic radiographs which differentiate between structures of only slightly different tissue densities. For example, bronchi and lung parenchyma with relatively low but slightly different tissue densities can then be distinguished from each other, as well as from pulmonary blood vessels, great veins, and aorta with slightly higher tissue densities. Fine differences in film density due to slightly different tissue densities are described as **tissue contrasts**; in this instance (lung and blood vessels) they would be referred to as soft tissue contrasts.

> High energy electromagnetic radiation selectively penetrates tissue of differing densities, and can be detected either on film or by other sensors. The high energy radiation of X-rays is produced by using a large potential difference to accelerate electrons between an anode and cathode in a vacuum tube. The impact of the electrons on the anode leads to emission of electromagnetic radiation.
>
> The main factors controlling contrast are the quantity and penetration of radiation. The *quantity* (exposure) is determined by the product of current and time (mA s). The *penetration* is determined by the potential difference (kilovoltage). The higher the kilovoltage the shorter the wavelength of the X-rays, and hence the greater their power of penetration. In principle, to obtain good contrast the penetration should be just sufficient to penetrate the part under examination; thus the kilovoltage is reduced for the less radiopaque parts of the body. The soft tissues of the thorax are particularly radiotranslucent. However, the fact that the thorax is surrounded by ribs raises a particular difficulty, in that a thoracic radiograph with perfect contrast for the soft structures would be largely obliterated by the ribs.

Various other factors also affect the production of a good radiograph. One which particularly impairs thoracic radiographs is *movement*, including the movement of breathing. The phase of breathing in which respiratory movement is minimal is usually end-expiration. However, an ideal thoracic radiograph should be taken at *full inspiration*, since the presence of air within the airways enhances the contrast between aerated and non-aerated tissues such as pulmonary blood vessels (see also Section 24.12). In general, when producing radiographs of soft tissues the radiographer has to deal with two contradictory factors. To obtain good contrast a low kilovoltage beam is needed, which entails an increase in exposure; however, to eliminate the effect of movement the exposure time must be as short as possible. The thoracic radiographer has the further difficulty of having to show soft tissues which are surrounded by a bony cage.

Thus a good thoracic radiograph has to be a compromise between several conflicting factors. Because of the difficulty of controlling these variables, the ability to obtain perfect thoracic radiographs depends on extensive experience and study.

Image intensification is a technique for increasing the brightness of the image while maintaining its sharpness. Calcium tungstate and rare-earth screens transform the invisible X-ray image into coloured light. This substantially reduces the exposure time. Rare-earth intensifying screens produce more intensification and are safer than calcium tungstate screens.

24.3 Thoracic radiography in domestic mammals

In veterinary practice, radiography of the thorax is carried out extensively in the dog and cat, but it is also a very useful diagnostic aid for foals, miniature horses, ponies, calves, and valuable sheep and goats. In many referral centres there are machines with sufficient capacity to radiograph the thorax of adult horses and cattle.

24.4 Positioning the body for thoracic radiography

The terms used for the position of the body during radiography indicate the direction of the X-ray beam. In a **dorsoventral radiograph** the beam enters the dorsal surface of the body and leaves the ventral surface; in a **ventrodorsal radiograph**, the beam enters through the ventral surface and exits through the dorsal surface. In a **lateral thoracic**

radiograph the beam enters one lateral surface of the body and goes out through the other.

Dorsoventral radiographs of the thorax of the **dog** and **cat** are generally taken while the animal is stretched out on its sternum and abdomen (sternal recumbency). For **ventrodorsal radiographs** the animal is, of course, placed on its back. **Lateral radiographs** are commonly taken while the animal is lying on either its left or its right side (**left** or **right lateral recumbency**); alternatively, the animal may be stretched out on its sternum and abdomen, or standing, or lying on its back with its feet in the air. When a lateral radiograph is taken with the animal lying on its side or on its back, the effects of *gravity* will modify the position of the movable organs, particularly of the heart and diaphragm, and this affects interpretation of the radiograph.

In the adult **horse** and **ox**, thoracic radiographs are only possible in lateral projection with the animal standing.

It is desirable to use constant radiographic positions as far as possible, since this makes it easier to detect abnormalities in the shapes and sites of the organs. Great care should be taken to ensure that the positions are always accurately placed. Thus it is essential that in **dorsoventral radiographs** the body should always be in as near the true upright position as possible, the vertebral column then being superimposed on the sternum (Fig. 24.1); if the body is not placed accurately in the upright position, the distortions due to gravity make it almost impossible to decide whether the shape and position of the heart are normal or abnormal. When lateral radiographs are taken with the animal lying on its side, the sternum must be supported by a bolster to ensure that the trunk is not rotated, since this would distort the effects of the caudal mediastinum and phrenicopericardiac ligament which tether the pericardium to the left half of the diaphragmatic cupola (Section 24.9.2).

It is a general rule that the tissue under investigation is as near the film as possible, and this may cause the radiographer to deviate from the standard procedure. For example, **dorsoventral radiographs** of the thorax are generally used to investigate the heart, but **ventrodorsal radiographs** may be preferred for investigations of the lungs. Similarly, **lateral radiographs** may be routinely taken with the animal lying on the right side, but for an examination of the left lung it may be preferred to place the animal on its left side. Furthermore, if a possible **pleural effusion** is to be investigated by a lateral radiograph, it would be best to place the animal in sternal recumbency, since the level of any fluid in the pleural cavity could then be assessed.

In the adult horse and ox, only lateral radiographs are feasible, even with very powerful apparatus. Furthermore, the size of the animal makes it impossible to image the entire thorax on a single film. A 450kg **horse** needs three or four films (Fig. 24.7) to cover a reasonable area of the lung, heart, and great blood vessels (Mair and Gibbs, 1990). In the **ox** (Section 24.11), useful thoracic radiographs can be obtained by centring the beam over the sixth rib midway between the caudal angle of the scapula and the olecranon process (Lee, 1974).

24.5 Viewing thoracic radiographs

Dorsoventral radiographs are generally viewed so that the ventral aspect of the body is facing the observer. In a dorsoventral radiograph, this puts the *left* side of the body on the *right* side of the viewing box.

Lateral radiographs should be viewed so that the long axis of the body is parallel with the ground. The head is usually placed on the left of the viewing box.

24.6 General difficulties in interpreting thoracic radiographs

24.6.1 *Breed variation*

The thoracic anatomy of the domestic mammals is remarkably constant in its *general principles*, much more so than abdominal anatomy for instance. Unfortunately, however, thoracic anatomy is also rather variable in its *details* especially within the breeds of dog. For example, in breeds like the greyhound, which have a narrow deep thorax, the heart is relatively slim in outline; furthermore its position is more in the midline in dorsoventral radiographs, and is less oblique (i.e. more upright) in lateral views. The opposite shapes and positions of the heart occur in barrel-chested breeds like the English bulldog which have a wide shallow thorax.

24.6.2 *Faulty positioning*

As already stated, if the animal is in an incorrect position when the radiograph is taken, the position of the main organs will be distorted. In particular, any degree of rotation of the body makes interpretation of the heart almost impossible in dorsoventral radiographs.

sible to see, and the heart may be virtually in the midline.

24.7 Dorsoventral thoracic radiographs of the dog and cat

The following structures can be observed in dorsoventral radiographs of the thorax of the normal dog (Fig. 24.1): the **heart, cranial vena cava, cranial mediastinal structures, diaphragm, caudal vena cava, pulmonary blood vessels** and **bronchi**, and **aorta**. Similar structures are seen in the **cat**, but less detail is visible than in the dog; the **aorta** and **caudal vena cava** are difficult or impos-

24.7.1 Heart

The heart is mainly on the left side of the thorax of the dog, the apex being substantially to the left of the midline (Fig. 24.1). The difference in the size of the heart shadow during **systole** and **diastole** is slight and often undetectable radiographically. The positions of the **atria** and **ventricles** can only be judged approximately (Fig. 24.2), but the apex is formed by the left ventricle, and the left and right edges of the cardiac shadow are formed by the left and right

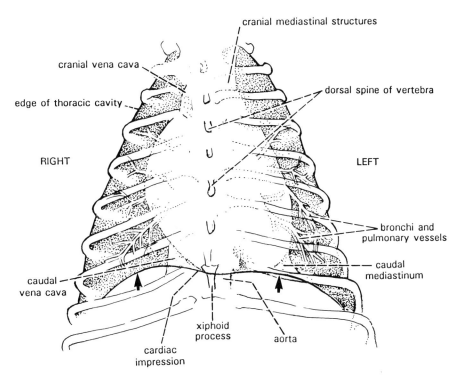

Fig. 24.1 Drawing of a dorsoventral radiograph of the thorax of a dog. The radiograph shows all the structures that are normally visible. The heart is predominantly on the left side. The apex of the heart is to the left of the midline. Large and medium sided bronchi accompany branches of the pulmonary vessels in a herring-bone pattern. The cupola of the diaphragm forms a sinuous and asymmetrical profile, a relatively common diaphragmatic pattern. It has two cranially directed bulges (arrows) of which the right one extends further cranially. Between the left and right bulges of the cupola is a slight cardiac impression caused by contact with the heart. The caudal mediastinum, reinforced by the phrenicopericardiac ligament, tethers the fibrous pericardium to the left side of the cupola. It is commonly, but not always, visible. The costodiaphragmatic and lumbodiaphragmatic recesses are not visible, since the aerated or fatty tissue needed for contrast is absent in those sites. The xiphoid process is in line with the thoracic vertebrae, showing that positioning is correct.

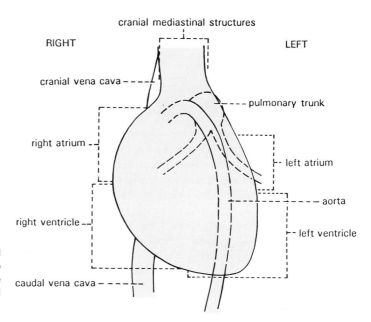

Fig. 24.2 Diagram of a dorsoventral radiograph of the normal heart of a dog, to show the approximate positions of the chambers of the heart and the great blood vessels.

chambers respectively. The **pulmonary trunk** is not visible on radiographs of the normal heart, although it contributes (Fig. 24.2) to the general opacity of the left cranial region of the cardiac shadow. If the right ventricle and pulmonary trunk are pathologically enlarged, this region of the cardiac shadow can become obviously larger and denser.

24.7.2 *Cranial vena cava*

The cranial vena cava is largely obscured by the general shadow of the **cranial mediastinal structures**, but its right lateral border can be seen in well exposed radiographs.

24.7.3 *Cranial mediastinal structures*

A broad but undetailed shadow (Fig. 24.1) is formed by the superimposition of the **brachiocephalic** and **subclavian vessels**, and of the **oesophagus** (and **thymus** in young animals).

24.7.4 *Diaphragm*

When correctly positioned, dorsoventral radiographs of the dog should show only the cupola (the dome) of the diaphragm and not the crura

(Section 8.11). The profile of the cupola varies greatly, but often takes the form of an asymmetrical sinuous line bulging cranially on either side of the midline (Figs 24.1, 24.3). The bulge of the cupola on the right side extends further cranially than the bulge on the left side. Between the two bulges, the midsection of the profile is flattened or faintly dished on its cranial surface to form a slight cardiac impression, caused by contact with the apex of the heart.

A definitive study of the radiographic anatomy of the canine diaphragm was made by Grandage (1974). Features that are potentially (though not always) recognizable on dorsoventral or ventrodorsal radiographs are summarized in Fig. 24.3. They include the cupola, the crura, the caudal vena cava, and the phrenicopericardiac ligament.

The profile of the **cupola** is always visible, but varies greatly in its shape (Fig. 24.4). The sinuous shape and degree of cranial projection of the cupola shown in Fig. 24.1 (and Fig. 24.4C) evidently constitute one of the commonest diaphragmatic profiles in dorsoventral or ventrodorsal radiographs of the dog. However, in deep-chested dogs the cupola projects cranially as a prominent median dome (Fig. 24.4A), whereas in barrel-chested dogs the profile of the cupola is much flatter (Fig. 24.4D). The **cardiac impression** ranges from being deep as in Fig. 24.4D to being absent as in Fig. 24.4A; it tends to be deep in puppies and chondrodystrophoid breeds.

The **caudal mediastinum**, probably reinforced by the

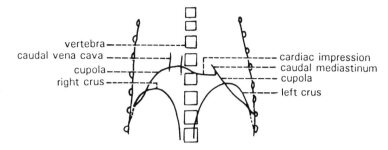

Fig. 24.3   Diagrammatic profile of the diaphragm of the dog, to show the components that theoretically may be visible in a dorsoventral or ventrodorsal thoracic radiograph. The cupola is always seen. The crura (augmented by the adjacent costal regions of the diaphragm) are only visible when the beam is aligned through the abdomen rather than through the thorax, so that rays pass obliquely over the crura. The caudal vena cava is always visible, passing through the right side of the cupola. The caudal mediastinum, reinforced by the phrenicopericardiac ligament, is commonly visible, running from the pericardium to the left side of the cupola; this attachment of the phrenicopericardiac ligament to the left side of the cupola causes the cardiac impression to be mainly on the left side of the cupola. Lacking the contrast of air and fat, the costodiaphragmatic recess (broken lines) is not visible. (Redrawn from Grandage (1974), with permission of the author and the British Veterinary Association; Grandage (personal communication, 1992) identified the caudal mediastinum as the cardiophrenic ligament.)

phrenicopericardiac ligament (Section 9.4), is commonly seen (Figs 24.1, 24.3), passing from the caudal part of the fibrous pericardium to the left side of the cupola (Grandage, 1974). The basal border of the lung is rarely visible.

The profile of the diaphragm depends, for contrast, on the air in the pulmonary exchange tissue or fatty tissue. Where such contrast is absent, as in the **costodiaphragmatic** and **lumbodiaphragmatic recesses**, the diaphragm is undetectable. Additional special techniques, such as **pleurography** (in which the parietal and visceral pleurae are coated with a contrast medium) or **pneumoperitoneum** (in which gas is intentionally introduced into the peritoneal cavity), are needed to demonstrate the whole of the diaphragm.

Occasionally the **crura** (augmented by the adjoining costal regions of the diaphragm) are also visible in dorsoventral radiographs. When seen they are superimposed on the dome of the cupola, producing the clover-leaf pattern shown in Figs 24.3 and 24.4F. These extra shadows are only present when the crura are silhouetted against the lungs. This can happen if the beam is aligned through the abdomen instead of the thorax, so that only oblique rays, travelling ventrocranially, pass over the crura.

24.7.5   Caudal vena cava

This great vein is nearly always distinct on the right side, passing between the caudal surface of the heart and the right aspect of the diaphragmatic cupola (Figs 24.1, 24.3).

24.7.6   Branches of the pulmonary vessels and bronchi

The relatively small branches of the pulmonary arteries and veins, accompanied by large and medium-sized bronchi, are visible in good radiographs as vague branching shadows, with much superimposition, in a herring-bone pattern (Fig. 24.1).

24.7.7   Aorta

Even in good radiographs, the aorta is only just visible, but in these it can be made out faintly as it passes the apex of the heart and approaches the cupola to the left of the midline (Fig. 24.1).

24.8   Major structures usually NOT seen in dorsoventral thoracic radiographs

Major structures which are usually *not* visible in dorsoventral radiographs of normal dogs and cats are the **trachea**, **oesophagus**, and **tracheobronchial lymph nodes**. The **crura** of the diaphragm are not visible in a correctly positioned dorsoventral radiograph.

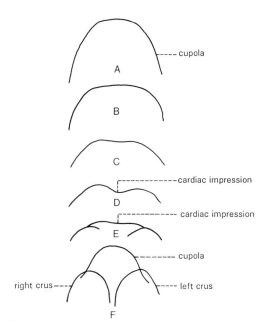

Fig. 24.4   Diagrams of the profile of the diaphragm of the dog as seen in a series of dorsoventral radiographs, to show the wide range of normal variation. Variant C is particularly common. The prominent dome in A is typical of deep-chested breeds; the shallow dome in D is typical of barrel-chested breeds. The cardiac impression may be absent, as in A and B. It tends to be deepest in chondrodystrophoid breeds and puppies, as in D, and is mainly on the left side of the cupola. The left and right crura (augmented by the adjacent costal regions of the diaphragm) are occasionally seen, forming a clover-leaf pattern as in E and F. These extra shadows are only seen when the crura are silhouetted against the lungs; this happens if the rays pass obliquely through the crura, as when the X-ray tube is positioned caudally, over the abdomen rather than over the thorax. (Redrawn from Grandage (1974), with permission of the author and the British Veterinary Association.)

As already stated, the crura may show as a clover leaf pattern (Figs 24.3, 24.4F) if oblique rays reach the thorax from a dorsoventral abdominal radiograph (Section 24.7.4).

24.9   Lateral thoracic radiographs of the dog and cat

The following structures can be seen in lateral radiographs of normal animals (Fig. 24.5): the **trachea**, the **heart**, **cranial vena cava**, and other **cranial mediastinal structures**, **diaphragm**, **caudal vena cava**, branches of **pulmonary vessels**, branches of the **bronchial tree**, and **aorta**.

24.9.1   *Trachea*

The trachea is always clearly visible as a translucent band for its whole course, both in the neck and in the thorax. After passing through the thoracic inlet, the thoracic trachea climbs somewhat dorsally over the base of the heart (Section 5.2), the general relationships of the organs being similar to those in Fig. 25.2. At the tracheal bifurcation, the trachea and the vertebral column diverge, making an angle which is open caudally.

At the **tracheal bifurcation** the two principal bronchi diverge caudolaterally. A lateral radiograph views these two great bronchi partly end-on. The result is a translucent oval which is often obvious in lateral radiographs of normal animals. This oval is wedged between the arch of the aorta and the base of the heart (Fig. 24.5). It provides an important landmark for interpreting the position of structures in thoracic radiographs. The oval is sometimes referred to as the carina, but this is a misnomer since the **carina** is the median vertical ridge of cartilage that splits the airway into the two principal bronchi (Section 5.3.1).

The topographical relationships of the caudal end of the trachea to the heart and vertebral column in the dog seem usually to resemble those in Fig. 25.2 (e.g. see Budras and Fricke, 1987, Figs 16A and 17A), but it is claimed (de Lahunta and Habel, 1986, p. 202) that the **angle of divergence between the end of the trachea and the vertebral column** varies with the breed of dog. The angle is nevertheless regarded as diagnostically important, because cardiac enlargement displaces the trachea dorsally and closes the angle. The angle can also be modified by space-occupying lesions (de Lahunta and Habel, 1986, p. 202).

24.9.2   *Heart*

In normal dogs and cats in the *standing position* the long axis of the heart is oblique in relation to the sternum, and consequently the heart is in extensive contact with the floor of the thoracic cage. In the dog in lateral recumbency, the heart makes contact with the diaphragm if the animal lies on its

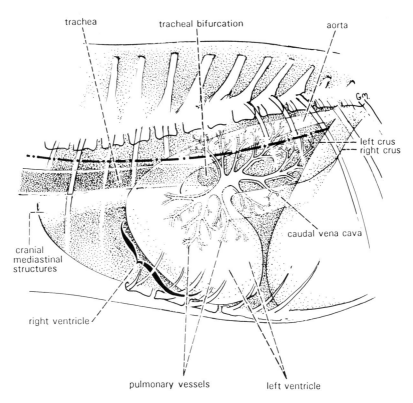

trachea   tracheal bifurcation   aorta

left crus
right crus

caudal vena cava

cranial
mediastinal
structures

right ventricle

pulmonary vessels   left ventricle

Fig. 24.5 Drawing of a lateral radiograph of the thorax of a dog in left lateral recumbency. All the structures normally visible are shown. The trachea is a broad translucent band passing over the base of the heart where it bifurcates at a translucent oval. Here it turns somewhat ventrally, forming a divergent angle with the vertebrae. When a dog is on its left side the heart is not quite in contact with the diaphragm. This is because in this position of the body the phrenicopericardiac ligament and caudal mediastinum, which tether the pericardium to the left aspect of the cupola, are no longer under tension; this allows the heart to move cranially away from the diaphragm. The cranial vena cava is obscured by other cranial mediastinal structures. The caudal vena cava slopes slightly dorsally as it joins the line of the right crus of the diaphragm. The left crus lies cranial to the right crus. Herring-bone patterns of pulmonary vessels accompanied by bronchi are visible. This radiograph could be identified as taken in left lateral recumbency, because the left crus is cranial to and then crosses the right crus, the heart has separated from the cupola, and the caudal vena cava is relatively ventral in the diaphragm. The broken line is the dorsal border of the oesophagus.

right side (Fig. 24.6A), but not if it lies on its left side (Figs 24.5, 24.6B); in the cat, the heart often is not in contact with the cupola.

There are no landmarks which precisely indicate the boundaries between the chambers of the heart, but the cranial edge of the cardiac shadow is formed by the right ventricle and the apex is formed by the left ventricle (Fig. 24.5). Changes in the contours of the heart may indicate pathological enlargement.

In lateral radiographs of the dog obtained with the animal lying on its *right side*, the **caudal mediastinum**

(reinforced by the **phrenicopericardiac ligament**; Section 9.4) tethers the heart to the left half of the cupola of the diaphragm; this maintains the heart in contact with the diaphragm, and gives a **cardiac impression** on the left part of the cupola (Fig. 24.6A, and see also Fig. 24.3). If the animal is lying on its *left side*, the caudal mediastinum and its supporting phrenicopericardiac ligament are slackened, allowing the heart to subside onto the left thoracic wall and lose its contact with the diaphragm (Figs 24.5, 24.6B) (Grandage, 1974; Barr, 1988).

The obliqueness of the long axis of the heart is less pronounced in deep-chested breeds such as the greyhound. In the cat the obliqueness is greater than in the dog.

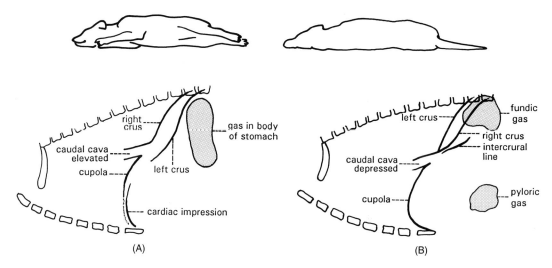

Fig. 24.6   Diagrams of the profile of the diaphragm of the dog as seen in lateral radiographs of the thorax. In all lateral radiographs the diaphragm shows three basic lines, formed by the cupola, the left crus, and the right crus (each crus includes the adjacent costal part of the diaphragm). If the animal is standing, or lying on its sternum, back, or side, the three basic lines are present.

A. **Right lateral recumbency.** The weight of the abdominal viscera forces the pendent crus (the right crus) cranial to the left crus. The cardiac impression is an extra line, but the cupola is indistinct. The cardiac impression is formed because the caudal mediastinum and phrenicopericardiac ligament, which tether the heart to the left aspect of the cupola, are under tension and thus pull the heart against the left side of the cupola. The caudal vena cava is elevated slightly dorsally, particularly at its cranial end but also at the caudal caval foramen. The single gas bubble is in the body of the stomach.

B. **Left lateral recumbency.** An additional intercrural line is formed by the deep cleft between the crura. The pendent crus (the left crus) is forced cranial to the right crus. There is no cardiac impression. This is because the heart droops to the left and therefore slackens the caudal mediastinum and phrenicopericardiac ligament, thus allowing the heart to move away from the cupola as in Fig. 24.5. The caudal vena cava is depressed somewhat ventrally, particularly at its cranial end. The dorsal and ventral gas bubbles respectively are in the fundic and pyloric regions of the stomach. (Redrawn from Grandage (1974), with permission of the author and the British Veterinary Association.)

24.9.3   Cranial vena cava

The ventral edge of the cranial vena cava may just be visible, but most of this vessel is obscured by the other cranial mediastinal structures.

24.9.4   Cranial mediastinal structures

A dense but vague shadow is formed by the superimposed brachiocephalic vessels and oesophagus (Fig. 24.5). The muscles of the shoulder region also contribute to the cranial part of this shadow.

24.9.5   Diaphragm

In a lateral radiograph of the canine thorax, the profile of the diaphragm varies greatly. However, it always has at least three lines (Fig. 24.6A,B), which are formed by the **left crus**, the **right crus**,

and the **cupola**. In addition, the deep 'intercrural cleft' between the two crura sometimes forms a linear shadow, the '**intercrural line**', which is shorter than the crural lines and caudoventral to them (Fig. 24.6B). If the cupola is indented by the heart, the '**cardiac impression**' also forms a line (Fig. 24.6A).

Strictly, the **crus dextrum** and **crus sinistrum** of the diaphragm are the right and left components (crura) that arise from the right and left aspects of the bodies of the cranial lumbar vertebrae, and together constitute the pars lumbalis (lumbar part) of the diaphragm (Section 8.11.3). In this account, however, the definition of the term 'crus' is widened for radiological convenience to follow Grandage (1974), and refers to the dorsal half of the diaphragm. It therefore includes not only the lumbar part of the diaphragm, but also the adjacent right and left pars costalis (costal part) of the diaphragm.

The extraordinarily variable radiographic appearance

of the canine diaphragm, particularly in lateral projections, has been analysed by Grandage (1974), who estimated – not entirely in jest – a possible total of 51 840 combinations. The main factors that cause these variations are gravity, malpositioning, breed conformation, the point at which the X-ray beam is centred, and breathing.

The effects of *gravity* are particularly dominant. The weight of the abdominal viscera causes sagging of whatever part of the diaphragm is nearest to the ground. Therefore in the *standing animal* the cupola bulges cranially, but if the animal is *on its back* the **crura** bulge cranially. Being equally affected by gravity, the left and right crura tend to be close together. But when the animal is lying *on its side* the pendent crus always bulges cranial to the upper one. Thus, if the animal is on its *right side* (Fig. 24.6A), the right crus bulges cranial to and parallel with the left crus. Also the **caudal mediastinum** and **phrenicopericardiac ligament** (Section 9.4), which suspend the heart from the left side of the cupola, maintain the heart in contact with the cupola, so that a **cardiac impression** may be present (Fig. 24.6A). Furthermore, the level of the **caudal caval foramen** rises somewhat dorsally (Section 24.9.6). On the other hand, if the animal lies on its *left side* (Fig. 24.6B) the left crus bulges cranial to the right crus and crosses it. The caudal mediastinum is slackened, allowing the heart to lose its contact with the cupola and thus leaving the cupola silhouetted against the lung as a single sharp line devoid of a cardiac impression. Figure 24.5 is a lateral projection of a dog in left lateral recumbency, showing these features, i.e. the crura crossing over, the gap between the heart and cupola, and the relatively ventral level of the caudal vena cava.

These effects of gravity when the animal lies on its side show that it is usually possible to identify the side on which the animal was lying, without looking at the labels on a radiograph. More importantly, the powerful influence of gravity reveals the necessity of taking great care always to place the animal in exactly the correct position. For instance, in lateral recumbency the sternum must be supported in precisely the right position. Even a slight malposition, such as the common fault of allowing the sternum to rotate towards the table, can cause a pronounced change in the relationships between the diaphragm and the viscera, both abdominal as well as thoracic (Grandage, 1974).

24.9.6   *Caudal vena cava*

This great vein is normally visible in the dog and cat as a radiopaque band passing between the heart and the diaphragm, ascending slightly caudodorsally (Fig. 24.5). The caudal vena cava passes through the **caudal caval foramen** (Fig. 8.24), which is to the *right* of the midline in the tendinous centre of the diaphragm; consequently, in a lateral thoracic radiograph, the shadow of the caudal vena cava appears to be continuous with the line caused by the shadow of the right crus (Figs 24.5, 24.6).

When the diaphragm moves cranially in exspiration, the junction of the caudal vena cava with the diaphragm moves slightly dorsally, reaching a level about two thirds of the distance from the sternum to the vertebral column. The caudal cava also rises dorsally when the animal lies on its right side (Fig. 24.6A), and this natural elevation may be mistaken for evidence of cardiac enlargement (Grandage, 1974).

24.9.7   *Branches of the pulmonary arteries and veins*

These vessels are visible on good radiographs as irregular herring-bone patterns of fine radiopaque lines accompanying longitudinal bronchi, particularly in the caudodorsal region between the heart and diaphragm (Fig. 24.5).

24.9.8   *Bronchi*

Bronchi of small and medium size can be detected. Some of those lying at right angles to the beam (i.e. running in the long axis of the lung) are normally visible as mainly longitudinal translucent (dark) lines, often accompanying pulmonary vessels (Fig. 24.5). When a sizeable bronchus is seen end-on in a lateral radiograph it can produce a small but distinct circular translucent area, bounded by the relatively radiopaque cartilages which are also end-on and therefore cause a ring-like shadow. These encircled translucent areas can be mistaken for lesions in the lung.

The bronchial tree can be shown by instilling radiopaque fluid into the airways. **Bronchograms** obtained in this way clearly show at least the first three orders of bronchi, and can reveal pathological changes in the bronchi such as **bronchiectasis** (Douglas and Hall, 1959). Bronchiectasis is characterized by chronic inflammatory dilation or sacculation of bronchi, usually in pendent parts of the lung (Section 5.10.3).

24.9.9   *Aorta*

The aorta is clearly visible for most of its thoracic course (Fig. 24.5).

24.10 Major structures usually NOT seen in lateral thoracic radiographs

Major structures that are usually not visible in lateral thoracic radiographs of the normal dog and cat are the **oesophagus** and the **tracheobronchial lymph nodes**. Occasionally, however, a lateral radiograph catches a bubble of gas in transit down the normal oesophagus, causing an unexpected elongated translucent area. If necessary, the oesophagus can always be shown by giving a barium sulphate meal. This will reveal oesophageal dilation or obstruction, including **megaoesophagus** (Section 3.23.1). Tracheobronchial lymph nodes do become visible if pathologically enlarged or dense. The **pleural cavity** is normally not seen in radiographs.

> The **diseased oesophagus** is often relaxed, and contains gas, saliva, or ingesta, or a combination of these, all of which are visible on plain radiographs. It is therefore not always necessary to do a contrast study in order

to make a radiographic diagnosis of, for example, megaoesophagus.

24.11 Lateral thoracic radiographs of farm animals

Most of the structures seen in the dog and cat are visible in **foals**, **calves**, and the **adults** of **small ruminants**, although the heart is more vertical in position. In all young mammals the **thymus** may be large and dense enough to be discernible in the cranial mediastinum.

In large adult horses and cattle, the bones and muscles of the forelimb, particularly the triceps and deltoid muscles, inevitably obscure much of the cranial region of the thorax. In co-operative horses this can be partly overcome by drawing the limb cranially. In these large animals the structures identified on lateral radiographs from the dog will be visible, but the detail will often be relatively poor. Four fields are usually needed for the thorax of an adult large **horse** (Fig. 24.7).

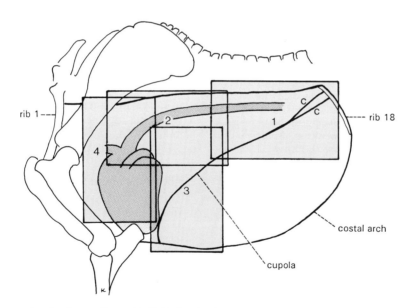

Fig. 24.7 Diagram showing four radiographic fields for the thorax of an adult horse. Field 1 shows an extensive area of lung tissue, and part of the left and right crura (c, c) and the cupola of the diaphragm. This is the best field for the assessment of peripheral lung tissue. Field 2 covers the dorsocaudal part of the heart, the great blood vessels that run dorsocaudally, the caudal end of the trachea, extensive lung tissue, and a small part of the cupola of the diaphragm. Field 3 is mainly occupied by the lung in the region of the hilus, the cupola of the diaphragm, and the caudal part of the heart. Field 4 is filled largely by the craniodorsal part of the heart, the cranial mediastinum, and the trachea. (Topographical data based on Mair and Gibbs, 1990.)

The **lung** of a large horse (Mair and Gibbs, 1990) is examined best in Fields 1 and 2 of Fig. 24.7. The herring-bone pattern of pulmonary vessels and longitudinal bronchi in peripheral lung tissue should be visible in Field 1. The bronchial cartilages are sometimes calcified, revealing the larger peripheral bronchi as fine dense linear or ring shadows. Pulmonary vessels up to the third generation can be evaluated here. Fine reticulolinear and nodular densities, perhaps partly caused by 'end-on' blood vessels, characterize the parenchyma of the normal equine lung, and are not a pathological infiltrate (Mair and Gibbs, 1990). The caudal end of the **trachea** and the major bronchi are detectable in Field 2. The region of the **hilus** of the lung, with some of the major bronchi in the form of 'end-on' rings, occurs in Field 3.

The **heart** and its **great blood vessels** are seen in Fields 2, 3, and 4. The base of the heart, aorta, and major pulmonary arteries and veins are visible in Field 2. The caudal part of the heart, including the left atrium, the larger pulmonary veins, and the caudal vena cava, are found in Field 3. The craniodorsal part of the heart and the root of the aorta are in Field 4.

The cupola of the **diaphragm** is included in Fields 1, 2, and 3, and the two crura are likely to be visible in Field 1. The **cranial mediastinum** is in Field 4.

Despite the importance of bovine respiratory disease, the radiology of the normal and diseased bovine lung seems to have received relatively little attention (Lee, 1974). Attempts to obtain radiographs of the whole of the cranial and middle lobes of the lung field have been of little value. However, fields aligned over rib 6 and half way between the caudal angle of the scapula and the olecranon process yield reasonable radiographs of the **caudal lobes** and the dorsal parts of the **middle** and **accessory lobes** (Lee, 1974). The main bronchi of the caudal and middle lobes are readily identifiable. Typical herring-bone patterns of longitudinal **bronchial branches** are visible, and these are accompanied by **pulmonary vessels** traceable to the second or third branch. The **aorta** and **caudal vena cava** can be identified. Fluid or gas may be seen in the oesophagus during eructation or regurgitation.

Bovine pulmonary diseases that induce radiographic changes (Lee, 1974) include parasitic bronchitis, bronchopneumonia, chronic pneumonia, and multiple pulmonary emboli.

Radiographs were obtained from over 100 adult standing cattle with a tentative diagnosis of **traumatic reticuloperitonitis** (Braun *et al.*, 1993). In those animals in which the diagnosis was subsequently found to be incorrect (i.e. they were apparently normal) the most cranial point of the cupola lay at or caudal to the seventh rib. A level at or cranial to the sixth rib was considered to be pathological. All these radiographs were taken just before maximum inspiration, and this may account for the rather caudal position (rib 7) of the normal diaphragm.

24.12 Recognition of pathological changes in thoracic radiographs

Abnormal radiodensity in the **lung**, either in small foci or large areas of the lung, indicates pulmonary disease. However, the recognition of abnormal density may not be easy. Nodular densities in the normal equine lung were mentioned in Section 24.11. In principle, the density of the lungs increases during normal **expiration**, and therefore the phase of the respiratory cycle (Section 24.2) should be taken into account (Grandage, 1974). Especially radiodense lungs have been reported in neonatal puppies at the end of expiration (Grandage, 1974), and this observation might be expected in **neonates** in general, during the period when the hitherto collapsed lungs undergo progressive inflation. Moreover, small carnivores in prolonged lateral recumbency because of anaesthesia or some morbid condition experience increased perfusion and thence increased radiodensity of the pendent lung, the mechanism being similar to that in the 'down' lung of large farm animals (Section 6.30.2).

Pneumothorax or **pleural effusion** can be identified.

Enlargement of one or more chambers of the **heart**, or of the **pulmonary trunk**, can be observed in various forms of **heart disease**. However, this requires interpretation of the general outline of the shadow of the heart, without the help of precise boundaries (Section 24.7.1).

Pericardial effusion may cause a generalized increase in the cardiac shadow, as opposed to a localized bulge involving a particular chamber of the heart.

Obstruction or dilation of the **oesophagus** can be detected by using a barium meal. Rupture of the **diaphragm** can be detected. **Neoplasms** tend to show as radiopaque areas.

24.13 Computed tomography

Computed tomography (computerized tomography, CT; computed axial tomography, CAT) is a development of conventional X-ray technology. A narrow beam of X-rays is passed through the tissues and impinges on a row of detectors. The source can rotate 360° around the subject, detectors being located around the full periphery. The machine looks like a huge doughnut, the subject being passed through its central aperture. Images of two-dimensional 'slices' through the body can be obtained. The detectors are also computer-processed to reconstruct adjacent two-dimensional slices into a composite three-dimensional image of a slice about 1 cm thick through the subject's body. The organs show more clearly than in conventional radiographs.

The images produced (**CT scans** or **CAT scans**) are cross-sections of the body, and are therefore similar to the views obtained by slicing the body with a band-saw (Figs 24.8, 24.9). The clinician needs a good knowledge of three-dimensional topographical relationships in order to interpret CT images.

The computation improves soft tissue contrasts and increases organ delineation, and therefore the images obtained by CT are better than those of plain radiographs. Furthermore, the region can be scanned slice by slice, often only 5 mm apart, enabling detailed analysis of an extensive region of the body. CT scanning tends to minimize the amount of radiation exposure. As in conventional radiography the images can be further enhanced by using contrast media. The equipment is usually designed for human medical use and cannot accommodate large animals such as horses and cattle, but is very useful for assessing foals, dogs and other small animals.

24.14   Ultrasonography

This imaging technique depends on the principle that high frequency sound waves selectively penetrate and are reflected by various tissues and surfaces of the body. The ultrasonic waves are emitted from a piezoelectric crystal, and confined to a narrow beam. When the beam strikes an interface between tissues of varying acoustic impedance (e.g. a boundary between muscle and blood) some or all of the sound waves are reflected back as echoes along the same plane as the beam. The echoes are converted into electrical impulses and displayed and/or recorded as images of the tissues essentially in cross-section or vertical section (**ultrasonograms**). These can be either 'stills', or continuous images of tissue movement which are particularly useful for studying cardiac function

(**echocardiograms**) (Section 24.15). Ultrasound scans conventionally display a tissue as a more or less white image on a black background.

Strong echoes appear white. **Bone** and **gas** reflect most of the sound waves at their surface, causing the surface of bone and gas to show as an intensely white line. There is no effective penetration of sound beyond this line, so structures deep to it are not imaged. Because gas cannot be penetrated, ultrasonography is not effective for the investigation of the lungs. Intermediate echoes are given by **soft tissues** in general, which therefore appear as various shades of grey, depending on the proportions of fat, fibrous tissue, and fluid. **Liquids** give no echoes at all (i.e. they are completely penetrated) and appear black. Highly reflective interfaces (bone and gas) are referred to as **echogenic** or **hyperechoic**. The moderately reflective interfaces (soft tissues) are described as **hypoechoic** or relatively **echolucent**. Non-reflective, completely penetrated, interfaces (liquids) are categorized as **echolucent** or **anechoic**.

The sound beam varies in shape, depending on the type of transducer. There are two main types of **transducer**, linear array and sector. A **linear array transducer** has crystals arranged in a line, and each crystal emits a pencil-like beam of ultrasound waves; the shape of the composite beam emitted by all the transducers together is therefore rectangular, and the entire beam is in one plane. A **sector transducer** (Fig. 24.10A) has only one crystal, which oscillates or rotates. The single crystal emits a single pencil-like beam of ultrasound one thousand times per second. The sound waves of the oscillating or rotating crystal are restricted to a fan-shaped beam in one plane, as in Fig. 24.10A; hence the term 'sector', i.e. a section of a circular area between two radii. The **plane of the beam** of either type of transducer can be selected by the operator, and is commonly horizontal (parallel to the ground) as in Fig. 24.10A, or vertical as in Fig. 24.11. For **echocardiography** a sector transducer is essential, in order to project the beam between the ribs.

The equipment incorporates sophisticated microcomputer components, as well as amplifiers for recording electrocardiograms (ECGs) and phonocardiograms (sound recordings). All the images are displayed on a video monitor. They can be recorded by a video recorder with

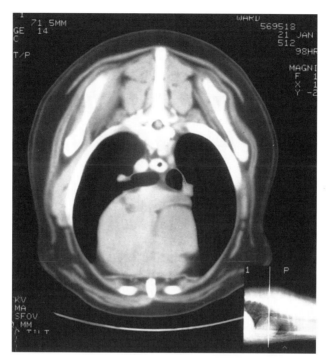

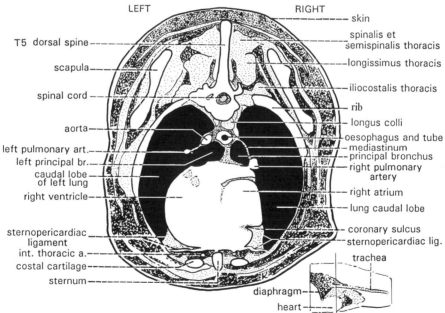

Fig. 24.8 Computed tomography scan through the thorax of a normal adult dog lying on its sternum. The craniocaudal level of the scan is shown by the vertical line on the drawing of the plain radiograph, lateral view, at bottom right. The beam has passed through the cranial third of the heart. The slice includes only the right-sided chambers of the heart, thus showing that the right and left ventricles are more craniocaudal than right–left in orientation. The space occupied by the right lung is larger than that of the left lung, reflecting the greater volume of the right lung. The heart is therefore more on the left side than the right. The tube in the oesophagus leads to an oesophageal balloon.

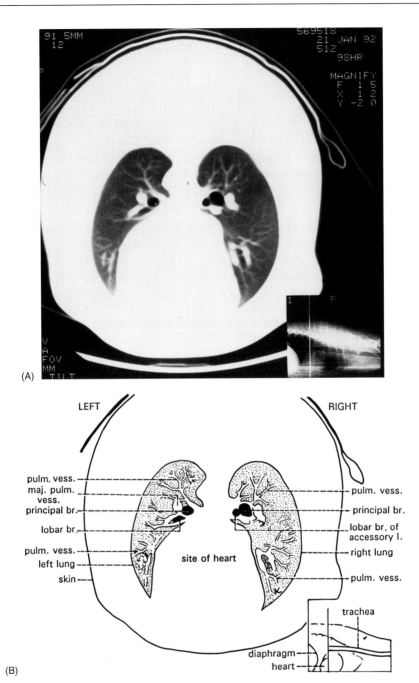

Fig. 24.9 Computed tomography scan through the thorax of the same normal dog as in Fig. 24.8. The craniocaudal level is about 4–5 cm caudal to Fig. 24.8 (see plain radiograph, the small diagram at bottom right). Computer processing has selected the lung, allowing the other tissues to be lost. The right lung is much larger than the left, displacing the heart to the left. The loop at top right is for holding the animal in the correct position. Abbreviations: br., bronchus; l., lobe; maj., major; pulm., pulmonary; vess., vessel.

freeze-frame facility for polaroid photography, or by a chart recorder using light- or heat-sensitive paper. Dimensions can be measured on photographs or chart recordings.

> The **ultrasonic waves** used for diagnosis are produced by the electrical stimulation of a **piezoelectric crystal**, which then becomes deformed and consequently emits high frequency sound waves (Barr, 1988). The crystal thus acts as a transducer or scanner. The ultrasound reflected back as echoes is detected and converted by the same transducer. The crystal emits sound in a short burst lasting only 1 μs (one millionth of a second) and is then silent for the next 999 μs while it receives the reflected sound waves; this cycle is repeated 1000 times per second. Because the time spent in transmission is so brief, very little energy is transferred to the tissues and this partly accounts for its non-injurious characteristics (O'Callaghan, 1987, p. 140).
>
> Both the *penetration of the beam* and the *quality of the image* depend on the **frequency of the sound waves**. Higher frequencies give sharper images but do not penetrate as deeply as lower frequencies. Most of the available instruments only permit imaging to depths of 20–25 cm. This is enough to examine the heart of a dog or cat, but in the horse the wall of the left ventricle may be 35–40 cm from the transducer. Therefore for the thorax of the horse, apparatus producing the lower range of frequency (2.5 MHz) is needed (O'Callaghan, 1987, p. 141).

24.15 Echocardiography

Echocardiography is the recording of the position of the walls and valves of the heart by ultrasonography. It enables the clinician to examine the walls and interior of the living heart, including the valves in motion. However, the accurate interpretation of echocardiographic images depends on being able to visualize the exact anatomy of the region of the heart through which the beam has passed.

The ultrasonic examination of the heart is obstructed by the ribs and lungs, the sound waves being unable effectively to penetrate bone and gas (Section 24.14). Therefore the beam has to be directed through an 'acoustic window'; an **intercostal space** is used to evade the ribs, and the lung can be avoided by using the **cardiac notch** (Section 5.6.2) or the **costomediastinal recess** (Section 5.7).

As stated in Section 24.14, two types of ultra-

sonic transducer are available for diagnostic purposes, namely a **linear array transducer** and a **sector transducer**. A sector transducer is essential for echocardiography in order to project the beam between the ribs. The *image* from both types of transducer can be displayed on a monitor screen in two standard forms, known as **two-dimensional scans** and **M mode images**. Both types of image can show movement by converting into **real time scans**.

24.15.1 *Two-dimensional scans (B mode)*

The image obtained by two-dimensional scans (B mode) is relatively easy to interpret, since it builds up a slice through the body in the plane of the beam. Thus a two-dimensional image of the heart resembles a complete anatomical cross-section of the heart, when the beam is horizontal as in Fig. 24.10B; if the beam is vertical, the image resembles a complete vertical slice through the heart as in Figs 24.11B and 24.15A,B. Since a sector transducer is always used for echocardiography, two-dimensional scans of the heart are also known as **sector scans**. The image on the videoscreen can be photographed with a polaroid camera, and the thickness of the ventricular walls, and/or the diameters of the ventricular lumens, can be measured on the photograph.

24.15.2 *Real time scans*

The heart changes its shape during each cardiac cycle, and this movement can be seen by continuously updating the two-dimensional (sector) images on the monitor screen. The updating of the two-dimensional images is known as **real time two-dimensional scanning** (or **real time sector scanning**), and this technique is in general use in medical and veterinary ultrasonography. The image can be arrested at any instant, and photographed with a polaroid camera. It can also be recorded on a video recorder or chart recorder.

24.15.3 *M mode scans*

The image obtained in **M mode** is more difficult to interpret, just as it is more difficult to understand how it is obtained. In essence, in M mode only a single beam is emitted. When a sector transducer

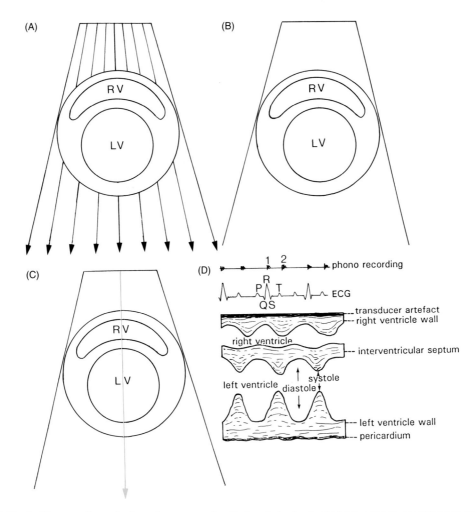

Fig. 24.10   A. Diagram of a sector transducer, scanning the heart of a dog in the horizontal plane in B mode. The scanner has a single crystal, which emits pencil-like ultrasonic beams (arrows) as it rotates. Each emission lasts 1 μs, and the crystal is then silent for 999 μs while it receives the echoes from the tissues. This cycle is repeated 1000 times per second. The beams transect the heart, and build up an anatomical image of the heart. RV, right ventricle; LV, left ventricle.

B. Diagram of the echocardiogram obtained by the scanner in A. The image is a sector (or two-dimensional) echocardiogram in the horizontal plane in B mode. It was based on a polaroid photograph of the arrested video display. It resembles an anatomical cross-section through the ventricles. RV, right ventricle; LV, left ventricle. A video display would show the movements of the ventricles during the cardiac cycle.

C. Diagram of a sector transducer scanning in M mode. As the crystal rotates in the horizontal plane, it emits a single beam of ultrasound but only when it reaches the position of the green line. RV, right ventricle; LV, left ventricle.

D. Diagram of the echocardiogram obtained by the scanner in C. The image is a sector echocardiogram in M mode in real time. The scanner is imaging the tissues only along the green line in C. Each recorded line is updated as the cycle of ventricular contractions proceeds. The updated lines are displayed adjacent to each other (as in Fig. 24.13), giving a record of the wave-like contractions of the walls of the right and left ventricles and the interventricular septum. The phonocardiogram has recorded the first and second heart sounds at the onset of ventricular systole and diastole. The diagram is based on a polaroid photograph of an arrested video display. (Diagrams A, B, and C are redrawn from Barr (1988), with permission of the author and the British Veterinary Association.)

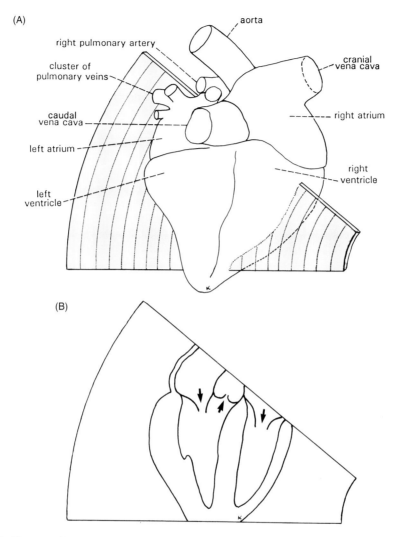

(A)

right pulmonary artery

cluster of
pulmonary veins

caudal
vena cava

left atrium

left
ventricle

aorta

cranial
vena cava

right atrium

right
ventricle

(B)

Fig. 24.11 A. **Diagram of a sector scanner, scanning a horse's heart in the vertical plane in B mode.** The vertical fan-shaped ultrasonic beam is green.

B. **Diagram of the echocardiogram obtained from the scanner in A.** The diagram was based on a polaroid photograph of the arrested video display. The image is a sector echocardiogram in the vertical plane in B mode. It resembles an anatomical section through the heart in the vertical plane. Down-going arrows, atrioventricular valves; up-going arrow, aortic valve. The video display showed the movements of the heart during the cardiac cycle. (Diagrams A and B are redrawn from material kindly supplied by M.W. O'Callaghan, 1987.)

is switched into M mode, its single crystal is allowed to emit waves at only one point on its arc of movement. This single beam is repeatedly emitted at the same point on its oscillation or rotation; such a beam is represented by the green line in Fig. 24.10C. (Similarly, when a linear array transducer is switched into M mode, only one of its crystals emits a beam and all the others are silenced.)

In Fig. 24.10C, the beam passes through the right and left ventricles at the same place at each oscillation or rotation. Wherever the beam hits tissues, it causes an echo which is recorded as a more or less bright spot depending on how echogenic that tissue happens to be. These echoes appear on the recording as a single line of bright spots. In this way, the beam from the sector transducer records the position (along the green line in Fig. 24.10C) of the tissues of the right ventricular wall, the interventricular septum, and the left ventricular wall.

But of course the ventricular walls are moving during each systole and diastole, and therefore the echo-generating points are constantly changing their position and being recorded afresh. Thus the positions of the bright spots representing the echo-generating points along the green line in Fig. 24.10C are being constantly updated. Once again, this is **real time scanning**, but this time in M mode. The apparatus displays the updated linear images adjacent to each other, as in Fig. 24.13, thus giving a picture of the movements of the tissues along this particular line throughout consecutive heart beats.

Real time M mode images in motion can be recorded on a tape or chart recorder. Those obtained in Fig. 24.10C would resemble Fig. 24.10D, and would consist of three parallel rows of saw-tooth waves. The waves represent the left and right ventricular walls and interventricular septum moving closer together during systole, and further apart during diastole. The thickness of the walls and the diameters of the heart chambers can be measured on polaroid photographs or chart recordings in M mode.

A phonocardiographic and electrocardiographic recording can be incorporated in the picture, as in Fig. 24.10D, thus enabling the cardiac cycle to be correlated with the wave-like images of the ventricular walls.

The **crucial difference between B mode and M mode** recordings is that B mode records an image of the *entire organ in section* (in this instance, the right and left ventricles in cross section): M mode

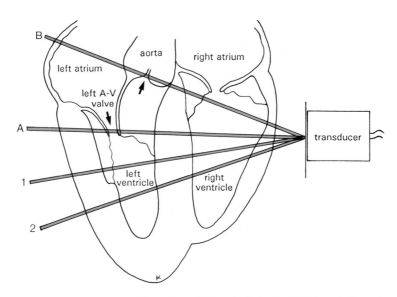

Fig. 24.12 Diagram of a sector scanner, scanning a horse's heart in the horizontal plane in M mode, with the ultrasonic beam (green) angled in four different positions. The transducer is placed on the right thoracic wall. Since the scan is in M mode, the crystal emits only a single pencil-like beam during each of its rotations, as in Fig. 24.10C. Beam A goes through the wall of the right ventricle, the interventricular septum, the two cusps of the left atrioventricular valve, and the wall of the left ventricle. This beam examines the movements of the left atrioventricular valve (Fig. 24.14A). Beam B passes through the wall of the right ventricle, the (septal) cusp of the right atrioventricular valve, the aortic valve (first through the septal semilunar valvule, and then through the left semilunar valvule), and finally through the wall of the left atrium. Beam B therefore allows the movements of the aortic valve to be observed (Fig. 24.14B). Beam 1 passes through the wall of the right ventricle, the interventricular septum, and then through the wall of the left ventricular wall; this beam is in the standard position for measuring ventricular dimensions. Beam 2 passes through the wall of the right ventricle, the interventricular septum, and finally through one or other of the two papillary muscles of the left ventricle. (Redrawn from material kindly supplied by M.W. O'Callaghan.)

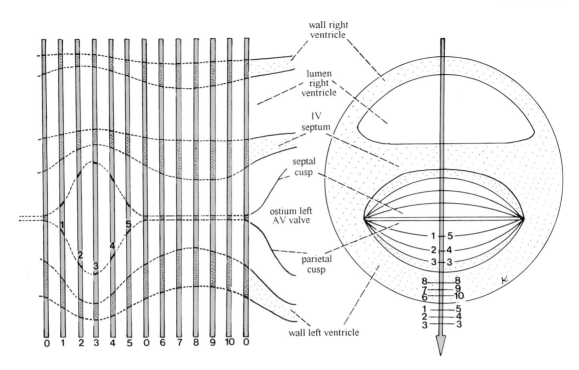

Fig. 24.13   Diagram to show how an M mode scan works. The diagram on the right shows a single M mode beam of ultrasound (green arrow), in the horizontal plane as in Fig. 24.10C. The orientation of the diagram is the same as in Figs 24.10 and 24.14, as shown by the arrows that indicate the direction of the beam in each figure. While the heart is beating, the beam is repeatedly projected along the line of the green arrow. The beam therefore enters the heart through the outer surface of the wall of the right ventricle, then goes through the lumen of the right ventricle, the interventricular septum, the septal cusp of the left A-V valve, the lumen of the left ventricle, the parietal cusp of the left A-V valve, and finally exits through the external surface of the outer wall of the left ventricle. Wherever the beam passes through the relatively thick tissue of the ventricular walls and interventricular septum, it records the echogenicity, and hence the changing positions, of this tissue (stippled areas along each of the beams in the figure on the left). It also records the changing positions of the free edges of the septal and parietal cusps.

The figure on the left is based on 13 beams projected successively during one cardiac cycle. Starting from the extreme left of the diagram, the first seven beams 0, 1, 2, 3, 4, 5, 0 occupy one ventricular diastole. These seven beams therefore record the positions of the tissues during the opening and closing of the atrioventricular valve. For example, in the diagram on the left, positions 0, 1, 2, 3 on the parietal cusp, and 0, 1, 2, 3 on the external surface of the left ventricle, record the progressive opening of the valve, whereas positions 4, 5, 0 on the parietal cusp, and 4, 5, 0 on the external surface of the left ventricle, record the progressive closing of the valve.

Beams 6, 7, 8, 9, 10, 0 on the left diagram occupy one ventricular systole. The actual orifice of the atrioventricular valve is closed throughout this part of the cardiac cycle. However, during ventricular systole the left ventricular wall at first progressively contracts and then begins to relax, so that its external surface moves slightly inwards and then outwards again. This systolic contraction of the ventricular wall is recorded in both the left and the right diagram by positions 6, 7, 8, which represent the changing positions of the external surface of the ventricle as it contracts inwards. The subsequent relaxation of the ventricular wall is represented by positions 8, 9, 10, as the external ventricular surface moves outwards.

The complete image in the left part of the diagram is built up by displaying the updated linear images, 0, 1, 2, 3, 4, 5, 0, 6, 7, 8, 9, 10, 0 adjacent to each other on the video screen. Thus image 0 is the first to appear on the screen, then image 1 is added alongside image 0, 2 is added alongside image 1, and so on.

When the emission rate of the beam is restored to the usual $1000\,s^{-1}$, the gaps between the tissues in the left diagram are filled in. The result then is an image like that shown in Fig. 24.14A, which displays the movements of the left atrioventricular valve. Polaroid photographs of the arrested video display can be taken, as in Figs 22.15A and 22.15C.

records the changing positions of *a single line of points in an organ* (in Fig. 24.10D, a line of points in the right ventricular wall, interventricular septum, and left ventricular wall).

A grasp of these general principles enables the potential of M mode echocardiography in diagnostic cardiology to be appreciated. Figure 24.12 shows the effects of altering the angle of a sector transducer, assuming that the sector is scanning in the horizontal plane. Positions 1 and 2 yield images essentially similar to Fig. 24.10B when in B mode, and Fig. 24.10D when in M mode. When the transducer is angled to position A in Fig.

24.12, the sector beam transects the two cusps of the left atrioventricular valve. The recorded images then resemble those in Fig. 24.10B when in B mode, and 24.14A when in M mode, thus revealing the opening and closing of the valve. When the transducer is in position B in Fig. 24.12 and in M mode, the beam transects the aortic valve and shows the movements of the left and septal semilunar valvules as the valve opens and closes (Fig. 24.14B). (The greater detail in Figs 24.14A and B, compared with that in Fig. 24.10D, is due to the faster speed of the chart recorder in Fig. 24.14A,B, which spreads out events in relation to

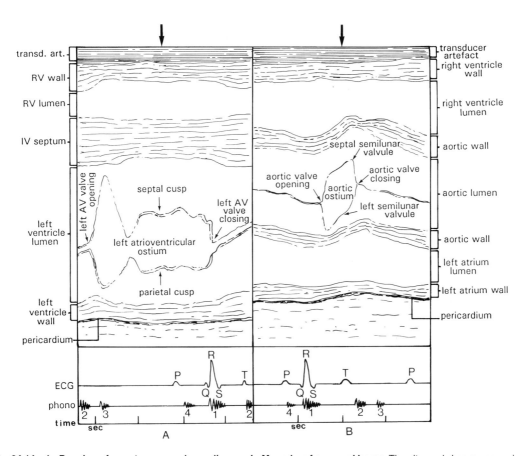

Fig. 24.14   A. Drawing of a sector scan echocardiogram in M mode, of a normal horse. The ultrasonic beam was projected in position A (horizontal plane) of Fig. 24.12. Viewed from left to right, the images reveal the opening and closing of the left atrioventricular valve. The electrocardiogram shows the timing of the cardiac cycle. The phonocardiogram records the four heart sounds (1–4). (Redrawn from a chart recording.)

   B. Sector scan echocardiogram in M mode, of a normal horse. The ultrasonic beam was projected as in position B (horizontal plane) of Fig. 24.12. Viewed from left to right, the images show the opening and closing of the aortic valve. The timing of the cardiac cycle is indicated by the electrocardiogram. The phonocardiogram records the four heart sounds (1–4). (Adapted from a chart recording kindly supplied by M.W. O'Callaghan.)

time, and of course the image is simpler in Figure 24.10D since the beam passes only through the body of the ventricles and misses the valves.) By imaging the heart from both sides of the thorax and varying the planes of the beam, it is possible to examine all the chambers, valves, and great vessels.

Abnormalities of the valves may then be detected, such as the common congenital anomaly of pulmonary stenosis. The right ventricular hypertrophy associated with pulmonary stenosis (Section 15.9) can also be observed. Acquired, as opposed to congenital, changes in cardiac dimensions can be seen and investigated by measurements. It is possible to link murmurs with abnormal valves.

Experience of echocardiography in the **dog** (Barr, 1988) shows that in this species the heart can be conveniently scanned by placing the transducer in an intercostal space over the apex beat (Section 23.11) on either the left or right side of the thorax. In this species the apex beat usually lies somewhere between the left fourth and left sixth intercostal spaces and the right fourth and fifth intercostal spaces, which would be in the general region of the **cardiac notch** on either side of the thorax (Section 5.6.2). Obstruction by the lung can be minimized by placing the dog on its left side, thus allowing the heart to subside onto the thoracic wall, and then imaging the heart from the 'down' side. In the **horse** (O'Callaghan, 1987), the recommended site for echocardiography is on the right side, at the fourth or fifth intercostal space at about the level of the olecranon process, the right leg being drawn cranially. It is found that in this position no lung tissue comes between the thoracic wall and the heart. Although this site only takes partial advantage of the right cardiac notch (which ends caudally at the fourth intercostal space), it is evidently far enough ventral to exploit the right **costomediastinal recess** (Section 9.6.2); it is conceivable that during resting breathing the ventral border of the lung would not enter this recess. The cardiac notch in the horse is considerably bigger on the left side (Section 5.6.2), but scanning the heart from the right side has the advantage of penetrating the relatively thin right ventricle before encountering the left ventricle (Fig. 24.10).

24.16 Clinical applications of echocardiography

An accurate knowledge of thoracic and cardiac anatomy is essential for obtaining and interpret-

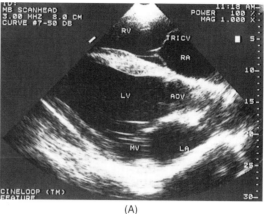

(A)

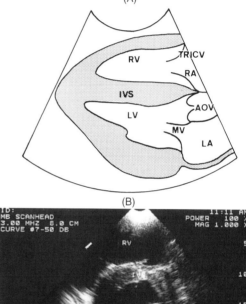

(B)

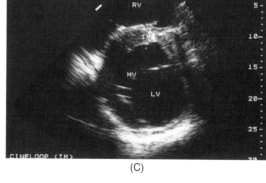

(C)

Fig. 24.15 Sector echocardiograms of the normal horse in B mode, projected from the right side of the heart. Polaroid photographs of the arrested videodisplay. AOV, aortic valve; IVS, interventricular septum; LA, left atrium; LV, left ventricle; MV, mitral valve; RA, right atrium; RV, right ventricle; TRICV, tricuspid valve. Scale, centimetres.

A. Scan in the vertical plane, as in Fig. 24.11B.

B. Diagram of the vertical scan shown in A.

C. Scan in the horizontal plane of line A in Fig. 24.12.

ing echocardiograms. **Acquired and congenital abnormalities** in all the chambers of the heart, in the valves, and in the great vessels can be examined. The Doppler effect can reveal the direction and volume of flow, as in mitral regurgitation. Pathological **cardiac dimensions** can be estimated. **Pericardial** and **pleural effusions** can be detected.

Considerable care in controlling the apparatus is needed to obtain images free of artefacts (Barr, 1988). Moreover the interpretation of images, especially in M mode, is very subjective, particularly in the measurement of dimensions (O'Callaghan, 1987, p. 147).

Congenital **aortic stenosis**, and congenital shortening and thickening of the **cusps** of the **atrioventricular valves**, can be recognised (Barr, 1988). The commonest congenital anomalies in the **dog** (Section 15.7), i.e. **pulmonary stenosis** and **patent ductus arteriosus**, are less easy to see, but the **right ventricular hypertrophy** with **pulmonary stenosis** and the **dilation of the left atrium and ventricle** which accompany a **patent ductus arteriosus** can be demonstrated (Barr, 1988). **Dilation** or **hypertrophy** of chambers can be demonstrated by direct measurements both in sector (two-dimensional) scans and in M mode scans (O'Callaghan, 1987, p. 145). Abnormal movements of the heart valves, and particularly of the cusps of the left atrioventricular valve, may be detectable. **Murmurs** can be correlated with vibration of the cusps of the left atrioventricular valve, or vibration of the valvules of the aortic valve. **Pericardial effusion** forms a conspicuous anechoic space between the ventricular wall and the strongly echogenic pericardium. **Pleural effusion** shows as an anechoic space unrelated to the contours of the heart (Barr, 1988).

The **Doppler effect** can be employed to demonstrate the actual flow of blood in arteries and veins (Blood and Studdert, 1988, p. 291; O'Callaghan, 1987, p. 142). Some of the sound waves are reflected back to the transducer by the moving blood cells. Because of the Doppler effect, the transmitted sound has a different pitch from the sound reflected from the moving blood cells, the difference being proportional to the velocity of the blood flow. The direction and flow characteristics of a blood stream can be represented on the video screen, and the volume of flow can also be estimated.

24.17   Thoracic scintigraphy

In scintigraphy (radionuclide scanning), **radioisotopes** (radionuclides) are injected intravenously, inhaled, or swallowed. The procedure is virtually risk-free for the subject, since the amount of radiation is minute.

The radioisotope emits **gamma rays**, which are detected by a gamma camera and displayed on an oscilloscope as bright dots. The resulting image, or **scintiscan**, therefore consists of an array of numerous small dots (Fig. 24.16A). Regional variations in the density and brightness of the dots correspond to regional variations in the intensity of the gamma emission. Furthermore, these variations can be quantified by computer analysis. The anatomical detail obtained by scintigraphy is inferior to that of other imaging techniques, but by revealing the distribution of the isotope and quantifying its concentration scintigraphy provides functional information that is unobtainable by the other methods of imaging.

Thoracic scintigraphy is used quite extensively to investigate the equine lung. **Lung ventilation** can be studied by introducing a radioisotope aerosol into the inspired air, and observing its distribution in a lung scintiscan; the density of dots will be relatively high where the lung is well-ventilated and relatively low at any site where ventilation is deficient (Fig. 24.16B). **Lung perfusion** can be examined in the same animal by the intravenous injection of radioactive particles of technetium. An example of a deficit in perfusion is shown in the scintiscan in Fig. 24.16C. Computer quantification of the radioactive count-rates of both ventilation and perfusion can give actual values for the **perfusion/ventilation ratio** (Section 6.29).

Although imaging by scintigraphy is of great diagnostic value in veterinary medicine, the expense of the equipment and radiation hazards are likely to confine it to the referral centre and research laboratory.

Technetium is the first element to be produced artificially and is now the most extensively used radioisotope in nuclear medicine (Blood and Studdert, 1988, pp. 898, 1015).

Photons of gamma energy are released from the radioisotope, and recorded by a gamma camera. The camera contains a large flat scintillation crystal that fluoresces at the point of each photon strike. Photomultiplier tubes behind the crystal respond to the glow by generating an electric pulse. By analysis of the strength of the signal from each tube the precise spatial origin of each photon is established. This point is displayed on an oscilloscope. Regional variations in the brightness of the image so obtained give a *qualitative* impression of the radioactivity of different regions of the lung. By computer analysis, the recorded data can be *quantified* as **count-rates**, thus giving a precise analysis of regional variations. Even the largest camera is unable to yield a single lateral view of the lung of a horse, but this difficulty can be overcome by recording a cranial and a caudal image and merging them by using a common marker on the skin (Fig. 24.16).

The value of scintigraphy in the study of **equine pulmonary disease** has been reviewed by O'Callaghan (1991a, b). It can provide functional information on **pulmonary ventilation** and **blood flow**, and hence **ventilation–perfusion matching**, and can do this over most of the surface of the lung. This is of diagnostic value in **exercise-induced pulmonary haemorrhage** (Section 17.28) and **chronic obstructive pulmonary disease** (Section 7.19). Scintigraphy can also investigate solute exchange in the **respiratory distress syndrome of the newborn** (Section 16.26.1), and **mucociliary clearance** (Section 7.17), as a complement to radiography and other lung function tests. Lung perfusion scintigraphy has been successfully used, in conjunction with plain radiography and blood-gas measurements, to demonstrate ventilation–perfusion mismatching in the cranioventral regions of the lungs in calves infected with bovine syncitial virus (Verhoeff *et al.*, 1992).

Ventilation imaging in the **horse** requires the recording of images at regular intervals while the animal inhales a technetium aerosol with particles 0.4–1.5 µm in diameter to ensure delivery to the alveoli, until equilibrium is reached; then, from equilibrium, the process is reversed until most of the gas has been eliminated. This reveals any areas of the lung with restricted ventilation and trapping of air. **Perfusion imaging** is performed by intravenous injection of albumin-aggregated technetium as particles 10–60 µm in diameter, most of which are caught in the alveolar blood capillaries. In **combined ventilation–perfusion scintigraphy**, the perfusion scans are carried out immediately after the last ventilation image has been acquired.

In most clinical cases in **horses**, the qualitative images

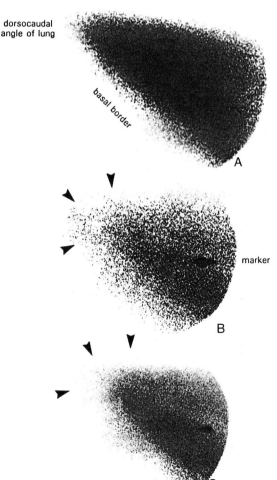

dorsocaudal angle of lung

basal border

marker

A

B

C

Fig. 24.16 A. **Scintiscan of the ventilation of the caudal part of the right lung of a normal horse.** The animal had breathed radioactive technetium aerosol with particles 0.5–1.5 µm in diameter. The head is to the right. A radioactive skin marker has enabled merging by computer of a caudal with a cranial image, to give a single image of the caudal part of the lung. The normality of the scan is evidenced by the uniform distribution of counts throughout the lung as a whole, the uniform distribution of counts along the basal border of the lung in particular, and the sharply defined distribution of counts at the dorsocaudal angle of the lung.

B. **Ventilation scintiscan of the caudal part of the right lung of a horse with a history of exercise induced pulmonary haemorrhage.** The horse had breathed a radioactive technetium aerosol, with merging of cranial and caudal images, as in A. Comparison with A shows that ventilation is deficient in the dorsocaudal angle and along the basal border of the lung.

C. **Perfusion scintiscan of the same lung as in B.** The pulmonary circulation was perfused with radioactive technetium–albumin aggregate of particle diameter 10–60 µm, with merging of cranial and caudal images as in A and B. Perfusion is deficient in the dorsocaudal angle of the lung, where ventilation is also deficient. (Scintiscans A, B, and C are from material kindly supplied by M.W. O'Callaghan.)

displaying ventilation and perfusion are sufficient for diagnosis. For example, Figs 24.16B and 24.16C, respectively, show deficient ventilation and deficient perfusion in the dorsocaudal region of the lung. However, the computer could calculate the actual ventilation/perfusion ratios, not only in this dorsocaudal region but over various parts of the surface of this lung, and display them as histograms. It is then possible to detect more subtle mismatching of regional perfusion and ventilation.

24.18   Thermography

Imaging by thermography depends on the detection of infrared radiation from the surface of the body. The instrument produces a **thermogram**, which is a map of the surface of the body using colour scales to indicate different temperatures. Areas of heat and cold may reflect relatively increased or reduced vascular perfusion. This technique has few if any applications in the diagnostic procedures on the thorax.

24.19   Magnetic resonance imaging

To perform magnetic resonance imaging (**MRI**), the body is inserted into a huge cylindrical electromagnet and exposed to short bursts of powerful magnetic fields and radio waves, which can be aimed at any selected plane of the body. The bursts stimulate protons in the hydrogen atoms of the tissues of the body to emit faint radio signals.

These radio signals are recorded and analysed by computer to produce a cross-sectional or three-dimensional image of the body, according to the strength of the signals emitted by the various tissues.

For diagnostic purposes, the signals for the images depend on the protons in the hydrogen atoms of water and on the protons in lipids and proteins. Tissues such as fat that contain a lot of hydrogen give a bright image, and those such as bone with little or no hydrogen appear black. The contrast between fat, muscle, cartilage, and bone, is good. The images resemble, in general, those obtained from CT scans, but usually give much greater contrast between normal and abnormal tissues. Again, accurate interpretation demands a good three-dimensional knowledge of topographical anatomy.

MRI equipment is very expensive to install and maintain, and is therefore unlikely to be widely used in veterinary medicine in the immediate future.

Normally the protons in the hydrogen atoms of body tissues are orientated at random, but in a powerful magnetic field they align themselves in the same direction as the magnetic lines of force. Application of the strong pulse of radio waves throws them out of alignment. After the pulse of radio waves is finished, the protons realign themselves. During realignment the protons emit faint radio signals, which are recorded by the scanner's radio wave detector and form the image.

MRI does not use ionizing radiation, and has no known adverse side effects even when performed repeatedly.

Chapter 25
Anatomical Principles of Surgical Approaches to the Thorax

25.1 Thoracocentesis

The insertion of a needle or cannula into the pleural cavity is known as thoracocentesis or pleurocentesis. The two main indications are the collection of diagnostic samples and the emergency removal from the pleural cavity of excess fluid (**pleural effusion**) or gas (**pneumothorax**). In principle, fluid is collected from the more ventral part of an intercostal space, and gas from the most dorsal available site. The site for puncturing the thoracic wall is selected (a) to minimize the risk of puncturing the pericardium or heart, (b) to maximize the chances of entering the pleural cavity, (c) to avoid penetrating the peritoneal cavity, and (d) to prevent damage to the intercostal vessels.

The sites lie from the sixth to the ninth intercostal spaces, the more caudal sites being used on the left side in order to avoid the heart (see Section 25.2). It is essential to introduce the needle craniodorsal to the **costodiaphragmatic line of pleural reflection** (Figs 23.2–23.4), since insertion caudoventral to this line will enter the peritoneal cavity (Section 23.8). The instrument is generally inserted midway between the two ribs to avoid the **intercostal nerve** and **intercostal blood vessels** (Section 8.16.2). To avoid laceration of the lungs or heart, insertion is oblique to the thoracic wall rather than at right angles.

In a standing horse the site on the right side is the seventh intercostal space, 5–10 cm dorsal to the level of the proximal end of the olecranon process. On the left a similar site is used, but at the eighth or ninth intercostal space; since the heart lies more on the left than on the right side, this more caudal site on the left avoids it. It is as well to be aware of the presence of the **superficial thoracic vein** (Section 25.3).

In the dog and cat (Rutgers, 1989) the sixth to the eighth intercostal spaces are used. With the animal standing or sternally recumbent, fluid is collected most efficiently from the ventral third of the space, and gas from the dorsal third. If the animal has to be laterally recumbent, gas is collected from the highest point on the thoracic wall.

In the dog, and sometimes in other species, the *ventral intercostal vessels* are double (Fig. 8.34), following both the cranial and the caudal borders of the distal ends of the ribs (Schummer *et al.*, 1981, Fig. 85). Therefore the intercostal space is generally pierced midway between the ribs (de Lahunta and Habel, 1986, p. 188).

In the dog and cat, **pneumothorax** is usually bilateral, but **pleural effusions** including pyothorax may be unilateral (Rutgers, 1989). Care is necessary to avoid creating an iatrogenic pneumothorax. Natural fenestrations in the mediastinum have been regarded as an explanation of bilateral pneumothorax and bilateral pleural effusions; despite controversy, it seems that very small fenestrations do occur normally in the adult dog and cat (Section 9.4).

25.2 Pericardiocentesis

Pericardiocentesis is the surgical entry into the **pericardial cavity**. This is done to collect fluid for diagnostic purposes, or to withdraw excess fluid and thereby relieve pressure within the **pericardial sac**.

Entry can be made through the ventral extremity of the left fifth intercostal or interchondral space; the interchondral space is the space between the *costal* cartilages (Fig. 5.5). In most species (though probably not the ox, see advanced text) this site utilizes the **cardiac notch**, which is larger on the left side than the right and is centred typically on the ventral quarter of the fourth rib or fourth intercostal space (Section 5.6.2, Fig. 5.5). The intercostal nerve and vessels are avoided as in thoracocentesis (Section 25.1).

Abnormal accumulations of fluid can occur in the pericardial cavity from many causes, including infections, the presence of neoplasms, and the rupture of blood vessels. The **pericardial sac** may be markedly distended, so that the **visceral** and **parietal pericardia** are widely separated by fluid. Usually the area of contact of the pericardium with the thoracic wall is then greatly increased, and this can be demonstrated by percussion, radiography, and ultrasonography. In chronic cases, the fluid may become very viscous or even solidified. The parietal pericardium may be greatly thickened.

In the ox, in which **traumatic pericarditis** is an important condition (Section 25.4), pericardiocentesis is done at the left fifth interchondral space (de Lahunta and Habel, 1986, p. 199). The observations on the **cardiac notch** by Hare (1975, p. 932) indicate that this site would be too far caudal to utilize the cardiac notch.

The accumulation of fluid in the pericardial sac tends to compress the heart by *tamponade* (Section 20.2). This may interfere with the action of the heart, leading to congestive heart failure and sudden death (Blood and Studdert, 1988, p. 895).

25.3   Thoracotomy

Thoracotomy means surgical entry into the thoracic cavity. This procedure is indicated for a variety of purposes including repair of penetrating wounds caused by slivers of wood or fractured ribs, cardiac surgery, pulmonary surgery, surgery on the oesophagus, and repair of a ruptured diaphragm.

The surgical approach is generally lateral via an intercostal space, from either the left or the right side. The intercostal space chosen depends on the organ to be approached. The cutaneus trunci, latissimus dorsi, and serratus ventralis muscles are transected. In some cases where good surgical access is needed, a part of a rib may be resected to allow the incision to be spread wider. Thoracotomy by the surgical removal of a rib is known as **thoracectomy**.

Occasionally a midline approach may be indicated, and this is done by splitting the sternum along its length, a **median sternotomy**. This provides a good bilateral view. It is indicated in some pericardial conditions, for cranial and bilateral exposure of the mediastinum and pleural cavity, and for some cranial abdominal problems such as repairing a diaphragmatic hernia, though rarely (Section 25.13).

In large animals (Fowler, 1973), the skin incision is parallel with the caudal border of triceps, beginning near the caudal border of the scapula and extending ventrally for about 45 cm. The vertical incision continues through the **cutaneus trunci** and **latissimus dorsi muscles**, which are therefore transected at right angles through their muscle fibres; the vertical incision through the **serratus ventralis**, however, is made parallel to its muscle fibres. Surgical entry through the thoracic wall causes **pneumothorax**, and a positive pressure pump (ventilator) to maintain breathing is incorporated into the circuit for gaseous anaesthesia.

In the horse, the **superficial thoracic vein** is large and runs caudodorsally across the thoracic wall, covered only by the cutaneus trunci muscle (Section 8.16.2). It is easily transected if an incision is made in the ventral quarter of the thoracic wall (Fowler, 1973). Its collateral circulation allows this vein to be ligated, if necessary. When intact, it can be used for intravenous injections in the horse. The superficial thoracic vein should also be avoided in thoracotomy in the ox.

25.4   Pericardiotomy

Pericardiotomy is the surgical incision of the **parietal pericardium**, and is sometimes required for extensive drainage and lavage (washing) of the **pericardial sac**, especially in the ox. Pericardiotomy in the ox may require *thoracectomy* (Section 25.3) of the distal part of the left fifth rib and its costal cartilage (Fig. 5.5), in order to enable a large enough opening to be made in the pericardial sac for lavage and drainage.

The anatomical relationships between the heart, diaphragm, and reticulum in the ox (Fig. 23.4) predispose to suppurative **traumatic pericarditis**. Thus the concave caudal border of the **heart** closely follows the dome of the diaphragm, and the **reticulum** is in direct contact with the caudal surface of the diaphragm; therefore the reticulum and the caudal wall of the parietal pericardium are only separated by a centimetre or two. Cattle can quite easily swallow a sharp object such as a nail or a piece of wire, which may then penetrate the reticulum and diaphragm and pierce the parietal pericardium, thus infecting the pericardial sac.

After being swallowed by a cow, a nail or piece of wire gravitates to the ventral floor of the reticulum. This can lead to **traumatic reticulitis** (Section 20.2). The powerful contractions of the reticulum that normally mix and move the ingesta can also drive a sharp object cranially into the wall of the reticulum and through the diaphragm to penetrate the parietal pericardium, particularly in the pregnant cow. The tissues are thus inoculated with a mixture of reticular ingesta and microorganisms, leading to a severe chronic infection of the pericardial sac which may cause death by a combination of congestive heart failure and bacterial toxaemia (Blood and Studdert, 1988, p. 686). Pericardiotomy may be attempted to drain and lavage the pericardial sac.

25.5   Intracardiac injection in the dog and cat

Direct injection into one of the chambers of the heart can be used for euthanasia of dogs and cats, if an intravenous injection is not possible. The **right ventricle** can be satisfactorily entered through the **fifth intercostal space** on the **right side** (Fig. 25.1).

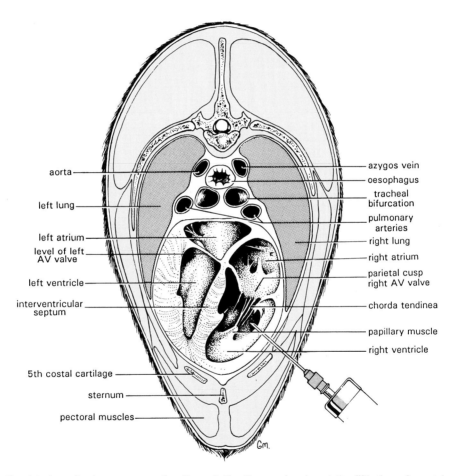

aorta

left lung

left atrium

level of left AV valve

left ventricle

interventricular septum

5th costal cartilage

sternum

pectoral muscles

azygos vein

oesophagus

tracheal bifurcation

pulmonary arteries

right lung

right atrium

parietal cusp right AV valve

chorda tendinea

papillary muscle

right ventricle

Fig. 25.1 Caudal view of a transverse section through the thorax of a dog at the fifth thoracic vertebra, showing injection of the right ventricle through the fifth intercostal space. The relatively thin wall of the right ventricle makes it easier to enter the right ventricle than the left. The needle is inserted rather obliquely in a craniodorsal direction, in the region of the costochondral junction as close as possible to the sternum. The right lung has a greater volume than the left, thus displacing the heart somewhat to the left side. The area of the heart that is in contact with the thoracic wall is therefore greater on the left side than the right, giving a larger area of cardiac dullness on the left side. The right atrioventricular valve is at a slightly more ventral level than the left valve, and this may be related to the audibility of lesions of the right valve near the costochondral junction of the right intercostal space. (Based on Habermehl (1964), with permission of the author.)

The anatomical grounds for regarding the **right ventricle** as the most easily entered chamber, and the technique for injecting it, have been carefully surveyed by Habermehl (1964). It is often said that the injection is best made into the **left ventricle**. This approach has the advantage that the heart is more on the left than the right side, and also the position of the left ventricle can often be gauged directly by feeling the apex beat. However, the left ventricle has a very thick wall and the point of the needle tends to lodge in the wall rather than the lumen. The **right ventricle**, on the other hand, has a much thinner wall (Fig. 25.1). The **atria** also have thin walls, but being more dorsal than the ventricles are deeper within the thorax and therefore less accessible. Hence the right ventricle is the best choice.

Despite the close relationship of the ventricles to the sternum, a direct ventral approach is not satisfactory. This is because the pectoral muscles are so thick ventrally that palpation of the space between the costal cartilages is very difficult. In both the dog and the cat a good place to enter the right ventricle is through the right **fifth intercostal space**, near the **costochondral junction** as close to the sternum as possible (Fig. 25.1). The needle is inserted obliquely, in a **craniodorsal** direction. A dog should be standing, or lying on its left side, but the cat is usually restrained on its left side. The fifth intercostal space may be most easily identified by counting the ribs from the thirteenth forward, especially in cats. Furthermore, in the cat the **olecranon process** is particularly close to the fifth costochondral junction, and this provides an additional landmark if the limb is placed in the normal standing position. In both the dog and cat it is also possible to enter the right ventricle through the right sixth intercostal space, but the needle must then be directed more cranially.

The length of the needle for dogs varies greatly with the breed and thinness of the animal. A length of 2–3 cm is needed for miniature dogs, about 4 cm for small, 5 cm for average, and 6 cm for large dogs, with at least 1 cm more for very fat animals. In cats it should be 4–5 cm long.

25.6   Tracheotomy: tracheal intubation

Tracheotomy in the horse is performed at tracheal rings 4–6, where the divergence of the left and right sternocephalic muscles facilitates palpation of the trachea (see Section 5.4.1). Excision of parts of two adjacent rings, rather than a complete segment of one ring, reduces the risk of tracheal collapse (Dyce *et al.*, 1987, p. 484); do not drop the bits into the trachea.

Endotracheal intubation for balanced anaesthesia is in general use in both small and large

animals. The required length of the tube depends critically on the site of the tracheal bifurcation, and the site of the tracheal bronchus in the pig and ruminants (see Section 5.4.2). The caudal end of the tube must not reach either of these sites; to do so would seal off the tracheal bronchus or (worse still) one of the two principal bronchi, thus preventing ventilation of these bronchi and creating a major venous-to-arterial shunt (Section 6.30).

25.7   Transtracheal aspiration

Samples of secretions in the trachea can be obtained by transtracheal aspiration in all the domestic species. These secretions have been transported by the **mucociliary escalator** (Section 7.2), and it has therefore been assumed that their constituents may have come from any part of the lower respiratory tract from the trachea to the alveoli. Examination of the cytological, microbiological, and physical characteristics of such secretions has therefore been regarded as of diagnostic value in diseases of the lung itself, but experiments suggest that tracheal aspirates may not represent bronchoalveolar characteristics.

The procedure for aspirating tracheal secretions is based on the insertion of a needle, or in large animals a trocar and cannula, into the cervical trachea in the midline, towards the cranial end of the neck where the trachea is relatively easy to palpate (Section 5.4). It is important to penetrate through an **annular ligament** (Section 5.3.2) and not to traumatize any cartilages, since this can lead to proliferative and hence obstructive changes in the cartilage. A catheter is passed through the needle or trocar and down the trachea as far as the **tracheal bifurcation**, which is related to about the fifth rib or fifth intercostal space (Section 5.2). Saline is introduced through the catheter into the trachea, immediately cranial to the bifurcation. The catheter is then withdrawn to the thoracic inlet; here the trachea is at its most ventral level (Section 5.2; Fig. 25.2). Therefore the fluid pools in this pendent part of the trachea, and can be aspirated from it. An alternative site for inserting the needle is through the **cricothyroid ligament**. This has the advantage of avoiding closure of the catheter by being nipped between tracheal rings.

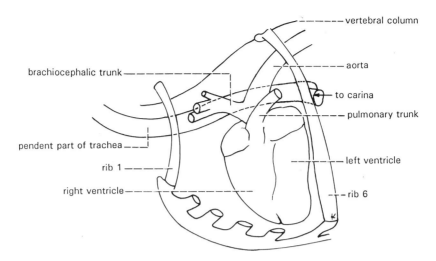

Fig. 25.2   Diagram of the thoracic trachea of the horse, showing its curvature and relations to the ribs and heart. The most ventral part of the trachea occurs almost at the thoracic inlet, a little distance cranial to the first rib. Caudal to this point, the thoracic trachea rises dorsally to lie on the dorsal aspect of the base of the heart. At about the level of the fifth or sixth intercostal space it divides at the carina into the left and right principal bronchi. In transtracheal aspiration, the catheter is advanced until it strikes the carina. It is then withdrawn slightly and the lavage fluid is released. The fluid runs cranially down the sloping trachea and pools in the most pendent part, from which it can then be aspirated.

The validity of the assumption that the cytology of a transtracheal aspirate represents the cell population of the airways within the lung itself has been questioned, at least for the horse. It has been found that the cell population of transtracheal aspirates is not representative of the cell population revealed by **bronchoalveolar lavage** in the same horses (Derksen *et al.*, 1989). It was therefore concluded that the cytological examination of transtracheal aspirates is of limited diagnostic value in horses with chronic lung disease, but bronchoalveolar lavage (Section 25.8) may be a useful diagnostic aid in such cases.

25.8   Bronchoscopy: bronchoalveolar lavage: bronchial biopsy: removal of bronchial foreign bodies

Advances in fibre optics have led to the development of flexible endoscopes, specially designed as **bronchoscopes**, which can be inserted down the trachea for examining the interior of the **tracheobronchial tree** (Fig. 25.3) in large and small domestic mammals for diagnostic and therapeutic purposes (Section 5.10). The images are usually displayed on a video screen and can be recorded. The instrument can find **lesions**, and locate **foreign bodies** (Section 5.10.2). In the horse

the latter have ranged from a raspberry cane 70 cm long, to (reported in good faith, apparently) a live frog, though this may have got in as a tadpole. The bronchoscope can also be used to estimate the velocity of **mucociliary transport** (Section 7.4) by instilling a drop of dye on the mucus and measuring the rate of transit visually.

A bronchoscope can incorporate facilities for **transtracheal aspiration** at the caudal end of the trachea (as in Section 25.7). For **bronchoalveolar lavage** the tip of the bronchoscope is passed into a bronchus, and then used to infuse and aspirate saline. The cytological and other data obtained by bronchoalveolar lavage are likely to be particularly valuable in the diagnosis of pulmonary disease (Section 25.7).

The bronchoscope can also carry jaws for taking a **biopsy** of the **tracheobronchial mucosa**, and a snare for removing **foreign bodies**.

The bronchoscope is inserted through the laryngeal airway, but the procedure varies according to the availability or otherwise of space for the tube in the nasal cavity, and the remarkable differences in the **laryngeal reflexes** in the various domestic species (Section 4.15.1).

In the horse (D.C. Knottenbelt, personal communication, 1995; Derksen, 1990), there is plenty of space in the

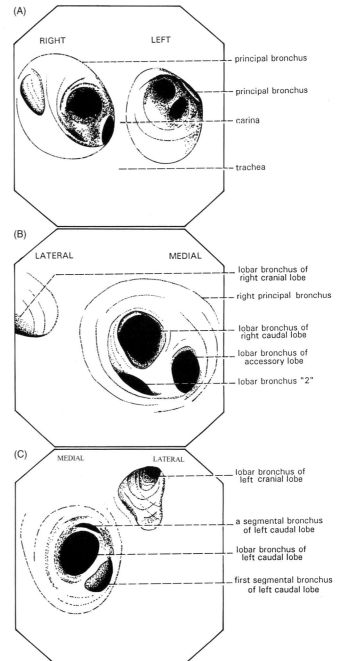

(A)

RIGHT   LEFT

— principal bronchus

— principal bronchus

— carina

— trachea

(B)

LATERAL   MEDIAL

— lobar bronchus of
right cranial lobe

— right principal bronchus

— lobar bronchus of
right caudal lobe

— lobar bronchus of
accessory lobe

— lobar bronchus "2"

(C)

MEDIAL   LATERAL

— lobar bronchus of
left cranial lobe

— a segmental bronchus
of left caudal lobe

— lobar bronchus of
left caudal lobe

— first segmental bronchus
of left caudal lobe

Fig. 25.3 Bronchoscope views obtained from a normal horse. Bear in mind that the bronchoscope sees the lung in a *caudal* direction, so that the right bronchus is on the viewer's left side.

A. **Division of the trachea into the right and left principal bronchi at the carina.** The total aperture of the right principal bronchus (including its cranial lobar bronchus) is substantially greater than that of the left. The left principal bronchus diverges obliquely from the carina.

B. **Right principal bronchus.** Lobar bronchus "2" goes *laterally* to the *caudal* lobe, and is bronchus (2) in Fig. 5.4. The 'lobar bronchus of right caudal lobe' is bronchus 3 in the right lung of Fig. 5.4. The 'lobar bronchus of right cranial lobe' is bronchus 1 of the right lung in Fig. 5.4.

C. **Left principal bronchus.**

ventral nasal meatus and therefore the bronchoscope passes easily through the nasal cavity. Moreover, the threshold of mechanoreceptor sensitivity of the laryngeal mucosa of the horse is so high that no anaesthesia is needed, local or general; the first and only response of the animal is a cough when the tip of the instrument strikes the **carina**, and at this point local anaesthetic can be sprayed from the tip onto the mucosa. In the ox, insertion through the nasal cavity is difficult because of lack of space, but it is possible. The mechanosensitivity of the bovine larynx is quite high, but the animal may cough and this can be relieved by a spray of local anaesthetic. In the pig the form of the nasal conchae leaves altogether insufficient space, so insertion through the nasal cavity is impossible. Insertion is therefore performed through the mouth under general anaesthesia. The laryngeal aditus of the pig is extremely sensitive, and hence the aditus is sprayed with local anaesthetic before laryngeal entry. In the dog and cat the bronchoscope is inserted through the oral cavity under general anaesthesia. In the cat, however, laryngeal mechanosensitivity is so extreme that the aditus must be sprayed with local anaesthetic before entering the larynx; otherwise dangerous laryngeal spasm is likely.

If a sample of tracheal secretions is taken, the procedure for infusing fluid is as for tracheal aspiration (Section 25.7), i.e. the saline should be released immediately cranial to the carina and collected at the pendent part of the trachea. **Bronchoalveolar lavage** is conducted (for example in the horse) by passing the bronchoscope through about twelve generations of bronchi, until the tip of the instrument jams in a bronchial lumen. This seals the entrance to a terminal component of the bronchial tree; as much as 300 ml of saline is then infused (Derksen *et al.*, 1989) and subsequently aspirated.

It has been found (McGorum *et al.*, 1993) that there are no regional variations within the lung in the volumes, cell counts, and concentrations of albumin or urea in samples of bronchoalveolar fluid of normal horses and horses with chronic obstructive respiratory disease. Therefore a single sample of bronchoalveolar fluid may be representative of the lungs as a whole.

The insertion of the bronchoscope through the nasal cavity in the largest species contaminates the instrument with nasal secretions, thereby obscuring the results of bronchoalveolar lavage. This difficulty can be overcome by introducing an endotracheal tube and then using this as a conduit for the bronchoscope.

The need for accurate identification of individual bronchi during bronchoscopy (Amis and McKiernan, 1986) has prompted a reconsideration of the terminology of **bronchi** in the dog (Section 5.10.1). Figure 9.3 shows the segmental bronchi of the dog as derived by these authors from their bronchoscopic observations.

The high mechanoreceptor threshold of the equine larynx presumably contributes to the entry of extraordinary foreign bodies into the tracheobronchial tree of horses. Brown and Collier (1983) reported the bronchoscopic finding and subsequent removal from the right principal bronchus of a 400 kg horse of a thorny raspberry cane '70 cm long'. Doubtless suspecting that 'cm' would be regarded as a misprint for 'mm', the authors wisely included a photograph of the cane, plus a ruler. They pointed out that, since the topographical relationship between the soft palate and larynx of the horse precludes mouth breathing, tracheobronchial foreign bodies presumably must enter via the nostril;

the thorns of the raspberry cane would act like a one-way ratchet, similar to the awns of the grain-sheath of grasses with well-known invasive powers. Evidently the owner of this horse was not in the habit of looking at it daily.

25.9 Pleuroscopy

Pleuroscopy is a diagnostic technique in which the **pleural cavity** is directly examined with a rigid or flexible endoscope. It provides details of pathological changes that may not be fully disclosed by radiography and ultrasonography. These include abscesses of the lung or pleura, pleural adhesions, intrathoracic tumours, and mycotic plaques, and presumably diaphragmatic hernia. It can also be used to take fluid samples or precise areas of lung or pleura for biopsy. Although not widely used in veterinary practice, the technique has been successfully employed on horses.

In the standing horse the thoracic wall is entered under local anaesthesia. An intercostal space is selected to reveal the site of a suspected lesion or to give a general view of the pericardium, diaphragm, and mediastinum. The tenth or eleventh intercostal space, at about the mid-point dorsoventrally, is suitable for a general examination of the pleural cavity. Entry is best made midway between the ribs, to avoid the **intercostal vessels and nerve** (Section 25.1). Air is admitted to collapse the lung on the operated side. Unilateral pneumothorax reveals the diaphragm, the heart beating within the pericardium, and the dorsal region of the caudal mediastinum containing the aorta, oesophagus, and dorsal and ventral vagal trunks. The visceral pleura and the surface of the lung can be examined. When a flexible endoscope is used, the objective can be turned to view the parietal pleura. If the lung is sufficiently collapsed, the thoracic inlet is visible cranially.

Pleuroscopy in the horse has been described by Mackey and Wheat (1985). The deliberate creation of a unilateral pneumothorax appears risky, because there are fenestrations in the mediastinum of the horse (Section 9.4). However, in a series of 15 horses, contralateral pneumothorax did not occur. At the end of the procedure the air is sucked out from the opened pleural cavity before the wound is closed.

25.10   Percutaneous lung biopsy

In percutaneous lung biopsy, a core of lung paren-chyma is obtained by inserting a suitable biopsy needle through the thoracic wall and into the lung. Histological details of pathological changes within the lung parenchyma itself can thus be obtained. This can be done in all the domestic species.

In the horse (Schatzmann *et al.*, 1974) the biopsy can be taken at the seventh or eighth left or right intercostal space, on or dorsal to the level of the shoulder joint (a point well dorsal to the **superficial thoracic vein**). This site yields a biopsy from the caudal third of the **caudal (diaphragmatic) lobe** of the lung.

After a small vertical incision through the skin under general or local anaesthesia, a trocar containing a stylet is inserted through the **intercostal muscle** and **parietal pleura**. While the end of the trocar is pressed against the **visceral pleura** to prevent **pneumothorax**, the stylet is removed and the hollow bit of the electric drill is introduced into the trocar. The bit has an internal diameter of about 5 mm, and is driven into the lung to a depth of up to 6 cm. After the drill is detached, a syringe is connected to the bit and the biopsy is aspirated. After some local haemorrhage, the biopsy site in the lung closes spontaneously by repair tissue in the parenchyma and pleura. Biopsy needles can avoid drills altogether.

25.11   Lung lobectomy

In species such as the dog, cat, and ox, in which the lobes of the lung are particularly well sepa-rated, a **lobar bronchus** and its accompanying **pulmonary artery** and **vein** (Section 5.6) can be isolated and ligated at the **hilus** (Section 5.5) and the whole lobe removed. In principle, surgery of the lung absolutely necessitates ligation of any severed bronchi, since an opened bronchus allows air to escape into the pleural cavity and causes **pneumothorax** (Section 10.3). Leaks through al-veoli and small bronchi seal themselves.

The indications for lobectomy include torsion of a lung lobe (Section 5.10.5), neoplasia, penetrating wounds, and abscesses.

Resection of pulmonary **segments**, as in man, is not a routine procedure in veterinary surgery (Section 5.10.4). However, partial lobectomy is possible in the large do-mestic mammals (Fowler, 1973), for example removal of the peripheral tip of a lobe. This requires ligation of the

bronchus and accompanying vessels at the point to be removed, followed by freeing of the parenchyma by dis-section along available **interlobular septa** (Section 5.8), ligating transected airways and blood vessels. Although lobectomy is not feasible in the horse due to the lack of discrete lobes, *partial* lobectomy of the **cranial (apical) lobe** is possible (Fowler, 1973).

Puncture wounds and lacerations of the lungs can be repaired (Fowler, 1973). The degree of bronchial involvement should be established by applying warm saline to the damaged surface of the lung to detect leaks; it may be necessary to dissect the area and ligate its bronchus. Lacerations of the borders of the lungs may require ligation of relatively large leaks; the incised lung margin can then be closed over by sutures to prevent further leakage. Despite the supposed thickness of the **visceral pleura** in both the horse and ox (Section 9.2), that of the horse is not strong enough to anchor simple sutures.

25.12   Transthoracic oesophagotomy

The sites at which large swallowed objects tend to stick in the oesophagus in the domestic species depend largely on anatomical factors. Potential bottlenecks are: (i) the junction between **pharynx** and oesophagus; (ii) the **thoracic inlet**, where all the structures entering and leaving the thorax must pass between the first pair of ribs; (iii) a point just cranial to the **base of the heart**, where the heart, great arteries and veins, trachea, and oesophagus all compete for space, and where the thorax itself is still narrow; and (iv) the **oesopha-geal hiatus** in the diaphragm (Fig. 8.24).

In the dog and cat, an obstruction of the tho-racic oesophagus can be relieved by exposing the oesophagus through the thoracic wall. The oesophagus goes through the **oesophageal hiatus** of the diaphragm (Section 8.11.6) in the midline at about the level of the dorsal quarter of the **tenth** rib. This site can be exposed between ribs 7 and 8 on the left side.

However, there are obvious anatomical difficul-ties in this approach. The oesophagus is deep within the thorax, and whilst this does not prevent incision of the oesophagus the subsequent sutur-ing of it is difficult. The dorsal and ventral **vagal trunks** (Section 3.11.1) are also major hazards, since these lie directly on the oesophagus here; cutting both of them can cause serious gastrointestinal disturbance (Section 3.15.3). A pump will have to be used to maintain breathing during the operation, and the expanding and contracting lung will get in the way.

Usually, obstruction of the thoracic oesophagus in these species is relieved by less heroic methods, such as pushing the obstruction onwards into the stomach or pulling it out through an incision in the base of the neck near the thoracic inlet. Surgery at the thoracic inlet requires attention to the relations of the oesophagus to the **common carotid artery**, **vagosympathetic trunk**, **recurrent laryngeal nerve**, and **internal jugular vein** (Fig. 5.1; Section 5.2), and to the presence of the **pleural cupola** (Section 9.6.5). The cupola may be entered accidentally during surgery at the thoracic inlet or by a penetrating wound, leading to pneumothorax and collapse of a lung.

In the ox and horse, the commonest sites of oesophageal obstruction in order of incidence are (i), (ii), and (iv), as above. The commonest sites in the dog are (iv) and (iii), followed by any part of the cervical oesophagus. The tendency for dogs to bolt their food, including large pieces of largely unchewed meat and hard materials such as pieces of bone, makes them liable to oesophageal obstruction (Dyce *et al.*, 1987, p. 387); dogs are particularly likely to do this if anyone tries to take these bits away, whereas cats usually take a more philosophical view of such inconsiderate human interference.

25.13   Diaphragmatic hernia

Diaphragmatic hernia occurs in all the domestic mammals. Usually it results from a sudden drastic increase in intra-abdominal pressure caused by trauma, and is then known as **traumatic diaphragmatic hernia**; the rupture is typically through a tear in the muscle of the diaphragm.

Congenital diaphragmatic hernias have been recorded, though relatively rarely, in calves, dogs, and cats. Three forms are recognized (Section 8.14), **pleuroperitoneal hernia**, **hiatus hernia**, and **pericardioperitoneal hernia**.

The developmental causes of the three conditions are considered in Section 8.15.

There are no pathognomonic clinical signs for diaphragmatic hernia, but the commonest sign is dyspnoea, since a breach in the diaphragm allows the fall in pressure in the pleural cavity during inspiration to be dispersed in the peritoneal cavity (Burton and White, 1997). In small animals the breach is usually the result of blunt trauma, which may directly damage the lung and may in itself produce ventilation–perfusion mismatching. However, in the dog and cat digestive disturbances may predominate, such as intermittent vomiting due to gastrointestinal entrapment or icterus due to biliary obstruction. In the ox the most common sign is *bloat*, due to herniation of the reticulum.

If the intra-abdominal pressure is severely raised, as when the wheel of a motor car passes over the abdomen of a dog or cat, the diaphragm may give way anywhere. However, the penetration by abdominal viscera usually occurs through the muscle of the diaphragm, rather than through its tendon or natural openings (the **aortic** or **oesophageal hiati**, and the **caval foramen**) (de Lahunta and Habel, 1986, p. 201). Tears in the muscle are usually ventral, and are either circumferential, radial, or both together (Burton and White, 1997). The liver is the organ most often herniated, but the stomach, small intestine, spleen, and great omentum are commonly included.

Surgical repair of a diaphragmatic hernia is possible via the thorax, but the access for suturing the diaphragm is rather restricted, even after removal of a rib or median sternotomy. In the dog and cat, repair is generally carried out through a midline incision in the abdominal wall (Burton and White, 1997). The approach may also be paracostal (Professor C.J. Gaskell, personal communication, 1995). In large farm animals the diaphragm can be repaired through a median sternotomy, though a simultaneous laparotomy may be needed for withdrawing viscera from the pleural cavity (Fowler, 1973).

Hiatus hernia is a common condition in man and is sometimes congenital, but otherwise develops from unknown causes in obese people. It also occurs in the dog.

References

Abbas, A.K., Lichtman, A.H. and Pober, E.S. (1994) *Molecular and Cellular Immunology*. Saunders, London.

Abdel-Magied, E.M. and King, A.S. (1978) The topographical anatomy and blood supply of the carotid body region of the domestic fowl. *J. Anat.* **126**, 535–546.

Abdel-Magied, E.M. and King, A.S. (1982) Effects of distal vagal ganglionectomy and midcervical vagotomy on the ultrastructure of axonal elements in the carotid body of the domestic fowl. *J. Anat.* **134**, 85–89.

Abdel-Magied, E.M., Tahaa, A.A.M. and King, A.S. (1982) An ultrastructural investigation of a baroreceptor zone in the common carotid artery of the domestic fowl. *J. Anat.* **135**, 463–473.

Abu-Hijleh, M.F. and Scothorne, R.J. (1996) Studies on haemolymph nodes. IV. Comparison of the route of entry of carbon particles into parathymic nodes after intravenous and intraperitoneal injection. *J. Anat.* **188**, 565–573.

Acker, H. and Xue, D. (1995) Mechanisms of O_2 sensing in the carotid body in comparison with other O_2-sensing cells. *News Physiol. Sci.* **10**, 211–216.

Ackerknecht, E. (1943) Das Eingeweidesystem. In *Ellenberger-Baum: Handbuch der Vergleichenden Anatomie der Haustiere*, 18th edn. (ed. O. Zietzschmann, E. Ackerknecht and H. Grau), Section IIIC. Springer, Berlin.

Adams, W.E. (1958) *The Comparative Morphology of the Carotid Body and Carotid Sinus*. Thomas, Springfield.

Adrian, E.D. (1933) Afferent impulses in the vagus and their effect on respiration. *J. Physiol.* **79**, 332–358.

Agostoni, E. (1964) Action of respiratory muscles. In *Handbook of Physiology: Respiration* (ed. W.O. Fenn and H. Rahn), Section 3, Vol. 1, Chapt. 12. American Physiological Society, Washington D.C.

Agostoni, E. and Mead, J. (1964) Statics of the respiratory system. In *Handbook of Physiology: Respiration* (ed. W.O. Fenn and H. Rahn), Section 3, Vol. 1, Chapt. 13. American Physiological Society, Washington D.C.

Akbar, S.J., Derksen, F.J., Billah, A.M. and Werney, U. (1994) Exercise induced pulmonary haemorrhage in racing camels. *Vet. Rec.* **135**, 624–625.

Alberts, B., Bray, D., Lewis, J., Raff, M., Roberts, K. and Watson J.D. (1983) *Molecular Biology of the Cell*. Garland Publishing, New York.

Allam, M.W., Lee, D.G., Nulsen, F.E. and Fortune, E.A. (1952) The anatomy of the brachial plexus of the dog. *Anat. Rec.* **114**, 173–180.

Amis, T.C. and McKiernan, B.C. (1986) Systematic identification of endobronchial anatomy during bronchoscopy in the dog. *Am. J. Vet. Res.* **47**, 2649–2657.

Amoroso, E.C., Bell, F.R., King, A.S. and Rosenberg, H. (1951) The aortic and sinus nerves of the lion and badger. *J. Anat.* **85**, 411.

Amory, H., Desmecht, D., Linden, A., McEntee, K., Rollin, F., Genicot, B., Beduin, J.-M. and Lekeux, P. (1993) Growth-induced haemodynamic changes in healthy Friesian calves. *Vet. Rec.* **132**, 426–434.

Anon. (1993). What was your diagnosis. *In Practice* **15**, 148.

Arey, L.B. (1958). *Developmental Anatomy* 6th edn. Saunders, Philadelphia.

Arthur, G.H., Noakes, D.E. and Pearson, H. (1982) *Veterinary Reproduction and Obstetrics* 5th edn. Baillière Tindall, London.

Ask-Upmark, E. (1935) The carotid sinus and the cerebral circulation. *Acta Psychiat. Neuro. Scand.* Suppl. VI.

Attwell, D. (1986) The physical chemistry of acid–base balance. In *Acid–Base Balance* (ed. R. Hainsworth), Chapt. 1. Manchester University Press, Manchester.

Atwal, O.S. and Minhas, K.J. (1992) In vivo interaction of cationised ferritin with the surface coat and endocytosis by pulmonary intravascular macrophages: a tracer kinetic study. *J. Anat.* **181**, 313–325.

Aviado, D.M. (1965) The bronchial circulation. In *The Lung Circulation: Physiology*. Vol. 1. Pergamon Press, London.

Baier, H. (1986) Functional adaptations of the bronchial circulation. *Lung* **164**, 247–257.

Bailey, C.S., Kitchell, R.L., Haghighi, S.S. and Johnson, R.D. (1984) Cutaneous innervation of the thorax and abdomen of the dog. *Am. J. Vet. Res.* **45**, 1689–1698.

Bal, H.S. (1977) The skin. In *Duke's Physiology of Domestic Animals* 9th edn. (ed. M.J. Swenson), Chapt. 38. Comstock, Ithaca.

Baldwin, B.A. and Bell, F.R. (1963) The anatomy of the cerebral circulation of the sheep and ox. The dynamic distribution of the blood supplies by the carotid and vertebral arteries to cranial regions. *J. Anat.* **97**, 203–215.

Banks, W.J. (1981) *Applied Veterinary Histology*. Williams and Wilkins, London.

Bannister, L.H. (1996) Haemolymphoid system. In *Gray's Anatomy* 38th edn. (ed. P.W. Williams, L.H. Bannister, M.M. Berry, P. Collins, M. Dyson, J.E. Dussek and M.W.J. Ferguson), Chapt. 9. Churchill Livingstone, Edinburgh.

Barclay, A.E., Franklin, K.J. and Prichard, M.M.L. (1944) *The Foetal Circulation and Cardiovascular System, and the Changes that they Undergo at Birth.* Blackwell, Oxford.

Baron, D.N. (ed.) (1994). *Units, Symbols, and Abbreviations* 5th edn. Royal Society of Medicine Press, London.

Baron, R., Jänig, W. and McLachlan, E.M. (1985) On the anatomical organization of the lumbosacral sympathetic chain and the lumbar splanchnic nerves of the cat – Langley revisited. *J. Autonom. nerv. Syst.* **12**, 289–300.

Barone, R. (1986) *Anatomie Comparée des Mammifères Domestique*, Vol. 1, Osteologie. Vigot, Paris.

Barone, R. (1996) *Anatomie Comparée des Mammifères Domestique*, Vol. 5, Angiologie. Vigot, Paris.

Barr, F. (1988) Diagnostic ultrasound in small animals. *In Practice* **10**, 17–25.

Barr, M.L. and Kiernan, J.A. (1983) *The Human Nervous System: an Anatomical Viewpoint.* Harper and Row, Philadelphia.

Bass, P., Code, C.F. and Lambert, E.H. (1961) Electric activity of gastroduodenal junction. *Am. J. Physiol.* **201**, 587–592.

Baumel, J.J. (1993) Systema cardiovasculare. In *Handbook of Avian Anatomy: Nomina Anatomica Avium* 2nd edn. (ed. J.J. Baumel, A.S. King, J.E. Breazile, H.E. Evans and J.C. Vanden Berge), Nuttall Ornithological Club, Cambridge, Mass.

Belardinelli, L. and Shryock, J.C. (1992) Does adenosine function as a retaliatory metabolite in the heart. *News Physiol. Sci.* **7**, 52–56.

Bellairs, A. d'A. and Attridge, J. (1975) *Reptiles.* Hutchinson, London.

Berry, M., Bannister, L.H. and Standring, S.M. (1995) Nervous system. In *Gray's Anatomy* 38th edn. (ed. P.W. Williams, L.H. Bannister, M.M. Berry, P. Collins, M. Dyson, J.E. Dussek and M.W.J. Ferguson), Chapt. 8. Churchill Livingstone, Edinburgh.

Bers, D.M. (1989) SR Ca loading in cardiac muscle preparations based on rapid cooling contractures. *Am. J. Physiol.* **256**, C109–120.

Bevan, J.A. (1967) The pulmonary artery baroreceptor region. In *Baroreceptors and Hypertension* (ed. P. Kezdi), pp. 69–73. Pergamon Press, Oxford.

Bezuidenhout, A.J. (1993) The lymphatic system. In *Miller's Anatomy of the Dog* 3rd edn. (ed. H.E. Evans), Chapt. 13. Saunders, Philadelphia.

Billman, G.E. (1992) Cellular mechanisms for ventricular fibrillation. *News Physiol. Sci.* **7**, 254–259.

Biscoe, T.J. and Duchen, M.R. (1990) Monitoring PO$_2$ by the carotid chemoreceptor. *News Physiol. Sci.* **5**, 229–233.

Biscoe, T.J., Lall, A. and Sampson, S.R. (1970) Electron microscopic and electrophysiological studies on the carotid body following intracranial section of the glossopharyngeal nerve. *J. Physiol.* **208**, 133–152.

Bishop, S.P. and van Vleet, J.F. (1979) Reaction of the myocardium to injury. In *Spontaneous Animal Models of Human Disease* (ed. E.J. Andrews, W.C. Ward and N.H. Altman), Vol. 1, Chapt. 20. Academic Press, New York.

Bland, P.W. and Whiting, C.V. (1993) Differential control of major histocompatibilty complex class-ii i- e-alpha-k protein expression in the epithelium and in subsets of lamina propria antigen-presenting cells of the gut. *Immunology* **79**, 107–111.

Blood, D.C. and Studdert, V.P. (1988) *Baillière's Comprehensive Veterinary Dictionary.* Baillière Tindall, London.

Bock, W.J. (1974) The avian skeletomuscular system. In *Avian Biology.* (ed. D.S. Farner and J.R. King), Vol. 1, Chapt. 3. Academic Press, New York.

Bocking, D. (1993) Effects of chronic hypoxaemia on circulatory control. In *Fetus and Neonate: Physiology and Clinical Applications.* Vol. 1, The Circulation (ed. M.A. Hanson, J.A.D. Spencer and C.H. Rodeck), Chapt. 9. Cambridge University Press, Cambridge.

Boehmer, H. von and Kisielow, P. (1991) How the immune system learns about self. *Sci. Am.* **265**, 74–81.

Booyse, F.M. and Rafelson, M.E. (1972) Regulation and mechanism of platelet aggregation. *Am. N.Y. Acad. Sci.* **201**, 37–60.

Bornemeier, W.C. (1960) Sphincter protecting haemorrhoidectomy. *Am. J. Proctol.* **11**, 48–52.

Boss, J. and Green, J.H. (1954) An histological investigation of six baroreceptor areas of the right common carotid artery in the cat. *J. Anat.* **88**, 569.

Bowsher, D. (1988) *Introduction to the Anatomy and Physiology of the Nervous System* (5th edn). Blackwell, Oxford.

Boyd, J.D. (1937) The development of the human carotid body. *Contrib. Embryol. Carnegie Inst.* **26**, 3–31 (cited by Comroe, 1964).

Brackenbury, J.H. (1984) Physiological responses of birds to flight and running. *Biol. Rev.* **59**, 559–575.

Braun, U., Fluckiger, M. and Nageli, F. (1993) Radiography as an aid in the diagnosis of traumatic reticuloperitonitis. *Vet. Rec.* **132**, 103–109.

Breazile, J.E. (1971) *Textbook of Veterinary Physiology.* Lea and Febiger, Philadelphia.

Breeze, R.G. and Wheeldon, E.B. (1977) The cells of the pulmonary airways. *Am. Rev. Resp. Dis.* **116**, 705–777.

Brodal, A. (1981) *Neurological Anatomy in Relation to Clinical Medicine* 3rd edn. Oxford University Press, New York.

Brodal, P. (1992) *The Central Nervous System: Structure and Function.* Oxford University Press, New York.

Brody, J.S., Klempfner, G., Staum, M.M., Vidyasagar, D., Kuhl, D.E. and Waldhausen, J.A. (1972) Mucociliary clearance after lung denervation and bronchial transection. *J. Appl. Physiol.* **32**, 160–164.

Broman, I. (1905) *Ergebn. Anat. Entwicklungsgesch.* **15**, 332–409 (cited by Arey, 1958).

Brooks, D.P. (1997) Endothelia: the 'prime suspect' in kidney disease. *News Physiol. Sci.* **12**, 83–89.

Brown, C.M. (1989) Limb and ventral edema. In *Problems*

in Equine Medicine (ed. C.M. Brown), Chapt. 11. Lea and Febiger, Philadelphia.

Brown, C.M. and Collier, M.A. (1983) Tracheobronchial foreign body in a horse. *J. Am. Vet. Med. Assoc.* **182**, 280–81.

Bruce, E.N. and Cherniak, N.S. (1987) Central chemoreceptors. *J. appl. Physiol.* **62**, 389–402.

Buchanan, M., Cousin, D.A.H., MacDonald, N.M. and Armour, D. (1991) Medical treatment of right-sided dilatation of the abomasum in cows. *Vet. Rec.* **129**, 111–112.

Budras, K-D. and Fricke, W. (1987) *Atlas der Anatomie des Hundes* 2nd edn. Schlütersche, Hannover.

Bülbring, E. and Kuriyama, H. (1972) The action of catecholamines on guinea-pig taenia coli. *Philos. Trans. R. Soc., London, Ser. B* **887**, 115–122.

Burnstock, G. (1985). Nervous control of smooth muscle by transmitters, cotransmitters and modulators. *Experientia* **41**, 869–874.

Burnstock, G. (1995) Autonomic nervous system. In *Gray's Anatomy* 38th edn. (ed. P.W. Williams, L.H. Bannister, M.M. Berry, P. Collins, M. Dyson, J.E. Dussek and M.W.J. Ferguson), pp. 1292–1309. Churchill Livingstone, Edinburgh.

Burton, C. and White, R. (1997) Surgical approach to a ruptured diaphragm in the cat. *In Practice* **19**, 298–305.

Butler, J. (1991) The bronchial circulation. *News Physiol. Sci.* **6**, 21–26.

Butler, W.F. (1967) Innervation of the horn region in domestic ruminants. *Vet. Rec.* **80**, 490–492.

Camner, P., Strandberg, K. and Philipson, K. (1974) Increased mucociliary transport by cholinergic stimulation. *Arch. Environ. Health* **29**, 220–224.

Campbell, E.J.M. (1964) Motor pathways. In *Handbook of Physiology: Respiration* (ed. W.O. Fenn and H. Rahn) Section 3, Vol. 1, Chapt. 21. American Physiological Society, Washington D.C.

Carpenter, R.E. (1985) Flight physiology of flying foxes (*Poliocephalus*). *J. Exp. Biol.* **114**, 619–647.

Carrig, C.B., Groenendyk, S. and Seawright, A.A. (1973) Dorsoventral flattening of the trachea in a horse and its attempted surgical correction. *J. Am. Vet. Radiology Soc.* **14**, 32–36.

Carter, A.M. (1993). Fetal placental circulation. In *Fetus and Neonate: Physiology and Clinical Applications*. Vol. 1 The Circulation (ed. M.A. Hanson, J.A.D. Spencer and C.H. Rodeck), Chapt. 5. Cambridge University Press, Cambridge.

Catchpole, H.R. (1966) The capillaries, veins and lymphatics. In *Physiology and Biophysics* 19th edn. (ed. T.C. Ruch and H.D. Patton) Chapt. 32. Saunders, Philadelphia.

Cervero, F. and Jänig, W. (1992) Visceral nociceptors: a new world order? *Trends Neurosci.* **15**, 374–378.

Chapleau, M.W., Hajduczok, G. and Abboud, F.M. (1991) Paracrine modulation of baroreceptor activity by vascular endothelium. *News Physiol. Sci.* **6**, 210–214.

Chapman, C.B. and Mitchell, J.H. (1974) The physiology of exercise. In *Vertebrate Structures and Functions* (ed. N.K. Wessells), Freeman, San Francisco.

Charan, N.B., Turk, G.M. and Dhand, R. (1984) Gross and subgross anatomy of bronchial circulation in sheep. *J. Appl. Physiol.* **57**, 658–664.

Chibuzo, G.H. (1979) The tongue. In *Miller's Anatomy of the Dog* 2nd edn. (ed. H.E. Evans and G.C. Christensen), pp. 423–445. Saunders, Philadelphia.

Chibuzo, G.H. (1993) The tongue. In *Miller's Anatomy of the Dog* 3rd edn. (ed. H.E. Evans), Chapt. 7. Saunders, Philadelphia.

Christensen, G.C. (1979) The urogenital apparatus. In *Miller's Anatomy of the Dog* 2nd edn. (ed H.E. Evans and G.C. Christensen), Chapt. 9. Saunders, Philadelphia.

Citters, R.L. van (1966) The coronary circulation: metabolism and nutrition of the heart; coronary disease. In *Physiology and Biophysics* 19th edn. (ed. T.C. Ruch and H.D. Patton), Chapt. 36. Saunders, Philadelphia.

Clark, W.E. Le Gros (1965) *The Tissues of the Body* 5th edn. Oxford University Press, Oxford.

Clements, J.A. (1974) Surface tension in the lungs. In *Vertebrate Structures and Functions* (ed. N.K. Wessells), Freeman, San Francisco.

Cohen, A.B. and Gold, W.M. (1975) Defense mechanisms of the lungs. *Ann. Rev. Physiol.* **37**, 325–350.

Coleridge, J.C.G. and Kidd, C. (1960) Electrophysiological evidence of baroreceptors in the pulmonary artery of the dog. *J. Physiol. (London)* **150**, 319–331.

Comroe, J.H. (1964) The peripheral chemoreceptors. In *Handbook of Physiology: Respiration* (ed. W.O. Fenn and H. Rahn), Section 3, Vol. 1, Chapt. 23. American Physiological Society, Washington D.C.

Comroe, J.H. (1975) *Physiology of Respiration* 2nd edn. Year Book Medical Publishers, Chicago.

Cook, R.D. and Burnstock, G. (1976). The ultrastructure of Auerbach's plexus in the guinea-pig. I. Neuronal elements. *J. Neurocytol.* **5**, 171–194.

Cordier, P. and Couloma, J. (1932) Recherches sur les nerfs du sinus carotidien et leurs variations. C.r. Ass. Anat. 27th réunion, 161–177.

Creed, K.E. (1979) Functional diversity of smooth muscle. *Brit. Med. Bull.* **35**, 243–247.

Crosby, E.C., Humphrey, T. and Lauer, E.W. (1962) *Correlative Anatomy of the Nervous System*. Macmillan, New York.

Crosfill, M.L. and Widdicombe, J.G. (1961) Physical characteristics of the chest and lungs and the work of breathing in different mammalian species. *J. Physiol.* **158**, 1–14.

D'Alccy, L.G. (1974) The cerebral circulation. In *Physiology and Biophysics* 20th edn. (ed. T.C. Ruch, H.D. Patton and A.M. Scher), Vol. 2, Chapt. 17. Saunders, Philadelphia.

Dalgleish, R. (1991) Differential diagnosis of respiratory disease in adult cattle. *In Practice* **13**, 237–241.

Daly, de B.D. and Hebb, C. (1966) *The Bronchial Circulation*. Butler and Arnold, London.

Darke, P.G.G. (1989) Congenital heart disease in the dog. *J. Small Anim. Pract.* **30**, 599–607.

Darke, P.G.G., Bonagura, J.D. and Kelly D.F. (1996) *Colour Atlas of Veterinary Cardiology.* Mosby-Wolfe, Turin.

Davis, C. and Kannan, M.S. (1987) Sympathetic innervation of human tracheal and bronchial smooth muscle. *Resp. Physiol.* **68**, 53–61.

Davis, D.D. and Story, H.E. (1943) Carotid circulation in the domestic cat. *Field Mus. Publ. (Zool.)* **28**, 5–47.

Dawes, G.S. (1961) Changes in the circulation at birth. *Br. Med. Bull.* **17**, 148–153.

Day, M.D. (1979) *Autonomic Pharmacology.* Churchill Livingstone, Edinburgh.

De Castro, F. (1926) Sur la structure et l'innervation de la glande intercarotidienne (glomus caroticum) de l'homme et des mammifères et sur un nouveau système d'innervation autonome du nerf glossopharyngien. *Trav. Lab. Rech. Biol.* **24**, 365.

De Castro, F. (1928) Sur la structure et l'innervation du sinus carotidienne de l'homme et des mammifères. *Trav. Lab. Rech. Biol.* **25**, 331.

Decramer, M. (1993) Respiratory muscle interaction. *News Physiol. Sci.* **8**, 121–124.

Dejours, P. (1981) *Principles of Comparative Respiratory Physiology* 2nd edn. Elsevier, Amsterdam.

de Lahunta, A. (1983) *Veterinary Neuroanatomy and Clinical Neurology* 2nd edn. Saunders, Philadelphia.

de Lahunta, A. and Habel, R.E. (1986) *Applied Veterinary Anatomy.* Saunders, Philadelphia.

Dennis, R. (1987) Radiographic examination of the canine spine. *Vet. Rec.* **121**, 31–35.

Derenne J., Macklem, P.T. and Roussos, C. (1978) The respiratory muscles: mechanics, control, and pathophysiology. Parts I and II. *Am. Rev. Resp. Dis.* **118**, 119–133, 373–390.

Derksen, F.J. (1990) Trachea and bronchi. In *Equine Endoscopy* (ed. J.L. Traub-Dargatz and C.M. Brown). Mosby, St. Louis.

Derksen, F.J., Brown, C.M., Sonea, I., Darien, B.J. and Robinson, N.E. (1989) Comparison of transtracheal aspirate and bronchoalveolar lavage cytology in 50 horses with chronic lung disease. *Eq. Vet. J.* **21**, 23–26.

Diana, J.N. and Fleming, B.P. (1979) Some current problems in microvascular research. *Microvasc. Res.* **18**, 144–152.

Dikranien, K., Loesch, A., and Burnstock, G. (1994) Localisation of nitric oxide synthase and its colocalisation with vasoactive peptides in coronary and femoral arteries. An electron microscope study. *J. Anat.* **184**, 583–590.

Dixon, J.B. (1993) *Immunological Reactions.* University of Liverpool, Liverpool.

Dixon, P.M. (1992) Respiratory mucociliary clearance in the horse in health and disease, and its pharmaceutical modification. *Vet. Rec.* **131**, 229–235.

Doidge, J.M. and Satchell, D.G. (1982) Adrenergic and non-adrenergic inhibitory nerves in mammalian airways. *J. Autonom. Nerv. Syst.* **5**, 83–99.

Dormans, J.A.M.A. (1985) The alveolar type III cell. *Lung* **163**, 327–335.

Douglas, S.W. and Hall, L.W. (1959) Bronchography in the dog. *Vet. Rec.* **71**, 901–903.

Drake, R.E. and Gabel, J.C. (1995) Pulmonary oedema fluid clearance pathways. *News Physiol Sci.* **10**, 107–111.

Dudel, J. (1978) Excitation of nerve and muscle. In *Fundamentals of Neurophysiology* 2nd edn. (ed. R.S. Schmidt), Chapt. 2. Springer, New York.

Duffin, J., Ezure, K. and Lipski, J. (1995) Breathing rhythm generation: focus on the rostral ventrolateral medulla. *News Physiol. Sci.* **10**, 133–140.

Dunnill, M.S. (1962) Quantitative methods in the study of pulmonary biology. *Thorax* **17**, 320–328.

Dunnill, M.S. (1979) Some aspects of pulmonary defence. *J. Path.* **128**, 221–236.

Dyce, K.M. (1958) The splanchnic nerves and major abdominal ganglia of the horse. *J. Anat.* **92**, 62–73.

Dyce, K.M., Sack, W.O. and Wensing, C.J.G. (1987) *Textbook of Veterinary Anatomy.* Saunders, Philadelphia.

Dyson, M. (1995) Urinary system. In *Gray's Anatomy* 38th edn. (ed. P.W. Williams, L.H. Bannister, M.M. Berry, P. Collins, M. Dyson, J.E. Dussek and M.W.J. Ferguson), Chapt. 13. Churchill Livingstone, Edinburgh.

Eckberg, D.L. and Fritsch, J.M. (1993) How should human baroreflexes be tested? *News Physiol. Sci.* **8**, 7–12.

Edvinson, L. and Uddman, R. (1993) *Vascular Innervation and Receptor Mechanisms.* Academic Press, London.

Edwards, D.A.W. and Rowland, E.N. (1986) Physiology of gastroduodenal junction. In *Handbook of Physiology: Alimentary Canal* (ed. C.F. Code), Vol. 4, Chapt. 97. American Physiological Society: Raven Press, New York.

Edwards, G.B. (1987) Equine dysautonomia: clinical picture and management. *J. small Animal Pract.* **28**, 364–368.

Eigenmann, U.J.E., Schoon, H.A., Jahn, D. and Grunert, E. (1984) Neonatal respiratory distress syndrome in the calf. *Vet. Rec.* **114**, 141–144.

Ellenberger, H.H. and Feldman, J.L. (1988) Monosynaptic transmission of respiratory drive to phrenic motoneurons from brainstem bulbospinal neurons in rats. *J. Comp. Neurol.* **269**, 47–57.

Elzinga, G. (1992) Starling's 'Law of the heart': rise and fall of the descending limb. *News Physiol. Sci.* **7**, 134–137.

Ettinger, S. (1971) Physical examination of the cardiovascular system. In *The Veterinary Clinics of North America* (ed. R.W. Kirk), Vol. 1, pp. 85–91, Saunders, Philadelphia.

Evans, D.L. (1994) In *The Athletic Horse: the Principles and Practice of Equine Sports Medicine* (ed. D.R. Hodgson and R.J. Rose), Chapt. 7. W.B. Saunders, Philadelphia.

Evans, H.E. (1993) In *Miller's Anatomy of the Dog* 3rd edn. (ed. H.E. Evans), Saunders, Philadelphia.

Evans, H.E. and Christensen, G.C. (1979) In *Miller's Anatomy of the Dog* 2nd edn. (ed. H.E. Evans and G.C. Christensen), Saunders, Philadelphia.

Ezure, K., Manabe, M. and Yamada, H. (1988) Distribution of medullary respiratory neurons in the rat. *Brain Res.* **455**, 262–270.

Fabiato, A. (1985) Time and calcium dependence of activation and inactivation of calcium-induced calcium release of calcium from the sarcoplasmic reticulum of a skinned cardiac Purkinje cell. *J. Gen. Physiol.* **85**, 247–290.

Fedde, M.R. (1990) High altitude bird flight: exercise in a hostile environment. *News Physiol. Sci.* **5**, 191–193.

Feigl, E.O. (1974) In *Physiology and Biophysics* 20th edn. (ed. T.C. Ruch, H.D. Patton and A.M. Scher), Vol. 2, Saunders, Philadelphia.

Fenn, W.O. (1964) Introduction to the mechanics of breathing. In *Handbook of Physiology: Respiration* (ed. W.O. Fenn and H. Rahn), Section 3, Vol. 1, Chapt. 10. American Physiological Society, Washington D.C.

Fidone, S.J., Zapata, P. and Stensaas, L.J. (1977) Axonal transport of labelled material into sensory nerve endings of cat carotid body. *Brain Res.* **124**, 9–29.

Fisher, E.W. (1972) Heart disease in the dog. *J. Small Anim. Pract.* **13**, 553–560.

Fowler, M.E., Crenshaw, G.L., Edwards, D.W., Holloway, C.K. and Whatley, J.L. (1963) Intrathoracic surgery in the horse. *Am. J. Vet. Res.* **24**, 766–771.

Fowler, M.E. (1973) Intrathoracic surgery in large animals. *J. Am. Vet. Med. Assoc.* **162**, 967–973.

Fox, E.L. (1984) *Sports Physiology* 2nd edn. Saunders, Philadelphia.

Franklin, K.J., Barclay, A.E. and Prichard, M.M.L. (1946) *The Circulation in the Foetus.* Blackwell, Oxford.

Freedman, B.J. (1972) The functional geometry of the bronchi. *Bull. Physio-pathol. Resp.* **8**, 545–551.

Frink, R.J. and Merrick, B. (1974) The sheep heart: coronary and conduction system anatomy with special reference to the presence of an os cordis. *Anat. Rec.* **179**, 189–200.

Gabella, G. (1979) Innervation of the gastrointestinal tract. *Int. Rev. Cytol.* **59**, 129–193.

Gabella, G. (1987) Structure of muscle and nerves in the gastrointestinal tract. *Physiology of the Gastrointestinal Tract* 2nd edn. (ed. L.R. Johnson), Chapt. 11. Raven Press, New York.

Gabella, G. (1996) Cardiovascular System. In *Gray's Anatomy* 38th edn. (ed. P.W. Williams, L.H. Bannister, M.M. Berry, P. Collins, M. Dyson, J.E. Dussek and M.W.J. Ferguson), Chapt. 7. Churchill Livingstone, Edinburgh.

Gallagher, J.T., Kent, P.W., Passatore, M., Phipps, R.J. and Richardson, P.S. (1975) The composition of tracheal mucus and the nervous control of its secretion in the cat. *Proc. R. Soc. London Ser. B* **192**, 49–76.

Gans, J.H. and Mercer, P.F. (1977) The kidneys. In *Duke's Physiology of Domestic Animals* 9th edn. (ed. M.J. Swenson), Chapt. 43. Cornell University Press, Ithaca.

Gardner, E., Gray, D.J. and O'Rahilly, R.O. (1960) The thorax: surface anatomy, physical examination. In *Anatomy: A Regional Study of Human Structure.* Saunders, Philadelphia.

Gasthuys, F., Verschooten, D., Parmentier, D., De Moor, A. and Steenhaurt, M. (1992) Laryngotomy as a treatment for chronic laryngeal obstruction in cattle: a review of 130 cases. *Vet. Rec.* **130**, 220–223.

Geelhaar, A. and Weibel, E.R. (1971) Morphometric estimation of pulmonary diffusion capacity, III. The effect of increased oxygen consumption in Japanese waltzing mice. *Resp. Physiol.* **11**, 354–366.

Gehr, P. and Schürch, S. (1992) Surface forces displace particles deposited in airways toward the epithelium. *News Physiol. Sci.* **7**, 1–5.

Gehr, P., Bachofen, M. and Weibel, E.R. (1978) The normal human lung: ultrastructure and morphometric estimation of diffusion capacity. *Resp. Physiol.* **32**, 121–140.

Gehr, P., Sehovic, S., Burri, P.H., Claassen, H. and Weibel, E.R. (1980) The lung of shrews: morphometric estimation of diffusion capacity. *Resp. Physiol.* **40**, 33–47.

Gehr, P., Mwangi, D.K., Amman, A., Maloiy, G.M.O., Taylor, C.R. and Weibel, E.W. (1981) Design of the mammalian respiratory system. V. Scaling morphometric pulmonary diffusing capacity to body mass: wild and domestic mammals. *Resp. Physiol.* **44**, 61–86.

Gentry, P.A. and Downie, H.G. (1977) Blood coagulation. In *Dukes' Physiology of Domestic Animals* 9th edn. (ed. M.J. Swenson), Chapt. 3. Comstock Publishing Associates, Ithaca.

Getty, R. (1975) In *Sisson and Grossman's Anatomy of the Domestic Animals.* 5th edn. (ed. R. Getty). Saunders, Philadelphia.

Gewirtz, H. (1991) The coronary circulation: limitations of current concepts of metabolic control. *News Physiol. Sci.* **6**, 265–268.

Ghoshal, N.G. (1975a) In *Sisson and Grossman's Anatomy of the Domestic Animals* (5th edn, ed. R. Getty). Saunders, Philadelphia.

Ghoshal, N.G. (1975b) Spinal nerves. In *Sisson and Grossman's Anatomy of the Domestic Animals* (5th edn, ed. R. Getty) Chapts. 24, 35, 57. Saunders, Philadelphia.

Ghoshal, N.G. (1975c) Abdominal, pelvic and caudal autonomic innervation. In *Sisson and Grossman's Anatomy of the Domestic Animals* (5th edn, ed. R. Getty). Chapts. 24, 35, and 57. Saunders, Philadelphia.

Gibson, E.A., Blackmore, R.J.L, Wijeratne, W.V.S. and Wrathall, A.E. (1976) The 'barker' (neonatal respiratory distress) syndrome in the pig: its occurrence in the field. *Vet. Rec.* **98**, 476–479.

Gillespie, J.R. and Tyler, W.S. (1967) Quantitative electron microscopy of the interalveolar septa of the horse lung. *Am. Rev. Resp. Dis.* **95**, 477–483.

Gillespie, J.R. and Tyler, W.S. (1969) Chronic alveolar emphysema in the horse. *Adv. Vet. Sci.* **13**, 59–99.

Gilmour, J.S. (1987) Equine dysautonomia: epidemiology and pathology. *J. Small Anim. Pract.* **28**, 373–380.

Glazier, B. (1987) Clinical aspects of equine cardiology. *In Practice* **9**, 98–104.

Godhino, H.P. and Getty, R. (1975) Cranial nerves. In *Sisson and Grossman's Anatomy of the Domestic Animals* 5th edn. (ed. R. Getty), Chaps. 24, 35. Saunders, Philadelphia.

Gompf, R.E. (1988) The clinical approach to heart disease: History and physical examination. In *Canine and Feline Cardiology* (ed. P.R. Fox). Churchill Livingstone, New York.

Gonzales, C., Almaraz, L., Obeso, A. and Rigual, R. (1992) Oxygen and acid chemoreception in the carotid body chemoreceptors. *Trends Neurosci.* **15**, 146–153.

Goodrich, E.S. (1930) *Studies on the Structure and Development of Vertebrates*. Macmillan, London. (Reprinted by Dover Publications.)

Gordon, A.M., Huxley, A.F. and Julian, F.J. (1966) The variation in isometric tension with sarcomere length in vertebrate muscle fibres. *J. Physiol.* **184**, 170–192.

Grandage, J. (1974) The radiology of the dog's diaphragm. *J. Small Anim. Pract.* **15**, 1–17.

Grandage, J. (1988) Appendix Anatomy. In *Baillière's Comprehensive Veterinary Dictionary* (ed. D.C. Blood and V.P. Studdert). Baillière Tindall, London.

Grau, H. (1943) Die peripheren Nerven. In *Ellenberger-Baum: Handbuch der Vergleichenden Anatomie der Haustiere* 18th edn. (ed. O. Zietzschmann, E. Ackerknecht and H. Grau), Section IIIC. Springer, Berlin.

Green, J.H. (1989) *An Introduction to Human Physiology* 4th edn. Oxford University Press, Oxford.

Greet, T.R.C. and Whitwell, K.E. (1987) Studies of oesophageal function. *J. Small Anim. Pract.* **28**, 369–372.

Grey, H.M., Sette, A. and Buus, S. (1989) How T cells see antigen. *Sci. Am.* Nov. 38–46.

Griffiths, I.R. and Pollin, M.M. (1987) Feline dysautonomia: pathology. *J. small Anim. Pract.* **28**, 347–349.

Guntheroth, W.G., Luchtel, D.L. and Kawabori, I. (1982) Pulmonary microcirculation: tubules rather than sheet and post. *J. Appl. Physiol.* **53**, 510–513.

Guthrie, D. (1945) *A History of Medicine*. Nelson, London.

Guyton, A.C. (1986) *Textbook of Medical Physiology* 7th edn. Saunders, Philadelphia.

Habel, R.E. (1970) *Guide to the Dissection of Domestic Ruminants*, 2nd edn. Habel, Ithaca.

Habel, R.E. (1975) Ruminant digestive system. In *Sisson and Grossman's Anatomy of the Domestic Animals* 5th edn. (ed. R. Getty), Chapt. 29. Saunders, Philadelphia.

Habel, R.E. (1992) Splanchnologia. In *Illustrated Veterinary Anatomical Nomenclature* (ed. O. Schaller, G.M. Constantinescu, R.E. Habel, W.O. Sack, P. Simeons and N.R. de Vos) pp. 234–414. Enke, Stuttgart.

Habel, R.E. and Biberstein, E.L. (1960) *Fundamentals of the Histology of the Domestic Animals*. Comstock, Ithaca.

Habermehl, K.H. (1964) Technique of intracardiac and intrapulmonary injection in carnivores. In *Blue Book for the Veterinary Profession* Vol. 8, pp. 6–16. Farbewerke Hoechst and Behringwerke AG.

Halliwell, R.E.W. (1993) Comment. *Vet. Rec.* **132**, 175.

Ham, A.W. (1974) *Histology* 7th edn. Lippincott, Philadelphia.

Hamilton, H.L. (1952) *Lillie's Development of the Chick* 3rd edn. Holt Rinehart & Winston, New York.

Hamlin, R.L., Muir, W.M., Gross, D.R. and Pipers, F.S. (1974) Right and left ventricular systolic intervals during ventilation and sinus arrhythmia in the dog: genesis of physiologic splitting of the second heart sound. *Am. J. Vet. Res.* **35**, 9–13.

Hamlin, R.L. and Smith R. (1977) In *Dukes' Physiology of Domestic Animals* 9th edn. (ed. M.J. Swenson), Comstock Publishing Associates, Ithaca.

Hammersen, F. (1976) Endothelial contractility – an undecided problem in vascular research. *Beitrg. Path. Bd.* **157**, 327–348.

Hance, A.J. and Crystal, R.G. (1975) The connective tissue of lung. *Am. Rev. Resp. Dis.* **112**, 657–711.

Hansen, H.J. (1952) A pathologic–anatomical study on disc degeneration in dog. *Acta Orthop. Scand.* Suppl. 11.

Hanson, M.A., Spencer, J.A.D. and Rodeck, C.H. (1993) *Fetus and Neonate: Physiology and Clinical Applications*, Vol. 1. The Circulation. Cambridge University Press, Cambridge.

Hanson, W.L., Emhardt, J.D., Bartek, J.P., Latham, L.P., Checkley, L.L., Capen, R.L. and Wagner, W.W. (1989) Site of recruitment in the pulmonary microcirculation. *J. Appl. Physiol.* **66**, 2079–2083.

Hare, W.C.D. (1955) The broncho-pulmonary segments in the sheep. *J. Anat.* **89**, 387–402.

Hare, W.C.D. (1975) Respiratory system. In *Sisson and Grossman's Anatomy of the Domestic Animals* 5th edn. (ed. R. Getty). W.B. Saunders, Philadelphia.

Harris, P. and Heath, D. (1962). *The Human Pulmonary Circulation*. Livingstone, Edinburgh.

Hartman, W. (1973) The pelvic outlet in female goats. Doctorate Thesis, University of Utrecht.

Harvey, W. (1628) *The Circulation of the Blood* (translated by K.J. Franklin, 1963). Everyman, London.

Hashim, M.A. and Waterman, A.E. (1991) Effects of thiopentone, propofol, alphaxalone–alphadolone, ketamine and xylazine–ketamine on lower oesophageal sphincter pressure and barrier pressure in cats. *Vet. Rec.* **129**, 137–139.

Hayek, H. von (1960) *The Human Lung* 2nd edn. Hafner, New York.

Hebb, C. (1969) Motor innervation of the pulmonary blood vessels of mammals. In *The Pulmonary Circulation and Interstitial Space* (ed. A.P. Fishman and H.H. Hecht). University of Chicago Press, Chicago.

Heinen, E. (1995) Follicular dendritic cells – phenotype, origin and functions. *Path. Biol.* **43**, 848–857.

Heymans, C., Bouckaert, J.J. and Regniers, P. (1933) *Le Sinus Carotidien et la Zone Homologue Cardio-aortique*. Doin, Paris.

Hildebrandt, J. (1974) Anatomy and physics of respiration. In *Physiology and Biophysics: Circulation, Respiration and Fluid Balance* 20th edn. (ed. T.C. Ruch, H.D. Patton and A.M. Scher), Vol. 2, Chapt. 20. Saunders, Philadelphia.

Hildebrandt, J. and Young, A.C. (1966). Anatomy and physics of respiration. In *Physiology and Biophysics* 19th edn. (ed. T.C. Ruch and H.D. Patton), Vol. 2, Chapt. 20. Saunders, Philadelphia.

Hirst, G.D.S., Gleria, S. de and Helden, D.F. van (1985) Neuromuscular transmission in arterioles. *Experientia* **41**, 874–879.

Hoerlein, B.F. (1953) Intervertebral disc protrusion in the dog. 1. Incidence and pathological lesions. *Am. J. Vet. Res.* **14**, 260–283.

Hoff, H.E. (1949) Cardiac output: regulation and estimation. In *Textbook of Physiology* 16th edn. (ed. J.F. Fulton), Chapt. 32. Saunders, Philadelphia.

Hoffman, B.B. (1989) Adrenoceptor-activating drugs. In *Basic and Clinical Pharmacology* 4th edn. (ed. B.G. Katzung). Prentice-Hall International, Englewood Cliffs.

Hoffman, J.I.E. (1995) Flow in coronary arteries – when and where? *News Physiol. Sci.* **10**, 191.

Hornbein, T.F. and Sørensen, S.C. (1974) The chemical regulation of ventilation. In *Physiology and Biophysics* 20th edn. (ed. T.C. Ruch, H.D. Patton and A.M. Scher), Vol. 2, Chapt. 23. Saunders, Philadelphia.

Hovelacque, A., Maes, J., Binet, L. and Gayet, R. (1930) Le nerf carotidien. Étude anatomique et physiologique. *Presse méd.* p. 449. (Cited by Ask-Upmark, 1935).

Hudlicka, O. (1985) Regulation of muscle flow. *Clin. Physiol.* **5**, 201–229.

Iggo, A. (1966) Physiology of visceral afferent systems. *Acta Neuoveg.* **28**, 121–134.

Iggo, A. (1977) Somesthetic sensory mechanisms. In *Duke's Physiology of Domestic Animals* 9th edn. (ed. M.J. Swenson), Chapt. 43. Cornell University Press, Ithaca.

Isaacs, A. (1971) *A Dictionary of Science*. Penguin Reference Books, London.

Iwamoto, H.S. (1993) Cardiovascular effects of acute fetal hypoxia and asphyxia. In *Fetus and Neonate: Physiology and Clinical Applications*. Vol. 1 The Circulation (ed. M.A. Hanson, J.A.D. Spencer and C.H. Rodeck), Chapt. 8. Cambridge University Press, Cambridge.

Jänig, W. and McLachlan, M. (1987) Organization of lumbar spinal outflow to distal colon and pelvic organs. *Physiol. Rev.* **67**, 1332–1404.

Jänig, W. and McLachlan, E.M. (1992) Characteristics of function-specific pathways in the sympathetic nervous system. *Trends Neurosci.* **15**, 475–481.

Jänig, W. and Morrison, J.F.B. (1986) Functional properties of spinal visceral afferents supplying abdominal and pelvic organs, with special emphasis on visceral nociception. *Progr. Brain Res.* **67**, 87–114.

Janssens, L.A.A. and Peeters, S. (1997) Comparisons between stress incontinence in women and sphincter mechanism incompetence in the female dog. *Vet. Rec.* **141**, 620–25.

Jeffery, P. and Reid, L. (1973) Intra-epithelial nerves in normal rat airways: a quantitative electron microscopic study. *J. Anat.* **114**, 35–45.

Jenkinson, D.M. (1969) Sweat gland function in domestic animals. In *The Exocrine Glands* (ed. S.Y. Bothelho, F.P. Brooks and W.B. Shelley). University of Pennsylvania Press, Philadelphia.

Jenkinson, D.M. (1973) Comparative physiology of sweating. *Br. J. Derm.* **88**, 397–406.

Jenkinson, D.M., Montgomery, I. and Elder, H.Y. (1978) Studies on the nature of the peripheral sudomotor control mechanism. *J. Anat.* **125**, 625–639.

Jenkinson, D.M., Montgomery, I. and Elder, H.Y. (1979) The ultrastructure of the sweat glands of the ox, sheep and goat during sweating and recovery. *J. Anat.* **129**, 117–140.

Jensen, A. and Berger, R. (1993) Regional distribution of cardiac output. In *Fetus and Neonate: Physiology and Clinical Applications*. Vol. 1 The Circulation (ed. M.A. Hanson, J.A.D. Spencer and C.H. Rodeck), Chapt. 2. Cambridge University Press, Cambridge.

Jericho, K.W.F. (1968) Pathogenesis of pneumonia in pigs. *Vet. Rec.* **82**, 507–517.

Jindal, S.K., Lakshminarayan, W.K. and Butler, J. (1984) Acute increase in anastomotic bronchial blood flow after pulmonary arterial obstruction. *J. Appl. Physiol.* **57**, 424–428.

Jokl, P. (1977) The role of exercise in medicine. In *Medicine and Sport* (ed. D. Brunner and E. Jokl), Vol. 10, pp. 13–35. Karger, Basel.

Jokl, E. and Jokl, P. (1977). Heart and sport. In *Medicine and Sport* (ed. D. Brunner and E. Jokl), Vol. 10, pp. 36–67. Karger, Basel.

Johnston, M. (1992) Equine colic – to refer or not to refer. *In Practice* **14**, 134–141.

Jones, J.H.B., Smith, B.L., Birks, E.K., Pascoe, J.R. and Hughes, T.R. (1992) Left atrial and pulmonary arterial pressures in exercising horses. *FASEB J.* **6**, A2020.

Junqueira, L.C. and Carneiro, J. (1983) *Basic Histology* (4th edn). Lange, Los Altos.

Karaosmanoglu, T., Muftuoglu, S., Dagderiven, A., Durgun, B., Aygun, B. and Ors, U. (1996) Morphological changes in the myenteric plexus of rat ileum after transection and end-to-end anastomosis. *J. Anat.* **188**, 323–331.

Karlsson, J.-A., Sant'Ambrogio, G. and Widdicombe, J.G. (1988) Afferent neural pathways in cough and reflex bronchoconstriction. *J. Appl. Physiol.* **65**, 1007–1023.

Katz, A.M. (1992) *Physiology of the Heart* (2nd edn). Raven, New York.

Keatinge, W.R. (1979) Blood vessels. *Br. Med. Bull.* **35**, 249–254.

Kelley, V.R. and Singer, G.G. (1993) The antigen presentation function of renal tubular epithelial-cells (APC). *Expl. Nephrol.* **1**, 102–111.

Kelly, D.F. (1989) Classification of naturally occurring arterial disease in the dog. *Toxicol. Pathol.* **17**, 77–93.

Kelly, D.F., Gaskell, C.J. and Lee, M.A. (1992) Arteriosclerosis of extramural coronary arteries in labradors with congestive heart failure. *J. Small Anim. Pract.* **33**, 437–442.

Kelly, K.A. (1981) Motility of the stomach and gastroduodenal junction. In *Physiology of the Gastrointestinal Tract* (ed. L.R. Johnson), Chapt. 3, pp. 393–410. Raven Press, New York.

Kienecker, E.W. and Knoche, H. (1978) Sympathetic innervation of the pulmonary artery, ascending aorta, coronary glomerula of the rabbit. *Cell Tiss. Res.* **188**, 329–333.

King, A.S. (1956a) An historical note on the discovery of the depressor nerve. *Br. J. Vet. Sci.* **112**, 353–356.

King, A.S. (1956b) The anatomy of disc protrusion in the dog. *Vet. Rec.* **68**, 939–944.

King, A.S. (1957) The cervical course of the aortic nerve in the horse. *J. Anat.* **91**, 228–236.

King, A.S. (1987) *Physiological and Clinical Anatomy of the Domestic Mammals: Central Nervous System*. Oxford University Press, Oxford.

King, A.S., King, D.Z., Hodges, R.D. and Henry, J. (1975) Synaptic morphology of the carotid body of the domestic fowl. *Cell Tiss. Res.* **162**, 459–473.

King, A.S. and McLelland, J. (1984) *Birds: Their Structure and Function* 2nd edn. Baillière Tindall, London.

King, A.S. and Smith, R.N. (1955) A comparison of the anatomy of the intervertebral disc in dog and man. *Br. Vet. J.* **111**, 135–149.

King, A.S. and Smith, R.N. (1958) Protrusion of the intervertebral disc in the cat. *Vet. Rec.* **70**, 509–512.

King, R.R., Raskin, R.E. and Rosbolt, J.P. (1990) Exercise-induced pulmonary haemorrhage in the racing greyhound dog. *J. Int. Med.* **4**, 130.

Kirchgessner, A.L. and Gershon, M.D. (1989) Identification of vagal efferent fibers and putative target neurons in the enteric nervous system of the rat. *J. Comp. Neurol.* **285**, 38–53.

Kirk, G.R., Smith, D.M., Hutcheson, D.P. and Kirkby, R. (1975) Postnatal growth of the dog heart. *J. Anat.* **119**, 461–469.

Kitchell, R.L. and Evans, H.E. (1993) The spinal nerves. In *Miller's Anatomy of the Dog* 3rd edn. (ed. H.E. Evans), Chapt. 17. Saunders, Philadelphia.

Knoche, H. and Addicks, K. (1976) Electron microscopic studies of the pressoreceptor fields of the carotid sinus of the dog. *Cell Tissue Res.* **173**, 77–94.

Knoche, H. and Kienecker, E.W. (1977) Sympathetic innervation of the carotid bifurcation in the rabbit and cat: blood vessels, carotid body and carotid sinus. *Cell Tissue Res.* **184**, 103–112.

Knoche, H., Wiesner-Menzel, L. and Addicks, K. (1980) Ultrastructure of baroreceptors in the carotid sinus of the rabbit. *Acta Anat.* **106**, 63–83.

Knowlton, G.C. and Larrabee, M.G. (1946) A unitary analysis of pulmonary volume receptors. *Am. J. Physiol.* **147**, 100–114.

Koch, E. (1931) *Die reflektorische Selbsteurung des Kreislaufes*. Steinkopff, Leipzig (cited by Comroe, 1964).

Koterba, A.M., Kosch, P., Beech, J. and Whitlock, T. (1988) Breathing strategy of the adult horse (*Equus cabellus*) at rest. *J. Appl. Physiol.* **64**, 337–346.

Kovách and Lefer, A.M. (1993) Endothelial dysfunction in shock states. *News Physiol. Sci.* **8**, 145–148.

Krahl, V.E. (1962) The glomus pulmonale: its location and microscopic anatomy. In Ciba Foundation Symposium on Pulmonary Structure and Function (ed. A.V.S. de Reuck and M. O'Connor). Churchill, London.

Krahl, V.E. (1964) Anatomy of the mammalian lung. In *Handbook of Physiology: Respiration* (ed. W.O. Fenn and H. Rahn), Section 3, Vol. 1, Chapt. 6. American Physiological Society, Washington D.C.

Krauhs, J.M. (1979) Structure of rat aortic baroreceptors and their relationship to connective tissue. *J. Neurocytol.* **8**, 401–414.

Krogh, A. (1941) *The Comparative Physiology of Respiratory Mechanisms*. (Reprinted in 1968 by Dover, New York.)

Krstic, R.V. (1984) *Illustrated Encyclopaedia of Human Histology*. Springer, Berlin.

Kuo L., Davis, M.J. and Chilian, W.M. (1992) Endothelial modulation of arteriolar tone. *News Physiol. Sci.* **7**, 5–9.

Kuwaki, T., Kurihara, Y., Kurihara, H., Yasaki, Y. and Kumada, M. (1995) Role of endothelin in central cardiorespiratory control: modern and classical approaches. *News Physiol. Sci.* **10**, 228–232.

Lackie, J.M. and Dow, J.A.T. (1989) *Dictionary of Cell Biology*. Academic Press, London.

Lahiri, S. (1994) Chromophores in O_2 chemoreception: the carotid body model. *News Physiol. Sci.* **9**, 161–165.

Laitinen, L.A. and Laitinen, A. (1987) Innervation of airway smooth muscle. *Am. Rev. Resp. Dis.* **136**, S38–S57.

Landis, S.C. (1990) Target regulation of neurotransmitter phenotype. *Trends Neurosci.* **13**, 344–350.

Langman, J. (1971) *Medical Embryology* 2nd edn. Williams and Wilkins, Baltimore.

Latshaw, W.K. (1987) *Veterinary Developmental Anatomy*. Decker, Toronto.

Lauweryns, J.M. and Baert, J.H. (1977) Alveolar clearance and the role of the pulmonary lymphatics. *Am. Rev. Resp. Dis.* **115**, 625–683.

Lauweryns, J.M., Cokelaere, M., Theunynck, P. and Deleersnyder, M. (1974) Neuroepithelial bodies in mammalian respiratory mucosa: light optical, histochemical and ultrastructural studies. *Chest* **65**, 22–29S.

Lauweryns, J.M., Cokelaere, M., Deleersnyder, M. and Liebens, M. (1977) Intrapulmonary neuro-epithelial bodies in newborn rabbits. *Cell Tissue Res.* **182**, 425–440.

Lechner, A.J. (1985) Pulmonary design in a micro-chiropteran bat (*Pipistrellus subflavus*) during hibernation. *Resp. Physiol.* **59**, 301–312.

Lee, R. (1974) Bovine respiratory disease: its radiological features. *J. Am. Radiol. Soc.* **15**, 42–48.

Leff, A.R. (1988) Endogenous regulation of bronchomotor tone. *Am. Rev. Resp. Dis.* **137**, 1198–1216.

Liebow, A.A., Hales, M.R., Harrison, W., Bloomer, W. and

Lindskog, G.E. (1950) The genesis and functional implications of collateral circulation of the lungs. *Yale J. Biol. Med.* **22**, 637–650.

Lodge, D. (1969) A survey of tracheal dimensions in horses and cattle in relation to endotracheal tube size. *Vet. Rec.* **85**, 300–303.

Lopez-Barneo, J. (1994) Oxygen-sensitive ion channels. *Trends Neurosci.* **17**, 133–135.

Lopez-Barneo, J., Benot, A.R. and Urena, J. (1993) Oxygen sensing and the electrophysiology of arterial chemoreceptor cells. *News Physiol. Sci.* **8**, 191–195.

Luisada, A.A., MacCanon, D.M., Kumar, S. and Feigen, L.P. (1974) Changing views on the mechanism of the first and second heart sounds. *Am. Heart J.* **88**, 503–514.

Lumsden, A. and Keynes, R. (1989) Segmental patterns of neuronal development in the chick hindbrain. *Nature* **337**, 424–428.

Lundberg, L.M., Alm, P., Wharton, J. and Polak, J.M. (1988) Protein gene product 9.5. A new neuronal marker visualizing the whole uterine innervation and pregnancy-induced and developmental changes in the guinea pig. *Histochemistry* **90**, 9–17.

Lüscher, T.F. and Dohi, Y. (1992) Endothelium-derived relaxing factor and endothelin in hypertension. *News Physiol. Sci.* **7**, 120–123.

Lutz, B.R. and Wyman, L.C. (1932a) The evolution of the carotid sinus reflex and the origin of vagal tone. *Science* **75**, 591 (cited by Adams, 1958).

Lutz, B.R. and Wyman, L.C. (1932b) Reflex cardiac inhibition of branchio-vascular origin in the elasmobranch, *Squalus acanthias. Biol. Bull., Woods Hole*, **622**, 10–16 (cited by Adams, 1958).

McArdle, W.D., Katch, F.E. and Katch, V.L. (1981) *Exercise Physiology: Energy, Nutrition and Human Performance.* Lea and Febiger, Philadelphia.

McCandlish, A.P., Nash, A.S. and Peggram, A. (1984) Unusual vascular ring in a cat: left aortic arch with right ligamentum arteriosum. *Vet. Rec.* **114**, 338–340.

McClure, R.C. (1979) The cranial nerves. In *Miller's Anatomy of the Dog* 2nd edn. (ed. H.E. Evans and G.C. Christensen), Chapt. 15. Saunders, Philadelphia.

McDonald, D.M. and Mitchell, R.A. (1975) The innervation of glomus cells, ganglion cells and blood vessels in the rat carotid body. *J. Neurocytol.* **4**, 177–230.

McGorum, B.C., Dixon, P.M., Halliwell, R.E.W. and Irving, P. (1993) Comparisons of cellular and molecular components of bronchoalveolar fluid harvested from different segments of the equine lung. *Res. Vet. Sci.* **55**, 57–59.

McHale, N.G. (1995) Role of the lymph pump and its control. *News Physiol. Sci.* **10**, 112–117.

McKibben, J.S. (1975) Cervical and thoracic autonomic innervation. In *Sisson and Grossman's Anatomy of the Domestic Animals* 5th edn. (ed. R. Getty), Chapt. 57. Saunders, Philadelphia.

McKibben, J.S. and Getty, R. (1968a) A comparative morphologic study of the cardiac innervation in domestic animals. I. The canine. *Am. J. Anat.* **122**, 533–544.

McKibben, J.S. and Getty, R. (1968b) A comparative morphologic study of the cardiac innervation in domestic animals. II. The feline. *Am. J. Anat.* **122**, 545–554.

McKibben, J.S. and Getty, R. (1969a) Innervation of heart of domesticated animals: horse. *Am. J. Vet. Res.* **30**, 193–202.

McKibben, J.S. and Getty, R. (1969b) Innervation of heart of domesticated animals: pig. *Am. J. Vet. Res.* **30**, 779–789.

McKibben, J.S. and Ghoshal, N.G. (1975) Cervical and thoracic autonomic innervation. In *Sisson and Grossman's Anatomy of the Domestic Animals* 5th edn. (ed. R. Getty), Chapt. 57. Saunders, Philadelphia.

McLaughlin, R.F., Tyler, W.S. and Canada, R.O. (1961) A study of the subgross pulmonary anatomy in various mammals. *Am. J. Anat.* **108**, 149–165.

Mackey, V.S. and Wheat, J.D. (1985) Endoscopic examination of the equine thorax. *Eq. Vet. J.* **17**, 140–142.

Magee, D.F. (1966) Secretions of the digestive tract. In *Physiology and Biophysics* 19th edn. (ed. T.C. Ruch and H.D. Patton), Chapt. 49. Saunders, Philadelphia.

Maina, J.N. and King, A.S. (1984) Correlations between structure and function in the design of the bat lung: a morphometric study. *J. Exp. Biol.* **111**, 43–61.

Maina, J.N., King, A.S. and King, D.Z. (1982) A morphometric analysis of the lung of a species of bat. *Resp. Physiol.* **50**, 1–11.

Maina, J.N., King, A.S. and Settle, G. (1989) An allometric study of pulmonary morphometric parameters in birds, with mammalian comparisons. *Philos. Trans. R. Soc. London, Ser. B* **326**, 1–57.

Maina, J.N., Thomas, S.P. and Hyde, D.M. (1991) A morphometric study of the lungs of different sized bats: correlations between structure and function of the chiropteran lung. *Philos. Trans. R. Soc. London, Ser. B* **333**, 31–50.

Mair, T. and Gibbs, C. (1990) Thoracic radiography in the horse. *In Practice* **12**, 8–10.

Mall, G., Klingel, K., Hasslacher, C., Mann, J., Mattfeldt, T., Baust, H. and Waldherr, R. (1987) Synergistic effects of diabetes mellitus and renovascular hypertension on the rat heart. Stereological investigations on papillary muscles. *Virchows Arch. Path. Anat. Physiol. A* **411**, 531.

Maly, F.E. and Schürer-Maly, C.C. (1995) How and why cells make superoxidase: the 'phagocytic' NADPH oxidase. *News Physiol. Sci.* **10**, 233–237.

Manohar, M., Hutchens, E. and Coney, E. (1993) Pulmonary haemodynamics in the exercising horse and their relationship to exercise-induced pulmonary haemorrhage. *Br. Vet. J.* **149**, 419–428.

Marshall, J.M. (1995) Skeletal muscle vasculature and systemic hypoxia. *News Physiol. Sci.* **10**, 274–280.

Mathias, C.J. (1987) Human dysautonomia: primary autonomic failure in man. *J. Small Anim. Pract.* **28**, 387–396.

Mattfeldt, T., Krämer, K., Zeitz, R. and Mall, G. (1985) Stereology of myocardial hypertrophy induced by physical exercise. *Virchows Arch. Path. Anat. Physiol. A* **409**, 473.

Mattfeldt, T. and Mall, G. (1987) Growth of capillaries and myocardial cells in the normal rat heart. *J. Mol. Cardiol.* **19**, 1237–1246.

Mayer, E.A. (1994) The physiology of gastric storage and emptying. In *Physiology of the Gastrointestinal Tract* (ed. L.R. Johnson), Chapt. 22. Raven Press, New York.

Mead, J. and Agostoni, E. (1964) Dynamics of breathing. In *Handbook of Physiology: Respiration* (ed. W.O. Fenn and H. Rahn), Section 3, Vol. 1, Chapt. 14. American Physiological Society, Washington D.C.

Mead, J. and Milic-Emili, J. (1964) Theory and methodology in respiratory mechanics with glossary of symbols. In *Handbook of Physiology: Respiration* (ed. W.O. Fenn and H. Rahn), Section 3, Vol. 1, Chapt. 11. American Physiological Society, Washington D.C.

Mead, J. and Whittenberger, J.L. (1964) Lung inflation and haemodynamics. In *Handbook of Physiology: Respiration* (ed. W.O. Fenn and H. Rahn), Section 3, Vol. 1, Chapt. 18. American Physiological Society, Washington D.C.

Meban, C. (1980) Thickness of the air–blood barriers in vertebrate lungs. *J. Anat.* **131**, 299–307.

Mellander, S. and Björnberg, J. (1992) Regulation of vascular smooth muscle tone and capillary pressure. *News Physiol. Sci.* **7**, 113–119.

Meyer, H.P., Rothuizen, G.J. and van den Ingh, T.S.G.A.M. (1995) Increasing incidence of hereditary intrahepatic portosystemic shunts in Irish wolfhounds in the Netherlands (1984 to 1992). *Vet. Rec.* **136**, 13–16.

Miller, W.S. (1947) *The Lung* (2nd edn). Thomas, Springfield.

Miller, Y.E. (1989) The pulmonary endocrine cell: a role in adult lung disease. *Am. Rev. Resp. Dis.* **140**, 283–284.

Miller, V.M. (1992) Interactions between neural and endothelial mechanisms in control of vascular tone. *News Physiol. Sci.* **6**, 60–63.

Mitchell, G.A.G. (1953) *Anatomy of the Autonomic Nervous System.* Livingstone, Edinburgh.

Monos, E. (1993) How does the vein wall respond to pressure. *News Physiol. Sci.* **8**, 124–128.

Morgan, M., Pack, R.J. and Howe, A. (1975) Nerve endings in rat carotid body. *Cell Tissue Res.* **157**, 255–272.

Muir, A.R. (1971) *The Mammalian Heart.* Oxford University Press, Oxford.

Murray, M. (1973) Local immunity and its role in vaccination. *Vet. Rec.* **93**, 500–504.

Nanda, B.S. (1975) Blood supply to brain. In *Sisson and Grossman's Anatomy of the Domestic Animals* 5th edn. (ed. R. Getty), Chapt. 44, Saunders, Philadelphia.

Nash, A.S. (1987) Clinical features and management. *J. Small Anim. Pract.* **28**, 339–342.

Nash, A.S., Griffiths, I.R. and Sharp, N.J.H. (1982) The Key–Gaskell syndrome – an autonomic polyganglionopathy. *Vet. Rec.* **111**, 307–308.

Navaratnam, V. (1975) *The Human Heart and Circulation.* Academic Press, London.

Neal, M.J. (1992). *Medical Pharmacology at a Glance.* Blackwell, Oxford.

Nickel, R., Schummer, A. and Seiferle, E. (1973) *The Anatomy of the Domestic Animals*, Vol. 2, The Viscera of the Domestic Mammals (translated and revised by W.O. Sack). Parey, Berlin.

Nicholas, T.E. (1993) Control of turnover of pulmonary surfactant. *News Physiol. Sci.* **8**, 12–18.

Niden, A.H. (1967) Bronchiolar and large alveolar cell in pulmonary phospholipid metabolism. *Science* **158**, 1323.

Noden, D.M. (1984) Craniofacial development: new views on old problems. *Anat. Rec.* **208**, 1–13.

Noden, D.M. and de Lahunta, A. (1985) *The Embryology of Domestic Animals. Developmental Mechanisms and Malformations.* Williams & Wilkins, Baltimore.

Nomina Anatomica (1977) 4th edn. (ed. R. Warwick), Excerpta Medica, Amsterdam.

Nomina Anatomica (1989) 6th edn. (ed. R. Warwick and M. Brookes), Churchill Livingstone, Edinburgh.

Nomina Anatomica Veterinaria (1983) 3rd edn. (ed. R.E. Habel, J. Frewein and W.O. Sack), World Association of Veterinary Anatomists, Ithaca.

Nomina Anatomica Veterinaria (1994) 4th edn. (ed. J. Frewein, R.E. Habel and W.O. Sack), World Association of Veterinary Anatomists, Zürich.

Nomina Embryologica Veterinaria (1992) (ed. W.O. Sack, J. Frewein and R.E. Habel) World Association of Veterinary Anatomists, Zurich. 1st edn.

Nomina Embryologica Veterinaria (1994) 1st edn. (ed. W.O. Sack, J. Frewein and R.E. Habel). World Association of Veterinary Anatomists, Zürich and Ithaca.

Nomina Histologica (1977) 1st edn. (ed. T.E. Hunt). Excerpta Medica, Amsterdam.

Nomina Histologica (1983) 2nd edn. (ed. I.R. Telford and R.L. Hullinger), World Association of Veterinary Anatomists, Ithaca.

Nomina Histologica (1989) 3rd edn. (ed. I.R. Telford and R.L. Hullinger). Churchill Livingstone, Edinburgh.

Nomina Histologica (1994) Revised 2nd edn. (ed. R.L. Hullinger, J. Frewein, and W.O. Sack) World Association of Veterinary Anatomists, Zürich and Ithaca.

Nonidez, J.F. (1937) Distribution of the aortic nerve fibres and the epithelioid bodies (supracardial paraganglia) in the dog. *Anat. Rec.* **69**, 299–317.

Nowell, J.A., Gillespie, J.R. and Tyler, W.S. (1971) Scanning electron microscopy of chronic pulmonary emphysema: a study of the equine model. *Scanning Electron Microscopy*: Proc. Fourth Annual Scanning Electron Microscope Symposium pp. 297–304.

O'Callaghan, M.W. (1987) Echocardiography. In *Current Therapy in Equine Medicine* (ed. N.E. Robinson), Vol. 2, Section 3 (ed. C.M. Brown) pp. 139–147. Saunders, Philadelphia.

O'Callaghan, M.W. (1989) Bleeding from the nose. In *Problems in Equine Medicine* (ed. C.M. Brown) Chapt. 9. Lea and Febiger, Philadelphia.

O'Callaghan, M.W. (1991a) Scintigraphic imaging of lung disease. In *Equine Respiratory Disorders* (ed. J. Beech), Chapt. 9. Lea and Febiger, Malvern.

O'Callaghan, M.W. (1991b) Nuclear imaging techniques for equine respiratory disease. In *Veterinary Clinics of North America Equine Practice* (ed. R.W. Kirk), Vol. 7, no. 2, pp. 417–433.

O'Callaghan, M.W., Pascoe, J.R., Tyler, W.S. and Mason, D.K. (1987a) Exercise-induced pulmonary haemorrhage in the horse: results of a detailed clinical, post mortem and imaging study. II. Gross lung pathology. *Equine Vet. J.* **19**, 389–393.

O'Callaghan, M.W., Pascoe, J.R., Tyler, W.S. and Mason, D.K. (1987b) Exercise-induced pulmonary haemorrhage in the horse: results of a detailed clinical, post mortem and imaging study. III. Subgross findings in lung subjected to latex perfusions of the bronchial and pulmonary arteries. *Equine Vet. J.* **19**, 394–404.

O'Callaghan, M.W., Pascoe, J.R., Tyler, W.S. and Mason, D.K. (1987c) Exercise-induced pulmonary haemorrhage in the horse: results of a detailed clinical, post mortem and imaging study. VIII. Conclusions and implications. *Equine Vet. J.* **19**, 428–434.

Oparil, S. and Wyss, J.M. (1993) Atrial natriuretic factor in central cardiovascular control. *News Physiol. Sci.* **8**, 223–228.

Otis, A.B. (1964) The work of breathing. In *Handbook of Physiology: Respiration* (ed. W.O. Fenn and H. Rahn), Section 3, Vol. 1, Chapt. 17. American Physiological Society, Washington D.C.

Pack, R.J. and Richardson, P.S. (1984) The aminergic innervation of the human bronchus: a light and electron microscopic study. *J. Anat.* **138**, 493–502.

Paintal, A.S. (1995) Sensations from J receptors. *News Physiol. Sci.* **10**, 238–243.

Palmer, A.C. and Rossdale, P.D. (1976) Neuropathological changes associated with the neonatal maladjustment syndrome in the Thoroughbred foal. *Res. Vet. Sci.* **20**, 267–275.

Partridge, L.D. and Swandulla, D. (1988) Calcium-activated non-specific cation channels. *Trends Neurosci.* **11**, 68–72.

Patten, B.M. (1948) *Embryology of the Pig* (3rd edn). Blakiston, Toronto.

Patten, B.M. (1958) *Foundations of Embryology.* McGraw-Hill, New York.

Patton, H.D. (1966) The autonomic nervous system. In *Physiology and Biophysics* 19th edn. (ed. T.C. Ruch and H.D. Patton), Chapt. 10. Saunders, Philadelphia.

Peao, M.N.D., Arguas, A.P., de Sa, C.M. and Grande, N.R. (1993) Anatomy of Clara cell secretion: surface changes observed by scanning electron microscopy. *J. Anat.* **183**, 377–388.

Petersen, E.S. (1987) The control of breathing pattern. In *The Control of Breathing in Man* (ed. B.J. Whipp), Chapt. 1. Manchester University Press, Manchester.

Phillipson, A.T. (1977) Ruminant digestion. In *Duke's Physiology of Domestic Animals* 9th edn. (ed. M.J. Swenson), Chapt. 22. Cornell University Press, Ithaca.

Piani, D., Constam, D.B., Frei, K. and Fontana, A. (1994) Macrophages in the brain: friends or enemies. *News Physiol. Sci.* **9**, 80–84.

Popesko, P. (1972) *Atlas of Topographical Anatomy of the Domestic Animals.* Saunders, Philadelphia.

Porter, K.R. (1972) *Herpetology.* Saunders, Philadelphia.

Proctor, D.F. (1964) Physiology of the upper airway. In *Handbook of Physiology: Respiration.* (ed. W.O. Fenn and H. Rahn), Section 3, Vol. 1, Chapt. 8. American Physiological Society, Washington D.C.

Radford, E.P. (1964) Static mechanical properties of mammalian lungs. In *Handbook of Physiology: Respiration* (ed. W.O. Fenn and H. Rahn), Section 3, Vol. 1, Chapt. 15. American Physiological Society, Washington D.C.

Randall, D.J., Burggren, W.W., Farrell, A.P. and Haswell, M.S. (1981) *The Evolution of Air Breathing in Vertebrates.* Cambridge University Press, Cambridge.

Reeves, J.T. (1995) Brunton's use of amyl nitrite in angina pectoris: an historic root of nitric oxide research. *News Physiol. Sci.* **10**, 141–144.

Reif, J.S. (1971) Physical examination of canine respiratory system. In *The Veterinary Clinics of North America* (ed. R.W. Kirk), Vol. 1, pp. 71–84. Saunders, Philadelphia.

Renkin, E.M. (1978) Transport pathways through capillary endothelium. *Microvasc. Res.* **15**, 123–135.

Renkin, E.M. and Tucker, V.L. (1996) Atrial natriuretic peptide as a regulator of transvascular fluid balance. *News Physiol. Sci.* **11**, 138–143.

Rhodin, J.A.G. (1974) *Histology: a Text and Atlas.* Oxford University Press, New York.

Richards, D.W. (1953) Nature of cardiac and pulmonary dyspnoea. *Circulation* **7**, 15–29.

Romanoff, A.L. (1960) *The Avian Embryo.* Macmillan, New York.

Romer, A.S. (1962) *The Vertebrate Body* 3rd edn. Saunders, Philadelphia.

Ross, J.A. and McIntire, L.V. (1995) Molecular mechanisms of mural thrombosis under dynamic flow conditions. *News Physiol. Sci.* **10**, 117–122.

Rossdale, P.D. (1972) Modern concepts of neonatal disease in foals. *Equine Vet. J.* **4**, 117–128.

Rossdale, P.D. and Mahaffey, L.W. (1958) Parturition in Thoroughbred mare with particular reference to blood deprivation in the new-born. *Vet. Rec.* **70**, 142–152.

Rowell, L.B. (1974) In *Physiology and Biophysics* 20th edn. (ed. T.C. Ruch, H.D. Patton and A.M. Scher), Vol. 2, Saunders, Philadelphia.

Ruch, T.C. (1966) Pathophysiology of pain. In *Physiology and Biophysics* 19th edn. (ed. T.C. Ruch and H.D. Patton), Chapt. 16, Saunders, Philadelphia.

Ruch, T.C. (1974) The urinary bladder. In *Physiology and Biophysics* 20th edn. (ed. T.C. Ruch, H.D. Patton and A.M. Scher), Vol. 2, Chapt. 28. Saunders, Philadelphia.

Rudolph, A.M. and Heymann, M.A. (1974) Fetal and

neonatal circulation and respiration. *Annu. Rev. Physiol.* **36**, 187–207.

Rushmer, R.F. (1966) In *Physiology and Biophysics* 19th edn. (ed. T.C. Ruch and H.D. Patton), Saunders, Philadelphia.

Ruskell, G.L. (1971) The distribution of autonomic postganglionic nerve fibres in the lacrimal gland in the rat. *J. Anat.* **109**, 229–242.

Ruskoaho, H. and Vuolteenaho, O. (1993) Regulation of atrial natriuretic peptide secretion. *News Physiol. Sci.* **8**, 261–266.

Russell, J.A. (1966) The adrenals. In *Physiology and Biophysics* 19th edn. (ed. T.C. Ruch and H.D. Patton), Chapt. 59, Saunders, Philadelphia.

Rutgers, H.C. (1989) Thoracocentesis in the dog and cat. *In Practice* **11**, 14–16.

Saar, L.I. and Getty, R. (1975) Lymphatic system. In *Sisson and Grossman's Anatomy of the Domestic Animals* 5th edn. (ed. R. Getty), Vols. 1 and 2, Chapts. 23, 34, 45, 56. Saunders, Philadelphia.

Salmons, S. (1995) Muscle. In *Gray's Anatomy* 38th edn. (ed. P.W. Williams, L.H. Bannister, M.M. Berry, P. Collins, M. Dyson, J.E. Dussek and M.W.J. Ferguson), Chapt. 7. Churchill Livingstone, Edinburgh.

Schaller, O., Constantinescu, G.M., Habel, R.E., Sack, W.O., Simeons, P. and Vos, N.R. de (1992) *Illustrated Veterinary Anatomical Nomenclature.* Enke, Stuttgart.

Schaper, W., Görge, G., Winkler, B. and Schaper, J. (1988) The collateral circulation of the heart. *Prog. Vasc. Dis.* **31**, 57–77.

Schatzmann, U., Straub, R. and Gerber, H. (1974) Percutaneous lung biopsy in the horse. *Vet. Rec.* **94**, 588–590.

Scher, A.M. (1966) In *Physiology and Biophysics* 19th edn. (ed. T.C. Ruch and H.D. Patton), Saunders, Philadelphia.

Scher, A.M. (1974) In *Physiology and Biophysics* 20th edn. (ed. T.C. Ruch, H.D. Patton and A.M. Scher), Vol. 2, Saunders, Philadelphia.

Schmid-Schönbein, G.W. and Zweifach, B.J. (1994) Fluid pump mechanisms in initial lymphatics. *News Physiol. Sci.* **9**, 67–71.

Schmidt, C.F. (1938) Respiration. In *Macleod's Physiology in Modern Medicine* 8th edn. (ed. P. Bard), pp. 469–619 (cited by Comroe, 1964).

Schmidt-Nielsen, K. (1990) *Animal Physiology: Adaptation and Environment* 4th edn. Cambridge University Press, Cambridge.

Schnorr, B. (1985) *Embryologie der Haustiere.* Enke, Stuttgart.

Schraufnagel, D.E. (1987) Microvascular corrosion casting of the lung. A state-of-the-art review. *Scanning Microsc.* **1**, 1733–1747.

Schrauwen, E., Ham, L. van, Maenhout, T. and Desmidt, M. (1991) Canine dysautonomia a case report. *Vet. Rec.* **128**, 524–525.

Schummer, A., Wilkens, H., Vollmerhaus, B. and

Habermehl, K.H. (1981) *Nickel, Schummer, and Seiferle's Anatomy of the Domestic Animals*, Vol. 3, *Circulatory System, Skin, and Cutaneous Organs of the Domestic Mammals.* (translated by W.G. Siller and P.A.L. Wight). Parey, Berlin.

Schwartz, C.J. (1989) Perspectives on coronary artery disease: aetiology, pathogenesis and unresolved problems. In *Histopathology Seminar on the Cardiovascular System of Laboratory Animals.* International Life Sciences Institute of Hannover Medical School.

Schwartz, C.J., Sprague, E.A., Valente, A.J., Kelley, J.L. and Edwards, E.H. (1989) Cellular mechanisms in the response of the arterial wall to injury and repair. *Tox. Path.* **17**, 66–71.

Schwartz, J.H. (1979) Axonal transport: components, mechanisms, and specificity. *Annu. Rev. Neurosci.* **2**, 467–504.

Scott, E.M. (1986) *Cardiovascular Physiology: an Integrated Approach.* Manchester University Press, Manchester.

Scott, J.S., Garon, H., Broadstone, R.V., Derksen, F.J. and Robinson, N.E. (1988) Adrenergic-induced airway obstruction in ponies with recurrent pulmonary disease. *J. Appl. Physiol.* **65**, 687–692.

Segal, S.S. (1992) Communication among endothelial and smooth muscle cells coordinates blood flow control during exercise. *News Physiol. Sci.* **7**, 152–156.

Sellers, A.F. (1977) Neurohumeral regulation of gastrointestinal function. In *Duke's Physiology of Domestic Animals* 9th edn. (ed. M.J. Swenson), Chapt. 20. Cornell University Press, Ithaca.

Sernka, T.J. and Jacobson, E.D. (1983) *Gastrointestinal Physiology* 2nd edn. Williams and Wilkins, Baltimore.

Sexton, A.J., Turmaine, M. and Burnstock, G. (1996) A sudy of the ultrastructure of developing human umbilical vessels. *J. Anat.* **188**, 75–85.

Sharp, N.J.H. (1987) Factors relating to the aetiology and pathogenesis of feline and equine dysautonomias. *J. Small Animal Pract.* **28**, 397–403.

Sheehan, D. and Pick, J. (1943) The rami communicantes in the rhesus monkey. *J. Anat.* **77**, 125–139.

Shepro, D. (1988) Endothelial cells, inflammatory oedema, and the microvascular barrier: comments by a free radical. *Microvasc. Res.* **35**, 247–264.

Sherman, J.L. (1963) Normal arteriovenous anastomoses. *Medicine (Baltimore)* **42**, 247–267.

Shields, S.A., MacDowell, K.A., Fairchild, S.B. and Campbell, M.L. (1987) Is mediating of sweating cholinergic, adrenergic, or both? A comment on the literature. *Psychophysiology* **24**, 312–319.

Siegwart, B., Gehr, P., Gil, J. and Weibel, E.R. (1971) Morphometric estimation of pulmonary diffusion capacity. IV. The normal dog lung. *Resp. Physiol.* **13**, 141–159.

Simoens, P. (1992) Angiologia. In *Illustrated Veterinary Anatomical Nomenclature* (ed. O. Schaller, G.M. Constantinescu, R.E. Habel, W.O. Sack, P. Simoens and N.R. de Vos), pp. 234–414. Enke, Stuttgart.

Sinclair, J.D. (1987) Respiratory drive in hypoxia: carotid body and other mechanisms compared. *News Physiol. Sci.* **2**, 57–60.

Sisson, S. (1975) In *The Anatomy of the Domestic Animals*, 5th edn. (ed. R. Getty), Vol. 1, Saunders, Philadelphia.

Sisson, S. and Grossman, J.D. (1969) *The Anatomy of the Domestic Animals* 4th edn. Saunders, Philadelphia.

Sisson, S. and Grossman, J.D. (1975) *The Anatomy of the Domestic Animals* 5th edn. (ed. R.G. Getty). Saunders, Philadelphia.

Smetzer, D.L., Hamlin, R.L. and Smith, C.R. (1977) Cardiovascular sounds. In *Dukes' Physiology of Domestic Animals* 9th edn. (ed. M.J. Swenson), Chapt. 8. Comstock Publishing Associates, Ithaca.

Smiesko, V. and Johnson, P.C. (1993) The arterial lumen is controlled by flow-related shear stress. *News Physiol. Sci.* **8**, 34–38.

Smith, C.R. and Hamlin, R.L. (1977) In *Dukes' Physiology of Domestic Animals* 9th edn. (ed. M.J. Swenson), Comstock Publishing Associates, Ithaca.

Smith, P., Heath, D. and Moosavi, H. (1974) The Clara cell. *Thorax* **29**, 147–163.

Smith, P.G. and Mills, E. (1981) Time course of Wallerian degeneration in the carotid body after carotid sinus nerve transection. In *Arterial Chemoreceptors*, Proc. VI International Meeting (ed. C. Belmonte, D.J. Pallot, H. Acker and S. Fidone), pp. 430–439.

Snow, D.H. (1985) Horse and dog, elite athletes why and how. *Proc. Nutr. Soc.* **44**, 267–272.

Sonea, I. (1989) The sick neonatal foal. In *Problems in Equine Medicine* (ed. C.M. Brown), Chapt. 19. Lea and Febiger, Philadelphia.

Sossin, W.S., Sweet-Cordero, A. and Scheller, R.H. (1990) Dale's hypothesis revisited: different neuropeptides derived from a common prohormone are targeted to different processes. *Proc. Natl. Acad. Sci. USA* **87**, 4845–4848.

St. Clair, L.E. (1975) Carnivore myology. In *Sisson and Grossman's The Anatomy of the Domestic Animals* 5th edn. (ed. R.G. Getty), Chapt. 50. Saunders, Philadelphia.

St. John, W.M. (1986) Diffuse pathways convey efferent activity from rostral pontile pneumotaxic center to medullary respiratory regions. *Exp. Neurol.* **94**, 155–165.

Sternini, C. (1988) Structural and chemical organization of the myenteric plexus. *Annu. Rev. Physiol.* **50**, 81–93.

Steward, A., Allot, P.R. and Mapleson, W.W. (1975) Organ weights in the dog. *Res. Vet. Sci.* **19**, 341–342.

Stokes, C. and Bourne, J.F. (1989) Mucosal immunity. In *Veterinary Clinical Immunology* (ed. R.E.W. Halliwell and N.T. Gorman). Saunders, Philadelphia.

Stromberg, M.W. (1993) The autonomic nervous system. In *Miller's Anatomy of the Dog* 3rd edn. (ed. H.E. Evans), Chapt. 15. Saunders, Philadelphia.

Suda, T., Sato, A., Sugiura, W. and Chida, K. (1995) Induction of mhc class ii antigens on rat bronchial epithelial-cells by interferon-gamma and its effect on antigen presentation. *Lung* **173**, 127–137.

Sved, A.F. and Gordon, F.J. (1994) Amino acids as central neurotransmitters in the baroreceptor reflex pathway. *News Physiol. Sci.* **9**, 243–246.

Swenson, M.J. (1977) Physiological properties and cellular and chemical constituents of blood. In *Duke's Physiology of Domestic Mammals* 9th edn. (ed. M.J. Swenson), Chapt. 2. Cornell University Press, Ithaca.

Taha, A.A.M. and King, A.S. (1986) Aortico-pulmonary bodies in the domestic fowl: ultrastructure, innervation and secretion. *J. Anat.* **149**, 41–53.

Taira, N. (1972) The autonomic pharmacology of the bladder. *Annu. Rev. Pharmacol.* **12**, 197–208.

Taylor, P.M. (1988) Report on Yorkshire BSAV Course on Anaesthesia by J.S. Baxter, *Vet. Practice* **20**, 1–4.

Tenney, S.M. (1977) Respiration in mammals. In *Dukes' Physiology of Domestic Mammals* 9th edn. (ed. M.J. Swenson), Chapt. 15. Comstock Publishing Associates, Ithaca.

Tenney, S.M. (1991) Who discovered the discoverers? *News Physiol. Sci.* **7**, 287–289.

Tenney, S.M. (1993) Inhibition and facilitation of visceral afferent information. *News Physiol. Sci.* **8**, 288.

Tenney, S.M. and Remmers, J.E. (1963) Comparative quantitative morphology of the mammalian lung: diffusing area. *Nature* **197**, 54–56.

Thomas, S.T. and Suthers, R.A. (1972) The physiology and energetics of bat flight. *J. Exp. Biol.* **57**, 317–335.

Thompson, J.W. (1961) The nerve supply to the nictitating membrane of the cat. *J. Anat.* **95**, 371–384.

Thornburg, K.L. and Morton, M.J. (1993) Growth and development of the heart. In *Fetus and Neonate: Physiology and Clinical Applications*, Vol. 1. The Circulation (ed. M.A. Hanson, J.A.D. Spencer and C.H. Rodeck), Chapt. 6. Cambridge University Press, Cambridge.

Tietz, W.J. and Hall, P. (1977) Autonomic nervous system. In *Duke's Physiology of Domestic Animals* 9th edn. (ed. M.J. Swenson), Chapt. 48. Comstock Publishing Associates, Ithaca.

Tucker, V.A. (1968) Upon the wings of the wind. *New Sci.* **38**, 694–696.

Tyler, W.S., McLaughlin, R.F. and Canada, R.O. (1967) Structural analogues of the respiratory system. *Arch. Environ. Health* **14**, 62–69.

Tyler, W.S., Gillespie, J.R. and Nowell, J.N. (1971) Symposium on pulmonary and cardiac function: modern functional morphology of the equine lung. *Equine Vet. J.* **3**, 1–11.

Vaillant, C. (1987) Feline dysautonomia: regulatory peptides. *J. Small Anim. Pract.* **28**, 355–363.

Van As, A. and Webster, I. (1974) The morphology of mucus in mammalian pulmonary airways. *Environ. Res.* **7**, 1–12.

Veit, H.G. and Farrell, R.L. (1978) The anatomy and physiology of the bovine respiratory system relating to pulmonary disease. *Cornell Vet.* **68**, 555–581.

Verhoeff, J., Brom, W.E. van den, Dik, K.J., Ingh, T.S.G.A.M. van den and Hartman, E.G. (1992) Radiographic and radionucleide lung perfusion imaging in healthy calves and calves naturally infected with bovine respiratory syncitial virus. *Vet. Rec.* **131**, 477–480.

Verna, A. (1973) Terminaisons nerveuses afférentes et efférentes dans le glomus carotidien du lapin. *J. Microsc.* **16**, 299–308.

Vidyadaran, M.K., King, A.S. and Kassim, H. (1987) Deficient anatomical capacity for oxygen uptake of the developing lung of the female domestic fowl when compared with the Red Jungle Fowl. *Schweiz. Arch. Tierheilk.* **129**, 225–237.

Vidyadaran, M.K., King, A.S. and Kassim, H. (1990) Quantitative comparisons of lung structure of adult domestic fowl and Red Jungle Fowl with reference to broiler ascites. *Avian Pathol.* **19**, 51–58.

Vincent, S.R. and Hope, B.T. (1992) Neurons that say NO. *Trends Neurosci.* **15**, 108–113.

Walker, A.M. (1993) Circulatory transitions at birth and the control of the neonatal circulation. In *Fetus and Neonate: Physiology and Clinical Applications.* Vol. 1. The Circulation (ed. M.A. Hanson, J.A.D. Spencer and C.H. Rodeck), Chapt. 7. Cambridge University Press, Cambridge.

Wang, N.-S. (1975) The preformed stomas connecting the pleural cavity and the lymphatics in the parietal pleura. · *Am. Rev. Resp. Dis.* **111**, 12–20.

Wang, S.C. and Ngai, S.H. (1964) General organization of central respiratory mechanisms. In *Handbook of Physiology: Respiration* (ed. W.O. Fenn and H. Rahn), Section 3, Vol. 1, Chapt. 19. American Physiological Society, Washington D.C.

Waterman, A.E. and Hashim, M.A. (1991) Measurement of the length and position of the lower oesophageal sphincter by correlation of external measurements and radiographic estimations in dogs. *Vet. Rec.* **129**, 261–264.

Wearn, J.T. (1940) The coronary circulation. *Harvey Lect.* **35**, 243–270.

Weibel, E.R. (1984) *The Pathway for Oxygen: Structure and Function in the Mammalian Respiratory System.* Harvard University Press, Cambridge.

Weibel, E.R. and Gomez, D.M. (1962) A principle for counting tissue structures on random sections. *J. Appl. Physiol.* **17**, 343–348.

Weibel, E.R., Taylor, C.R., Gehr, P., Hoppeler, H., Mathieu, O. and Maloiy, G.M.O. (1981) Design of the mammalian respiratory system. IX. Functional and structural limits for oxygen flow. *Resp. Physiol.* **44**, 151–164.

Weiner, N. and Taylor, O. (1985) Neurohumeral transmission: the autonomic and somatic nervous systems. In *The Pharmacological Basis of Therapeutics* 7th edn. (ed. A.G. Gilman, T.W. Rall and F. Murid), Chapt. 4. Macmillan, New York.

West, J.B. (1975) *Respiratory Physiology: The Essentials.* Williams & Wilkins, Baltimore.

West, J.B. and Mathieu-Costello, O. (1994) Stress failure of pulmonary capillaries as a mechanism for exercise in-

duced pulmonary haemorrhage in the horse. *Equine. Vet. J.* **26**, 441–447.

West, J.B., Mathieu-Costello, O., Jones, J.H., Birks, E.K., Logemann, R.B., Pascoe, J.R. and Tyler, W.S. (1993) Stress failure of pulmonary capillaries in racehorses with exercise-induced pulmonary haemorrhage. *J. Appl. Physiol.* **75**, 1097–1109.

Weyns, A.A.L.M. (1988) *The Enteric Nervous System in the Ruminant Stomach (Ovis aries).* Doctorate Thesis, University of Antwerp.

White, C.J., Ramee, S.R., Card, H.G., Abrahams, L.A., Svinarich, J.T., Wade, C.E., Rodkey, W.G. and Virmani, R. (1988) Laser angioplasty: an atherosclerotic swine model. *Lasers Surg. Med.* **8**, 318–321.

White, J.C., Smithwick, R.H. and Simeone, F.A. (1952) *The Autonomic Nervous System.* Macmillan, New York.

White, R.A.S. and Pomeroy, C.J. (1989) Phenylpropanolamine: an α-adrenergic agent for the management of urinary incontinence in the bitch associated with urethral sphincter mechanism incompetence. *Vet. Rec.* **125**, 478–480.

Whitwell, K.E. (1975) Morphology and pathology of the equine umbilical cord. *J. Reprod. Fert.* **Suppl. 23**, 599–603.

Whitwell, K.E. and Greet, T.R.C. (1984) Collection and evaluation of tracheobronchial washes in the horse. *Equine Vet. J.* **16**, 499–508.

Widdicombe, J.G. (1964) Respiratory reflexes. In *Handbook of Physiology: Respiration* (ed. W.O. Fenn and H. Rahn), Section 3, Vol. I, Chapt. 24. American Physiological Society, Washington D.C.

Widdicombe, J.G. (1977) Studies on afferent airway innervation. *Am. Rev. Resp. Dis.* **115**, 99–105.

Widdicombe, J.G. (1986a) Reflexes from the upper respiratory tract. In *Handbook of Physiology: The Respiratory System II* (ed. Cherniack and J.G. Widdicombe), Chapt. 11. American Physiological Society, Washington D.C.

Widdicombe, J.G. (1986b) Sensory innervation of the lungs and airways. In *Progress in Brain Research* (ed. F. Cervero and J.F.B. Morrison). Elsevier, Amsterdam.

Wiedeman, M.P., Tuma, R.F. and Mayrovitz, H.N. (1976) Defining the precapillary sphincter. *Microvasc. Res.* **12**, 71–75.

Wiederhielm, C.A. (1974) The capillaries, veins and lymphatics. In *Physiology and Biophysics* 20th edn. (ed. T.C. Ruch, H.D. Patton and A.M. Scher), Vol. 2, Chapt. 9. Saunders, Philadelphia.

Wiggers, C.J. (1974) The heart. In *Vertebrate Structures and Functions*, Chapt. 9. Freeman, San Francisco.

Williams, P.L., Warwick, R., Dyson, M. and Bannister, L.H. (1989) *Gray's Anatomy* 37th edn. Churchill Livingstone, Edinburgh.

Williams, P.L., Bannister, L.H., Berry, M.M., Collins, P., Dyson, M., Dussek, J.E. and Ferguson, M.W.J. (1995) *Gray's Anatomy* 38th edn. Churchill Livingstone, Edinburgh.

Willison, H. (1996) An unwanted defence: anti-ganglioside

antibodies and limb paralysis. *Wellcome Trust Review 1996.*

Williston, S.W. (1925) *The Osteology of the Reptiles.* Harvard University Press, Cambridge.

Winaver, J., Hoffman, A., Abassi, Z. and Haramati, A. (1995) Does the heart's hormone, ANP, help in congestive heart failure. *News Physiol. Sci.* **10**, 247–253.

Winkler, G.C. (1988) Pulmonary intravascular macrophages in domestic animal species: Review of structural and functional properties. *Am. J. Anat.* **181**, 217–234.

Wira, C.R. and Rossoll, R.M. (1995) Antigen-presenting cells in the female reproductive tract – influence of the estrous-cycle on antigen presentation by uterine epithelial and stromal cells. *Endocrinology* **136**, 4526–4534.

Wood, C.E. (1993) Local and endocrine factors in the control of the circulation. In *Fetus and Neonate: Physiology and Clinical Applications.* Vol. 1 The Circulation (ed. M.A. Hanson, J.A.D. Spencer and C.H. Rodeck), Chapt. 4. Cambridge University Press, Cambridge.

Wood, J.D. (1987) Physiology of the enteric nervous system. *Physiology of the Gastrointestinal Tract* 2nd edn.(ed. L.R. Johnson), Vol. 1, Chapt. 3. Raven Press, New York.

Woodbury, D.M. (1974) Physiology of body fluids. In *Physiology and Biophysics* 20th edn. (ed. T.C. Ruch, H.D. Patton and A.M. Scher), Vol. 2, Chapt. 26. Saunders, Philadelphia.

Yamada, H., Ezure, K. and Manabe, M. (1988) Efferent projections of inspiratory neurons of the ventral respiratory group. A dual labeling study in the rat. *Brain Res.* **455**, 283–294.

Young, A.C. (1974) Neural control of respiration. In *Physiology and Biophysics* 20th edn. (ed. T.C. Ruch, H.D. Patton and A.M. Scher), Vol. 2, Chapt. 22. Saunders, Philadelphia.

Young, J.Z. (1962) *The Life of Vertebrates* 2nd edn. Clarendon, Oxford.

Zaagsma, J., Amsterdam, R.G.M. van, Brouwer, F., Heijden, P.J.C.M. van, Schaar, M.W.G. van, Verwey, W.M. and Veenstra, V. (1987) Adrenergic control of airway function. *Am. Rev. Resp. Dis.* **136**, S45–S50.

Zeitzschmann, O. (1943) Die Arterien. In *Ellenberger-Baum: Handbuch Der Vergleichenden Anatomie der Haustiere* 18th edn. (ed. O. Zietzschmann, E. Ackerknecht and H. Grau), Section IVB, IV. Springer, Berlin.

Zweifach, B.W. (1959) The microcirculation of the blood. *Vertebrate Structures and Functions: Readings from Scientific American* (ed. N.K. Wessells), Chapt. 10, pp. 107–113.

Index

Page numbers in **bold print** are the main sources